Multi-Detector CT Imaging Handbook

Multi-Detector CT Imaging

Abdomen, Pelvis, and CAD Applications

Multi-Detector CT Imaging Handbook

Multi-Detector CT Imaging: Principles, Head, Neck, and Vascular Systems

Multi-Detector CT Imaging: Abdomen, Pelvis, and CAD Applications

Multi-Detector CT Imaging

Abdomen, Pelvis, and CAD Applications

edited by

Luca Saba • Jasjit S. Suri

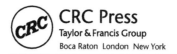

CRC Press
Taylor & Francis Group
Boca Raton London New York

CRC Press is an imprint of the
Taylor & Francis Group, an **informa** business

CRC Press
Taylor & Francis Group
6000 Broken Sound Parkway NW, Suite 300
Boca Raton, FL 33487-2742

First issued in paperback 2017

© 2014 by Taylor & Francis Group, LLC
CRC Press is an imprint of Taylor & Francis Group, an Informa business

No claim to original U.S. Government works

ISBN-13: 978-1-4398-9397-5 (hbk)
ISBN-13: 978-1-138-07252-7 (pbk)

Library of Congress Cataloging-in-Publication Data

Multi-detector CT imaging : principles, head, neck, and vascular systems / editors, Luca Saba and Jasjit S. Suri.
   p. ; cm.
   Includes bibliographical references and index.
   ISBN 978-1-4398-9380-7 (alk. paper)
   I. Saba, Luca. II. Suri, Jasjit S.
   [DNLM: 1. Multidetector Computed Tomography--methods. 2. Brain Diseases--radiography. 3. Neck--radiography. 4. Vascular Diseases--radiography. WN 206]

616.07'5722--dc23
                                    2012048761

Visit the Taylor & Francis Web site at
http://www.taylorandfrancis.com

and the CRC Press Web site at
http://www.crcpress.com

Luca Saba dedicates this book to his parents

Giovanni Saba and Raffaela Polla for their love.

Jasjit S. Suri dedicates this book to his children

Harman Suri and Neha Suri for their love.

Contents

Section I Gastro-Intestinal and Abdomen

Section II Urogenital

Section III Muscle and Skeleton

Section IV Special Applications

Section V CAD Applications

Foreword

Medical imaging, and computed tomography (CT) in particular, have revolutionized medical care over the past four decades in ways unimaginable prior to the introduction of CT. The impact of CT extends over virtually every clinical field and region of the body, and through all aspects of care including screening, diagnosis and problem solving, monitoring disease progression and treatment responses, and directing minimally invasive procedural interventions. It is no wonder then, with the critical role CT plays, and with the rapid innovations in computer technology, that advances in the capabilities and complexity of CT imaging continue to evolve. An up-to-date complete and authoritative educational and reference volume covering the entire spectrum of CT is a difficult task to accomplish and lacking in the radiology literature. *Multi-Detector CT Imaging*, edited by Dr. Luca Saba and Dr. Jasjit Suri, excels in meeting this need.

Drs. Saba and Suri have brought together an outstanding collection of international authors recognized worldwide as leaders in their fields. Their extensive clinical experience and practical knowledge are logically presented, well organized, and brilliantly visualized. The two books in this set are amazingly complete in content, depth, and quality, yet read easily as an educational introduction or as a reference source.

The value of these books will be appreciated by readers in many ways. They cover all aspects of CT imaging, with technical principles and postprocessing methodologies comprehensibly presented, and extensive clinical specialty chapters easily searchable for specific information without need of an index. The value goes far beyond just a "how-to" or an encyclopedia of findings, however. The authors have uniformly put techniques, clinical findings, pathologic disease presentations, and clinical implications of imaging findings in practical perspective. The organization of the chapters is a wonderful progression that actually follows how the radiologist approaches unknown cases. Most chapters start with a review of imaging techniques for the organ or disease process. This is often followed with a practical discussion reviewing the spectrum of abnormal CT findings and their significance and differential diagnosis, followed subsequently by thorough material organized around understanding disease processes. Helpful correlative material with MRI and PET imaging is frequently presented to illustrate how these modalities complement each other.

This resource is a remarkable tool that will be of value to imaging professionals from every clinical vantage point and will serve well those experienced with CT or those using it to first learn about CT. I personally look forward to using this resource and having it available for our trainees, not only as an essential educational tool, but knowing that it will stimulate our community to further push the frontiers of CT imaging.

Richard L. Baron, MD
Dean for Clinical Practice
Professor of Radiology
University of Chicago Pritzker School of Medicine

Preface

The introduction of multi-detector row computed tomography (CT) in the early 1990s resulted in a fundamental and far-reaching improvement of CT imaging. For the first time, volumes of data could be acquired without misregistration of anatomical details, which indicated the development of 3D image processing techniques. In the last 20 years, CT technology has further improved with the introduction of systems up to 320-detector rows and with the development of dual-source and multispectral technology.

From these developments, the diagnostic potential of CT has impressively improved with an exceptional spatial resolution and the possibility to analyze with an exquisite level of detail several kinds of pathology. Thanks to the development of CT perfusion technique, functional brain imaging as well as liver imaging is now possible.

The purpose of this book is to cover clinical and engineering benefits in the diagnosis of human pathologies. It discusses the protocols and potential of advanced computed tomography scanners, explaining easily, but with an adequate level of detail, the role and potential of CT.

Acknowledgments

It is not possible to overstate our gratitude to the many individuals who helped to produce this book. In particular, Luca Saba would like to thank Professors Giorgio Mallarini and Giancarlo Caddeo, who first taught him the principles of computed tomography. Dr. Saba also thanks Stefano Marcia, Paolo Siotto, and Giovanni Argiolas and his many colleagues, residents, students, and friends for their continuous exchanges during these years. A special thanks also to Carlo Nicola de Cecco for his help. Finally, Dr. Saba would like to acknowledge the patience and understanding displayed by Tiziana throughout his work. Without her continuous encouragement, this book would not have been completed.

Jasjit S. Suri acknowledges Dr. Luca Saba for his continuous dedication in the field of computer tomography imaging and his willingness to participate in successfully launching this project. Dr. Suri also thanks his family, Malvika, Harman, and Neha, who are always a source of shine and laughter. Special thanks to all his friends and collaborators around the world who helped commercialize medical devices and healthcare imaging products over the course of years.

Both editors have received considerable support and cooperation from individuals at CRC/Taylor & Francis, particularly Michael Slaughter, Jessica Vakili, Joette Lynch, Michele Smith and from Dennis Troutman at diacriTech, each of whom helped to minimize the obstacles that the editors encountered.

Editors

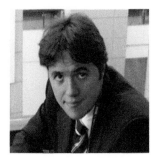

Luca Saba earned his MD from the University of Cagliari, Italy, in 2002. Today, he works in the University of Cagliari School of Medicine. His research fields are focused on multi-detector row computed tomography, magnetic resonance, ultrasound, neuroradiology, and diagnostics in vascular sciences.

His works, as lead author, have appeared in more than 100 high impact factor, peer-reviewed journals such as the *American Journal of Neuroradiology, European Radiology, European Journal of Radiology, Acta Radiologica, Cardiovascular and Interventional Radiology, Journal of Computer Assisted Tomography, American Journal of Roentgenology, Neuroradiology, Clinical Radiology, Journal of Cardiovascular Surgery,* and *Cerebrovascular Diseases.* He is a well-known speaker and has spoken over 45 times at national and international levels.

Dr. Saba has won 12 scientific and extracurricular awards during his career. He has presented more than 430 papers and posters at national and international congresses (RSNA, ESGAR, ECR, ISR, AOCR, AINR, JRS, SIRM, AINR). He has written eight book chapters, and he is currently serving as an editor of four books in the field of cardiovascular and neurodegenerative imaging.

He is a member of the Italian Society of Radiology, European Society of Radiology, Radiological Society of North America, American Roentgen Ray Society, and European Society of Neuroradiology.

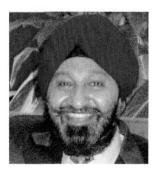

Jasjit S. Suri earned his MS in neurological MRI from the University of Illinois, a PhD in cardiac imaging from the University of Washington and an MBA from the Weatherhead School of Management, Case Western Reserve University. He has worked as scientist, manager, senior director, vice president, and chief technology officer at IBM, Siemens Medical, Philips Healthcare, Fisher, and Eigen Inc.

He has written over 400 publications, 60 patents, 4 FDA clearances, and more than 25 books in medical imaging and biotechnologies (diagnostic and therapeutic). Dr. Suri has had a leadership role in releasing products in the men's and women's market in the fields of cardiology, neurology, urology, vascular, ophthalmology, and breast cancer.

Dr. Suri has received the President's Gold Medal and Fellow of American Institute of Medical and Biological Engineering from the National Academy of Sciences. He has won over 50 awards during his career. Dr. Suri is also a strategic advisory board member for more than half a dozen industries and international journals focused on biomedical imaging and technologies.

Contributors

Behnoush Abdollahi
BioImaging Laboratory
Bioengineering Department
and
Computer Engineering and
    Computer Science Department
University of Louisville
Louisville, Kentucky

Mohamed Abou El-Ghar
Urology and Nephrology Department
University of Mansoura
Mansoura, Egypt

Rita Agarwala
Department of Radiology
John H. Stroger Hospital of Cook
    County
Chicago, Illinois

Hirotaka Akita
Department of Diagnostic
    Radiology
Keio University School of
    Medicine
Tokyo, Japan

Luis Guzmán Álvarez
Department of Radiology
Hospital of Traumatology
Granada, Spain

Garyfalia Ampanozi
Institute of Forensic Medicine
University of Zurich
Zurich, Switzerland

J. Dámaso Aquerreta
Servicio de Radiología
Clínica Universidad de Navarra
Navarra, Spain

Davide Bellini
Department of Radiological
    Sciences, Oncology and
    Pathology
Sapienza University of Rome—
    Polo Pontino
Rome, Italy

Jonathan W. Berlin
Department of Radiology
North Shore University Health
    System
University of Chicago
Evanston Hospital
Evanston, Illinois

Ashu Seith Bhalla
Department of Radiology
All India Institute of Medical
    Sciences
New Delhi, India

Michael A. Blake
Division of Abdominal Imaging
    and Interventional Radiology
Massachusetts General Hospital
Boston, Massachusetts

Carlo Catalano
Department of Radiological
    Sciences
Sapienza University of Rome
Rome, Italy

Heang-Ping Chan
Department of Radiology
University of Michigan
Ann Arbor, Michigan

Ali Cahid Civelek
Radiology Department
School of Medicine
University of Louisville
Louisville, Kentucky

Ian Crosbie
Department of Radiology
Mater Misercordiae University
    Hospital
Dublin, Ireland

Carlo Nicola De Cecco
Department of Radiological
    Sciences, Oncology and
    Pathology
Sapienza University of Rome—
    Polo Pontino
Rome, Italy

and

Department of Radiology &
    Radiological Sciences
Medical University of South
    Carolina
Charleston, South Carolina

Maurizio Del Monte
Department of Radiological
    Sciences
Sapienza University of Rome
Rome, Italy

Michele DiMartino
Department of Radiological
    Sciences
Sapienza University of Rome
Rome, Italy

Rossella DiMiscio
Department of Radiological
    Sciences
Sapienza University of Rome
Rome, Italy

Lars C. Ebert
Institute of Forensic
    Medicine
University of Zurich
Zurich, Switzerland

Ayman El-Baz
BioImaging Laboratory
Bioengineering Department
University of Louisville
Louisville, Kentucky

Jorge Elias Jr.
Abdominal Imaging Section
University of Sao Paulo at
    Ribeirao Preto School of
    Medicine
Ribeirao Preto, Brazil

Ahmed Elnakib
BioImaging Laboratory
Bioengineering Department
University of Louisville
Louisville, Kentucky

Robert Falk
Medical Imaging Division
Jewish Hospital
Louisville, Kentucky

Elliot K. Fishman
Department of Radiology
Johns Hopkins University School of
    Medicine
Baltimore, Maryland

Patricia M. Flach
Institute of Forensic Medicine
University of Zurich
and
Institute of Diagnostic and
    Interventional Radiology
University Hospital Zurich
Zurich, Switzerland

Thomas Flohr
Siemens Healthcare Computed
    Tomography
Forchheim, Germany

and

Institute for Diagnostic Radiology
Eberhard Karls University Tübingen
Tübingen, Germany

Jurgen J. Fütterer
Department of Radiology
Radboud University Nijmegen
    Medical Centre
Nijmegen, the Netherlands

María del Mar Castellano García
Department of Radiology
Hospital of Traumatology
Granada, Spain

Daniel Gieger
Department of Radiological Sciences
Sapienza University of Rome
Rome, Italy

Georgy Gimel'farb
Department of Computer Science
University of Auckland
Auckland, New Zealand

Ajit H. Goenka
Imaging Institute
Cleveland Clinic
Cleveland, Ohio

Richard M. Gore
Department of Radiology
North Shore University Health
    System
University of Chicago
Evanston Hospital
Evanston, Illinois

Ali Guermazi
Department of Radiology
Boston University School of
    Medicine
Boston, Massachusetts

Pankaj Gupta
Department of Radiology
All India Institute of Medical
    Sciences
New Delhi, India

Lubomir Hadjiiski
Department of Radiology
University of Michigan
Ann Arbor, Michigan

Daichi Hayashi
Boston University School of
    Medicine
Boston, Massachusetts

Matthew T. Heller
Division of Abdominal Imaging
University of Pittsburgh Medical
    Center
Pittsburgh, Pennsylvania

Franco Iafrate
Department of Radiological
    Sciences, Oncology and
    Pathology
Sapienza University of Rome—
    Polo Pontino
Rome, Italy

Mohamed Jarraya
Department of Radiology
Boston University School of
    Medicine
Boston, Massachusetts

R. Brooke Jeffrey
Department of Radiology
Stanford University Medical
    Center
Stanford, California

Masahiro Jinzaki
Department of Diagnostic
    Radiology
Keio University School of Medicine
Tokyo, Japan

Satomi Kawamoto
Department of Radiology
Johns Hopkins University School of
    Medicine
Baltimore, Maryland

Eiji Kikuchi
Department of Urology
Keio University School of Medicine
Tokyo, Japan

Karin Knesaurek
Department of Radiology
Division of Nuclear Medicine
Mount Sinai School of Medicine
New York, New York

Lale Kostakoglu
Department of Radiology
Division of Nuclear Medicine
Mount Sinai School of Medicine
New York, New York

Sachio Kuribayashi
Department of Diagnostic
    Radiology
Keio University School of
    Medicine
Tokyo, Japan

Andrea Laghi
Department of Radiological
    Sciences, Oncology and
    Pathology
Sapienza University of Rome—
    Polo Pontino
Rome, Italy

Katherine Leung
Department of Radiology and
    Diagnostic Imaging
University of Alberta
Edmonton, Alberta, Canada

Xiao-Feng Li
Radiology Department
School of Medicine
University of Louisville
Louisville, Kentucky

Concetta Lombardo
Department of Radiological
    Sciences
Sapienza University of Rome
Rome, Italy

Gavin Low
Department of Radiology and
    Diagnostic Imaging
University of Alberta
Edmonton, Alberta, Canada

Fabiano Lucchesi
Radiology Department
Barretos Cancer Hospital
Barretos, Brazil

John E. Madewell
Department of Diagnostic
    Radiology
University of Texas MD Anderson
    Cancer Center
Houston, Texas

Joaquín Martín
Sección de Radiología
Hospital Reina Sofía de Tudela
Navarra, Spain

Shaunagh McDermott
Division of Abdominal Imaging
    and Interventional Radiology
Massachusetts General Hospital
Boston, Massachusetts

Uday K. Mehta
Department of Radiology
North Shore University Health
    System
University of Chicago
Evanston Hospital
Evanston, Illinois

José M. Mellado
Sección de Radiología
Hospital Reina Sofía de Tudela
Navarra, Spain

Valdair Muglia
Abdominal Imaging Section
University of Sao Paulo at
    Ribeirao Preto School of
    Medicine
Ribeirao Preto, Brazil

Giuseppe Muscogiuri
Department of Radiological
    Sciences, Oncology and
    Pathology
Sapienza University of Rome—
    Polo Pontino
Rome, Italy

Geraldine M. Newmark
Department of Radiology
North Shore University Health
    System
University of Chicago
Evanston Hospital
Evanston, Illinois

Owen J. O'Connor
Division of Abdominal Imaging
    and Interventional Radiology
Massachusetts General Hospital
Boston, Massachusetts

Paul O'Sullivan
Department of Diagnostic Imaging
Bons Secours Hospital
Cork, Ireland

Evangelos N. Perdikakis
Department of Radiology
412 General Military Hospital
212 Mobile Army Surgical Hospital
Xanthi, Greece

Jonelle M. Petscavage-Thomas
Department of Radiology
Penn State Milton S. Hershey
    Medical Center
Hershey, Pennsylvania

Laura Pérez del Palomar
Servicio de Radiología
Hospital Royo Villanova
Zaragoza, Spain

Mark Pisaneschi
Department of Radiology
John H. Stroger Hospital of Cook
    County
Chicago, Illinois

Prabhakar Rajiah
Cardiovascular Imaging
    Laboratory
Cleveland Clinic
Cleveland, Ohio

Erick M. Remer
Imaging Institute
Cleveland Clinic
Cleveland, Ohio

Marco Rengo
Department of Radiological
    Sciences, Oncology and Pathology
Sapienza University of Rome—
    Polo Pontino
Rome, Italy

Pedram Rezai
Department of Radiology
John H. Stroger Hospital of Cook
    County
Chicago, Illinois

Frank Roemer
Department of Radiology,
University of Erlangen
Erlangen Germany

and

Department of Radiology
Boston University School of
    Medicine
Boston, Massachusetts

Fernando Ruiz Santiago
Department of Radiology
Hospital of Traumatology
Granada, Spain

Bernhard Schmidt
Siemens Healthcare Computed
    Tomography
Forchheim, Germany

Amar B. Shah
Department of Radiology
New York Medical College
Valhalla, New York

Shetal N. Shah
Imaging Institute
Cleveland Clinic
Cleveland, Ohio

Martin J. Shelly
Division of Abdominal
    Imaging and Interventional
    Radiology
Massachusetts General Hospital
Boston, Massachusetts

Robert I. Silvers
Department of Radiology
North Shore University Health
    System
University of Chicago
Evanston Hospital
Evanston, Illinois

Susana Solanas
Sección de Radiología
Hospital Reina Sofía de Tudela
Navarra, Spain

Erich Sorantin
Division of Paediatric Radiology
Department of Radiology
Medical University of Graz
Graz, Austria

Kalyanasundaram Srinivasan
Department of Radiology
All India Institute of Medical Sciences
New Delhi, India

Damien L. Stella
Department of Radiology
University of Melbourne
Royal Melbourne Hospital
Melbourne, Australia

Jasjit S. Suri
Biomedical Technologies, Inc.
Roseville, California

Kiran H. Thakrar
Department of Radiology
North Shore University
    Health System
University of Chicago
Evanston Hospital
Evanston, Illinois

Michael J. Thali
Institute of Forensic Medicine
University of Zurich
Zurich, Switzerland

Diana Tran
Department of Radiology
Bankstown Hospital
Sydney, Australia

Sabine Weissensteiner
Division of Paediatric Radiology
Department of Radiology
Medical University of Graz
Graz, Austria

Daniel R. Wenzke
Department of Radiology
North Shore University Health
    System
University of Chicago
Evanston Hospital
Evanston, Illinois

Minoru Yamada
Department of Diagnostic
    Radiology
Keio University School of Medicine
Tokyo, Japan

Yoshitake Yamada
Department of Diagnostic
    Radiology
Keio University School of Medicine
Tokyo, Japan

Section I

Gastro-Intestinal and Abdomen

1

Liver

Michele DiMartino, Rossella DiMiscio, Daniel Gieger, Maurizio
Del Monte, Concetta Lombardo, and Carlo Catalano

CONTENTS

1.1 Introduction

Hepatic imaging is an important component of abdominal computed tomography (CT) examination and is crucial for a wide range of clinical applications: detection and characterization of primary or metastatic hepatic lesions, diagnosis of diffuse liver diseases, assessment of vascular and biliary patency or obstruction, tumor staging, monitoring treatment response, and pre- and postoperative evaluation for surgical resection. The introduction in clinical practice of multi-detector computed tomography (MDCT) from four detector row through 64 and more significantly improves the role of CT in the evaluation of liver disease. The main advantages of MDCT are the routine use of thinner sections that yield higher spatial resolution and decrease of gantry rotation time, which result in a significant reduced scan time. Reducing acquisition scan time makes it possible to acquire the entire liver volume with a multiphasic CT protocol during different vascular phases in a single, comfortable, breath hold. Sixteen and more slice CT scanners allow the acquisition of datasets of images with nearly isotropic voxels for multiplanar reconstruction, useful for a better evaluation of liver disease. In this chapter, we discuss the segmental and vascular anatomy of the live, technical parameters, contrast media application, and acquisition protocol of liver examination. In addition, CT imaging findings of main focal and diffuse liver disease are reviewed.

1.2 Liver Anatomy

The knowledge of segmental liver is useful for communicating the CT findings to the surgeon. The system proposed by Coinaud [1–2] and later modified by Bismuth provides the details needed for surgery and is easily applicable to axial imaging techniques such as CT, magnetic resonance imaging and ultrasound. The liver is divided into eight segments, except the caudate lobe and medial segment of the left lobe, segments are defined not only by the three vertical fissures described by the three major hepatic veins, but also by a transverse plane through the left and right portal-venous branches. The segment I is the caudate lobe, segments II–VIII are numbered clockwise looking at the liver ventrally (Figure 1.1). Each segment has an independent blood supply and biliary drainage. The amendment made by Bismuth IV divides the segment into subsegments higher (IVa) and lower (IVb).

The most common anatomic variation is the Riedel lobe, which is an extended, tongue-like, right lobe of the liver. It is not pathological; it is a normal anatomical variant and may extend into the pelvis. It is often mistaken for a distended gallbladder or liver tumor.

A liver located on the left is found in a full or partial situs viscerum inversus.

1.3 Vascular Anatomy and Variants

The hepatic artery carries only 25%–30% of the blood, which is related to the liver.

The common hepatic artery usually originates from the celiac trunk. After gastroduodenal artery originated behind the pylorus, it becomes the proper hepatic artery, which passes into the hepatoduodenal ligament to the anteromedial portal vein and anterior to the bile duct. At hepatic hilum, it divides into left and right branch. The middle hepatic artery that supplies the segment IV with equal frequency originates from the left or right hepatic artery (Figure 1.2).

The classical distribution of the hepatic arteries is only slightly more than half of the subjects, whereas 45% have one or more variants. The most common variants include the left hepatic branch that originates from the left gastric artery (10%–25%) (Figure 1.3) and the right hepatic branch that originates from the superior mesenteric artery (11%–17%) (Figure 1.4).

The Michel classification of hepatic artery variant anatomy is shown in Table 1.1 [3].

The portal vein divides at the hilum into two branches, right and left, which run next to the hepatic arteries and the bile ducts.

In the parenchyma of the right lobe, the right portal vein divides into anterior and posterior branches, which go to the corresponding liver segments (Figure 1.5).

The portal system can be affected by anatomical variants, such as the trifurcation of the portal vein hilum (8%–10%), other anomalies can be also recognized including agenesis or atrophy of one of the two main branches, with atrophy of the liver parenchyma (Figure 1.6).

In the classic anatomy, three main hepatic veins drain into the inferior vena cava (IVC) the left hepatic vein drains segment II and III, the middle hepatic vein drains segment IV, V, and VIII, and the right hepatic vein drains V, VI, and VII. In approximately 60% of the population, the middle and left hepatic veins join to form a common trunk (Figure 1.7).

The most common variant seen is an accessory right hepatic vein draining the segment VI directly into the IVC (Figure 1.8) [4].

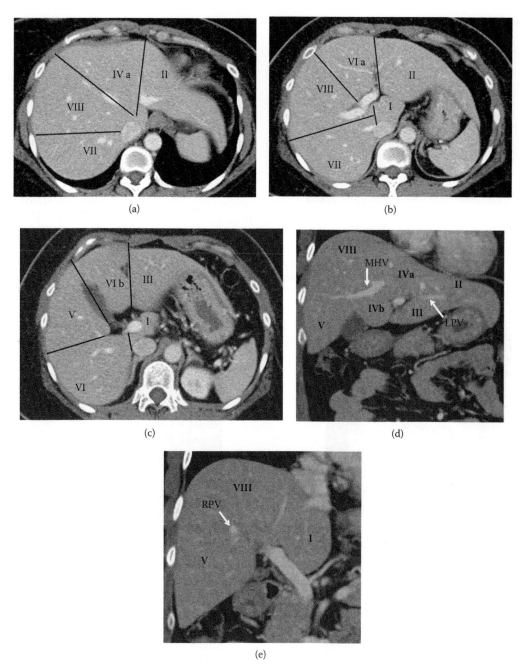

FIGURE 1.1
Segmental anatomy. (a–c) CT axial images show liver segment distribution according to the anatomic segmentation schemes of Couinaud and Bismuth. Falciform ligament plane separates medial (IV segment) from lateral (II—III segments) left lobe. Segmental anatomy. (d and e) CT coronal images show liver segment distribution according to the anatomic segmentation schemes of Couinaud and Bismuth.

1.4 Acquisition Parameters

As the number of detector channels increases, application of thin collimation has become a routine part of MDCT. The minimum section collimation of 16-, 32-, and 64-slice scanners range between 0.5 and 0.625 mm. This submillimeter feature allows for isotropic data acquisition. An isotropic voxel is cubic, having equal dimensions in the x-, y-, and z-axes. Since the x- and y-axes are determined by both field of view (FOV) and matrix size, isotropic voxel can be acquired only when slice thickness z-axis measures 0.75 mm or less. The major advantage of these nearly isotropic datasets is the ability to reformat images in multiplanar manner, with spatial resolution similar to that of axial images. Recent studies have shown the usefulness of multiplanar reformatted images in the detection of hepatocellular

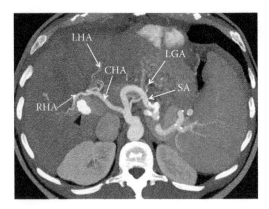

FIGURE 1.2
Normal hepatic arterial anatomy. Axial MIP image shows the normal anatomy of the hepatic artery: common hepatic artery (CHA), left hepatic artery (LHA), right hepatic artery (RHA), superior mesenteric artery (SMA), and splenic artery (SA). Note the presence of transjugular intrahepatic portosystemic shunt (TIPS) in patients with portal hypertension (arrowhead).

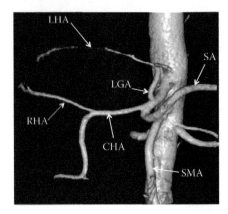

FIGURE 1.3
Variant hepatic arterial anatomy. Three-dimensional (3D) volume-rendered image from a multi-detector CT (MDCT) shows the left hepatic artery (LHA) arising from the left gastric artery (LGA). SA = splenic artery, CHA = common hepatic artery, SMA = superior mesenteric artery, RHA = right hepatic artery.

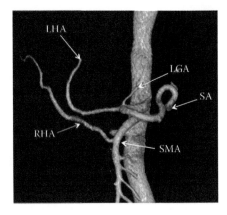

FIGURE 1.4
Variant hepatic arterial anatomy. Three-dimensional volume-rendered image from MDCT shows the right hepatic artery (RHA) arising from superior mesenteric artery (SMA). LGA = left gastric artery, LHA = left hepatic artery, SA = splenic artery.

TABLE 1.1

Hepatic Arterial Variants According to the Michel Classification

Type	Frequency	Description
I	55	RHA, MHA, and LHA arise from the CHA
II	10	RHA, MHA, and LHA arise from the CHA; replaced LHA from the LGA
III	11	RHA and MHA arise from the CHA; replaced RHA from the SMA
IV	1	Replaced RHA and LHA
V	8	RHA, MHA, and LHA arise from the CHA; accessory LHA from the LGA
VI	7	RHA, MHA, and LHA arise from the CHA; accessory RHA
VII	1	Accessory RHA and LHA
VIII	4	Replaced RHA and accessory LHA or replaced LHA and accessory RHA
IX	4.5	Entire hepatic trunk arise from the SMA
X	0.5	Entire hepatic trunk arise from the LGA

CHA = common hepatic artery, RHA = right hepatic artery, LHA = left hepatic artery, MHA = middle hepatic artery, SMA = superior mesenteric artery, LGA = left gastric artery.

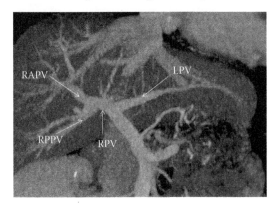

FIGURE 1.5
Normal portal vein (PV) anatomy. Coronal MIP image shows the PV branching into the left PV (LPV) and right PV. The latter divides into the right anterior (RAPV) and right posterior (RPPV) PV.

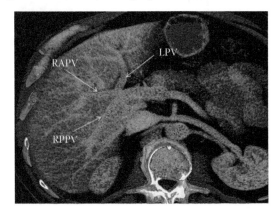

FIGURE 1.6
Portal vein (PV) trifurcation. 3D volume rendered (VR) from CT postcontrast image shows trifurcation of the PV into right anterior (RAPV), right posterior portal vein (RPPV), and left portal vein (LPV).

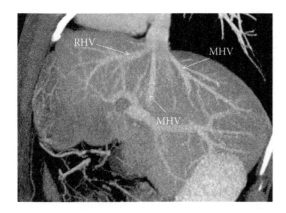

FIGURE 1.7
Normal hepatic veins anatomy. Coronal MIP image shows the confluence into inferior vena cava of the left hepatic vein (LHV), middle hepatic vein (MHV), and right hepatic vein (RHV).

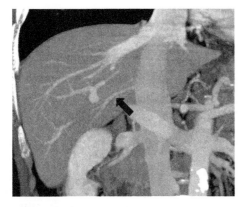

FIGURE 1.8
Accessory hepatic vein. Maximum intensity projection (MIP) from CT postcontrast image shows the presence of an accessory inferior right hepatic veinc (RHV) draining the VI segment directly into the inferior vena cava (IVC).

carcinoma (HCC) [5–6]. Owing to increased spatial resolution and reduced partial volume averaging, thinner-slice collimation also results in an improved ability to detect small hepatic lesion. However, no improvement in lesion detection was found with a collimation width less than 2.5 mm. Furthermore, hepatic imaging with thinner sections caused an increase in image noise, with significantly lower performance in the detection of hepatic lesions [7].

The typical acquisition parameters for liver MDCT are summarized in Table 1.2.

1.5 Contrast Administration

Contrast enhancement of the liver is affected by numerous factors, such as contrast medium volume and concentration, rate and type of injection, scan delay time, and body weight [8–10]. The magnitude of hepatic parenchymal enhancement is directly and almost linearly related to the amount of total iodine mass administered (i.e., total contrast medium volume times concentration) [11–12]. The most important patient-related factor affecting the magnitude of hepatic enhancement is body weight, which shows a near-linear inverse relationship with the magnitude of enhancement: as body weight increases, the magnitude of hepatic parenchymal enhancement decreases. Therefore, when imaging large patients, the total iodine load should be increased to achieve a constant degree of hepatic enhancement. The iodine load can be increased by increasing the contrast medium concentration or volume or injection rate [13–14].

Insufficient hepatic parenchymal enhancement results in diminished conspicuity of a lesion [12]. With MDCT, 50 HU is commonly considered to be a diagnostically appropriate level of hepatic phase enhancement at abdominal CT. Iodine mass required to achieve this enhancement can be estimated by considering patient weight (i.e., maximum hepatic enhancement of 96 HU ± 19 per gram of iodine per kilogram of body weight). This suggests that approximately 0.5 g of iodine per kilogram is needed to achieve the maximum hepatic enhancement of 50 HU (35 g of iodine for a 70-kg patient). For routine abdominal CT (scanning at the portal-venout phase only), injection rates of 3 mL/s are sufficient. Improved lesion-to-liver contrast may be obtained either by a faster injection rate (e.g., 4–6 mL/s) or by an increased iodine concentration. Fast injections increase the magnitude of arterial enhancement and contribute to the increased separation (both time and magnitude) between the arterial and hepatic parenchymal enhancement phases. As a result, fast injections are desirable for multiphase hepatic imaging and the detection of hypervascular liver masses.

Abdominal and hepatic CT imaging has been commonly performed with a fixed-rate injection protocol regardless of the patient's weight [12–14]. This protocol, however, results in inconsistent degrees of contrast enhancement in patients of varying body sizes. This limitation can be overcome by use of contrast material injection protocol, having a fixed injection duration but with individually weight-adapted injection rates. The fixed injection duration protocol facilitates the achievement of consistent arterial and hepatic enhancements and the standardization of scan timing, and perhaps improves the depiction of hypervascular HCCs [15–17]. Iodine dose adjusted to patient weight of 0.5 g of iodine per kilogram injected over 25–30 seconds seems appropriate for dual-phase hepatic CT imaging, resulting in aortic enhancements of more than 250 HU and hepatic enhancements of 50 HU [17]. This protocol involves adjusting the iodine dose and injection rate to the patient's body weight

TABLE 1.2

MDCT Acquisition Parameters for Liver Examination

	4-slice MDCT	16-slice MDCT	64-slice MDCT
Detector configuration (mm)	$4 \times 1.5/1$	$16 \times 1.5/0.7$	64×0.625
kVp	120	120	120
Effective mAs	165	180	240[a]
Reconstruction algorithm	Soft tissue (B 30f)	Soft tissue (B 20f)	Soft tissue (B 20f)
Slice thickness (mm)	3 mm	3 mm	3 mm
Pitch	1.5	0.9	0.9
Rotation time (s)	0.5	0.5	0.5
Table speed (mm/rotation)	12.5	22/11	17.3

[a] By using CARE dose system Scan parameters using 4-, 16, and 64 slice MDCT (developed for Siemens scanner).

while fixing the total duration of the injection (e.g., for a 70-kg patient, 100 mL of 350 mg of iodine per milliliter of contrast material injected at 4 mL/s for 25 seconds). The recent development of double-syringe mechanical power injectors simplified the saline flush technique. Immediate injection of a saline bolus after contrast agent administration has been shown to increase the efficiency of contrast medium use by avoiding dispersion of contrast material within the injection tubing and venous system [18].

1.6 CT Protocol

The increasing speed of MDCT scanners has improved the ability to perform multiphasic examinations of the liver. Before contrast medium administration, the acquisition of precontrast scan is useful and recommended. First of all it is helpful to distinguish fluid lesions from solid tumors; moreover it is indicated for the diagnosis of acute hemorrhage of the liver, the valuation of diffuse liver disease (steatosis, hemochromatosis, detection and calcification of hepatic calcification (calcified metastases, hydatid cysts). Contrast-enhanced MDCT of the liver is regulated by a dual blood supply (75% from the portal vein and 25% from the hepatic artery), resulting in various phase enhancement. Following an intravenous bolus of contrast material, the hepatic artery enhances first approximately 15 seconds and reaches peak attenuation at 30 seconds. The contrast agent returns to the liver from the intraperitoneal organs through the portal system after 30 seconds. Liver parenchyma peak enhancement range from 60 to 70 seconds. The equilibrium phase, when the contrast agent is equally divided between intra- and extracellular space, occurs after almost 3 minutes. According to the different enhancement curves of the hepatic artery, portal vein, and hepatic parenchyma, four phases can be

distinguished: early arterial, late arterial, portal venous, and delayed (Figure 1.9).

The early arterial phase begins with the arrival of contrast medium in the hepatic artery and ends before portal vein enhancement. The diagnostically useful early arterial phase with sufficient contrast enhancement begins 5–10 seconds after aortic contrast material arrival. The early arterial phase is useful primarily for angiographic imaging of abdominal arterial anatomy and is infrequently obtained for a diagnostic purpose. The late arterial phase is the preferred imaging phase for detecting hypervascular primary or metastatic neoplasms [19–23]. During this phase, hypervascular hepatic lesions enhance maximally, whereas hepatic parenchyma remains relatively unenhanced, commensurate with the relatively small contribution of the hepatic artery to the total hepatic blood supply. The acquisition of images during two arterial contrast phases does not seem to provide additional benefit for the detection of hypervascular focal liver lesion, so late arterial phase alone could be sufficient to reach this topic.

Portal-venous phase started after 60–70 seconds after contrast material injection, when the liver parenchyma reaches its peak enhancement. This phase is useful to well delineate portal and hepatic veins and bile ducts dilatation. Hypovascular tumors are well detected on this phase because of the maximum difference in liver-to-lesion contrast.

Delayed phase (or equilibrium) appears approximately after 180 seconds postcontrast agent administration, when the contrast diffuses into the liver parenchyma and the difference attenuation between vessels and liver parenchyma is minimal. Delayed imaging phase is useful for detecting and characterizing HCCs [24] and for characterizing cholangiocarcinoma (CCC) [25]. During this phase, HCCs typically appear as hypoattenuating, whereas CCCs often show delayed contrast enhancement relative to the background hepatic parenchyma.

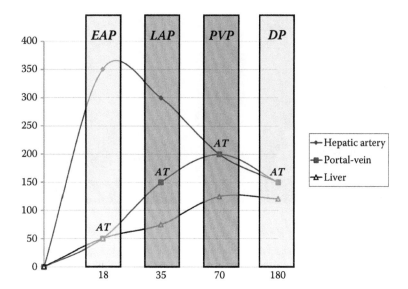

FIGURE 1.9
Different enhancement of hepatic artery, portal vein, and liver parenchyma after contrast medium administration and relative acquisition time of four different vascular phases. EAP = early arterial phase, LAP = late arterial phase, PVP = portal-venous phase, DP = delayed phase AT = acquisition time.

1.7 Reconstruction Parameters

As previously described, with the adventure of 16-slice and more scanners, it became possible to acquire images with a resolution of 1 mm or less, resulting in a nearly isotropic dataset. This three-dimensional (3D) volume can be used for two-dimensional (2D) or 3D post-processing. The most important techniques adopted for liver imaging are multiplanar reformation (MPR), maximum intensity projection (MIP), minimum intensity projection, and volume rendering (VR) [18].

MPR, representing a 2D reformatted plane other than the axial plane, is used to better visualize anatomic and pathologic findings (Figure 1.1a–e).

MIP is routinely used to evaluate hepatic arteries, portal vein and hepatic veins, since the projections display the greatest attenuation difference between vessels and adjacent tissue (Figure 1.2).

The VR technique allows the user to view the entire volume dataset in an appropriate 3D context, including a range type of abdominal tissue. These images are well appreciated by surgeons, since they offer true 3D view of vascular anatomy (Figures 1.3 and 1.4)

1.8 Dual-Energy CT

Dual-energy CT (DECT) is a novel CT technique that is becoming available in most advanced referral diagnostic units and it implies the application of two different energies to add, to the classic single energy MDCT study, information yielded from material differentiation because of the interaction between tissues and different energy levels [26]. DECTs deliver the two energy spectra by a dual tube configuration working at different voltages with intersecting radiation beams or by a single tube able of fast voltage switching. DECT is presently offered by major vendors and is transitioning from first generation apparatuses to second generation ones. Latest generation models overcome some limitations of the first-generations ones; for example, some of the earlier models had smaller FOV of the lower energy tube. As a matter of fact, from first experimental applications in the early 80s, DECT has undergone major technical advances in combination to CT technologic improvements [27,28], that made it suitable for the abdominal region investigation [29–32]. The application of this technique in liver CT imaging, although still under investigation, already showed advantages in the clinical setting.

DECT of the liver (Figure 1.10) can be considered as an interesting strategy to reduce radiation dose delivery to the patients, suitable especially in liver diseased populations undergoing multiple exams because of liver chronic illnesses. This concept is fundamental in a clinical scenario where cumulative exposure from CT ionized radiation is increasing [33] and reduction of patient dose delivery is a mandatory issue [34] to improve patient safety [35]. Dose reduction from DECT can be achieved by taking advantage of the possibility of virtual noncontrast (VNC) images (Figure 1.11) generation from a dual-energy acquired dataset applying a specific three-point algorithm that differentiates soft tissues,

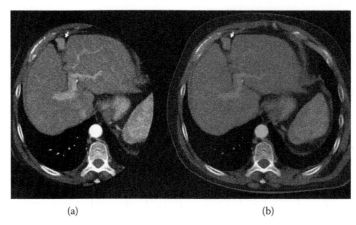

(a)   (b)

FIGURE 1.10
Dual-energy late arterial phase liver axial images in a cirrhotic patient. On the left (a) the low energy (80 kVp) and on the right (b) the higher energy (140 kVp) acquisitions. Note the left liver hypertrophy and the recanalized paraumbilical vein (arrow), the latter as signs of cirrhosis and portal hypertension.

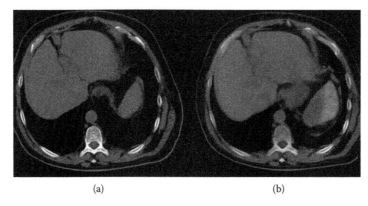

(a)   (b)

FIGURE 1.11
Liver unenhanced (a) and virtual noncontrast (b) axial images. Note in the VNC image that the algorithm applies only to the area of superimposed energies. Therefore, because of the smaller field of view of the low-kVp tube, part of the volume, external to the liver area, is excluded.

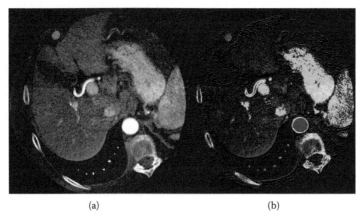

(a)   (b)

FIGURE 1.12
Iodine only axial images. Color coding (b) can be applied to enhance liver vasculature or parenchymal lesions.

iodine, and fat. VNC images can therefore simulate true nonenhanced acquisitions. Investigations by Barrett et al. [36] and Zhang et al. [37] showed a 24.8% and 33% dose reduction, respectively, if the above technique is applied in a DECT of the liver. In addition, by the same algorithm, it is possible to achieve an iodine-only image dataset that eventually could be color coded, depicting the iodine distribution in the liver parenchyma, therefore, enhancing hypervascular liver lesions detection (Figure 1.12).

Advantage of a dual-energy liver acquisition is also the potential benefit arising from the acquisition of the low-kVp dataset, derived from one of the CT tubes, both in the identification and characterization of hypervascular liver tumors [38]. To understand the latter concept, the reader needs to keep in mind that kilovoltage (kVp) and milliampere second (mAs) are two important factors to be considered; mAs shares a linear relation with effective radiation dose, whereas kVp and effective radiation dose share an exponential one [39]. Iodine has specific K-edge characteristics presenting a spike at 33 keV (Figure 1.13). This intrinsic property can be taken in advantage to enhance hypervascular lesion conspicuity arising from the low-kVp acquisitions, although the latter benefit has a drawback in high image noise that needs to be compensated with higher mAs tube current values. To solve the latter drawback, different authors investigated low-kVp imaging of the liver and its ability to enhance hypervascular liver lesions in combination with iterative reconstruction (IR) methods, to lower the dose maintaining at the same time a good image quality. Presently, major CT manufacturers offer IR techniques (ASIR, MBIR, IRIS, AIDR, iDose) showing a significant lowering of patient dose delivery, up to 65%, when using a low-kVp iteratively reconstructed abdominal CT protocol [40–44]. We expect that this techniques combination (low-kVp protocols + IR) and the application of IR techniques to low-kVp acquisitions derived from DECT will be standard in the next future, for abdominal CT acquisitions.

Also DECT ability to evaluate iron deposition in a noninvasive manner is one of the interesting applications that are being investigated and showed positive results in recent literature both in phantom models [45] and in human liver transplant recipients [46].

The application of different energy spectra to the liver is a challenging and stimulating topic that is presently being investigated and in combination to future,

technological advancements will yield different information that will help our diagnostic daily challenges and open new diagnostic frontiers in liver CT.

1.9 Cystic Focal Lesions

1.9.1 Hepatic Cyst

Simple hepatic cyst is benign developmental lesion that do not communicate with the biliary tree. The current theory regarding the origin of true hepatic cyst is that they originate from hamartomatous tissue [47]. Hepatic cysts are common lesions and presume to be present in almost 5% of the population; they are more often discovered in women, almost always asymptomatic. Simple hepatic cysts can be solitary or multiple, with the latter being the more typical scenario. At histopathologic analysis, true hepatic cysts contain serous fluid and are lined by a nearly imperceptible wall consisting of cuboidal ephitelium, identical to that of bile ducts, and a thin rim of fibrous tissue. At unenhanced MDCT, hepatic cysts appear as a homogeneous hypoattenuated lesion (HU < 20), typical round or oval in shape and with well-defined wall, without contrast enhancement after contrast medium injection (Figure 1.14) [48].

1.9.2 Polycystic Disease

Autosomal dominant polycystic liver disease (ADPLD) is often found in association with renal polycystic disease. It is thought to result from progressive dilation of the abnormal ducts in biliary hamartomas as part of a ductal plate malformation at the level of the small intrahepatic bile ducts. The small bile ducts have lost continuity with the remaining biliary tree, which explains the noncommunicating nature of the cysts.

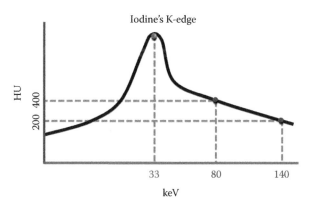

FIGURE 1.13
Graph representing the relation between iodine and different energy spectra. Note the iodine's K-edge at 33 keV.

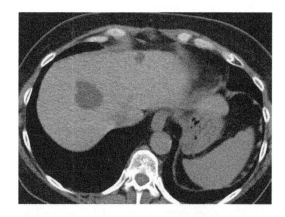

FIGURE 1.14
Simple cyst. Postcontrast CT image shows two homogeneous, rounded, well-defined, nonenhancing cystic lesions, which are consistent with simple bile duct cysts.

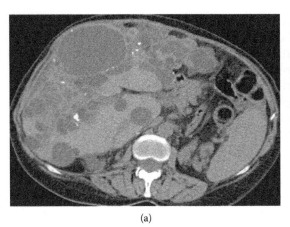
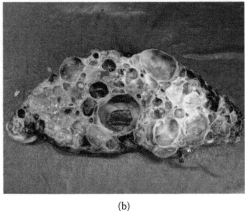

(a)   (b)

FIGURE 1.15
Autosomal dominant polycystic liver disease. Precontrast CT image (a) shows multiple hepatic cysts with thin wall and regular margin; some wall calcifications may also be appreciable. Photograph of the hepatic specimen (b) shows numerous cysts that replace the hepatic parenchyma.

At imaging, it typically manifests as an enlarged and diffusely cystic liver, with the cysts varying from less than 1 cm to more than 10 cm in diameter. Calcification of the cystic walls has been reported (Figure 1.15) [49].

The leading complications in ADPLD are infection, compression, bleeding, or rupture of the cysts. Malignant degeneration is extremely rare. In selected cases of diffuse bilobar polycystic disease with massive hepatomegaly, percutaneous interventional alcohol ablation is as useful as an alternative to partial liver resection for liver transplantation [47].

Although the diagnosis of polycystic is easily made with CT, MRI is more sensitive for the detection of complicated cysts.

1.9.3 Cystic Metastases

Most hepatic metastases are solid but some have partially or complete cystic appearance. In general, two different pathologic mechanisms can explain the cyst-like appearance of hepatic metastases [50]. Hypervascular metastatic with rapid growth tumors may lead to necrosis and cystic degeneration (neuroendocrine tumor, melanoma, certain subtype of lung and breast carcinoma). Cystic metastases may also be seen in mucinous adenocarcinomas such as colorectal or ovarian carcinoma (Figure 1.16) [51]. Ovarian metastases commonly spread by means of peritoneal seeding rather than blood vessels; therefore, they appear as cystic serosal implants on the liver surface rather than intraparenchymal lesions.

1.9.4 Hepatic Abscesses

1.9.4.1 Pyogenic Abscess

Pyogenic abscesses may be caused by ascending cholangitis, gastrointestinal infection via the portal vein, disseminated sepsis via the hepatic artery, superinfection of necrotic tissue [52–53]. The clinical manifestations

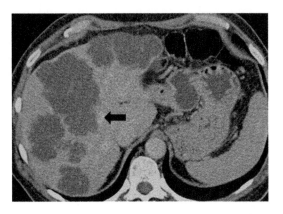

FIGURE 1.16
Cystic metastases. Postcontrast CT image acquired on portal-venous phase shows multiple cystic lesions from mucinous colorectal adenocarcinoma. In the central lesion, it is also visible a peripheral enhancing nodule (arrow).

of pyogenic abscesses are highly variable. Patients may present with high fever, right-side abdominal pain, and rigors. Hepatic biochemical abnormalities are nonspecific, including slightly elevated total bilirubin and aminotransferase levels [52,54]. Early diagnosis and percutaneous treatment have markedly reduced the mortality rates [55].

Pyogenic abscesses appear as a solitary or multiple lesions ranging from few millimeters to several centimeters in diameter; when multiple may appear to cluster, or aggregate, in a pattern that suggested the beginning coalescence into a single larger abscess cavity [56].

At CT microabscesses appear as multiple hypoattenuated well-defined lesions. Faint rim enhancement and perilesional edema may be seen, findings that help differentiate them from hepatic cysts.

Large abscesses are generally well defined and hypoattenuating; they can be unilocular with smooth margins or complex with internal septa and irregular contour (Figure 1.17). Rim enhancement and presence of gas are relatively uncommon.

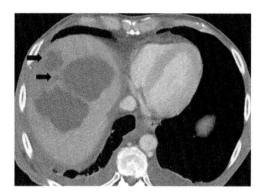

FIGURE 1.17
Hepatic pyogenic abscess. Postcontrast enhanced CT image shows a large multiloculated lesion in the right lobe of the liver surrounded by other smaller areas (arrows).

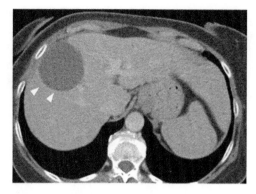

FIGURE 1.18
Amebic abscess. Contrast-enhanced CT scan shows a large, rounded, well-defined cystic mass in the right hepatic lobe. Note the slightly enhancement of the thin wall of the lesion (arrowheads).

Despite it has some characteristic finding, CT appearance of hepatic abscess is not specific and sometimes difficult to distinguish from hepatic metastases.

1.9.4.2 Amebic Abscess

Amebic liver abscess is the most common extraintestinal complication of amebiasis, occurring in 3%–9% of the cases. Patients usually show high fever and right-side abdominal pain. Histologic features of amebic liver abscesses include scant inflammatory reaction at the margins and a shaggy fibrin lining. Because of hemorrhage into the cavities, the abscesses are sometimes filled with a chocolate-colored, pasty material known as "anchovy paste." Secondary bacterial infection may make these abscesses purulent [57]. CT findings of amebic abscess are aspecific. It usually appears as a solitary oval or round mass located near the liver capsule [58]. At contrast-enhanced CT, amebic abscesses usually appear as rounded, well-defined lesions with attenuation values that indicate the presence of complex fluid (10–20 HU) [54]. An enhancing wall is common and somewhat characteristic for this lesion (Figure 1.18). The central abscess cavity may show multiple septa or fluid–debris levels and, rarely, air bubbles or hemorrhage [59–60]. Extra hepatic extension of amebic abscess is relatively common, and involvement of the chest wall, pleural cavity, pericardium, and adjacent viscera has been reported.

1.9.5 Echinococcus Disease

Hepatic echinococcosis is a severe and common parasitic disease that is endemic to the Mediterranean basin and in other countries such as Australia, New Zealand, Canada. It is generally caused by *Echinococcus granulosus*. The ingested embryos invade the intestinal mucosal wall and proceed to the liver through the portal vein system. Although the liver filters most of these embryos, those that are not destroyed become hydatid cysts [61].

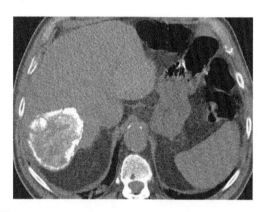

FIGURE 1.19
Hidatyd cyst. Unenhanced CT image shows a well-defined, rounded lesion, in the right lobe of the liver with wall calcifications.

Maturation of a cyst is characterized by the development of daughter cysts in the periphery as a result of endocyst invagination. At CT, hydatid cysts appear as a hypoattenuating uni- or multilocular cyst, with well-defined margins and thin or thick walls [62–64]. Generally, calcifications of the walls and/or septa may be seen [64] (Figure 1.19).

Treatment of hydatid cyst is often surgical because of the inadequate efficacy of medicine therapy.

1.9.6 Bile Duct Hamartoma

Biliary Hamartoma, also known as Von Meyenburg complex, are composed of one or more dilated bile duct-like structures lined by epithelium accompanied by a variable amount of fibrous stroma [49]. At pathologic analysis they appear as grayish-white nodular lesions that do not communicate with the biliary tree and are scattered throughout the liver parenchyma. They are typically multiple, round or oval, and small in size (less than 1.5 cm). It is difficult to distinguish them from simple cysts or microabscess (Figure 1.20) [65]. They also may be confused with liver metastases, however, the latest are more heterogeneous in size and attenuation.

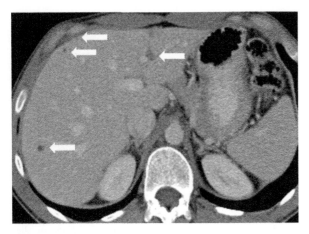

FIGURE 1.20
Biliary hamartoma. Postcontrast CT image during the portal-venous phase shows cystic-like lesion in the liver parenchyma without peripheral contrast enhancement (arrows).

At MDCT, biliary hamartomas are discovered as hypoattenuated small focal lesions, without contrast enhancement, although a peripheral enhancing rim has been described [66].

1.9.7 Biliary Cystadenoma and Cystadenocarcinoma

Biliary cystadenomas are rare, usually low growing, multilocular cystic tumors, that represent less than 5% of intrahepatic cystic lesions. They usually develop in middle-aged women and are considered premalignant lesions. They are single or multiple and the fluid within the lesion may be mucinous, serous, or hemorrhagic [67].

Polypoid, peduncolated masses are seen most commonly in cystadenocarcinoma than in cystadenoma. The MDCT features of cystadenoma and cyst-adenocarcinoma are: well-defined cystic lesions, with fibrous capsule, internal septa and rarely calcification (Figure 1.21). Wherever present, solid mass within the lesion shows enhancement after contrast medium injection [48–68].

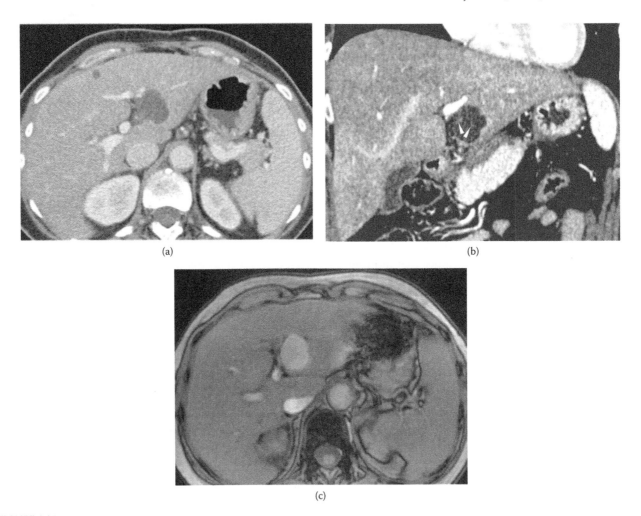

(a)

(b)

(c)

FIGURE 1.21
Biliary cystadenoma. Postcontrast CT images acquired on axial and coronal planes (a and b) show low-attenuation rounded lesion with regular margins and thin septa within the lesion (arrowheads). (c) Axial T1-weighted MR image shows proteinaceous content within the lesion.

1.10 Benign Focal Lesions

1.10.1 Focal Nodular Hyperplasia

Focal nodular hyperplasia (FNH) is a benign tumor caused by a hyperplastic response to a localized vascular abnormality and it is the second most common benign tumor after hemangioma [69]. FNH is common in young and middle-aged women; it's not associated to the assumption of oral contraceptives, but they have a trophic effect on growth.

The lesion is usually solitary, peripherally located, small in size (generally less than 5 cm) and sometimes with a cenral scar related to the presence of fibrous septa. Multiple FNHs are associated with multiorgan vascular malformations and such brain neoplasms [70].

The lesion is composed of hepatocytes, Kupffer's cells, and bile ducts, which are located in an abnormal order.

At unenhanced MDCT, FNH is usually either hypoattenuating or isoattenuating to the surrounding liver parenchyma. On the late arterial phase, FNH shows a strong enhancement because of its arterial supply. During the portal-venous and equilibrium phases the lesion is isodense to the surrounding liver [71]. The central scar, when present, shows delayed enhancement and washout because of the presence of mixomatous stroma (Figure 1.22) [72]. Sometimes, FNH presents a pseudocapsule related to the effective mass of the liver parenchyma and the inflammatory reaction [73]. In large lesions may be seen multiple feeding arteries, with central and septal vessels, and also ectatic draining veins (Figure 1.23) [74,75]. The differential diagnosis of FNH includes other hypervascular liver lesions such as hepatocellular adenoma, HCC, and hypervascular metastases. Therefore, distinction between FNH and other hypervascular tumors is crucial to ensure proper therapy.

1.10.2 Hepatocellular Adenoma

Hepatic Adenoma (HA) is a benign tumor which is often seen in young women with use of oral contraceptive. It arises from hepatocytes arranged in sheets of proliferated cells, with few Kupffer cells and absence of bile ducts [76]. Hepatocellular adenoma cells could present lipid and glycogen storage. It is typically a capsulated solitary lesion, although multiple lesions have been reported, with a tendency to spontaneous hemorrhage [77]. Since these lesions may also undergo malignant transformation to an HCC, it is considerate surgical [78] .

Unenhanced MDCT image may provide important clues such as fat or hemorrhage content (respectively hypo- or hyperattenuated areas) (Figure 1.24).

During the late arterial phase, hepatic adenoma enhances rapidly more than surrounding liver parenchyma. During the portal-venous phase and delayed phase, adenoma appearance is variable and not specific; most of them are nearly isoattenuating compared with surrounding liver parenchyma (Figures 1.24 and 1.25). Despite HA shows similar postcontrast pattern compared with FNH, the enhancement during the late arterial phase is higher for FNH [79]. With the introduction

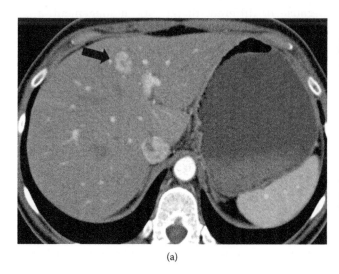

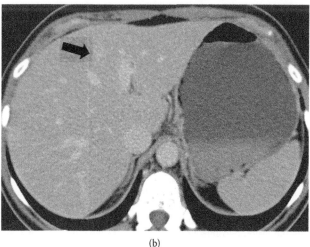

(a)   (b)

FIGURE 1.22

Focal nodular hyperplasia. Postcontrast CT image acquired during the arterial phase (a) shows hypervascular lesion with a central scar (arrow). After 3 minutes during the delayed phase (b), the lesion is isoattenuating to the surrounding liver parenchyma with a slight enhancement of the central scar (arrow).

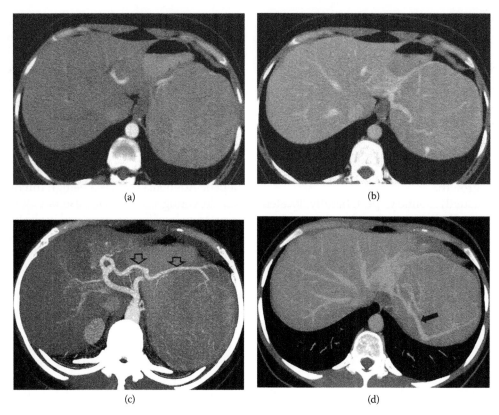

(a)   (b)

(c)   (d)

FIGURE 1.23
Focal nodular hyperplasia. Postcontrast images (a and b) acquired during the arterial and portal-venous phases show a hypervascular large mass on liver segment II (a), which becomes isoattenuating to the liver parenchyma on the delayed phase (b). Maximum intensity projection (MIP) images (c and d) show the abnormal arterial vascular supply (open arrows in c) of the lesion and a large drainage vein (arrow in d).

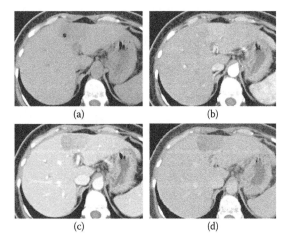

(a)   (b)

(c)   (d)

FIGURE 1.24
Hepatic adenoma. (a) Unenhanced CT image shows a rounded hypoattenuating area related to the presence of lipid storage (asterisk). On an arterial-phase CT scan (b), the tumor shows heterogeneous enhancement. (c and d) On a portal-venous and delayed CT scans the lesion becomes hypoattenuating to the surrounding liver parenchyma.

in clinical practice of liver specific contrast agent, MRI significantly increases its diagnostic performance in the differentiation of FNH from HA. Because of the

presence of functional hepatocytes, FNH is hyper- to isointense on hepatobiliary phase, whereas because the absence of bile ductules, hepatic adenoma does not show uptake of the contrast agent (Figure 1.26) [80]. Because of different therapeutic management, a correct diagnosis is crucial between FNH and hepatic adenoma.

Large HAs may be heterogeneous than smaller lesions, and their CT appearance is less specific. Multiple adenomas in adenomatosis or glycogen disease may have a wide variety of imaging appearance, but CT characteristics of individual lesions are similar to those reported for solitary adenomas (Figure 1.27).

1.10.3 Hepatic Hemangioma

Hepatic hemangioma is a benign tumor composed of multiple vascular channels lined by a single layer of endothelial cells supported by a thin fibrous stroma [81].

Its vascular supply arises from a branch of the hepatic artery and presents slow flow. Most hemangiomas are asymptomatic, particularly those that are less than 4 cm. However, lesions greater than 4 cm can cause sign and symptoms sufficiently severe to require surgical treatment [82].

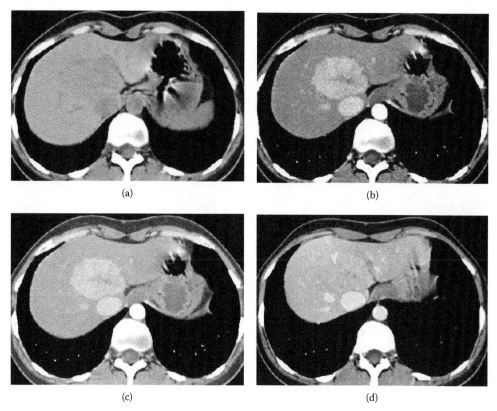

(a)   (b)

(c)   (d)

FIGURE 1.25
Hepatic adenoma. Unenhanced CT image (a) shows a large rounded hypoattenuating mass in liver segment VIII. An Arterial-phase CT scan shows a heterogeneous hypervascular mass that becomes less evident on portal-venous and delayed phase (c and d).

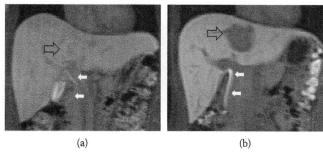

(a)   (b)

FIGURE 1.26
Comparison of focal nodular hyperplasia (FNH) and hepatic adenoma (HA) during the MR imaging hepatobiliary phase. On the coronal T1-weighted MR image, FNH (open arrow in a) is iso- to hyperintense because of the presence of functional hepatocytes and bile structure nodule, whereas HA (open arrow in b) does not show uptake of contrast agent because the absence of bile ducts. Note the clear visualization of the main biliary duct on both images (arrows).

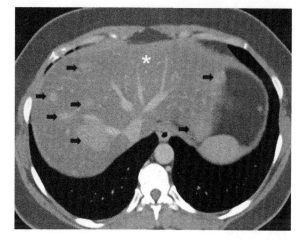

FIGURE 1.27
Hepatic adenomatosis. Postcontrast CT image on portal-venous phase shows multiple adenomas (arrowheads). The lesions appear hyperattenuating because of the underlying liver steatosis (asterisk).

At noncontrast MDCT, hemangioma shows the same clues that of vascular structures; it is hypodense to the surrounding liver parenchyma; but it should be iso- to hyperdense when liver steatosis is present [83]. Postcontrast images of hepatic hemangioma show a typical peripheral enhancement with slow progressive centripetal trend (Figures 1.28 and 1.29) [84]. Small flash-filling hemangiomas appear as high hypervascular lesion, which tends to become isoattenuating to the surrounding parenchyma on portal-venous and delayed phase, they could be misdiagnosed as arterial-portal shunt (Figure 1.30) [85].

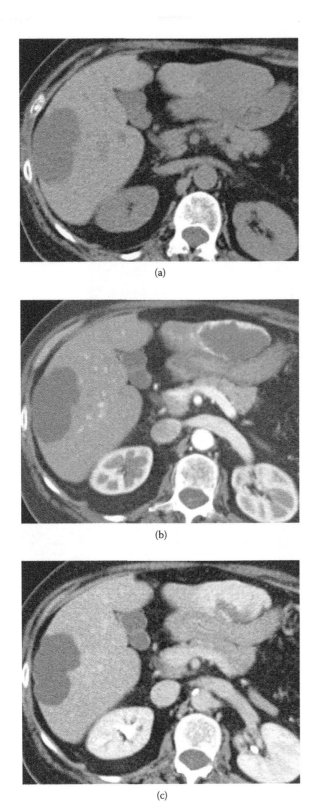

FIGURE 1.28
Hepatic hemangioma. (a) Unenhanced CT image reveals a focal liver lesion with an attenuation similar to that of vessels. (b) On arterial-phase CT scan the mass shows peripheral globular enhancement; (c) during the delayed phase the lesion is totally enhanced.

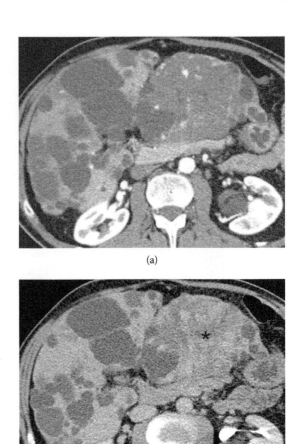

FIGURE 1.29
Hepatic hemangioma. Postcontrast CT images acquired on arterial (a) and delayed (b) phases show a large mass with typical peripheral enhancement with slow progressive centripetal enhancement. Note a central area because of the presence of fibrous tissue (asterisk).

1.11 Rare Benign Lesions

Primary leiomyoma of the liver is a rare benign tumor that affects both young and adults, with increased incidence in patients with acquired immunodeficiency syndrome or immunosuppressed state after organ transplantation [86]. It is composed of interlacing bundles of smooth muscle fibers. Clinical presentation may range from small incidentally discovered lesions to large palpable, upper abdominal masses. Although primary leiomyoma rarely degenerates into malignant lesion, liver resection is often required to yield a definite diagnosis. Results of imaging studies reported a marked enhancement of leiomyoma during the arterial phase, despite specific findings have not been shown (Figure 1.31). Further, hindering definitive diagnosis is the wide range of either

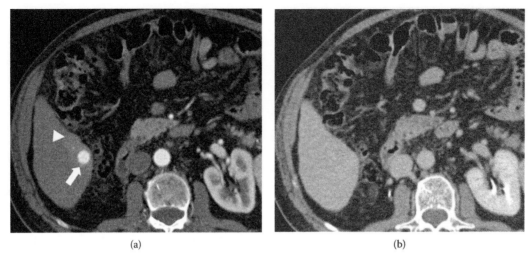

FIGURE 1.30

Flash-filling hemangioma. (a) Postcontrast CT image acquired during the arterial phase show a hypervascular rounded small lesion with an attenuation similar to that of aorta (arrow). Note a tiny hypervascular area near the lesion related to an arteroportal shunt (arrowheads). (b) On the corresponding delayed phase the lesion becomes isoattenuating to the surrounded liver parenchyma.

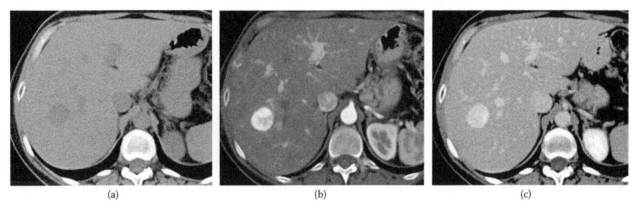

FIGURE 1.31

Leiomyoma. (a) Precontrast CT image shows a well-defined, rounded, hypodense lesion in the right hepatic lobe. (b and c) Postcontrast CT images acquired during the arterial and delayed phase show a hypervascular lesion with prolonged enhancement.

benign or malignant hypervascular liver lesions that could be included in any differential diagnosis [86–88].

Angiomylipoma is a benign, unencapsulated mesenchymal tumor that is composed of varying proportions of three elements: smooth muscle cells, thick-walled blood vessels, and mature adipose tissue. Angiomyolipoma can be classified on the basis of fat content into mixed, lipomatous, myomatous, and angiomatous types. At CT precontrast scan, it appears with a peripheral angiomyomatous tissue and a fatty component. Postcontrast images shows enhancement of both angiomyomatous and fatty components (Figure 1.32). It is difficult to distinguish angiomyolipoma from HCC with fatty infiltration; however, washout sign during delayed phase, typical of HCC, helps to the right characterization [89–90].

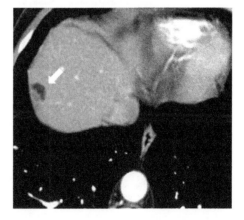

FIGURE 1.32

Angiomyolipoma. CT postcontrast image shows a well-circumscribed lesion with fat component (arrow).

1.12 Malignant Focal Lesions

1.12.1 Hepatocellular Carcinoma

HCC is the most common primary tumor of the liver and is the fourth most common tumor in men and the fifth most common in women [91,92]. It occurs primarily in subjects who have chronic liver disease or liver cirrhosis and is the primary cause of death among this group. The development of HCC may arise from de novo hepatocarcinogenesis or by means of a multistep progression from regenerative nodules, through dysplastic nodules to HCC.

Unfortunately, despite numerous technological developments and improvements in recent years, the sensitivity and specificity of MDCT in patients with cirrhosis is still relatively low, ranging between 33% and 70% [93–97]. The relatively poor diagnostic performance for the detection of HCC in cirrhotic liver is due principally to overlapping imaging features and thus, difficulties in differentiating dysplastic nodules from small HCC and to problems associated with diagnosing arterially enhancing nodules smaller than 2 cm in diameter.

The CT appearance of HCC is extremely variable and depends on growth pattern (solitary, multifocal masses or infiltrating neoplasm) (Figures 1.33 through 1.35), size, and histologic composition. Up to 36% of HCC are associated with fatty infiltration, which may aid the identification on unenhanced (Figure 1.36) [98].

The majority of HCCs are hypoattenuating on precontrast scan: although unenhanced images seem to not add significant advantage in terms of HCC detection, they could play an important role in the differentiation of uncertain lesions such as siderotic nodules, focal confluent fibrosis, and focal sparing of fatty infiltration [99].

Typically, HCC is hypervascular during the arterial phase: small lesions show more homogeneous enhancement compared with larger neoplasms that are heterogeneous because of the presence of necrosis and hemorrhage. During the portal-venous phase, HCC becomes iso- to hypoattenuating to the surrounding liver. On delayed phase, the tumors washout more rapidly than hepatic parenchyma. Based on recent guidelines, these diagnostic criteria are sufficient for a noninvasive diagnosis of HCC (Figure 1.33).

Several studies recommended the utility of delayed phase in a CT protocol of cirrhotic liver because of its ability to significantly improve the detection and characterization of HCC, especially, for smallest nodules [99–102].

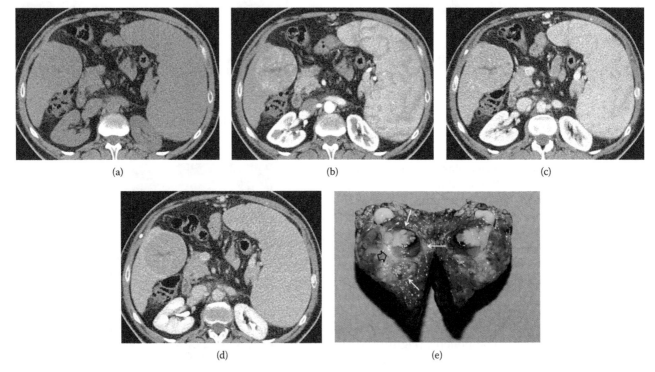

(a) (b) (c)

(d) (e)

FIGURE 1.33
Hepatocellular carcinoma (HCC). Unenhanced CT image (a) shows a hypoattenuating lesion in liver segment five. (b) Postcontrast CT images reveal during the late arterial phase a hypervascular lesion which becomes isoattenuating during the portal-venous phase (c) phase and hypodense during delayed phase (d). The lesion shows the so called "wash-out" sign that is typical for HCC. (e) Photograph of the gross specimen shows an encapsulated lesion (arrows) within fibrous septum (open arrow). (Courtesy of M. Rossi, MD.)

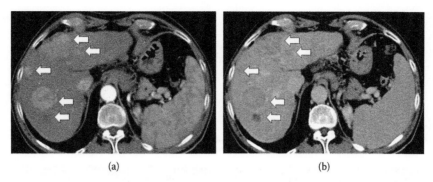

FIGURE 1.34
Multifocal hepatocellular carcinoma. (a and b) Postcontrast CT images acquired during arterial and delayed phase reported multiple hypervascular masses with washout after three minutes of contrast medium injection typical for HCCs (arrows).

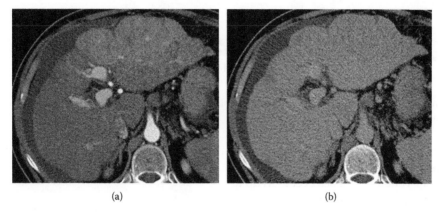

FIGURE 1.35
Infiltrative hepatocellular carcinoma. (a) Postcontrast CT images acquired during arterial phase show a large hypervascular area that englobes all the left liver lobe, modifying its anterior surface, which shows irregular margins. (b) On delayed phase this area is slightly hypoattenuating to the right liver lobe.

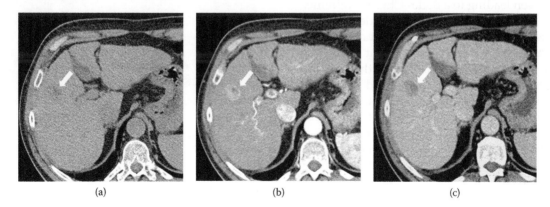

FIGURE 1.36
Hepatocellular carcinoma. (a–c) Pre- and postcontrast CT images reveal typical HCC in liver segment five with a small area of adipose tissue density. Generally, presence of fat tissue within the tumor is associated to well-differentiated neoplasm.

HCC could also present atypical findings such as ipervascular lesion without washout or hypovascular tumor (Figure 1.37). Hypovascular nodules are not uncommon and they usually represent early stages like displastic nodules with focal HCC or well-differentiated small HCCs. They show little or any enhancement during the arterial phase. They may also be poorly visualized on later scans as iso- to hypodense lesion. It has been recently shown that hypervascular HCCs without washout represent almost 45% of hypervascular nodules encountered in cirrhotic liver. As well as, of 12% of large (>2 cm) hypovascular nodules discovered in explanted liver, 66% are HCCs [103].

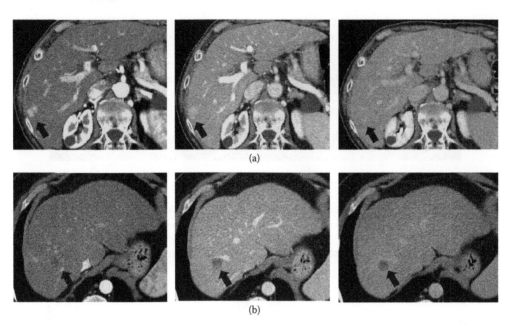

(a)

(b)

FIGURE 1.37
Hepatocellular carcinoma with atypical findings. (a) Pre- and postcontrast CT images of hypervascular HCC without washout sign. (b) Pre- and postcontrast CT images of hypovascular HCC.

Moreover, HCC could present a tumor capsule, which may be visible on delayed phase.

Thrombosis of portal-venous branches occurs in up to 40% of HCCs and is frequently caused by direct tumor invasion: these tumor thrombi are only moderately hypoattenuating and enhance irregularly after contrast administration during the arterial phase (Figure 1.38). The invasion of the hepatic veins is less common and may cause occlusion leading to a Budd–Chiari syndrome.

Despite, HCC develops mainly in patients with cirrhosis caused by virus B and C infection or alcohol abuse; it has been recently shown that nonalcoholic fatty liver disease (NAFLD) is one of the most common causes of liver chronic disease and it has a high risk to develop HCC. Recently, CT imaging findings of HCC in this particular patients' population have been described [104]. The neoplasm usually manifests as a large, hypervascular, solitary mass characterized by smooth and capsulated margins and central necrotic area (Figure 1.39).

1.12.2 Intrahepatic Cholangiocarcinoma

CCC is the most common primary tumor of the bile ducts. Patients usually present painless and jaundice due to biliary obstruction. It should be classified as peripheral or hilar. A tumor originating from the primary bile duct branches is considered at the hilum; moreover a lesion that arises at the confluence of the left and right hepatic ducts is referred as a Klatskin tumor. Predisposing factors for CCC include

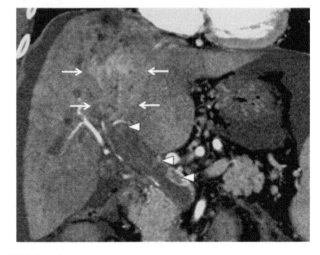

FIGURE 1.38
Diffuse hepatocellular carcinoma with neoplastic involvement of portal vein (PV). Coronal postcontrast CT image show a diffuse ill-defined hypervascular mass in liver segment VIII (arrows) with thrombus into the PV. Note the enlargement of the PV and its tiny enhancement (arrowheads).

ulcerative colitis, Caroli disease, sclerosing cholangitis, and congenital biliary abnormalities. The role of MDCT imaging is to establish tumor extension and its resectability. The CT appearance of intrahepatic CCC is classified into three types: mass-forming, periductal infiltrating, and intraductal. Peripheral tumors usually appear as well-defined or irregular mass-forming lesion along the course of dilated intrahepatic ducts, usually with liver capsule retraction. On CT, during

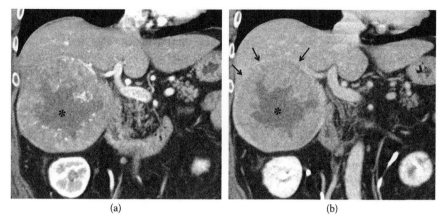

(a)   (b)

FIGURE 1.39
Hepatocellular carcinoma in nonalcoholic fatty liver disease (NAFLD). (a) Postcontrast CT image during arterial phase shows a faintly hyperattenuating mass with a central hypoattenuating necrotic area (asterisk). (b) Contrast-enhanced image during delayed phase shows washout of the solid component and a peripheral capsule (arrows).

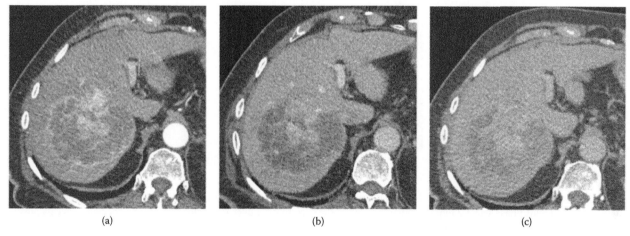

(a)   (b)   (c)

FIGURE 1.40
Peripheral cholangiocarcinoma. (a and b) Postcontrast CT image during arterial and portal-venous phases show a low-attenuation mass with rim enhancement. (c) On delayed phase CT scan, the mass looks smaller because of the enhancement of the central zone.

both late arterial and portal-venous phase, CCC shows as a hypoattenuating mass with incomplete peripheral rim enhancement [105–107]. The central portion of the tumor may show prolonged enhancement and be hyperattenuating on delayed phase (10 minutes) because of slow washout related to the large amount of fibrous tissue (Figure 1.40) [108]. Hilar CCC typically takes one of the three shapes: infiltrative, exophytic, or polypoid (Figure 1.41). The most common type is the periductal infiltrating form. Postcontrast CT images of infiltrating hilar CCC may detect focal duct wall thickening, which appears hyperattenuating relative to liver parenchyma during the portal-venous phase or delayed [109]. A supplementary CT finding of hilar carcinomas includes lobar atrophy because of either severe or long-standing ductal obstruction.

1.12.3 Metastases

One of the major indications for hepatic MDCT is the detection of metastatic liver disease, which is by far the most common malignant tumor in patients without cirrhosis. The CT image appearance of liver metastases may vary widely depending on the histologic nature of the lesion, size presence of necrosis or calcification. The type of MDCT protocol for depiction of liver metastases depends on the degree of primary tumor vascularization.

Most hepatic metastases are hypovascular and arise from primary tumor of gastrointestinal tract, pancreas, urothelium, lung, head, and neck, as well as gynecologic tumors. During the portal-venous phase, these lesions are typically hypoattenuating owing to superior enhancement of adjacent liver parenchyma, so most authorities recommend a single-CT scan during

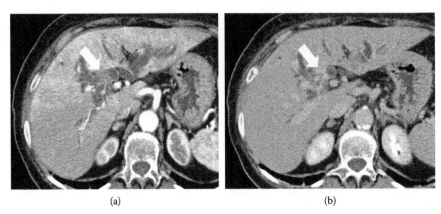

(a)   (b)

FIGURE 1.41
Polypoid hilar cholangiocarcinoma. (a) Postcontrast CT image during the arterial phase shows a hypoattenuating mass at the hepatic hilum, mainly in segment IV (arrow). Both intrahepatic ducts are dilated. (b) Postcontrast CT image during delayed phase (8 minutes) show an enhancement of the lesion because of the presence of fibrous stroma.

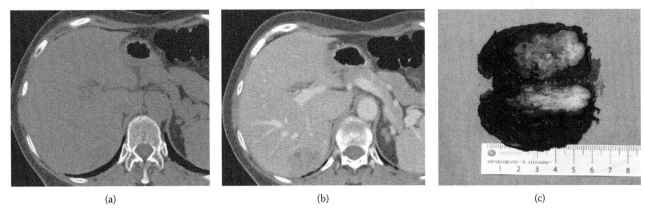

(a)   (b)   (c)

FIGURE 1.42
Hypovascular metastasis. (a) Precontrast image shows a hypoattenuating subcapsular lesion in liver segment VII. (b) Postcontrast CT images during the portal-venous phase shows a hypoattenuating lesion to the surrounding liver. (c) Photograph of liver specimen reveals the malignant nature of the lesion. (Courtesy of M. Rossi, MD.)

the portal-venous phase for evaluation of hypovascular metastases (Figure 1.42). In the periphery of these metastases, there may be increased enhancement during either arterial or portal-venous phase, represented by a hypervascular rim or halo, which is been recently showed in almost 85% of hypovascular metastases (Figure 1.43) [110]. Several studies have shown that the additional use of precontrast or hepatic arterial phase does not improve the detection of hypovascular liver metastases [111–113]. The reported detection rate of hypovascular liver metastases for CT is ranging between 85% and 91% [110–114]. Precontrast images are useful in the detection of hemorrhage or calcification within the lesion: calcified metastases are more commonly associated with mucinous colorectal cancer; however, a wide variety of other primary tumors are associated with calcified liver metastases (renal cell carcinoma, breast carcinoma, chondrosarcoma) [115]. These calcifications may be central or peripheral in location and are founded in areas of reduced attenuation (Figure 1.44).

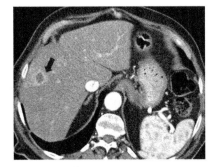

FIGURE 1.43
Hypovascular metastasis with rim enhancement. Transverse arterial phase CT scan of metastasis from a colo-rectal cancer depicts ring enhancement (arrows) with well-defined smooth inner margins surrounding central regions of low attenuation.

Few studies investigated the usefulness of smaller slice thickness in the identification of liver metastases: no more benefits have been reported for a slice thickness of 2.5 cm compared with 5 mm. It should suggest that lot of small lesions (≤15 mm) are benign [116]. However,

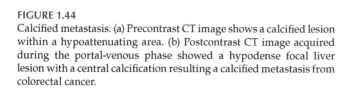

(a)

(b)

FIGURE 1.44
Calcified metastasis. (a) Precontrast CT image shows a calcified lesion within a hypoattenuating area. (b) Postcontrast CT image acquired during the portal-venous phase showed a hypodense focal liver lesion with a central calcification resulting a calcified metastasis from colorectal cancer.

further studies should be conducted to assess the optimal slice thickness for the identification of liver metastases.

Primary tumor that tend to be associated with hypervascular metastases include neuroendocrine tumors, renal cell carcinoma, thyroid carcinoma, melanoma, and occasionally breast cancer. The imaging protocol for hypervascular metastases is significantly different from hypovascular. Hypervascular lesions are typically hyperattenuating during the late arterial phase because of an earlier and increased contrast media uptake compared with adjacent liver parenchyma and becomes isoattenuating to liver parenchyma on subsequent vascular phases (Figure 1.45) [117,118]. These lesions are sometimes misinterpreted as FNH, hemangiomas, and focal fatty infiltration.

In the detection of liver metastases, CT and MRI have been shown to be effective for the detection and characterization of liver metastases, with slight, albeit nonsignificant, tendency for better overall diagnostic

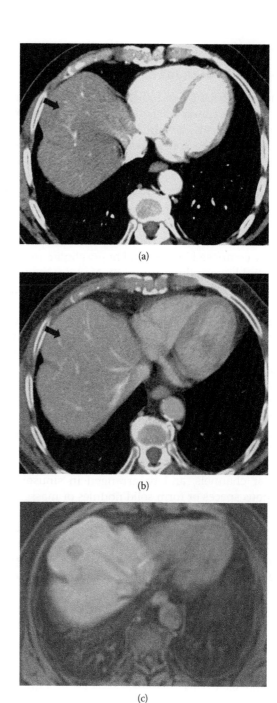

(a)

(b)

(c)

FIGURE 1.45
Hypervascular metastasis. (a) Postcontrast CT image acquired during the arterial phase show a hypervascular lesion in liver segment VIII. (b) On delayed phase, the lesion in slightly hypoattenuating compared to the surrounding liver parenchyma. (c) MR imaging acquired during the hepatobiliary phase helps to correctly characterize this lesion, indeed it shows a hypointense lesion to the surrounding parenchyma, which is a sign of absence of functional hepatocytes.

performance for the latter technique. Moreover, the introduction in clinical practice of hepatobiliary contrast agent significantly improves the diagnostic performance of MR in the detection of liver metastases (Figure 1.45) [119–121].

1.13 Rare Malignant Lesions

Epithelioid hemangioendothelioma is a primary malignant vascular tumor of the liver, characterized by the epithelioid appearance with neoplastic cells [122].

It should not be confused with infantile epithelioid hemangioendothelioma, which is benign and occurs exclusively in young children and resolves spontaneously in many cases [123]. Two-thirds of the patients are women; the clinical course is unpredictable and variable; however, most of the 40% have an extended survival at 5 years. It is usually constituted by multiple peripheral nodules, composed by a central hypocellular area and a peripheral hypercellular rim zone. Nodules may merge into a large mass; they often determine liver capsule retraction and rare calcifications may be present [124].

Unenhanced MDCT images show an area of homogeneous low attenuation compared to the surrounding liver. Postcontrast images show a central area of low density with peripheral rim enhancement. Some lesions have a second more peripheral hypodense zone that correlated with a thin avascular rim visible at histopathologic examination (Figure 1.46) [125].

Primary angiosarcoma of the liver is a malignant spindle cell tumor of endothelial cell derivation that can form poorly organized vessels, grow along performed vascular channels, and be arranged in sinusoidal or cavernous spaces or form solid nodules or masses [126]. It has an example of malignant transformation secondary to environmental exposure and has been associated with multiple chemical carcinogens including thorium dioxide, vinyl chloride, and arsenic [127]. The prognosis at the time of the diagnosis is infausted, with a median survival of only 6 months.

It could be present as a single large mass, multiple, or both; peripheral located nodules or mass may produce hemoperitoneum.

Nonenhanced CT shows a hypoattenuated lesion with iso- to hyperdense area because of the presence of hemorrhagic areas. After contrast agent administration, angiosarcoma reported a heterogeneous patchy enhancement; however, it has been also described in literature a vascular pattern similar to that of hepatic hemangioma [128]. Combined interpretation of pre- and postcontrast images helps to well characterize angiosarcoma from hemangioma; moreover, hemangioma show a centripetal wash-in, whereas nodular enhancement of angiosarcoma are generally central and irregular. Multiple nodular patterns should be mistaken as hypervascular metastases [129].

Primary lymphoma of the liver is a rare tumor, but its incidence is increasing. It is generally a non-Hodgkin type. It develops as a single, large, multilobulated mass (Figure 1.47).

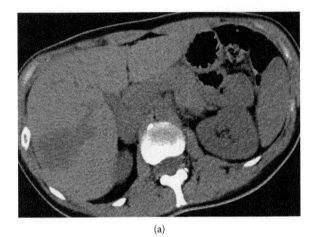

(a)

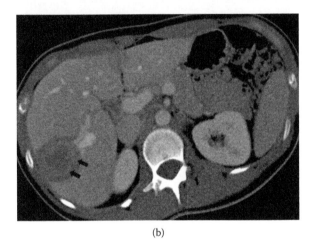

(b)

FIGURE 1.46
Hepitheliod hemangioendothelioma. (a) Unenhanced CT image shows a homogeneous hypoattenuating peripheral located lesion with tiny capsular retraction. Postcontrast CT image (b) shows tumor nodule with complex enhancement pattern consisting of a nonenhancing center, hypervascular rim, and low-attenuation outer halo (arrows).

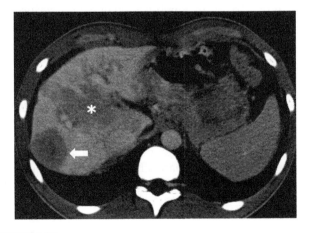

FIGURE 1.47
Hepatic lymphoma. Postcontrast CT image shows a large hypodense mass in the liver segment VII. Note a diffuse and heterogeneous area in the central segments because of the presence of acute hepatitis (asterisk).

Un-enhanced CT images show a hypoattenuting lesion; postcontrast scans reveal a hypodense mass. Sometimes thin rim enhancement or calcifications may be present.

Secondary liver lymphoma can have a greater variety of appearances and is more likely to be multiple or diffusely infiltrating lesions than a solitary lesion [131].

1.14 Vascular and Perfusion Disorders

1.14.1 Budd–Chiari Syndrome

Budd–Chiari syndrome is an uncommon disorder resulting from an obstructed hepatic venous outflow tract. The obstruction lesion is situated in the main hepatic veins, in the IVC or in both. It is classified as primary when it is caused by an intrinsic luminal web or thrombus, and secondary when it is caused by an extraluminal compression or neoplasm invasion [132]. Membrane or web arises from the wall of the vessels and may obliterate the lumen completely or partially. This type of lesion is believed to be a sequel of long-standing thrombosis. Hematologic abnormalities (factor V Leiden mutation, myeloproliferative disorders, antiphospholipid syndrome, etc.) are responsible for the majority of cases of Budd–Chiari syndrome [133]. The other factors include pregnancy immediate postpartum and use of oral contraceptives.

The secondary Budd–Chiari syndrome is caused by an extraluminal compression of a space occupying lesion or luminal invasion of malignant neoplasia (renal cell carcinoma, adrenal carcinoma, and HCC, primary leiomyosarcoma of IVC. As the hepatic vein constitutes the sole efferent vascular drainage of the liver, obstruction or increased pressure within these vessels result in an increased sinusoidal pressure, which leads in a delayed or reversed portal-venous outflow.

The portal-venous stasis and congestion cause hypoxemic damage in adjacent hepatocytes. Afterward, centrilobular fibrosis, nodular regenerative hyperplasia, and ultimately cirrhosis occur.

At unenhanced MDCT, acute form of Budd–Chiari syndrome show diffuse hypodensity of enlarged liver. Hepatic veins are narrowed and hyperdense thrombus may be seen [134]. Postcontrast MDCT images show an early enhancement of caudate lobe and central parenchyma around IVC with decreased liver enhancement peripherally (Figures 1.48 and 1.49). On delayed phase it could be observed a late enhancement of the previously hypodense areas leading to an almost homogenous areas or a hyperdensity of the peripheral parenchyma (flip-flop sign) (Figure 1.49b). In chronic stage, caudate lobe is often enlarged and main hepatic veins cannot be seen. The presence of regenerative nodules leads to a progression to cirrhosis and so the risk to develop HCC. Of about 40% of cases, the enhancement pattern of the liver is almost homogeneous; this is because of the more stable hepatic perfusion that occurs after the formation of intra- and extrahepatic collateral veins [135–136].

1.14.2 Passive Hepatic Congestion

Passive hepatic congestion is caused by stasis of blood within liver parenchyma because of a compromised venous drainage. It is a common complication of congestive heart failure and constrictive pericarditis, wherein elevated central venous pressure is directly transmitted from the right atrium to the hepatic veins [137].

On contrast-enhanced MDCT, liver parenchyma may present an inhomogeneous mottled, reticulated-mosaic pattern. Retrograde hepatic venous opacification on the initial bolus scans is also a transient finding indicative of elevated right heart pressure (Figure 1.50). Moreover, IVC and hepatic veins are enlarged (Figure 1.51) [138].

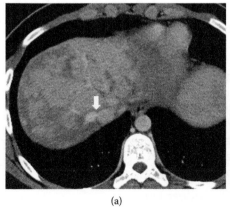
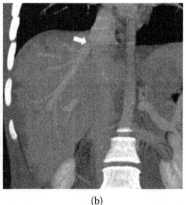

(a)   (b)

FIGURE 1.48
Budd–Chiari syndrome. (a and b) Axial and coronal postcontrast CT images during the portal-venous phases show an inhomogeneous enhancement of liver parenchyma because of the obstruction of left and median hepatic veins. Note a diaphragm at the origin of the right hepatic vein (arrow).

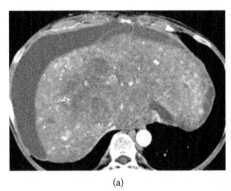
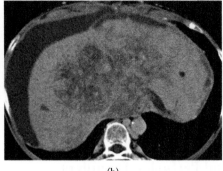

(a)   (b)

FIGURE 1.49
Budd–Chiari syndrome. Axial postcontrast CT image acquired during the arterial phase (a) shows multiple hypervascular nodules in an enlarged liver. Postcontrast axial image acquired during the delayed phase (b) shows a low attenuation of the central part of the liver with accumulation of the contrast material from the capsular veins (flip-flop sign).

Other collateral nonspecific findings that could be present are cardiomegaly, ascites, and pleural effusions.

The parenchyma enhancement pattern is similar to that of Budd–Chiari syndrome but in this latest case the IVC and hepatic veins are not opacificated, and large regenerative nodules may be present [139].

1.14.3 Hereditary Hemorrhagic Telangiectasia (Osler–Weber–Rendu Syndrome)

Hereditary hemorragic telenagectasia (HHT) is a rare autosomal dominant, multisystem vascular disorder affecting many organ systems and occurring in approximately 10–20 individuals per 100,000 [140,141]. It is characterized by angiodysplastic lesions, in which there is direct communication between arteries and veins of varying sizes without an intervening capillary network [142].

Hepatic vascular lesions range from tiny telangiectases to transient perfusion abnormalities and large confluent vascular masses [143,144].

Focal hepatic lesions are often associated with arteriovenous, arterioportal, or portovenous shunts. Telangiectases are the most commonly seen hepatic lesion and can be focal or diffuse. They are hypervascular rounded masses, usually measuring only few millimeters in size. Coronal MIP images are helpful in appreciating telangiectases, especially when they exist in proximity to the large vessels.

Large confluent vascular masses are defined as large areas of multiple telangiectases that coalesce or large shunts that are directly visible; any enhancing lesion with a diameter larger than 10 mm is so called [143]. These lesions usually show early enhancement that is seen during arterial and portal-venous phases (Figure 1.52).

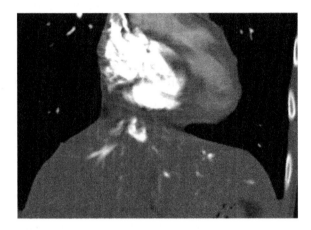

FIGURE 1.50
Hepatic congestion. Postcontrast coronal reformatted image acquired for the study of the pulmonary vessels shows retrograde enhancement of the inferior vena cava and the hepatic veins, which is a sign of elevated right heart pressure.

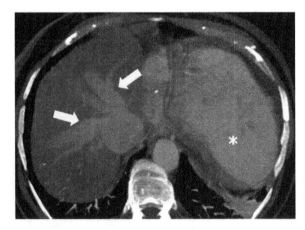

FIGURE 1.51
Hepatic congestion. Axial maximum intensity projection (MIP) image show the great dilatation of the inferior vena cava and the hepatic veins (arrows). Note the great volume of the heart (asterisk).

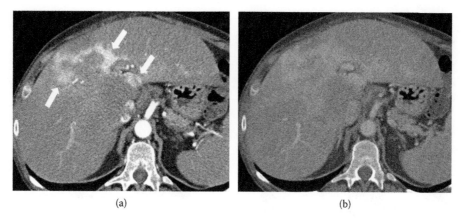

(a)   (b)

FIGURE 1.52
Hereditary hemorragic telangiectasia: (a and b) Postcontrast CT images during arterial and portal-venous phase show large confluent vascular masses (arrows). The masses show delayed and persistent enhancement.

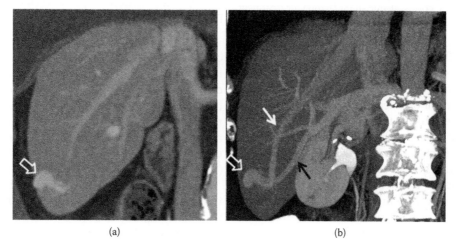

(a)   (b)

FIGURE 1.53
Hereditary hemorragic telangiectasia. Coronal MPR and MIP images obtained in the portal-venous phase show porto-hepatic venous shunting, with the dilated portal vein (black arrow) communicating with the median hepatic vein (white arrow) through a focal vascular mass (open arrow).

Hepatic perfusion abnormalities are identified as an inhomogeneous attenuating pattern within the liver parenchyma. They are best seen during the early and late arterial phase, almost always disappearing in the hepatic parenchyma becoming homogeneous. In contrast to that seen in HHT, the perfusion abnormalities in the setting of cirrhosis usually are more focal, peripherally located, and wedge-shaped configuration on either coronal or axial projections.

With HHT, the perfusion abnormalities are frequently more diffuse and inhomogeneous or ill-defined [144–145].

Three types of hepatic vascular shunts exist in HHT: arteriovenous, arterioportal, and portovenous. Arteriovenous and arterioportal shunts are artery to vein shunts with early enhancement draining vein

connecting to the hepatic vein or portal vein. Both are detected during the early arterial phase, with latter phases being less diagnostic. Portovenous shunts are seen in the hepatic phase, with a dilated portal vein branch (during the portal-venous phase) communicating with the large hepatic vein (Figure 1.53) [146].

1.14.4 Hepatic Infarction

Hepatic infarction is defined as areas of coagulation necrosis from hepatocyte death cells caused by local ischemia because of the obstruction of the circulation of the affected area by a thrombus or embolus.

It is uncommon because of the dual vascular supply from the hepatic artery and portal vein. Hepatic infarction may be iatrogenic (transarterial chemoembolization)

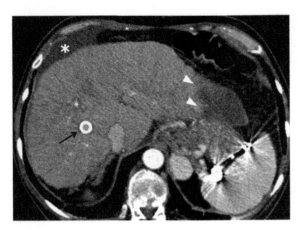

FIGURE 1.54
Hepatic infarction after HCC transarterial chemoembolization. Postcontrast CT image acquired during the arterial phase shows a hypodense, peripheral wedge-shaped area (arrowheads). Note a transjugular intrahepatic portosystemic shunt (arrow) for treatment of intractable ascites (asterisk).

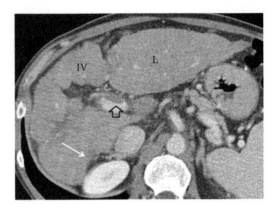

FIGURE 1.55
Cirrhosis. Postcontrast CT during portal-venous phase show the enlargement of hilar periportal space because of atrophy of medial segment of left lobe (IV). Liver also present irregular margins, enlargement of the left lobe (L) and a notch in posterior segments (arrow). Note the presence of portal vein thrombosis, which is a complication of liver cirrhosis (open arrow).

or posttraumatic (laceration of hepatic artery or portal vein). It can occur as a complication of liver transplantation; it may be secondary to vasculitis or infection [126]. Hepatic artery thrombosis leading to infarction most often occurs after liver transplantation has been reported in almost 3% of adult transplant recipients.

Unenhanced CT shows peripheral wedge-shaped, rounded, or irregularly shaped area of low attenuation of the liver. Bile leaks may be seen as a late sequel of large infarcts from ischemia necrosis of bile ducts epithelium. Gas formation has been described in sterile infarcts as well as infected ones [147].

Postcontrast images show a better defined area of lower attenuation to the surrounding liver (Figure 1.54). It manifests as perfusion defects in a geographic or segmental pattern with or without defined margins. Its enhancement pattern is patchy or heterogeneous because of nondisplaced vessels in the infarcted areas. Preservation of portal tracts is a feature worthy of emphasis because it helps to differentiate infarction from other causes of hypoattenuating foci (abscess, biloma) [139].

Focal steatosis is also included in the differential diagnosis; however, it develops in specific site and vascular structures are preserved.

1.15 Diffuse Liver Disease

1.15.1 Cirrhosis

Liver cirrhosis is a chronic response to repetitive hepatic insult, which is characterized by regenerative nodules and fibrosis [148]. The changes of cirrhosis occur cyclically with episodes of impaired circulation, injury inflammation, fibrosis, and regeneration. Obstruction of intrahepatic vascular bed by fibrosis and regenerative nodules results in portal hypertension. Liver cirrhosis could be classified into (1) micronodular, with nodule less than 3 mm and thin septa; (2) macronodular, with nodules more than 3 mm and thick septa, (3) mixed.

The main causes of liver cirrhosis include viral infection, such as hepatitis B and C and alcohol abuse. Secondary causes should be hemochromatosis, biliary obstruction, biliary primary cirrhosis, metabolic disorder, and storage disease. Complications of liver cirrhosis result in portal hypertension and development of hepatofugal portal flow via multiple portosystemic venous collateral channels, which lead to hepatic encephalopathy and variceal hemorrhage [149].

MDCT of the liver in cirrhotic patient should evaluate changes in liver morphology, complications of portal hypertension and exclude the risk of liver hepatocarcinogenesis.

A primary morphologic change on liver parenchyma is the enlargement of hilar periportal space because of atrophy of medial segment of left lobe (IV segment) [150]. Morphologic changes in advanced cirrhosis include the atrophy of the right lobe, the enlargement of the left and caudate lobe, a nodular liver contour, and widened fissures between liver segments, this latter aspect is detectable especially on alcoholic cirrhosis [151,152] (Figure 1.55).

Fifteen percent of patients with advanced cirrhosis develop an area of confluent fibrosis. CT appearance is a wedge-shaped area of lesser attenuation than adjacent liver parenchyma at pre-and postcontrast CT images (Figure 1.56)

CT extrahepatic findings of liver cirrhosis include portal vein thrombosis, ascitis, splenomegaly and portosystemic shunts (Figures 1.55 through 1.57).

Cirrhosis-associated hepatocellular nodules result from the localized proliferation of hepatocytes and their supporting stroma [153]. Most are benign regenerative nodules; however, regenerative nodules may progress along a well-described carcinogenic pathway to become dysplastic nodules or HCCs [154]. The imaging evaluation of cirrhosis-associated hepatocellular nodules therefore is important for their optimal management. There are four classes of lesions that are characteristically found in the cirrhotic liver; regenerative nodules, dysplastic foci, dysplastic nodules, and HCC. Regenerative nodules also may be classified according to size as either micronodules (<3 mm) or macronodules (≥3 mm). Giant regenerative nodules with a diameter of 5 cm have been described, but they are rare. Lesions with dysplastic features that do not satisfy the histologic criteria for malignancy or invasion are described as either (1) dysplastic foci (<1 mm in diameter) or (2) dysplastic nodules (≥1 mm in diameter). Dysplastic nodules usually occur in the setting of cirrhosis and may be classified as low or high grade, according to the degree of dysplasia. According to the latest guidelines from the American Association for the Study of Liver Diseases, dysplastic nodules should not be treated or managed as cancers, and patients with known or suspected dysplastic nodules should not be monitored more aggressively than patients without such nodules [155]. Regenerative nodules and low-grade dysplastic nodules are predominantly portally perfused and, after contrast medium administration, show enhancement similar to that of the surrounding liver (Figure 1.58) [156,157]. As dedifferentiation progresses within these nodules, angiogenic pathways are activated that induce new vessel formation, which manifests as an increased density of unpaired arteries and capillary units [156]. This development leads to an increasing shift from predominant venous perfusion to predominant arterial perfusion as low-grade dysplastic nodules and HCCs become high-grade lesions (Figure 1.59) [155].

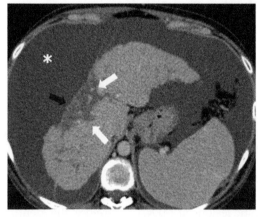

FIGURE 1.56
Confluent hepatic fibrosis in liver cirrhosis. Postcontrast CT scan shows wedge-shaped lesion (white arrow) of lower attenuation than adjacent liver parenchyma in the anterior segment of the right lobe. Deep retraction of liver capsule is seen (black arrow). Note the lot amount of intra-abdominal fluid (asterisk).

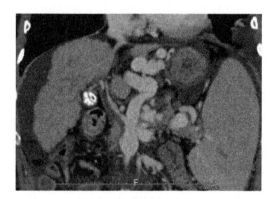

FIGURE 1.57
Complications in liver cirrhosis. Postcontrast CT image show portal hypertension signs such as thrombosis of portal vein, splenomegaly, and portosystemic venous collateral channels.

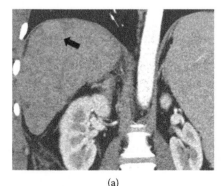 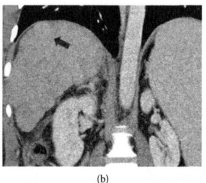

(a) (b)

FIGURE 1.58
Regenerative nodule. (a and b) Postcontrast CT images acquired during arterial and portal-venous phase show a tiny hypervascular subcapsular lesion in liver segment VIII with prolonged enhancement during the portal-venous phase (arrow).

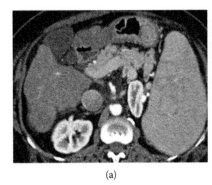
(a)

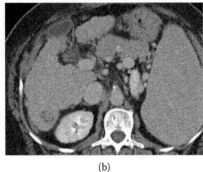
(b)

FIGURE 1.59
Dysplastic nodule. (a) Postcontrast CT image during arterial phase reveals any focal live lesion. (b) Postcontrast CT image during delayed phase (3 minutes) show a hypoattenuating focal liver lesion in liver segment V, which was confirmed to be a dysplastic nodule at liver biopsy.

The increasingly dedifferentiated nodules appear more markedly enhanced on early arterial phase images obtained after the intravenous injection of a contrast agent, with more pronounced washout on venous phase images and equilibrium phase images [158]. The major shift in angiogenesis typically occurs during the transition from low-grade to high-grade dysplasia.

Although the term siderotic nodule is not included in the International Working Party lexicon, it is mentioned here because it appears commonly in the radiology literature. The term was coined by radiologists to describe cirrhosis-associated nodules with high levels of endogenous iron.

1.15.2 Steatosis

Steatosis or fatty change is an excessive accumulation of triglycerides within the hepatocytes [159]. Several toxic and metabolic disorders may produce it such as alcohol abuse, obesity, diabetes mellitus, hepatitis, and drugs. This is generally a reversible change, but it is often undetectable at clinical or laboratory examination.

Fatty change can have a correspondingly variable appearance on images with patterns of fatty liver such as diffuse and uniform, focal, multifocal, and confusing.

At unenhanced MDCT, fatty infiltration results in a lowering of the liver attenuation. The normal liver has an attenuation of about 8 HU greater than that of the spleen [160,161]. Mild steatosis can be diagnosed when the liver attenuation is slightly less than that of the spleen; marked steatosis leads in an attenuation value lower than that of the intrahepatic blood vessels (Figure 1.60).

Although fatty change may be diagnosed also on contrast-enhanced MDCT, postcontrast images evaluation is less reliable and specific. After contrast medium administration, significant fatty infiltration can be depicted if liver attenuation in less than that of muscle or if it has an attenuation value of at least 25 HU lower than that of the spleen [162].

Focal fatty infiltration, perivascular fat distributions, and residual foci of unaffected liver parenchyma

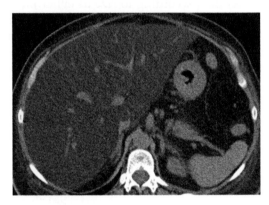

FIGURE 1.60
Liver steatosis. Unenhanced CT image shows a lower attenuation of liver parenchyma compared to that of spleen. Note the clear visualization of intrahepatic liver vessels.

surrounded by fatty infiltration may all be confused with neoplastic lesions at MDCT. Therefore, the identification of specific findings is crucial to achieve a correct diagnose.

Focal fatty infiltration commonly has a segmental or lobar distribution. These often irregularly shaped lesions typically extend to liver capsule, without associated bulging of liver contour. Moreover, vessels coursing through the area of abnormality are not displaced common locations or fatty infiltrations are in the anterior part of the segment IV, adjacent to the falciform ligament [163].

1.15.3 Hemochromatosis

The term hemochromatosis refers to iron overload disorders; it can be classified as (1) primary, when it origins from a genetic disturbance [human leukocyte antigen) that promotes the increase of iron absorption, or (2) secondary to chronic disease or multiple transfusions. Hemochromatosis can lead to chronic liver disease, cirrhosis, and often HCC [164]. Basically, iron is stored in the reticuloendothelial cells; an iron overload is accumulated within the hepatocytes producing inflammation and liver damage. Unenhanced MDCT shows a homogenous increase in the attenuation of the hepatic parenchyma to 70 HU or more (Figure 1.61) [165,166]. CT has low sensitivity (63%) and high specificity (96%) for the diagnosis of iron over load. Certain conditions, such as associated steatosis, can reduce the sensitivity still further reducing the hepatic parenchyma attenuation [167]. Other factors, such as Wilson disease, colloidal gold treatment, and long-term administration of amiodarone, also increase the liver attenuation, which decrease the diagnostic specificity of CT. It has been shown that a positive linear correlation exists between CT attenuation and iron overload at both "single energy" CT and "dual energy CT." Moreover, because of the high atomic number of iron, the increase of hepatic parenchyma attenuation can be better appreciated with a lower kVp (80) than conventional kVp (120). [168] In advanced stage of hemocrhomatosis, liver shows typical pattern of cirrhosis, postcontrast acquisitions are useful to avoid the presence of liver neoplasms.

1.15.4 Wilson Disease

Hepatolenticular degeneration, more commonly known as Wilson disease, is an autosomal recessive disorder characterized by increased intestinal uptake of copper and subsequent deposition in the liver, basal ganglia, cornea (Kayser–Fleischer rings), and other tissues. It can manifest as acute and even fulminant hepatitis or with rapid progression to liver cirrhosis: progression to HCC is extremely rare. Patients with Wilson disease present low level of ceruloplasmin. As well as liver hemochromatosis, deposition of copper in the liver determines an increasing of liver attenuation. This finding is variable, however, in part because the associated fatty infiltration decreased liver attenuation, preventing any appreciable increase in attenuation. Spectrum of imaging injury is nonspecific; changes of fatty infiltration or cirrhosis are indistinguishable from those of other entities [126,169,170].

1.16 Local Treatment

Local-regional treatment play a key role in the management of HCC and recently also for treatment of liver metastases. Image-guided tumor ablation is recommended in patients with early stage HCC; moreover, it has been shown that it is the treatment of choice for lesion smaller than 2 cm compared to liver resection [171]. Radiofrequency (RF) ablation has shown superior response and greater survival benefit to other percutaneous technique such as ethanol injection.

After the procedure, CT examination reveals a well-defined, delineated, rounded hypodense area without contrast enhancement after contrast material injection. The area of RF-induced coagulated tissue forms a necrotic "scar" that usually shrinks with time, but most often very slowly (Figure 1.62) [172].

During the arterial phase, a thin peripheral rim related to inflammatory alteration is usually visible, sometimes a wedge-shaped peripheral area due to a transitory arteroportal shunt is also appreciable. Local regrowth shows the same radiological findings of primary tumor (Figure 1.63) [173].

Transcatheterarterial chemoembolization (TACE) is the standard of care for patients with multinodular HCC out of criteria for liver transplantation in an intermediate stage of disease. A limit of CT in the evaluation of HCC post-TACE is the high density of high-iodized oil within the tumor and its artifact. Embolic microspheres, which

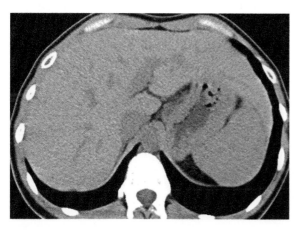

FIGURE 1.61
Liver hemochromatosis. Unenhanced CT image shows diffuse, marked increased attenuation (higher than that of the spleen) secondary to iron deposition.

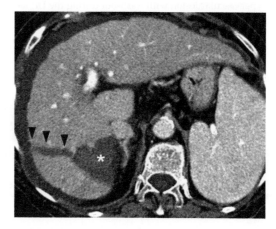

FIGURE 1.62
Radiofrequency ablation of HCC. Postcontrast image acquired on portal-venous phase shows a large hypoattenuating area in liver segment VI without contrast enhancement. Note the "ghost" of the lesion (asterisk) and the track released by the needle (arrowheads). (Courtesy of M. Bezzi, MD.)

have the ability to release a drug in a controlled and sustained fashion, have been shown to substantially increase the safety and efficacy of TACE in comparison to conventional ethiodized oil-based regimens (Figure 1.64).

1.17 Complication Post-Liver Transplantation

Liver transplantation is currently an accepted first-line treatment in patients with end-stage acute or chronic liver disease, but postoperative complications may limit the long-term success of transplantation. It is important for the radiologist to be aware of the most common anastomotic techniques and expected postoperative imaging findings [174,175].

Posttransplantaion complications are broadly classified into vascular, biliary, and other disorders. Vascular complications include hepatic artery thrombosis-stenosis,

pseudoaneurysm, hepatic infarct, and portal vein, IVC or hepatic veins thrombosis-stenosis. After rejection, vascular complications are the most common cause of graft failure and should be considered in patients with liver failure, bile leak, and abdominal bleeding septicemia [176]. Biliary complications include bile duct obstruction, anastomotic and nonanastomotis stenosis, bile leak, biloma, cholangitis, and biliary necrosis. Other complications of liver transplantation include hematoma, abscess, infection, recurrent malignancy, and lymphoproliferative disorder. Hepatic artery stenosis-thrombosis is the most common vascular complication occurring in 2%–12% of cases, vascular stenosis is usually seen at anastomotic level as a focal narrowing [177,178]. Three-dimensional reconstruction of CT angiographic data allows reliable identification of this finding (Figure 1.65). Hepatic artery thrombosis and stenosis can lead to biliary ischemia, since the hepatic artery is the only vascular supply to bile ducts. Hepatic artery pseudoaneurysm is an uncommon complication that generally develops at the site of anastomosis or a complication of angioplasty. Treatment options for an extrahepatic pseudoaneurysm include surgical resection, embolization, and exclusion with stent placement. Contrast-enhanced CT shows a focal lesion with central enhancement that followed arterial blood-pool attenuation (Figure 1.66).

Portal vein complications following liver transplantation are relatively unusual, occurring in 1%–3% of cases and results from faulty surgical technique, vessel misalignment, and differences in caliber of anastomoted vessels.

Although in less graphic manner compared with MR-cholangiopancreatography, CT can also show biliary complications, which occur in an estimated 25% of liver transplantation recipients, usually within the first 3 months after transplantation.

Biliary complications include leak, stricture, obstruction, and stone formation (Figure 1.67). Transplant recipients have external biliary drainage catheters (T-tube) in the

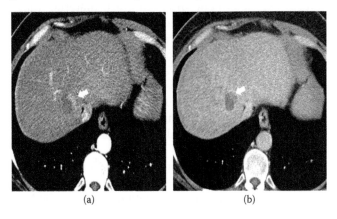

FIGURE 1.63
Hepatocellular carcinoma recurrence after RF ablation. (a and b) CT images acquired during the arterial and delayed phases (DPs) show a tiny hypervascular lesion with wash-out during the DP, located in the medial margin of the treated lesion.

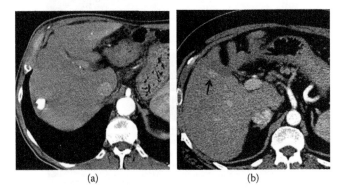

FIGURE 1.64
Hepatocellular carcinoma treated with TACE. (a) Postcontrast CT image of HCC treated with iodized oil show the high attenuation of the lesion where is difficult detect disease recurrence. (b) TACE performed with DC-beads allows the identification of a small hypervascular peripheral lesion due to disease recurrence.

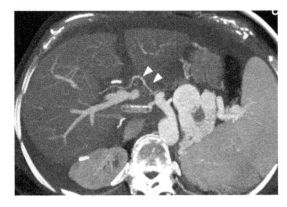

FIGURE 1.65
Complication of liver transplantation. Axial MIP image shows marked stenosis of the transplant hepatic artery at the anastomosis (arrowheads).

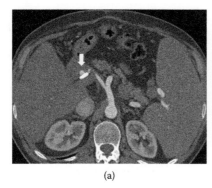
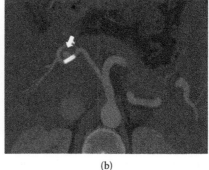

(a)   (b)

FIGURE 1.66

Complication of liver transplantation. (a and b) Postcontrast CT image during the arterial phase and its MIP reconstruction on axial plane revealed an extrahepatic artery pseudoaneurysm at vascular anastomosis treated with endovascular stent. Note that the aneurysm is not completely excluded (arrow).

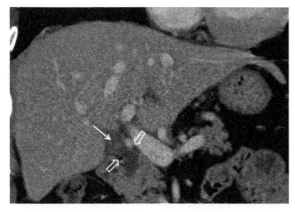

FIGURE 1.67

Complication of liver transplantation. Coronal postcontrast CT image shows a biliary stricture at anastomosis level (open arrows). Note the presence of a bile duct stone (arrow).

postoperative period, so it is fast and easy to perform cholangiography to determine the state of the biliary system when a complication is suspected. The choledochocholedochostomy is the type of biliary anastomosis that is most frequently employed, accompanying a cholecystectomy.

Patients are also at increased risk for developing malignancy, especially non–Hodgkin lymphoma and squamous cell skin cancer because of immunosuppressive therapy [3]. Lymphoma can involve any organ, including the liver graft itself, where it is seen as multiple hypoattenuating nodules. In patients with a neoplasm treated with liver transplantation (HCC, CCC) the primary tumor can recur in the graft or at any other location.

References

1. Couinaud C. *The Liver: Anatomical and Surgical Studies.* Paris, France: Masson, 1957; 9–12.
2. Bismuth H. Surgical anatomy and anatomical surgery of the liver. *World J Surg* 1982; 6: 3–8.
3. Catalano OA, Singh AH, Uppot RN et al. Vascular and biliary variants in the liver: implications for liver surgery. *Radiographics* 2008; 28: 359–378.
4. Makuuchi M, Hasegawa H, Yamazaki S et al. The inferior right hepatic vein ultrasonic demonstration. *Radiology* 1983; 148: 213–217.
5. Marin D, Catalano C, De Filippis G et al. Detection of hepatocellular carcinoma in patients with cirrhosis: added value of coronal reformations from isotropic voxel with 64-MDCT. *Am J Roentgenol* 2009; 192: 180–187.
6. Maetani YS, Ueda M, Haga H et al. Hepatocellular carcinoma in patients undergoing living-donor liver transplantation. *Intervirology* 2008; 51: 46–51.
7. Abdelmoumene A, Chevallier P, Charlon M et al. Detection of liver metastases under 2 cm: comparison of different acquisition protocols in four row multidetector-CT (MDCT). *Eur Radiol* 2005; 15: 1881–1887.
8. Bae KT. Intravenous contrast medium administration and scan timing at CT. consideration and approaches. *Radiology* 2010; 256: 32–61.
9. Heiken JP, Brink JA, McClennan BL et al. Dynamic incremental CT: effect of volume and concentration of contrast material and patient weight on hepatic enhancement. *Radiology* 1995; 195(2): 353–357.
10. Yamashita Y, Komohara Y, Takahashi M et al. Abdominal helical CT: evaluation of optimal doses of intravenous contrast material—a prospective randomized study. *Radiology* 2000; 216(3): 718–723.
11. Kondo H, Kanematsu M, Goshima S et al. Abdominal multidetector CT in patients with varying body fat percentages: estimation of optimal contrast material dose. *Radiology* 2008; 249(3): 872–877.
12. Tello R, Seltzer SE, Polger M et al. A contrast agent delivery nomogram for hepatic spiral CT. *J Comput Assist Tomogr* 1997; 21(2): 236–245.
13. Yanaga Y, Awai K, Nakaura T et al. Optimal contrast dose for depiction of hypervascular hepatocellular carcinoma at dynamic CT using 64-MDCT. *AJR Am J Roentgenol* 2008; 190(4): 1003–1009.
14. Foley WD, Mallisee TA, Hohenwalter MD et al. Multiphase hepatic CT with a multirow detector CT scanner. *AJR Am J Roentgenol* 2000; 175(3): 679–685.

15. Goshima S, Kanematsu M, Kondo H et al. MDCT of the liver and hypervascular hepatocellular carcinomas: optimizing scan delays for bolus-tracking techniques of hepatic arterial and portal venous phases. *AJR Am J Roentgenol* 2006; 187(1): W25–W32.

16. Yanaga Y, Awai K, Nakayama Y et al. Optimal dose and injection duration (injection rate) of contrast material for depiction of hypervascular hepatocellular carcinomas by multidetector CT. *Radiat Med* 2007; 25(6): 278–288.

17. Sultana S, Awai K, Nakayama Y et al. Hypervascular hepatocellular carcinomas: bolus tracking with a 40-detector CT scanner to time arterial phase imaging. *Radiology* 2007; 243(1): 140–147.

18. Schindera ST, Nelson RC. Hepatobiliary imaging by MDCT Springer, 2008.

19. Baron RL. Understanding and optimizing use of contrast material for CT of the liver. *AJR Am J Roentgenol* 1994; 163(2): 323–331.

20. Hollett MD, Jeffrey RB Jr, Nino-Murcia M et al. Dual-phase helical CT of the liver: value of arterial phase scans in the detection of small (< or = 1.5 cm) malignant hepatic neoplasms. *AJR Am J Roentgenol* 1995; 164(4): 879–884.

21. Oliver JH 3rd, Baron RL. Helical biphasic contrast-enhanced CT of the liver: technique, indications, interpretation, and pitfalls. *Radiology* 1996; 201(1): 1–14.

22. Oliver JH 3rd, Baron RL, Federle MP, Rockette HE Jr. Detecting hepatocellular carcinoma: value of unenhanced or arterial phase CT imaging or both used in conjunction with conventional portal venous phase contrast-enhanced CT imaging. *AJR Am J Roentgenol* 1996; 167(1): 71–77.

23. Mitsuzaki K, Yamashita Y, Ogata I et al. Multiple-phase helical CT of the liver for detecting small hepatomas in patients with liver cirrhosis: contrast-injection protocol and optimal timing. *AJR Am J Roentgenol* 1996; 167(3): 753–757.

24. Lim JH, Choi D, Kim SH et al. Detection of hepatocellular carcinoma: value of adding delayed phase imaging to dual-phase helical CT. *AJR Am J Roentgenol* 2002; 179(1): 67–73.

25. Lacomis JM, Baron RL, Oliver JH 3rd et al. Cholangiocarcinoma: delayed CT contrast enhancement patterns. *Radiology* 1997; 203(1): 98–104.

26. Johnson TR, Krauss B, Sedlmair M et al. Material differentiation by dual energy CT: initial experience. *Eur Radiol* 2007 Jun; 17(6): 1510–1517.

27. Kalender WA. CT: the unexpected evolution of an imaging modality. *Eur Radiol* 2005 Nov; 15 Suppl 4: D21–D24.

28. Kalender WA, Perman WH, Vetter JR, Klotz E. Evaluation of a prototype dual-energy computed tomographic apparatus. I. Phantom studies. *Med Phys* 1986 May–Jun; 13(3): 334–339.

29. Graser A, Johnson TR, Chandarana H et al. Dual energy CT: preliminary observations and potential clinical applications in the abdomen. *Eur Radiol* 2009 Jan; 19(1): 13–23. Review.

30. Coursey CA, Nelson RC, Boll DT et al. Dual-energy multidetector CT: how does it work, what can it tell us, and when can we use it in abdominopelvic imaging? *Radiographics* 2010 Jul-Aug; 30(4): 1037–1055.

31. Yeh BM, Shepherd JA, Wang ZJ et al. Dual-energy and low-kVp CT in the abdomen. *AJR Am J Roentgenol* 2009 Jul; 193(1): 47–54. Review.

32. Silva AC, Morse BG, Hara AK et al. Dual-energy (spectral) CT: applications in abdominal imaging. *Radiographics* 2011 Jul-Aug; 31(4): 1031–1046; discussion 1047–1050.

33. Mettler FA Jr, Huda W, Yoshizumi TT et al. Effective Doses in Radiology and diagnostic nuclear medicine: a Catalog; Fred. *Radiology* 2008 Jul; 248(1): 254–263.

34. ICRP. *Recommendations of the International Commission on Radiological Protection (Users Edition).* ICRP Publication 103. Ann. ICRP 2007; 37: 2–4.

35. Marin D, Nelson RC, Rubin GD et al. Body CT: technical advances for improving safety. *AJR Am J Roentgenol* 2011 Jul; 197(1): 33–41.

36. Barrett T, Bowden DJ, Shaida N et al. Virtual unenhanced second generation dual-source CT of the liver: is it time to discard the conventional unenhanced phase? *Eur J Radiol* 2012; 81: 1438–45.

37. Zhang LJ, Peng J, Wu SY et al. Liver virtual non-enhanced CT with dual-source, dual-energy CT: a preliminary study. *Eur Radiol* 2010 Sep; 20(9): 2257–2264.

38. Marin D, Nelson RC, Samei E et al. Hypervascular liver tumors: low tube voltage, high tube current multidetector CT during late hepatic arterial phase for detection—initial clinical experience. *Radiology* 2009 Jun; 251(3): 771–779.

39. McNitt-Gray MF. AAPM/RSNA physics tutorial for residents: topics in CT, radiation dose in CT, Michael F. *RadioGraphics* 2002; 22: 1541–1553.

40. Hara AK, Paden RG, Silva AC et al. Iterative reconstruction technique for reducing body radiation dose at CT: feasibility study. *AJR Am J Roentgenol* 2009 Sep; 193(3): 764–771. Erratum in: *AJR Am J Roentgenol* 2009 Oct; 193(4): 1190.

41. Martinsen ACT, Sæther HK. Iterative reconstruction reduces abdominal CT dose. *EURR-5493*; 1–5.

42. Mitsumori LM, Shuman WP, Busey JM et al. Adaptive statistical iterative reconstruction versus filtered back projection in the same patient: 64 channel liver CT image quality and patient radiation. *Eur Radiol.* doi 10.1007/s00330-011-2186-3.

43. Schindera ST, Diedrichsen L, Müller HC et al. Iterative reconstruction algorithm for abdominal multidetector CT at different tube voltages: assessment of diagnostic accuracy, image quality, and radiation dose in a phantom study. *Radiology* 2011 Aug; 260: 454–62.

44. Marin D, Nelson RC, Schindera ST et al. Low-tube-voltage, high-tube-current multidetector abdominal CT: improved image quality and decreased radiation dose with adaptive statistical iterative reconstruction algorithm, initial clinical experience. *Radiology* 2010 Jan; 254(1): 145–153.

45. Fischer MA, Reiner CS, Raptis D et al. Quantification of liver iron content with CT-added value of dual-energy. *Eur Radiol* 2011 Aug; 21(8): 1727–1732. Epub 2011 Apr 7.

46. Joe E, Kim SH, Lee KB et al. Feasibility and accuracy of dual-source dual-energy CT for noninvasive determination of hepatic iron accumulation. *Radiology* 2012 Jan; 262(1): 126–135. Epub 2011 Nov 21.

47. Van Sonnenberg E, Wroblicka JT, D'Agostino HB et al. Symptomatic hepatic cysts. Percutaneous drainage and sclerosis. *Radiology* 1994; 190: 387–392.

48. Mortelè KJ, Ros PR. Cystic focal liver lesions in the adult: differential CT and MR imaging features. *Radiographics* 2001; 21: 895–910.

49. Brancatelli G, Federle MP, Vilgrain V et al. Fibroplolycystic liver disease: CT and MR imaging findings. *Radiographics* 2005; 25: 659–670.

50. Lewis KH, Chezmar JL. Hepatic metastases. *Magn Reson Imaging Clin N Am* 1997; 5: 241–253.

51. Sugawara Y, Yamamoto J, Yamasaki S et al. Cystic liver metastases from colorectal cancer. *J Surg Oncol* 2000; 74: 148–152.

52. Barnes PF, DeCock KM, Reynolds TN, Ralls PW. A comparison of amebic and pyogenic abscess of the liver. *Medicine* 1987; 66: 472–483.

53. Huang CJ, Pitt HA, Lipsett PA et al. Pyogenic hepatic abscess. *Ann Surg* 1996; 223: 600–609.

54. Mortele KJ, Segatto E, Ros PR. The infected liver: radiologic-pathologic correlation *Radiographics* 2004; 24: 937–955.

55. Pitt HA. Surgical management of hepatic abscesses. *World J Surg* 1990; 14: 498–504.

56. Jeffreey RB Jr, Tolentino CS, Chang CF, Federle MP. CT of small pyogenic hepatic abscesses: the cluster sign. *Am J Roentgenol* 1988; 151: 487–489.

57. Van Sonnenberg E, Mueller PR, Schiffman HR et al. Intrahepatic amebic abscesses: indications for and results of percutaneous catheter drainage. *Radiology* 1985; 156: 631–635.

58. Samuelson J, Von Lichtenberg F. Infectious diseases. In: Cotran RS, Kumar V, Robbins SL eds. *Pathologic Basis of Disease*. 5th ed. Philadelphia, PA: Saunders, 1994; 305–377.

59. Radin DR, Ralls PW, Colletti PM, Halls JM. CT of amebic liver abscess. *AJR Am J Roentgenol* 1988; 150: 1297–1301.

60. Suwan Z. Sonographic findings in hydatid disease of the liver: comparison with other imaging methods. *Ann Trop Med Parasitol* 1995; 89: 261–269.

61. Mergo PG, Ros PB. MR Imaging of inflammatory disease of the liver. *Magn Reson Imaging Clin N Am* 1997; 5: 367–376.

62. Beggs I. The radiology of hydatid disease. *Am J Roentgenol* 1985 145: 539–548.

63. Kalovidouris A, Pissiotis C, Pontifex G et al. CT characterization of multivesicular hydatid cysts. *J Comput Assisted Tomogr* 1986; 10: 428–431.

64. Pedrosa I, Saiz A, Arrazola J et al. Hydatid disease. Radiologic and pathologic features and complications. *Radiographics* 2000; 20: 795–817.

65. Horton KM, Bluemke DA, Hrban RH et al. CT and MR imaging of benign hepatic and biliary tumors. *Radiographics* 1999; 19: 431–451.

66. Semelka R, Hussain SM, Marcos HB, Woosley JT. Biliary hamartomas: solitary and multiple lesion shown on current MR technique including gadolinium enhancement. *J Magn Reson Imaging* 1999; 10: 196–201.

67. Choi BI, Lim JH, Han MC et al. Biliary cystadenoma and cystadenocarcinoma: CT and ultrasonography findings. *Radiology* 1989; 171: 57–61.

68. Palacios E, Shannon M, Solomon C, Guzman M. Biliary cystadenoma: ultrasound, CT, and MRI. *Gastrointest Radiol* 1990; 15: 313–316.

69. Craig J, Peters R, Edmonson H. *Tumors of the Liver and Intrahepatic Bile Ducts (Second Series)*. Atlas of tumor pathology, vol fascicle 26. Washington, DC: Armed Forces Institute of Pathology, 1989.

70. Hussain SM, Terkivatan T, Zondervan PE et al. Focal nodular hyperplasia: findings at state-of-art MR imaging, US, CT, and pathologic analysis. *Radiographics* 2004; 24: 3–17.

71. Welch TJ, Sheedy PF II, Johnson CM et al. Focal nodular hyperplasia and hepatic adenoma: comparison of angiography, CT, US and scintigraphy. *Radiology* 1985; 156: 593–595.

72. Mortele KJ, Praet M, Van Vlierberghe H et al. CT and MR imaging findings in focal nodular hyperplasia of the liver: radiologic-pathologic correlation. *AJR Am J Roentgenol* 2000; 175: 687–692.

73. Shamsi K, De Shepper A, Degryse H, Deckers F. Focal nodular hyperplasia of the liver: radiologic findings. *Abdom Imaging* 1993; 18: 32–38.

74. Brancatelli G, Federle MP, Katyal S, Kapoor V. Hemodinamic characterization of focal nodular hyperplasia using three-dimensional volume-rendered multidetector CT angiography. *AJR Am J Roentgenol* 2002; 179: 81–85.

75. Choi CS, Freeny PC. Triphasic helical CT of hepatic focal nodular hyperplasia: incidence of atypical findings. *AJR Am J Roentgenol* 1998; 170: 391–395.

76. Kerlin P, Davis GL, McGill DB et al. Hepatic adenoma and focal nodular hyperplasia: clinical, pathologic, and radiologic features. *Gastroenterology* 1983; 84: 994–1002.

77. Ichikawa T, Federle MP, Grazioli L, Nalesnik M. Hepatocellular adenoma: multiphasic CT and histopathologic findings in 25 patients. *Radiology* 2000; 214: 861–868.

78. Grazioli L, Federle MP, Brancatelli G et al. Hepatic adenoma: imaging and pathologic findings. *Radiographics* 2001; 21: 877–892.

79. Ruppert-Kholmayr AJ, Uggowitzer MM, Kugler C et al. Focal nodular hyperplasia and hepatocellular adenoma of the liver, differentiation with multiphasic helical CT. *AJR Am J Roentgenol* 2001; 176: 1493–1498.

80. Grazioli L, Morana G, Kirchin MA, Schneider G. Accurate differentiation of focal nodular hyperplasia from hepatic adenoma at gadobenate dimeglumine-emhanced MR imaging: prospective study. *Radiology* 2005; 236: 166–177.

81. Wright TL, Venook AP, Millward-Sadler GH. Hepatic tumors. In: Millward-Sadler GH, Wright R, Arthur MJOP, eds. *Wrght's Liver and Biliary Disease*. vol 2, 3rd ed. Philadelphia, PA: WB Saunders, 1992; 1079–1121.

82. Belli L, De Carlis L, Beati S et al. Surgical treatment of syntomatic giant hemangiomas of the liver. *Surg Gynecol Obstet* 1992; 174: 474–478.

83. Whitehouse RW. Computed tomography attenuation measurements for the characterization of hepatic hemangiomas. *Br J Radiol* 1991; 64: 1019–1022.

84. Quinn SF, Benjamin GG. Hepatic cavernous hemangiomas: simple diagnostic sign with dynamic bolus CT. *Radiology* 1992; 182: 545–548.

85. Hanafusa K, Ohashi I, Himeno Y et al. Hepatic hemangioma: findings with two phase CT. *Radiology* 1995; 196: 465–469.

86. Wachsberg RH, Cho KC, Adekosan A. Two leiomyomas of the liver in an adult with AIDS: CT and MR appearance. *J Comput Assist Tomogr* 1994; 18: 156–157.

87. Marin D, Catalano C, Rossi M et al. Gadobenate dimeglumine-enhanced MR imaging of primary leiomyoma of the liver. *J Magn Reson Imag* 2008; 28: 755–758.

88. Herzberg AJ, MacDonald JA, Tucker JA et al. Primary leiomyoma of the liver. *Am J Gastroenterol* 1990; 85: 1642–5.

89. Bergeron P, Oliva VL, Lalonde L et al. Liver angiomyolipoma: classic and unusual presentations. *Abdom Imaging* 1994; 19: 543–545.

90. Chang JC, Lee YW, Kim HJ. Preoperative diagnosis of angiomyolipoma of the liver. *Abdom Imaging* 1994; 19: 546–548.

91. World Health Organization. mortality database. Available from: http//www.who.int/whosis/en (2010)

92. Bosch FX, Ribes J, Diaz M, Cleries R. Primary liver cancer: worldwide incidence and trends. *Gastroenterology* 2004; 127: 5–16.

93. Libbrecht L, Bielen D, Verslype C et al. Focal lesions in cirrhotic explant livers: pathological evaluation and accuracy of pretransplantation imaging examinations. *Liver Transpl* 2002; 8: 749–761.

94. Boone JM. Multidetector CT: opportunities, challenges, and concerns associated with scanners with 64 or more detector rows. *Radiology* 2006; 241: 334–337.

95. Marin D, Catalano C, De Filippis G et al. Detection of hepatocellular carcinoma in patients with cirrhosis: added value of coronal multiplanar reformations from isotropix voxel with 64-MDCT. *AJR Am J Roengenol* 2009; 192: 775–782.

96. Bruix J, Sherman M, Llovet JM et al. EASL panel of experts on HCC. Clinical management of hepatocellular carcinoma. Conclusions of the Barcelona-2000 EASL conference. European association for the study of the liver. *J Hepatol* 2001; 35: 421–430.

97. Baron RL, Oliver JH III, Confer S et al. Screening cirrhosis for hepatocellular carcinoma (HCC) with helical contrast CT: specificity. *Radiology* 1997; 2005: 143.

98. Kutami R, Nakashima Y, Nakashima O et al. Pathomorphologic study on the mechanism of fatty change in small hepatocellular carcinoma of humans. *J Hepatol* 2000; 33: 282–289.

99. Iannaccone R, Laghi A, Catalano C et al. Hepatocellular carcinoma of unenhanced and delayed phase multi detector row helical CT in patients with cirrhosis. *Radiology* 2005; 234: 460–467.

100. Lim JH, Choi D, Kim SH et al. Detection of hepatocellular carcinoma: value of adding delayed phase to dual-phase helical CT. *AJR Am J Roentgenol* 2002; 179: 67–73.

101. Hawang GJ, Kim MJ, Yhoo HS, Lee JT. Nodular hepatocellular carcinomas: detection with arterial-, portal- and delayed-phase images at spiral CT. *Radiology* 1997; 202: 383–388.

102. Kim SE, Lee HC, Shim JH et al. Noninvasive diagnostic criteria for hepatocellular carcinoma in hepatic masses larger than 2 cm in a hepatitis B virus-endemic area. *Liver Int* 2011; 31: 1469–1477.

103. Luca A, Caruso S, Milazzo M et al. Multidetector-row computed tomography (MDCT) for the diagnosis of hepatocellular carcinoma in cirrhotic candidates for liver transplantation: prevalence of radiological vascular pattern and histological correlation with liver explants. *Eur Radiolo* 2010; 20: 898–907.

104. Iannaccone R, Piacentini F, Murakami T et al. Hepatocellular carcinoma in patients with nonalcoholic fatty liver disease: helical CT and MR findings with clinical pathologic comparison. *Radiology* 2007; 243: 422–430.

105. Kim TK, Choi BI, Han JK et al. Peripheral cholangiocarcinoma of the liver: two phase Ct findings. *Radiology* 1997; 204: 539–543.

106. Vallas C, Guma A, Puig I et al. Intrahepatic cholangiocarcinoma: CT evaluation 2000. *Abdom Imaging* 2000; 25: 490–496.

107. Keogan MT, Seabourn JT, Paulson EK et al. Contrast-enhanced CT of intrahepatic and hilar cholangiocarcinoma: delay time for optimal imaging. *AJR Am J Roentgenol* 2004; 169: 1493–1499.

108. Han JK, Choi BI, Kim AY et al. Cholangiocarcinoma: pictorial essay of CT and cholangiographic findings. *Radiographics* 2002; 22: 173–187.

109. Menias OC, Venkastewar RS, Srinivasa RP et al. Mimics of cholangiocarcinoma: spectrum of disease. *Radiographics* 2008; 28: 1115–1129.

110. Nino-Murcia M, Olcott EW, Jeffrey RB Jr et al. Focal liver lesions: pattern-based classification scheme for enhancement at arterial phase. *Radiology* 2000; 215: 746–751.

111. Soyer P, Poccard M, Boudiaf M et al. Detection of hypovascular metastases at triple phase helical CT: sensitivities of phases and comparison with surgical and histopathologic findings *Radiology* 2004; 231: 413–420.

112. Miller FH, Butler FS, Hoff FL et al. Using triphasic helical CT to detect focal hepatic lesions in patient with neoplasms. *AJR Am J Roentgenol* 1998; 171: 643–649.

113. Ch'en IY, Katz DS, Jeffrey RB Jr et al. Do arterial phase improve detection and characterization of colorectal liver metastases? *J Comput Assist Tomogr* 1997; 21: 391–397.

114. Valls C, Andia E, Sanchez A et al. Hepatic metastases from colorectal cancer: preoperative detection and assessment of respectability with helical CT. *Radiology* 2001; 218: 55–60.

115. Stoupis C, Taylor HM, Paley MR et al. The rocky liver: radiologic pathologic correlation of calcified hepatic masses. *Radiographics* 1998; 18: 675–685.

116. Khalil HI, Patterson SA, Panicek DM. Hepatic lesions deemed to small to characterize at CT: prevalence and importance in women with breast cancer. *Radiology* 2005; 235: 872–878.

117. Blake SP, Wersinger K, Atkins MB, Raptopoulos V. Liver metastases from melanoma: detection with multiphasic contrast-enhanced CT. *Radiology* 1999; 213: 92–96.

118. Bressler EL, Alpern MB, Glazer GM et al. Hypervascular hepatic metastases: CT evaluation. *Radiology* 1987; 162: 49–51.

119. Ward J, Robinson PJ, Guthrie A et al. Liver metastases in candidates for hepatic resection: comparison of helical CT and gadolinium and SPIO-enhanced MR Imaging. *Radiology* 2005; 237: 170–180.

120. Del Frate C, Bazzocchi M, Mortele KJ et al. Detection of liver metastases: comparison of gadobenate dimeglumine–enhanced and ferumoxides-enhanced MR imaging examinations. *Radiology* 2002; 225(3): 766–772.

121. Petersein J, Spinazzi A, Giovagnoni A et al. Focal liver lesions: evaluation of the efficacy of gadobenate dimeglumine in MR imaging—a multicenter phase III clinical study. *Radiology* 2000 June; 215(3): 727–736.

122. Weis JC, Enzinger FM. Epithelioid hemangioendothelioma: a vascular tumor often mistaken for a carcinoma. *Cancer* 1982; 50: 970–981.

123. Keslar PJ, Buck JL, Selby DM. Infantile hemangioendothelioma revisited. *Radiographics* 1993; 13: 657–670.

124. Buetow PC, Buck JL, Ros PR, Goodman Z. Malignant vascular tumors of the liver: radiologic pathologic correlation. *Radiographics* 1994; 14: 153–166.

125. Miller JW, Dodd GD III, Federle MP, Baron RL. Epithelioid Hemangioendothelioma of the liver: imaging findings with pathologic correlation. *AJR Am J Roentgenol* 1992; 159: 53–7

126. Federle MP. *Diagnostic Imaging. Abdomen.* Salt Lake City, Utah: Amirsys, 2004.

127. Locker GY, Doroshow JH, Zwelling LA et al. The clinical features of hepatic angiosarcoma: a report a for cases and e review of the English literature. *Medicine* 1979; 58: 48–64.

128. Itai Y, Teraoka T. Angiosarcoma of the liver mimicking cavernous hemangioma on dynamic CT. *J Comput Assist Tomogr* 1989; 13: 910–912.

129. Koyama T, Fletcher JG, Johnson CD et al. Primary hepatic angiosarcoma: findings at CT and MR imaging. *Radiology* 2002; 24: 87–104.

130. Sanders ML, Botet JF, Straus DJ et al. CT of primary lymphoma of the liver. *AJR Am J Roentgenol* 1989; 152: 973–976.

131. Gazelle GS, Lee MJ, Hahan PF et al. US, CT and MRI of primary and secondary lymphoma of the liver. *J Comput Assist Tomogr* 1994; 18: 412–415.

132. Janssen HL, Garcia-Pagan JC, Elias E et al. Budd-Chiari syndrome; a review by an expert panel. *J Hepatol* 2003; 38: 364–371.

133. Bogin V, Marcos A, Shaw-Stiffel T. Budd-Chiari syndrome: in evolution. *Eur J Gastroenterol Hepatol* 2005; 17: 33–35.

134. Mathieu D, Vasile N, Menu Y et al. Budd-Chiari syndrome: dynamic CT. *Radiology* 1987; 165: 409–413.

135. Brancatelli G, federle MP, Grazioli L et al. Benign regenerative nodules in Budd-Chiari syndrome and other vascular disorders of the liver: radiologic-pathologic and clinical correlation. *Radiographics* 2002; 22: 847–862.

136. Erden A. Budd-Chiari syndrome: a review of imaging findings. *Eur J Radiolo* 2007; 61: 44–56.

137. Moulton JS, Miller BL, Dood III GD et al. Passive hepatic congestion in heart failure: CT abnormalities. *Am J Roentgenol* 1988; 151: 939–942.

138. Gore RM, Mathieu DG, White EM et al. Passive hepatic congestion: cross-sectional imaging features. *Am J Roentgenol* 1994; 162: 71–75.

139. Torabi M, Hosseinzaldeh K, Federle MP. CT of non neoplastic hepatic vascular and perfusion disorders. *Radiographics* 2008; 28: 1967–1982.

140. Kjeldsen AD, Vase P, Green A. Hereditary haemorrhagic telangiectasia: a population-based study of prevalence and mortality in Danish patients. *J Intern Med* 1999;245:31–33.

141. Dakeishi M, Shioya T, Wada Y et al. Genetic epidemiology of hereditary hemorrhagic telangiectasia in a local community in the northern part of Japan. *Hum Mutat* 2002; 19: 140–148.

142. Guttmacher AE, Marchuk DA, White RI Jr. Hereditary hemorrhagic telangiectasia. *N Engl J Med* 1995; 333: 918–924.

143. Memeo M, Stabile Ianora MM, Scardapane A et al. Hepatic involvement in hereditary hemorrhagic telangiectasia: CT findings. *Abdom Imaging* 2004; 29: 211–220.

144. Yu JS, Kim KW, Sung KB et al. Small arterial-portal venous shunts: cause of pseudolesions at hepatic imaging. *Radiology* 1997; 203: 737–742.

145. Kim TK, Choi BI, Han JK et al. Non tumorous arterio-portal shunt mimicking hypervascular tumor in cirrhotic liver: two phase spiral CT findings. *Radiology* 1998; 208: 597–603.

146. Siddiki H, Doherty MG, Fletcher JG et al. Abdominal findings in hereditary hemorrhagic Telangiectasia: pictorial essay in 2D and 3D findings with isotropic multiphase CT. *Radiographics* 2008 Jan-Feb; 28(1): 171–184.

147. Holbert BL, Baron RL, Dodd GD 3rd. Hepatic infarction caused by arterial insufficiency: spectrum and evolution oc CT findings. *AJR Am J Roentgenol* 1996; 166: 815–820.

148. Brenner DA, Atcom JM. Pathogenesis of hepatic fibrosis. In: Kaplowitz, ed. *Liver and biliary disease.* Baltimore, MD: Williams & Wilkins, 1992; 118–129.

149. Waller RM, Olive TW, McCain AH et al. Computed tomography and sonography of hepatic cirrhosis and portal hypertension. *Radiology* 1984; 4: 677–715.

150. Ito K, Mitchell DG, Gabata T et al. Enlargement of hiler periportal space: a sign of early cirrhosis in MR imaging. *J Magn Reson Imag* 2000; 11: 136–140.

151. Okazaki H, Ito K, Fujita K et al. Discrimination of alcoholic from virus-induced cirrhosis on MR imaging. *Am J Roentgenology* 2000; 175: 1677–1681.

152. Harbin WP, Robert NJ, Ferrucci JT. Diagnosis of cirrhosis based on regional changes in hepatic morphology. *Radiology* 1980; 135: 273–283.

153. Terminology of nodular hepatocellular lesions. International working party. *Hepatology* 1995; 22: 983–993.

154. Coleman WB. Mechanisms of human hepatocarcinogenesis. *Curr Mol Med* 2003; 3: 573–588.

155. Bruix J, Scherman M. Management of hepatocellular carcinoma: an update. *Hepatolgoy* 2011; 53: 1020–1022.

156. Roncalli M, Roz E, Coggi G et al. The vascular profile of regenerative and dysplastic nodules of the cirrhotic liver: implications for diagnosis and classification. *Hepatology* 1999; 30: 1174–1178.

157. Choi BI, Han JK, Hong SH et al. Dysplastic nodules of the liver: imaging findings. *Abdom Imaging* 1999; 24: 250–257.

158. Park YN, Yang CP, Fernandez GJ et al. Neoangiogenesis and sinusoidal "capillarization" in dysplastic nodules of the liver. *Am J Surg Pathol* 1998; 22: 656–662.

159. Alpers DH, Sabesin M. Fatty liver: biochemical and clinical aspects. In: Shiff L, Schiff ER, eds. *Disease of the Liver*. Philadelphia, PA: JB Lippincott Co, 1982; 813.

160. Piekarsky J, Goldberg HI, Royal SA et al. Difference between liver and spleen CT numbers in the normal adult: its usefulness in predicting the presence of diffuse liver disease. *Radiology* 1980; 137: 727–729.

161. Stephens DH, Sheedy PF, Hattery RR et al. Computed tomography of the liver. *AJR Am J Roentgenol* 1977; 128: 579–590.

162. Alpern MB, Lawson TL, Foley WD et al. Focal hepatic masses and fatty infiltration detected by enhanced dynamic CT. *Radiology* 1986; 158: 45–49.

163. Hamer OW, Aguirre DA, Casola G, Sirlin CB. Imaging features of perivascular fatty infiltration of the liver: initial observations. *Radiology* 2005; 237: 159–169.

164. Bradbear RA, Bain C, Siskind V et al. Cohort study of internal malignancy in genetic hemochromatosis and other chronic nonalcoholic diseases. *J Natl Cancer Inst* 1985; 75: 81–84.

165. Chezmar JL, Nelson RL, Malko JA et al. Hepatic iron overload: diagnosis and quantification by non invasive imaging. *Gastrointest Radiol* 1990; 15: 27–31.

166. Guyader D, Gandon Y, Dugnier Y et al. Evaluation of computed tomography in the assessment of hepatic iron overload. *Gastroenterology* 1989; 97: 747–753.

167. Howard JM, Ghent CN, Carey LS et al. Diagnostic efficacy of hepatic computed tomography in the detection of iron overload. *Gastroenterology* 1983; 84: 209–215.

168. Baron RL, Gore RM. Diffuse liver disease. In: Gore RM, Levine MS, eds. *Testbook of Gastrointestinal Radiology*. 1994; 191: 123–128.

169. Boll TD, Merkel EM. Diffuse liver disease: strategies for hepatic CT and MR imaging. *Radiographics* 2009; 29: 1591–1614.

170. Mergo PJ, Ros PR, Buetow PC. Diffuse disease of the liver: radiologic-pathologic correlation. *Radiographics* 1994; 14: 1291–1307.

171. Livraghi T, Meloni F, Di Stasi M et al. Sustained complete response and complications rates after radiofrequency ablation of early hepatocellular carcinoma in cirrhosis: is resection still the treatment of choice? *Hepatology* 2008; 47: 82–89.

172. Dromain C, de Baere T, Elias D et al. Hepatic tumors treated with percutaneous radio-frequency ablation: CT and MR imaging follow up. *Radiology* 2002; 223: 255–262.

173. Lencioni R, Crocetti L. Local-regional treatment of hepatocellular carcinoma. *Radiology* 2012; 262: 43–58.

174. Caiado AHM, Blasbalg R, Marcelino ASZ et al. Complications of liver transplantation: multimodality imaging approach. *Radiographics* 2007; 27: 1401–1417.

175. Singh AK, Nachiappan AC, Verma HA et al. Postoperative imaging in liver transplantation what radiologists should know. *Radiographics* 2010; 30: 339–351.

176. Nghiem HV. Imaging of hepatic transplantation. *Radiol Clin North Am* 1998; 36(2): 429–443.

177. Ito K, Siegelman ES, Stolpen AH, Mitchell DG. MR imaging of complication after liver transplantation. *AJR Am J Roentgenol* 2000; 175: 1145–1149.

178. Quiroga S, Sebastià MC, Margarit C et al. Complication after orthotopic liver transplantation: spectrum of findings with helical CT. *Radiographics* 2001; 21: 1085–1102.

2

Gallbladder and Bile Ducts

R. Brooke Jeffrey

CONTENTS

2.1 Introduction and Clinical Overview

Disorders of the gallbladder and bile ducts are among the most prevalent diseases in the developed world, and each year in the United States, cholecystectomy is among the most common of all abdominal surgical procedures [1]. Nevertheless, a broad spectrum of inflammatory, neoplastic, traumatic, and congenital disorders may involve the gallbladder and bile ducts. A tailored diagnostic approach is required for optimal diagnosis, using a variety of noninvasive and invasive imaging techniques. Fortunately, there are multiple imaging modalities that may provide clinically important information regarding biliary abnormalities, and each has its own strengths and limitations in the assessment of biliary pathology. These modalities include ultrasound, computed tomography (CT), magnetic resonance imaging (MRI), magnetic resonance cholangiopancreatography (MRCP), biliary scintigraphy, endoscopic retrograde cholangiopancreatography (ERCP), transhepatic cholangiography, and positron emission tomography.

The most common indication for biliary imaging is the investigation of the patient with right upper quadrant (RUQ) pain and possible biliary colic or cholecystitis.

In this clinical setting, ultrasound is the diagnostic imaging method of choice, due to its high accuracy in detecting gallstones and abnormal thickening of the gallbladder wall [2,3]. Similarly, in patients with jaundice, ultrasound of the bile ducts is often performed as a screening study to differentiate biliary obstruction from cholestasis related to hepatocellular disease. In many instances, however, further diagnostic information beyond that provided by screening sonography must be obtained to appropriately manage the patient. Not uncommonly, a combination of CT, biliary scintigraphy, and MRCP is used to provide additional diagnostic information, particularly in patients with common duct stones, complex cholecystitis, pericholecystic abscesses, and/or gallbladder perforation [4–7].

In patients with suspected gallbladder or biliary tract neoplasms, CT, MR, and ERCP are the mainstays of diagnosis to accurately stage the full extent of intrahepatic and extrahepatic diseases [8–10]. CT and MRI are particularly valuable in identifying liver metastases and periportal or retroperitoneal adenopathy. In patients with biliary neoplasms who have been treated surgically, CT is the mainstay for diagnosis of postoperative surveillance and identification of complications such as RUQ and perihepatic abscesses [8–10].

In patients with inflammatory diseases of the intraheptic or extrahepatic bile ducts, MRCP and ERCP play primary roles in identifying areas of strictures or associated cholangiocarcinomas [11–13]. CT may detect discontinuous areas of ductal obstruction to suggest the diagnosis, but is often inadequate to provide precise anatomic detail of the subtle ductal abnormalities [14–16].

2.2 Normal Biliary Anatomy on CT

The gallbladder is a pear-shaped organ that lies in the main lobar fissure of the liver, dividing the right and left lobes [17,18]. Anatomists and surgeons typically divide the gallbladder into four segments: fundus, body, infundibulum (Hartmann's pouch), and neck. The cystic duct containing spiral valves attaches the gallbladder to the common bile duct. In a fasting patient, the gallbladder typically contains 40–50 mL of bile, which on CT is equal attenuation to water (<10 Hounsfield units [HU]).

On CT, the normal gallbladder wall is less than 3 mm and is of uniform soft-tissue attenuation. Anatomic variations in the configuration of the gallbladder fundus are common and include a folding over the fundus, known as the Phrygian cap. Anatomic variations in the cystic duct insertion to the common duct are important surgically, particularly the long junction of the cystic duct that runs in a parallel course to the common hepatic duct, enveloped by the hepatoduodenal ligament [19]. Stones impacted in this long cystic duct may result in secondary common hepatic duct obstruction, known as the Mirizzi syndrome [20].

The blood supply to the gallbladder is derived from the cystic artery, which is a branch of the right hepatic artery. The cystic artery terminates into superficial and deep branches, which arborize into capillaries at the gallbladder fundus [21]. Because the fundus has the poorest blood supply, it is most often the site of gallbladder ischemia and perforation with prolonged cystic duct obstruction and gangrenous cholecystitis [21]. On CT, the gallbladder is normally surrounded by pericholecystic fat and omentum. An important secondary sign of gallbladder inflammation is fat stranding in the adjacent pericholecystic fat and omentum. Often, the inflamed omentum will act to "wall off" gallbladder perforations and prevent pericholecystic abscesses from leading to generalized peritonitis.

One unique anatomic feature of the gallbladder is that its wall is comprised histologically of a mucosa, lamina propria, smooth muscular layer, and perimuscular connective tissue without a discrete submucosal layer. Furthermore, there is no serosal layer at its point of attachment to the liver along the undersurface of the liver. These two anatomic features facilitate direct invasion of the liver by gallbladder carcinoma.

On CT with thin collimation (3 mm or less), the normal proximal branches of the right and left main bile ducts can be visualized and typically measure less than 2 mm [22]. The common duct on CT in the normal patient is generally less than 7 mm, but may slightly increase with age, and in patients over 50, it is not uncommon to see cross-sectional measurements of 8 mm in patients without biochemical evidence of biliary obstruction. While in most patients the dimensions of the bile duct do not change after cholecystectomy, in a small percentage of patients, the bile duct can measure normally up to 10 mm in cross-sectional diameter, most likely due to loss of intramural elastic tissue [23].

2.3 Optimization of CT Technique for Imaging of the Gallbladder and Bile Ducts

Both the imaging modality selected and precise protocol used in scanning should be tailored to the patient's clinical presentation. To optimally image the liver and biliary system, intravenous contrast is essential for state-of-the-art multi-detector CT. The rate and volume of contrast injection, however, will vary with the clinical indication. In patients whose screening ultrasound examination suggests complicated cholecystitis, CT was performed with a uniphasic acquisition during the portal venous phase [60–70 seconds following onset of intravenous injection) and at an injection rate of 2–4 cc/s, for a total of 120–150 m of nonionic contrast. Thin collimation (0.625–1.25 mm) with either a 16- or 64-slice multi-detector CT is essential to provide a high-quality diagnostic study [6,7]. The thin-collimation scans (0.625 mm) are the foundation of an isotropic data set that is ideal for the performance of sophisticated 2D and 3D reformations, including 3D volume rendering and curved planar reformations.

In patients presenting with jaundice and potential pancreaticobiliary neoplasms, however, a dedicated dual-phase acquisition is performed with both a late arterial scan of the upper abdomen (25–35 seconds after ingestion) and the standard portal venous phase [24–27]. The entire liver and upper abdomen is scanned using a rapid bolus of 4–5 cc/s of contrast injected with a power injector. The arterial-phase acquisition is particularly useful to opacify the hepatic and peripancreatic vasculature to identify hypervascular pancreatic neoplasms such as neuroendocrine tumors and to demonstrate hypervascular liver metastasis. Portal venous phase acquisitions are essential to identify hypovascular liver metastasis, such as with ductal adenocarcinoma, and venous encasement or occlusion with resultant collateral varices [24,25].

Scirrhous lesions such as cholangiocarcinomas characteristically demonstrate delayed retention of intravenous contrast. A triphasic study comprising late arterial, portal venous, and delayed acquisition is performed in these patients. Delayed imaging at approximately 10 minutes after the onset of intravenous injection is particularly valuable in demonstrating progressive enhancement of intrahepatic extension of a cholangiocarcinoma [24]. This late retention of contrast in areas of intrahepatic extension is thought to be related to the slow diffusion of contrast into the tumor's interstitium and surrounding fibrous tissue [25].

2.4 Pathology of the Gallbladder and Bile Ducts

2.4.1 Calculus Disease

Cholelithiasis is endemic in the Western world and its incidence among adults increases with age. There are significant gender differences, and it is estimated that 20% of women and 8% of men over the age of 40 have gallstones [1]. Overall, it is estimated that 25 million individuals have gallstones in the United States [1].

Sonography is the imaging method of choice to detect gallstones and has been reported to have an accuracy of 96% [26,27]. CT appears to be substantially less sensitive than sonography, particularly for the identification of predominantly cholesterol stones, and has been reported to have a sensitivity of only 75% [6,28,29,30]. Gallstones on CT have a variable size and appearance, largely due to their variable composition of cholesterol, calcium and bilirubin salts, as well as bile acids, fatty acids, and inorganic salts [29]. Gallstones may have a calcified rim, may contain gas, or be of low attenuation on CT. Cholesterol stones may not be visible on CT (Figures 2.1 through 2.3). However, in patients with higher-attenuation biliary sludge, cholesterol stones may be identified as low attenuation, rounded or faceted lesions within the gallbladder. Degeneration of stones with nitrogen gas release that collects in central fissures may result in the "Mercedes Benz" sign, which can be readily appreciated on CT. Overall, because of its lower sensitivity and associated radiation, CT is generally not employed as a primary imaging modality for detection of gallstones.

FOCUS POINTS: VARIABLE CT APPEARANCE OF GALLSTONES

- Pure cholesterol stones invisible in 25% of patients
- Predominantly cholesterol stones may be lower attenuation than biliary sludge
- Gallstones may have homogeneous or rim calcification
- Mixed composition or pigment stones may be of soft-tissue density
- Gas with stones results in "Mercedes Benz" sign

In addition to stones, both sonography and CT may detect viscous bile related to cholestasis, also referred to as sludge (Figure 2.4). Sludge forms when there is precipitation of calcium bilirubinate and cholesterol crystals from a supersaturated solution of bile. Invariably this is related to stasis of the biliary tree in patients who experience prolonged fasting or in patients receiving intravenous total parenteral nutrition who lack a cholecystokinin stimulus to empty their gallbladder. Sludge may result in a fluid–fluid level within the gallbladder, or aggregation of sludge may result in "tumefactive sludge," which appears as an avascular soft-tissue mass [30]. On CT, sludge appears higher than water density depending on the degree of calcium bilirubinate admixture within the sludge and is often greater than 15 HU [6].

Choledocholithiasis in the Western world is almost entirely related to passage of gallstones into the cystic duct and common bile duct. In some patients, this may be entirely symptomatic; however, in other patients it may lead to significant complications such as bacterial cholangitis and/or gallstone pancreatitis. Unlike stones in the gallbladder, stones within the common duct are seen far less frequently with ultrasound, with reported sensitivities ranging from 20% to 75% [31,32]. CT has only slightly higher sensitivity, and thus, if common duct stones are suspected, either MRCP or direct ERCP should be performed [33,34]. It should be noted that small stones may not result in significant biochemical abnormalities or abnormal liver function tests; thus, small stones within the common duct may be entirely asymptomatic [34]. In general, if common duct stones are suspected clinically, unenhanced CT appears to have a higher sensitivity, as the stones appear to be slightly higher in attenuation than adjacent bile (Figure 2.2). Common duct stones may have either a "rim" sign configuration, a "crescent" sign (Figure 2.3), or appear as focal areas of discrete hyperattenuation, particularly on noncontrast scans [33,34]. Contrast-enhanced CT

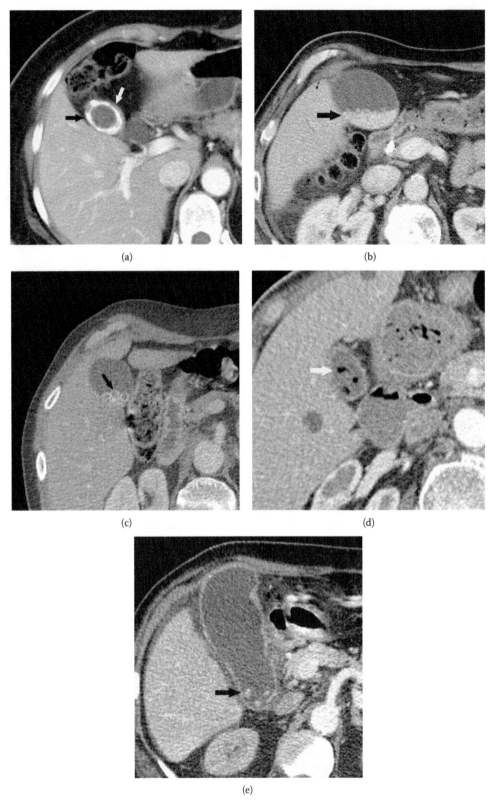

FIGURE 2.1
Variable CT appearance of gallstones. (a) Note large gallstone with calcified peripheral rim (black arrow). Patient had chronic cholecystitis with completely collapsed gallbladder (white arrow = gallbladder wall). (b) Gallstones appear as layer of calcified microliths. Note high-attenuation foci layering dependently in gallbladder from small, calcified stones (arrow). (c) Multiple small, rim-like calcified stones in gallbladder (arrow). (d) Multiple gas-containing stones are identified as low-attenuation foci within gallbladder (arrow). (e) Multiple small, soft-tissue attenuation stones (arrow) are identified in dependent portion of distended gallbladder.

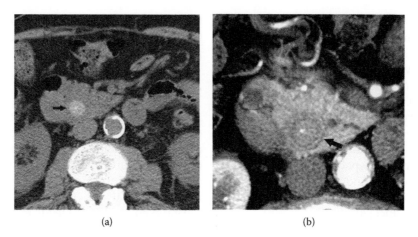

(a) (b)

FIGURE 2.2
Distal common bile duct stone. (a) Noncontrast scan demonstrating high-attenuation stone in distal common bile duct (arrow). (b) Following contrast enhancement stone appears to be of soft-tissue attenuation relative to pancreas, with high-attenuation peripheral rim (arrow) in distal common bile duct.

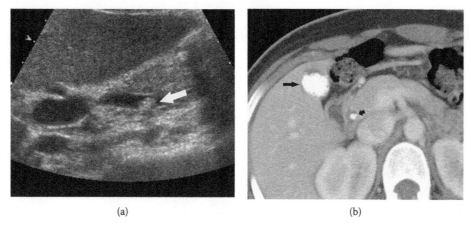

(a) (b)

FIGURE 2.3
Calcified common bile duct stone. (a) Parasagittal sonogram demonstrating common duct stone (arrow). (b) Note on CT multiple calcified gallstones (long black arrow) and calcified distal common duct stone (short black arrow).

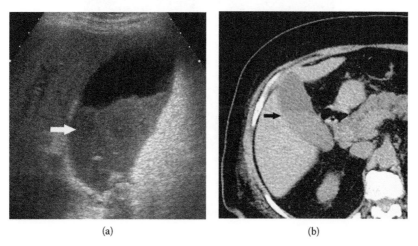

(a) (b)

FIGURE 2.4
Gallbladder sludge on ultrasound and CT. (a) Sagittal sonogram of gallbladder demonstrating layer of particulate debris in dependent portion of gallbladder, representing sludge (arrow). (b) Noncontrast CT in same patient demonstrating higher-attenuation sludge layering dependently in gallbladder (arrow).

cholangiography has been performed, particularly in evaluation of donor anatomy before liver transplantation. Although there are reports that this technique may provide a high sensitivity for detection of common duct stones, there appears to be no significant advantage over MRCP in this regard [35].

In patients with impacted stones in either the neck of the gallbladder or an unusually long cystic duct, secondary mass effect or inflammation may result, causing obstruction of the common hepatic duct. This entity is known as Mirizzi syndrome and, if not diagnosed preoperatively, may lead to intraoperative injury or ligation of the common hepatic duct [20].

Gallstones may erode into the small bowel and obstruct either the second duodenum (Bouveret) or distal small bowel (gallstone ileus). In patients with gallstone ileus on CT, there is evidence of gas in the gallbladder and/or

biliary tree and a distal small bowel obstruction [36]. Often, the obstructing gallstone can be identified at the point of obstruction (Figure 2.5).

2.4.2 Cholecystitis

Acute cholecystitis is one of the most common causes of the acute abdomen resulting in surgery [1]. In 95% of patients, the etiology is related to calculous obstruction of the cystic duct with resultant gallbladder distension and elevated intraluminal pressure, ultimately resulting in mucosal ischemia. Ischemia and sloughing of the gallbladder mucosa leads to chemical injury involving the lamina propria and muscular layers caused by exposure to bile salts and ultimately leading to superimposed bacterial infection. This inflammatory process generally results in acute RUQ pain, leukocytosis, and

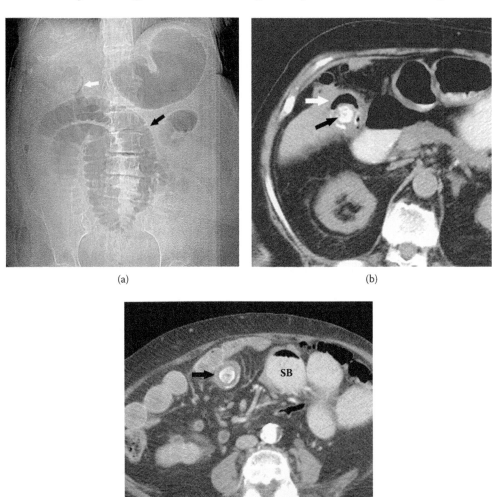

(a)

(b)

(c)

FIGURE 2.5
Gallstone ileus on CT. (a) Digital scout radiograph of abdomen demonstrating gas within gallbladder (white arrow) and dilated distal small bowel (black arrow). (b) Note gas within gallbladder from enteric fistula (white arrow) as well as residual calcified stone in gallbladder (black arrow). (c) Note distal calcified gallstone causing obstruction of small bowel. SB = dilated small bowel.

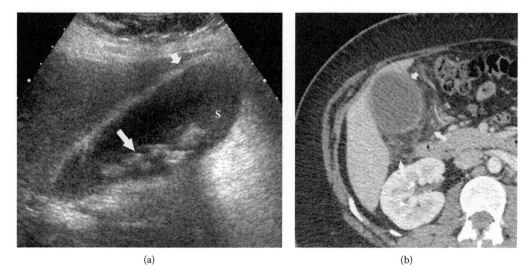

(a) (b)

FIGURE 2.6
Acute calculous cholecystitis. (a) Parasagittal ultrasound of gallbladder demonstrating stones (long arrow), sludge ("S"), and thickened wall (short arrow). Patient had received pain medication and sonographic Murphy's sign was negative. (b) CT in same patient demonstrating uniformly enhancing thickened wall (short arrow) and prominent pericholecystic inflammation in surrounding fat (white arrows).

low-grade fever. Ultrasound is the initial diagnostic method of choice for patients with suspected acute cholecystitis [37–39]. When ultrasound demonstrates gallstones, gallbladder wall thickening greater than 3 mm, and a positive sonographic Murphy's sign (focal tenderness directly over gallbladder elicited with pressure from ultrasound transducer), there is a 92% positive predictive value for the diagnosis [3]. In patients who have received pain medication before sonography, it may not be possible to detect a true sonographic Murphy's sign. Similarly, patients with gangrenous cholecystitis may not have a sonographic Murphy's sign, due to infarction of the afferent sympathetic nerve fibers to the gallbladder. In patients with uncomplicated cholecystitis, CT is rarely of clinical value. However, in some patients, CT may be performed before sonography because of confusing signs and symptoms.

The CT findings in patients with acute cholecystitis include the presence of gallstones, gallbladder distension, mural thickening (>3 mm), and, most importantly, stranding and soft-tissue infiltration of the pericholecystic fat indicative of pericholecystic inflammation [5,6,40,41] (Figure 2.6). This last finding is the most specific for acute cholecystitis, as chronic cholecystitis may result in mural thickening. With uncomplicated acute cholecystitis, the gallbladder wall enhances uniformly without patches or global areas of mucosal ischemia characteristic of gangrenous change.

2.4.3 Acalculous Cholecystitis

In 5%–10% of patients, inflammation of the gallbladder occurs in the absence of cystic duct obstruction [41]. A variety of predisposing factors have been attributed to this disease, such as diabetes, major surgical procedures, hyperalimentation, AIDS, and patients who are critically ill following trauma or burns [41]. Common predisposing factors are prolonged gallbladder distension, bile stasis, and mucosal ischemia from lowflow states [41–43]. The absence of gallstones makes the diagnosis difficult with ultrasound. Similarly, as patients are often critically ill and receiving pain medication or on ventilators, the sonographic Murphy's sign is often unreliable. CT may be of value in the diagnosis of acute acalculous cholecystitis by demonstrating pericholecystic inflammation, fluid, and mural thickening of the gallbladder wall [42,43] (Figure 2.7). Following intravenous contrast, there may be adjacent hyperemia seen transiently in the liver on late arterial phase images [43].

2.4.4 Complicated Cholecystitis

Unless promptly treated, acute cholecystitis may evolve and result in a variety of complications including gangrene, hemorrhage, and emphysematous cholecystitis [44]. Many of these complications occur in elderly patients with either diabetes or advanced atherosclerosis [44]. The end result may cause perforation and/or pericholecystic abscess formation with high morbidity from sepsis. Once complications occur from acute cholecystitis, CT plays an increasingly important role, as ultrasound often has significant limitations in this subset of patients [45–47]. Ultrasound can suggest the diagnosis of gangrenous cholecystitis, when there is asymmetric wall thickening relating to ulceration, hemorrhage, and intramural necrosis with microabscess formation. In addition to the mural

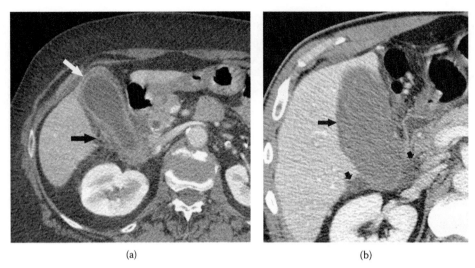

(a)   (b)

FIGURE 2.7
Acalculous cholecystitis in two patients. (a) Gallbladder wall thickening (white arrow) and stranding in pericholecystic fat (black arrow).
Patient had acalculous cholecystitis confirmed at surgery. In another patient (b), complete lack of mucosal enhancement of gallbladder wall
indicating gangrenous change (long black arrow). Note surrounding pericholecystic inflammatory stranding (short black arrow), indicative of
gangrenous acalculous cholecystitis. This was confirmed at surgery.

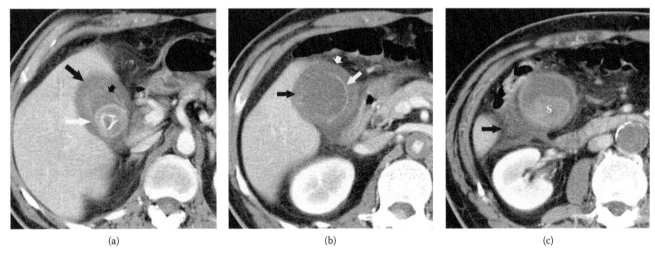

(a)   (b)   (c)

FIGURE 2.8
Gangrenous cholecystitis with lack of mural enhancement. (a) Note large gallstone in neck of gallbladder (white arrow). There is lack of mucosal enhancement of gallbladder fundus (short black arrow) with associated gallbladder wall thickening (long black arrow). (b) Note areas of
normal mucosal enhancement seen immediately along gallbladder wall (long white arrow). Note lack of mucosal enhancement along lateral
gallbladder wall, indicating gangrenous change (black arrow; short white arrow indicates marked gallbladder wall thickening). (c) Note large
amount of dependent sludge in gallbladder ("S") and marked pericholecystic inflammation in hepatorenal fossa (black arrow).

changes, intraluminal membranes related to fibrin-
ous debris and/or strands of clot may also be present
sonographically.

CT, however, has proven to be more specific in the diagnosis of gangrenous cholecystitis [45–47]. Intravenous
contrast is essential to identify focal and/or diffuse areas
of mucosal ischemia because of lack of enhancement
(Figure 2.8). Intraluminal hemorrhage can be suggested
when attenuation is greater than 25 HU (Figure 2.9). CT
is similarly more accurate in demonstrating loculated
fluid collections representing pericholecystic abscess

formation (Figure 2.10). In patients with emphysematous cholecystitis, intraluminal and intramural gas may
be detected at sonography; however, CT is more accurate for the identification of minute gas bubbles to confirm the diagnosis (Figures 2.11 and 2.12).

Gallbladder perforation can be diagnosed on CT when
there is focal lack of mural enhancement with an associated complex fluid collection, often with mass effect, in
the pericholecystic space [48]. Defining the true extent
of pericholecystic abscesses is critical to direct patients
to appropriate therapy (Figure 2.10). When localized to

the immediate pericholecystic area, CT-directed catheter drainage is often the diagnostic method of choice. However, if there is extensive perihepatic abscess formation, open surgical drainage is required.

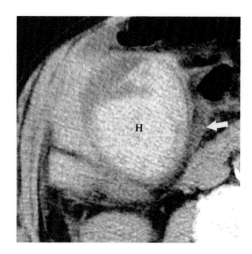

FOCUS POINT: CT IN ACUTE CHOLECYSTITIS

- Uncomplicated: Gallbladder distended with uniformly enhancing thickened wall, pericholecystic fat stranding
- Gangrenous cholecystitis: Areas of mucosal nonenhancement indicating ischemia; adjacent abscesses if perforated
- Hemorrhagic cholecystitis: Intraluminal blood >25 HU
- Emphysematous cholecystitis: Gas in gallbladder lumen, wall, or both

FIGURE 2.9
Hemorrhagic cholecystitis. Noncontrast CT demonstrates high-attenuation hemorrhage ("H") that measured 47 HU. Note pericholecystic inflammatory changes (white arrow), indicative of gangrenous hemorrhagic cholecystitis.

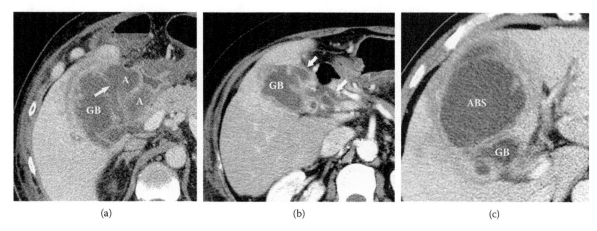

(a)   (b)   (c)

FIGURE 2.10
Gallbladder perforation with pericholecystic abscesses in three different patients. (a) Note focal disruption of gallbladder wall (arrow; GB = gallbladder). Note surrounding pericholecystic abscesses ("A"). (b) Another patient with gallbladder perforation (GB = gallbladder) and multiple loculated pericholecystic abscesses (arrows). (c) Different patient with large, rounded pericholecystic abscess ("ABS") adjacent to decompressed gallbladder ("GB").

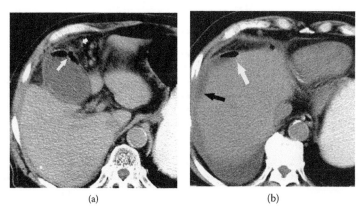

(a)   (b)

FIGURE 2.11
Emphysematous cholecystitis with perforation. (a) Note intraluminal gas within distended gallbladder (long white arrow). Note pericholecystic inflammatory changes adjacent to gallbladder (short white arrow). (b) Note free air in subhepatic space (white arrow) and adjacent pus in perihepatic spaces (black arrow).

2.4.5 Inflammatory Disorders of the Biliary Tract

Bacterial cholangitis results from obstruction and stasis of the biliary tract with secondary infection [49,50]. In a high percentage of patients, there is either a biliary stricture or obstruction related to common duct stones. While in most patients this is primarily a clinical diagnosis, the detection of dilated ducts in a septic patient is often the most typical clinical presentation. On ultrasound, there may be complex fluid with pus and debris located within the dilated common bile duct. This may be difficult to appreciate on CT, but there may be abnormal mural enhancement of the common duct in association with significant intrahepatic dilatation as well as intraductal stones and debris (Figure 2.13).

2.4.6 Primary Sclerosing Cholangitis

Primary sclerosing cholangitis (PSC) is an idiopathic disorder resulting in inflammation and periductal fibrosis of the intrahepatic and extrahepatic bile ducts [51]. About 70% of patients are male, and approximately 70% of patients also have inflammatory bowel disease [51]. PSC is most often associated ulcerative colitis, but PSC has also been rarely reported in Crohn's disease. Not infrequently, the PSC findings precede the clinical onset of ulcerative colitis [51]. In its early stages, histologic sections of the liver may show periductal fibrosis and inflammation confined to the periportal areas [51]. As the disease extends, septal or bridging necrosis develops, ultimately resulting in end-stage liver disease and cirrhosis. End-stage liver disease from PSC is most commonly treated with liver transplantation.

In approximately 80% of patients, the disease involves primarily the main intrahepatic and extrahepatic ductal branches [51]. In a small percentage of cases, the disease is limited to small intrahepatic and hilar ducts. The most feared complication of PSC is the development of cholangiocarcinoma [52], which may be exceedingly difficult to diagnose on the basis of imaging alone, but may be suggested when there is progressive ductal dilatation or the development of a periductal mass [52].

The most specific imaging findings of early PSC are best demonstrated on ERCP or MRCP with the

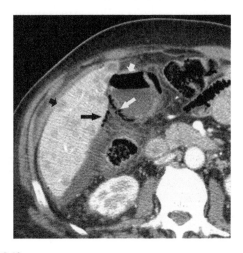

FIGURE 2.12
Emphysematous cholecystitis with perforation in patient with metastatic melanoma. Note intramural gas in gallbladder (long white arrow) as well as intraluminal gas in nondependent portion of gallbladder (short white arrow). Note ectopic gas in hepatorenal fossa (long black arrow) and multiple low-attenuation liver metastases (short black arrow).

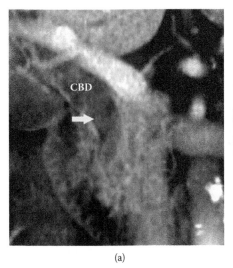

(a)

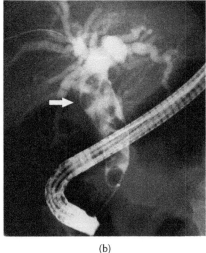

(b)

FIGURE 2.13
Bacterial cholangitis. (a) Coronal volume-rendered image demonstrating dilatation of common bile duct ("CBD") and numerous soft-tissue filling defects (arrow). (b) ERCP in same patient demonstrating multiple common duct stones. Pus was observed coming from duct after sphincterotomy, confirming cholangitis.

identification of multifocal, irregular strictures of the intrahepatic and extrahepatic ductal systems [53]. Often, the ducts have a beaded appearance related to the short and focal alternating strictures and slightly dilated segments (Figure 2.14). Ultrasound findings in PSC are often quite subtle but may demonstrate mild mural thickening, particularly of the common bile duct. On contrast-enhanced CT, the most suggestive features include scattered areas of ductal dilatation in early stages [54] (Figure 2.15). As the disease progresses, there are characteristic morphologic changes of the liver with the PSC-associated cirrhosis that can be identified with CT. Often, there is marked atrophy of the posterior segment of the right lobe and the lateral segment of the left lobe, with secondary hypertrophy of the caudate lobe [54] (Figure 2.16). This often results in a distinctive "rounded" morphology to the liver. When these findings are seen in conjunction with scattered intrahepatic dilated ducts, the diagnosis of PSC can be suggested. Other secondary findings on contrast CT include capsular retraction, increased mural enhancement of the extrahepatic ducts, and alternating areas of narrowing and saccular dilatation of the common duct to produce a beaded appearance. Bile stasis from long-standing strictures may result in intrahepatic stone formation (Figure 2.17). The clinical outcome in PSC is unpredictable, but most patients have slowly progressive disease with a mean survival of 12 years without hepatic transplantation [54].

2.4.7 Recurrent Pyogenic Cholangitis

Unlike calculous disease in the Western world, in which cholesterol and calcium bilirubinate stones form primarily in the gallbladder, endemic in certain Asian populations is the development of pigment stones primarily in the intrahepatic and extrahepatic bile ducts. This entity

> **FOCUS POINT: CT OF PRIMARY SCLEROSING CHOLANGITIS**
>
> - ERCP and MRCP demonstrate early changes of subtle beading and stricturing of bile ducts
> - CT reveals asymmetric and often discontinuous biliary dilatation
> - End-stage disease results in marked atrophy of right lobe and caudate lobe hypertrophy causing "rounded" appearance to liver

is referred to as recurrent pyogenic cholangitis (RPC). The gallbladder is typically uninvolved in patients with RPC [55]. Invariably, these patients are colonized with bacteria, often with *Escherichia coli* or other gram-negative bacteria, and experience multiple episodes of recurrent bacterial cholangitis. Predisposing factors to RPC include parasitic infections with clonorchis sinensis or ascaris lumbricoides, malnutrition, and prior episodes of portal venous bacteremia [56].

In some patients with RPC, the left biliary ductal system appears to be disproportionately affected, and when that is the only site of disease, left hepatic resection may be curative [56]. More commonly, both the right and left ductal systems have numerous stones often larger than 1.5 cm. In some patients, massive dilatation of the common bile duct by pigment stones is seen (Figure 2.18). Noncontrast CT is often particularly valuable in these patients to demonstrate the higher attenuation bilirubinate stones [56]. Intravenous contrast, however, is useful to detect complications of RPC such as associated intrahepatic abscesses. Periductal inflammatory changes often result in the "arrowhead" appearance that has been described cholangiographically [56].

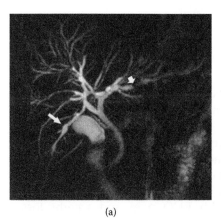
(a)

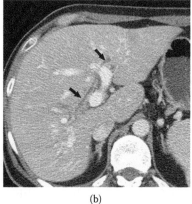
(b)

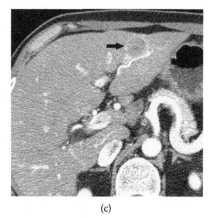
(c)

FIGURE 2.14
Early changes of sclerosing cholangitis complicated by intrahepatic cholangiocarcinoma. (a) MRCP demonstrating beading (long arrow) and strictures (short arrow) of intrahepatic ducts. (b) Note minimal dilatation of right and left hepatic bile ducts (black arrows). (c) Note solid enhancing mass in lateral segment of left lobe, surgically proven to be intrahepatic cholangiocarcinoma.

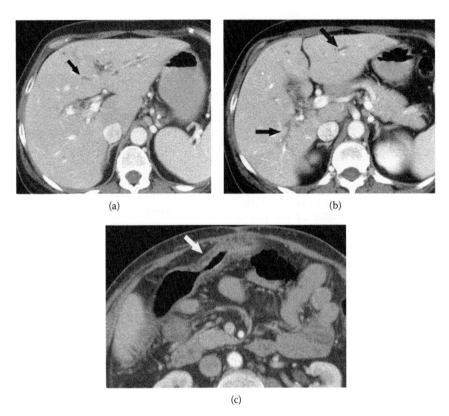

FIGURE 2.15
CT of primary sclerosing cholangitis associated with ulcerative colitis. (a) Note intrahepatic biliary dilatation in medial segment of left lobe (arrow). (b) There are scattered, discontinuous, peripherally dilated ducts in both right and left lobes (black arrows). (c) Note colonic wall thickening of hepatic flexure with submucosal fat deposition, consistent with chronic ulcerative colitis.

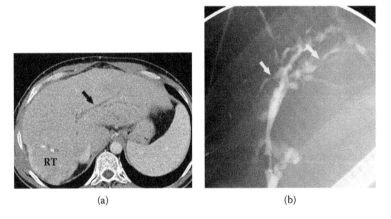

FIGURE 2.16
End-stage sclerosing cholangitis with marked atrophy of right lobe. (a) Note dilated biliary radical and hypertrophied left lobe. Note marked atrophy of right lobe (RT = right lobe). (b) ERCP demonstrates marked intrahepatic ductal pruning and extensive stricture formation (white arrows).

2.4.8 Neoplasms of the Gallbladder and Bile Duct

2.4.8.1 Gallbladder Carcinoma

Adenocarcinoma of the gallbladder is largely a disease of elderly women and is responsible for at least 3000 deaths per year in the United States [57]. A number of predisposing factors have been associated with an increased risk for gallbladder carcinoma, including the presence of gallstones, porcelain gallbladder,

underlying gallbladder adenomas, and exposure to carcinogenic chemicals [58].

Adenocarcinomas of the gallbladder have a variety of clinical presentations often mimicking acute cholecystitis with RUQ pain and weight loss [58]. Unfortunately, the most common radiologic finding in carcinoma of the gallbladder is a mass replacing the entire gallbladder fossa [58–60] (Figure 2.19). This has been reported to occur in 70% of patients with

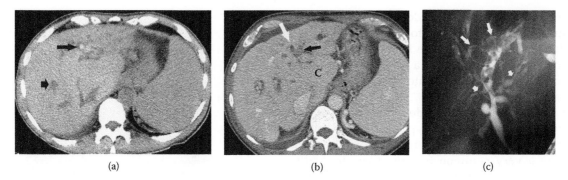

FIGURE 2.17
Intrahepatic calculi complicating primary sclerosing cholangitis. (a) Noncontrast CT demonstrating high-attenuation stones within left hepatic ducts (long arrow). Areas of scattered dilated right hepatic ducts are noted as well (short black arrow). (b) Contrast-enhanced scan of same patient demonstrating hypertrophy of caudate lobe ("C"), as well as dilated biliary radicals (white arrow). Note appearance of intrahepatic ductal calculi in left lobe (black arrow). (c) ERCP demonstrating multiple intrahepatic filling defects representing stones (white arrows). Note areas of intrahepatic stricture formation (short white arrows).

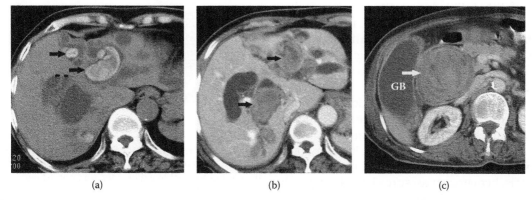

FIGURE 2.18
CT of recurrent pyogenic cholangitis. (a) Note massively dilated intrahepatic ducts with multiple high-attenuation intraductal calculi (black arrows). (b) Contrast-enhanced CT demonstrates extensive intrahepatic bilirubinate stones within massively dilated intrahepatic ducts (arrows). (c) CT scan at level of common duct demonstrating massive common bile duct dilatation with intrahepatic stone formation (arrow). Gallbladder ("GB") is normal.

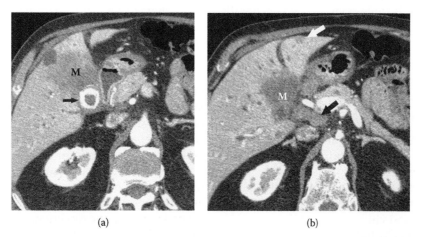

FIGURE 2.19
Gallbladder carcinoma replacing gallbladder fossa. (a) Note hypodense mass ("M") in main lobar fissure replacing gallbladder. There is calcified stone at base of gallbladder (arrow), but no recognizable gallbladder wall. (b) Note both hepatic metastases (white arrow) and periportal lymphadenopathy (black arrow) from gallbladder mass ("M").

adenocarcinoma of the gallbladder. Not infrequently the infiltrating mass extends into the main lobar fissure to invade both lobes of the liver. When there is hepatic invasion, the disease has a very poor prognosis because of the invariably associated nodal and peritoneal metastasis.

About 25% of patients with adenocarcinoma of the gallbladder present with a polypoid mass on ultrasound or CT [61]. Although benign polyps of the gallbladder are a very common finding, they generally are small (<1 cm). Any mucosal polyp larger than 1 cm should be considered at risk for carcinoma and treated with prophylactic cholecystectomy. The only hope for cure in patients with gallbladder carcinoma is to detect the disease at an early stage, when the cancer is confined to the gallbladder mucosa without extramural extension to the liver. A third presentation of gallbladder carcinoma is either diffuse or focal thickening of the gallbladder wall. At times, when the carcinoma is limited to the fundus, it may mimic adenomyomatosis [60]. Generalized gallbladder-wall thickening is often mistaken for chronic cholecystitis unless regional lymphadenopathy or liver metastasis is identified [60].

Until late in the clinical course, gallbladder carcinoma spreads locally, often directly invading the liver and hepatoduodenal ligament, as well as the hepatic flexure and the second duodenum [58–60] (Figure 2.20). Lymphatic spread to periportal and retroperitoneal nodes is quite common, as is hematogenous spread to the liver. In addition, there may be peritoneal metastasis with omental caking and peritoneal implants. Owing to delay in clinical diagnosis due to lack of symptoms, gallbladder carcinoma at the time of presentation has often spread beyond the confines of the gallbladder fossa to involve the liver or periportal nodes in the majority of patients (stage T3) [58–60]. The overall prognosis of patients with gallbladder carcinoma is quite poor, and it is generally felt that only 15% of patients survive 5 years with this disease [58].

FOCUS POINTS: CT OF GALLBLADDER CARCINOMA

- Most common CT finding is mass replacing gallbladder fossa invading right and left lobes of liver
- Other CT findings include focal or diffuse gallbladder wall thickening, or mucosal polypoid mass >1 cm
- Pattern of spread includes direct liver invasion, periportal nodes, peritoneal implants, and hematogenous liver metastases

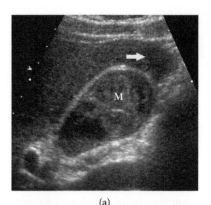

(a)

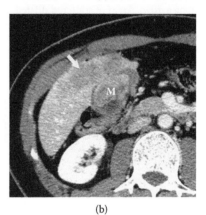

(b)

FIGURE 2.20
Gallbladder carcinoma with hepatic invasion. (a) Sagittal sonogram demonstrating intra-gallbladder mass ("M"). Note subtle hypoechoic liver lesion adjacent to gallbladder. (b) Contrast-enhanced scan demonstrating enhancing mass ("M") with direct invasion into liver, making patient unresectable for cure (white arrow = liver metastases).

2.4.8.2 Cholangiocarcinoma

Cholangiocarcinomas are adenocarcinomas arising from the biliary ductal epithelium. Predisposing factors include PSC, choledochal cysts, familial polyposis, congenital hepatic fibrosis, chronic biliary calculous disease, underlying infection with liver flukes (clonorchis sinensis), and prior exposure to thorium dioxide (thorotrast) [61].

Classifications of cholangiocarcinomas may be based on morphologic appearance as well as their anatomic location. Anatomically, there are three main forms of cholangiocarcinoma, related to their site of origin: (1) intrahepatic lesions; (2) hilar, or confluence, lesions; and (3) extrahepatic common bile duct lesions [62]. The surgical approach and subsequent clinical management is often quite different for these three subtypes, as peripheral intrahepatic cholangiocarcinomas are treated with hepatic resection, while confluence lesions, the so-called hilar Klatskin tumors, are generally managed with hepatectomy and roux-en-Y hepaticojejunostomy [63]. Extrahepatic cholangiocarcinomas of the common bile duct are treated similarly to pancreatic and ampullary malignancies and undergo Whipple's resection with pancreaticoduodenectomy. The most common form of cholangiocarcinoma involves the extrahepatic ducts, accounting for 65% of cholangiocarcinomas. Approximately 25% are hilar confluence Klatskin tumors, and 10% are peripheral intrahepatic cholangiocarcinomas [64] (Figure 2.21).

In addition to these anatomic locations, cholangiocarcinomas may be further subdivided by their morphologic appearance [62]. These include the mass-forming type, the periductal infiltrating type, and the polypoid or intraductal mass lesion. Peripheral intrahepatic cholangiocarcinomas characteristically result in a large mass that on CT has a characteristic peripheral rim enhancement on arterial-phase images, with areas of heterogeneous central necrosis (Figure 2.21). Hilar confluence types often result in periductal infiltration and fibrosis and a biliary stricture [62]. There is often a very small mass on CT that occludes the hilar confluence (Figure 2.22). There may be intrahepatic invasion that is

best displayed on delayed enhancement, as the fibrous tissue associated with hepatic invasion often results in delayed retention of contrast. Other CT findings include enhancement of the thickened ductal wall and, when present, regional lymphadenopathy in the hepatoduodenal ligament, porta hepatis, and adjacent retroperitoneum. These types of malignant strictures are often quite difficult to diagnose cytologically with ERCP and brushings and often the diagnosis is established by characteristic imaging findings of hilar confluence biliary obstruction, with or without an associated mass. Not infrequently, there are subtle areas of biliary ductal wall thickening and abnormal enhancement associated with the tumor (Figure 2.22). The extrahepatic type of cholangiocarcinoma may show an enhancing area of focal thickening of the common bile duct wall (Figure 2.23) or an actual polypoid intraluminal mass (Figure 2.24).

Cystic biliary neoplasms may arise from small peripheral intrahepatic ducts or more central biliary radicals [65]. Biliary cystadenomas often appear as complex cysts with

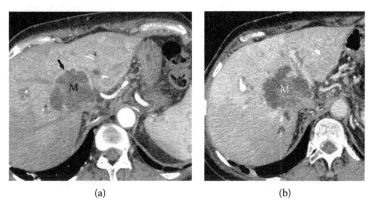

(a)　　　　　　　　　　(b)

FIGURE 2.21
Intrahepatic mass forming cholangiocarcinoma. (a) Note peripheral rim enhancement of mass ("M") during arterial-phase image. (b) Venousphase image demonstrating necrotic irregular mass ("M").

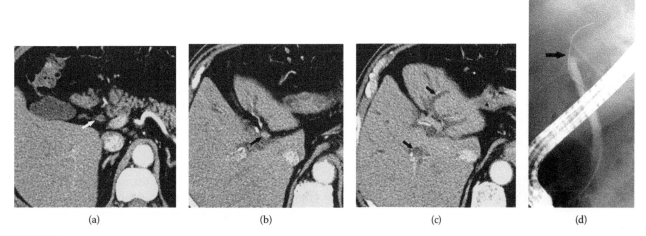

(a)　　　　　　(b)　　　　　　(c)　　　　　　(d)

FIGURE 2.22
Hilar confluence cholangiocarcinoma. (a) Note subtle asymmetric mural thickening of proximal common bile duct (arrow) due to tumor infiltration. (b) Note small enhancing mass at hilar confluence (arrow). (c) Moderately dilated intrahepatic bile ducts (arrows). (d) ERCP demonstrating obstruction at hilar confluence (arrow).

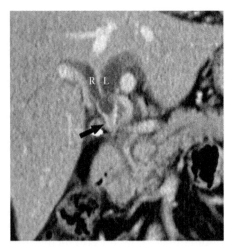

FIGURE 2.23
Extrahepatic, infiltrating type of cholangiocarcinoma. Coronal scan through extrahepatic bile duct demonstrates thickening and abnormal enhancement of infiltrating mural mass (arrow). (R = right lobe bile duct; L = left bile duct).

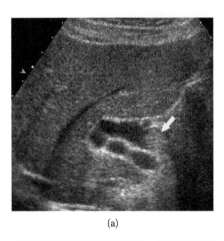

(a)

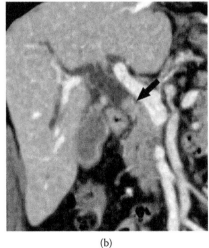

(b)

FIGURE 2.24
Polypoid type of cholangiocarcinoma. (a) Sagittal scan of bile duct demonstrating echogenic polypoid mass (arrow). (b) Coronal CT demonstrating enhancing mass within common bile duct (arrow).

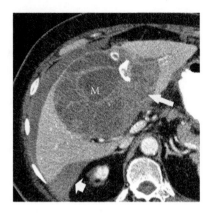

FIGURE 2.25
Ruptured biliary cystadenocarcinoma. Note large complex mass with solid internal tissue (long arrow). Lesion has ruptured into peritoneal cavity and perihepatic blood is present (short arrow) in the hepatorenal fossa.

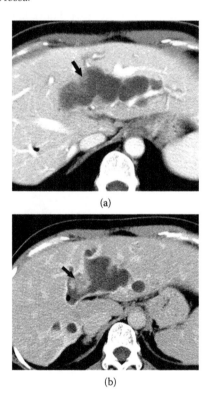

(a)

(b)

FIGURE 2.26
Malignant intraductal papillary mucinous tumor of left main bile duct. (a) Note marked distention of left main duct (arrow). (b) A 10-minute delayed scan reveals enhancing intraductal mass (arrow), confirmed to be adenocarcinoma at pathology.

thin septations. Malignant transformation results in solid enhancing tissue within the cyst, similar to ovarian carcinomas. These tumors may present with vague pain or rarely acute symptoms secondary to rupture (Figure 2.25). Intraductal biliary neoplasms are often mucinous tumors, similar to intraductal papillary mucinous tumors of the pancreas, and may result in extensive mucinous dilatation of the ductal system [65] (Figure 2.26).

FOCUS POINTS: CT OF CHOLANGIOCARCINOMA

- Morphologic classification: Mass forming, periductal infiltrating, and intraductal polypoid forms
- Anatomic classification: Peripheral intrahepatic (10%), hilar confluence or Klatskin tumor (25%), and extrahepatic (65%)

References

1. Greenberger NJ, Paumgartner G, "Chapter 305. Diseases of the Gallbladder and Bile Ducts." In Fauci AS, Braunwald E, Kasper DL et al. (eds): *Harrison's Principles of Internal Medicine*, 17e: http://www.accessmedicine.com/content.aspx?aID=2874111.
2. Ralls PW, Colletti PM, Halls JM et al. Prospective evaluation of 99mTc-IDA cholescintigraphy and gray-scale ultrasound in the diagnosis of acute cholecystitis. *Radiology* 1982; 144:369–71.
3. Ralls PW, Colletti PM, Lapin SA et al. Real-time sonography in suspected acute cholecystitis. *Radiology* 1985; 155:767–71.
4. Brook OR, Kane RA, Tyagi G et al. Lessons learned from quality assurance: errors in the diagnosis of acute cholecystitis on ultrasound and CT. *AJR Am J Roentgenol* 2011; 196:597–604.
5. Fidler J, Paulson EK, Layfield L. CT evaluation of acute cholecystitis: findings and usefulness in diagnosis. *AJR Am J Roentgenol* 1996; 166:1085–8.
6. Paulson EK. Acute cholecystitis: CT findings. *Semin Ultrasound CT MR* 2000; 21:56–63.
7. Shakespear JS, Shaaban AM, Rezvani M. CT findings of acute cholecystitis and its complications. *AJR Am J Roentgenol* 2010; 194:1523–9.
8. Aljiffry M, Walsh MJ, Molinari M. Advances in diagnosis, treatment and palliation of cholangiocarcinoma: 1990–2009. *World J Gastroenterol* 2009; 15(34):4240–62.
9. Charbel H, Al-Kawas FH. Cholangiocarcinoma: epidemiology, risk factors, pathogenesis, and diagnosis. *Curr Gastroenterol Rep* 2011; 13(2):182–7.
10. Akamatsu N, Sugawara Y, Hashimoto D. Surgical strategy for bile duct cancer: advances and current limitations. *World J Clin Oncol* 2011; 10(2):94–107.
11. Gotthardt D, Stiehl A. Endoscopic retrograde cholangiopancreatography in diagnosis and treatment of primary sclerosing cholangitis. *Clin Liver Dis* 2010; 14(2):349–58.
12. Dave M, Elmunzer BJ, Dwamena BA et al. Primary sclerosing cholangitis: meta-analysis of diagnostic performance of MR cholangiopancreatography. *Radiology* 2010; 256(2):387–96.
13. Weber C, Kuhlen cordt R, Grotelueschen R et al. Magnetic resonance cholangiopancreatography in the diagnosis of primary sclerosing cholangitis. *Endoscopy* 2008; 40(9):739–45.
14. Macchi V, Floreani A, Marchesi P et al. Imaging of primary sclerosing cholangitis: preliminary results by two new non-invasive techniques. *Dig Liver Dis* 2004; 36(9):614–21.
15. Campbell WL, Peterson MS, Federle MP et al. Using CT and cholangiography to diagnose biliary tract carcinoma complicating primary sclerosing cholangitis. *AJR Am J Roentgenol* 2001; 177(5):1095–100.
16. Campbell WL, Ferris JV, Holbert BL et al. Biliary tract carcinoma complicating primary sclerosing cholangitis: evaluation with CT, cholangiography, US, and MR imaging. *Radiology* 1998; 207(1):41–50.
17. Friedman AC, Sachs L. Embryology, anatomy, histology and radiologic anatomy. In Friedman AC (ed): *Radiology of the Liver, Biliary Tract, Pancreas and Spleen*. Baltimore, Williams & Wilkins, 1987, pp. 305–332.
18. Balfe DM, Molmenti EP, Bennett HF. Normal abdominal and pelvic anatomy. In Lee JKT, Sagel SS, Stanley RJ et al. (eds): *Computed Body Tomography with MRI Correlation*, 3rd ed. Philadelphia, Lippincott-Raven, 1998, pp. 573–635.
19. Turner MA, Fulcher AS. The cystic duct: normal anatomy and disease processes. *Radiographics* 2001; 21(1):3–22.
20. Yun EJ, Choi CS, Yoon DY et al. Combination of magnetic resonance cholangiopancreatography and computed tomography for preoperative diagnosis of the Mirizzi syndrome. *J Comput Assist Tomogr* 2009; 33(4):636–40.
21. Wang X, Shah RP, Maybody M et al. Cystic artery localization with a three-dimensional angiography vessel tracking system compared with conventional two-dimensional angiography. *J Vasc Interv Radiol* 2011; 22(10):1414–9.
22. Bret PM, de Stempel JV, Atri M et al. Intrahepatic bile duct and portal vein anatomy revisited. *Radiology* 1988; 169:405–7.
23. Horrow MM, Horrow JC, Naikosari A et al. Is age associated with size of adult extrahepatic bile duct? Sonographic study. *Radiology* 2001; 221:411–4.
24. Lacomis JM, Baron RL, Oliver JH 3rd et al. Cholangiocarcinoma: delayed CT contrast enhancement patterns. *Radiology* 1997; 203(1):98–104.
25. Vasanawala SS, Desser T. Value of delayed imaging in MDCT of the abdomen and pelvis. Pictorial essay. *AJR Am J Roentgenol* 2006; 187:154–63.
26. Cooperberg P. Imaging of the gallbladder. *Radiology* 1987; 163:605.
27. McIntosh DM, Penney HF. Gray-scale ultrasonography as a screening procedure in the detection of gallbladder disease. *Radiology* 1980; 136:725–7.
28. Barakos JA, Ralls PW, Lapin SA et al. Cholelithiasis: evaluation with CT. *Radiology* 1987; 162:415–18.
29. Baron RL, Rohrmann CA, Lee SP et al. CT evaluation of gallstones in vitro: correlation with chemical analysis. *AJR Am J Roentgenol* 1988; 151:1123–8.
30. Kelly IM, Lees WR, Russell RC. Tumefactive biliary sludge: a sonographic pseudotumour appearance in the common bile duct. *Clin Radiol* 199 3; 47(4):251–4.
31. Dong B, Chen M. Improved sonographic visualization of choledocholithiasis. *J Clin Ultrasound* 1987; 15:185–90.
32. Laing FC, Jeffrey RB, Wing VW. Improved visualization of choledocholithiasis by sonography. *AJR Am J Roentgenol* 1984; 143:949–52.

33. Baron RL. Common bile duct stones: reassessment of criteria for CT diagnosis. *Radiology* 1987; 162:419–24.

34. Baron RL. Diagnosing choledocholithiasis: how far can we push helical CT? *Radiology* 1997; 203:601–3.

35. Yeh BM, Coakley FV, Westphalen AC et al. Predicting biliary complications in right lobe liver transplant recipients according to distance between donor's bile duct and corresponding hepatic artery. *Radiology* 2007; 42(1):144–51.

36. Delabrousse E, Batholomot B, Sohm O et al. Gallstone ileus: CT findings. *Eur Radiol* 2000; 10(6):938–40.

37. Laméris W, van Randen A, van Es HW et al. Imaging strategies for detection of urgent conditions in patients with acute abdominal pain: diagnostic accuracy study. *BMJ* 2009 June 26; 338:b2431.

38. Laing FC, Federle MP, Jeffrey RB Jr et al. Ultrasonic evaluation of patients with acute right upper quadrant pain. *Radiology* 1981; 140:449–55.

39. van Randen A, Laméris W, van Es HW et al. A comparison of the accuracy of ultrasound and computed tomography in common diagnoses causing acute abdominal pain. *Eur Radiol* 2011; 21(7):1535–45.

40. Kane RA, Costello P, Duszlak E. Computed tomography in acute cholecystitis: new observations. *AJR Am J Roentgenol* 1983; 141:697–701.

41. Mariat G, Mahul P, Prevot N et al. Contribution of ultrasonography and cholescintigraphy to the diagnosis of acute acalculous cholecystitis in intensive care patients. *Intensive Care Med* 2000; 26:1658–63.

42. Blankenberg F, Wirth R, Jeffrey RB et al. Computed tomography as an adjunct to ultrasound in the diagnosis of acute acalculous cholecystitis. *Gastrointest Radiol* 1991; 16:149–53.

43. Mirvis SE, Whitley NO, Miller JW. CT diagnosis of acalculous cholecystitis. *J Comput Assist Tomogr* 1987; 11:83–7.

44. Wu Ch, Chen CC, Wang CJ et al. Discrimination of gangrenous from uncomplicated acute cholecystitis: accuracy of CT findings. *Abdom Imaging* 2011; 36(2):174–8.

45. Bennett GL, Rusinek H, Lisi V et al. CT findings in acute gangrenous cholecystitis. *AJR Am J Roentgenol* 2002; 178(2):275–81.

46. Singh AK, Sagar P. Gangrenous cholecystitis: prediction with CT imaging. *Abdom Imaging* 2005; 30(2):218–21.

47. De Vargas Macciucca M, Lanciotti S, De Cicco ML et al. Ultrasonographic and spiral CT evaluation of simple and complicated acute cholecystitis: diagnostic protocol assessment based on personal experience and review of the literature. *Radiol Med* 2006; 111(2):167–80.

48. Tsai MJ, Chen JD, Tiu CM et al. Can acute cholecystitis with gallbladder perforation be detected preoperatively by computed tomography in ED? Correlation with clinical data and computed tomography features. *Am J Emerg Med* 2009; 27(5):574–81.

49. Agarwal N, Sharma BC, Sarin SK. Endoscopic management of acute cholangitis in elderly patients. *World J Gastroenterol* 2006; 12(40):6551–5.

50. Bornman PC, van Beljon JI, Krige JE. Management of cholangitis. *J Hepatobiliary Pancreat Surg* 2003; 10(6):406–14.

51. Fleming KA. The hepatobiliary pathology of primary sclerosing cholangitis. *Eur J Gastroenterol Hepatol* 1992; 4:266–71.

52. Sugiura T, Nishio H, Nagino M et al. Value of multidetector-row computed tomography in diagnosis of portal vein invasion by perihilar cholangiocarcinoma. *World J Surg* 2008; 32(7):1478–84.

53. Unno M, Okumoto T, Katayose Y et al. Preoperative assessment of hilar cholangiocarcinoma by multidetector row computed tomography. *J Hepatobiliary Pancreat Surg* 2007; 14(5):434–40.

54. Dodd GD, Baron RL, Oliver JH et al. End-stage primary sclerosing cholangitis: CT findings of hepatic morphology in 36 patients. *Radiology* 1999; 211:357–62.

55. van Sonnenberg E, Casola G, Cubberley DA et al. Oriental cholangiohepatitis: diagnostic imaging and interventional management. *AJR Am J Roentgenol* 1986; 146:327–31.

56. Chan FL, Man SW, Leong LLY et al. Evaluation of recurrent pyogenic cholangitis with CT: analysis of 50 patients. *Radiology* 1989; 170:165–9.

57. Jemal A, Siegel R, Ward E et al. Cancer statistics, 2007. *CA Cancer J Clin* 2007; 57:43–66.

58. Kumaran V, Gulati S, Paul B et al. The role of dual-phase helical CT in assessing resectability of carcinoma of the gallbladder. *Eur Radiol* 2002; 12(8):1993–9.

59. Ohtani T, Shirai Y, Tsukada K et al. Carcinoma of the gallbladder: CT evaluation of lymphatic spread. *Radiology* 1993; 189(3):875–80.

60. Ohtani T, Shirai Y, Tsukada K et al. Spread of gallbladder carcinoma: CT evaluation with pathologic correlation. *Abdom Imaging* 1996; 21(3):195–201.

61. Henson DE, Albores-Saavedra J, Corle D. Carcinoma of the extrahepatic bile ducts: histologic types, stage of disease, grade, and survival rates. *Cancer* 1992; 70:1498–1501.

62. Lim JH. Cholangiocarcinoma: Morphologic classification according to growth pattern and imaging findings. *AJR Am J Roentgenol* 2003; 181:819–27.

63. Choi BI, Lee JM, Han JK. Imaging of intrahepatic and hilar cholangiocarcinoma. *Abdom Imaging* 2004; 29:548–57.

64. Han JK, Choi BI, Kim AY et al. Cholangiocarcinoma: pictorial essay of CT and cholangiographic findings. *RadioGraphics* 2002; 22:173–87.

65. Korobkin M, Stephens DH, Lee JKT et al. Biliary cystadenoma and cystadenocarcinoma: CT and sonographic findings. *AJR Am J Roentgenol* 1989; 153:507–11.

3

Spleen

Satomi Kawamoto and Elliot K. Fishman

CONTENTS

3.1 Introduction

The spleen is a functionally complex organ, and is responsible for initiating immune reactions and for filtering the blood of foreign material and old or damaged red blood cells. In comparison to other parenchymal organs, it is not a common site of primary disease. However, a wide variety of pathologic process can occur in the spleen including congenital, inflammatory, neoplastic, and traumatic lesions. In addition, certain normal variants may occur in the spleen. Most of these anatomical variants have no clinical significance, however, it is important for radiologists to recognize these findings correctly.

Computed tomography (CT) can easily and rapidly image the spleen, and is valuable in the diagnosis of splenic lesions. Multi-detector (MD) CT plays an important role in the detection and characterization of the splenic lesions. The advantages of MDCT includes improved temporal resolution, improved spatial resolution in the z axis, increased concentration of intravascular contrast material, decreased image noise, efficient x-ray tube use, and longer anatomic coverage [1]. These factors improve evaluation of splenic lesions, especially in the detection of subtle parenchymal disease and vascular pathology, and have helped to increase the diagnostic confidence for radiologists. This chapter will discuss CT evaluation of a wide variety of pathological processes involving the spleen.

3.2 Technique

In most cases, the spleen is evaluated on CT in conjunction with the other abdominal organs such as the liver and pancreas. The spleen is usually imaged using the same parameters as described for liver [2]. Typically, 100–120 mL of nonionic iodinated intravenous contrast is administered at a rate of 2–3 mL per second. Rates higher than this are occasionally used when the examination is targeted for vascular mapping and for evaluation of traumatic injury, but in the routine patient such rapid injection rates are not necessary. Typically, scanning begins usually at 60–70 seconds. If necessary, an arterial phase scanning may also be obtained for a dedicated examination of splenic vasculature, splenic masses, and perisplenic and splenic hilar lesions.

In the early arterial phase, the spleen enhances heterogeneously (Figure 3.1). This early heterogeneous enhancement should not be misinterpreted as splenic pathology. After a minute or more, the splenic parenchyma achieves homogeneous contrast enhancement. Delayed scans (obtained several minutes after injection) may be useful in cases of confusing splenic pathology or

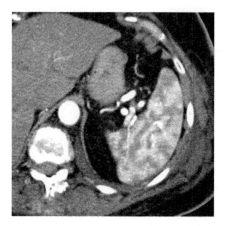

FIGURE 3.1
Normal early heterogeneous contrast enhancement of the spleen. Axial arterial phase computed tomography CT shows heterogeneous, archiform distribution of contrast enhancement.

to help differentiate a heterogeneously enhancing normal spleen from an abnormal spleen.

The advent of volume acquisition of MDCT data sets in conjunction with improvement in three-dimensional software markedly improves three-dimensional and multiplanar imaging capabilities [3]. Three-dimensional and multiplanar reconstructions are very helpful in demonstrating splenic and perisplenic processes [2]. Sagittal and coronal reconstructions can be routinely generated and help clarify confusing cases where the origin of a particular mass or lesion is uncertain. Curved reconstruction may allow for further assessment. Certain processes, such as splenic vascular pathology, splenic infarcts, and lacerations, are at times better shown with additional views. The reconstructed images can be reviewed in real time using an interactive display format.

3.3 The Normal Spleen

3.3.1 Development and Anatomy of the Spleen

The spleen begins to develop during the fifth week of fetal life in the dorsal mesogastrium from a mass of mesenchymal cells that migrate between the leaves of the mesentery and coalesce. During the next 4–5 weeks, the dorsal mesogastrium swings to the left due to enlargement and rotation of the stomach to the left, and that of the liver to the right. Subsequently, the most posterior part of dorsal mesogastrium lies against and fuses with posterior peritoneum to form short splenorenal ligament [4]. Failure of this fusion leads to a long splenic mesentery and a wandering spleen [4]. The tail of the pancreas is commonly located within the splenorenal ligament and abuts the splenic hilum [4].

The spleen is an intraperitoneal organ and almost surrounded by peritoneum, which is firmly adherent to the capsule [5]. It is located deep in the left upper quadrant of the abdomen, closely abutting the left hemidiaphragm. The hilum is usually directed anteromedially, and the splenic artery and vein enters the spleen in this region. The lateral and superior border along the abdominal wall has a smooth, convex surface margin. The medial surface is concave, and faces the posterior wall of the stomach anteriorly and the upper part of the left kidney posteriorly. The splenorenal and gastrosplenic ligaments are the two folds of peritoneum that hold the spleen in its position. The splenic vessels enter the spleen through the splenorenal ligament.

3.3.2 Microscopic Anatomy and Circulation of the Spleen

Histologically, the spleen is divided into two compartments; white pulp and red pulp, separated by an ill-defined interphase known as the marginal zone. The white pulp consists of lymphatic tissue, and contains germinal centers, similar to those in lymph nodes [6]. The white pulp is the site of the spleen's immunological and cytopoietic functions. The red pulp consists of a complex network of sinusoids and splenic cords. The sinusoids and splenic cords of the red pulp contain macrophages and function as a filter and blood flow regulator. The red pulp is responsible for erythrocyte storage and macrophage proliferation and differentiation. There is slow circulation in the splenic sinuses in the red pulp allowing maximal interaction of antigenic material such as bacteria, antibody-coated blood cells, and structurally abnormal red cells with macrophages [6].

3.3.3 Normal CT Appearance of the Spleen

The spleen is optimally evaluated using intravenous contrast material. CT attenuation values of the normal spleen on noncontrast CT are in the range of 40–65 Hounsfield units (HU), normally slightly lower (5–10 HU) than those for the normal liver [7,8].

Following bolus intravenous contrast administration, the normal spleen enhances heterogeneously [9–11]. This transient pattern of heterogeneous contrast enhancement of the spleen is thought to be related to the unique anatomic structure of the spleen, with variable rates of blood flow through the cords of the red and white pulp of the spleen [10,11]. Some of the flow reaches the splenic veins after traversing through arteriole to the splenic cords to venules, resulting in relatively slow flow and delayed enhancement. The remaining flow directly reaches the splenic veins through arteriole to venule connection without intervening flow through the splenic cords, resulting in prompt enhancement [10–12]. Contrast material

flowing through the rapid pathway will enhance particular portions of the spleen before others. In combination, these variable pathways contribute to overall heterogeneous enhancement of normal spleen following bolus contrast administration [10–12]. This effect is transient and can only be appreciated for a brief time following a rapid injection. After a minute or more, the splenic parenchyma achieves the uniform, homogeneous contrast enhancement. At least 50% of normal spleens show inhomogeneous enhancement on dynamic CT [10]. This heterogeneous enhancement is more pronounced with faster injection rates, or when scanning begins soon after the initiation of contrast administration (arterial phase) [9].

The pattern of normal splenic enhancement can vary greatly among patients. A serpentine, cordlike, archiform distribution of enhancement seen homogeneously throughout the splenic tissue is the most common pattern (Figure 3.1) [9,12]. Peripheral opacification of the spleen with relatively delayed enhancement of the central splenic tissue (Figure 3.2) may also be seen in

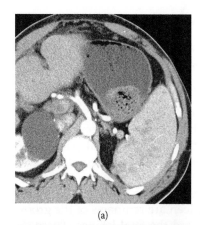

(a)

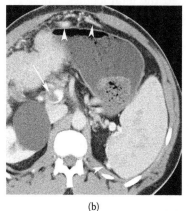

(b)

FIGURE 3.2
A 56-year-old man with history of hepatitis C cirrhosis and metastatic colorectal cancer. Heterogeneous contrast enhancement with delayed transit. (a) Axial arterial and (b) portal venous phase contrast-enhanced CT show heterogeneous enhancement and delayed transit of contrast. The patient has portal hypertension and portal vein thrombosis (white arrow). Note cirrhotic appearance of the liver and collateral veins (arrowheads).

patients with portal hypertension [12]. Occasionally, the spleen enhances irregularly in a manner that is difficult to further characterize. Delayed images of the spleen are very helpful to differentiate normal heterogeneous contrast enhancement from a pathologic process when uncertainty persists. Diffuse forms of normal splenic heterogeneity are transient and typically disappear on delayed imaging.

Normal heterogeneous splenic enhancement can also be exaggerated in patients with decreased cardiac output or heart failure [12]. Delayed transit of contrast material can also result from splenic vein occlusion, portal hypertension, or portal vein thrombosis (Figure 3.2) [11,12]. When a patient with exaggerated heterogeneous enhancement is encountered, the region of the splenic vein and pancreas should be carefully evaluated to exclude a vascular thrombosis or occlusion from an adjacent pancreatic tumor [2].

3.4 Normal Variant and Congenital Anomalies

3.4.1 Splenic Clefts and Lobulations

The fetal spleen is lobulated. Splenic lobules normally disappear before birth; however, splenic lobulations may persist along the medial part of the spleen [13]. Lobulations usually occur along the medial part of the spleen, and may be supplied by an early branch of the splenic artery [4]. The clefts on the superior border of the adult spleen are remnants of the grooves that originally separated the fetal lobules. These clefts are occasionally as deep as 2–3 cm, and can mimic lacerations (Figure 3.3) [13]. Clefts usually occur on the superior diaphragmatic surface of the spleen [4].

3.4.2 Accessory Spleen

Accessory spleen is a congenital abnormality consisting of normal splenic tissue in ectopic sites. Accessory spleen is found in 10%–20% of individuals at autopsy examination [14,15]. They arise as a result of failure of fusion of some of the multiple buds of splenic tissue in the dorsal mesogastrium during the early embryologic life [16]. They are usually smooth, round, or ovoid mass, and their size varies from a few millimeters to several centimeters in diameter (Figure 3.4). The blood supply to an accessory spleen is usually derived from the splenic artery, with drainage occurring into the splenic vein. Supplying vascular branches arising from the splenic artery may be visualized on CT (Figure 3.4) [16].

The most common location of an accessory spleen is in the vicinity of the splenic hilum [4,16], and the second most common site is within the tail of the pancreas [14,15]. In autopsy studies, 11%–17.8% of accessory spleens were located in the tail of the pancreas [14,15]. Rarely, they occur in unusual location including in the wall of the stomach or bowel, in the greater omentum or mesentery, or in the pelvis or scrotum [13]. In most patients, they have no clinical significance; however, occasionally it is confused with tumor when the location is atypical [13]. In particular, an accessory spleen is located within the tail of the pancreas (Figure 3.5); it can be mistaken for other mass-forming lesions in the pancreas, particularly nonfunctioning pancreatic neuroendocrine tumors [17,18].

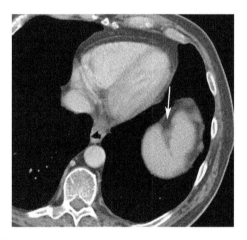

FIGURE 3.3
Cleft on the superior border of the spleen. Axial contrast-enhanced CT shows linear cleft on the superior border of the spleen, normal anatomical variant, which may simulate laceration.

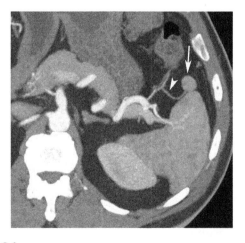

FIGURE 3.4
Accessory spleen. Axial contrast-enhanced volume rendered image shows a small accessory spleen anterior to the spleen (arrow). A small vascular branch arises from the splenic artery supplying the accessory spleen (arrowhead).

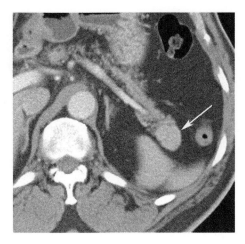

FIGURE 3.5
A 73-year-old man with history of prostate cancer. Intrapancreatic accessory spleen. Axial contrast-enhanced CT shows well-defined oval soft tissue mass (arrow) within the tip of the tail of the pancreas, which is isodense to the spleen. Tc-99m sulfur colloid scan confirmed that it represents an accessory spleen.

Similar attenuation of the lesion to the spleen on noncontrast, and postcontrast CT at different phases is helpful to make diagnosis of an accessory spleen. If a mass fails to enhance to the same degree as to the splenic parenchyma, it should not be considered an accessory spleen, and other etiology such as lymphadenopathy or tumors of other organs should be considered [13]. In problematic cases, nuclear scintigraphy with technetium-99m sulfur colloid scan or heat-damaged tagged red blood cell study, or superparamagnetic iron oxide (SPIO)-enhanced magnetic resonance imaging (MRI) may be useful [18].

Complications involving an accessory spleen have been reported, including torsion [19], infarction, and spontaneous rupture with bleeding [20]. An accessory spleen can also be involved with a congenital (epidermoid) cyst [21].

3.4.3 Splenosis

In patients with previous splenectomy, accessory spleens can significantly enlarge. In patients with hypersplenism from a hematologic disorder, growth of accessory splenic tissue can lead to a relapse of hypersplenism [22]. Therefore, awareness of the presence of an accessory spleen is important in a patient evaluated by CT prior to splenectomy.

Splenosis is ectopic splenic tissue caused by autotransplantation of splenic cells resulting from traumatic disruption of the splenic capsule via trauma or surgery. Splenosis is more numerous and widespread than accessory spleens (Figure 3.6) [23]. Splenosis nodules are typically found incidentally within the abdomen or pelvis adjacent to the small-bowel serosa, greater omentum,

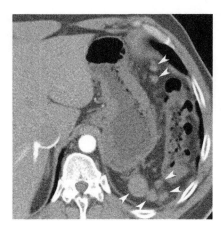

FIGURE 3.6
A 43-year-old man with remote history of splenectomy secondary to trauma. Round nodules (arrowheads) in the left upper quadrant representing splenosis.

parietal peritoneum and along the diaphragm [16]. However, unusual locations including subcutaneous, intrahepatic, and intracranial splenosis have been reported [23]. Similar to accessory spleens, splenosis can simulate malignancy. However, different from the accessory spleens, which is of embryologic origin, blood supply to splenosis derives from neovascularization and may have limited blood supply [16,23].

3.4.4 Wandering Spleen

Wandering spleen results from congenital deficiency or acquired laxity of the splenic suspensory ligaments [24]. The wandering spleen has a long vascular pedicle that allows the spleen to migrate from its normal position in the left upper quadrant to move about in the abdomen, and is at risk of torsion around the vascular pedicle [24,25]. It is a rare condition, and mainly affects children [24,26]. Among adults, it most frequently affects women of reproductive age [24,26]. Clinically, patients with wandering spleen may present with a spectrum of clinical findings ranging from an asymptomatic abdominal or pelvic mass, mild discomfort, or intermittent abdominal pain secondary to intermittent torsion, to an acute abdomen secondary to compromised vascular supply, and leading to splenic ischemia or infarction [24]. CT can confirm the absence of the spleen in its expected location and the presence of wandering spleen in the abdomen or pelvis seen as a soft-tissue density mass (Figure 3.7). In splenic torsion, CT shows minimal or no splenic enhancement (Figure 3.7) [24,25]. A whirled appearance of unenhancing splenic vessels may also be observed closely to the spleen (Figure 3.7) [24]. If the pancreatic tail is involved in the torsion, a whorled appearance of the pancreatic tail and adjacent fat may be observed on CT (Figure 3.7) [27].

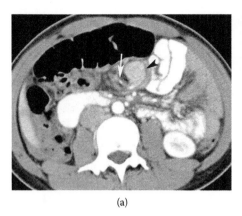

(a)

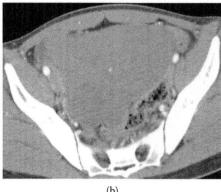

(b)

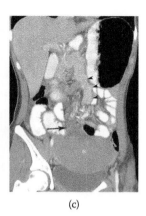

(c)

FIGURE 3.7
Torsed wandering spleen with infarction. A 16-year-old woman with two days history of severe lower abdominal pain. (a) and (b) Contrast-enhanced axial, and (c) coronal multiplanar reformation CT images show torsed wandering spleen within the pelvis (white asterisk), which is enlarged and poorly enhanced. Note splenic artery (white allows) extends inferiorly, with absent flow within the torsed pedicle (black arrows) near the spleen. Pancreas head is in normal position, but the body and tail (black arrowheads) extends inferiorly with splenic artery. Small ascites is present in the right paracolic gutter. The patient underwent laparoscopic splenectomy. Pathological exam of the spleen revealed hemorrhagic infarct.

3.4.5 Polysplenia and Asplenia

Situs ambiguous, or heterotaxy, refers to visceral mal-position and dysmorphism associated with indeterminate atrial arrangement, and includes polysplenia syndrome and asplenia syndrome [28]. Polysplenia is a rare, complex syndrome and consists of situs ambiguous with features of left isomerism (bilateral left-sidedness). The pattern of abnormalities in this syndrome involves various organ systems, although typical anomalies can occasionally be found only in one organ system [29]. Polysplenia is more common in females. In most cases, multiple spleens are present in either the right or left upper quadrant (Figure 3.8). However, patients with polysplenia may have a single, lobulated spleen or even a normal spleen [28]. Other abdominal anomalies include anomalous positions of abdominal viscera, short pancreas, and abnormal rotation of the bowel [30]. In an autopsy series of 146 patients with polysplenia, heterotaxy of abdominal viscera was seen in 56% and cardiovascular anomalies over 50% including bilateral superior vena cava, interruption of the inferior vena cava with azygos continuation (Figure 3.8), ventricular septal defect, and ostium primum defect [29]. However, many patients have no or mild congenital heart disease [29]. The associated abnormalities may be discovered as an incidental finding on CT during adulthood [31].

Asplenia is characterized by an absent spleen, situs ambiguous, and multiple anomalies including cardiovascular anomalies, intestinal malrotation, and genitourinary tract anomalies. The spleen is absent in virtually all patients with asplenia, although a rudimentary spleen may rarely be detected [32]. Asplenia occurs more frequently in males. The cardiovascular

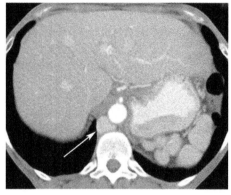

FIGURE 3.8
Polysplenia. A 41-year-old woman with left isomerism with polysplenia, congenital malrotation of the bowel, and azygos continuation of the intrahepatic vena cava, which were incidentally found on CT several years ago during work up for abdominal pain. Axial contrast-enhanced CT shows multiple small spleens in the left upper quadrant. Note the absence of hepatic segment of the inferior vena cava with dilated azygos vein (arrow).

anomalies are typically more complex than those seen with polysplenia, and account for much of the high mortality [32]. Children with asplenia syndrome also have a significantly greater incidence of sepsis.

3.5 Splenic Size

3.5.1 Normal Splenic Size

Splenic size can vary in different individuals and in the same individuals under different conditions. In the adult, it typically weighs approximately 150 g and measures approximately 12 cm in length, 3–4 cm in thickness, and 7 cm in width [5]. Various indices have been described for calculating splenic size [33,34]. In practice, however, most observers assess splenic volume by subjective evaluation of the CT based on experience [35]. More accurate approach to the assessment of the splenic volume has been performed using computer programs with a volume data of CT. In some studies, the splenic weight decreased with age and increased with body weight, and is slightly smaller in women [36,37], however, these tendencies were not found in other studies [38].

3.5.2 Splenomegaly

A wide variety of disease processes can lead to splenomegaly. They include hematologic, vascular, neoplastic, infectious, immunologic disorders, and storage disease. The CT can provide information as to whether the spleen is enlarged and on the degree of enlargement. However, splenomegaly alone is often nonspecific in appearance on CT. Clinical correlation is essential for accurate diagnosis in these cases.

Liver cirrhosis with portal hypertension with altered splenic blood flow is one of the most common causes of splenic enlargement. When characteristic alterations in the size and shape of the liver along with ascites and collateral venous channels are observed, the diagnosis of cirrhosis and portal hypertension is easily made at CT. When splenomegaly is caused by isolated splenic vein thrombosis or occlusion as seen in patients with pancreatitis or pancreatic carcinoma, CT can also suggest an underlying cause for splenomegaly in these cases.

Most hematological malignancies can affect the spleen, including various types of lymphomas, leukemias, and plasma cell malignancies [39]. Presence of abdominal lymph node enlargement may suggest lymphoma or leukemia. Chronic lymphocytic leukemia can result in massive splenomegaly.

Splenomegaly can also result from many infectious processes. These include bacterial infections such as endocarditis and viral infections such as infectious mononucleosis. Granulomatous infection such as tuberculosis or histoplasmosis may cause splenomegaly in the acute phase but more typically presents with a normal-sized spleen with scattered granulomata. Patients with acquired immunodeficiency syndrome (AIDS) will frequently show splenomegaly, often the result of superimposed infection [40]. Splenomegaly in AIDS patients may also result from diffuse involvement of lymphoma, and it can be extremely difficult to differentiate infectious splenomegaly from malignant splenomegaly in these patients.

Systemic processes such as sarcoidosis and Gaucher's disease can present with splenomegaly with focal masses simulating malignant tumors, and the CT appearance may mimic lymphoma. If ancillary findings of pulmonary sarcoidosis are present, diagnosis of sarcoidosis is suggested. In Gaucher's disease, discrete areas of low attenuation corresponding to local deposits of glucocerebroside within the reticuloendothelial cells in the spleen along with splenomegaly can be seen.

3.6 Neoplasm

Both benign and malignant primary splenic neoplasms are uncommon. They can arise from lymphatic tissue (white palp) that gives rise to lymphoid neoplasms, and vascular element (red pulp) that gives rise to vascular neoplasms [41]. Splenic metastasis is unusual, and is typically seen in patients with widespread metastatic disease.

3.6.1 Hematological Malignancies

Lymphoma is the most common malignancy involving the spleen [42]. Splenic involvement in lymphoma as part of disseminated disease is common, and the spleen is involved in up to 40% of patients with Hodgkin's disease and non-Hodgkin's lymphoma [43]. Splenic involvement is considered nodal in Hodgkin's disease and extranodal in non-Hodgkin's lymphoma [44]. Accurate assessment of splenic involvement in lymphoma is important because it may alter tumor staging, influence treatment options, and determine the overall prognosis [39,43].

The CT finding of splenic involvement in lymphoma include a homogemeous enlargement of the spleen without a discrete mass, diffuse infiltration with miliary lesions, multiple focal nodular lesions (1–10 cm), and a large solitary mass [7,39,43].

Splenomegaly alone (Figure 3.9) is not sensitive or specific to determine splenic involvement of lymphoma. The size of the spleen is normal in up to one-third of patients with splenic involvement in lymphoma [45,46]. Moreover, in up to 30% of patients with lymphoma, splenic enlargement is not due to lymphoma unless the spleen is markedly enlarged (>400 g) [45].

Focal lymphomatous deposits occur in both normal-sized and enlarged spleens [39,43]. On CT, focal lymphomatous deposits (Figure 3.10) are seen as homogeneous mass or masses, which are hypodense than the normal spleen, and best seen in late venous phase CT [39]. Markedly hypodense, cyst-like masses or fluid-like component within masses can represent areas of liquefactive necrosis or hypovascular solid tumor [43]. Calcification is unusual but has been reported in aggressive lesions [47] and after therapy [39,43]. Ancillary

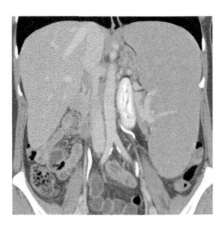

FIGURE 3.9
A 52-year-old woman with left abdominal fullness. Splenomegaly was found clinically. Bone marrow biopsy revealed low-grade B cell lymphoma. Contrast-enhanced coronal CT image shows markedly enlarged spleen. No discrete nodule is identified within the spleen. The left kidney is displaced medially because of the enlarged spleen.

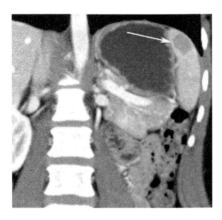

FIGURE 3.10
A 29-year-old woman with recurrence of Hodgkin's disease, nodular sclerosis type. The patient was in remission after her initial treatment, and developed recurrence. Contrast-enhanced coronal CT image shows a small solitary hypodense nodule (arrow) in the spleen. Splenectomy revealed Hodgkin's disease.

findings of adenopathy in the chest or abdomen can help in suggesting the diagnosis of lymphoma. In patients with non-Hodgkin's lymphoma, splenic involvement is associated with para-aortic adenopathy in approximately 70% of patients [48].

Primary splenic lymphoma is rare and constitutes approximately 1%–2% of all lymphomas at presentation [49,50], most commonly diffuse large B-cell lymphoma [39]. Primary splenic lymphoma is defined as lymphomatous involvement of the spleen with or without splenic hilar lymphadenopathy [39]. Primary splenic lymphoma usually presents as a single large mass (Figure 3.11) or multiple focal masses, rather than splenomegaly alone [51]. In a study of primary splenic lymphoma, 17 of 21 cases presented as a solitary large mass (>5 cm), 4 cases as multifocal masses of varying size (1–10 cm), and no

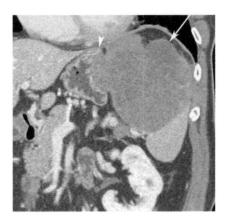

FIGURE 3.11
Primary splenic lymphoma (Large B-cell lymphoma). A 64-year-old man with left upper quadrant abdominal pain. Contrast-enhanced coronal CT image shows a large heterogeneous hypodense mass (arrow) with lobulated contour, which involves the short gastric arteries and greater curvature of the stomach (arrowhead). The patient underwent splenectomy and partial gastrectomy.

cases presented with splenomegaly alone or with miliary masses [51]. Primary splenic lymphoma may be bulky, and transgress the splenic capsule, and involve the adjacent organs (Figure 3.11) [7].

18-FDG PET/CT has established a definite role in staging and follow-up for patients with lymphoma [52]. In a recent study, CT and PET/CT for detection of splenic involvement in lymphoma at initial staging was evaluated in 111 patients with malignant lymphoma [53]. Using follow-up PET/CT to confirm splenic involvement in lymphoma, the sensitivity and specificity of CT, PET, and PET/CT were 91% and 96%, 75% and 99%, and 100% and 95%, respectively [53]. CT criteria for splenic involvement in this study were defined as splenic enlargement according to the described criteria, or the presence of splenic nodules (an area with lower attenuation than adjacent normal splenic parenchyma on contrast-enhanced CT at portal venous phase).

In patients with leukemia, CT may show splenomegaly and lymphadenopathy [39]. Rarely, leukemic deposits in the spleen can be seen as tiny low attenuation splenic nodules [39].

3.6.2 Tumors Arising from Vascular Elements

3.6.2.1 Hemangioma

Splenic hemangioma is the most common benign splenic neoplasm [54]. Its prevalence at autopsy ranges from 0.3% to 14% [41]. Splenic hemangiomas are mostly solitary, but may be multiple, and also be a part of systemic angiomatosis [55]. Splenic hemangiomas can vary in size from a few millimeters to several centimeters, but most lesions are less than 2 cm in size (Figure 3.12) [56]. They are usually asymptomatic, and found incidentally on

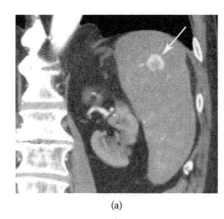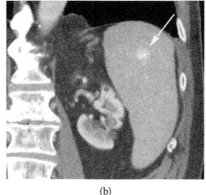

(a)　　　　　　　　　　　　　　　(b)

FIGURE 3.12
Presumed hemangioma. 76-year-old man with history of colon cancer and liver metastasis. (a) Arterial and (b) portal venous phase coronal CT images show a small round mass (arrow) with dense contrast enhancement on arterial phase, with persistent centripetal enhancement on portal venous phase.

imaging studies; however, may present with abdominal pain or mass [54]. In patients with Klippel–Trenauney–Weber syndrome, multiple splenic hemangiomas or hemangiomas in other organs may occur [41].

Splenic hemangiomas are thought to be congenital in origin, arising from sinusoidal epithelium [41]. Histologically, they are composed of endothelial lined blood-filled spaces of varying size ranging from capillary to cavernous size [41]. Central, punctate calcifications can be seen in the solid portions, and curvilinear calcifications may be seen in the periphery of the cystic areas [41,55].

There is considerable variation of CT appearances of hemangiomas following intravenous (IV) contrast administration reflecting the proportion of cavernous and capillary features [54]. Some lesions, such as capillary hemangiomas, show immediate homogeneous enhancement. Others may show centripetal enhancement from the periphery with persistence on delayed images (Figure 3.12) [54]. Other lesions, typically large lesions, may have a variable combination of solid and cystic spaces, and only solid component display contrast enhancement [57]. These large lesions may show mottled enhancement with areas remaining hypodense relative to the normal spleen in the late phase of contrast enhancement rather than centripetal enhancement. This enhancement pattern is different from hepatic cavernous hemangiomas [57], probably reflecting presence of cystic spaces filled with serous or hemorrhagic fluid that may be seen in large cavernous hemangioma of the spleen due to necrosis [41].

3.6.2.2 Lymphangioma

Splenic lymphangiomas are composed of endothelium-lined cystic spaces, containing proteinaceous fluid instead of blood as seen in hemangiomas [41,43]. These

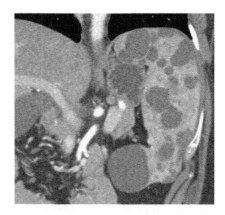

FIGURE 3.13
Cystic lymphangiomatosis. A 46-year-old woman with splenic mass found on laparoscopy during hysterectomy for uterine leiomyomas. Contrast-enhanced coronal CT image shows multiple thin-walled, well-marginated cysts of variable size throughout the enlarged spleen. Some cysts are exophytic. The patient underwent laparoscopic splenectomy for increasing left upper quadrant discomfort and pain. Pathology revealed cystic lymphangiomatosis.

are classified as capillary, cavernous, and cystic based on the size and location of the vascular channels [41]. There is no firm consensus, but splenic lymphangioma may represent a hamartomatous rather than a neoplastic lesion [41]. Splenic lymphangiomas are uncommon, and usually asymptomatic and found incidentally [41]. Lymphangioma can be single or multiple. Lymphangiomatosis is a syndrome in which multiple organs can be involved including the mediastinum, retroperitoneum, axilla, and neck, often seen in children [41,57].

On CT, splenic lymphangiomas are seen as discrete thin-walled, well-marginated cysts without contrast enhancement within normal-sized or enlarged spleen. Lymphangiomas are often located in a subcapsular region (Figure 3.13) [41,58]. Unlike the random localization seen with hemangiomas, lymphangioma often

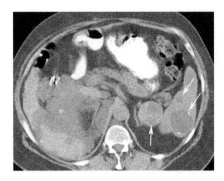

FIGURE 3.14
68-year-old woman with history of retroperitoneal lymphangiomas diagnosed by surgical biopsy of the right retroperitoneal mass in the past. Noncontrast CT shows large cystic masses in the retroperitoneum (asterisk) and in the liver and spleen (arrows), representing lymphangiomas. Small peripheral calcifications are seen in the splenic lymophangiomas. The spleen is lobulated in contour.

involves the capsule and trabeculae of the spleen, where lymphatics are normally concentrated [41]. Curvilinear peripheral mural calcifications may be seen (Figure 3.14). CT attenuation measurements vary from 15–35 HU [58].

3.6.2.3 Hamartoma

Splenic hamartoma is also called splenoma or nodular hyperplasia of the spleen. They are rare, benign splenic lesions. Hamartomas may occur at any age with equal gender predilection. They are usually single nodule, but may manifest as multiple nodules [41]. Splenic hamartoma is a malformation composed of an anomalous mixture of normal splenic red pulp elements. Histologically, they contain a mixture of unorganized vascular channels lined by endothelial cells and surrounded by fibrotic cords of predominant splenic red pulp [41].

On noncontrast CT, splenic hamartomas appear as well-circumscribed iso- or hypodense masses, and occasionally contain calcifications and cystic components [54,57]. After intravenous contrast material administration, they often appear nearly iso-attenuating relative to normal spleen [41], or show moderate heterogeneous contrast enhancement [54,57]. On delayed phase images, persistent hyperenhancement has been described [59].

3.6.2.4 Hemangiopericytoma

Hemangiopericytoma has a variable biologic behavior. The high rate of local recurrence (36%) has been reported [57], with the most common site of recurrence is local, followed by lung and bone for distant metastasis [60]. CT findings in hemangiopericytoma include a large splenic mass with polylobular contours and smaller disseminated lesions throughout the spleen [57]. Speckled calcification may be seen on CT

scans [57]. Contrast-enhanced studies show discrete hyperattenuation of solid portions and septations. These tumors often bleed because of their hypervascular nature and expansile growth [57].

3.6.2.5 Littoral Cell Angioma

Littoral cell angioma of the spleen is a recently recognized primary vascular lesion of the spleen, which was first described by Falk et al. [61] in 1991. This neoplasm is thought to arise from littoral cells, which normally line the splenic sinuses of the red pulp, and is unique to the spleen. These tumors were originally thought to be benign, however, there have been several reports of littoral cell angioma with malignant features [41]. Radiologically, littoral cell angioma usually presents as multiple nodules within the spleen [62] and rarely as a solitary mass [63,64]. The most common CT manifestation of littoral cell angioma is splenomegaly with innumerable masses [62]. Although several reports have described the imaging appearances of littoral cell angioma, they are nonspecific, requiring pathology for a definitive diagnosis [65]. The differential diagnosis for littoral cell angioma with multiple hypodense splenic lesions on CT includes both neoplastic and inflammatory conditions [41,65].

3.6.2.6 Angiosarcoma

Although rare, angiosarcoma is the most common malignant primary nonlymphoid tumor of the spleen [57]. Typically, patients present with splenomegaly, abdominal pain, fever, fatigue, and weight loss. Anemia, thrombocytopenia, or other coagulopathy may also be present [66]. Splenomegaly is common, and spontaneous rupture can be associated with 15%–30% of patients [41,57]. Distant metastases are common in angiosarcoma, and it has a poor prognosis.

The most common CT appearance of splenic angiosaroma is a complex mass or masses in an enlarged spleen (Figure 3.15) [67]. The mass may show heterogeneous contrast enhancement containing low attenuation areas suggesting necrosis [67]. Scattered punctate calcifications may occasionally be seen. Hemoperitoneum can be seen in patients with spontaneous rupture [41,57]. Hypervascular metastasis to the liver and other organs are well shown on CT [41].

Previous exposure to chemical agents, such as thorium dioxide (Thoratrast), vinyl chloride, and arsenic, is associated with an increased risk of hepatic angiosarcoma, however, splenic angiosarcoma has no documented association with exposure to these agents [66]. However, there is a reported case of splenic angiosarcoma associated with Thoratrast [68].

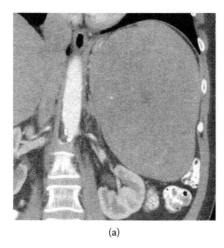
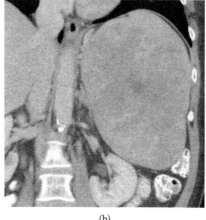

(a) (b)

FIGURE 3.15
Epithelioid angiosarcoma. A 54-year-old woman presented with thrombocytopenia, splenomegaly and left upper quadrant pain. (a) Arterial and (b) late venous phase coronal CT images show a large, heterogeneous mass with moderate contrast enhancement in the enlarged spleen.

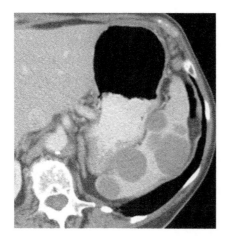

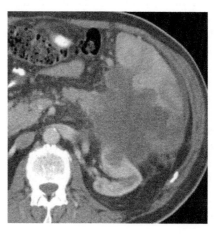

FIGURE 3.16
Metastatic melanoma. A 78-year-old woman with history of malignant melanoma on her face. Contrast-enhanced axial CT shows multiple hypodense masses in the spleen representing metastases, which are nearly cystic in appearance.

FIGURE 3.17
Direct invasion from pancreatic cancer. A 70-year-old man presented with diffuse abdominal pain and weight loss. Axial contrast-enhanced CT shows a large lobulated hypodense mass involving the tail of the pancreas, spleen, and left kidney. Pathology revealed adenocarcinoma of the pancreas with squamous differentiation.

3.6.3 Metastases

Metastatic lesions to the spleen are uncommon despite the fact that the spleen has a rich blood supply. Splenic involvement by metastases occurs in up to 7% of cancer patients [69,70]. Although cases of isolated metastasis have been reported, they are usually seen in patients with widespread metastases. Common primary sites for splenic metastasis include breast, lung, ovary, stomach, malignant melanoma, and prostate gland [70,71]. On CT, splenic metastases typically appear as hypoattenuating solid or cystic masses with homogeneous or occasionally heterogeneous contrast enhancement (Figure 3.16) [7]. Cystic metastasis may occur from internal necrosis in rapidly growing lesions such as melanoma (Figure 3.16), or from the mucinous primary tumor such as ovarian carcinoma [54].

Serosal implants to the spleen are seen with peritoneal carcinomatosis, most commonly from primary tumors of the ovary, but also seen in association with gastrointestinal adenocarcinoma and pancreatic cancer. CT shows solid or cystic implant tumors at the surface of the spleen, which cause scalloping of the surface of the spleen [7]. Peritoneal implants may occasionally intrude into the splenic parenchyma [7]. Direct invasion of the spleen is uncommon but can occur from a large adjacent primary tumor of the stomach, colon, pancreas, or left kidney (Figure 3.17) [7].

3.7 Cysts

3.7.1 Congenital Cyst

Congenital cyst, also called epithelial, epidermoid, mesothelial, primary, or true cyst, is congenital in origin, and is defined by the presence of an inner epithelial lining. This epithelial lining is thought to originate from infolding of peritoneal mesothelium or collections of peritoneal mesothelial cells trapped within the splenic parenchyma during development [72]. Congenital epithelial cysts are typically seen as a large, unilocular, fluid density mass with imperceptible walls on CT (Figure 3.18) [7]. The borders are sharply defined and there is no appreciable rim enhancement following contrast administration.

3.7.2 False Cysts

False cyst or nonepithelial cysts are thought to result from previous trauma, infarction, or infection of the spleen. Histologically, they lack a cellular lining. It is often difficult to distinguish a true cyst from a false cyst radiologically and histologically [7]. On CT, false cysts appear as spherical, well-defined cystic lesions with attenuation equal to that of water, with no rim enhancement (Figure 3.19). Cyst wall trabeculation or peripheral septations are uncommon in false cysts, but common in congenital cysts in one series [73]. Cyst wall calcification is more common in false cysts, and CT reportedly shows cyst wall calcifications in 50% of false cysts [73].

3.7.3 Echinococcal Cysts

Echinococcal cysts remain the common health problem in large areas of the world, but are distinctly unusual in most Western countries. The splenic involvement of echinococcal infection occurs in less than 2% of cases of all patients with hydatid disease [7]. Splenic echinococcal cyst generally develops by means of systemic dissemination or intraperitoneal spread from a ruptured liver cyst [74]. Isolated splenic involvement is very uncommon [74]. On CT, echinococcal cysts are well-circumscribed, round or ovoid mass that has attenuation in the range of that of water that may enlarge the spleen [72]. Splenic echinococcal cysts are usually solitary, and their imaging characteristics are similar to those of hepatic echinococcal cysts [74]. Cyst wall calcification is common, seen in 70% of patients in one series [75]. A splenic echinococcal cyst should be treated surgically [76].

3.7.4 Intrasplenic Involvement of Pancreatic Pseudocysts

Pancreatic pseudocysts may present as a cystic lesion adjacent to or within the spleen (Figure 3.20). It may extend beneath the splenic capsule or into the splenic parenchyma [54]. Intrasplenic involvement of pancreatic pseudocyst associated with pancreatitis has been reported to occur in 1%–5% of patients with pancreatitis [77,78]. Pseudocysts can become quite large and completely surround and engulf the spleen. Associated findings of acute or chronic pancreatitis are usually present to help establish the diagnosis. Pancreatitis often occludes the splenic vein and may result in areas of splenic infarction [79]. Patients with splenic pseudocysts are prone to splenic rupture with even minor trauma and, thus, should be monitored closely [80].

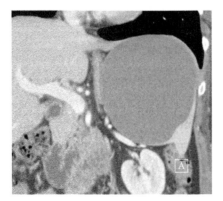

FIGURE 3.18
True cyst. A 21-year-old woman with a large cystic mass incidentally found on CT during evaluation for renal stone. Contrast-enhanced coronal CT image shows a large, unilocular, fluid density mass with imperceptible wall, representing a true cyst.

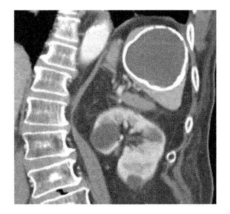

FIGURE 3.19
Presumed false cyst. A 78-year-old man with history of lung cancer. Contrast-enhanced coronal CT image shows a spherical, well-defined cystic mass with dense, linear rim calcification. It is stable for 6 years, and thought to represent old hematoma.

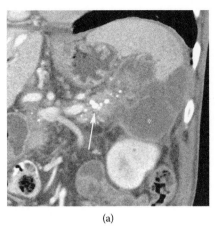
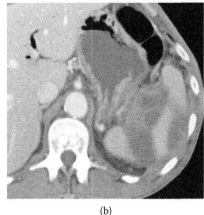

(a)   (b)

FIGURE 3.20
Intrasplenic extension of pancreatic pseudocyst. A 59-year-old man, status after Whipple procedure for complicated chronic pancreatitis 1 year ago. (a) Coronal and (b) axial contrast-enhanced CT show large, multiloculated cysts (asterisk) around the tail of the pancreas, also involving the spleen. Multiple calcifications in the pancreas (arrow) representing underlying chronic pancreatitis.

3.8 Infection

3.8.1 Splenic Abscess

Splenic abscess is a rare yet potentially lethal disease process. The high morbidity is in part due to vague clinical symptoms, which often lead to a delay in diagnosis. Patients predisposed to splenic abscess formation include immunosuppressed status in cancer, transplant, AIDS, diabetes mellitus, alcoholism, or intravenous drug abuse, and hematologic disorders including sickle cell disease. Endocarditis, splenic trauma, splenic infarction, or contiguous infection from adjacent organs can also result in a splenic abscess. Splenic abscesses may be solitary or multiple. Unilocular abscesses have most likely a bacterial etiology [81]. Multiple abscesses are more common among immunocompromised patients and are usually associated with abscesses in other viscera [56].

CT is sensitive in detecting splenic abscesses [81–83], but its specificity is limited [83]. Splenic infarct, cysts, tumors, and hematomas may simulate abscess. Clinical information combined with imaging findings is important, but ultrasound-guided fine needle aspiration may be needed for a definitive diagnosis [83]. On CT, splenic abscess typically appears as a focal low-attenuating lesion and may show rim enhancement when a capsule has developed (Figure 3.21) [7]. The presence of gas in an intrasplenic collection is diagnostic for an abscess (Figure 3.21) [7]. However, gas formation in the abscess is seen only up to 22% of patients [82,83].

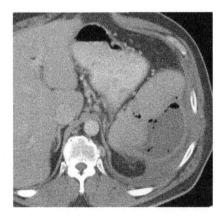

FIGURE 3.21
A 44-year-old man with splenic abscess, developed after splenic laceration. Axial contrast-enhanced CT shows focal fluid density lesion with rim enhancement containing bubbles of air. Small ascites is seen around the spleen.

3.8.2 Fungal, Mycobacterial, and other Infection

Fungal infection in immunocompromised hosts can have a specific appearance. Multiple small (<2 cm), typically 5–10 mm, hypoattenuating lesions can suggest the diagnosis of fungal microabscesses, usually due to candidiasis [84,85]. Occasionally, a central focus of higher attenuation may be observed [7]. Systemic fungal infection is a serious complication in patients with hematological malignancies who have neutropenia after chemotherapy. The spleen is the second most common solid organ after the liver involved with systemic fungal infection. Distinguishing between splenic infection and lymphoma or leukemia can be difficult on imaging findings alone. When significant perisplenic lymphadenopathy is present, it is not a feature

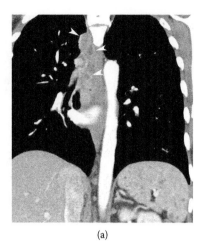
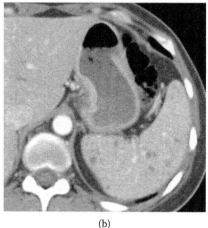

(a)   (b)

FIGURE 3.22
A 38-year-old woman with history of acquired immunodeficiency syndrome (AIDS). Mycobacterium avium-intracellulare infection diagnosed by biopsy of mediastinal adenopathy. (a) Coronal and (b) axial contrast-enhanced CT shows multiple small nodules of low attenuation in the spleen. There are multiple enlarged mediastinal lymph nodes with central low-attenuation and peripheral enhancement (arrowheads).

of splenic infection and more likely lymphoma [43]. Lymphomatous deposits in the spleen are typically larger and less uniform compared to splenic microabscesses [43].

Patients with immunosuppression, particularly with AIDS, may develop small hypodense lesions in the liver and spleen due to disseminated tuberculosis infection or mycobacterium avium-intracellulare (MAI) infection (Figure 3.22) [86,87]. Hepatosplenic lesions are, however, usually in a fine miliary pattern and often below the resolving capacity of CT. Therefore, patients with hepatosplenic tuberculosis and MAI infection most commonly present with nonspecific hepatosplenomegaly [86,87]. When infectious deposits coalesce into larger areas of involvement, small nodules of low attenuation appear in the liver and spleen on CT [7]. Low-density adenopathy with peripheral enhancement is a supportive finding for mycobacterial infection central low-attenuation within adenopathy is more commonly seen with mycobacterium tuberculosis infection than MAI infection [87]. However, patients with AIDS also have an increased risk of splenic involvement in lymphoma, and noninfectious etiology should be also considered as differential diagnosis [43].

Certain viral illnesses, such as infectious mononucleosis, can result in splenomegaly without frank abscess formation. CT in such cases usually reveals nonspecific splenic enlargement.

3.9 Other Nonneoplastic Conditions

3.9.1 Sarcoidosis

Sarcoidosis is a systemic disease of unknown etiology, characterized by multiple noncaseating granulomas in almost any organ. Splenic involvement is frequently

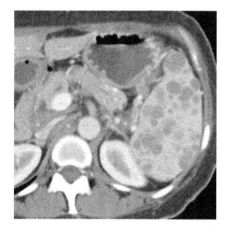

FIGURE 3.23
45-year-old woman with sarcoidosis. Axial contrast-enhanced CT shows multiple small hypodense nodules in the enlarged spleen. There are also enlarged lymph nodes (asterisk) in the retroperitoneum and near the splenic hilum. Biopsy finding of perisplenic lymph node was consistent with sarcoidosis.

observed at microscopic examination in approximately 24%–59% of patients [88,89]. Splenic involvement in sarcoidosis is usually asymptomatic. Splenomegaly is the most common finding on CT, seen in approximately one-third of patients [90]. Splenic nodules corresponding to aggregated granulomata are visible on CT in approximately 6%–33% of sarcoid patients, and range in size from 1–2 mm to 2 cm, usually diffusely distributed throughout the spleen [90]. On contrast-enhanced CT, splenic nodules appear hypodense relative to background spleen (Figure 3.23). The spleen may be normal in size or enlarged. Nodular lesions tend to become confluent with increasing in size. Approximately 50% of patients with splenic nodules will also show hepatic nodules on CT [90]. Coexistent abdominal lymphadenopathy is noted frequently in patients with splenomegaly. The appearance and presentation may mimic lymphoma, granulomatous infection or other process associated with splenic nodules and/or splenomegaly. Sarcoidosis should be considered as a differential diagnosis for multiple splenic nodules with or without splenomegaly.

3.9.2 Inflammatory Pseudotumor of the Spleen

Inflammatory pseudotumors are rare, benign lesions consisting of a polymorphous inflammatory cell infiltrate with varying amounts of granulomatous reaction, fibrosis, and necrosis. The etiology of inflammatory pseudotumor remains uncertain. Speculated etiologies include infectious and autoimmune origin. They are usually well-circumscribed solitary mass, but rarely multiple splenic lesions have been reported [91]. On noncontrast CT, they usually appear as a rounded heterogeneous hypodense mass (Figure 3.24) [7,92]. Peripheral or stippled calcification may be present in the mass [7,92]. After administration of intravenous contrast material, splenic pseudotumor may show mild to moderate heterogeneous contrast enhancement, with a progressive opacification of the lesion in some cases [7,92]. Central hypodense area may be observed on post-contrast CT in a reported case, which corresponded to central stellate fibrotic area [92].

3.9.3 Sclerosing Angiomatous Nodular Transformation of the Spleen

Sclerosing angiomatous nodular transformation of the spleen is a recently recognized, rare benign vascular splenic lesion of uncertain etiology, first characterized by Martel et al. in 2004 [93]. It is most commonly encountered in middle-aged adults, with a mean age of presentation of 48 years. Reported female-to-male ratio is 2:1 [93]. The size of reported lesions ranges from 3 to 17 cm in diameter; all reported cases have been solitary, and splenectomy is curative [94]. Most reported cases are clinically silent and found incidentally [93]. The spleen is often normal in size or mildly enlarged. The mass is isodense to minimally hypodense on noncontrast CT (Figure 3.25). After administration of intravenous contrast, peripheral nodular contrast enhancement may be initially seen in arterial phase. In venous phase and delayed phase, progressive enhancement from the periphery to the center of the mass approaching the attenuation of surrounding splenic tissue has been described [94–97]. Radiating hypodense bands may be seen in delayed phase, which correspond to stellate-shaped fibrotic stroma separating hemorrhagic angiomatoid nodules [94–96].

3.9.4 Sickle Cell Disease

Sickle cell disease is one of the most common human hereditary disorders [98]. Patients with homozygous gene disorder of sickle cell disease (sickle cell anemia) affects 1 of every 400–500 African-American newborns in the United States [6]. Doubly heterozygous sickle trait is found in 8%–10% of the African-American population, and includes sickle beta thalassemia and sickle-C hemoglobinopathy [6]. The pathophysiology and clinical severity of sickle beta thalassemia is very similar to those of sickle cell anemia. Sickle-C hemoglobinopathy is clinically milder and associated with prolonged splenomegaly and relative preservation of splenic function [6].

Patients with sickle cell anemia often have loss of splenic function in early childhood. The spleen becomes smaller, containing diffuse, microscopic deposits of calcium and iron due to repeated episodes of splenic

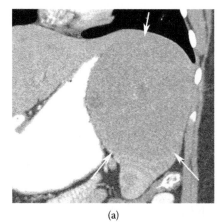
(a)

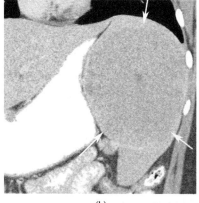
(b)

FIGURE 3.24
Inflammatory pseudotumor. A 15-year-old woman with abdominal pain and abdominal distention. Ultrasound at outside institution revealed splenic mass. (a) Arterial and (b) late venous phase coronal images show a large round mass (arrows) with small central and peripheral hypodense areas in the enlarged spleen. Slightly increased enhancement of the mass on late venous phase compared to arterial phase.

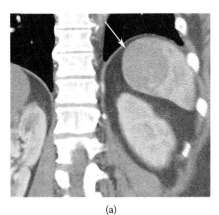
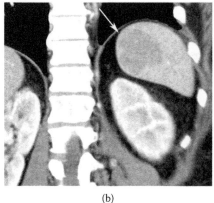

(a)   (b)

FIGURE 3.25
Sclerosing angiomatous nodular transformation. A 49-year-old man with history of pancreatic mass. The splenic mass was incidentally found during the workup for pancreatic mass. (a) Contrast-enhanced coronal CT in arterial phase shows well-circumscribed hypodense mass (arrow) in the spleen with areas of peripheral enhancement. (b) On venous phase, increasing peripheral contrast enhancement of the mass is seen.

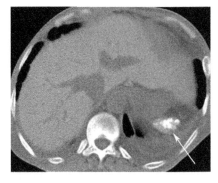

FIGURE 3.26
Autosplenectomy. A 52-year-old woman with sickle cell anemia. Axial noncontrast CT shows severe atrophy of the spleen with calcifications (arrow). Small bilateral pleural effusions and dilated inferior vena cava and hepatic veins, suggestive of right-sided cardiac failure.

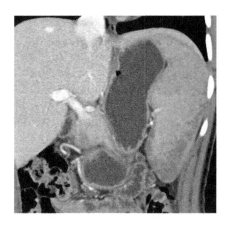

FIGURE 3.27
Splenic sequestration. A 23-year-old woman with heterozygous sickle cell disease (Sickle-C disease) with sudden onset left upper quadrant pain. Contrast enhanced coronal CT shows moderate splenomegaly with peripheral ill-defined hypodensities representing sequestration. Her hemoglobin/hematocrit dropped from 12.4 (g/dL)/34.3 (%) to 7.2 (g/dL)/20.7 (%) for 4 days.

infarction, and is eventually replaced by fibrous tissue, termed "autosplenectomy" (Figure 3.26) [6,98].

Acute splenic sequestration is often a catastrophic event, characterized by sudden trapping of a large amount of blood in the spleen, resulting in sudden splenic enlargement and a rapid decrease in hematocrit and hypovolemic shock [6]. It almost exclusively occurs during infancy and childhood in patients with homozygous sickle cell disease, but may occur at any age in patients with heterozygous sickle cell disease [7]. This diagnosis is usually clinical, based on the enlargement of the spleen with a drop in hemoglobin level by >2g/dL [99], and it is rare that imaging studies are ordered. However, for patients who present with nonspecific findings of an acute abdomen, it is important to recognize the appearance of sequestration on imaging studies [99]. Two distinct patterns of CT findings are reported; multiple peripheral

nonenhancing low-density areas (Figure 3.27), or large, diffuse areas of low density in the majority of the splenic tissue [99].

Secondary hemochromatosis (also referred to as hemosiderosis) results from iron overload, as in patients who have undergone multiple blood transfusions. Secondary hemochromatosis is characterized initially by reticuloendothelial cell iron deposition. Later, it may become pathologically and clinically indistinguishable from primary hemochromatosis. CT shows increased attenuation in the spleen secondary from iron deposition in the reticuloendothelial system as well as calcification (Figure 3.28).

Infarction may be encountered in adults with heterozygous sickle cell disease. The spleen is generally enlarged, and there are peripheral segmental areas of

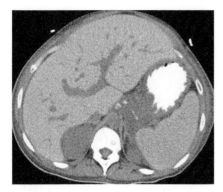

FIGURE 3.28
Hemosiderosis. A 21-year-old woman with sickle cell anemia requiring monthly blood transfusions. Axial noncontrast CT shows increased attenuation in the liver and spleen from iron deposition. Liver core biopsy showed marked hepatocellular and Kupffer cell iron accumulation.

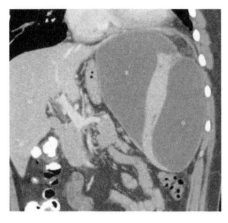

FIGURE 3.29
Large chronic subcapsular splenic hematoma. A 39-year-old man with heterozygous sickle cell disease (sickle-beta thalassemia) who presented with worsening left upper quadrant pain for 3 weeks and decreased hemoglobin. Coronal contrast-enhanced CT shows large subcapsular collection (asterisk) with compressed, distorted splenic parenchyma, presumably representing chronic subcapsular hematoma.

hypoattenuation [7]. Splenic rupture is a rare complication of sickle cell disease that occurs in an enlarged spleen. Intrasplenic or subcapsular hemorrhage may also be seen (Figure 3.29).

3.10 Splenic Artery Aneurysm/ Pseudoaneurysm

The splenic artery is the third most common site of intra-abdominal aneurysms after aneurysms of the abdominal aorta and the iliac arteries [100]. Although rupture of splenic artery aneurysm is a rare event, its consequences can be devastating. The predisposing

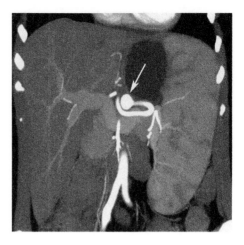

FIGURE 3.30
Splenic artery aneurysm. A 56-year-old woman with history of myelofibrosis. Coronal arterial phase CT shows markedly enlarged spleen. Tortuous splenic artery with 2 cm splenic artery aneurysm (arrow).

conditions of splenic artery aneurysm are pregnancy, multiparity, systemic and portal hypertension, liver transplantation, and atherosclerotic disease [101,102]. Most aneurysms are saccular, and located in the distal third of the splenic artery [102,103].

A splenic artery aneurysm usually appears as a well-defined and homogeneous contrast-enhanced mass on CT (Figure 3.30). Peripheral calcifications or a mural thrombus may also be visible. Indication for treatment include an aneurysm greater than 2.5 cm, symptomatic, found in pregnant women or women of childbearing age, the presence of portal hypertension, and planned liver transplantation [103]. Splenic artery aneurysm can be managed by interventional radiological techniques (arterial stent or percutaneous angiographic embolization) or by surgery (operative occlusion, resection, or arterial bypass) [103].

Pseudoaneurysm of the splenic artery can be associated with acute or chronic pancreatitis, peptic ulcer disease, trauma, iatrogenic and postoperative causes, and neoplasm [103]. In the setting of pancreatitis, splenic artery pseudoaneurysm may result from weakening of wall by pancreatic enzymes [102]. It is important to discriminate between aneurysms and pseudoaneurysms because they require different therapeutic approaches [102,103].

Aneurysm or pseudoaneurysm enhances to similar degree to arteries following IV contrast administration. An intensely enhancing structure contiguous with a pancreatic or peripancreatic artery or within or adjacent to a pancreatic pseudocyst is highly indicative of a pseudoaneurysm [104]. Surrounding the enhancing lumen of pseudoaneurysm, thrombus or hematoma may be seen as a hyperdense, unenhanced structure (Figure 3.31) [102]. Pseudoaneurysm of any size should be treated [103].

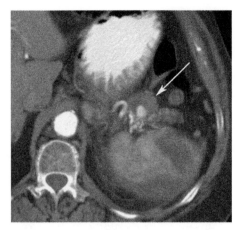

FIGURE 3.31
Splenic artery pseudoaneurysm. A 66-year-old woman with history of chronic pancreatitis, presented with abdominal pain. Contrast-enhanced CT shows densely enhanced pseudoaneurysm arising from the distal splenic artery, surrounded by hematoma (arrow). Splenic infarct is also seen.

3.11 Infarction

Splenic infarcts are relatively common and usually result from embolic occlusion of the splenic artery (e.g., bacterial endocarditis and mitral valve disease). Other causes include local thrombosis, hematological disorders (e.g., sickle cell anemia, myelofibrosis, leukemia, and lymphoma), vasculitis, pancreatic disease, and splenic artery aneurysm [7]. Splenomegaly itself may result in infarction due to functional ischemia [105]. Patients with splenomegaly with portal hypertension also have increased risk of splenic infarct. Areas of splenic infarcts are known to predispose to splenic rupture and superimposed infection [7].

Classic CT appearance of splenic infarcts is wedge-shaped zones of decreased attenuation that extend to the surface of the spleen (Figure 3.32). However, infarcts may also appear as heterogeneous, poorly marginated low-attenuation lesions that may be indistinguishable from other splenic lesions such as abscesses, hematomas, or tumors [105]. In areas of hemorrhagic infarct, focal areas of increased attenuation may be seen (Figure 3.32) [105]. The appearance of infarcts can vary depending on age. They usually become less dense and better defined with time [105]. Infarcts may completely disappear or heal with fibrosis and form multiple scars, which can be appreciated on CT as notching of the splenic contour.

Global infarct can result in diffuse hypodensity and can mimic splenic abscess or tumor [12]. In cases of global infarction, peripheral enhancement, so-called "rim sign," may be visualized because of perfusion from capsular vessels (Figure 3.33) [105]

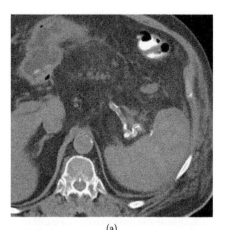

(a)

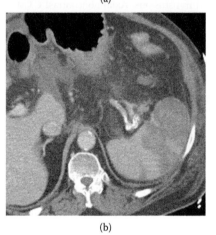

(b)

FIGURE 3.32
Splenic infarct. A 69-year-old man with endocarditis. (a) Axial non-contrast and (b) portal venous phase CT images show a wedge-shaped zones of decreased attenuation that extend to the surface of the spleen, representing infarct. Heterogeneous high attenuation on noncontrast CT, suggesting hemorrhagic infarct.

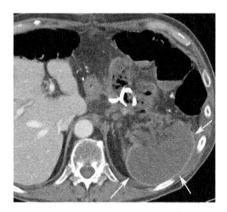

FIGURE 3.33
Global splenic infarct. An 80-year-old man status post esophagectomy. Percutaneous drainage placement for abdominal fluid collection. Venous phase axial CT shows diffuse hypodensity of the spleen with peripheral enhancement ("rim sign") (arrows) due to perfusion from capsular vessels. Splenic infarct is secondary to celiac artery occlusion. The liver is spared because of replaced origin of the common hepatic artery from the superior mesenteric artery.

3.12 Spontaneous Splenic Rupture

Patients with splenomegaly are more prone to spontaneous splenic rupture. Splenic rupture is an uncommon but life-threatening complication of leukemias and lymphomas (Figure 3.34). Spontaneous splenic rupture can also be associated with infection such as malaria or infectious mononucleosis, or mass-forming lesions in the spleen such as abscess, intrasplenic involvement of pancreatic pseudocyst, and tumor involvement.

3.13 Trauma

The spleen is the most frequently injured organ in blunt abdominal trauma [106]. Contrast-enhanced CT scanning is currently the diagnostic imaging tool of choice for the assessment of hemodynamically stable patients with spleen injury [107]. The most widely used CT-grading system for splenic injury in trauma patients is based on the American Association for the Surgery of Trauma scale [108]. CT can be used to detect and distinguish different patterns of blunt splenic injuries.

Subcapsular hematoma is located between the splenic capsule and splenic parenchyma, which typically causes compression of the splenic parenchyma. Intrasplenic hematoma appears as a hypodense area within normally perfused splenic parenchyma. Parenchymal splenic laceration appears as linear defects (Figures 3.35 through 3.37)

[107]. A subcapsular and a perisplenic hematoma appear as hyperdense fluid collection along the surface of the spleen. However, because the splenic capsule cannot usually be visualized, it is sometimes difficult to distinguish between a subcapsular and a perisplenic hematoma [107].

Even if a splenic laceration is not seen, the presence of focal hyperdense (>60 HU), perisplenic clotted blood should suggest the diagnosis of splenic trauma. It is often referred to as the "sentinel clot" sign [109]. Active arterial hemorrhage appears as area of focal or diffuse high attenuation, which is isodense to adjacent major arterial structures (Figure 3.37). Area of active hemorrhage is often surrounded by high-attenuation fluid representing hematoma [110]. Contrast extravasation occurs in approximately 17.7% of patients with splenic injury. The extravasation can be used to localize anatomic sites of hemorrhage and to guide angiographic or surgical intervention [106]. It is a significant predictor of nonsurgical management failure [106].

The normal early heterogeneous contrast enhancement of the spleen should not be mistaken for splenic trauma. If uncertainty about splenic enhancement persists, delayed scans of the spleen can be performed. A normal spleen will show a homogeneous appearance on delayed scans.

Delayed splenic rupture is a well-recognized, potentially dangerous clinical entity, occurring at least 48 hours after trauma [111]. Delayed splenic rupture has been reported to occur in approximately 5%–6% of nonsurgically managed adults [111]. Delayed rupture of a subcapsular hematoma, or free rupture of an initially confined perisplenic hematoma into the

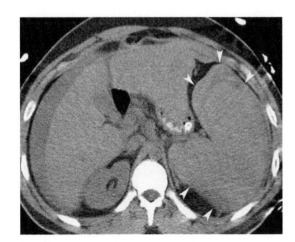

FIGURE 3.34
Spontaneous splenic rupture secondary to aggressive B-cell lymphoma. A 30-year-old man with history of human immunodeficiency virus (HIV) infection who had rapidly growing lump under the left axilla, thrombocytopenia, and petechia. Axial noncontrast CT shows enlarged spleen with surrounding subcapsular and perisplenic hemorrhage (arrowheads), and moderate hemoperitoneum.

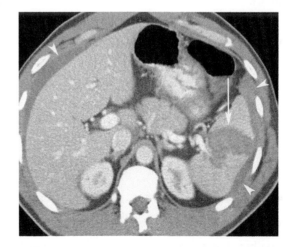

FIGURE 3.35
Splenic laceration, hemoperitoneum. A 47-year-old man with history of scooter accident presented a week later with abdominal pain. Axial contrast-enhanced CT shows a large splenic laceration (arrow) extending to the hilum with hemoperitoneum (arrowheads). No evidence of active extravasation. Patient was treated with coil embolization of the splenic artery.

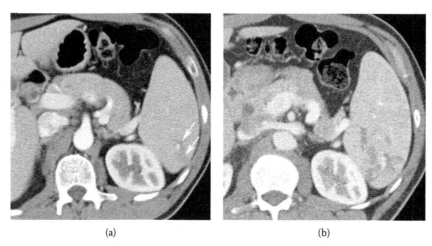

(a)   (b)

FIGUR1E 3.36
Splenic laceration. A 43-year-old man who was a restrained passenger of a motor vehicle collision. (a) Initial contrast-enhanced axial CT shows a small laceration with small focus of contrast enhancement (arrows) suggesting small vascular injury. (b) Contrast-enhanced axial CT obtained after 28 hours (a) shows increasing size of laceration and focus of contrast enhancement. The patient was closely monitored, and follow-up CT obtained 4 days later showed healing of laceration.

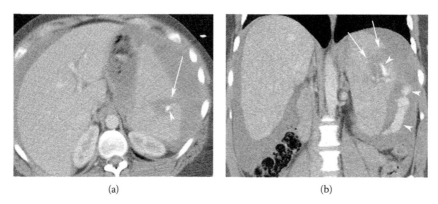

(a)   (b)

FIGURE 3.37
Liver laceration with active bleeding. A 34-year-old woman, status post blunt abdominal trauma. (a) axial and (b) coronal contrast-enhanced CT show splenic laceration (arrows). There is active contrast extravasation within the laceration, with hemorrhage extending lateral to the spleen (arrowheads). Large hemoperitoneum is present.

peritoneal cavity are suspected mechanisms for this complication [111]. Posttraumatic pseudocysts were reported in 0.44% of splenic injury patients [112]. Splenic abscess formation and pseudoaneurysm are rare complications of blunt trauma.

References

1. Rydberg J, Buckwalter KA, Caldemeyer KS et al. Multisection CT: scanning techniques and clinical applications. *Radiographics* 2000;20:1787–1806.
2. Kawamoto S, Fishman EK. MDCT Evaluation of the Spleen. In: Fishman EK, Brooke JR, eds. *Multidetector CT: Principles, Techniques, and Clinical Applications*. Philadelphia, PA: Lippincott Williams & Wilkins; 2003:255–270.
3. Ros PR, Ji H. Special focus session: multisection (multidetector) CT: applications in the abdomen. *Radiographics* 2002;22:697–700.
4. Dodds WJ, Taylor AJ, Erickson SJ, Stewart ET, Lawson TL. Radiologic imaging of splenic anomalies. *American Journal of Roentgenology* 1990;155:805–810.
5. Standring S, ed. The anatomical bases of clinical practice. In: *Gray's Anatomy*, 40th ed. Philadelphia, PA: Churchill Livingstone; Elsevier; 2008:1191–1195.
6. Khatib R, Rabah R, Sarnaik SA. The spleen in the sickling disorders: an update. *Pediatric Radiology* 2009;39:17–22.
7. Rabushka LS, Kawashima A, Fishman EK. Imaging of the spleen: CT with supplemental MR examination. *Radiographics* 1994;14:307–332.
8. Nelson RC, Chezmar JL, Peterson JE, Bernardino ME. Contrast-enhanced CT of the liver and spleen: comparison of ionic and nonionic contrast agents. *American Journal of Roentgenology* 1989;153:973–976.

9. Donnelly LF, Foss JN, Frush DP, Bisset GS, 3rd. Heterogeneous splenic enhancement patterns on spiral CT images in children: minimizing misinterpretation. *Radiology* 1999;210:493–497.

10. Glazer GM, Axel L, Goldberg HI, Moss AA. Dynamic CT of the normal spleen. *American Journal of Roentgenology* 1981;137:343–346.

11. Miles KA, McPherson SJ, Hayball MP. Transient splenic inhomogeneity with contrast-enhanced CT: mechanism and effect of liver disease. *Radiology* 1995;194:91–95.

12. Urban BA, Fishman EK. Helical CT of the spleen. *American Journal of Roentgenology* 1998;170:997–1003.

13. Gayer G, Zissin R, Apter S, Atar E, Portnoy O, Itzchak Y. CT findings in congenital anomalies of the spleen. *The British Journal of Radiology* 2001;74:767–772.

14. Halpert B, Gyorkey F. Lesions observed in accessory spleens of 311 patients. *American Journal of Clinical Pathology* 1959;32:165–168.

15. Wadham BM, Adams PB, Johnson MA. Incidence and location of accessory spleens. *The New England Journal of Medicine* 1981;304:1111.

16. Mortele KJ, Mortele B, Silverman SG. CT features of the accessory spleen. *American Journal of Roentgenology* 2004;183:1653–1657.

17. Kawamoto S, Johnson PT, Hall H, Cameron JL, Hruban RH, Fishman EK. Intrapancreatic accessory spleen: CT appearance and differential diagnosis. *Abdominal Imaging* 2012: 37;812–827.

18. Kim SH, Lee JM, Han JK et al. Intrapancreatic accessory spleen: findings on MR Imaging, CT, US and scintigraphy, and the pathologic analysis. *Korean Journal of Radiology* 2008;9:162–174.

19. Impellizzeri P, Montalto AS, Borruto FA et al. Accessory spleen torsion: rare cause of acute abdomen in children and review of literature. *Journal of Pediatric Surgery* 2009;44:e15–18.

20. Coote JM, Eyers PS, Walker A, Wells IP. Intra-abdominal bleeding caused by spontaneous rupture of an accessory spleen: the CT findings. *Clinical Radiology* 1999;54:689–691.

21. Motosugi U, Yamaguchi H, Ichikawa T et al. Epidermoid cyst in intrapancreatic accessory spleen: radiological findings including superparamagnetic iron oxide-enhanced magnetic resonance imaging. *Journal of Computer Assisted Tomography* 2010;34:217–222.

22. Ambriz P, Munoz R, Quintanar E, Sigler L, Aviles A, Pizzuto J. Accessory spleen compromising response to splenectomy for idiopathic thrombocytopenic purpura. *Radiology* 1985;155:793–796.

23. Fremont RD, Rice TW. Splenosis: a review. *Southern Medical Journal* 2007;100:589–593.

24. Raissaki M, Prassopoulos P, Daskalogiannaki M, Magkanas E, Gourtsoyiannis N. Acute abdomen due to torsion of wandering spleen: CT diagnosis. *European Radiology* 1998;8:1409–1412.

25. Bakir B, Poyanli A, Yekeler E, Acunas G. Acute torsion of a wandering spleen: imaging findings. *Abdominal Imaging* 2004;29:707–709.

26. Bouassida M, Sassi S, Chtourou MF et al. A wandering spleen presenting as a hypogastric mass: case report. *The Pan African Medical Journal* 2012;11:31.

27. Parker LA, Mittelstaedt CA, Mauro MA, Mandell VS, Jaques PF. Torsion of a wandering spleen: CT appearance. *Journal of Computer Assisted Tomography* 1984;8:1201–1204.

28. Applegate KE, Goske MJ, Pierce G, Murphy D. Situs revisited: imaging of the heterotaxy syndrome. *Radiographics* 1999;19:837–852; discussion 834–853.

29. Peoples WM, Moller JH, Edwards JE. Polysplenia: a review of 146 cases. *Pediatric Cardiology* 1983;4:129–137.

30. Gayer G, Apter S, Jonas T et al. Polysplenia syndrome detected in adulthood: report of eight cases and review of the literature. *Abdominal Imaging* 1999;24:178–184.

31. Winer-Muram HT, Tonkin IL, Gold RE. Polysplenia syndrome in the asymptomatic adult: computed tomography evaluation. *Journal of Thoracic Imaging* 1991;6:69–71.

32. Fulcher AS, Turner MA. Abdominal manifestations of situs anomalies in adults. *Radiographics* 2002;22:1439–1456.

33. Bezerra AS, D'Ippolito G, Faintuch S, Szejnfeld J, Ahmed M. Determination of splenomegaly by CT: is there a place for a single measurement? *American Journal of Roentgenology* 2005;184:1510–1513.

34. Rezai P, Tochetto SM, Galizia MS, Yaghmai V. Splenic volume model constructed from standardized one-dimensional MDCT measurements. *American Journal of Roentgenology* 2011;196:367–372.

35. Warshauer DM. Spleen. In: Lee JK, Sagel SS, Stanley RJ, Heiken JP, eds. *Computed Body Tomography with MRI Correlation.* 4th ed. Philadelphia, PA: Lippincott Williams & Wilkins; 2005:973–1006.

36. Harris A, Kamishima T, Hao HY et al. Splenic volume measurements on computed tomography utilizing automatically contouring software and its relationship with age, gender, and anthropometric parameters. *European Journal of Radiology* 2010;75:e97–101.

37. DeLand FH. Normal spleen size. *Radiology* 1970;97:589–592.

38. Prassopoulos P, Daskalogiannaki M, Raissaki M, Hatjidakis A, Gourtsoyiannis N. Determination of normal splenic volume on computed tomography in relation to age, gender and body habitus. *European Radiology* 1997;7:246–248.

39. Saboo SS, Krajewski KM, O'Regan KN et al. Spleen in haematological malignancies: spectrum of imaging findings. *The British Journal of Radiology* 2012;85:81–92.

40. Jeffrey RB, Jr., Nyberg DA, Bottles K et al. Abdominal CT in acquired immunodeficiency syndrome. *American Journal of Roentgenology* 1986;146:7–13.

41. Abbott RM, Levy AD, Aguilera NS, Gorospe L, Thompson WM. From the archives of the AFIP: primary vascular neoplasms of the spleen: radiologic-pathologic correlation. *Radiographics* 2004;24:1137–1163.

42. Shirkhoda A, Ros PR, Farah J, Staab EV. Lymphoma of the solid abdominal viscera. *Radiologic Clinics of North America* 1990;28:785–799.

43. Bhatia K, Sahdev A, Reznek RH. Lymphoma of the spleen. *Seminars in ultrasound, CT, and MR* 2007;28:12–20.

44. Paes FM, Kalkanis DG, Sideras PA, Serafini AN. FDG PET/CT of extranodal involvement in non-Hodgkin lymphoma and Hodgkin disease. *Radiographics* 2010;30:269–291.

45. Kadin ME, Glatstein E, Dorfman RF. Clinicopathologic studies of 117 untreated patients subjected to laparotomy for the staging of Hodgkin's disease. *Cancer* 1971;27:1277–1294.

46. Kim H, Dorfman RF. Morphological studies of 84 untreated patients subjected to laparotomy for the staging of non-Hodgkin's lymphomas. *Cancer* 1974;33:657–674.

47. Marti-Bonmati L, Ballesta A, Chirivella M. Unusual presentation of non-Hodgkin lymphoma of the spleen. *Canadian Association of Radiologists Journal (Journal l'Association Canadienne des Radiologists)* 1989;40:49–50.

48. Veronesi U, Musumeci R, Pizzetti F, Gennari L, Bonadonna G. Proceedings: the value of staging laparotomy in non-Hodgkin's lymphomas (with emphasis on the histiocytic type). *Cancer* 1974;33:446–459.

49. Ahmann DL, Kiely JM, Harrison EG, Jr., Payne WS. Malignant lymphoma of the spleen. A review of 49 cases in which the diagnosis was made at splenectomy. *Cancer* 1966;19:461–469.

50. Brox A, Bishinsky JI, Berry G. Primary non-Hodgkin lymphoma of the spleen. *American Journal of Hematology* 1991;38:95–100.

51. Dachman AH, Buck JL, Krishnan J, Aguilera NS, Buetow PC. Primary non-Hodgkin's splenic lymphoma. *Clinical Radiology* 1998;53:137–142.

52. Schaefer NG, Hany TF, Taverna C et al. Non-Hodgkin lymphoma and Hodgkin disease: coregistered FDG PET and CT at staging and restaging— do we need contrast-enhanced CT? *Radiology* 2004;232:823–829.

53. de Jong PA, van Ufford HM, Baarslag HJ et al. CT and 18F-FDG PET for noninvasive detection of splenic involvement in patients with malignant lymphoma. *American Journal of Roentgenology* 2009;192:745–753.

54. Warshauer DM, Hall HL. Solitary splenic lesions. *Seminars in ultrasound, CT, and MR* 2006;27:370–388.

55. Ros PR, Moser RP, Jr., Dachman AH, Murari PJ, Olmsted WW. Hemangioma of the spleen: radiologic-pathologic correlation in ten cases. *Radiology* 1987;162:73–77.

56. Robertson F, Leander P, Ekberg O. Radiology of the spleen. *European Radiology* 2001;11:80–95.

57. Ferrozzi F, Bova D, Draghi F, Garlaschi G. CT findings in primary vascular tumors of the spleen. *American Journal of Roentgenology* 1996;166:1097–1101.

58. Pistoia F, Markowitz SK. Splenic lymphangiomatosis: CT diagnosis. *American Journal of Roentgenology* 1988;150:121–122.

59. Ramani M, Reinhold C, Semelka RC et al. Splenic hemangiomas and hamartomas: MR imaging characteristics of 28 lesions. *Radiology* 1997;202:166–172.

60. Enzinger FM, Smith BH. Hemangiopericytoma. An analysis of 106 cases. *Human Pathology* 1976;7:61–82.

61. Falk S, Stutte HJ, Frizzera G. Littoral cell angioma. A novel splenic vascular lesion demonstrating histiocytic differentiation. *The American Journal of Surgical Pathology* 1991;15:1023–1033.

62. Levy AD, Abbott RM, Abbondanzo SL. Littoral cell angioma of the spleen: CT features with clinicopathologic comparison. *Radiology* 2004;230:485–490.

63. Arber DA, Strickler JG, Chen YY, Weiss LM. Splenic vascular tumors: a histologic, immunophenotypic, and virologic study. *The American Journal of Surgical Pathology* 1997;21:827–835.

64. Tan YM, Chuah KL, Wong WK. Littoral cell angioma of the spleen. *Annals of the Academy of Medicine, Singapore* 2004;33:524–526.

65. Venkatanarasimha N, Hall S, Suresh P, Williams MP. Littoral cell angioma in a splenunculus: a case report. *The British Journal of Radiology* 2011;84:e11–13.

66. Falk S, Krishnan J, Meis JM. Primary angiosarcoma of the spleen. A clinicopathologic study of 40 cases. *The American Journal of Surgical Pathology* 1993;17:959–970.

67. Thompson WM, Levy AD, Aguilera NS, Gorospe L, Abbott RM. Angiosarcoma of the spleen: imaging characteristics in 12 patients. *Radiology* 2005;235:106–115.

68. Levy DW, Rindsberg S, Friedman AC et al. Thorotrast-induced hepatosplenic neoplasia: CT identification. *American Journal of Roentgenology* 1986;146:997–1004.

69. Morgenstern L, Rosenberg J, Geller SA. Tumors of the spleen. *World Journal of Surgery* 1985;9:468–476.

70. Berge T. Splenic metastases. Frequencies and patterns. *Acta Pathologica et Microbiologica Scandinavica Section A, Pathology* 1974;82:499–506.

71. Marymont JH, Jr., Gross S. Patterns of metastatic cancer in the spleen. *American Journal of Clinical Pathology* 1963;40:58–66.

72. Urrutia M, Mergo PJ, Ros LH, Torres GM, Ros PR. Cystic masses of the spleen: radiologic-pathologic correlation. *Radiographics* 1996;16:107–129.

73. Dawes LG, Malangoni MA. Cystic masses of the spleen. *The American Surgeon* 1986;52:333–336.

74. Polat P, Kantarci M, Alper F, Suma S, Koruyucu MB, Okur A. Hydatid disease from head to toe. *Radiographics* 2003;23:475–494; quiz 536–477.

75. Culafic DM, Kerkez MD, Mijac DD et al. Spleen cystic echinococcosis: clinical manifestations and treatment. *Scandinavian Journal of Gastroenterology* 2010;45:186–190.

76. Durgun V, Kapan S, Kapan M, Karabicak I, Aydogan F, Goksoy E. Primary splenic hydatidosis. *Digestive Surgery* 2003;20:38–41.

77. Malka D, Hammel P, Levy P et al. Splenic complications in chronic pancreatitis: prevalence and risk factors in a medical-surgical series of 500 patients. *The British Journal of Surgery* 1998;85:1645–1649.

78. Siegelman SS, Copeland BE, Saba GP, Cameron JL, Sanders RC, Zerhouni EA. CT of fluid collections associated with pancreatitis. *American Journal of Roentgenology* 1980;134:1121–1132.

79. Fishman EK, Soyer P, Bliss DF, Bluemke DA, Devine N. Splenic involvement in pancreatitis: spectrum of CT findings. *American Journal of Roentgenology* 1995;164:631–635.

80. Warshaw AL, Chesney TM, Evans GW, McCarthy HF. Intrasplenic dissection by pancreatic pseudocysts. *The New England Journal of Medicine* 1972;287:72–75.

81. Nelken N, Ignatius J, Skinner M, Christensen N. Changing clinical spectrum of splenic abscess. A multicenter study and review of the literature. *American Journal of Surgery* 1987;154:27–34.

82. Chang KC, Chuah SK, Changchien CS et al. Clinical characteristics and prognostic factors of splenic abscess: a review of 67 cases in a single medical center of Taiwan. *World Journal of Gastroenterology* 2006;12:460–464.

83. Tikkakoski T, Siniluoto T, Paivansalo M et al. Splenic abscess. Imaging and intervention. *Acta Radiology* 1992;33:561–565.

84. Shirkhoda A. CT findings in hepatosplenic and renal candidiasis. *Journal of Computer Assisted Tomography* 1987;11:795–798.

85. Pastakia B, Shawker TH, Thaler M, O'Leary T, Pizzo PA. Hepatosplenic candidiasis: wheels within wheels. *Radiology* 1988;166:417–421.

86. Pereira JM, Madureira AJ, Vieira A, Ramos I. Abdominal tuberculosis: imaging features. *European Journal of Radiology* 2005;55:173–180.

87. Koh DM, Burn PR, Mathews G, Nelson M, Healy JC. Abdominal computed tomographic findings of Mycobacterium tuberculosis and Mycobacterium avium intracellulare infection in HIV seropositive patients. *Canadian Association of Radiologists Journal (Journal l'Association Canadienne des Radiologists)* 2003;54:45–50.

88. Selroos O. Fine-needle aspiration biopsy of the spleen in diagnosis of sarcoidosis. *Annals of the New York Academy of Sciences* 1976;278:517–521.

89. Taavitsainen M, Koivuniemi A, Helminen J et al. Aspiration biopsy of the spleen in patients with sarcoidosis. *Acta Radiology* 1987;28:723–725.

90. Warshauer DM. Splenic sarcoidosis. *Seminars in ultrasound, CT, and MR* 2007;28:21–27.

91. Glazer M, Lally J, Kanzer M. Inflammatory pseudotumor of the spleen: MR findings. *Journal of Computer Assisted Tomography* 1992;16:980–983.

92. Franquet T, Montes M, Aizcorbe M, Barberena J, Ruiz De Azua Y, Cobo F. Inflammatory pseudotumor of the spleen: ultrasound and computed tomographic findings. *Gastrointestinal Radiology* 1989;14:181–183.

93. Martel M, Cheuk W, Lombardi L, Lifschitz-Mercer B, Chan JK, Rosai J. Sclerosing angiomatoid nodular transformation (SANT): report of 25 cases of a distinctive benign splenic lesion. *The American Journal of Surgical Pathology* 2004;28:1268–1279.

94. Subhawong TK, Subhawong AP, Kamel I. Sclerosing angiomatoid nodular transformation of the spleen: multimodality imaging findings and pathologic correlate. *Journal of Computer Assisted Tomography* 2010;34:206–209.

95. Zeeb LM, Johnson JM, Madsen MS, Keating DP. Sclerosing angiomatoid nodular transformation. *American Journal of Roentgenology* 2009;192:W236–238.

96. Thacker C, Korn R, Millstine J, Harvin H, Van Lier Ribbink JA, Gotway MB. Sclerosing angiomatoid nodular transformation of the spleen: CT, MR, PET, and (9)(9)(m)Tc-sulfur colloid SPECT CT findings with gross and histopathological correlation. *Abdominal Imaging* 2010;35:683–689.

97. Karaosmanoglu DA, Karcaaltincaba M, Akata D. CT and MRI findings of sclerosing angiomatoid nodular transformation of the spleen: spoke wheel pattern. *Korean Journal of Radiology* 2008;9 Suppl:S52–55.

98. Magid D, Fishman EK, Charache S, Siegelman SS. Abdominal pain in sickle cell disease: the role of CT. *Radiology* 1987;163:325–328.

99. Sheth S, Ruzal-Shapiro C, Piomelli S, Berdon WE. CT imaging of splenic sequestration in sickle cell disease. *Pediatric Radiology* 2000;30:830–833.

100. Trastek VF, Pairolero PC, Joyce JW, Hollier LH, Bernatz PE. Splenic artery aneurysms. *Surgery* 1982;91:694–699.

101. Selo-Ojeme DO, Welch CC. Review: spontaneous rupture of splenic artery aneurysm in pregnancy. *European Journal of Obstetrics, Gynecology, and Reproductive Biology* 2003;109:124–127.

102. Agrawal GA, Johnson PT, Fishman EK. Splenic artery aneurysms and pseudoaneurysms: clinical distinctions and CT appearances. *American Journal of Roentgenology* 2007;188:992–999.

103. Saba L, Anzidei M, Lucatelli P, Mallarini G. The multidetector computed tomography angiography (MDCTA) in the diagnosis of splenic artery aneurysm and pseudoaneurysm. *Acta Radiology* 2011;52:488–498.

104. Marshall GT, Howell DA, Hansen BL, Amberson SM, Abourjaily GS, Bredenberg CE. Multidisciplinary approach to pseudoaneurysms complicating pancreatic pseudocysts. Impact of pretreatment diagnosis. *Archives of Surgery* 1996;131:278–283.

105. Balcar I, Seltzer SE, Davis S, Geller S. CT patterns of splenic infarction: a clinical and experimental study. *Radiology* 1984;151:723–729.

106. Yao DC, Jeffrey RB, Jr., Mirvis SE et al. Using contrast-enhanced helical CT to visualize arterial extravasation after blunt abdominal trauma: incidence and organ distribution. *American Journal of Roentgenology* 2002;178:17–20.

107. Becker CD, Mentha G, Terrier F. Blunt abdominal trauma in adults: role of CT in the diagnosis and management of visceral injuries. Part 1: liver and spleen. *European Radiology* 1998;8:553–562.

108. Moore EE, Cogbill TH, Jurkovich GJ, Shackford SR, Malangoni MA, Champion HR. Organ injury scaling: spleen and liver (1994 revision). *The Journal of Trauma* 1995;38:323–324.

109. Orwig D, Federle MP. Localized clotted blood as evidence of visceral trauma on CT: the sentinel clot sign. *American Journal of Roentgenology* 1989;153:747–749.

110. Lubner M, Menias C, Rucker C et al. Blood in the belly: CT findings of hemoperitoneum. *Radiographics* 2007;27:109–125.

111. Hassan R, Abd Aziz A. Computed tomography (CT) imaging of injuries from blunt abdominal trauma: a pictorial essay. *The Malaysian Journal of Medical Sciences* 2010;17:29–39.

112. Kristoffersen KW, Mooney DP. Long-term outcome of nonoperative pediatric splenic injury management. *Journal of Pediatric Surgery* 2007;42:1038–1041; discussion 1032–1041.

4

Pancreas

Katherine Leung and Gavin Low

CONTENTS

4.1 Anatomy

The pancreas is a retroperitoneal organ that is stratified anatomically into the pancreatic head and uncinate process, neck, body, and tail (Figure 4.1). The gland has an oblique orientation within the upper abdomen with the pancreatic head located anteriorly adjacent to the doudenal C-loop and the pancreatic body and tail located posteriorly, superiorly, and to the left toward the splenic hilum. The following radiological relationships are observed: the pancreatic head is bordered anteriorly by the gastroduodenal artery, posteriorly by the common bile duct (CBD) and inferior vena cava, laterally by the second part of the duodenum, and inferiorly by the third part of the duodenum. The uncinate

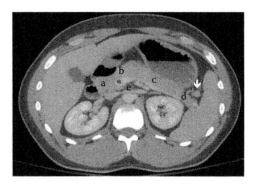

FIGURE 4.1
Normal pancreas on an axial contrast-enhanced computed tomography (CT) image. (a) Pancreatic head, (b) pancreatic neck, (c) pancreatic body, (d) pancreatic tail, (e) superior mesenteric artery, (arrow) splenule, (asterisk) portosplenic confluence.

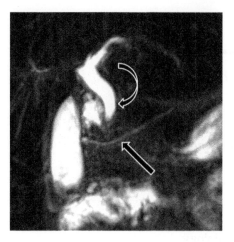

FIGURE 4.2
A coronal maximum intensity projection (MIP) MRCP image showing pancreatic divisum. The main pancreatic duct (straight arrow) enters the minor papilla. The common bile duct (curved arrow) does not communicate with the main pancreatic duct and enters the major papilla separately.

process lies inferior to the pancreatic head and the superior mesenteric vessels pass anterior to this portion of the gland. Furthermore, the superior mesenteric vessels demarcate the point of transition between the pancreatic head (to the right) and the pancreatic neck (to the left). The pancreatic body lies to the left of the midline and is bordered anteriorly by the stomach and lesser sac and posteriorly by the splenic vein. The pancreatic tail is the most peripheral portion of the pancreas and passes within the splenorenal ligament to lie adjacent to the splenic hilum [1]. The pancreas is fed from tributaries of the celiac axis and the superior mesenteric artery. The short branches of the splenic artery provide most of the arterial supply to the pancreas with additional contributions by the superior and inferior pancreatoduodenal arteries to the head and uncinate process [1,2].

4.2 Embryology and Variants

The pancreas is derived embryologically from the dorsal and ventral pancreatic buds. The dorsal pancreatic bud originates to the left of the duodenum and the ventral pancreatic bud originates to the right of the duodenum near the bile duct. The ventral bud then typically migrates anterior to the duodenum and inferior to the dorsal pancreatic bud, eventually developing into the inferior pancreatic head and uncinate process. The dorsal bud develops into the remainder of the pancreas. The pancreatic duct of the ventral pancreatic bud fuses with the distal dorsal pancreatic bud duct forming the main pancreatic duct (MPD) (of Wirsung). The MPD fuses with the CBD forming the ampulla of Vater, which drains into the second part of the duodenum.

Occasionally, the proximal dorsal pancreatic bud duct persists as the accessory pancreatic duct (of Santorini). The accessory pancreatic duct drains into the minor papilla, which enters the second part of the duodenum more anteriorly and proximally than the main duct [3]. The pancreatic ducts generally measure ≤2 mm in diameter.

The two most common embryological variants encountered clinically are pancreatic divisum and annular pancreas. In pancreatic divisum, the dorsal and ventral pancreatic buds fail to fuse creating two independent ductal systems (Figure 4.2). By convention, the accessory pancreatic duct of Santorini drains into the larger dorsal pancreatic bud (superior pancreatic head, neck, body, and tail) via the minor papilla. A shorter MPD of Wirsung drains into the ventral pancreatic bud (inferior pancreatic head and uncinate process) [3]. Historically, pancreatic divisum was believed to be an etiological factor in the development of acute pancreatitis [4]. However, recent evidence suggests that there is no significant difference in the incidence of acute pancreatitis in patients with pancreatic divisum compared to those with conventional ductal anatomy. The considerations are likely multifactorial but pancreatic divisum may represent a cofactor with certain genetic mutations, which may in turn predispose to the development of acute pancreatitis [5]. In annular pancreas, as the ventral pancreatic bud migrates anterior to the duodenum, a portion of the ventral pancreatic bud also migrates posterior to the duodenum forming a ring of pancreatic tissue around the second part of the duodenum (Figure 4.3). This may lead to duodenal obstruction.

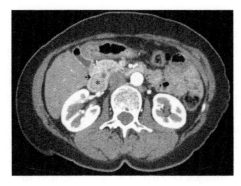

FIGURE 4.3
Annular pancreas on an axial contrast-enhanced CT image (courtesy of Dr. Maureen Hutson, Royal Alexandra Hospital, Edmonton). An ectopic ring of pancreatic tissue (arrow) circumferentially surrounds and narrows the second part of the duodenum (asterisk).

4.3 Physiology

The pancreas has both exocrine and endocrine functions. The majority of the gland contributes to the exocrine function by producing a myriad of digestive enzymes. These include digestive enzymes for proteins (trypsin, chymotrypsin, elastase, carboxypeptidase), fats (lipase), polysaccharides (amylase), and nucleic acids (ribonuclease and deoxyribonuclease). In addition, the pancreas secretes bicarbonate ions, which help to neutralize gastric acid secretions. The endocrine role of the pancreas is crucial in metabolism, producing insulin and glucagon within the islets of Langerhans [6]. The islets represent approximately 2% of the pancreatic glandular mass.

4.4 Imaging Techniques

4.4.1 Computed Tomography

Multi-detector contrast-enhanced computed tomography (CECT) is the standard workhorse for evaluating the pancreas. This is due to its widespread availability, speed, and accuracy. At our institution, a thin-collimation (1–3 mm slice thickness) triple-phase (noncontrast/arterial/portal venous) CECT examination is used for assessing the pancreas. Approximately 100 ml of non-ionic iodinated contrast media is administered intravenously by pump injection at a rate of 2–3 ml/s. The initial noncontrast phase is used primarily for localizing the pancreas and detecting calcifications. Following this, an arterial phase is performed on the upper abdomen at 20 seconds postinjection. This is performed primarily for detecting hypervascular pancreatic neoplasms such as neuroendocrine tumors.

Finally, a pancreatic parenchyma phase at 45 seconds postinjection is performed for the entire abdomen. The use of oral contrast is optional and based on the discretion of the practicing radiologist; however, approximately 500–1000 ml of negative oral contrast (usually water) is generally used. A second smaller oral bolus is often given when the patient is on the CT table to provide optimal distension of the duodenum.

4.4.2 Magnetic Resonance Imaging

Magnetic resonance imaging (MRI) provides inherently superior soft tissue resolution than CECT and has the further attraction of not utilizing ionizing radiation. The routine use of intravenous gadolinium chelate contrast agents improves lesion conspicuity/detection while permitting lesion characterization based on characteristic enhancement patterns. Innovations in both MR hardware (e.g., stronger gradient strengths and parallel imaging) and software (e.g., ultrafast pulse sequences) have led to improvements in both spatial resolution and temporal resolution.

At our institution, the standard pancreas protocol includes the following:

- Coronal FISP sequence (Fast Imaging with Steady-State Precession, Siemens) of the abdomen and pelvis.
- Axial dual gradient echo chemical shift T1 in-phase and opposed phase FLASH sequence (Fast Low-Angle Shot, Siemens).
- Axial fat-suppressed FLASH sequence of the pancreas.
- Axial T2 HASTE sequence (Half-Fourier Acquisition Single-Shot Turbo Spin Echo, Siemens) at Echo Time (TE) 90 and fat-suppressed TE 180.
- Axial Diffusion Weighted Imaging sequence with Prospective Acquisition Correction acquired at $b = 0$, 50, 150, and 500.
- Axial 6 mm collimation pre- and post-contrast fat-suppressed 3D gradient echo VIBE sequences (Volumetric Interpolated Breath Hold Examination, Siemens). Four post-contrast sequences are acquired at 0, 30, 60, and 300 seconds post-contrast injection.

Magnetic resonance cholangio-pancreatography (MRCP) is a valuable sequence that is often used to supplement the standard pancreas protocol. This is a heavily T2-weighted technique that offers excellent noninvasive multiplanar visualization of the ductal anatomy. At our institution, the MRCP technique involves performing a coronal 3D fat-suppressed Turbo Spin Echo sequence

(Siemens) of the MPD and biliary tree. This is followed by thick slab 3D maximum intensity projection reformats of the source dataset.

4.5 Hereditary Pancreatic Disorders

4.5.1 Cystic Fibrosis

Cystic fibrosis (CF) is the most common autosomal recessive disorder affecting Caucasians. While the majority of symptoms and fatalities are related to respiratory complications, the incidence of extrapulmonary involvement such as hepatobiliary and pancreatic disease is high. Pancreatic exocrine insufficiency due to pancreatic duct obstruction from inspissated secretions occurs in 85%–90% of patients with CF [7–10]. Furthermore, ductal obstruction predisposes to an increased risk of pancreatitis [11,12]. Endocrine dysfunction occurs in 30%–50% as a result of parenchymal fibrosis or glandular atrophy [7–9,12]. Progression to complete fatty replacement is recognized on CECT and MRI and has been referred to as "lipomatous pseudohypertrophy of the pancreas" [7,10,13] (Figure 4.4). This manifests as fat attenuation in the pancreas on CT (typically ranging from −30 to −100 Hounsfield units [HU]) and high T1 and T2 signal intensities on MRI with signal loss on fat-suppressed sequences [10]. In contrast, pancreatic fibrosis will appear as low T1 and T2 signal intensities [10]. Other findings in the pancreas in CF include pancreatic cysts, calcifications, ductal abnormalities, and increased risk of adenocarcinoma [7].

4.5.2 Hemochromatosis

Hemochromatosis is a disorder that is characterized by excessive parenchymal iron deposition. Primary or hereditary hemochromatosis is an autosomal recessive disorder, whereas secondary hemochromatosis is often iatrogenic typically as a result of multiple blood transfusions. Consequent to the increased iron deposition, the pancreas appears high attenuation on CT, a feature best depicted on a non-contrast phase. On chemical shift T1-weighted MR images, organs involved by iron deposition show signal intensity loss on the in-phase compared with the opposed phase due to increased T2* effects from the longer TE times associated with in-phase images (Figure 4.5). T2-weighted images also show low signal intensity in organs involved by iron deposition [14]. Primary hemochromatosis typically affects the liver, pancreas, thyroid, and myocardium. In contrast, secondary hemochromatosis typically affects organs containing reticuloendothelial cells such as the liver and spleen. Therefore, primary and secondary hemochromatosis may be differentiated on imaging based on the pattern of organs involved by the iron deposition.

4.5.3 Von Hippel–Lindau Disease

Von Hippel–Lindau (VHL) disease is an autosomal dominant inherited multiorgan neoplastic disorder resulting from a mutation in the *VHL* gene. The most common manifestations of VHL include retinal hemangioblastomas, craniospinal hemangioblastomas, renal cell carcinoma (RCC), renal cortical cysts, pancreatic tumors, and pancreatic cysts [15,16]. The incidence of pancreatic lesions ranges from 15% to 77% [16–19]. Approximately 90% of these lesions are simple epithelial pancreatic cysts while the remainders are neuroendocrine tumors or serous cystic neoplasms (SCNs) (Figure 4.6). Neuroendocrine tumors are typically hypervascular neoplasms best detected on the arterial phase of a cross-sectional imaging examination. Confirmatory tests may include endoscopic ultrasound (EUS) and somatostatin receptor scintigraphy (octreotide imaging).

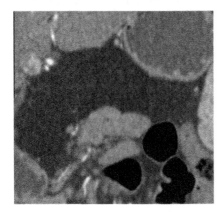

FIGURE 4.4
Lipomatous pseudohypertophy of the pancreas in cystic fibrosis on an axial contrast-enhanced CT image. The pancreas is completely fatty replaced and exhibits uniform fat attenuation.

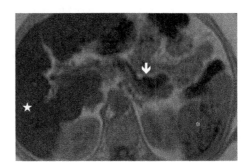

FIGURE 4.5
Hemochromatosis on an axial in-phase T1 weighted image. Low signal intensity is seen in the pancreas (arrow), spleen (asterisk) and liver (star)—organs involved by iron deposition.

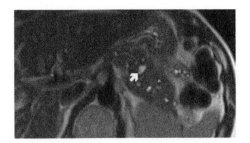

FIGURE 4.6
Von Hippel–Lindau (VHL) disease of the pancreas on an axial T2-weighted MRI image (courtesy of Dr. Iain Birchall, University of Alberta Hospital, Edmonton). Multiple simple pancreatic cysts (arrow) are present throughout the pancreas.

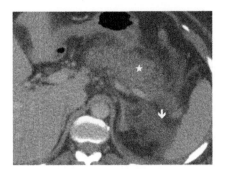

FIGURE 4.7
Acute interstitial edematous pancreatitis on an axial contrast-enhanced CT. The pancreatic parenchyma is swollen but exhibits normal enhancement (star). Note the acute peripancreatic fluid collection (arrow) posterior to the tail of the pancreas.

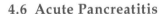

4.6 Acute Pancreatitis

Acute pancreatitis is an inflammatory disease of the pancreas and is a common cause for hospital admissions worldwide. There are many causes of acute pancreatitis; of these, gallstones and alcohol are by far the most common etiologies, particularly in Western society. Other important causes include drugs, viruses, and medical procedures such as endoscopic retrograde cholangio-pancreatography (ERCP). Classically, patients present with central abdominal pain that radiates to the back. In severe cases, patients may exhibit signs of shock. Areas of discoloration and ecchymosis in the periumbilical region and flanks are recognized clinical findings termed as Cullen's and Grey Turner's signs, respectively. These clinical stigmata reflect pancreatic necrotic exudates tracking in these areas [20]. An elevated serum amylase or lipase, usually greater than or equal to three times the normal limit, supports the diagnosis of acute pancreatitis [20,21].

According to the 2008 Revision of the Atlanta Classi-fication of Acute Pancreatitis, the classification of sever-ity is based on clinical findings (such as presence of shock or organ failure) during the first week of the acute event and then rests primarily on the imaging findings once this time period has elapsed [22]. The revised Atlanta criteria stratify acute pancreatitis into acute interstitial edematous pancreatitis and acute necrotizing pancreatitis. Interstitial edematous pan-creatitis is characterized on CECT by mild enlarge-ment of the pancreas with preserved parenchymal enhancement and mild peripancreatic fat inflamma-tion (Figure 4.7). On occasion, patchy enhancement of the pancreas may be present. In this scenario, a repeat CECT in 5 to 7 days may be helpful in differentiating pancreatic necrosis from interstitial edematous pancre-atitis that is associated with heterogeneity [22]. A nor-mally enhancing pancreas generally has a post-contrast

TABLE 4.1

CT Severity Index [23]

Prognostic Indicator	Points
Pancreatic inflammation	
Normal pancreas	0
Focal or diffuse enlargement of the pancreas	1
Intrinsic pancreatic abnormalities with inflammatory changes in the peripancreatic fat	2
Single, ill-defined fluid collection or phlegmon	3
Two or more poorly defined fluid collections or presence of gas in or adjacent to the pancreas	4
Pancreatic necrosis	
None	0
≤30%	2
>30%–50%	4
>50%	6

PANCREATITIS:
Mild, 0–3 points
Moderate, 4–6 points
Severe, 7–10 points

attenuation >80 HU. In contrast, features of severe acute pancreatitis on imaging include the presence of pan-creatic necrosis (non-enhancing foci in the pancreas) or more extensive free peripancreatic fluid. Pancreatic necrosis typically has an attenuation of ≤50 HU on CECT. Acute necrotizing pancreatitis may involve the pancreatic parenchyma and/or the peripancreatic tis-sues. In the acute setting, nonenhancement of ≤30% on CECT is indeterminate for pancreatic necrosis. In this scenario, a repeat CECT in 7 days time is suggested to clarify these equivocal findings. The extent of nonen-hancing parenchyma (≤30%, 30%–50% or ≥50%) is a helpful gauge for estimating the severity of necrosis [22]. The presence of solid material in a peripancreatic "fluid" collection aids in the diagnosis of peripancreatic tissue necrosis.

Both the CT Severity Index (CTSI) (Table 4.1) [23] and Modified CTSI (MCTSI) (Table 4.2) [24] may be used

TABLE 4.2

Modified CT Severity Index [24]

Prognostic Indicator	Points
Pancreatic inflammation	
Normal pancreas	0
Intrinsic pancreatic abnormalities with or without inflammatory changes in the peripancreatic fat	2
Pancreatic or peripancreatic fluid collection or peripancreatic fat necrosis	4
Pancreatic necrosis	
None	0
≤30%	2
>30%	4
Extra-pancreatic complications (one or more of pleural effusion, ascites, vascular complications, parenchymal complications, or gastrointestinal tract involvement)	2

PANCREATITIS:
Mild, 0–2 points
Moderate, 4–6 points
Severe, 8–10 points

to help determine the clinical severity of pancreatitis. Both scales are based on morphologic imaging features including the extent of pancreatic necrosis. The MCTSI also incorporates extra-pancreatic findings. According to Bollen et al., both imaging scales are comparable and correlate well with the clinical severity in conjunction with the Revised Atlanta Classification; each is superior to the clinical scale, APACHE II in predicting prognosis [25].

4.6.1 Peripancreatic Fluid Collections

Peripancreatic fluid collections are termed either acute (if <4 weeks of age) or chronic collections (if >4 weeks of age).

4.6.1.1 Acute Peripancreatic Fluid Collections

Acute peripancreatic fluid collections (APFCs) are common findings in acute pancreatitis affecting 30%–50% of patients [26–29]. APFCs are postulated to be a consequence of disruption of the pancreatic ductal system and are typically located either within the pancreas or in the adjacent peripancreatic tissues [22,26]. These collections are devoid of a solid component or a wall of granulation tissue. On CECT, APFCs typically appear as ill-defined fluid collections with indistinct margins that may show contiguity with the surrounding intra-abdominal structures [22,26]. In the acute setting, CECT may be used to help differentiate APFCs from postnecrotic pancreatic fluid collections (PNPFCs), because only the latter show foci of pancreatic necrosis. Occasionally, this distinction

can prove to be quite difficult to make necessitating repeat imaging within 2 weeks to confirm the presence or absence of pancreatic necrosis [26]. Inferring if an APFC is infected or sterile is a further radiological challenge. The presence of gas in a collection strongly suggests that it is infected. However, the absence of gas does not mean the APFC is sterile. If there is strong clinical suspicion for an infected collection, image-guided diagnostic aspiration ± therapeutic drainage can be performed. Most APFCs resolve spontaneously within a few days and clinically do not require drainage unless infected [26,30].

4.6.1.2 Pseudocyst

The term pseudocyst is used to describe a peripancreatic fluid collection that has persisted for >4 weeks and has developed a wall of fibrous granulation tissue. The pseudocyst fluid is typically rich in pancreatic enzymes such as amylase. Pseudocysts are found in 5%–16% of patients suffering from pancreatitis, with alcohol- or gallstone-induced pancreatitis, the two most common etiological factors [28,31,32]. Patients may present clinically with signs of abdominal pain, obstruction, mass effect, and occasionally, fever. The presence of fever or sepsis should raise the clinical suspicion for an infected pseudocyst.

CECT is a highly accurate modality for evaluating pancreatic pseudocysts—in determining the number, size, and location of the pseudocysts and for evaluating its effects on adjacent intra-abdominal structures. On CECT, a pseudocyst typically has a thin wall (<2 mm), low attenuation (<15 HU), and smooth regular margins [26]. MRI offers additional value in assessing complex pseudocysts and the pancreatic ductal system. The presence of hemorrhage in a pseudocyst is best evaluated on MRI as blood degradation products are associated with a characteristic set of MR signal intensities. Occasionally, hemorrhage in a pseudocyst may be recognized on noncontrast CT as foci of high attenuation within the fluid collection.

Overall, 50% of pseudocysts show spontaneous resolution. However, the presence or absence of ductal changes has been documented to affect resolution and treatment options [33]. A type 1 (normal), type 2 (stricture), type 3 (duct occlusion or "disconnected" duct) and type 4 ducts (chronic pancreatitis) have all been described. According to Nealon et al., 87% of pseudocysts that resolve spontaneously are of the type 1 duct variety. Percutaneous drainage is more successful in the type 1 and 2 ducts. Operative debridement is often needed in type 2 and 3 ducts, while persistent fistula after debridement occurs in 85% of type 3 ducts compared with 27% and 54% in types 1 and 2 ducts, respectively [33]. Percutaneous intervention is not recommended in asymptomatic pseudocysts as this may convert a sterile collection into an abscess.

4.6.1.2.1 Infected Pseudocyst

Patients with known pseudocysts that present with increasing abdominal pain, fever, and sepsis should undergo imaging for signs of an infected collection. The presence of gas is the most concerning radiologic sign for an infected pseudocyst [22,26]. However, presence of gas is not specific for infection as it is also seen in the presence of pseudocyst-enteric fistulas or cysto-gastrostomies or following recent percutaneous intervention [26]. Ultimately, gram stain and culture of a diagnostic aspirate from the pseudocyst is the most definitive method for confirming that a pseudocyst is infected. Pseudocyst evacuation is mandated in infected collections and this may be performed by image-guided percutaneous catheter insertion or via endoscopic cysto-gastrostomy or at surgery. As a general rule, patients with infected pseudocysts tend to be more stable than patients with infected walled-off pancreatic necrosis (WOPN). As such, patients with infected pseudocysts are often better candidates for tolerating a surgical or an endoscopic procedure [34].

4.6.1.2.2 Pseudocyst Mimics

Differentiating a pseudocyst from a cystic pancreatic neoplasm can be challenging radiologically. Typically, the former will have a preceding history of acute or chronic pancreatitis. In equivocal cases, EUS-guided cyst fluid aspiration (for biochemical and cytological analyses) is often helpful in reaching the correct diagnosis [35]. In pseudocysts, this analysis typically shows elevated levels of amylase, low levels of carcinoembryonic antigen (CEA), and absence of mucin.

4.6.1.3 Postnecrotic Pancreatic Fluid Collections

Fluid collections associated with pancreatic necrosis are termed postnecrotic pancreatic collection or PNPFC (Figure 4.8). The presence of solid material within the fluid collection in the presence of pancreatic necrosis confirms the diagnosis. MRI and ultrasound are more sensitive than CECT in detecting the presence of solid material [22,36–39]. As with all peripancreatic fluid collections, determining if the collection is infected is challenging. Unless there is gas present, diagnosing an infected PNPFC is a very difficult call and ultimately diagnostic aspiration may be required.

4.6.1.4 Walled-off Pancreatic Necrosis

When the PNPFC becomes well defined with a thickened wall, it is then termed WOPN. The solid necrotic

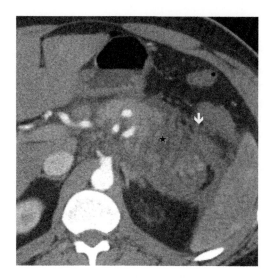

FIGURE 4.8
Post-necrotic pancreatic fluid collection on an axial contrast-enhanced CT. Focus of non-enhancement consistent with necrosis (star) is present in the pancreatic body/tail with surrounding anteriorly located peripancreatic fluid (arrow).

tissue within WOPN is sometimes difficult to appreciate on CECT. MRI, ultrasound, or EUS may prove more helpful in this regard. Although ductal involvement is important clinically, it is often not apparent on CECT. MRI or EUS may be utilized in these instances [39]. Features of WOPN that can help distinguish it from a pancreatic pseudocyst include a larger size (>10 cm), extension into the paracolic gutters, presence of fat debris, irregular wall definition, pancreatic deformity, and pancreatic discontinuity [40].

4.6.2 Vascular Complications

Extra-pancreatic vascular complications of acute pancreatitis are well assessed on CECT. The adjacent peripancreatic vascular structures and in particular the splenic vein and artery are most frequently involved. Splenic vein thrombosis occurs in approximately 25% of patients with acute pancreatitis and may be the result of either extrinsic compression from the pseudocyst or a sequalae of the inflammatory process [41]. Pseudoaneurysm is a serious complication of acute pancreatitis occurring in 3.5%–10% of patients [42,43]. The pseudoaneurysms may be a result of pseudocysts eroding into nearby arteries such as the splenic, gastroduodenal, or pancreaticoduodenal arteries. Pseudoaneurysm rupture (typically of a splenic pseudoaneurysm) may result in massive hemorrhage and hemodynamic instability and shock. In general, hemorrhage is a late complication of acute pancreatitis occurring in 1.3%–6.2% of patients [44,45].

4.7 Chronic Pancreatitis

Chronic pancreatitis has been defined as a progressive inflammatory disorder that belongs to a spectrum that includes acute pancreatitis [46]. More accurately, it represents the end stage of repeated attacks of acute pancreatitis leading to chronic and often irreversible glandular changes such as fibrosis, as identified histologically and on imaging. Clinically, patients typically present with central abdominal pain, malabsorption (from exocrine pancreatic insufficiency), and diabetes (from endocrine pancreatic insufficiency) [47]. In Western society, alcohol is the most common etiological factor. In the East (e.g., China, India, and to a lesser extent in Japan), chronic pancreatitis is most commonly idiopathic in origin. Other etiological factors include gallstones, drugs, and CF. Chronic pancreatitis is divided into three categories: (1) usual or calcifying chronic pancreatitis, (2) obstructive chronic pancreatitis, and (3) autoimmune chronic pancreatitis [48,49]. Usual or calcifying chronic pancreatitis is generally a consequence of recurrent episodes of acute pancreatitis and is typically associated with intraductal calcifications. Alcohol and cigarette smoking are reported risk factors [48,50–52]. Obstructive chronic pancreatitis is a secondary form of pancreatitis caused by tumors or benign strictures that cause ductal obstruction and upstream inflammation. Intraductal calcifications are rare. Autoimmune pancreatitis is discussed in the next section.

The imaging findings in chronic pancreatitis vary depending on the underlying etiology. In most cases, the pancreas shows glandular atrophy, coarse calcifications, and delayed and diminished parenchymal enhancement due to fibrosis [53] (Figure 4.9). The MPD is typically irregular in caliber and may show focal strictures with upstream main duct dilatation and side-duct ectasia. Pseudocysts may be seen in the pancreas or in the adjacent tissues. Associated extra-pancreatic finding include biliary dilatation (typically from external compression of the distal CBD), inflammatory gastrointestinal strictures (e.g., luminal narrowing of the second part of the duodenum), and vascular complications similar to that found in acute pancreatitis.

4.7.1 Autoimmune Pancreatitis

Autoimmune pancreatitis, also known as lymphoplasmacytic sclerosing pancreatitis, is a rare entity that may be misdiagnosed for pancreatic cancer radiologically [54]. Recent advances in pathophysiology, immunohistochemistry, and imaging have led to a better recognition and understanding of the disease process. Autoimmune pancreatitis is characterized by a lymphoplasmacystic infiltrate histologically, elevated serum IgG4 biochemically, and is associated with other autoimmune disease clinically (e.g., Sjogren's syndrome, inflammatory bowel disease, and primary sclerosing cholangitis). On imaging, autoimmune pancreatitis may show either diffuse pancreatic involvement or less commonly focal pancreatic involvement. The diffuse form of the disease typically causes uniform pancreatic enlargement ("sausage-shaped pancreas") associated with a circumferential peripancreatic halo (this typically shows low attenuation on CT and low T1 and T2 signal intensities on MRI) [55]. The focal form of autoimmune pancreatitis may appear mass like and may mimic pancreatic adenocarcinoma (Figure 4.10). A reduced caliber or normal caliber MPD is typically seen in autoimmune pancreatitis (in contrast, upstream ductal dilatation is typically seen in pancreatic adenocarcinoma) [54,56]. Acute peripancreatic inflammatory changes and pseudocysts are uncommon, unlike other forms of pancreatitis such as alcohol-induced pancreatitis. Furthermore, a myriad of recognized extra-pancreatic findings are reported in autoimmune pancreatitis.

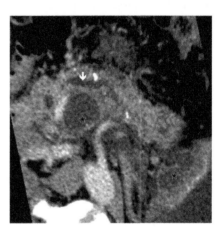

FIGURE 4.9
Chronic pancreatitis on an axial contrast-enhanced CT. The pancreatic parenchyma has heterogeneous attenuation, coarse calcifications, an irregularly dilated pancreatic duct (arrow) and a pseudocyst (star).

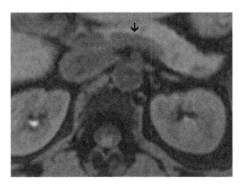

FIGURE 4.10
Autoimmune pancreatitis on an axial fat-suppressed T1 weighted image. A focal area of low signal intensity is present in the pancreatic body. This has been confirmed pathologically to represent focal autoimmune pancreatitis (arrow).

These include biliary tract strictures, gallbladder wall-thickening, parenchymal renal lesions, retroperitoneal fibrosis, sclerosing mesenteritis, adenopathy, sialadenitis, lung infiltrates, and so on [54,56]. Of clinical importance, autoimmune pancreatitis generally responds well to corticosteroid treatment with improvement in clinical and imaging findings (and even spontaneous resolution) reported in as early as a few weeks [56–59]. Untreated cases may show pancreatic fibrosis and intraductal calcifications [54].

4.8 Solid Neoplasms of the Pancreas

A variety of solid pancreatic neoplasms are encountered in clinical practice. These include pancreatic adenocarcinoma, neuroendocrine tumor, solid pseudopapillary tumor (SPT), and rare entities such as pancreatoblastoma, lymphoma, metastases to the pancreas, and acinar cell carcinoma. An understanding of these diseases including knowledge of relevant clinical and imaging finding facilitates appropriate lesion characterization and differentiation. These neoplasms are discussed in the following section.

4.8.1 Adenocarcinoma

Pancreatic adenocarcinoma accounts for 85%–95% of all pancreatic malignancies and is the fourth leading cause of cancer-related deaths [60,61]. Most patients are 60–80 years of age, and males are twice as commonly affected as females [60,61]. A total of 60%–70% of tumors are located in pancreatic head, 10%–20% in the body, and 5%–10% in the tail. Diffuse gland involvement occurs in 5%. Abdominal pain, weight loss, and jaundice are the main presenting complaints but generally occur late in the disease course. Prognosis is poor with a 1-year

survival rate of <20% and a 5-year survival rate of <5% [60,62]. Seventy-five percent of patients have unresectable disease at presentation, with metastases present in 85% of these, mainly to the liver and peritoneum [60,61]. Surgery is the only cure and offers a 5-year survival of 20% [60,61].

Thin collimation biphasic (arterial and portal) CECT is the most commonly used technique for evaluating pancreatic adenocarcinoma. The arterial/pancreatic phase (acquired 20–40 seconds post-contrast injection) provides the optimal display of the tumor and peripancreatic arteries. Maximal contrast between the hypovascular tumor and the normal pancreas renders maximal tumor conspicuity in this phase. Most tumors are hypoattenuating with a mean size of 3 cm (range 1.5–10 cm, average size in head 2.5–3 cm, in the body and tail 5–7 cm) [60,61]. The portal phase (acquired 50–70 seconds post injection) is the best phase for detecting liver metastases and evaluating patency of venous vessels. A pancreatic mass is occult in 10% of cases as the tumor appears isoattenuating with the pancreatic parenchyma [60,62] (Figures 4.11a and b). The mass is inferred from secondary signs such as mass effect, convex contour abnormality of the pancreas, ductal obstruction, and vascular invasion [60–62]. Tumors in the pancreatic head may cause dilatation of both CBD and MPD—double duct sign (Figure 4.11b) while tumors in the pancreatic body may cause upstream MPD dilatation. Atrophy of the pancreas proximal to the tumor is recognized in chronic obstruction. A circumferential soft tissue cuff around the peripancreatic vessels with loss of the perivascular fat plane denotes vascular invasion (Figure 4.12). Eighty-four percent sensitivity and 98% specificity for invasion is reported if the tumor is contiguous with greater than 50% of the vessel circumference [60,63]. Other features suggesting vascular invasion include vessel deformity, thrombosis, and

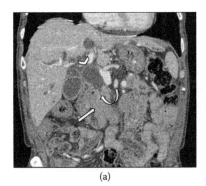
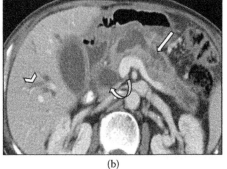

(a)   (b)

FIGURE 4.11

Isodense pancreatic adenocarcinoma. (a) Coronal portal phase post-contrast CT image shows an isodense tumor (straight arrow) in the pancreatic head causing proximal dilatation (arrowhead) and abrupt distal narrowing of the common bile duct (curved arrow). (b) Axial portal phase post-contrast CT image shows the double duct sign—simultaneous dilatation of main pancreatic duct (straight arrow) and common bile duct (curved arrow) due to an obstructing mass. Intrahepatic ductal dilatation (arrowhead) is also present. (From Low G, Panu A, Millo N, Leen E, *Radiographics*, Jul–Aug; 31(4), 2011. With permission.)

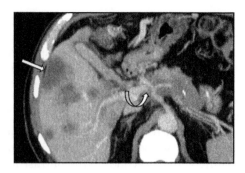

FIGURE 4.12
Irresectable adenocarcinoma with vascular invasion and liver metastases. Axial portal phase post-contrast CT image shows encasement of the celiac axis and occlusion of the portal vein by a diffuse hypodense pancreatic tumor (curved arrow). Multiple ill-defined hypodense liver metastases (straight arrow) are also present. (From Low G, Panu A, Millo N, Leen E, *Radiographics*, Jul-Aug; 31(4), 2011. With permission.)

development of collateral vessels. The tear drop superior mesenteric vein (SMV) sign refers to an alteration of the normal round shape of this vessel to a tear drop shape on axial images secondary to tumor infiltration or peritumoral fibrosis [60,64]. Cystic-necrotic degeneration is an uncommon feature of adenocarcinoma present in 8% of cases [60,65]. Metastases are most commonly found in the liver and peritoneum. CECT has an accuracy of 85%–95% for tumor detection, positive predictive value of 89%–100% for unresectability, and negative predictive value of 45%–79% for resectability [60,62]. On MRI, adenocarcinoma typically shows low T1 and T2 signal intensity. Similar to CECT, the hypovascular neoplasm enhances less than the normal pancreas although on MRI a thin peritumoral rim of greater enhancement is often observed, which may help establish disease focality. MRI has superior contrast resolution than CECT and is better at detecting small tumors and metastases. MRI has 90%–100% accuracy for adenocarcinoma [60,66].

EUS, a high-resolution imaging method, has a recognized role in the detection and staging of small tumors. It can detect masses as small as 0.2–0.3 cm. EUS can clarify equivocal findings on CT and/or MRI and allows biopsy of suspicious lesions. Adenocarcinoma appears as an ill-defined heterogeneous hypoechoic mass on EUS. DeWitt et al. [67] found EUS to be more sensitive than CECT for detecting adenocarcinoma (98% vs. 86%) and more accurate for tumor staging (67% vs. 47%). EUS does have certain limitations. It is highly operator dependent with a relatively steep learning curve. It also suffers from a narrow field of view, so it is limited in the assessment of locoregional invasion or vessel involvement other than the portal vein.

Positron emission tomography (PET) is an emerging technique for characterizing tissue based on functional rather than morphologic information. The principle of ^{18}F-fluoro-2-deoxy-D-glucose (^{18}FDG)-PET imaging is that malignant tissues have a higher uptake and retention of ^{18}FDG compared to normal tissue due to enhanced glucose metabolism. Pancreatic adenocarcinoma generally shows an intense focal ^{18}FDG uptake. The biggest potential impact of ^{18}FDG-PET is in the detection of small metastases, an area where CECT (45%–79% negative predictive value of resectability) and MRI generally underperform. Frohlich et al. [68] found that ^{18}FDG-PET detected 97% of liver metastases greater than 1 cm and 43% of metastases smaller than 1 cm, with a specificity of 95%.

4.8.2 Neuroendocrine Tumor

Pancreatic neuroendocrine tumors, a component of gastroenteropancreatic neuroendocrine tumors according to World Health Organization (WHO) classification, were previously referred to as islet cell tumors, as these were thought to have arisen from the islets of Langerhans; however, recent evidence suggests that these tumors originate from pluripotential stem cells in ductal epithelium [60,69]. They account for 1%–5% of all pancreatic tumors, possess equal sex distribution, and typically present at a mean age of 51–57 years. Most cases are sporadic, but association with syndromes such as multiple endocrine neoplasia type 1 (MEN1), VHL, neurofibromatosis type 1, and tuberous sclerosis is recognized. Neuroendocrine tumors are classified into functioning (if they produce symptoms related to excessive hormone production) and nonfunctioning tumors. Functioning tumors account for 15%–70% [60,70] of all tumors and are subdivided according to the hormones they produce. The features of functioning and nonfunctioning neuroendocrine tumors are presented in Table 4.3 [60].

A variable spectrum of imaging appearances exists. Tumors tend to be multiple especially when associated with syndromes such as MEN1 and VHL. Single lesions are the norm in insulinoma (single in 90%) while multiple lesions are present in 20%–40% of gastrinomas [60]. Tumor size is variable. In general, functioning tumors present early in the course of disease when the tumors are small due to the clinical manifestations of excessive hormone production while nonfunctioning tumors present when they are large due to mass effect. Risk of malignancy increases with tumor size (especially if >5 cm) with 90% of nonfunctioning tumors being malignant at presentation [70]. Tumor morphology is variable. Small tumors are generally solid and homogeneous. Larger tumors are heterogeneous and may show cystic/necrotic degeneration and calcifications [70]. Malignant tumors may show features of local spread, vascular invasion, lymph node involvement, and organ metastases.

Neuroendocrine tumors share some common features that permit their distinction [60]. On MRI, these tumors generally have longer T1 and T2 relaxation times than the normal pancreas and most other pancreatic neoplasms. Consequently, most neuroendocrine tumors show low

TABLE 4.3

Features of Pancreatic Neuroendocrine Tumors

Tumor	Size	Malignancy	Location	Symptoms	Survival
Insulinoma (50% of tumors)	90% <2 cm, 66% <1.5 cm, 40% <1 cm	10% malignant	90% in pancreas, equal gland distribution	Hypoglycemic attacks, atypical seizure	Resection generally curative
Gastrinoma (20% of tumors)	Mean size 4 cm	60% Malignant; metastases in up to 60%	25%–60% in pancreas. 90% occur in gastrinoma triangle (junction between bile duct and cystic duct superiorly, body of pancreas medially and duodenum inferiorly)	Zollinger Ellison syndrome with peptic ulceration and diarrhea	90% 10-year survival following complete resection
Glucagonoma (1% of tumors)	Most are 2–6 cm	70% malignant; metastases in up to 60%	>90% in pancreas with predilection for body and tail	Necrolytic migratory erythema, weight loss, diabetes, diarrhea	More favorable with complete resection; prolonged even with liver metastases
Vipoma (3% of tumors)	Mean size 5 cm	Up to 75% malignant; metastases in up to 70%	90% in pancreas (mainly tail), 10%–20% are extrapancreatic most commonly in retroperitoneal sympathetic chain and adrenals	Werner-Morrison syndrome with watery diarrhea and hypokalaemia	5-year survival of 95% with complete resection; with metastases 60%
Somatostatinoma (<1% of tumors)	Often >5 cm	50% malignant; metastases in up to 50%	50% in pancreas; 50% in duodenum	Gallstones, weight loss, diarrhea, steatorrhea, diabetes	5-year survival of 95% with complete resection, with metastases 60%
Nonfunctioning tumors (15%–50% of tumors)	30% >10 cm; range 3–24 cm	90% malignant; metastases in up to 50%	Predilection for pancreatic head	Symptoms from mass effect (e.g. abdominal pain and distension, jaundice, weight loss, etc.	5-year survival of >50% with complete resection

Source: Low G, Panu A, Millo N, Leen E, *Radiographics*, Jul-Aug; 31(4), 2011. With permission.

signal on T1-weighted MRI sequence and intermediate to high signal on T2-weighted MRI sequence relative to the normal pancreas. The most discriminating feature for neuroendocrine tumors is their behavior on contrast-enhanced imaging. Neuroendocrine tumors have a rich vascular supply. For this reason, they show avid enhancement during the arterial phase of imaging, enhancing more rapidly and intensely than the normal pancreas [70] (Figure 4.13). Homogeneous enhancement is typical for small tumors <2 cm while larger lesions tend to show heterogeneous enhancement, which can be ring like [70]. Capturing this vascular blush is essential for diagnosis of small tumors such as insulinoma, which often do not distort the contour of the pancreas [60]. On the portal phase of imaging, tumors may be hyper-, iso-, or hypo-enhancing compared to the normal pancreas. Some tumors have atypical delayed enhancement, so they are best appreciated on portal-phase imaging [70]. Metastases to lymph nodes and solid organs such as

the liver may have a similar enhancement pattern as the primary tumor. For clinically suspected neuroendocrine tumor, CT or MRI should be performed using high-resolution dual phase imaging to maximize tumor detection, characterization, and staging. Gouya et al. [71] found that thin-section biphasic CECT had a sensitivity of 94.4%, biphasic CECT without thin section 57%, and sequential CECT 28.6% for diagnosing insulinomas. MRI has a sensitivity of 85%–94% [72,73].

EUS and indium[111] octreotide play a role in evaluating neuroendocrine tumors. Gouya et al. [71] found that the sensitivity of EUS for diagnosing insulinoma was 93.8%, and the overall combined sensitivity for thin-slice dual-phase CECT and EUS was 100%. Indium[111]-radiolabelled octreotide (a somatostatin analogue) is taken up by somatostatin receptors 2 and 5 found in most neuroendocrine tumors except insulinoma. Insulinomas rarely express somatostatin receptors, thus limiting sensitivity to 10%–50% [74]. In practice, the main advantage of

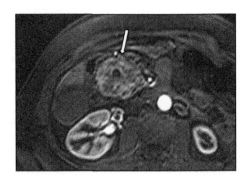

FIGURE 4.13
Malignant neuroendocrine tumor. Axial arterial phase post-contrast T1-weighted MRI image shows heterogeneous hyper-enhancement of the pancreatic tumor (arrow). (From Low G, Panu A, Millo N, Leen E, *Radiographics*, Jul-Aug; 31(4), 2011. With permission.)

octreotide imaging is the capability to perform whole body scanning to detect small tumors and metastases especially in areas not under clinical suspicion [60]. [18]FDG-PET may have a role in the assessment of poorly differentiated neuroendocrine tumors that are generally octreotide negative. These tumors exhibit increased uptake on [18]FDG-PET as they possess a high proliferative rate, unlike well-differentiated tumors that show poor uptake due to low proliferative rates [60].

It is important to differentiate neuroendocrine tumors from other tumors of the pancreas, particularly adenocarcinoma as prognosis (more favorable for neuroendocrine tumor) and treatment options are different. Features that aid in differentiation from adenocarcinoma include the following [60,70]:

1. Enhancement (adenocarcinoma is a hypovascular tumor while neuroendocrine tumor is hypervascular).

2. Calcifications (2% of adenocarcinomas show calcifications as opposed to 20% of neuroendocrine tumors).

3. Vascular involvement (adenocarcinoma is associated with vascular encasement while malignant neuroendocrine tumors may show vascular infiltration with tumor thrombus).

4. Ductal involvement (adenocarcinoma has a high propensity for ductal obstruction but this is uncommon in neuroendocrine tumors).

5. Necrosis and cystic degeneration is more common in neuroendocrine tumor than adenocarcinoma.

4.8.3 Solid Pseudopapillary Tumor

It has been originally described by Frantz in 1959 [75] that this entity has been called by many different names, including solid cystic papillary epithelial tumor, papillary

cystic tumor, and solid and cystic tumor [60]. In 1996, the WHO renamed it as SPT [76]. SPT accounts for 1%–2% of pancreatic tumors. It is most common in females (female to male ratio [F:M] = 9:1), young adults (mean age 25 years, range 10–74 years) [77], and African and Asian racial groups. SPT has a low malignant potential with excellent prognosis following complete resection. Metastases are uncommon, occurring in 7%–9% of cases, and mostly to the liver, omentum, and peritoneum [78]. The most common presenting complaints are pain and an abdominal mass, but it may be asymptomatic in up to 15% of cases.

SPT is typically a large (mean size, 9 cm), slow-growing, well-encapsulated mass [60,77,79]. It most commonly occurs in the pancreatic tail, followed closely by the pancreatic head [60]. It has a tendency to displace rather than invade surrounding structures and rarely causes bile or pancreatic duct obstruction [60]. The pseudocapsule (composed of compressed pancreatic tissue and reactive fibrosis) shows low attenuation on CECT and low T1 and T2 signal intensities on MRI. Internal hemorrhagic and cystic degeneration is the hallmark of SPT due to the fragile vascular network of the tumor. These imaging features are best appreciated on MRI [60] (Figures 4.14a through d). Subacute hemorrhage may show high T1 signal intensity and variable T2 signal intensity while chronic hemorrhage shows low T1 and T2 signal intensities. A fluid–fluid level or a fluid–debris level is detected in 10%–18% of cases due to the hematocrit effect [77]. Peripheral calcification is present in 30% of cases [77]. The typical enhancement pattern of SPT is peripheral heterogeneous enhancement during the arterial phase followed by progressive non-uniform enhancement thereafter, with enhancement being generally lower than that of the normal pancreas [60,80]. The main differential consideration for SPT is cystic neuroendocrine tumor [60]. Features that help distinguish the two entities include age at presentation (neuroendocrine tumors rarely occur in patients younger than 30 years), the signal intensity on T1-weighted MRI sequences (neuroendocrine tumor shows low signal while SPT containing hemorrhage shows high signal), and the tumor enhancement characteristics (neuroendocrine tumors are more vascular and demonstrate either diffuse or ring hyperenhancement) [60].

4.8.4 Miscellaneous Solid Neoplasms

These rare neoplasms include the following:

- PANCREATOBLASTOMA

  This is the most common pancreatic neoplasm of young children (accounting for 0.2% of all pancreatic tumors) [81]. The mean age is 5 years. Typically slow growing, pancreatoblastoma

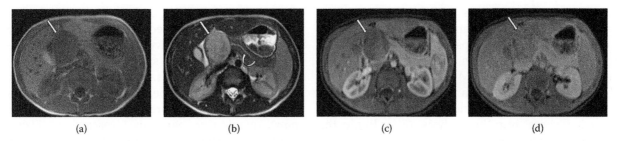

FIGURE 4.14
Solid pseudopapillary tumor. (a) Axial T1-weighted MRI image, (b) axial T2-weighted MRI image, (c) axial arterial phase post-contrast T1-weighted MRI image, and (d) axial portal phase post-contrast T1-weighted MRI image show a well-encapsulated solid tumor (straight arrow) in the head of the pancreas that has low signal on T1- and intermediate to high signal on corresponding T2-weighted images. The tumor shows mild heterogeneous arterial enhancement with progressive non-uniform fill-in during the portal phase. Despite its large size, the tumor does not obstruct the main pancreatic duct (curved arrow), which is of normal caliber. (From Low G, Panu A, Millo N, Leen E, *Radiographics*, Jul-Aug; 31(4), 2011. With permission.)

generally presents as an asymptomatic large mass (mean size, 10 cm; range, 1.5–20 cm) [81]. On imaging, it is not possible to identify the organ of origin in 50% of cases due to the large size of the mass at presentation [82]. Biopsy is generally required to establish diagnosis. Aggressive behavior with local and distant spread is recognized. In some cases, pancreatoblastoma may appear as a circumscribed, lobulated mass (with a predilection for the pancreatic head) with solid and cystic components and/or calcification [60]. Despite its size, it rarely causes biliary or duodenal obstruction as the tumor has a soft gelatinous consistency [60].

- LYMPHOMA

Pancreatic lymphoma is most commonly a B-cell subtype of Non-Hodgkin's lymphoma (NHL) and is classified as either primary or secondary. Secondary lymphoma (found in 30% of NHL patients with widespread disease) is the dominant form [83]. Primary pancreatic lymphoma is rare representing <2% of extranodal lymphoma and 0.5% of pancreatic tumors [60,83]. Two morphological patterns of pancreatic lymphoma are recognized [60,84]: a focal well-circumscribed form, and a diffuse form. The focal form occurs in the pancreatic head in 80% of cases and has a mean size of 8 cm (range 2–15 cm) [85]. The diffuse form is infiltrative leading to gland enlargement and ill definition, features that can simulate the appearance of acute pancreatitis [60].

- METASTASES TO THE PANCREAS

Pancreatic metastases have an autopsy incidence of 2%–11% and account for 2%–5% of malignant neoplasms [86]. Metastases are most frequently

from RCC and lung carcinoma, followed by breast carcinoma, colorectal carcinoma, and melanoma [86]. Three morphological patterns of involvement are recognized—solitary (50%–70% of cases), multifocal (5%–10%), and diffuse (15%–44%) [60,86,87]. On CT and MRI, appearances of pancreatic metastases closely resemble that of the primary cancer [60]. In most cases, the medical history of cancer aids in achieving a correct diagnosis [60]. Equivocal cases should be biopsied.

- ACINAR CELL CARCINOMA

Acinar cell carcinoma accounts for approximately 1% of all exocrine pancreatic neoplasms. Most patients are in the 5th to 7th decades of life and the mean age is 60 years. Lipase hypersecretion from the tumor may result in subcutaneous fat necrosis, subcutaneous nodules, polyarthropathy, and bone infarcts [60]. The tumor is typically large (mean size = 10 cm), hypovascular, and heterogeneous with internal cystic-necrotic degeneration.

4.9 Cystic Neoplasms of the Pancreas

Pancreatic cystic lesions are a modern phenomenon due to an explosion in the volume of imaging performed and the increased sensitivity of state-of-the-art imaging technologies available. The vast majority of these lesions are small asymptomatic cysts discovered on imaging performed for unrelated clinical indications. The prevalence of pancreatic cysts in the literature varies depending on the study design and the imaging modalities employed. Kimura et al. [88], Zhang et al. [89], and Spinelli et al. [90] evaluated the prevalence of pancreatic cysts in study cohorts that did not discriminate against patients with known pancreatic disease. The prevalence of pancreatic cysts was found to be 24.3% (*n* = 300 autopsies) in Kimura's study [88], 19.6% (*n* = 1444 MRIs) in Zhang's study [89], and 1.2% (*n* = 24,039 combined MRIs & CTs) in Spinelli's study [90]. In contrast, Laffan et al. [91], de Jong et al. [92], and Lee et al. [93] excluded patients with known pancreatic disease from the analysis. Accordingly, the prevalence of pancreatic cysts was 2.6% in Laffan's study [91] (*n* = 2,832 CTs), 2.4% in de Jong's study [92] (*n* = 2,803 MRIs), and 13.5% in Lee's study [93] (*n* = 616 MRIs). The high prevalence of pancreatic cysts in the general population has raised the clinical dilemma on how to optimally manage these incidentalomas. Traditional dogma advocates that pseudocysts account for the vast majority of pancreatic cysts found in clinical practice. However, over the last few decades, it has become increasingly clear that a large proportion of pancreatic cysts are neoplastic in origin. Of these; SCNs, mucinous cystic neoplasms (MCNs), and intraductal papillary mucinous neoplasms (IPMNs) account for approximately 90%. Furthermore, the mucinous tumors, MCNs, and IPMNs harbor underlying malignant potential. Solid pseudopapillary tumor and solid neoplasms with cystic-necrotic degeneration such as pancreatic adenocarcinoma, neuroendocrine tumors, acinar cell carcinoma, and pancreatic metastases account for the remaining 10%. Surgical ethos dictates that resection for curative intent is ideally performed while lesions are small and noninvasive with worsening prognosis when lesions become large and invasive.

Nevertheless, this must be balanced with the knowledge that most cystic neoplasms are indolent tumors with low-grade aggressiveness while pancreatic resections constitute major surgery with its recognized attendant complications. Current recommendations are that lesions may be risk-stratified according to clinical findings (the presence or absence of symptoms), imaging appearances (presence or absence of suspicious findings of malignancy), and biochemical cyst fluid analysis. While the optimal management of these cysts remains unclear and there is absence of uniform clinical consensus, there will be variability in the clinical work-up of the disease. Unquestionably, the understanding and management of the disease is very much a work in progress. To try and address some of these uncertainties, the American College of Radiology (ACR) commissioned the ACR's Incidental Findings Committee to provide guidance for practicing radiologists. The recommendations of the committee for the imaging work-up of asymptomatic pancreatic cysts are included in Figure 4.15 [94,95]. In the following section, we discuss the three most common causes of cystic pancreatic neoplasms; SCNs, MCNs, and IPMNs focusing on relevant clinical, pathological, and radiological findings.

4.9.1 Serous Cystic Neoplasm

SCNs are characterized pathologically by serous fluid-filled cysts lined by a single layer of uniform cuboidal epithelial cells with centrally located round nuclei and

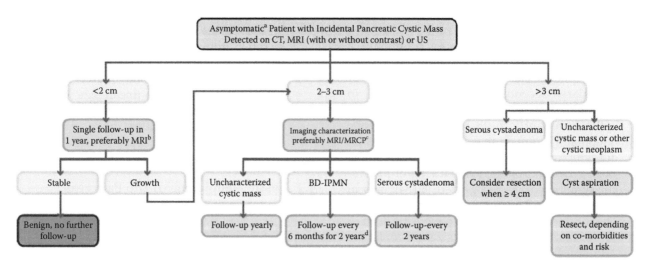

FIGURE 4.15
Flow chart for imaging work-up of incidental pancreatic masses in asymptomatic patients.
[a]Signs and symptoms include hyperamylasemia, recent onset diabetes, severe epigastric pain, weight loss, steatorrhea or jaundice.
[b]Consider decreasing interval if younger, omitting with limited life expectancy. Recommend limited T2-weighted MRI for routine follow-ups.
[c]Recommend pancreas-dedicated MRI + MRCP. If no growth after 2 years, follow yearly.
[d] If growth or suspicious features develop, consider resection. (From Berland LL, Silverman SG, Gore RM et al., *J Am Coll Radiol*, 2010 Oct;7(10), 2010. With permission.)

a glycogen-rich cytoplasm [96,97]. Previously termed "serous cystadenomas," SCNs generally have an indolent biologic behavior and excellent prognosis. A malignant form of SCNs, serous cystadenocarcinomas is reported in approximately 3% [98,99]. However, for practical and management purposes, SCNs are regarded clinically as benign neoplasms [96,97]. SCNs account for 20%–30% of all cystic pancreatic neoplasms [96,97,100]. Most affected patients are in the 7th decade of life (average age 62 years, range 35–84 years) and there is a female preponderance (F:M = 3–4:1) [96,97]. VHL accounts for 15%–30% of cases [97,18]. VHL-associated SCNs affect both sexes equally and typically involve the pancreas diffusely [97,101]. Most patients with SCNs are asymptomatic and the disease is usually discovered incidentally on imaging. Symptoms are typically nonspecific in nature and are mainly due to mass effect (e.g., abdominal pain, abdominal fullness, nausea, vomiting, and weight loss). Biliary obstruction and jaundice are rare. The likelihood of symptoms increases with increasing tumor size. Tseng et al. [102] found that tumors >4 cm were 3 times more likely to be symptomatic than tumors smaller than 4 cm. Furthermore, tumors < 4 cm were found to grow at a rate of 0.6 cm/year and tumors >4 cm at 0.12 cm/year [102].

SCNs show a mild geographic predilection for the pancreatic head [96,97]. The average tumor size is approximately 5–7 cm (range 2–25 cm) [96,97,102,103]. SCNs do not show ductal communication and rarely obstruct the MPD. Rather, larger tumors may displace the pancreatic duct. Upstream parenchymal atrophy is uncommon. On imaging, SCNs are typically well-circumscribed lobulated tumors composed of a constellation of microcystic locules (Figure 4.16) [104]. Individual cystic locules are generally <2 cm and more commonly <1 cm in size (locules <2 cm are termed "microcystic" while locules >2 cm are termed "macrocystic") and most tumors are composed of more than six locules [96,97,104]. An enhancing stellate fibrous stroma is typically present, and central "sunburst" calcification (a characteristic

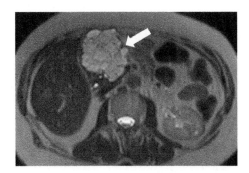

FIGURE 4.16
Serous cystic neoplasm. Axial T2-weighted MR image show the lobulated cystic tumor (arrow) of the pancreatic head which is composed of innumerable microcysts simulating a "honeycomb" appearance.

radiological finding) is found in 20% [96,97,104]. The walls of the tumor and the internal septations are thin (<2 mm) and show little if any enhancement. On MRI, the cystic locules show low T1 signal intensity and high T2 signal intensity while the fibrous stroma and calcifications show low T1 and T2 signal intensities. In 20%, SCNs exhibits a "honeycomb" spongy appearance as a result of the large quantity of microcystic locules [96,97,104]. These tumors can be misdiagnosed as solid appearing lesions on US, and CECT as the locules are often too small and numerous to clearly resolve on these modalities. In such cases, MRI (with its superior soft tissue resolution) can correctly decipher the true cystic nature of these lesions. In 10%, SCNs have an atypical oligocystic or macrocystic morphology [96,97,104]. These tumors pose a diagnostic challenge as imaging features overlap with pseudocysts and MCNs.

As SCNs are benign, asymptomatic cases may be managed conservatively with periodic imaging surveillance. Surgery should be considered for symptomatic tumors, tumors that show rapid growth and tumors that are of uncertain etiology [96,97]. SCNs located in the pancreatic head are generally treated by pylorus-sparing pancreatoduodenectomy while tumors in the body or tail are treated by distal pancreatectomy. Enucleation is not typically an option due to tumor size.

4.9.2 Mucinous Cystic Neoplasm

MCNs are characterized pathologically by mucin-secreting columnar epithelium, viscous cystic fluid, and ovarian-type stroma. Unlike IPMNs, MCNs do not show communication with the pancreatic duct. MCNs have inherent malignant potential and account for approximately 50% of all cystic pancreatic neoplasms [105]. Pathologically, MCNs show a spectrum of histological variability even within a single lesion (e.g., cellular atypia, dysplasia, carcinoma in situ, and invasive carcinoma). The WHO has classified MCNs into three categories: mucinous cystadenoma, mucinous cystadenoma with moderate dysplasia, and mucinous cystadenocarcinoma (infiltrating or non-infiltrating). Approximately 6%–36% of cases show invasive cancer [97,106]. On average, patients with malignant tumors are 15 years older than those with benign tumors suggesting a time-dependent malignant transformation [97,107].

Most patients are in the 4th and 5th decades of life and the average age is approximately 45–47 years (patients with MCNs are generally younger than patients with SCNs and IPMNs) [106,108]; 95% of patients are female [97,105,106]. Up to 76% of cases are symptomatic [106]. Symptoms are most commonly secondary to mass effect, although pancreatitis, new-onset diabetes, and a palpable mass are also reported findings. The presence of symptoms should raise the suspicion of underlying malignancy. However, the absence of symptoms does not guarantee that the tumor is benign. In asymptomatic cases, early or invasive cancer is found in 18% and potential malignancy in 42% [109]. On imaging, MCNs are typically well-circumscribed round cystic tumors located in the pancreatic body or tail in 90–95% of cases [97,105,106,110] (Figure 4.17). Most tumors measure 8–10 cm, although tumors as large as 25 cm are reported [105]. MCNs are most commonly unilocular with 20% being multilocular (with <6 locules) [105]. Individual locules measure >2 cm (macrocystic). This macrocystic appearance helps to differentiate MCNs from SCNs, which are typically microcystic in appearance. MCNs generally have thick walls and internal septations >2 mm in thickness. Unilocular MCN may be differentiated from pseudocysts by the absence of a history of pancreatitis or imaging features to suggest this. Debris or hemorrhage may be present in the cyst fluid, although typically the fluid appears anechoic on US, hypoattenuating on CECT, and low T1 signal intensity and high T2 signal intensity on MRI. Alternatively, the cyst fluid may show high T1 signal intensity due to mucin or hemorrhage. Peripheral "eggshell" calcification is a characteristic finding found in <20% [97]. In the absence of objective evidence of cancer (e.g., local invasion or metastases), radiologic features suspicious for malignancy include a large size, a solid component, thick cyst walls, mural nodules, and calcifications [105]. In a study of 163 resected MCNs, Crippa et al. [108] found that all malignant neoplasms were >4 cm while malignant lesions (both carcinoma in-situ and invasive cancer) were larger than benign lesions (on average 8 cm vs. 4.5 cm). MRI is superior to CT for demonstrating the complex architecture and morphological features of MCNs. Calcifications are best appreciated on CT compared with MRI. EUS with its superior spatial resolution is particularly useful for assessing MCNs—its

walls and septations and the presence of mural nodules. In addition, EUS permits fine needle aspiration (FNA) of the tumor wall and diagnostic aspirate of the cyst fluid. Cytological analysis is generally unhelpful as it suffers from sampling error and poor diagnostic yield. Biochemical analysis is typically positive for mucin and shows low amylase levels due to absence of ductal communication and high levels of CEA. Brugge et al. [111] found that CEA was more accurate than the combination of cytology, cyst morphology, and CA 19–9. Although there is no standardized cut-off level for CEA, many centers use a cut-off of 192 ng/ml for differentiating mucinous from non-MCNs (75% sensitivity, 84% specificity, 79% accuracy) [111]. Furthermore, a CEA level of <5 ng/ml has 50%–100% sensitivity and 77%–95% specificity for excluding a mucinous neoplasm, whereas CEA levels >800 ng/ml are 48% sensitive and 98% specific for MCNs [112,113].

The definitive treatment for MCNs is surgical resection, given the innate malignant potential of the entity. Tumors in the pancreatic body and tail are typically treated by distal pancreatectomy (±splenectomy), while tumors in the head are treated by pancreatoduodenectomy. The 5-year survival rate following surgery is ≥90% for non-invasive MCNs and 50%–75% for invasive MCNs [104,108]. However, recent evidence suggests a worse prognosis for invasive MCNs (15%–33% 5-year survival) than was initially reported [97,103,104,108].

4.9.3 Intraductal Papillary Mucinous Neoplasm

IPMN was first described by Ohhashi et al. in 1982 as "mucinous secreting cancer of the pancreas" [105,114]. In 1996, the WHO recognized intraductal papillary mucinous tumor as a distinct clinical entity separate from MCNs. In the revised WHO classification of 2000, the disease was renamed as IPMN. In essence, this refers to an intraductal mucin-producing neoplasm with tall columnar mucin-containing epithelium with or without papillary projections involving the MPD and/or the branch ducts, and lacking ovarian stroma characteristic of MCNs [105,115]. IPMNs account for approximately 25% of all cystic pancreatic neoplasms [105]. Most patients are in the 6th and 7th decade of life (mean age, 65 years) and males are more commonly affected than females [110,105]. IPMNs are associated with extrapancreatic malignancies such as gastric cancer and colorectal cancer [116]. IPMNs show a spectrum of histological variability ranging from benign lesions (e.g., intraductal papillary mucinous adenoma) to borderline lesions (e.g., IPMN with moderate dysplasia) to frankly malignant neoplasms (e.g., intraductal papillary mucinous carcinoma, noninfiltrating or infiltrating). IPMNs are believed to undergo a step-wise malignant transformation with a lag time of 5–7 years observed between

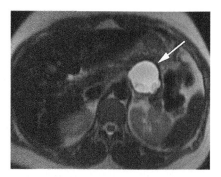

FIGURE 4.17
Axial T2-weighted MR image shows a round thick-walled cystic structure (arrow) in the pancreatic tail consistent with a mucinous cystadenoma. (From Kalb B, Sarmiento JM, Kooby DA, Adsay NV, Martin DR, *Radiographics*, Oct;29(6), 2009. With permission.)

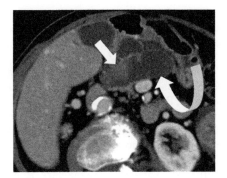

FIGURE 4.18
Main-duct IPMN. An axial post-contrast CT image shows gross dilatation of the main pancreatic duct (curved arrow) with associated ductal-based soft tissue tumor (arrow).

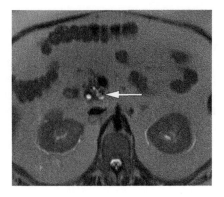

FIGURE 4.19
Axial T2-weighted MR image demonstrates focal dilatation of ductal side branches in the pancreatic head (arrow), findings that represent a small side branch IPMN. (From Kalb B, Sarmiento JM, Kooby DA, Adsay NV, Martin DR, *Radiographics*, Oct;29(6), 2009. With permission.)

benign and malignant manifestations of the disease [97].

There are three distinct forms of IPMN: main-duct IPMN, branch-duct IPMN, and mixed/combined IPMN. Main-duct IPMN is characterized by diffuse or segmental dilatation of the MPD and an aggressive biologic behavior (Figure 4.18). Approximately 5%–10% of IPMNs involve the pancreas diffusely [117]. Mixed- or combined-type IPMNs show both main duct and branch duct forms of the disease, and they have a biologic behavior similar to main duct IPMNs. A pooled analysis of nine studies found malignancy in approximately 70% of main duct IPMNs and invasive cancer in approximately 43% [118]. In 30% on ERCP, a protruding and patulous papilla of Vater ("fish-mouth" papilla) is identified with copious mucus extruding from the orifice [97,105]. Additional ERCP findings include a dilated MPD with associated intraductal filling defects due to mural nodules or mucus plugs. MRI is the modality of choice for evaluating IPMNs due to the exquisite sensitivity of MRCP in evaluating the pancreatic duct and for determining the relationship of tumors to the ductal system. Dilatation of the MPD, ductal wall thickening, and intraductal mural nodules are recognized findings on MRCP. The mural nodules can be differentiated from mucus plugs on contrast-enhanced MRI as the former show enhancement unlike the latter. Biliary obstruction can occur from mucus plugging or extrinsic compression of the distal CBD or ampulla. Ductal obstruction from mucus plugging may cause repeated attacks of pancreatitis. This can ultimately give rise to imaging features of chronic pancreatitis such as glandular atrophy and parenchymal fibrosis (manifest on MRI as loss of high T1 signal intensity in the pancreas with associated delayed and diminished parenchymal enhancement).

Branch-duct IPMNs may be unifocal or multifocal (in 30%) and most commonly involve the pancreatic head and uncinate process (Figure 4.19) [105]. In general, these tumors are smaller in size and have a less-aggressive behavior than main-duct IPMNs. Malignancy is found in approximately 25% of branch-duct IPMNs and invasive cancer in 15% [118]. On cross-sectional imaging, branch-duct IPMNs have a pleomorphic segmental cystic morphology often described as a "cluster of grapes" appearance. Unlike MCNs that have a "cyst within a cyst" configuration, the cysts in branch-duct IPMNs have a "side by side" configuration [117]. Presence of ductal communication is essential for establishing a diagnosis of branch-duct IPMN and is best performed on thin collimation multiplanar MRCP. Often times, the MPD remains nondilated in branch-duct IPMN. In IPMNs, EUS-guided cyst fluid analysis is typically positive for mucin and shows elevated amylase and CEA levels. This helps to differentiate IPMNs from MCNs (low amylase levels, high CEA levels) and pseudocysts (high amylase levels, low CEA levels).

The risk factors for malignancy in IPMNs include age >70 years, the presence of symptoms (e.g., abdominal pain, jaundice, weight loss, new-onset diabetes), dilatation of the MPD >1 cm, mural nodules, main-duct disease, and cysts >3 cm in size [105]. Main-duct and mixed/combined-duct IPMNs should be treated by surgical resection, given the high incidence of malignancy in these tumors. The recommendations for branch-duct IPMNs are less clear. Asymptomatic tumors <3 cm with an MPD ≤ 6 mm and no mural nodules may be managed conservatively by periodic imaging surveillance [118]. Tumors that do not fulfill this criterion should be considered for surgery. The optimal frequency and duration of follow up is unclear although the International Association of Pancreatology proposes annual follow up for tumors <1 cm, 6–12 monthly follow up for tumors measuring 1–2 cm, and 3–6 monthly follow up for tumors >2 cm [118]. In invasive IPMNs, Chari et al. [119] and Jang et al. [120] found comparable recurrence rates for total pancreatectomy compared to partial pancreatectomy, given that most recurrences were due to extra-pancreatic metastases. Given that total pancreatectomy does not confer a survival advantage compared to partial pancreatectomy but is associated with increased morbidity including pancreatic insufficiency, current guidelines advocate performing oncologic partial pancreatic resections for IPMNs reserving total pancreatectomy for main-duct IPMNs with diffuse pancreatic involvement. The 5-year survival rate following surgery is >70% for noninvasive IPMNs and 30%–50% for invasive IPMNs [105].

4.10 Conclusions

A wide range of benign and malignant, diffuse and focal disease entities affect the pancreas. This chapter provides a review of some of these pathologies focusing on their clinical and imaging findings and the imaging techniques used to optimize disease characterization and differentiation.

References

1. Mitchell AWM, Dick R. Liver, gall bladder pancreas and spleen. In: Butler P, Mitchell A, Ellis H, eds. *Applied Radiological Anatomy*. Cambridge: Cambridge University Press; 1999:253–6.
2. Drake R, Vogl W, Mitchell, A. *Gray's Anatomy for Students*. 1st ed. Canada: Elsevier; 2005.
3. Sadler TW. *Langman's Medical Embryology*. 9th ed. United States of America: Lippincott Williams & Wilkins; 2004.
4. Dhar A, Goenka MK, Kochhar R, Nagi B, Bhasin DK, Singh K. Pancrease divisum: five years' experience in a teaching hospital. *Indian J Gastroenterol*. 1996;15:7–9.
5. Bertin C, Pelletier AL, Vullierme MP et al. Pancreas divisum is not a cause of pancreatitis by itself but acts as a partner of genetic mutations. *Am J Gastroenterol*. 2012 Feb;107(2):311–7.
6. Widmaier E, Raff H, Strang K. *Vander, Sherman and Luciano's Human Physiology: The Mechanisms of Body Function*. 9th ed. United States of America: McGraw-Hill; 2004.
7. Robertson MB, Choe KA, Joseph PM. Review of the abdominal manifestations of cystic fibrosis in the adult patient. *Radiographics*. 2006 May-Jun;26(3):679–90.
8. Lugo-Olivieri CH, Soyer PA, Fishman EK. Cystic fibrosis: spectrum of thoracic and abdominal CT findings in the adult patient. *Clin Imaging*. 1998 Sep-Oct;22(5):346–54.
9. Agrons GA, Corse WR, Markowitz RI, Suarez ES, Perry DR. Gastrointestinal manifestations of cystic fibrosis: radiologic-pathologic correlation. *Radiographics*. 1996 Jul;16(4):871–93.
10. King LJ, Scurr ED, Murugan N, Williams SG, Westaby D, Healy JC. Hepatobiliary and pancreatic manifestations of cystic fibrosis: MR imaging appearances. *Radiographics*. 2000 May-Jun;20(3):767–77.
11. Boat TF. Cystic fibrosis. In: Behrman RE, Klieg-man RM, Jenson HB, eds. *Nelson Textbook of Pediatrics*. 17th ed. Philadelphia, PA: Saunders; 2004:1437–50.
12. Gilljam M, Ellis L, Corey M, Zielenski J, Durie P, Tullis DE. Clinical manifestations of cystic fibrosis among patients with diagnosis in adulthood. *Chest*. 2004 Oct;126(4):1215–24.
13. Nakamura M, Katada N, Sakakibara A et al. Huge lipomatous pseudohypertrophy of the pancreas. *Am J Gastroenterol*. 1979; 72:171.
14. Jäger HJ, Mehring U, Götz GF et al. Radiological features of the visceral and skeletal involvement of hemochromatosis. *Eur Radiol*. 1997;7(8):1199–206.
15. Lonser RR, Glenn GM, Walther M et al. von Hippel-Lindau disease. *Lancet*. 2003 Jun 14;361(9374):2059–67.
16. Mohr VH, Vortmeyer AO, Zhuang Z et al. Histopathology and molecular genetics of multiple cysts and microcystic (serous) adenomas of the pancreas in von Hippel–Lindau patients. *Am J Pathol*. 2000;157:1615–21.
17. Neumann HP, Dinkel E, Brambs H et al. Pancreatic lesions in the von Hippel–Lindau syndrome. *Gastroenterology*. 1991 Aug;101(2):465–71.
18. Hammel PR, Vilgrain V, Terris B et al. Pancreatic involvement in von Hippel–Lindau disease. The Groupe Francophone d'Etude de la Maladie de von Hippel-Lindau. *Gastroenterology*. 2000 Oct;119(4):1087–95.
19. Hough DM, Stephens DH, Johnson CD, Binkovitz LA. Pancreatic lesions in von Hippel–Lindau disease: prevalence, clinical significance, and CT findings. *AJR Am J Roentgenol*. 1994 May;162(5):1091–4.
20. Frossard JL, Steer ML, Pastor CM. Acute pancreatitis. *Lancet*. 2008 Jan 12;371(9607):143–52.
21. Matull WR, Pereira SP, O'Donohue JW. Biochemical markers of acute pancreatitis. *J Clin Pathol*. 2006;59:340–44.
22. Acute Pancreatitis Classification Working Group. Revision of the Atlanta classification of acute pancreatitis 2008. Available at: www.pancreasclub.com/resources/AtlantaClassification.pdf (accessed 15/12/11).
23. Balthazar EJ, Robinson DL, Megibow AJ, Ranson JH. Acute pancreatitis: value of CT in establishing prognosis. *Radiology*. 1990 Feb;174(2):331–6.
24. Mortele KJ, Wiesner W, Intriere L et al. A modified CT severity index for evaluating acute pancreatitis: improved correlation with patient outcome. *AJR Am J Roentgenol*. 2004 Nov;183(5):1261–5.
25. Bollen TL, Singh VK, Maurer R et al. Comparative evaluation of the modified CT severity index and CT severity index in assessing severity of acute pancreatitis. *AJR Am J Roentgenol*. 2011 Aug;197(2):386–92.
26. Brun A, Agarwal N, Pitchumoni CS. Fluid collections in and around the pancreas in acute pancreatitis. *J Clin Gastroenterol*. 2011 Aug;45(7):614–25.
27. Siegelman SS, Copeland BE, Saba GP, Cameron JL, Sanders RC, Zerhouni EA. CT of fluid collections associated with pancreatitis. *AJR Am J Roentgenol*. 1980;134:1121–32.

28. Bradley EL, Gonzalez AC, Clements JL Jr. Acute pancreatic pseudocysts: incidence and implications. *Ann Surg.* 1976;184:734–7.

29. Johnson CD. Timing of intervention in acute pancreatitis. *Postgrad Med J.* 1993;69:509–515.

30. Stringfellow G, Vansonnenberg E, Casola G et al. Management of fluid collections in acute pancreatitis. In: *The Pancreas: An Integrated Textbook of Basic Science, Medicine and Surgery.* 2nd ed. Malden, MA: Blackwell Publishing Limited; 2009:344–55.

31. Maringhini A, Uomo G, Patti R et al. Pseudocysts in acute nonalcoholic pancreatitis: incidence and natural history. *Dig Dis Sci.* 1999;44:1669–73.

32. London NJ, Neoptolemos JP, Lavelle J, Bailey I, James D. Serial computed tomography scanning in acute pancreatitis: a prospective study. *Gut.* 1989;30:397–403.

33. Nealon WH, Bhutani M, Riall TS, Raju G, Ozkan O, Neilan R. A unifying concept: pancreatic ductal anatomy both predicts and determines the major complications resulting from pancreatitis. *J Am Coll Surg.* 2009;208:790–9;discussion 799–801.

34. Cannon JW, Callery MP, Vollmer CM Jr. Diagnosis and management of pancreatic pseudocysts: what is the evidence? *J Am Coll Surg.* 2009 Sep;209(3):385–93.

35. Cizginer S, Turner B, Bilge AR, Karaca C, Pitman MB, Brugge WR. Cyst fluid carcinoembryonic antigen is an accurate diagnostic marker of pancreatic mucinous cysts. *Pancreas.* 2011 Oct;40(7):1024–8.

36. Bollen TL, van Santvoort HC, Besselink MG, van Es WH, Gooszen HG, van Leeuwen MS. Update on acute pancreatitis: ultrasound, computed tomography, and magnetic resonance imaging features. *Semin Ultrasound CT MR.* 2007 Oct;28(5):371–83.

37. Morgan DE, Baron TH, Smith JK, Robbin ML, Kenney PJ. Pancreatic fluid collections prior to intervention: evaluation with MR imaging compared with CT and US. *Radiology.* 1997;203(3):773–8.

38. Ward J, Chalmers AG, Guthrie AJ, Larvin M, Robinson PJ. T2-weighted and dynamic enhanced MRI in acute pancreatitis: comparison with contrast enhanced CT. *Clin Radiol.* 1997;52(2):109–14.

39. Morgan DE. Imaging of acute pancreatitis and its complications. *Clin Gastroenterol Hepatol.* 2008 Oct;6(10):1077–85.

40. Takahashi N, Papachristou GI, Schmit GD et al. CT findings of walled-off pancreatic necrosis (WOPN): differentiation from pseudocyst and prediction of outcome after endoscopic therapy. *Eur Radiol.* 2008 Nov;18(11):2522–9.

41. Butler JR, Eckert GJ, Zyromski NJ, Leonardi MJ, Lillemoe KD, Howard TJ. Natural history of pancreatitis-induced splenic vein thrombosis: a systematic review and meta-analysis of its incidence and rate of gastrointestinal bleeding. *HPB (Oxford).* 2011 Dec;13(12):839–45.

42. Mallick IH, Winslet MC. Vascular complications of pancreatitis. *JOP.* 2004 Sep 10;5(5):328–37.

43. White AF, Baum S, Buranasiri S. Aneurysms secondary to pancreatitis. *AJR Am J Roentgenol.* 1976 Sep;127(3):393–6.

44. Balthazar EJ, Fisher LA. Hemorrhagic complications of pancreatitis: radiologic evaluation with emphasis on CT imaging. *Pancreatology.* 2001;1(4):306–13.

45. Sharma PK, Madan K, Garg PK. Hemorrhage in acute pancreatitis: should gastrointestinal bleeding be considered an organ failure? *Pancreas.* 2008 Mar;36(2):141–5.

46. Braganza JM, Lee SH, McCloy RF, McMahon MJ. Chronic pancreatitis. *Lancet.* 2011 Apr 2;377(9772):1184–97.

47. Witt H, Apte MV, Keim V, Wilson JS. Chronic pancreatitis: challenges and advances in pathogenesis, genetics, diagnosis, and therapy. *Gastroenterology.* 2007 Apr;132(4):1557–73.

48. Chari ST. Chronic pancreatitis: classification, relationship to acute pancreatitis, and early diagnosis. *J Gastroenterol.* 2007 Jan;42 Suppl 17:58–9.

49. Sainani N, Catalano O, Sahani D. Pancreas. In: Haaga J, Dogra V, Forsting M, Gilkeson R, Ha HK, Sundaram M, eds. *CT and MRI of the Whole Body.* 5th ed. China: Mosby Elsevier; 2009.

50. Yadav D, Whitcomb DC. The role of alcohol and smoking in pancreatitis. *Nat Rev Gastroenterol Hepatol.* 2010;7:131–45.

51. Wittel UA, Hopt UT, Batra SK. Cigarette smoke-induced pancreatic damage: experimental data. *Langenbecks Arch Surg.* 2008;393:581–88.

52. Hao J-Y, Li G, Pang B. Evidence for cigarette smoke-induced oxidative stress in the rat pancreas. *Inhalation Toxicol.* 2009;21:1007–12.

53. Choueiri NE, Balci NC, Alkaade S, Burton FR. Advanced imaging of chronic pancreatitis. *Curr Gastroenterol Rep.* 2010 Apr;12(2):114–20.

54. Kawamoto S, Siegelman SS, Hruban RH, Fishman EK. Lymphoplasmacytic sclerosing pancreatitis (autoimmune pancreatitis): evaluation with multidetector CT. *Radiographics.* 2008 Jan-Feb;28(1):157–70.

55. Irie H, Honda H, Baba S et al. Autoimmune pancreatitis: CT and MR characteristics. *AJR Am J Roentgenol.* 1998;170(5):1323–7.

56. Finkelberg DL, Sahani D, Deshpande V, Brugge WR. Autoimmune pancreatitis. *N Engl J Med.* 2006 Dec 21;355(25):2670–6.

57. Ito T, Nakano I, Koyanagi S et al. Autoimmune pancreatitis as a new clinical entity: three cases of autoimmune pancreatitis with effective steroid therapy. *Dig Dis Sci.* 1997;42:1458–68.

58. Saito T, Tanaka S, Yoshida H et al. A case of autoimmune pancreatitis responding to steroid therapy: evidence of histologic recovery. *Pancreatology.* 2002;2:550–6.

59. Kojima E, Kimura K, Noda Y, Kobayashi G, Itoh K, Fujita N. Autoimmune pancreatitis and multiple bile duct strictures treated effectively with steroid. *J Gastroenterol.* 2003;38:603–7.

60. Low G, Panu A, Millo N, Leen E. Multimodality imaging of neoplastic and nonneoplastic solid lesions of the pancreas. *Radiographics.* 2011 Jul-Aug;31(4):993–1015.

61. Ros PR, Mortele KJ. Imaging features of pancreatic neoplasms. *JBR–BTR.* 2001;84:239–49.

62. Brennan DD, Zamboni GA, Raptopoulos VD, Kruskal JB. Comprehensive preoperative assessment of pancreatic adenocarcinoma with 64 section volumetric CT. *Radiographics.* 2007;27:1653–66.

63. Lu DS, Reber HA, Krasny RM, Kadell BM, Sayre J. Local staging of pancreatic cancer: criteria for unresectability of

major vessels as revealed by pancreatic phase, thin section helical CT. *AJR Am J Roentgenol.* 1997;168(6):1439–43.

64. Haugh TJ, Raptopoulos V, Siewert B, Matthews JB. Teardrop superior mesenteric vein: CT sign for unresectable carcinoma of the pancreas. *AJR Am J Roentgenol.* 1999;173(6):1509–12.

65. Kosmahl M, Pauser U, Anlauf M, Kloppel G. Pancreatic ductal adenocarcinomas with cystic features: neither rare nor uniform. *Mod Pathol.* 2005;18(9):1157–64.

66. Hanbidge AE. Cancer of the pancreas: the best image for early detection – CT, MRI, PET or US? *Can J Gastroenterol.* 2002;16(2):101–5.

67. DeWitt J, Devereaux B, Chriswell M et al. Comparison of endoscopic ultrasonography and multidetector computed tomography for detecting and staging pancreatic cancer. *Ann Intern Med.* 2004;141(10):753–63.

68. Frohlich A, Diederichs CG, Staib L, Vogel J, Beger HG, Reske SN. Detection of liver metastases from pancreatic cancer using FDG-PET. *J Nucl Med.* 1999;40(2):250–5.

69. Oberg K, Eriksson B. Endocrine tumors of the pancreas. *Best Pract Res Clin Gastroenterol.* 2005;19(5):753–81.

70. Noone TC, Hosey J, Firat Z, Semelka RC. Imaging and localization of islet cell tumors of the pancreas on CT and MRI. *Best Pract Res Clin Endocrinol Metab.* 2005;19(2):195–211.

71. Gouya H, Vignaux O, Angui J et al. CT, endoscopic sonography and a combined protocol for preoperative evaluation of pancreatic insulinomas. *AJR Am J Roentgenol.* 2003;181(4):987–92.

72. Owen NJ, Sohaib SA, Peppercorn PD et al. MRI of pancreatic neuroendocrine tumors. *Br J Radiol.* 2001;74(886):968–73.

73. Thoeni RF, Mueller-Lisse UG, Chan R, Do NK, Shyn PB. Detection of small functional islet cell tumors in the pancreas: selection of MR imaging sequences for optimal sensitivity. *Radiology.* 2000;214(2):483–90.

74. Ricke J, Klose KJ, Mignon M, Oberg K, Wiedenmann B. Standardisation of imaging in neuroendocrine tumors: results of a European Delphi process. *Eur J Radiol.* 2001;37(1):8–17.

75. Frantz VK. Tumors of the pancreas. In: *Atlas of Tumor Pathology: FASC* 27–28, ser 7. Washington, DC: Armed Forces Institute of Pathology; 1959:32–3.

76. Adams AL, Siegal GP, Jhala NC. Solid pseudopapillary tumor of the pancreas: a review of salient clinical and pathologic features. *Adv Anat Pathol.* 2008;15(1):39–45.

77. Buetow PC, Buck JL, Pantongrag-Brown L, Beck KG, Ros PR, Adair CF. Solid and papillary epithelial neoplasm of the pancreas: Imaging-pathologic correlation on 56 cases. *Radiology.* 1996;199(3):707–11.

78. Al-Qahtani S, Gudinchet F, Laswed T et al. Solid pseudopapillary tumor of the pancreas in children: typical radiological findings and pathological correlation. *Clin Imaging.* 2010;34(2):152–6.

79. Yao X, Ji Y, Zeng M, Rao S, Yang B. Solid pseudopapillary tumor of the pancreas: cross-sectional imaging and pathologic correlation. *Pancreas.* 2010;39(4):486–91.

80. Cantisani V, Mortele KJ, Levy A et al. MR imaging features of solid pseudopapillary tumor of the pancreas in adult and pediatric patients. *AJR Am J Roentgenol.* 2003;181(2):395–401.

81. Chung EM, Travis MD, Conran RM. Pancreatic tumors in children: radiologic-pathologic correlation. *Radiographics.* 2006;26(4):1211–38.

82. Montemarano H, Lonergan GJ, Bulas DI, Selby DM. Pancreatoblastoma: imaging findings in 10 patients and review of the literature. *Radiology.* 2000;214(2):476–82.

83. Zucca E, Roggero E, Bertoni F, Cavalli F. Primary extranodal non Hodgkin's lymphomas. Part 1: Gastrointestinal, cutaneous and genitourinary lymphomas. *Ann Oncol.* 1997;8(8):727–37.

84. Merkle EM, Bender GN, Brambs HJ. Imaging findings in pancreatic lymphoma: differential aspects. *AJR Am J Roentgenol.* 2000;174(3):671–5.

85. Nayer H, Weir EG, Sheth S, Ali SZ. Primary pancreatic lymphomas: a cytopathologic analysis of a rare malignancy. *Cancer.* 2004;102(5):315–21.

86. Tsitouridis I, Diamantopoulou A, Michaelides M, Arvanity M, Papaioannou S. Pancreatic metastases: CT and MRI findings. *Diagn Interv Radiol.* 2010;16(1):45–51.

87. Muranaka T, Teshima K, Honda H, Nanjo T, Hanaka K, Oshiumi Y. Computed tomography and histologic appearance of pancreatic metastases from distant sources. *Acta Radiol.* 1989;30(6):615–9.

88. Kimura W, Nagai H, Kuroda A, Muto T, Esaki Y. Analysis of small cystic lesions of the pancreas. *Int J Pancreatol.* 1995;18(3):197–206.

89. Zhang XM, Mitchell DG, Dohke M, Holland GA, Parker L. Pancreatic cysts: depiction on single-shot fast spin-echo MR images. *Radiology.* 2002 May;223(2):547–53.

90. Spinelli KS, Fromwiller TE, Daniel RA et al. Cystic pancreatic neoplasms: observe or operate. *Ann Surg.* 2004 May;239(5):651–7; discussion 657–9.

91. Laffan TA, Horton KM, Klein AP et al. Prevalence of unsuspected pancreatic cysts on MDCT. *AJR Am J Roentgenol.* 2008 Sep;191(3):802–7.

92. de Jong K, Nio CY, Hermans JJ et al. High prevalence of pancreatic cysts detected by screening magnetic resonance imaging examinations. *Clin Gastroenterol Hepatol.* 2010 Sep;8(9):806–11.

93. Lee KS, Sekhar A, Rofsky NM, Pedrosa I. Prevalence of incidental pancreatic cysts in the adult population on MR imaging. *Am J Gastroenterol.* 2010 Sep;105(9):2079–84.

94. Megibow AJ, Baker ME, Gore RM, Taylor A. The incidental pancreatic cyst. *Radiol Clin North Am.* 2011 Mar;49(2):349–59.

95. Berland LL, Silverman SG, Gore RM et al. Managing incidental findings on abdominal CT: white paper of the ACR incidental findings committee. *J Am Coll Radiol.* 2010 Oct;7(10):754–73.

96. Sakorafas GH, Smyrniotis V, Reid-Lombardo KM, Sarr MG. Primary pancreatic cystic neoplasms revisited. Part I: serous cystic neoplasms. *Surg Oncol.* 2011 Jun;20(2):e84–92.

97. Tran Cao HS, Kellogg B, Lowy AM, Bouvet M. Cystic neoplasms of the pancreas. *Surg Oncol Clin N Am.* 2010 Apr;19(2):267–95.

98. Strobel O, Z'graggen K, Schmitz-Winnenthal FH et al. Risk of malignancy in serous cystic neoplasms of the pancreas. *Digestion.* 2003;68(1):24–33.

99. Yoshimi N, Sugie S, Tanaka T et al. A rare case of serous cystadenocarcinoma of the pancreas. *Cancer.* 1992 May 15;69(10):2449–53.

100. Sarr MG, Kendrick ML, Nagorney DM, Thompson GB, Farley DR, Farnell MB. Cystic neoplasms of the pancreas: benign to malignant epithelial neoplasms. *Surg Clin North Am.* 2001 Jun;81(3):497–509.

101. Klöppel G, Kosmahl M. Cystic lesions and neoplasms of the pancreas. The features are becoming clearer. *Pancreatology.* 2001;1(6):648–55.

102. Tseng JF, Warshaw AL, Sahani DV, Lauwers GY, Rattner DW, Fernandez-del Castillo C. Serous cystadenoma of the pancreas: tumor growth rates and recommendations for treatment. *Ann Surg.* 2005 Sep;242(3):413–9; discussion 419–21.

103. Sakorafas GH, Sarr MG. Cystic neoplasms of the pancreas: What a clinician should know. *Cancer Treat Rev.* 2005 Nov;31(7):507–35.

104. Sahani DV, Kadavigere R, Saokar A, Fernandez-del Castillo C, Brugge WR, Hahn PF. Cystic pancreatic lesions: a simple imaging-based classification system for guiding management. *Radiographics.* 2005 Nov-Dec;25(6):1471–84.

105. Sakorafas GH, Smyrniotis V, Reid-Lombardo KM, Sarr MG. Primary pancreatic cystic neoplasms revisited. Part III. Intraductal papillary mucinous neoplasms. *Surg Oncol.* 2011 Jun;20(2):e109–18.

106. Goh BK, Tan YM, Chung YF et al. A review of mucinous cystic neoplasms of the pancreas defined by ovarian-type stroma: clinicopathological features of 344 patients. *World J Surg.* 2006 Dec;30(12):2236–45.

107. de Calan L, Levard H, Hennet H, Fingerhut A. Pancreatic cystadenoma and cystadenocarcinoma: diagnostic value of preoperative morphological investigations. *Eur J Surg.* 1995 Jan;161(1):35–40.

108. Crippa S, Salvia R, Warshaw AL et al. Mucinous cystic neoplasm of the pancreas is not an aggressive entity: lessons from 163 resected patients. *Ann Surg.* 2008 Apr;247(4):571–9.

109. Fernández-del Castillo C, Targarona J, Thayer SP, Rattner DW, Brugge WR, Warshaw AL. Incidental pancreatic cysts: clinicopathologic characteristics and comparison with symptomatic patients. *Arch Surg.* 2003 Apr;138(4):427–3; discussion 433–4.

110. Kalb B, Sarmiento JM, Kooby DA, Adsay NV, Martin DR. MR imaging of cystic lesions of the pancreas. *Radiographics.* 2009 Oct;29(6):1749–65.

111. Brugge WR, Lewandrowski K, Lee-Lewandrowski E et al. Diagnosis of pancreatic cystic neoplasms: a report of the cooperative pancreatic cyst study. *Gastroenterology.* 2004 May;126(5):1330–6.

112. Hutchins GF, Draganov PV. Cystic neoplasms of the pancreas: A diagnostic challenge. *World J Gastroenterol.* 2009;15(1):48–54.

113. van der Waaij LA, van Dullemen HM, Porte RJ. Cyst fluid analysis in the differential diagnosis of pancreatic cystic lesions: a pooled analysis. *Gastrointest Endosc.* 2005 Sep;62(3):383–9.

114. Ohhashi K, Murakimi Y, Maruyama M et al. Four cases of mucin producing cancer of the pancreas on specific findings of the papilla of Vater. *Prog Dig Endosc.* 1982;20:348–51.

115. Fasanella KE, McGrath K. Cystic lesions and intraductal neoplasms of the pancreas. *Best Pract Res Clin Gastroenterol.* 2009;23(1):35–48.

116. Yoon WJ, Ryu JK, Lee JK et al. Extrapancreatic malignancies in patients with intraductal papillary mucinous neoplasm of the pancreas: prevalence, associated factors, and comparison with patients with other pancreatic cystic neoplasms. *Ann Surg Oncol.* 2008 Nov;15(11):3193–8.

117. Bhosale P, Balachandran A, Tamm E. Imaging of benign and malignant cystic pancreatic lesions and a strategy for follow up. *World J Radiol.* 2010 Sep 28;2(9):345–53.

118. Tanaka M, Chari S, Adsay V et al. International Association of Pancreatology. International consensus guidelines for management of intraductal papillary mucinous neoplasms and mucinous cystic neoplasms of the pancreas. *Pancreatology.* 2006;6(1–2):17–32.

119. Chari ST, Yadav D, Smyrk TC et al. Study of recurrence after surgical resection of intraductal papillary mucinous neoplasm of the pancreas. *Gastroenterology.* 2002 Nov;123(5):1500–7.

120. Jang JY, Kim SW, Ahn YJ et al. Multicenter analysis of clinicopathologic features of intraductal papillary mucinous tumor of the pancreas: is it possible to predict the malignancy before surgery? *Ann Surg Oncol.* 2005 Feb;12(2):124–32.

5

Adrenal Gland

Shaunagh McDermott, Owen J. O'Connor,
Martin J. Shelly, and Michael A. Blake

CONTENTS

5.1 CT Techniques

5.1.1 Unenhanced CT

This test is based on the premise that unenhanced CT can detect intracytoplasmic fat and uses the fact that around 70% of adrenal adenomas contain significant intracellular lipid, in contrast to almost all malignant lesions that do not. Korobkin et al. [1] showed an inverse relationship between the intracytoplasmic fat content and the CT density value. Nonadenomatous lesions typically have higher CT density values because their cytoplasm is relatively lipid poor, except for myelolipomatous lesions.

Lee et al. first reported that unenhanced CT densitometry could effectively differentiate many adrenal adenomas from nonadenomatous disease. They found that the mean attenuation of adenomas (−2.2 Hounsfield unit [HU] ± 16) was significantly lower than that of nonadenomas (28.9 HU ± 10.6). By using a threshold of 0 HU, these lesions could be differentiated with sensitivity and specificity of 47% and 100%, respectively [2]. A meta-analysis of published studies found that if the CT attenuation threshold is raised to 10 HU, the test sensitivity becomes far higher (71%) while high specificity (98%) is maintained [3]. Therefore in clinical practice, 10 HU is the most widely used threshold value for the diagnosis of a lipid-rich adrenal adenoma (Figure 5.1).

A caveat to unenhanced CT densitometry is that two independent studies reported that different single-detector and multi-detector helical scanners produce slightly different but statistically significant unenhanced

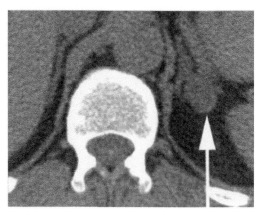

FIGURE 5.1
A 50-year-old man diagnosed with melanoma. A 2 cm left adrenal lesion (arrow) identified on staging computed tomography (CT). On a follow-up noncontrast study, the attenuation measured 8 HU consistent with a lipid-rich adenoma. This lesion was stable on follow-up imaging.

attenuation levels [4,5], which sometimes could conceivably lead to erroneous categorization.

5.1.2 CT Washout

Washout refers to the reduction of attenuation values from a peak value in the adrenal lesion at CT during a variable period after intravenous injection of a bolus of contrast material. A study by Korobkin et al. [6] found that adrenal adenomas show a much earlier and more rapid washout of contrast enhancement than do nonadenomas.

However, as delayed CT densitometry measurements may depend on the type, total dose, and injection rate of intravenous contrast material, as well as on the cardiac output of the patient, an absolute attenuation measurement on a delayed scan was not found to be very useful [7–10]. Fortuitously, it was observed that the ratio of adrenal attenuation measurements on the washout-delayed scan when compared with the initial dynamic enhanced study could help characterize adrenal lesions with great precision [8,11]. The percentage washout represents the percentage of the initial wash-in of enhancement that is washed out at the time of delayed scanning [6–8]. If an unenhanced scan has been obtained, an absolute percentage washout (APW) can be calculated. If no unenhanced·scan is available, it has proved just as useful in clinical practice to calculate the relative percentage washout (RPW). These percentage washouts are easy to calculate using the following equations:

$$APW = \{(EHU - DHU)/(EHU - UHU)\} \times 100$$
$$RPW = \{(EHU - DHU)/(EHU)\} \times 100$$

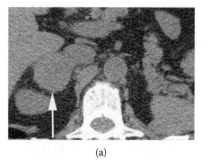

(a)

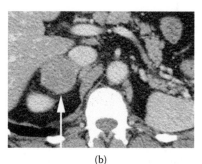

(b)

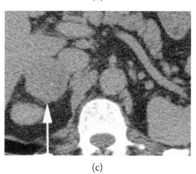

(c)

FIGURE 5.2
A 64-year-old man with an enlarging right adrenal mass (arrow), now measuring 4.5 cm. It measured 26 HU on the noncontrast study (a), 64 HU on the enhanced study (b), and 44 HU on the 15-minute delayed study (c). The calculated absolute percentage washout (APW) was 53%, consistent with a nonadenomatous lesion. Follow-up biopsy confirmed metastatic high-grade carcinoma.

Applying a percentage washout threshold to the data set makes it possible to determine an optimal level that permits sufficient sensitivity and specificity for the test to be useful. Controversy exists as to whether to use a 5-, 10-, or 15-minute contrast-enhanced delayed images to calculate the washout fraction.

If a 15-minute delay after contrast administration protocol is used, an absolute washout of 60% or higher has reported sensitivity of 86%–88% and specificity of 92%–96% for the diagnosis of adenoma (Figure 5.2) [6,9]. After 15 minutes, if a RPW of 40% or higher is achieved, sensitivity is 96% and specificity is 100% for the diagnosis of an adenoma [9].

In similar fashion, if a 10-minute delayed protocol is used, sensitivity of 100% and specificity of 98% has been obtained for a threshold APW value of 52%. Also if a 10-minute protocol is used, an RPW of greater than

37.5% had reported sensitivity and specificity of 100% and 95%, respectively, for the detection of malignant lesions (Figure 5.3) [12].

However, Sangwaiya et al. published a study on reassessing the accuracy of the 10-minute delay imaging protocol in characterizing adrenal lesions in a large cohort of patients. They concluded that the 10-minute delayed adrenal contrast washout protocol has reduced sensitivity for the detection of adenomas compared with results from prior studies, and the test sensitivity appears to be clinically suboptimal [13].

Kamiyama et al., however, have recently recommended a 5-minute delayed imaging protocol. They demonstrated that a combination of diagnostic parameters (tumor size, unenhanced attenuation, 35-second and 5-minute enhanced attenuation, wash-in and washout attenuation, percentage enhancement washout ratio, and relative percentage enhancement washout ratio) yielded diagnostic results comparable with those of longer scanning times [14]. Foti et al. assessed the accuracy of quadriphasic contrast-enhanced CT also with 5-minute delays in distinguishing adenomas from nonadenomas. They proposed a three-step algorithm: step one, unenhanced attenuation ≤10 HU; step two, maximum attenuation reached during the delayed phase; step three, RPW using

a ≥30% threshold. This algorithm reported an accuracy of 97.1% [15].

Furthermore, Parks et al. have assessed adrenal incidentalomas detected and characterized by triphasic helical CT using a modified relative percentage of the enhancement washout (mRPEW) values at a still shorter delay after contrast administration. The mRPEW was defined as: ([attenuation value at portal phase CT – attenuation value at delayed phase CT at 3 minutes]/ [attenuation value at portal phase CT]) × 100. With a cutoff value >25%, the positive predictive value and specificity were 100%. With a cutoff value >5%, the negative predictive value and sensitivity for adenomas was 100%, but the accuracy was only 57%. If an adrenal mass had an mRPEW value of >25% or ≤5%, the mass was diagnosed as an adenoma or a metastasis, respectively, on triphasic helical CT including 3-minute delays [16].

5.1.3 Perfusion CT

The basis for the use of perfusion CT (PCT) in oncology is that the microvascular changes in angiogenesis are reflected by increased tumor perfusion in vivo [17]. PCT shows a more linear relationship between attenuation and contrast concentration, and thus provides absolute quantitative information about various perfusion parameters, such as blood volume (BV), blood flow (BF), mean transit time, and permeability surface area production (PS). These parameters can be used to demonstrate the hemodynamic changes in tumor tissues, in which neovascularization of tumors produces a high microvessel density (MVD). Increasing MVD leads to an increase in BF, BV, and the surface area of vessel walls. The elevation of vascular endothelial growth factor production in tumor tissues is likely to increase the permeability of these vessel walls [18].

Qiao et al. performed first-pass PCT imaging in 32 patients with adrenal masses. They reported that the perfusion parameters such as BV, BF, and PS were statistically different between the two groups, with adenomas showing higher mean BV (12.18 vs. 3.86), BF (97.51 vs. 45.99), and PS (21.73 vs. 10.93) compared with metastases [19]. A more recent study by Qin et al. also found that PCT imaging can be used to differentiate between adenomas and nonadenomas, primarily using BV measurement. In addition, PS in adenomas was significantly higher that than in nonadenomas [20].

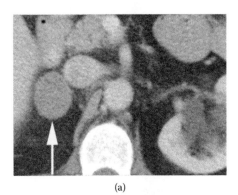

(a)

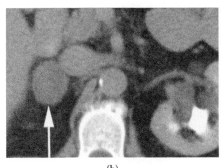

(b)

FIGURE 5.3
A 61-year-old man with a history of bladder cancer being investigated for anemia. CT demonstrated a 3.5 cm right adrenal mass (arrow), which measured 58 HU on the enhanced scan (a) and 26 HU on the 10-minute delayed scan (b). The relative percentage washout was calculated as 55%, consistent with an adrenal adenoma. The mass was stable on follow-up imaging.

5.1.4 Dual-Energy CT

Dual-energy CT uses two rotating tubes to acquire both high- and low-voltage images. Since the images are dependent on the attenuation of the x-ray beam, which depends on the voltage applied across the tube, each image acquired is energy dependent. Attenuation is also dependent on the density of the material through which the beam passes, and knowing the energy of the beam allows assumptions to be made about the attenuating material based on the spectral properties of the detected radiation.

Results of studies on the appearance of adrenal adenomas at low (e.g., 80 kVp) and high (e.g., 140 kVp) energies have been mixed. In a preliminary investigation of the attenuation values of adrenal adenomas, Kalra et al. [21] reported a decrease in mean attenuation of 20 ± 5.5 HU (range 0–38) at 80 kVp from that at 140 kVp (n = 17 adenomas in 16 patients). In a follow-up study of 69 adenomas in 58 patients imaged at 80 and 120 kVp, the authors reported a decrease in mean attenuation of only 3.3 HU (range 0–25 HU) (Figure 5.4) [22]. Gupta et al. reported

that of 26 adenomas, half (n = 13) demonstrated a mean decrease of 5.5 ± 2.9 HU at 80 kVp from that at 140 kVp. The other half demonstrated a mean increase of 6.3 ± 4.5 HU at 80 kVp. The variable appearance of adrenal adenomas at dual-energy CT may be due to varying amounts of intracellular lipids. In addition, Gupta et al. [23] reported that all metastases (n = 5) demonstrated a mean increase of 9.2 + 4.3 HU at 80 kVp. Larger studies are needed to determine if a decrease in attenuation at 80 kVp is a specific (but not a sensitive) sign of adenoma (Figure 5.5). The use of virtual unenhanced images also may help characterize some adrenal lesions as benign adenomas, which would have been characterized as indeterminate if only enhanced images were available.

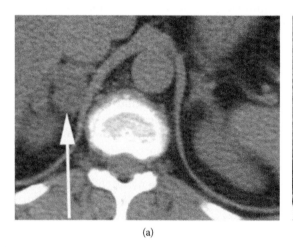
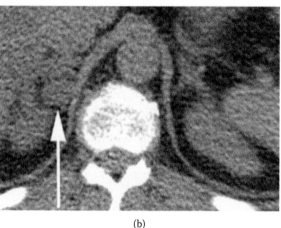

(a)　　　　　　　　　　　　　　　　　　(b)

FIGURE 5.4

A 51-year-old woman with a diagnosis of multiple endocrine neoplasia type 1. A dedicated adrenal washout CT identified a 2.3 cm right adrenal mass (arrow) but was inconclusive in characterizing the mass. On dual-energy CT, the mass measured 20 HU on the 120 kVp scan (a) and 13 HU on the 80 kVP scan (b), consistent with an adenoma. This was confirmed on chemical shift magnetic resonance imaging (CS-MRI), and the lesion was stable on follow-up imaging.

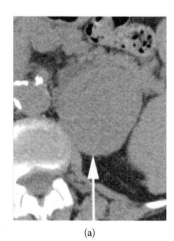
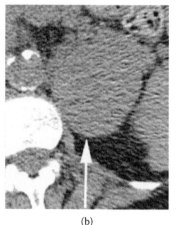

(a)　　　　　　　　　(b)

FIGURE 5.5

An 81-year-old woman with a left adrenal mass found on CT for constipation underwent a dual-energy CT. The mass measured 39 HU on the 120 kVp scan (a) and 45 HU on the 80 kVp scan (b), with the increase between the 120 and 80 kVp outruling an adenoma. Percutaneous biopsy was positive for metastatic small cell carcinoma.

5.1.5 CT Histogram Analysis

Mean CT attenuation results in averaging of tissue density over the CT pixels. Tissue heterogeneity, therefore, may result in inadequate information being obtained about densities present in a smaller volume from a region of interest where the mean CT attenuation is measured. CT histogram analysis provides objective insight into the varying CT densities and the number of pixels with these densities.

Histogram analysis for the evaluation of adrenal masses was first reported by Bae et al. [24]. Subsequent studies have shown that the sensitivity and specificity of this technique can be improved if a threshold of more than 5%–10% negative pixels is applied for diagnosis of an adenoma [25–30]. Ho et al. concluded that CT histogram analysis was superior to mean CT attenuation analysis for the evaluation of adrenal nodules. They reported a sensitivity of 85% and specificity of 100% for the diagnosis of an adenoma using an unenhanced CT threshold of more than 10% negative pixels. This compared favorably with using an unenhanced CT mean attenuation threshold of less than 10 HU, which yielded a sensitivity of 68% and a specificity of 100% [28]. Halefoglu also found that 10% negative pixel threshold had a higher sensitivity than mean attenuation threshold of less than 10 HU on unenhanced CT (90.9% vs. 77.2%). But with contrast-enhanced CT, although 100% specificity was maintained, the sensitivities obtained for both methods were very poor (28.8% and 12.1%, respectively). Nonetheless, even if infrequent, such confident recognition of an adenoma on a contrast-enhanced scan would be helpful in such cases to avoid the need for additional testing for the individual patient. An earlier study by Halefoglu et al. also found that CT histogram analysis method using a 10% negative pixel threshold

on unenhanced CT gave a high sensitivity (91%) and a perfect specificity for the diagnosis of adrenal adenoma. However, in spite of the good results obtained with the CT histogram analysis method, chemical shift (CS) magnetic resonance imaging (MRI) using adrenal-to-spleen CS ratio and adrenal signal intensity index formulas had a higher sensitivity [29].

5.2 Other Imaging Modalities Used in the Imaging of the Adrenal Glands

5.2.1 Magnetic Resonance Imaging

The principle magnetic resonance (MR) technique used in adrenal evaluation is CS imaging obtained as dual-echo breath-hold gradient echo acquisition. Similar to CT density measurement, this technique depends on the presence of intracytoplasmic lipid in adenomas to separate them from nonadenomas [31,32]. The theory behind CS-MRI is that lipid and water protons precess at different frequencies in a given magnetic field, and the signal from these protons can be either additive or subtractive, depending on the TE (Echo Time) chosen. CS-MRI uses the decrease in signal on out-of-phase images to identify intracellular lipid (Figure 5.6). It has been demonstrated that qualitative evaluation of this drop-off on the MR image is sufficient to diagnose a lipid-rich adenoma [33], but some prefer to use a quantitative method to demonstrate the fractional signal drop-off from the in-phase to the out-of-phase image. A signal drop-off of 16.5% is generally considered to indicate a lipid-rich adenoma [34]. An important caveat to be aware of, however, is that adrenal cortical carcinoma, pheochromocytoma, and

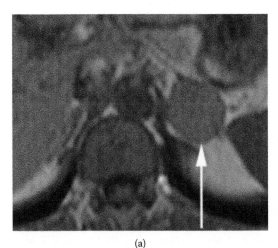

(a)

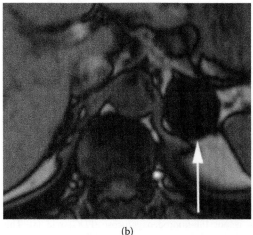

(b)

FIGURE 5.6
A 54-year-old man who had an incidental 3.4 cm left adrenal lesion (arrow) on a CT performed because of abdominal pain. There is a homogenous drop out between the in-phase (a) and out-of-phase (b), consistent with a lipid-rich adenoma.

clear cell renal cell carcinoma metastasis can all sometimes show signal loss on out-of-phase images.

5.2.2 Positron Emission Tomography (PET)

PET and PET–CT using 18F-fluorodeoxyglucose (FDG) is becoming a standard step in the evaluation for metastasis in many oncology patients. In general, metastases have increased FDG uptake because of increased glucose metabolism, and most adrenal metastases show increased activity relative to the liver, whereas most benign adenomas do not. PET-CT further improves diagnostic performance through incorporating CT density measurement analysis of an adrenal mass and allowing its accurate localization. PET and PET-CT can be used to differentiate benign from malignant adrenal masses in patients with cancer, with a sensitivity and specificity ranging from 93% to 100% and 90% to 100%, respectively (Figure 5.7) [35–38]. A 5% false-positive rate for PET-CT has been reported secondary to a variety of

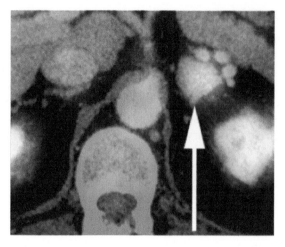

FIGURE 5.8
A 67-year-old man who underwent a PETCT to investigate a degenerative neurological condition. PETCT identified a 2.2 cm FDG-avid left adrenal mass (arrow). This was unchanged in size from a prior CT performed 7 years ago. The mass was excised and pathology confirmed an adrenal adenoma.

causes including significant FDG uptake in some adrenal adenomas (Figure 5.8), adrenal endothelial cysts, and inflammatory and infectious causes [37]. Furthermore, false-negative findings may be seen in adrenal lesions with hemorrhage or necrosis, small (<10 mm) metastatic nodules, and metastases from primary carcinomas that are not FDG avid, including carcinoid tumors and pulmonary brochoalveolarcarcinoma [37].

5.2.3 Single Photon Emission CT

A number of agents have been used in the radionuclide imaging of pheochromocytoma. Iodine-131 or ^{123}I metaiodobenzylguanidine (MIBG) scintigraphy is often useful when clinically suspected pheochromocytoma cannot be localized to confirm that a mass is a pheochromocytoma (Figure 5.9) or to exclude metastatic disease. MIBG has almost 100% specificity but limited sensitivity [39]. Somatostatin receptor scintigraphy performed with octreotide, an analogue of somatostatin, provides another method for localizing pheochromocytoma. However, a conventional dose of octreotide enables localization of pheochromocytoma in less than 30% of cases [40].

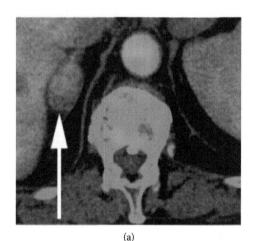

(a)

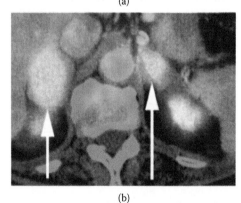

(b)

FIGURE 5.7
An 80-year-old woman with a history of breast cancer. Positron emission tomography CT (PETCT) demonstrated a 3 cm right adrenal lesion (arrow), which is not 18F-fluorodeoxyglucose (FDG)-avid (a). This lesion also demonstrated drop in signal in CS-MRI, consistent with an adenoma. A 78-year-old man with a history of lung cancer. PETCT demonstrated bilateral FDG-avid adrenal lesions (arrows) (b). Biopsy of the right adrenal lesion confirmed metastatic adenocarcinoma.

5.3 Specific Adrenal Entities on CT Imaging

5.3.1 Hyperplasia

In a study performed with 10 mm CT sections, it was reported that normal adrenal limbs should be ≤5 mm [41]. Another study performing CT with both 10 mm and 3 to 5 mm sections showed that slightly but significant

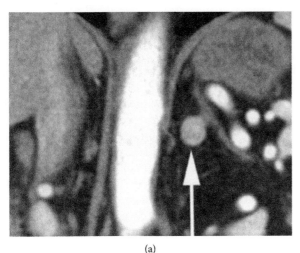

(a)

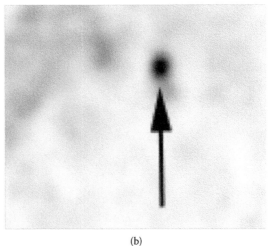

(b)

FIGURE 5.9
A 57-year-old man involved in a MVA (motor vehicle accident) had a CT chest on which a 1.2 cm, avidly enhancing left adrenal nodule (arrow) was identified (a). There was a focus of intense tracer uptake (arrow) on ^{123}I metaiodobenzylguanidine body scan, which correlated with the left adrenal mass (b) and was confirmed on the fused image. This was confirmed as a pheochromocytoma on resection.

larger measurements were obtained using the thinner sections (mean limb width, $\gtrsim$15%) [42]. Another study showed that normal adrenal shape varies, even in the same patient at different levels [43]. The right side can be linear, an inverted V (with or without asymmetric limbs), horizontally linear, or K-shaped. The left adrenal gland has been described as an inverted V, an inverted Y, triangular, or linear [42,43].

Hormonal abnormalities related to the adrenal gland include hypercortisolism (Cushing's syndrome) and hyperaldosteronism (Conn's syndrome).

Hypercortisolism is adrenocorticotropic hormone (ACTH) dependent in 80%–85% of cases: of pituitary origin or in Cushing's disease in 80%–85% and due to an ectopic ACTH-secreting tumor in 10%–15% [42,44]; ACTH-independent Cushing's syndrome is due to either adrenal adenoma or carcinoma in most cases [44]. The adrenal enlargement is most commonly diffuse but can be nodular or mixed. In patients with ACTH-dependent hyperplasia, Sohaib et al. [42] showed that ectopic tumor ACTH produced adrenal hyperplasia in a higher percentage of cases (90%) than pituitary ACTH hypersecretion. In those patients with hyperplasia due to ectopic ACTH production, the adrenal gland morphology was lobular in 40% and either smooth or nodular in 30% each. In the setting of pituitary-induced hyperplasia, 62% of adrenals were enlarged, most commonly smooth (55%), followed by lobular (28%) or nodular (17%) [42].

In the setting of hyperaldsteronism (Conn's syndrome), the absence of an adenoma traditionally suggested adrenal hyperplasia as the cause. With improved CT resolution, gland measurements have proven useful. Lingam et al. [45] revealed that the medial and lateral limbs were significantly larger in hyperplasia. A cutoff of 5 mm was 47% sensitive and 100% specific; using a 3 mm cutoff, sensitivity was 100% and specificity was 54%. In comparison, the absence of an adenoma at imaging was 93.3% sensitive and 84.6% specific.

5.3.2 Myelolipoma

Myelolipoma is a benign tumor composed of mature fat and interspersed hematopoietic elements that resemble bone marrow. Most commonly, myelolipomas originate in an otherwise normal adrenal gland. A review of incidental adrenal lesions in patients with no known malignancy confirmed that 6% of these lesions were myelolipomas [46]. CT allows for accurate quantification of fat content in myelolipomas (Figure 5.10). In the AFIP series of 86 myelolipomas, adrenal myelolipomas contained 50%–90% fat, had an average size of 10 cm, majority (75%) had a pseudocapsule, and calcifications, which were usually small or punctate, were identified in 24% of adrenal myelolipomas [47]. The soft tissue component may enhance following the administration of contrast material.

5.3.3 Adrenal Cyst

The most common adrenal cyst is reportedly a pseudocyst, believed to be a sequela of previous hemorrhage (or possible infection) (Figure 5.11). Wang et al. [48] correlated CT appearances with pathology in seven pseudocysts. Only 43% (3/7) were predominantly cystic, with mixed or solid lesions reflecting organized hematoma; the predominantly cystic lesions contained liquefied hemorrhage (86%). Pseudocysts may be unilocular or multilocular; calcification—mural, septal, or central—was identified in 43%. In 6 of the 32 pseudocysts analyzed by Erickson et al. [49], associated tumors were

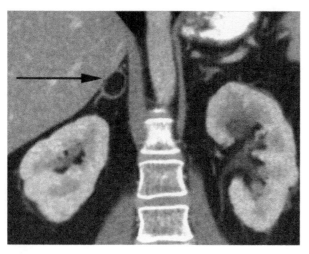

FIGURE 5.10
A 49-year-old woman with a fat-containing lesion of the right adrenal gland (arrow), consistent with a myelolipoma.

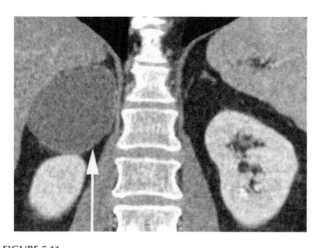

FIGURE 5.11
A 57-year-old man with a history of a gastric gastrointestinal stromal tumor. Staging CT demonstrated a large (8.5 cm), homogenous right adrenal mass with an attenuation of 6 HU (arrow). There is no evidence of enhancement and no FDG uptake on PET. Findings are consistent with an adrenal cyst.

identified, including pheochromocytoma, adenoma, and adrenocortical carcinoma (ACC).

Other adrenal cysts include endothelial cysts, and less commonly, epithelial and parasitic cysts (i.e., echinococcus) [50]. Roznblit et al. [51] reported that pseudocysts were more likely to be unilocular (81%) with calcification (74%); multilocularity and calcification was identified in 44% of endothelial cysts. They also noted that the wall was generally imperceptible in benign cystic masses but measured 4 mm in a cystic pheochromocytoma and >6 mm in a cystic ACC. In addition, the cyst fluid attenuation was higher in tumors (22–25 HU) than in benign nonhemorrhagic cysts (5–17 HU); two hemorrhagic cysts measured 67 and 75 HU.

5.3.4 Hemorrhage

Adrenal injury occasionally occurs in the setting of severe trauma. The prevalence of radiographically detected abnormalities is 2% [52], although the adrenal injury has been reported in 28% of patients studied at autopsy who had sustained significant abdominal trauma [53]. The injury occurs in the right side in up to 90% of cases [54]. CT is the modality of choice for detecting adrenal injury, especially hematoma. The most common CT feature of adrenal injury is a round to oval adrenal hematoma (83% of cases), followed by diffuse irregular hemorrhage obliterating the gland (9%) and uniform adrenal enlargement (9%) [52]. Periadrenal hemorrhage is usually present and is evidenced by an ill-defined adrenal margin, periadrenal stranding, and asymmetric thickening of the diaphragmatic crus. Hematomas vary in attenuation depending on their age. Acute to subacute adrenal hematomas have increased attenuation ranging from 50 to 90 HU. They gradually diminish in size, and there is a corresponding decrease in attenuation at follow-up CT. Calcification may develop a few months after adrenal hemorrhage [55].

Spontaneous adrenal hemorrhage is usually associated with anticoagulant therapy or with stress caused by surgery, sepsis, or hypotension [56]. Nontraumatic adrenal hematomas can be either unilateral or bilateral. Like traumatic hematomas, they are round or oval and may contain periadrenal hemorrhage. The attenuation of these lesions at CT depends on the age of the hematoma. Spontaneous unilateral adrenal hemorrhage may be idiopathic but has been reported to be associated with an underlying adrenal condition such as a cyst, adenoma, hemangioma, myelolipoma, or metastasis [57,58].

5.3.5 Infection

Among infectious disorders, both tuberculosis (TB) and histoplasmosis can involve the adrenal gland [59–63]. The appearance of the gland on CT depends on the chronicity of the infection and whether it has been treated. Most patients have bilateral gland enlargement, mass-like in 50%–65% and adreniform in 35%–50% [59,60,62]. Unenhanced CT shows attenuation to be more commonly homogenous, but one-third is heterogeneous [62]. After contrast injection, the classic appearance of peripheral enhancement with central necrosis is seen in 40%–50% of cases; alternatively, the glands may enhance heterogeneously [59,62]. Untreated TB causes adrenal calcification in 40%–60% of patients [59,62]. Atrophy and calcification both develop after treatment [60,61].

Although *Pneumocystis carinii* is usually considered a respiratory pathogen, in immunocompromised patients such as those with acquired immunodeficiency syndrome, generalized dissemination of *P. carinii* infection from the lungs may occur as a result of failure to achieve adequate blood levels of aerosolized pentamidine. Unenhanced abdominal CT may reveal punctate or coarse calcifications in the adrenal glands as well as in the spleen, liver, kidneys, and lymph nodes [64].

5.3.6 Adenoma

The prevalence of adrenal adenoma is age related. Kloos et al. [65] reported the frequency of unsuspected adenoma according to age, citing 0.14% for patients aged 20–29 years and 7% in those older than 70 years. The majority of adenomas are not functioning although endocrinologists believe that they may be responsible for more subclinical hypercortisolism than was previously appreciated. Although CT does not allow differentiation of functioning from nonfunctioning masses, the presence of contralateral adrenal atrophy suggests that a lesion may be functioning because ACTH secretion is suppressed by elevated cortisol levels [66]. Adenomas are typically well-defined and often homogenous in attenuation, on both noncontrast and postcontrast images [67,68]. The precontrast attenuation varies according to the presence or absence of lipid, with mean attenuation in the range of –2 to 10 HU in lipid-rich adenomas (Figure 5.12) [6,10,11,67,69–71] and higher attenuation (11–25 HU) seen in the setting of lipid-poor adenomas [9,27,72]. Lipid-poor adenomas represent 10%–40% of adenomas [9,72].

5.3.7 Pheochromocytoma

Pheochromocytomas may be homogeneous or heterogeneous, solid or cystic complex masses and may show calcification (Figure 5.13). Smaller tumors tend to have a more uniform attenuation. Most pheochromocytomas have an attenuation higher than 10 HU; rarely, do they contain sufficient intracellular fat to have an attenuation of less than 10 HU [73]. Still, some pheochromocytomas could be incorrectly categorized as adenomas by CT densitometry [3]. Pheochromocytomas with macroscopic fat may also rarely be seen. Conversely, some pheochromocytomas may demonstrate very high attenuation due to hemorrhage. Pheochromocytomas typically enhance avidly, which can be a diagnostic tip-off but can be heterogeneous or show regions of no enhancement due to cystic changes. Pheochromocytomas can demonstrate different and variable washout patterns and may again therefore be confused with either adenomas or metastases [9,11,73,74]. Ten percent of pheochromocytomas are malignant. Metastatic spread or direct local involvement of adjacent structures are the only reliable criteria for the diagnosis of malignant pheochromocytoma.

5.3.8 Adrenocortical Carcinoma

ACC has a bimodal peak (first and fourth decades). A review of 15 published series revealed that on average 55% (range 26%–94%) were functional, manifesting as Cushing syndrome, feminization virilization, or mixed Cushing syndrome—virilization. Hypertension is common in all syndrome types [75]. Alternatively, patients may have pain, a palpable mass, or gastrointestinal complaints.

With respect to size and appearances, ACC is typically a larger mass, with the literature quoting a range from 3 to 25 cm in diameter [76–78]. Fishman et al. reported CT findings in 38 patients and noted that larger masses compressed the kidney posteriorly and the pancreas and stomach anteriorly. Tumors

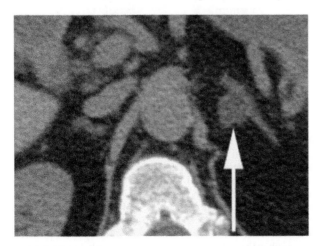

FIGURE 5.12
A 65-year-old man who underwent CT to investigate abnormal liver function tests was found to have a 1.5 cm left adrenal nodule (arrow). This measured 4 HU on the noncontrast study, consistent with a lipid-rich adenoma.

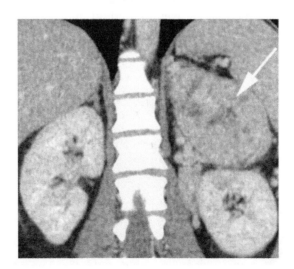

FIGURE 5.13
A 27-year-old man who was found to have high blood pressure of routine preoperative workup. CT demonstrated a 13 cm, heterogeneous left adrenal mass (arrow). The mass was excised and pathology came back as pheochromocytoma.

were inhomogeneous at nonenhanced CT, particularly masses larger than 6 cm, owing to the presence of necrosis. After contrast material infusion, ACC enhances heterogeneously, often peripherally, with a thin rim of enhancing capsules seen in some cases [78]. Studies of lesion washout have reported that ACC typically has a RPW of less than 40% [71,79]. Invasion of the inferior vena cava (IVC) is a well-known complication of ACC (Figure 5.14); however, other lesions can invade the IVC. Cuevas et al. [80] reviewed 21 cases and found that, in addition to leiomyosarcoma of the IVC, IVC involvement occurred with renal cell carcinoma, leiomyosarcoma of the adrenal, hepatocellular carcinoma, and a retroperitoneal metastasis. Some benign tumors can invade the IVC, such as uterine leiomyomas [81]; in addition, reports indicate that pheochromocytoma rarely invades the IVC [82].

5.3.9 Lymphoma

Lymphoma can involve the adrenal gland secondarily or arise as a primary adrenal tumor (uncommon); the latter lesion is frequently bilateral (Figure 5.15). Adrenal involvement by non-Hodgkin lymphoma has been reported to range from 4% to 25% [83,84]. Primary adrenal lymphomas usually manifest as large, well-defined, soft tissue masses replacing the adrenal gland with homogeneous or slightly inhomogeneous enhancement. Large tumors especially tend to infiltrate adjacent structures [85].

5.3.10 Metastases

In a review of 30 years experience at one institution, adrenal metastases were found at autopsy in 3% of patients and were bilateral in 49% of cases [86] (Figure 5.16). In this study, 90% of adrenal metastases were carcinoma (lung, gastric, esophageal, hepatic–biliary,

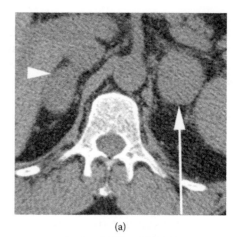
(a)

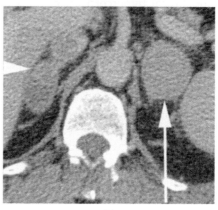
(b)

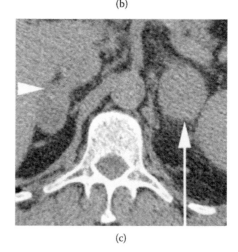
(c)

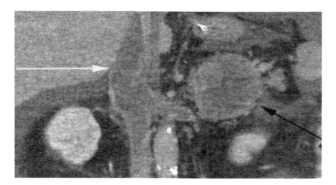

FIGURE 5.14
A 66-year-old man with a 6 cm heterogeneous left adrenal mass (black arrow) with tumor thrombus extending into the left renal vein and inferior vena cava (white arrow). This was resected and confirmed to be ACC.

FIGURE 5.15
A 53-year-old man who was found to have bilateral adrenal masses on a CT to further assess a right lower limb deep vein thrombosis. Follow-up dedicated adrenal CT is shown. There is a 4.4 cm left adrenal mass (arrow), which measures 41 HU on the noncontrast study (a), 70 HU on the enhanced scan (b), and 62 HU on the 10-minute delayed scan (c). There is also a heterogeneous right adrenal mass, which has a low attenuation nonenhancing component posteriorly and an enhancing soft tissue component anteriorly (arrowhead). This component measured 39 HU on the noncontrast scan, (a), 64 HU on the enhanced scan (b), and 53 HU on the 10-minute delayed scan (c). The APW was 28% for the left adrenal lesion and 44% for the right, consistent with nonadenomatous masses. Biopsy of the left adrenal lesion was positive for diffuse large B-cell lymphoma.

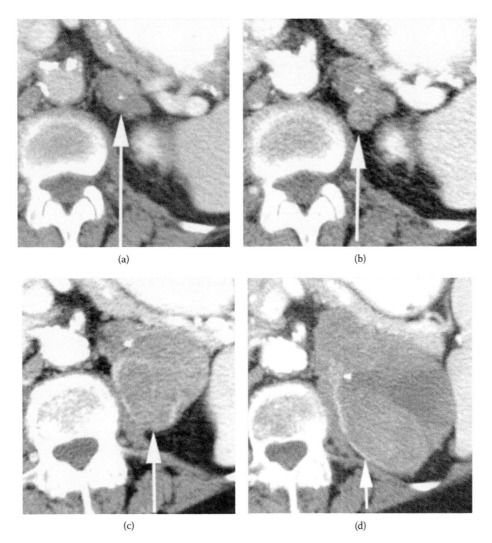

(a)

(b)

(c)

(d)

FIGURE 5.16
An 84-year-old man with a history of small cell lung cancer. CT images demonstrate a left adrenal mass (arrow), which increases dramatically in size over a 2 year period (a through d).

pancreatic, colon, renal, breast). Of these, 56% were adenocarcinomas and 15% were squamous cell carcinomas; the remainder included hematopoietic tumors, sarcomas, and melanomas. Hypervascular metastases may enhance similarly to pheochromocytomas, in particular metastases from renal cell carcinomas [87]. After contrast material administration, metastases usually demonstrate slower washout at delayed imaging than do adenomas [71,88].

5.4 An Imaging Algorithm

The American College of Radiology recently published a white paper on the management of incidental findings on abdominal CT [89]. They developed a flowchart,

which reflects the most commonly encountered imaging scenarios and attempts to diagnose both leave-alone masses and those that warrant further treatment (Figure 5.17).

5.5 Conclusion

Adrenal lesions are commonly detected at cross-sectional imaging. The majority of these masses can be characterized into benign adenomatous disease or nonadenomatous disease on imaging alone. Radiologists should therefore be familiar with the principles and techniques of CT and other imaging modalities that are used to detect and characterize adrenal lesions.

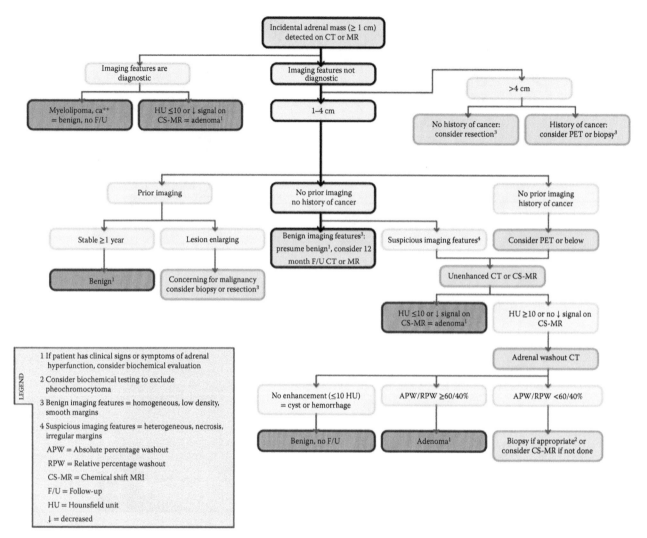

FIGURE 5.17
Flowchart for incidental adrenal mass detected on CT or magnetic resonance. (Reprinted from *Journal of the American College of Radiology,* 7(10), Berland, L.L. et al., Managing incidental findings on abdominal CT: White paper of the ACR Incidental Findings Committee, 754–773, Copyright 2010, with permission from Elsevier.)

References

1. Korobkin M, Giordano TJ, Brodeur FJ, Francis IR, Siegelman ES, Quint LE et al. Adrenal adenomas: Relationship between histologic lipid and CT and MR findings. *Radiology.* 1996;200(3):743–7.
2. Lee MJ, Hahn PF, Papanicolaou N, Egglin TK, Saini S, Mueller PR et al. Benign and malignant adrenal masses: CT distinction with attenuation coefficients, size, and observer analysis. *Radiology.* 1991;179(2):415–8.
3. Boland GW, Lee MJ, Gazelle GS, Halpern EF, McNicholas MM, Mueller PR. Characterization of adrenal masses using unenhanced CT: An analysis of the CT literature. *AJR Am J Roentgenol.* 1998;171(1):201–4.
4. Hahn PF, Blake MA, Boland GW. Adrenal lesions: attenuation measurement differences between CT scanners. *Radiology.* 2006;240(2):458–63.

5. Stadler A, Schima W, Prager G, Homolka P, Heinz G, Saini S et al. CT density measurements for characterization of adrenal tumors ex vivo: variability among three CT scanners. *AJR Am J Roentgenol.* 2004;182(3):671–5.
6. Korobkin M, Brodeur FJ, Francis IR, Quint LE, Dunnick NR, Londy F. CT time-attenuation washout curves of adrenal adenomas and nonadenomas. *AJR Am J Roentgenol.* 1998;170(3):747–52.
7. Dunnick NR, Korobkin M. Imaging of adrenal incidentalomas: current status. *AJR Am J Roentgenol.* 2002;179(3):559–68.
8. Korobkin M. CT characterization of adrenal masses: the time has come. *Radiology.* 2000;217(3):629–32.
9. Caoili EM, Korobkin M, Francis IR, Cohan RH, Platt JF, Dunnick NR et al. Adrenal masses: Characterization with combined unenhanced and delayed enhanced CT. *Radiology.* 2002;222(3):629–33.

10. Pena CS, Boland GW, Hahn PF, Lee MJ, Mueller PR. Characterization of indeterminate (lipid-poor) adrenal masses: Use of washout characteristics at contrast-enhanced CT. *Radiology*. 2000;217(3):798–802.

11. Szolar DH, Kammerhuber FH. Adrenal adenomas and nonadenomas: assessment of washout at delayed contrast-enhanced CT. *Radiology*. 1998;207(2):369–75.

12. Blake MA, Kalra MK, Sweeney AT, Lucey BC, Maher MM, Sahani DV et al. Distinguishing benign from malignant adrenal masses: Multi-detector row CT protocol with 10-minute delay. *Radiology*. 2006;238(2):578–85.

13. Sangwaiya MJ, Boland GW, Cronin CG, Blake MA, Halpern EF, Hahn PF. Incidental adrenal lesions: Accuracy of characterization with contrast-enhanced washout multidetector CT—10-minute delayed imaging protocol revisited in a large patient cohort. *Radiology*. 2010;256(2):504–10.

14. Kamiyama T, Fukukura Y, Yoneyama T, Takumi K, Nakajo M. Distinguishing adrenal adenomas from nonadenomas: Combined use of diagnostic parameters of unenhanced and short 5-minute dynamic enhanced CT protocol. *Radiology*. 2009;250(2):474–81.

15. Foti G, Faccioli N, Mantovani W, Malleo G, Manfredi R, Mucelli RP. Incidental adrenal lesions: Accuracy of quadriphasic contrast enhanced computed tomography in distinguishing adenomas from nonadenomas. *Eur J Radiol*. 2012;81(8):1742–50.

16. Park BK, Kim CK, Kim B. Adrenal incidentaloma detected on triphasic helical CT: Evaluation with modified relative percentage of enhancement washout values. *Br J Radiol*. 2008;81(967):526–30.

17. Miles KA, Charnsangavej C, Lee FT, Fishman EK, Horton K, Lee TY. Application of CT in the investigation of angiogenesis in oncology. *Acad Radiol*. 2000;7(10):840–50.

18. Yi CA, Lee KS, Kim EA, Han J, Kim H, Kwon OJ et al. Solitary pulmonary nodules: Dynamic enhanced multidetector row CT study and comparison with vascular endothelial growth factor and microvessel density. *Radiology*. 2004;233(1):191–9.

19. Qiao ZW, Xia CM, Zhu YB, Shi WP, Miao F. First-pass perfusion computed tomography: Initial experience in differentiating adrenal adenoma from metastasis. *Eur J Radiol*. 2010;73(3):657–63.

20. Qin HY, Sun HR, Li YJ, Shen BZ. Application of CT perfusion imaging to the histological differentiation of adrenal gland tumors. *Eur J Radiol*. 2012;81(3):502–7.

21. Kalra M, Blake M, Sahani D, Hahn P, Mueller P, Boland G. Dual energy CT for characterization of adrenal adenomas (abstr). In: *Radiological Society of North America Scientific Assembly and Annual Meeting*. Oak Brook, IL: Radiological Society of North America. 2007, p. 347.

22. Boland G, Jagtiani M, Kambadakone Ramesh A, Hahn P, Sahani D, Kalra M. Characterization of lipid poor adrenal adenomas: Accuracy of dual energy CT (abstr). In: *Radiological Society of North America Scientific Assembly and Annual Meeting*. Oak Brook, IL: Radiological Society of North America. 2008, p. 390.

23. Gupta RT, Ho LM, Marin D, Boll DT, Barnhart HX, Nelson RC. Dual-energy CT for characterization of adrenal nodules: Initial experience. *AJR Am J Roentgenol*. 2010;194(6):1479–83.

24. Bae KT, Fuangtharnthip P, Prasad SR, Joe BN, Heiken JP. Adrenal masses: CT characterization with histogram analysis method. *Radiology*. 2003;228(3):735–42.

25. Jhaveri KS, Wong F, Ghai S, Haider MA. Comparison of CT histogram analysis and chemical shift MRI in the characterization of indeterminate adrenal nodules. *AJR Am J Roentgenol*. 2006;187(5):1303–8.

26. Remer EM, Motta-Ramirez GA, Shepardson LB, Hamrahian AH, Herts BR. CT histogram analysis in pathologically proven adrenal masses. *AJR Am J Roentgenol*. 2006; 187(1):191–6.

27. Jhaveri KS, Lad SV, Haider MA. Computed tomographic histogram analysis in the diagnosis of lipid-poor adenomas: Comparison to adrenal washout computed tomography. *J Comput Assist Tomogr*. 2007;31(4):513–8.

28. Ho LM, Paulson EK, Brady MJ, Wong TZ, Schindera ST. Lipid-poor adenomas on unenhanced CT: Does histogram analysis increase sensitivity compared with a mean attenuation threshold? *AJR Am J Roentgenol*. 2008;191(1):234–8.

29. Halefoglu AM, Yasar A, Bas N, Ozel A, Erturk SM, Basak M. Comparison of computed tomography histogram analysis and chemical-shift magnetic resonance imaging for adrenal mass characterization. *Acta Radiol*. 2009;50(9):1071–9.

30. Halefoglu AM, Bas N, Yasar A, Basak M. Differentiation of adrenal adenomas from nonadenomas using CT histogram analysis method: A prospective study. *Eur J Radiol*. 2010;73(3):643–51.

31. Mitchell DG, Crovello M, Matteucci T, Petersen RO, Miettinen MM. Benign adrenocortical masses: Diagnosis with chemical shift MR imaging. *Radiology*. 1992;185(2):345–51.

32. Outwater EK, Siegelman ES, Radecki PD, Piccoli CW, Mitchell DG. Distinction between benign and malignant adrenal masses: Value of T1-weighted chemical-shift MR imaging. *AJR Am J Roentgenol*. 1995;165(3):579–83.

33. Mayo-Smith WW, Lee MJ, McNicholas MM, Hahn PF, Boland GW, Saini S. Characterization of adrenal masses (<5 cm) by use of chemical shift MR imaging: Observer performance versus quantitative measures. *AJR Am J Roentgenol*. 1995;165(1):91–5.

34. Fujiyoshi F, Nakajo M, Fukukura Y, Tsuchimochi S. Characterization of adrenal tumors by chemical shift fast low-angle shot MR imaging: Comparison of four methods of quantitative evaluation. *AJR Am J Roentgenol*. 2003;180(6):1649–57.

35. Metser U, Miller E, Lerman H, Lievshitz G, Avital S, Even-Sapir E. 18F-FDG PET/CT in the evaluation of adrenal masses. *J Nucl Med*. 2006;47(1):32–7.

36. Kumar R, Xiu Y, Yu JQ, Takalkar A, El-Haddad G, Potenta S et al. 18F-FDG PET in evaluation of adrenal lesions in patients with lung cancer. *J Nucl Med*. 2004;45(12):2058–62.

37. Chong S, Lee KS, Kim HY, Kim YK, Kim BT, Chung MJ et al. Integrated PET-CT for the characterization of adrenal gland lesions in cancer patients: Diagnostic efficacy and interpretation pitfalls. *Radiographics*. 2006;26(6):1811–24;discussion 24–6.

38. Boland GW, Blake MA, Holalkere NS, Hahn PF. PET/CT for the characterization of adrenal masses in patients with cancer: Qualitative versus quantitative

accuracy in 150 consecutive patients. *AJR Am J Roentgenol.* 2009;192(4):956–62.

39. Tenenbaum F, Lumbroso J, Schlumberger M, Mure A, Plouin PF, Caillou B et al. Comparison of radiolabeled octreotide and meta-iodobenzylguanidine (MIBG) scintigraphy in malignant pheochromocytoma. *J Nucl Med.* 1995;36(1):1–6.

40. van der Harst E, de Herder WW, Bruining HA, Bonjer HJ, de Krijger RR, Lamberts SW et al. [(123)I]metaiodoben-zylguanidine and [(111)In]octreotide uptake in begnign and malignant pheochromocytomas. *J Clin Endocrinol Metab.* 2001;86(2):685–93.

41. Vincent JM, Morrison ID, Armstrong P, Reznek RH. The size of normal adrenal glands on computed tomography. *Clin Radiol.* 1994;49(7):453–5.

42. Sohaib SA, Hanson JA, Newell-Price JD, Trainer PJ, Monson JP, Grossman AB et al. CT appearance of the adrenal glands in adrenocorticotrophic hormone-dependent Cushing's syndrome. *AJR Am J Roentgenol.* 1999;172(4):997–1002.

43. Wilms G, Baert A, Marchal G, Goddeeris P. Computed tomography of the normal adrenal glands: Correlative study with autopsy specimens. *J Comput Assist Tomogr.* 1979;3(4):467–9.

44. Doppman JL, Chrousos GP, Papanicolaou DA, Stratakis CA, Alexander HR, Nieman LK. Adrenocorticotropin-independent macronodular adrenal hyperplasia: An uncommon cause of primary adrenal hypercortisolism. *Radiology.* 2000;216(3):797–802.

45. Lingam RK, Sohaib SA, Vlahos I, Rockall AG, Isidori AM, Monson JP et al. CT of primary hyperaldosteronism (Conn's syndrome): The value of measuring the adrenal gland. *AJR Am J Roentgenol.* 2003;181(3):843–9.

46. Song JH, Chaudhry FS, Mayo-Smith WW. The incidental indeterminate adrenal mass on CT (> 10 H) in patients without cancer: Is further imaging necessary? Follow-up of 321 consecutive indeterminate adrenal masses. *AJR Am J Roentgenol.* 2007;189(5):1119–23.

47. Kenney PJ, Wagner BJ, Rao P, Heffess CS. Myelolipoma: CT and pathologic features. *Radiology.* 1998;208(1):87–95.

48. Wang LJ, Wong YC, Chen CJ, Chu SH. Imaging spectrum of adrenal pseudocysts on CT. *Eur Radiol.* 2003;13(3):531–5.

49. Erickson LA, Lloyd RV, Hartman R, Thompson G. Cystic adrenal neoplasms. *Cancer.* 2004;101(7):1537–44.

50. Pradeep PV, Mishra AK, Aggarwal V, Bhargav PR, Gupta SK, Agarwal A. Adrenal cysts: An institutional experience. *World J Surg.* 2006;30(10):1817–20.

51. Rozenblit A, Morehouse HT, Amis ES, Jr. Cystic adrenal lesions: CT features. *Radiology.* 1996;201(2):541–8.

52. Burks DW, Mirvis SE, Shanmuganathan K. Acute adrenal injury after blunt abdominal trauma: CT findings. *AJR Am J Roentgenol.* 1992;158(3):503–7.

53. Sevitt S. Post-traumatic adrenal apoplexy. *J Clin Pathol.* 1955;8(3):185–94.

54. Sivit CJ, Ingram JD, Taylor GA, Bulas DI, Kushner DC, Eichelberger MR. Posttraumatic adrenal hemorrhage in children: CT findings in 34 patients. *AJR Am J Roentgenol.* 1992;158(6):1299–302.

55. Kenney PJ, Stanley RJ. Calcified adrenal masses. *Urol Radiol.* 1987;9(1):9–15.

56. Wolverson MK, Kannegiesser H. CT of bilateral adrenal hemorrhage with acute adrenal insufficiency in the adult. *AJR Am J Roentgenol.* 1984;142(2):311–4.

57. Hoeffel C, Legmann P, Luton JP, Chapuis Y, Fayet-Bonnin P. Spontaneous unilateral adrenal hemorrhage: Computerized tomography and magnetic resonance imaging findings in 8 cases. *J Urol.* 1995;154(5):1647–51.

58. Kawashima A, Sandler CM, Ernst RD, Takahashi N, Roubidoux MA, Goldman SM et al. Imaging of nontraumatic hemorrhage of the adrenal gland. *Radiographics.* 1999;19(4):949–63.

59. Yang ZG, Guo YK, Li Y, Min PQ, Yu JQ, Ma ES. Differentiation between tuberculosis and primary tumors in the adrenal gland: Evaluation with contrast-enhanced CT. *Eur Radiol.* 2006;16(9):2031–6.

60. Liatsikos EN, Kalogeropoulou CP, Papathanassiou Z, Tsota I, Athanasopoulos A, Perimenis P et al. Primary adrenal tuberculosis: Role of computed tomography and CT-guided biopsy in diagnosis. *Urol Int.* 2006;76(3):285–7.

61. Guo YK, Yang ZG, Li Y, Ma ES, Deng YP, Min PQ et al. Addison's disease due to adrenal tuberculosis: Contrast-enhanced CT features and clinical duration correlation. *Eur J Radiol.* 2007;62(1):126–31.

62. Ma ES, Yang ZG, Li Y, Guo YK, Deng YP, Zhang XC. Tuberculous Addison's disease: Morphological and quantitative evaluation with multidetector-row CT. *Eur J Radiol.* 2007;62(3):352–8.

63. Kumar N, Singh S, Govil S. Adrenal histoplasmosis: Clinical presentation and imaging features in nine cases. *Abdom Imaging.* 2003;28(5):703–8.

64. Radin DR, Baker EL, Klatt EC, Balthazar EJ, Jeffrey RB, Jr., Megibow AJ et al. Visceral and nodal calcification in patients with AIDS-related Pneumocystis carinii infection. *AJR Am J Roentgenol.* 1990;154(1):27–31.

65. Kloos RT, Gross MD, Francis IR, Korobkin M, Shapiro B. Incidentally discovered adrenal masses. *Endocr Rev.* 1995;16(4):460–84.

66. Reznek RH, Armstrong P. The adrenal gland. *Clin Endocrinol (Oxf).* 1994;40(5):561–76.

67. Ctvrtlik F, Herman M, Student V, Ticha V, Minarik J. Differential diagnosis of incidentally detected adrenal masses revealed on routine abdominal CT. *Eur J Radiol.* 2009;69(2):243–52.

68. Mayo-Smith WW, Boland GW, Noto RB, Lee MJ. State-of-the-art adrenal imaging. *Radiographics.* 2001; 21(4):995–1012.

69. Israel GM, Korobkin M, Wang C, Hecht EN, Krinsky GA. Comparison of unenhanced CT and chemical shift MRI in evaluating lipid-rich adrenal adenomas. *AJR Am J Roentgenol.* 2004;183(1):215–9.

70. Park BK, Kim B, Ko K, Jeong SY, Kwon GY. Adrenal masses falsely diagnosed as adenomas on unenhanced and delayed contrast-enhanced computed tomography: Pathological correlation. *Eur Radiol.* 2006;16(3):642–7.

71. Szolar DH, Korobkin M, Reittner P, Berghold A, Bauernhofer T, Trummer H et al. Adrenocortical carcinomas and adrenal pheochromocytomas: Mass and enhancement loss evaluation at delayed contrast-enhanced CT. *Radiology.* 2005;234(2):479–85.

72. Caoili EM, Korobkin M, Francis IR, Cohan RH, Dunnick NR. Delayed enhanced CT of lipid-poor adrenal adenomas. *AJR Am J Roentgenol*. 2000;175(5):1411–5.

73. Blake MA, Krishnamoorthy SK, Boland GW, Sweeney AT, Pitman MB, Harisinghani M et al. Low-density pheochromocytoma on CT: A mimicker of adrenal adenoma. *AJR Am J Roentgenol*. 2003;181(6):1663–8.

74. Park BK, Kim CK, Kwon GY, Kim JH. Re-evaluation of pheochromocytomas on delayed contrast-enhanced CT: Washout enhancement and other imaging features. *Eur Radiol*. 2007;17(11):2804–9.

75. Wajchenberg BL, Albergaria Pereira MA, Medonca BB, Latronico AC, Campos Carneiro P, Alves VA et al. Adrenocortical carcinoma: Clinical and laboratory observations. *Cancer*. 2000;88(4):711–36.

76. Ng L, Libertino JM. Adrenocortical carcinoma: Diagnosis, evaluation and treatment. *J Urol*. 2003;169(1):5–11.

77. Copeland PM. The incidentally discovered adrenal mass. *Ann Surg*. 1984;199(1):116–22.

78. Fishman EK, Deutch BM, Hartman DS, Goldman SM, Zerhouni EA, Siegelman SS. Primary adrenocortical carcinoma: CT evaluation with clinical correlation. *AJR Am J Roentgenol*. 1987;148(3):531–5.

79. Slattery JM, Blake MA, Kalra MK, Misdraji J, Sweeney AT, Copeland PM et al. Adrenocortical carcinoma: Contrast washout characteristics on CT. *AJR Am J Roentgenol*. 2006;187(1):W21–4.

80. Cuevas C, Raske M, Bush WH, Takayama T, Maki JH, Kolokythas O et al. Imaging primary and secondary tumor thrombus of the inferior vena cava: Multi-detector computed tomography and magnetic resonance imaging. *Curr Probl Diagn Radiol*. 2006;35(3):90–101.

81. Bender LC, Mitsumori LM, Lloyd KA, Stambaugh LE, 3rd. AIRP best cases in radiologic-pathologic correlation: Intravenous leiomyomatosis. *Radiographics*. 2011;31(4):1053–8.

82. Kandpal H, Sharma R, Gamangatti S, Srivastava DN, Vashisht S. Imaging the inferior vena cava: A road less traveled. *Radiographics*. 2008;28(3):669–89.

83. Paling MR, Williamson BR. Adrenal involvement in non-Hodgkin lymphoma. *AJR Am J Roentgenol*. 1983;141(2):303–5.

84. Case records of the Massachusetts General Hospital. Weekly clinicopathological exercises. Case 35-2000. An 82-year-old woman with bilateral adrenal masses and low-grade fever. *N Engl J Med*. 2000; 343(20):1477–83.

85. Zhou L, Peng W, Wang C, Liu X, Shen Y, Zhou K. Primary adrenal lymphoma: Radiological, pathological, clinical correlation. *Eur J Radiol*. 2010;81(3): 401–5.

86. Lam KY, Lo CY. Metastatic tumours of the adrenal glands: A 30-year experience in a teaching hospital. *Clin Endocrinol (Oxf)*. 2002;56(1):95–101.

87. Scatarige JC, Sheth S, Corl FM, Fishman EK. Patterns of recurrence in renal cell carcinoma: Manifestations on helical CT. *AJR Am J Roentgenol*. 2001;177(3):653–8.

88. Boland GW, Hahn PF, Pena C, Mueller PR. Adrenal masses: Characterization with delayed contrast-enhanced CT. *Radiology*. 1997;202(3):693–6.

89. Berland LL, Silverman SG, Gore RM, Mayo-Smith WW, Megibow AJ, Yee J et al. Managing incidental findings on abdominal CT: White paper of the ACR Incidental Findings Committee. *J Am Coll Radiol*. 2010; 7(10):754–73.

6

Pathology of the Stomach and Small Bowel

Richard M. Gore, Daniel R. Wenzke, Robert I. Silvers, Geraldine M. Newmark,
Kiran H. Thakrar, Uday K. Mehta, and Jonathan W. Berlin

CONTENTS

6.1 Introduction

Traditionally, upper gastrointestinal (GI) endoscopy, upper GI series and small bowel follow through examinations, and more recently video capsule endoscopy have been the preferred means of evaluating gastric, duodenal, and small bowel pathology. These tests provide exquisite mucosal detail but are inadequate in evaluating extramucosal pathology. Computed tomography (CT) has become the premier imaging technique for evaluating the mural, mesenteric, and omental components of GI tract pathology [1].

The development of multi-detector CT (MDCT) technology affords high-resolution imaging of the entire abdomen in one breath hold, obviating motion artifacts. The imaging data can be acquired with near isotropic voxels that allow for high-quality and clinically useful volume imaging. The CT data can be viewed in any plane, and three-dimensional (3D) techniques can be used to effectively and graphically display large data sets in a user-friendly format that is understandable to referring physicians [1]. This chapter discusses the current status of MDCT of the stomach, duodenum, and small bowel; gives an overview of the technique and different oral preparation methods possible; and discusses normal anatomy and the most common diseases as detected and characterized with MDCT.

6.2 Technique

6.2.1 Lumen Opacification

Proper distention and marking of the bowel lumen is vital in detecting mural thickening and excluding mural masses and mesenteric and omental pathology. There are several methods available to accomplish this goal, and the choice depends on the clinical setting [2].

In the emergent setting in which bowel obstruction or intestinal ischemia is suspected, the intrinsic secretions and gas within the gut are usually sufficient to highlight the lumen. Orally administered contrast may be vomited and may remain in the stomach because of absent or diminished GI motility [3].

As part of a general survey examination of patients with no localizing signs or symptoms, a study performed with positive intraluminal contrast is often obtained. As a caveat, the assessment of mural and mucosal enhancement of the gut will be compromised with positive contrast [4]. In addition, positive intraluminal contrast will interfere with CT angiography and some 3D techniques. Air or carbon dioxide as intraluminal contrast agents are used in the setting of CT gastrography (CTG) [5].

Positive contrast opacification of the gut is accomplished by administering either 1%–2% barium suspensions or 2%–3% solution of iodinated water-soluble agents. The low percentage of barium requires commercial preparations made specifically for CT, in which additives are used to ensure that the barium remains in suspension. In most patients, contrast material will reach the distal ileum within 45 minutes after initiation of drinking [6].

The choice between oral barium suspensions and water-soluble agents is dictated by the experience and preference of the radiologist. Water-soluble agents are recommended for patients with abdominal trauma or suspected perforated viscus, for those who have a high likelihood of immediate surgery, and as an aid in percutaneous CT biopsy or other interventional procedures.

Neutral contrast agents have several advantages over positive contrast agents for evaluating mucosal, mural, and serosal pathology. They allow excellent depiction of mural enhancement of the gut without the algorithm undershoot or overshoot that accompanies intraluminal high-density positive contrast and low-density gas. Neutral contrast agents are the preferred means of opacifying the bowel for CT enterography [7–11]. Neutral contrast agents also facilitate the performance of CT angiography for vascular assessment; GI bleeding studies; and staging and preoperative evaluation of hepatic, biliary, and pancreatic malignancies. Neutral contrast agents include water, milk, a 0.1% solution of barium (Volumen E-Z-EM; Lake Success, New York), and water mixed with mannitol or polyethelene glycol.

Gaseous distention of the stomach is important when evaluating mucosal and mural pathology. Gastric distention with gas has been used with great success in CTG for the diagnosis and staging of upper GI tract malignancies [12–14].

6.2.2 Vascular Opacification

Opacification of the blood vessels is essential for complete evaluation of inflammatory, infectious, neoplastic, vascular, and traumatic diseases of the stomach and small bowel. Obviously, this cannot be performed in all clinical settings (e.g., poor renal function and poor venous access). For general diagnostic cases, 100–150 cc (depending on concentration) of nonionic contrast is administered at a rate of at least 3 $mL \cdot s^{-1}$ with a power injector. If CT angiography or other 3D techniques are to be performed, the rate is increased to 5 $mL \cdot s^{-1}$ [15].

One of the advantages of MDCT is that multiple data sets can be acquired with a single bolus of intravenous contrast material. The following is a list of possible imaging times that may be used when scanning the abdomen and pelvis: unenhanced, early arterial phase (20 seconds), late arterial-enteric phase (40 seconds), portal venous phase (70–90 seconds), equilibrium phase (210 seconds), and delayed phase (5–20 minutes).

For general survey abdominal imaging, obtaining scans during the portal venous phase is adequate. When assessing the viability of bowel, searching for a source of GI hemorrhage, evaluating the cirrhotic liver, and searching for hypervascular metastases, it is useful to obtain noncontrast scans as well as scans during the later hepatic arterial phase and portal venous phase. When performing CT angiography, scans should be obtained during the early arterial phase [16].

6.3 Normal Bowel Wall on Multi-Detector Computed Tomography

Virtually, all pathology of the bowel wall results in mural thickening that is often accompanied by changes in the density of the bowel wall because of edema, hemorrhage, tumor, fat, or gas. One of the most common pitfalls in interpreting CT examinations of the gut is confusing an insufficiently distended loop of bowel for pathologic thickening or mistaking a poorly opacified or nonopacified bowel loop for an abdominal mass.

6.3.1 Normal Stomach

The stomach is a functionally and anatomically dynamic organ and its appearance depends on the degree of luminal distention and gastric location. For the well-distended, nondependent gastric fundus and body, wall thickness of up to 5–10 mm is considered normal. The mural thickness of the antrum, however, is affected by anatomic and functional factors that make it normally thicker than other portions of the stomach [17].

When the normal stomach is distended with neutral contrast, enhancement of the mucosa may be seen highlighted against the lower attenuation mucosa and muscularis propria. Up to one quarter of patients show linear submucosal low attenuation or mural stratification in the antrum on contrast-enhanced MDCT examinations. This may be in part because of deposition of fat in the submucosa [18].

6.3.2 Normal Small Bowel

The normal small bowel is approximately 22 ft long and is suspended by a mesenteric root that measures 6–9 in. and courses from the level of the ligament of Treitz caudal to the level of the ileocecal valve. As with conventional barium small bowel examinations, the valvulae conniventes are more prominent in the jejunum than in the ileum. Reversal of this pattern can be seen in patients with celiac disease.

The normal small bowel wall measures between 1 and 2 mm when the lumen is well distended with positive, neutral, or gas contrast media. When collapsed, the normal mural thickness of the small bowel measures between 2 and 3 mm.

When scanning patients during the enteric phase (40–60 seconds following contrast injection), collapsed bowel segments have greater attenuation than distended bowel segments. Also the jejunum has greater attenuation than the ileum. Because collapsed small bowel loops have increased attenuation that is similar to that of inflamed bowel loops, secondary findings of infectious or inflammatory small bowel disease (e.g., engorged vasa recta, creeping fat of the mesentery, and enlarged lymph nodes) should be considered [19].

6.4 Bowel Wall: Pathologic Changes on Multi-Detector Computed Tomography

Mural thickening is the pathologic hallmark of GI disease on MDCT. When evaluating the abnormal gut, the following features should be carefully analyzed: mural attenuation and enhancement patterns, the degree of mural thickening, the symmetry of bowel wall thickening, and the length of the diseased segment. Wittenberg et al. have described a classification system for the abnormal bowel wall as depicted on MDCT (Figure 6.1) [20].

6.4.1 White Attenuation Pattern

When the diseased segment of gut shows contrast enhancement to a degree equal or greater than that of venous opacification on the same scan, this indicates abnormal enhancement. Avid mural contrast enhancement is probably related to vasodilation and/or injury to intramural vessels with interstitial leakage of the contrast medium.

This pattern of enhancement is seen most commonly in patients with acute inflammatory and infectious bowel disease, reflecting the hyperemic and hypervascular state found with acute inflammation and infection. Vascular disorders such as shock bowel also may manifest with the white attenuation pattern (Figure 6.2). The increased vascular permeability and slowed perfusion that accompanies hypoperfusion permit the interstitial leakage of molecules of contrast material. Delayed venous drainage and altered vascular permeability are also responsible for this sign in patients with bowel ischemia. On noncontrast enhanced scans, intramural hemorrhage will produce a hyperdense bowel wall [21].

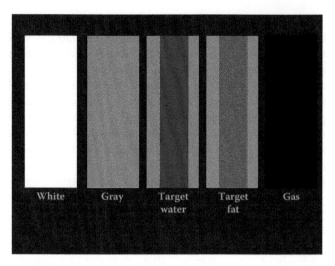

FIGURE 6.1
Classification scheme for mural thickening of the gastrointestinal (GI) tract. White pattern: inflammatory bowel disease, shock bowel, reperfused ischemia. Gray pattern: cicatrizing Crohn's disease, neoplasm, ischemia. Target pattern with submucosal edema: active inflammatory bowel disease, infection, ischemia, post radiation, angiotensin converting enzyme inhibitors. Target pattern with submucosal fat: chronic inflammatory bowel disease, celiac disease, chemotherapy, obesity. Gas pattern: ischemia, infection, trauma, mucosal disruption.

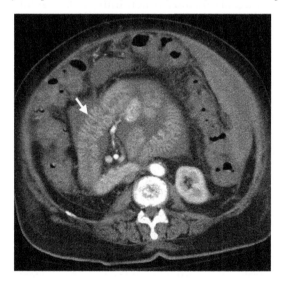

FIGURE 6.2
White pattern: shock bowel. There is diffuse mural hyperenhancement (arrow) of the mid small bowel in this patient with massive abdominal hemorrhage and hypovolemia.

6.4.2 Gray Attenuation Pattern

In this pattern, thickened bowel wall shows little enhancement and a homogeneous attenuation comparable with that of enhanced muscle. This pattern should only be diagnosed if the intravascular contrast levels are adequate. Malignancy should be suspected in significantly thickened segments of gut that show minimal enhancement and do not exhibit mural stratification [22].

Adenocarcinomas of the gut usually show the uniform, gray-enhancement pattern unless there are focal regions of necrosis. Lymphomas typically show a greater degree of wall thickening and are more homogeneous in attenuation as well.

Ischemic bowel to arterial compromise will also show poor "gray" enhancement relative to other segments of bowel (Figure 6.3).

GI stromal tumors (GISTs) and metastases often cause mural thickening but are typically inhomogeneous in attenuation. In patients with Crohn's disease, the presence of a thick, nonenhancing segment suggests the fibrotic cicatrizing stage of the disease.

6.4.3 Water Halo Pattern

This is the most commonly seen pattern and is observed in patients with active infectious, inflammatory, ischemic disorders of the GI tract. It can also be seen in angioedema related to angiotensin converting enzyme inhibitors (Figure 6.4) [23]. The bowel, when viewed in the axial plane, has a target or "bull's-eye" appearance. An enhancing central higher density mucosal layer is surrounded by a water-density submucosa, which in turn is surrounded by a higher density muscularis propria [1].

6.4.4 Fat Halo Pattern

Fat in the submucosa of the gut produces the fat halo pattern (Figure 6.5). It has lower attenuation than the grayer tone of the water halo sign. When visualized in the small bowel, chronic Crohn's disease should be suspected. Rapid accumulation of submucosal fat has also been reported in patients undergoing cytoreductive surgery for lymphoproliferative and myeloproliferative disorders and graft versus host disease.

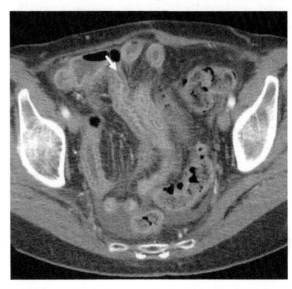

FIGURE 6.4
Water halo pattern: angiotensin converting enzyme inhibitors. The angioedema caused by these antihypertensive drugs can cause mural thickening and submucosaledema (arrow) of the small bowel. There is also a small amount of intraperitoneal fluid.

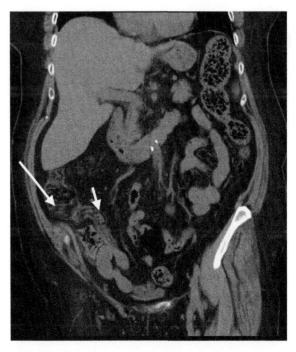

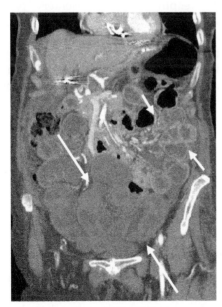

FIGURE 6.3
Gray pattern: mesenteric ischemia because of superior mesenteric artery embolism. Coronal multiplanar reformation images show poor, "gray" enhancement of the ileal loops (large arrows) compared to the normally enhancing jejunum (small arrows).

FIGURE 6.5
Fat halo pattern: chronic Crohn's disease. Coronal multiplanar reformation image shows deposition of fat in the terminal ileum (small arrow) and proximal colon (large arrow).

In patients with fat isolated to the duodenum and proximal jejunum, celiac disease needs to be excluded [24]. Submucosal fat deposition in the stomach, duodenum, small bowel, and colon is now understood to be a fairly common, benign finding in obese individuals. In a patient without GI symptoms in whom the fat is found incidentally, further evaluation is usually not needed [25].

6.4.5 Black Attenuation Pattern

Pneumatosis of the gut should always be considered as part of an acute ischemic, infectious, or traumatic injury to the gut. Any disease process that compromises the integrity of the mucosa can introduce intramural gas. The presence of intramural gas can herald an abdominal catastrophe (Figure 6.6) and must be viewed with suspicion. It can be seen as a benign process in patients with pneumatosis cystoides intestinalis, scleroderma, or other connective tissue diseases that weaken the integrity of the bowel wall and the setting of enteral catheters. It is not only important to detect small intramural collections of gas but to avoid confusing them with pseudopneumatosis. Follow-up scanning and correlation with serum lactic acid levels and white blood cell count should also be considered in these cases [26,27].

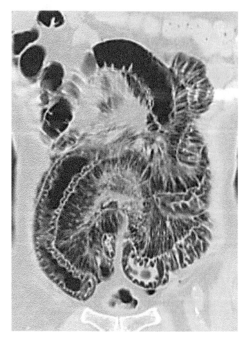

FIGURE 6.6
Intramural gas pattern: mesenteric infarction. Coronal multiplanar reformation image displayed with lung windows shows diffuse pneumatosis intestinalis of the small bowel.

6.5 Mesenteric and Omental Fat Pathology

Careful evaluation of the attenuation, vascularity, and lymph nodes of the fat within the subperitoneal spaces surrounding the gut provides important information about pathology in the adjacent abnormal bowel segment.

6.5.1 Blood Vessels

When a thickened segment of gut is supplied by engorged blood vessels (vasa recta), the pathology most likely is infectious or inflammatory. In the small bowel, mural thickening can be seen in Crohn's disease and lymphoma. If the vasa recta supplying the affected segment are engorged (the comb sign), then the disease is most likely Crohn's disease [28].

6.5.2 Serosal and Subperitoneal Fat Density

Comparing the degree of fat stranding surrounding an abnormal segment of gut and the associated mural thickening is an important clue in evaluating patients with the acute abdomen. Inflammatory conditions are associated with disproportionate fat stranding. In other words, the amount of fat stranding is greater than the degree of mural thickening. In malignancies, the degree of fat stranding is typically much less impressive than the degree of mural thickening [29].

So called "creeping fat of the mesentery" is a common finding in patients with Crohn's disease. This abnormal fat often shows prominent lymph nodes and engorged vasa recta and causes separation of bowel loops. Carcinoid tumors of the small bowel induce an intense desmoplastic reaction, creating a retractile appearance on CT [30].

Neoplasms also produce changes in the subperitoneal fat of the adjacent mesentery or omentum. Tumor invasion into the peri-intestinal fat results in more sharply defined and thicker dense strands than in those found with inflammation and infection. Spike-like densities correlate with pathologic findings of tumor extension through the serosa into perienteric fat.

6.5.3 Lymph Nodes

The evaluation of mesenteric and omental lymph nodes is an important part of assessing abnormal bowel pathology. As a general rule, when lymph node size is disproportionately greater than the mesenteric or omental inflammatory response, a malignancy should be considered.

Patients with Crohn's disease often have mildly enlarged lymph nodes in the mesentery adjacent to the involved segment of gut. GI infections and mesenteric adenitis often produce mildly enlarged lymph nodes as well. The adenopathy, however, is less impressive than that found in patients with lymphoma. The degree of mural thickening is often greater in patients with lymphoma, and coexistent retroperitoneal adenopathy is often present.

Carcinomas of the stomach and small bowel may only infiltrate a lymph node without necessarily increasing its size. Accordingly, any normal-sized lymph nodes, especially if three or more in number, near a GI tract malignancy must be viewed with suspicion. Local adenopathy associated with carcinoid tumors may calcify [31].

6.5.4 Calcifications

Omental and mesenteric calcifications can develop in several benign and malignant disorders of the abdomen and pelvis. Carcinoid tumor often presents with a calcified mass in the mesentery associated with tethering of adjacent small bowel loops. The vasoactive peptides secreted by these tumors cause a local desmoplastic reaction with retraction of the mesentery, kinking of the adjacent loops, and mural thickening. Foci of mesenteric and omental calcifications can also be seen in patients with metastatic mucinous ovarian and GI neoplasms [32].

6.6 Gastritis and Peptic Ulcer Disease

Inflammation of the upper GI tract mucosa may be acute or chronic. Acute gastritis is usually seen in the setting of excessive alcohol consumption, nonsteroidal anti-inflammatory drugs, smoking, and the severe stress that accompanies trauma, burns, and surgery. Superficial mucosa erosions and hemorrhage are seen pathologically. In ulcer disease, there is a full-thickness destruction of the mucosa with ulcer craters extending into the submucosa, serosa, or beyond. In the majority of cases of chronic gastritis and ulcer disease, there is associated *H pylori* infection [33].

Upper GI endoscopy and upper GI barium series are the primary means of establishing the diagnosis of gastritis and peptic ulcer disease. In the acute setting, patients with peptic ulcer disease often present with nonlocalizing signs and symptoms indistinguishable from those of acute pancreatitis or cholecystits, and MDCT is often the first examination ordered. The most common CT manifestation of gastritis is thickening of the gastric folds (Figure 6.7) and wall. In severe cases, the gastric wall will show submucosal edema and hyperenhancement of the gastric mucosa. Gastritis may not involve the stomach diffusely and thus may appear as focal or segmental thickening that can simulate cancer. Because the CT appearances of gastritis and tumors

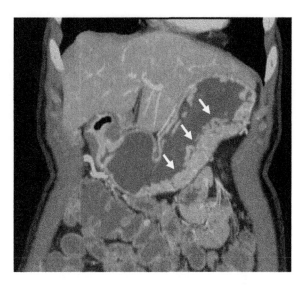

FIGURE 6.7
Gastritis because of *H. pylori.* Coronal multiplanar reformation image of the stomach with water distention shows thickening of the rugal folds (arrows) predominantly along the greater curvature aspect of the gastric body and proximal antrum.

can overlap, endoscopy is often necessary for definitive diagnosis [17].

Most gastric ulcers are superficial and consequently are not visible on CT. Deep ulcers or ulcers that have penetrated or perforated the gastric wall, however, can be detected. Actual extravasation of contrast material (Figure 6.8) or extraluminal gas bubbles and pneumoperitoneum may be seen, but more commonly there is mural thickening of the stomach, inflammatory change in adjacent soft tissue, in addition to gastric wall thickening [34].

Emphysematous gastritis is an uncommon, life-threatening disorder with a high mortality rate that is usually caused by invasion of the gastric wall by gas-producing organisms, typically *Escherichia coli.* CT shows mural thickening of the stomach and air within the layers of the wall (Figure 6.9). Air within the gastric wall may rarely occur after caustic ingestion or gastric infarction [17].

Gastric emphysema, a relatively benign and more common entity, can simulate the appearance of emphysematous gastritis; however, patients with benign gastric emphysema are asymptomatic, and the condition tends to resolve [17].

Ménétrier's disease is a rare, idiopathic, chronic, gastric disorder that is characterized by grossly thickened lobulated folds of the gastric fundus and body with relative antral sparing. The greatest degree of fold thickening occurs on or near the greater curvature. Focally enlarged folds can be mistaken for polypoid carcinomas. The most important differential diagnosis is lymphoma [35].

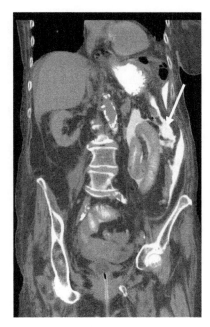

FIGURE 6.8
Perforated gastric ulcer. Coronal multiplanar reformation image shows contrast extravasation along the greater curvature aspect of the gastric body. The contrast material is seen extending into the left paracolic gutter (arrow) and into the mesenteric leaves surrounding the jejunum.

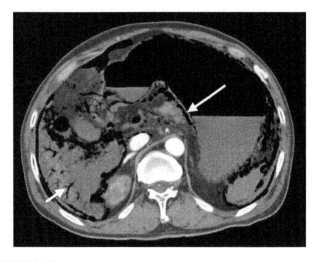

FIGURE 6.9
Emphysematous gastritis. There is intramural gas (long arrow) within the stomach as well as gas in the intrahepatic (small arrow) and extrahepatic portal venous system.

6.7 Benign Polyps of the Stomach and Small Bowel

6.7.1 Gastric Polyps

Gastric polyps may be adenomatous, hamartomatous, or hyperplastic, with the later accounting for 80%–90% of cases. Hyperplastic polyps are non-neoplastic

lesions, whereas gastric adenomas are true neoplasms, morphologically similar to those seen in the colon. Both hyperplastic and adenomatous polyps are seen in patients with chronic atrophic gastritis and familial adenomatous polyposis (FAP). Although most polyps are asymptomatic, anemia because of chronic blood loss, iron deficiency, or malabsorption of vitamin B12 may be present [36].

Hyperplastic polyps are often seen in the setting of chronic gastritis, atrophic gastritis, or bile reflux gastritis. On MDCT, most hyperplastic gastric polyps are smooth, sessile, round, or oval lesions, ranging from 5 to 10 mm in diameter. They usually occur as multiple lesions of similar size, clustered in the gastric body or fundus on the posterior gastric wall [17].

Adenomatous polyps of the stomach are rare in the general population. They are larger (about 2 cm in diameter) than hyperplastic polyps and more commonly pedunculated. As in the colon, the malignant potential of a gastric adenoma is related to size with up to 50% of adenomas >2 cm in size containing a focus of carcinoma. Adenomatous polyps are solitary and occur adjacent to the antrum. They may appear sessile or pedunculated and tend to have a more lobulated appearance [37].

Neural tumors constitute about 5%–10% of benign gastric tumors. The majority are nerve sheath tumors (neurinomas, schwannomas [Figure 6.10], or neuromas). Most nerve sheath tumors are benign, but sarcomatous changes in these lesions have occasionally been reported. Neural tumors in the stomach usually appear on CT scans as submucosal masses (with or without ulceration) that are indistinguishable from other mesenchymal tumors [36].

6.7.2 Small Bowel Polyps

Benign neoplasms are found throughout the small bowel, but some patterns are apparent. Adenomas are evenly distributed; however, there is a slightly higher

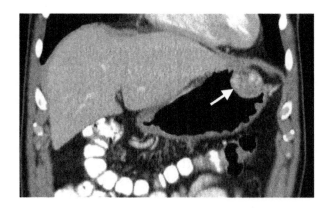

FIGURE 6.10
Gastric schwannoma. Coronal multiplanar reformation image shows an inhomogeneous fundal mass (arrow) that was found incidentally.

frequency of these lesions in the duodenum and ileum. Fibromas and lipomas are more common in the ileum, and 80%–90% of hemangiomas and neurofibromas are distributed evenly between the jejunum and ileum. Adenomas arise from mucosal glands and though they begin as sessile tumors, they become polypoid when sufficiently large. Adenomas account for nearly one-third of all benign small bowel neoplasms and, as in the colon, can be divided into tubular, villous, and tubulovillous on the basis of histological exam. Villous adenomas are not as common as tubular neoplasms but are usually larger, more often sessile, and typically are located in the second portion of the duodenum. On MDCT, these adenomas tend to enhance and their visibility depends on their size and the nature of the contrast material within the bowel lumen [38,39].

6.8 Adenocarcinoma

6.8.1 Adenocarcinoma of the Stomach

Adenocarcinoma is the most common malignancy of the stomach, accounting for nearly 90% of gastric tumors. It is responsible for approximately 700,000 deaths worldwide each year and is second only to lung cancer in overall cause of cancer-related mortality. The majority of gastric cancers in Western countries are detected at an advanced stage owing to the insidious nature of the onset of symptoms and their similarity in early states to benign causes of dyspepsia. Without early diagnosis and surgical treatment, the prognosis of this tumor remains poor [40].

Recent advances in MDCT, endoscopic ultrasound, magnetic resonance imaging, and positron emission tomography-CT (PET-CT) have dramatically improved the accuracy of preoperative staging of patients with gastric cancer and have provided a more accurate means of assessing tumor response to therapy and detecting recurrent disease [13].

Histologically, gastric cancer is divided into two main types: well-differentiated, intestinal type and undifferentiated, diffuse type. The latter occurs in the setting of diffuse gastritis without atrophy. This histologic type is seen throughout the world, whereas intestinal type occurs in areas with a high incidence of gastric cancer and follows a predictable stepwise progression of cancer development from metaplasia. In 1994, the International Agency for Research on Cancer and The World Health Organization classified *Helicobacter pylori* as a type I carcinogen, but the exact mechanism leading to gastric carcinoma is not clearly understood [40].

On MDCT, advanced gastric cancer presents with mural thickening and abnormal mucosal enhancement.

Early gastric cancer can also be visualized, albeit with less sensitivity, but detection is improved with CTG and multiplanar reformation (MPR) techniques (Figure 6.11). The imaging features depend on the histologic type of tumor and the size and depth of invasion. A high degree of contrast enhancement is significantly more common in signet ring cancer than with nonsignet ring cancers [41].

Initial reports found close agreement between T staging as determined by CT and pathologic staging [42]. Subsequent reports have been less sanguine so that endoscopic ultrasound is currently the most reliable method for preoperative determination of earlier T stage disease. On CT, T1 (see Figure 6.11) and T2 (Figure 6.12) lesions, in which tumor invasion is limited to the gastric wall, the outer border of the stomach, is typically smooth. With T3 lesions, the serosal contours become blurred, and strand-like areas of increased density are often seen extending into the perigastric fat (Figure 6.13). In T4 lesions (Figure 6.14), there is frank tumor extension into the subperitoneal spaces of the various ligaments and omenta and ultimately into the adjacent organs and/or the peritoneal cavity. The spleen may be invaded by the gastrosplenic ligament, the liver via the lesser omentum, the pancreas via the lesser sac, and the colon via the gastrocolic ligament [13].

It is very important to differentiate between T3 and T4 lesions because invasion of adjacent structures makes surgery very difficult. If a gastric mass abuts an adjacent organ on CT and there is absence of a fat plane between the mass and the organ, tumor invasion should be suspected, but this finding is not diagnostic for invasion. Several studies using MPR images have shown improved accuracy when compared to axial images alone [43].

On MDCT, the diagnosis of tumor-related adenopathy depends on size criteria based on short-axis diameter. Lymph nodes in the upper abdomen vary between 6 and 11 mm in size, depending on their location. Lymph nodes in the gastrohepatic ligament (Figure 6.15) are considered abnormal if they exceed 8 mm in diameter. Lymph node size, however, is not a reliable indicator for lymph node metastases in patients with gastric cancer [44].

Liver metastases are present in up to 25% of patients with advanced gastric cancer at the time of presentation. The presence of ascites usually indicates peritoneal seeding although depiction of a solitary small peritoneal deposit may be beneath the spatial resolution of CT. Laparoscopy is more sensitive than CT in the detection of small peritoneal deposits [45].

Gastric cancer spreads beyond the confines of the stomach via a variety of routes: direct extension, intraperitoneal seeding, lymphangitic invasion, and hematogenous metastases (Figure 6.16). The mesenteric reflections and ligaments provide an important natural pathway for direct extension of gastric cancer into the

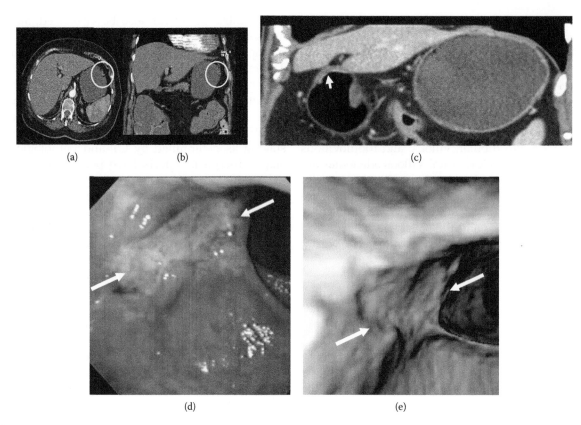

(a)   (b)   (c)

(d)   (e)

FIGURE 6.11
T1 gastric cancer. Axial (a) and coronal multiplanar reformation (MPR) (b) images show a focal mucosal mass along the greater curvature aspect of the gastric fundus (circles). In a different patient, coronal MPR (c), endoscopic (d), and virtual gastroscopy (e) images show a small antral neoplasm (arrows).

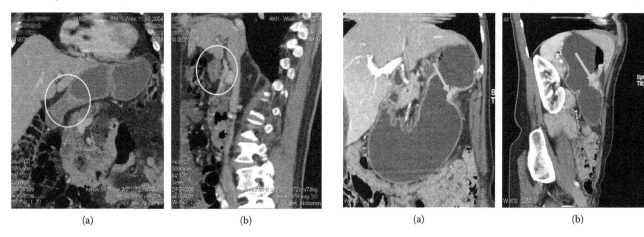

(a)   (b)   (a)   (b)

FIGURE 6.12
T2 gastric cancer. Coronal (a) and sagittal (b) multiplanar reformation images show diffuse circumferential wall thickening of the gastric antrum (arrows). The perigastric fat is intact.

FIGURE 6.13
T3 gastric cancer. Coronal (a) and sagittal (b) multiplanar reformation images show transmural thickening along the greater curvature of the stomach with infiltration of the perigastric fat (arrows).

liver, colon, pancreas, and spleen. The lesser omentum is a frequent site of tumor invasion from gastric and esophageal cancers as well as those arising from the gastroesophageal junction. Gastric cancers can extend down to the subperitoneal space of the gastrocolic ligament and involve the superior haustral row of the transverse colon that becomes fixed and straightened with

selective loss of haustral sacculations. Cancers of the greater curvature of the gastric body and fundus typically spread into the gastrosplenic ligament [32].

Gastric cancer commonly invades adjacent lymphatics, and identification of specific nodal groups is an important part of the staging process. These metastases generally follow lymphatic pathways in the adjacent

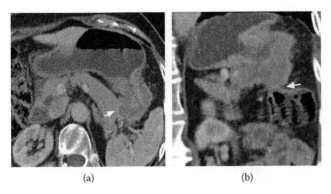

FIGURE 6.14
T4 gastric cancer. (a) Axial scan shows invasion of the pancreatic tail (arrow). (b) Coronal multiplanar reformation shows invasion (arrow) of the transverse mesocolon and superior aspect of the transverse colon.

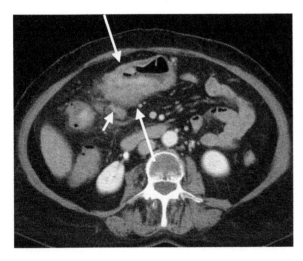

FIGURE 6.15
Perigastric adenopathy in gastric cancer. Axial scan shows marked mural thickening (large arrows) of the gastric antrum with inhomogeneous attenuation. Perigastric adenopathy (small arrow) is present.

peritoneal ligaments, subperitoneal spaces, mesenteries, and omenta [13].

The liver and gut are common sites of hematogenous metastases. The spread of malignant gastric tumor cells in the peritoneal cavity is determined by several factors: the presence of ligaments, mesenteries, and omenta; intraperitoneal fluid pressure gradients; cell type and mitotic rate; and the presence of adhesions and previous surgery. Malignant gastric cells grow where natural flow allows the affected ascites to pool. Ovarian involvement, also known as Krukenberg tumors, may occur via three pathways: hematogenous spread, peritoneal dissemination, and lymphatic invasion [32].

6.8.2 Adenocarcinoma of the Duodenum

Adenocarcinoma is the most frequent primary small bowel tumor, accounting for 40% of these neoplasms. More than half of small bowel adenocarcinomas arise in the duodenum, even though this organ comprises only 4% of the entire length of the small bowel. The majority of adenocarcinomas of the small bowel are located within 25 cm of the ligament of Treitz, either distally or proximally. Adenocarcinomas account for about 80% of all malignant tumors of the duodenum and are slightly more common in men than in women by a factor of 1.2–1.5. A smaller percentage of tumors arise in the jejunum, particularly in the first 30 cm distal to the ligament of Treitz. Ileal adenocarcinomas are the least common, except in patients with Crohn's disease [46].

Primary adenocarcinoma of the duodenum is a rare disease with a poorly defined natural history. It represents less than 0.5% of all GI tract malignant neoplasms but accounts for up to 45% of small bowel cancers. The disease is usually diagnosed at an advanced stage but reported 5 year survivals range as high as 50% [46].

The remarkable feature of duodenal carcinoma is the striking tendency to be associated with several disorders including FAP, Peutz–Jegher's syndrome, Torre's syndrome, neurofibromatosis, and colon carcinoma. Duodenal adenocarcinoma can develop within adenomatous polyps and villous adenocarcinomas in which case it is usually cured by limited excision. There is also an association between celiac disease and Crohn's disease with these neoplasms. Adenocarcinomas of the duodenum most frequently develop in the seventh decade but may develop in individuals under the age of 30 [46].

Duodenal carcinomas are classified according to their relationship to the ampulla of Vater. Infra-ampullary tumors account for about 50%; 40% are ampullary or periampullary, and the remaining 10% are suprampullary. When associated with FAP, they have a strong tendency to develop in the ampullary region. FAP patients have a 100–300 fold increased lifetime risk for developing duodenal or periampullary cancer compared with the general population. Indeed, periampullary adenocarcinoma is the most common extracolonic neoplasm in FAP, and patients with known FAP should undergo surveillance for the purpose of biopsy of normal appearing duodenal and ampullary mucosa to identify early precancerous lesions [47,48].

On CT, duodenal carcinomas present as a discrete polypoid mass or mass-like thickening of the duodenal wall (Figure 6.17). When local adenopathy is present, it may be difficult to differentiate duodenal carcinoma from an adjacent duodenal neoplasm. Concentric or asymmetric narrowing of the duodenal lumen may be present, and the tumor is usually heterogeneous in attenuation and may show moderate contrast enhancement following intravenous contrast administration. Features such as tumor necrosis and ulceration are readily identified. When CT shows an exophytic or intramural mass containing central necrosis and ulceration, this

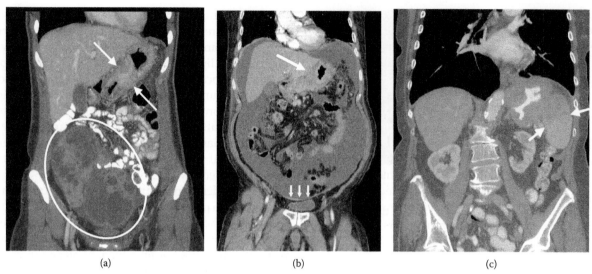

(a)   (b)   (c)

FIGURE 6.16
Advanced gastric cancer in three different patients: patterns of disease spread on multi-detector computed tomography (MDCT). (a) Coronal multiplanar reformation (MPR) images show mural thickening of the stomach (arrows) with bilateral, large ovarian metastases (circle), so called Krukenberg tumors. (b) Coronal MPR shows mural thickening of the stomach with invasion of the gastohepatic ligament (large arrow), malignant ascites, and peritoneal implants (small arrows). (c) Coronal MPR image shows invasion of the gastosplenic ligament (arrows).

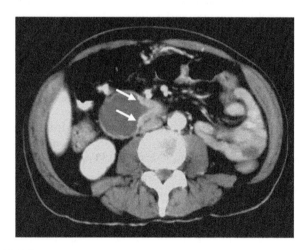

FIGURE 6.17
Duodenal adenocarcinoma. Axial image shows concentric mural thickening (arrows) of the duodenum.

combination of findings is reported to have a sensitivity of 100% and an accuracy of 86% for the detection of malignant tumor [39].

Additional CT findings, such as invasion of retroperitoneal fat planes or surrounding organs, lymph node enlargement, vascular encasement, and distant metastases, help in predicting tumor resectability [49].

6.8.3 Adenocarcinoma of the Small Bowel

On CT, small bowel carcinomas present as a discrete polypoid mass, an annular narrowing with abrupt concentric or irregular "overhanging edges," or an ulcerative

lesion. The tumor is usually heterogeneous in attenuation and may show moderate contrast enhancement following intravenous contrast administration. Features such as tumor necrosis and ulceration are readily identified. Duodenal adenocarcinomas tend to be papillary or polypoid, whereas more distal lesions tend to be annular. Typically, only a short segment of the bowel is involved, and gradual narrowing of the lumen leads to partial or complete small bowel obstruction (SBO) [50].

6.9 Gastric and Small Bowel Lymphoma

The GI tract is the most common extranodal site of involvement by systemic lymphoma, and more than 50% of patients with non-Hodgkin's lymphoma (NHL) have GI tract involvement [51].

6.9.1 Gastric Lymphoma

The stomach is the most common primary site of GI lymphoma followed by the small intestine, the ileocecal region, and the colon. Primary gastric lymphomas are those tumors without systemic involvement until very late in the disease. Confirmatory criteria for primary gastric lymphoma include no palpable adenopathy, normal peripheral blood smear and bone marrow examination, no mediastinal adenopathy, lymphoma limited to the stomach, and no hepatic or splenic involvement except by direct extension [52].

The commonest lymphomas encountered in the stomach are extranodal marginal zone B cell lymphoma of mucosa-associated lymphoid tissue (MALT) type and diffuse B cell lymphomas. The stomach may also be infiltrated in up to 25% of nodal type of lymphomas [53].

MALT lymphoma is a distinctive type of lymphoma that manifests as localized disease and generally has a favorable prognosis. The gastric mucosa normally does not contain lymphatic tissue, and MALT lymphoma is associated with follicular gastritis caused by *H pylori*. CT is useful in differentiating high-grade from low-grade MALT lymphomas. Most low-grade lymphomas show superficial spreading lesions with mucosal nodularity, shallow ulcers, and minimal fold thickening. Most high-grade lymphomas show mass-forming lesions or severe fold thickening [54,55].

Gastric wall thickening is the most common CT finding in NHL (Figure 6.18). Mural thickness is generally greater than 1 cm, and the mean thickness ranges from 2.9 to 5 cm. Thickening affects the wall of the entire stomach in 50% of cases. Lesions in the proximal part of the stomach are often of the segmental form, whereas antral involvement is of the diffuse form. Mural thickening typically involves more than half the circumference of the gastric lumen, and more than one region of the stomach is involved. These findings typify the submucosal spread of gastric lymphoma [56].

In gastric lymphoma, the mural thickening usually is homogeneous but may be inhomogeneous because of the presence of necrosis, hemorrhage, submucosal edema, or infarction. The outer gastric margin is usually smooth or lobulated, whereas the inner gastric wall is frequently irregular in contour representing distortion of the thickened gastric rugae [57].

On CT, gastric lymphoma may be indistinguishable from adenocarcinomas. Features that favor gastric lymphoma over adenocarcinoma include marked gastric wall thickening, more than one lesion, no gastric outlet obstruction, and adenopathy that extends below the level of the renal hila [58].

In patients with known or suspected gastric lymphoma, 2D MPR and CTG may allow both depiction of a gastric lesion and staging of generalized lymphoma in the abdomen. Because the most frequent finding in both gastric lymphoma and gastric MALT lymphoma is mural thickening, careful attention to technique is needed. CTG and two-dimensional (2D) MPR images provide clear visualization of the gross morphology of gastric lymphoma, including change in the dimensions of the gastric lumen, the gastric wall, and the perigastric adenapthy. CTG affords better evaluation of the mucosal changes. CTG can show mucosal nodularity, a shallow or deep ulcer, single or multiple masses, rugal thickening, and enlarged areae gastricae. CTG and 2D MPR may permit early diagnosis of disease progression in patients undergoing therapy and follow-up for low-grade MALT lymphoma [59].

6.9.2 Small Bowel Lymphoma

NHL is the third most common small bowel malignancy representing approximately 10%–15% of these tumors. Most primary malignant lymphomas of the small intestine occur in the terminal ileum but on rare occasion may originate in the duodenum. Men are affected three times more frequently than women, with a peak age of the fifth decade [60].

Reflecting the diverse morphology of the disease, small bowel lymphoma has a great variety of radiologic appearances: an infiltrating form, a polypoid form, multiple nodular defects, and an endoenteric-exoenteric form with ulceration and fistula formation [61].

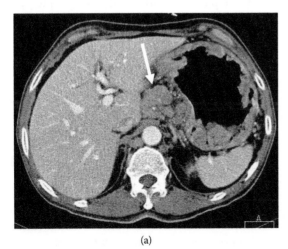

(a)

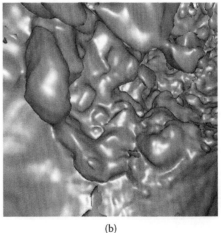

(b)

FIGURE 6.18

Gastric lymphoma. (a) Coronal multiplanar reformation image shows marked thickening of the rugal folds of the stomach as well as retrocrural and gastrohepatic ligament (arrow) adenopathy. (b) Endoluminal view from computed tomography gastroscopy (CTG).

Circumferentially, infiltrating lymphoma involves a variable length of small bowel with thickening and later effacement of folds. The lumen is more often widened than narrowed, so called "aneurysmal dilatation." This implies a localized, nonobstructive dilatation of the bowel caused by destruction of the muscle wall and myenteric plexus by infiltrating tumor.

On CT, lymphoma of the small bowel typically presents as a homogenous density mass causing mural thickening and separation of adjacent small bowel loops (Figure 6.19). These lesions tend to be more homogenous and show less contrast enhancement than other malignant tumors. In the cavitary endoenteric form of the disease, there is deep ulceration within a large lymphomatous mass arising from the small bowel. NHL of the small bowel does not evoke a desmoplastic reaction so that bowel obstruction is rare even though the associated tumor mass may be large compared to adenocarcinoma or carcinoid [56].

Infiltrating lymphomas manifest with diffuse wall thickening and destruction of the normal small bowel folds without obstruction. This type of lymphoma commonly infiltrates the muscular layer and disrupts the myoenteric plexus, leading to so called "aneurysmal dilation" of the affected segment in up to 50% of cases [61].

The fourth pattern of small bowel lymphoma is an exophytic mass that can ulcerate simulating adenocarcinoma, GIST, and metastases [62].

Small bowel lymphomas commonly present with mesenteric adenopathy as well. As the tumor grows, the mesenteric vessels and small bowel loops may become encased but not obstructed. Following intravenous contrast administration, the vascular encasement of the

normal vessels coursing through the adenopathy can produce the so called sandwich sign [63].

6.10 Gastrointestinal Stromal Tumors

GIST is a neoplasm that arises in the smooth muscle pacemaker cells of Cajal. GISTs constitute the majority of all GI mesenchymal tumors. Formerly classified as leiomyomas and leiomyosarcomas, GISTs are now recognized as a distinct class of mesenchymal tumors that is separate from true smooth muscle tumors of the GI tract. They have a different etiology, immunohistology, and clinical course [64].

GISTs arise within the muscularis propria of the GI wall and can occur anywhere in the GI tract from the esophagus to the rectum but arise most frequently in the stomach (60%), followed by the small intestine (20%–30%), the colon, the rectum, and the esophagus. GISTs are submucosal in origin with a predilection for extraluminal involvement. They are highly vascular neoplasms with a tendency to undergo necrosis that explains their heterogeneous appearance on imaging [65].

These tumors express the c-kit protooncogene protein, a cell membrane receptor with tyrosine kinase activity. A mutation in the c-kit protooncogene results in activation of the Kit receptor tyrosine kinase, which leads to unchecked cell growth and resistance to apoptosis. The development of a Kit tyrosine kinase inhibitor, imatinibmesylate (Gleevac), has made it vital to distinguish GISTs from other mesenchymal tumors of the GI tract [66].

GISTs are rare in patients younger than 40 years, occurring predominantly in middle-aged patients. Most patients with GIST are symptomatic and bleeding because mucosal ulceration is the most common symptom. Surgery remains the mainstay of treatment in patients with localized GISTs [67].

Unlike most GI epithelial tumors, the majority of GISTs (76%) are exophytic in growth so that obstruction is uncommon even in the setting of very large tumors. These tumors may undergo extensive necrosis and fistula formation, resulting in the formation of a cavity within the mass and bleeding. GISTs that have a fistulous tract to the gut may show an air-fluid level. Orally administered positive contrast material may also be seen within the mass. After the intravenous administration of contrast material, large tumors show heterogeneous enhancement, whereas small tumors may show homogeneous enhancement [68,69].

The presence of focal areas of low attenuation in GISTs is a nonspecific finding that can be seen in a variety of pathologic conditions such as hypocellular tumor,

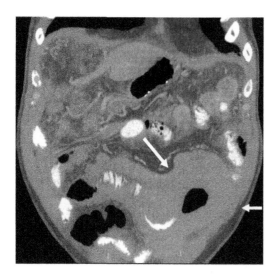

FIGURE 6.19
Small bowel lymphoma: MDCT findings. Coronal multiplanar reformation image shows relatively homogeneous, marked mural thickening of the ileum (arrow) with aneurysmal dilation.

hemorrhage, necrosis, cystic degeneration, and fluid in an ulcer. Accordingly, these low-density areas in small GISTs are not predictors of malignant potential [70].

GISTs are usually detected on MDCT examinations and are often found incidentally. Small tumors manifest as intramural masses. [71] As the tumor grows, the overlying mucosa can ulcerate (Figure 6.20). Imaging features that suggest malignancy include a large tumor size, an exophytic mass, and a mass containing areas of central necrosis or calcification. When tumors are large and exophytic, it may be difficult to identify the organ of origin (Figure 6.21). It is unusual to find adenopathy in patients with GISTs [72].

With the new generation of molecularly target agents such as Gleevac, apparently the conventional objective response criteria such as lesion size are no longer sufficient to assess tumor response to therapy. The difference in metabolic activity after even a single dose of imatinibmesylate can be dramatic on PET-CT, whereas little or no change may be seen on the corresponding CT scan. The best metrics are the optimized PET standardized uptake values threshold of 3.4 at 1 month [73,74].

6.11 Carcinoid and Other Neuroendocrine Tumors

Carcinoid tumors are rare tumors of neuroendocrine cells that can arise in the GI tract or bronchial tree. All carcinoids are considered to have malignant potential and are typically slow growing. They most commonly occur in the small bowel, but the incidence of gastric carcinoid is increasing. [75] Tumor location and patient age are the main predictors of pathologic behavior. Patients greater than 60 years have a poorer prognosis [76].

6.11.1 Gastric Carcinoid Tumors

Type I and I enterochromaffin-like cell gastric carcinoids are multifocal, smoothly marginated, 1–2 cm mural masses located in the gastric body and fundus. They may appear as an enhancing mucosal or submucosal mass. Irrespective of cell type and biologic potential, larger carcinoids may have mucosal ulcerations on the surface of the mass. In the setting of Zollinger–Ellison

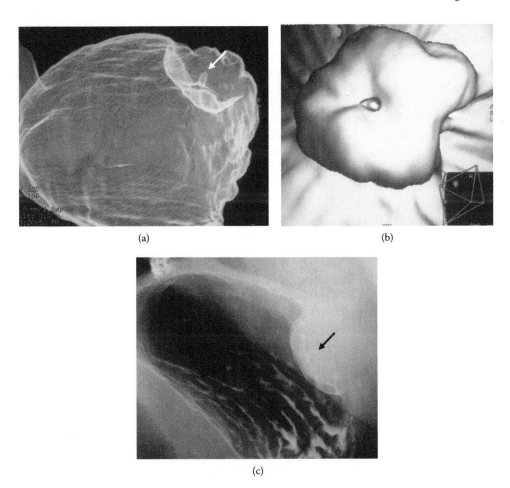

(a)

(b)

(c)

FIGURE 6.20
Benign gastric gastrointestinal stromal tumor (GIST). Shaded surface display (a), endoluminal view (b), and barium study (showing) and ulcerating mass (c) (arrows) along the greater curvature aspect of the stomach.

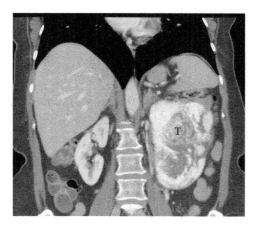

FIGURE 6.21
Hypervascular gastric GIST. Coronal multiplanar reformation image shows an inhomogeneously, robustly enhancing tumor (T) in the left upper quadrant.

syndrome and multiple endocrine neoplasia-type 1, marked mural thickening of the stomach and innumerable nodular mucosal and mural masses may be present that show enhancement during the hepatic arterial phase. In patients with hypergastrinemia and suspected gastric carcinoids, gastric distention is important and scans should be obtained during the hepatic arterial and portal venous phases to maximize detection of the primary gastric lesions as well as liver metastases [77,78].

Type III enterochromaffin-like cell carcinoids are solitary, large mural masses in the body and fundus of the stomach that may be ulcerated. Because these lesions have a distinct malignant potential, imaging studies should be scrutinized for the presence of perigastric adenopathy and liver metastases [77,79].

6.11.2 Duodenal Carcinoid and Other Neuroendocrine Tumors

Considerable evidence has accumulated indicating that carcinoid and endocrine tumors of the duodenum are so closely related that they represent variants of the same category of neoplasm. Although they originate from a common neuroectodermal precursor cell that is related to the argentaffin cell, they have various names depending on histologic features, histochemistry, immunocytochemistry and ultrastructure, and secreted peptide: carcinoid, glandular carcinoid, carcinoid-islet cell tumor, gastrinoma, somatostatinoma, and insulinoma [80].

Many duodenal neuroendocrine tumors manifest as smooth, tan-yellow, submucosal polypoid masses. Incidentally discovered masses that become symptomatic secondary to the elaboration of hormones are generally small, <2 cm. Large lesions may reach several

centimeters in diameter and present with symptoms related to mass lesions such as recurrent abdominal pain, painless jaundice, and GI hemorrhage [81].

Three GI neuroendocrine tumors have a predicilition for the duodenum: somatostatinoma, gangliocytic paraganglioma, and gastrinoma [82–84].

On CT, neuroendocrine tumors typically are well marginated and hypervascular (Figure 6.22). If they actively secrete peptides, they are usually found at an earlier stage and as a consequence may be small. If endocrinologically inactive or hypoactive, they can attain a large size. Hepatic metastases from these neoplasms are typically hypervascular [85].

CT findings include asymmetrical mural thickening that seldom causes obstruction, a large polypoid mass with necrosis or cavitation, similar to GIST. Additional visceral or retroperitoneal adenopathy as well as splenomegaly also suggest the diagnosis [13,86].

6.11.3 Small Bowel Carcinoids

The majority of GI carcinoids are found within 2–3 ft of the ileocecal valve: 50% in the appendix and 33% in the small bowel. Small bowel carcinoids that come

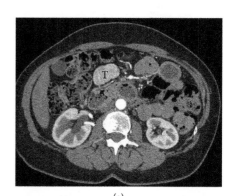

(a)

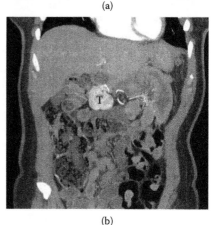

(b)

FIGURE 6.22
Duodenal neuroendocrine tumor. Axial (a) and coronal multiplanar reformation (b) images show a strikingly vascular duodenal mass (T).

to surgery are usually small, 1–2 cm, submucosal-intramural tumors that bulge slightly into the lumen. As they enlarge, they can become polypoid and cause intussusception or obstruction. Tumors <2 cm in size are usually discovered incidentally. They appear as smooth, rounded, 1–2 cm elevations in the distal ileum. The tumors may be mucosal or submucosal in appearance, without desmoplastic changes, and be indistinguishable from other tumors such as GISTs, lipomas, adenomas, submucosal metastases, and lymphoma. When submucosal carcinoids ulcerate, they produce a "target" or "bull's-eye" appearance that can be seen with metastatic melanoma or breast cancer, lymphoma, and Kaposi's sarcoma [87].

Small bowel carcinoids begin as small polypoid masses but have a tendency to invade into the submucosa and eventually infiltrate the muscularispropria, serosa, and then invade mesenteric lymph nodes. Small carcinoid tumors when confined to the bowel wall can be difficult to detect on routine CT scans. These lesions present as small, robustly enhancing masses, and detection is improved when water or other neutral contrast is given as an intraluminal contrast agent and MPR images obtained [88].

MDCT is superb in depicting the mesenteric extension of carcinoid tumors, the presence of adenopathy and liver metastases. A stellate, spiculated, and infiltrative mesenteric mass (Figure 6.23) is usually identified, and calcifications are identified in up to 70% of cases. The spiculation does not necessarily indicate tumor invasion but more commonly reflects the desmoplastic changes that occur in the mesentery in response to secretion of serotonin and tryptophan. The mesenteric vessels may be involved directly by tumor encasement and narrowing or indirectly as a result of the vasoactive hormones than affect the vessel wall [89].

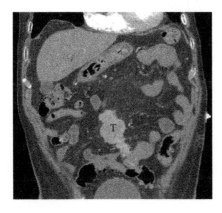

FIGURE 6.23
Small bowel carcinoid. Coronal multiplanar reformation image shows a spiculated mesenteric mass (T).

6.12 Metastases to the Stomach and Small Bowel

6.12.1 Gastric Metastases

Gastric metastases are uncommon, found at autopsy in less than 2% of patients who die of malignancy. The majority of lesions are hematogenous metastases from malignant melanoma or carcinoma of the breast or lung. These lesions are typically submucosal in origin. Breast cancer metastases may cause diffuse mural thickening of the gastric wall indistinguishable from infiltrative gastric adenocarcinoma [90].

Contiguous tumor invasion into the stomach may occur from tumors that arise in neighboring structures: pancreatic cancer may invade the posterior wall of the gastric body and antrum via the transverse mesocolon; colon cancer arising in the transverse colon may invade the stomach via the gastrocolic ligament, and carcinoma of the distal esophagus can invade the gastric cardia [32].

6.12.2 Small Bowel Metastases

Metastases may spread to the small bowel hematogeonously, by direct extension or by intraperitoneal seeding. Mucinous tumors of the ovary, pancreas, appendix, and colon may seed the peritoneum, leading to multiple small nodular metastases along the serosa, mesentery, and omentum. The clinical history is often needed to distinguish metastatic lesions from multiple primary small bowel tumors such as lymphomas and adenocarcinomas. Ovarian tumors are the most common cause of disseminated serosal implants [38].

Hematomgeonous metastases from bronchogenic carcinoma and breast or malignant melanoma may develop into a large bulky mesenteric mass. MDCT is helpful in determining the extent of metastatic involvement and identifying the primary tumor. As in primary adenocarcinoma, metastases may cause mural thickening. Metastates may also involve the mesenteric or retroperitoneal fat with diffuse infiltration or increase density. Duodenal metastases may also cause biliary and pancreatic ductal obstruction [91].

6.13 Small Bowel Obstruction

SBO is responsible for nearly 20% causes of acute abdominal surgical conditions. Most are due to adhesions (50%), hernias (30%), and neoplasms (5%). Less common causes include inflammatory bowel disease, trauma, gallstones, abscesses associated with appendicitis and diverticulitis, foreign bodies, and endometriosis. MDCT has replaced conventional contrast studies because it can more reliably answer several key questions: is obstruction present?; what is the level of the obstruction?; what is the cause of the obstruction?; what is the severity of the obstruction?; is the obstruction simple or closed loop?; and is strangulation or ischemia present? It is important to differentiate between simple and closed-loop obstruction because the later requires prompt surgical intervention while the former may respond to conservative measures [92,93].

The hallmark of bowel obstruction is the delineation of a transition zone between dilated and decompressed bowel. Careful inspection of the transition zone and luminal contents often reveals the underlying cause of the obstruction. On MDCT, there are several clues that are helpful for finding the point of obstruction. The so called "small bowel feces sign" (Figure 6.24) is the presence of mottled, feculent-appearing, intraluminal small bowel contents [94]. This usually develops closest to the point of obstruction. The lumen of small bowel proximal to the obstruction also becomes progressively more dilated, the closer to the level of the obstruction. If positive contrast material is given orally, it typically becomes more dilute approaching the obstruction. Also, it is important to search for incisions and port sites along the anterior abdominal and pelvic wall as adhesions often occur at these locations [95–98].

6.13.1 Simple Bowel Obstruction

In simple SBO, there is typically a single transition zone between dilated and nondilated segments of small bowel (Figure 6.25). The dilatation of the small bowel proximal to the level of the obstruction tapers gradually toward the

ligament of Trietz. The obstructed loops have a meandering course that mirrors the course of the root of the small bowel mesentery. No ischemic changes are present [99].

6.13.2 Closed-Loop Obstruction and Strangulation

Closed-loop, SBO is a high-grade mechanical obstruction in which a segment of bowel is occluded at two points along its course by a single constricting lesion occluding the small bowel lumen. CT findings in closed-loop obstruction depend on the length, degree of distention, and orientation of the closed loop in the abdomen (Figure 6.26). When a closed small bowel loop is horizontally oriented, it has a U- or C-shaped configuration. A radial configuration, simulating a peacock's tail, with stretched mesenteric vessels converging toward the site of torsion may be detected depending on the orientation of the small bowel loops [100]. At the site of obstruction, the collapsed loops are round, oval, or triangular. The "beak sign" seen at the site of torsion appears as a fusiform tapering at longitudinal bowel imaging. A tightly twisted mesentery may be present in patients with volvulus producing the so called "whirl sign" [101].

When ischemia develops, the bowel wall may thicken and have a target appearance caused by submucosal edema. Enhancement of the bowel segment in the closed loop may be diminished or delayed. Fluid and hemorrhage may collect in the mesentery, bowel wall, and lumen of the involved segment. The mesentery becomes hazy in appearance, and ascites may develop. Closed-loop obstruction is most commonly seen in patients with volvulus and internal and external hernias [102,103].

The reported prevalence of strangulating SBO ranges from 5% to 42%, and its mortality rate ranges from 20% to 37%. Although strangulation can be seen with adhesive obstruction, it most commonly occurs in patients

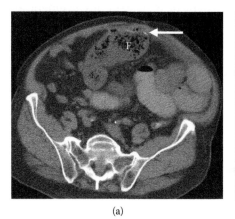 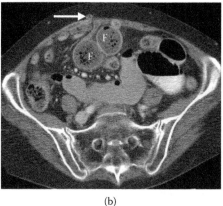 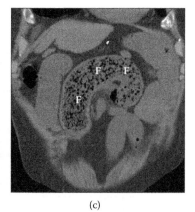

(a)   (b)   (c)

FIGURE 6.24
Small bowel feces sign in three different patients. (a) Axial scan shows an adhesion associated with herniorrhaphy mesh (arrow) as the cause of obstruction. Note the small bowel feces (F) sign. (b) Port site hernia (arrow) leading to small bowel obstruction and the small bowel feces (F) sign. (c) Coronal multiplanar reformation image shows the small bowel feces sign (F). The case of the obstruction was a small carcinoid tumor not visualized on the scan.

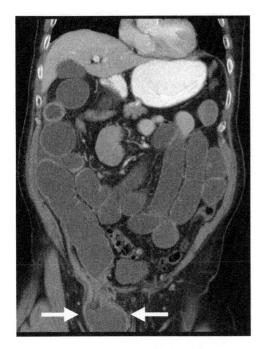

FIGURE 6.25
Simple small bowel obstruction on MDCT. Coronal multiplanar reformation image shows a right inguinal hernia (arrows) causing the obstruction.

with internal or external hernias. CT findings include high-grade SBO, a circumferentially thickened loop with high attenuation within the wall, the "target sign," and congestion or hemorrhage in the mesentery attached to the closed loop. With worsening strangulation, pneumatosis intestinalis may develop. Ascites is also a suspicious finding for ischemia and strangulation [61,104,105].

6.13.3 Gastric Outlet Obstruction

Peptic ulcer disease is responsible for two-thirds of gastric outlet obstructions in adults. An annular constricting carcinoma of the distal antrum or pylorus is the second leading cause (30%–35% of cases), but other infiltrating primary malignant tumors or metastatic lesions can also produce gastric outlet obstruction. CT shows a massively dilated, secretion-and/or food-filled stomach. Benign versus malignant causes of the gastric outlet obstruction can be differentiated by observing a mass in the region of the gastric outlet or by demonstration of inflammatory disease in adjacent structures [17].

6.13.4 Extrinsic Causes of Small Bowel Obstruction

6.13.4.1 Adhesions

Adhesions develop in more than 90% of patients who have had prior abdominal and pelvic surgery. It is therefore not surprising that adhesions are responsible for

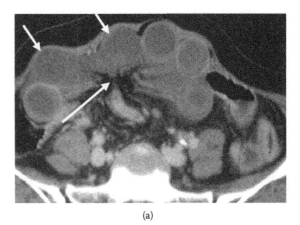

(a)

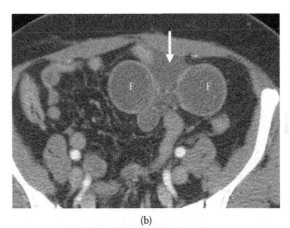

(b)

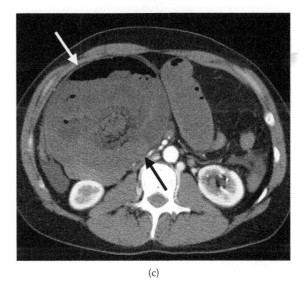

(c)

FIGURE 6.26
Closed-loop obstruction in three different patients. (a) There is a cluster of small bowel loops that converge to a single point (large arrow), arrayed-like a peacock's tail. Note the poorly perfused, ischemic segments (small arrows) and mesenteric edema in this patient with a transomental hernia. (b) There is a short segment of markedly distended fluid filled (F) small bowel associated with mesenteric fluid (arrow) in this patient with a transmesenteric internal hernia. (c) Right paraduodenal hernia with a poorly perfused segment of jejunum (arrows) causing high-grade small bowel obstruction and mural and mesenteric edema and hemorrhage.

some 50%–80% of SBOs. The adhesion(s) can be seen either at the site of surgery or remotely in the peritoneal cavity. Less common causes of adhesions include prior peritoneal inflammation and endometriosis. The diagnosis of adhesive obstruction is primarily one of exclusion because adhesive bands are not seen typically identified at CT. More commonly, an abrupt change in the caliber of the bowel is seen without any associated mass lesion, significant inflammation, mesenteric twist, or bowel wall thickening at the transition point. These findings combined with a history of abdominal surgery and associated kinking and tethering of the adjacent nonobstructed bowel usually suggests the diagnosis [106].

6.13.4.2 Hernias

Hernias are the second most common cause of SBO, responsible for 10% of cases. They are classified according to the anatomic location of the orifice through which the bowel protrudes and further categorized as external or internal types. An external hernia results from a defect in the abdominal and pelvic wall at sites of congenital weakness or previous surgery. Internal hernias, which are less common, develop when there is protrusion of bowel through a portion of the peritoneum, omentum, or mesentery and into a compartment within the abdominal cavity. Diagnosis of an internal hernia is almost always made radiologically, whereas many external hernias are apparent on physical examination [107].

MPR images are often helpful in assessing the size and location of the hernia defect; its contents; and depicting adverse features such as ischemia, strangulation, infection, or inflammation. Inguinal, femoral, obturator, spigelian, ventral, hiatal, lumbar, Bochdalek, and Morgagni hernias are well depicted on MDCT with MPR images. [108].

6.13.4.3 Tumors

SBO is one of the major manifestations of carcinoid tumor. It usually results from the intense desmoplastic disease in the adjacent mesentery. CT shows the mesenteric metastasis as a nodular mass in association with retraction of surrounding bowel loops with mural thickening [109].

NHL produces a small bowel lesion that is soft and tends to produce early cavitation. Obstruction is rare, even when they are annular. Nodal NHL, however, may arise in the mesentery and grow to invade small bowel segments, causing obstruction by compression, kinking, and infiltration.

Metastases are the most common form of malignant SBO (Figure 6.27). Carcinomatosis and serosal involvement is typically found with a mesenteric or omental mass in the transition zone causing obstruction [110].

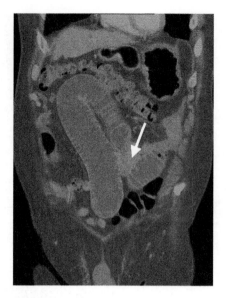

FIGURE 6.27
Small bowel obstruction because of recurrent colon cancer. Peritoneal tumor (arrow) is producing small bowel obstruction on the coronal multiplanar reformation image.

When a small bowel adenocarcinoma causes SBO, it is usually at an advanced stage and shows pronounced, asymmetric, and irregular mural thickening at the transition point. Adenocarcinoma of the cecum or ileocecal valve is the colonic cause of SBO. An obstruction located anywhere in the colon can lead to small bowel dilation and obstruction, if the ileocecal valve is competent and obstructed colonic contents reflux and decompress into the small bowel [93].

6.13.4.4 Appendicitis, Colonic Diverticulitis, and Meckel's Diverticulum

Appendicitis, colonic diverticulits, and Meckel's diverticulum complications are under appreciated causes of SBO. MDCT is superb in depicting both the primary pathologic process and the obstruction. SBO usually occurs in the setting of a complicating phlegmon, abscess, or peritonitis. The bowel loops become trapped within the inflammatory process, resulting in fixation and narrowing [111,112].

Intestinal obstruction is the second most common complication of Meckel's diverticulum; however, the diagnosis is rarely made preoperatively. The CT diagnosis of Meckel's diverticulitis relies on the identification of a blind-ending, tubular, round, or oval structure in the right lower quadrant or periumbilical region with surrounding inflammation. The diverticulum may contain an air-fluid level, fluid only, or fecal-like material. Inflammatory changes such as mural thickening and hyperenhancement may be observed. Softtissue stranding and adjacent fluid collections are also suggestive features of diverticulitis. Enteroliths will occasionally be present within the inflamed diverticulum [113]. Other helpful diagnostic features include the presence of a pouch-like structure attached to the adjacent small bowel and visualization of a normal appendix [114].

6.13.5 Intrinsic Causes of Small Bowel Obstruction

6.13.5.1 Intussusception

A variety of intrinsic and less commonly extrinsic or intraluminal processes may cause obstructing small bowel intussusception. In this disorder, there is invagination of a more proximal small bowel loop and part of its mesentery into the lumen of the more distal small bowel or colon (Figure 6.28). Nonobstructing transient intussusception is the most common type of intussusception found in adults. Transient intussusceptions as a general rule do not need to be further evaluated; if the patient is otherwise asymptomatic, the intussusception is in the jejunum and is less than 3.5 cm in length, and there is no associated proximal dilation of bowel [115].

Benign or malignant polypoid tumors are the most common cause of obstructing small bowel intussusception in adults. Intussusception may occur in extrinsic disorders such as adhesions or duplications. On MDCT, intussusception displays one of three patterns depending on the severity and duration of the disease and the scanning plane: the target sign, a sausage-shaped mass with alternating layers of low and high attenuation, and a reniform mass. When sufficiently large, the lead point can be depicted on CT [116].

6.13.5.2 Crohn's Disease

In the advanced cicatrizing phase of Crohn's disease, patients frequently present with recurrent episodes of partial SBO and, less commonly, high-grade obstruction. CT is extremely useful for determining the site, level, and cause of SBO secondary to Crohn's disease. This is discussed more fully later [30].

6.13.5.3 Adenocarcinoma

Adencarcinoma of the small bowel is an uncommon cause of SBO and usually manifests as mural thickening with luminal narrowing at the transition point. CT also depicts the presence of tumor extension into the adjacent mesentery or organs and the presence of local or distant metastases [93].

6.13.6 Intraluminal Causes

Gallstone ileus is caused by migration of a large gallstone through a biliary-intestinal fistula with

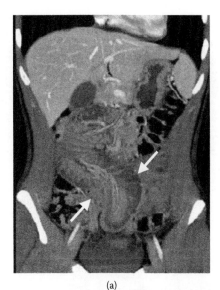

(a)

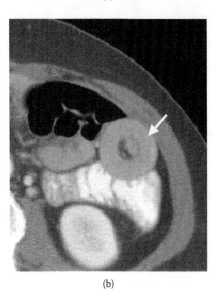

(b)

FIGURE 6.28
Intussusception: MDCT findings. (a) Coronal reformatted multiplanar reformation image shows an intussusception producing a sausage-like appearance (arrows) because of lymphoma. (b) Transient intussusceptions are typically nonobstructing, occur in the jejunum, extend <3.5 cm in length, and create a target appearance (arrow) on axial images. These usually are of little clinical significance.

subsequent impaction in the small bowel. CT findings are pathognomonic, corresponding to the radiographic triad of pneumobilia, ectopic gallstone, and SBO (Figure 6.29) [93].

Bezoars as a cause of SBO are increasing in number as more patients are undergoing gastric bypass surgery. This surgery prevents adequate digestion of vegetable fibers, which become impacted, causing the obstruction. Bezoars appear as an intraluminal mass with an ovoid shape and a mottled gas pattern on MDCT [93].

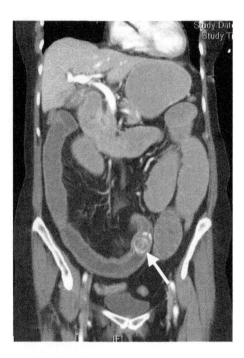

FIGURE 6.29
Gallstone ileus. A lamellated gallstone (arrow) is causing moderately high-grade small bowel obstruction on this coronal multiplanar reformation image.

6.14 Crohn's Disease

Crohn's disease is an idiopathic inflammatory disease that can affect any part of the GI tract from the mouth to the anus. The small bowel is involved in 80% of patients with the terminal ileum by far the most common location. Symptomatic patients may have active inflammatory disease, chronic changes, or pathology unrelated to Crohn's disease. The purposes of imaging are to detect the presence, severity, and extent of disease; assess disease activity and response to therapy; and depict extraintestinal complications such as abscesses, fistula, and obstruction [30,117].

Traditionally, the small bowel barium examination has been the primary means of evaluating patients with known or suspected Crohn's disease. MDCT, particulary, CT enterography (CTE) with MPR images have gained acceptance as the primary means of depicting the mural and mesenteric manifestations of Crohn's disease [19,118,119].

Four subtypes of Crohn's disease have been identified that are useful for guiding medical and surgical management: active inflammatory, fistulizing-perforating, fibrostenosing, and reparative-regenerative [120,121].

6.14.1 Active Inflammatory Subtype

Focal inflammation, superficial or deep ulceration, and activation of lymphoid tissue characterize the active inflammatory subtype of Crohn's disease. MDCT at this early stage may show hyperenhancement of the mucosa with minimal mural thickening (Figure 6.30a). These findings are more readily appreciated with neutral intraluminal contrast agents. With more extensive disease, mural stratification producing a target appearance of the small bowel becomes apparent. There is an inner ring of thickened, inflamed-enhancing mucosa, a middle low-density ring because of submucosa edema, and an outer soft-tissue density ring formed by the muscularis propria. Other features include local mesenteric hypervascularity (comb sign); mesenteric fat stranding (creeping fat of the mesentery); and detection of extraluminal findings such as adenopathy, mesenteric abscess, and subperitoneal and free intraperitoneal fluid [122].

These signs, either alone or in combination, correlate well with clinical disease activity and symptoms. Mesenteric changes, such as including dilated and tortuous vessels, supplying the inflamed segment strongly correlate with disease activity. Prominent lymph nodes and fibrofatty proliferation of the mesentery are increased in active disease. Thickening of the bowel wall alone does not predict disease activity, but the combination of mural thickening, mucosal hyperenhancement, and mural stratification shows a significant correlation to disease activity [123].

6.14.2 Fistulizing-Perforative Subtype

This subtype is characterized by active inflammation with progression of the deep ulcers through the bowel wall, resulting in sinus tracts or fistulae formation. On MDCT, the following features are seen: deep fissuring ulcers and sinus tracts; fistulae to adjacent bowel loops (Figure 6.30b) or other organs; abscess formation; and extraintestinal disease [124].

6.14.3 Fibrosteontic Subtype

Fibrostenosing Crohn's disease usually develops in patients with long standing disease. Mural thickening and lumen narrowing are present that leads to SBO and prestenotic dilation (Figure 6.30c). The stenotic wall may only show mild enhancement because of the fibrous nature of the disease. The degree of stenosis is variable, ranging from mild to severe. This subtype can cause SBO that needs to be differentiated from SBO secondary to spasm and submucosal edema associated with active disease [125].

6.14.4 Reparative or Regenerative Disease Subtype

The regenerative-reparative subtype of Crohn's disease is histologically consistent with inactive CD. It may be associated with other phases of Crohn's disease located in different locations in the small bowel. On MDCT, submucosal fat deposition may be found (Figure 6.30d). Also, loss of mural stratification because of transmural fibrosis

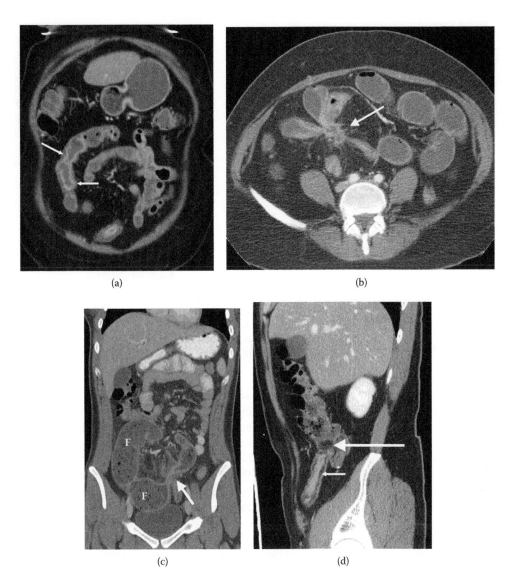

(a)

(b)

(c)

(d)

FIGURE 6.30
The four subtypes of Crohn's disease: MDCT features. (a) Active inflammatory subtype. Coronal reformatted multiplanar reformation (MPR) shows mural thickening and mucosal hyperenhancement (arrows) of several segments of mid ileum. (b) Fistulizing-perforative subtype. Enteroenteral fistulae are associated with a small mesenteric abscess (arrow). (c) Fibrostenotic subtype. Coronal reformatted MPR image shows stenosis (arrow) of the proximal ileum causing partial small bowel obstruction and the small bowel feces sign (F). (d) Reparative-regenerative subtype. Sagital MPR image shows mural thickening with submucosal fat (small arrow) in this patient with chronic Crohn's disease. There is fatty infiltration of the ileocecal valve (large arrow).

may also be seen. There may be a decrease in lumen caliber, postinflammatory pseudopolyps, but there should be no active inflammation seen in affected segment [126].

In many patients, different segment of small bowel will show different phases of disease activity (Figure 6.31).

6.15 Mesenteric Ischemia

Patients with intestinal ischemic disorders most often present with abdominal pain and other nonspecific symptoms such as nausea, vomiting, diarrhea, and bloating [127]. The diagnosis of mesenteric ischemia is often one of exclusion after more common possibilities including bowel obstruction, appendicitis, diverticulitis, cholelithiasis, peptic ulcer disease, and gastroenteritis have been excluded. Intestinal ischemia accounts for approximately 1% of patients presenting with the acute abdomen and 0.1% of all hospital admissions [128,129].

GI tract ischemia can threaten bowel viability with potentially catastrophic consequences including intestinal necrosis and gangrene. Dramatic improvements in MDCT as well as other cross-sectional imaging techniques have the potential to afford earlier and

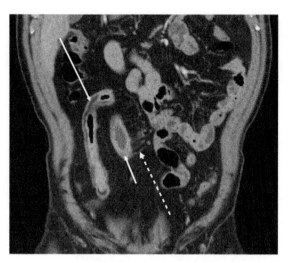

FIGURE 6.31
Spectrum of mural involvement by Crohn's disease in the same patient. Hyperenhancement of the mucosa (short solid arrow) and engorged vasa recta (long broken arrow) indicate active inflammatory disease. Submucosal fat deposition (long solid arrow) is seen in another segment indicating reparative-regenerative disease.

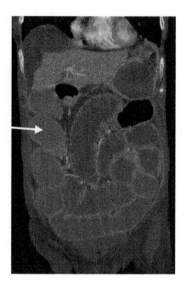

FIGURE 6.32
Bowel changes in superior mesenteric artery embolism. Coronal reformatted multiplanar reformation image shows diffuse small bowel dilation with a large amount of intraluminal fluid. The fluid in the distal ileal loop is somewhat hyperdense (arrow) because of hemorrhage.

more precise diagnosis, key to reducing morbidity and mortality of this potentially fatal condition [130].

The principle causes of small bowel ischemic disorders are as follows: superior mesenteric artery embolism (SMAE)—50%; nonocclusive mesenteric ischemia (NOMI)—20%–30%; superior mesenteric artery thrombosis (SMAT)—15%–25%; and superior mesenteric vein thrombosis (SMVT)—5% [131].

MDCT has become the preferred imaging technique for the evaluation of patients with suspected acute and chronic intestinal ischemia [132]. It can be performed quickly in critically ill patients and is less dependent on operator skill and patient factors than on other imaging examinations. CT angiography can visualize even tiny distal vascular segments and depict stenoses and their causes: atherosclerotic plaque, thrombus, anatomic abnormalities (e.g., bowel obstruction), and tumor [130,133].

6.15.1 Superior Mesenteric Artery Embolism

The wide caliber and narrow take off angle of the superior mesenteric artery (SMA) off the aorta make it particularly vulnerable to embolic events. The embolism usually lodges in the proximal SMA, 3–10 cm from its origin, in a tapered segment just distal to the middle colic artery branch, although some 15% of emboli will cause occlusion at the origin of the SMA. Multiple emboli are present in 20% of cases [134].

The initial immediate response to vascular injury of the gut is spasm of the involved segments. MDCT may show increased intraluminal secretions within the involved segments (Figure 6.32). With persistent

arterial occlusion, there is disruption of the microvascular integrity of the bowel wall. This increases mucosal permeability so that the remaining blood may extravasate causing hemorrhagic foci in the thinned bowel wall. MDCT shows these findings as a "paper thin" bowel wall with decreased mural enhancement. (see Figure 6.3) If reperfusion does not occur, transmural bowel necrosis may ensue and intramural air may dissect into the necrotic mucosa and from there intramurally, subperitoneally, into the peritoneal cavity, and ultimately spread through the mesenteric and portal venous system [135].

If the arterial blood flow compromise is alleviated, reperfusion of the gut is associated with several radiographic findings best seen with MDCT. Blood plasma, contrast material, and/or red blood cells may extravasate through the disrupted vascular wall into the mucosa and submucosa causing mural thickening and bloody fluid filling the intestinal lumen. The thickened submucosa may be hyperdense because of hemorrhage. Following contrast administration, the mucosa may show hyperenhancement with submucosal edema and hypodensity. Mural stratification typically is preserved. Poor inner-layer enhancement of MDCT is consistent with sloughed or necrotic mucosa [136].

The distribution of pneumatosis intestinalis is useful in differentiating early and nontransmural mesenteric ischemia from full-thickness and irreversible transmural infarction. Linear pneumatosis is more often seen than bubbly pneumatosis in patients with transmural bowel infarction. Pneumatosis intestinalis that accompanies portomesenteric venous gas correlates strongly with transmural bowel infarction, whereas pneumatosis without evidence of portomesenteric gas is more commonly seen in the setting of ischemia [27].

6.15.2 Nonocclusive Mesenteric Ischemia

The diagnosis of NOMI is made by excluding other causes for intestinal ischemia such as atherosclerosis, arterial or venous thrombosis, embolism, or vasculitis. NOMI is seen in the setting of splanchnic vasoconstriction precipitated by hypoperfusion from acute myocardial infarction, congestive heart failure, arrhythmias, shock, cirrhosis, sepsis, hypovolemia, chronic renal disease, medications, and the use of splanchnic vasoconstrictors [116].

On MDCT, the so called "shock bowel" appearance (see Figure 6.2) is caused by prolonged hypoperfusion because of hypovolemic shock. This is a transient phenomenon that resolves with restoration of normotension. Shock bowel causes increased permeability of the bowel wall to macromolecules, and the mural thickening and intraluminal fluid is due to failure of fluid resorption. Other findings include small bowel mural and mucosal thickening (Figure 6.33), increased luminal fluid, lumen dilation, increased mural enhancement, and a normal appearing colon. There is decreased caliber of the abdominal aorta and inferior vena cava and moderate to large peritoneal fluid collections. Hyperenhancing adrenal glands are another feature of shock bowel. The mural changes are due to increased mucosal permeability related to oxygen hypoperfusion, failed resorption capacity, slow flow, and interstitial leakage of contrast material [15].

6.15.3 Superior Mesenteric Artery Thrombosis

SMAT may have a somewhat more insidious onset than SMAE. The acute ischemic event is commonly superimposed on chronic mesenteric ischemia, and 20%–50% of these patients have a history of postprandial abdominal pain, food aversion, and weight loss during the weeks to months before the seminal event. Because of the antecedent stenosing atherosclerosis, patients with SMAT usually tend to develop symptoms more subacutely than those patients with SMAE. The imaging findings are similar to those seen in patients with same.

6.15.4 Superior Mesenteric Vein Thrombosis

SMVT occurs as an acute, subacute (weeks to months), or chronic disorder. The location of the primary thrombus within the mesenteric venous circulation is dependent on the cause. SMVT because of cirrhosis, neoplasm, or operative injury begins at the site of obstruction and propagates peripherally. Thrombosis because of

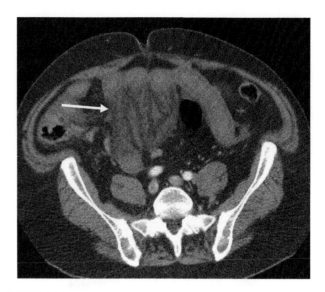

FIGURE 6.33
Nonocclusive mesenteric ischemia because of septic shock. There is diffuse thickening of the small bowel on this axial image as well as mesenteric edema (arrow).

hypercoagulable states starts in smaller branches and propagates into the major trunks. SMVT is associated with an extremely wide clinical spectrum, ranging from a relatively asymptomatic patient in whom the thrombosis is diagnosed incidentally to an acute, severe, life-threatening disease [137].

MDCT shows thrombus in the SMV or at the portal vein confluence associated with mural thickening of the involved segments of bowel (Figure 6.34). The intramural blood volume increases as arterial blood keeps flowing into the bowel wall in patients with venous compromise. This leads to increased intravascular hydrostatic pressure that dilates the blood vessels and widens the fenestrations between the vascular endothelial cells. This leads to extravasation of plasma, contrast material, and/or red blood cells into the bowel wall or lumen. Tension in the submucosal extravascular compartment or prolonged stasis-induced thrombosis of the microvasculature may interrupt arterial blood flow. The imaging findings at this stage of disease are related to mural thickening, intramural hemorrhage, and submucosal edema [138].

On MDCT, the ischemic gut shows a target appearance with an inner, hyperdense ring because of surface mucosal hypervascularity, hemorrhage, and ulceration; a middle hypodense edematous submucosa; and a normal or slightly thickened muscularis propria. The damage to the gut may be reversible at this stage of impaired venous drainage because the integrity of the deeper mural layers is preserved. If the vascular compromise persists, three possible outcomes may ensue: healing, chronic ischemia, or progression to intestinal infarction. Healing may lead to stricture formation because of

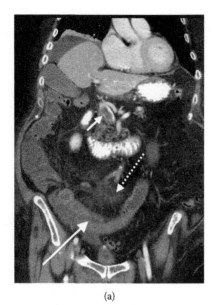

(a)

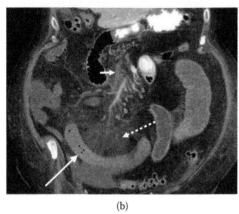

(b)

FIGURE 6.34
Superior mesenteric vein thrombosis: MDCT findings. Coronal multiplanar reformation images (a, b) show intravenous thrombus (short arrow), mesenteric edema (long broken arrow), and mesenteric edema (long solid arrow).

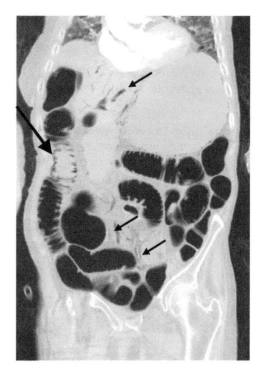

FIGURE 6.35
Ischemic infarction of the small bowel. Coronal multiplanar reformation image displayed with lung windows, shows mesenteric and portal venous gas (short arrows) and ileal pneumatosis intestinalis (long arrow).

evident in the mesenteric and portal veins, bowel wall, and subperitoneal or peritoneal space [128,139].

circumferential granulation tissue formation and fibrosis in response to parietal layer damage [128].

Persistent venous thrombosis leads to mesenteric vascular engorgement and edema with the formation of venous collateral blood vessels. This stage produces imaging findings typical of patients with chronic venous impairment. CT shows mural thickening of the involved segments, peritoneal fluid, and mesenteric engorgement [128].

Frank intestinal infarction initially causes progressive submucosal hemorrhage and edema. The cyanosis leads to loss of integrity of the intestinal wall with necrosis and peritonitis. Intramural and mesenteric venous gas (Figure 6.35). may be apparent associated with subperitoneal, or intraperitoneal serosanguineous, or bloody fluid. On CT, venous thrombosis, absence of mural enhancement, and the presence of fluid and gas may be

6.16 Gastrointestinal Hemorrhage

GI hemorrhage is a major clinical problem that is responsible for more than 400,000 hospitalizations annually in the United States. It varies in severity from life-threatening exsanguination to slow insidious bleeding that produces only iron deficiency anemia. The utility of MDCT in the diagnosis of active and occult sources of GI hemorrhage has becoming increasingly accepted. When specifically searching for a bleeding source, the patient should drink the neutral contrast material previously discussed. An unenhanced scan is initially obtained to reveal intraluminal blood. Intravascular contrast material is then infused at a high rate (5 mL·s⁻¹) with a power injector. MDCT scans are subsequently obtained during the arterial dominant phase (25 second delay) and then the venous dominant phase (70 second delay). Coronal and sagittal MPR images are very helpful in showing the origin of the hemorrhage. When the examination is positive, conventional angiography, guided by the results, can be performed [123,140].

References

1. Gore RM. 2008. Multidetector-row computed tomography of the gastrointestinal tract: Principles of interpretation. In *Textbook of Gastrointestinal Radiology*, 3rd ed. Ed. RM Gore, MS Levine, 81–90. Philadelphia, PA: Saunders Elsevier.

2. Stoker J, van Randen A, Laméris W, Boermeester MA. 2009. Imaging patients with acute abdominal pain. *Radiology*. 253:31–46.

3. Atri M et al. 2009. Multidetector helical CT in the evaluation of acute small bowel obstruction: comparison of nonenhanced (no oral, rectal or IV contrast) and IV enhanced CT. *Eur J Radiol*. 71:135–40.

4. Blachar A et al. 2011. Radiologists' performance in the diagnosis of acute intestinal ischemia, using MDCT and specific CT findings, using a variety of CT protocols. *Emerg Radiol*. 18:385–94.

5. Furukawa K et al. 2011. Diagnosis of the invasion depth of gastric cancer using MDCT with virtual gastroscopy: comparison with staging with endoscopic ultrasound. *AJR Am J Roentgenol*. 197:867–75.

6. Pilleul F, Penigaud M, Milot L, Saurin JC, Chayvialle JA, Valette PJ. 2006. Possible small-bowel neoplasms: contrast-enhanced and water-enhanced multidetector CT enteroclysis. *Radiology*. 241:796–801.

7. Patak MA, Mortele KJ, Ros PR. 2005. Multidetector row CT of the small bowel. *Radiol Clin North Am*. 43:1063–77.

8. Maglinte DD. 2006. Small bowel imaging—a rapidly changing field and a challenge to radiology. *Eur Radiol*. 16:967–71.

9. Paulsen SR et al. 2006. CT enterography as a diagnostic tool in evaluating small bowel disorders: review of clinical experience with over 700 cases. *Radiographics*. 26:641–57.

10. Elsayes KM, Al-Hawary MM, Jagdish J, Ganesh HS, Platt JF. 2010. CT enterography: principles, trends, and interpretation of findings. *Radiographics*. 30:1955–70.

11. Zamboni GA, Raptopoulos V. 2010. CT Enterography. *Gastrointest Endosc Clin N Am*. 20:347–66.

12. Chen CY et al. 2008. MDCT for differentiation of category T1 and T2 malignant lesions from benign gastric ulcers. *AJR Am J Roentgenol*. 190:1505–11.

13. Gore RM, Kim JH, Chen C-Y. 2010. MDCT, EUS, PET/CT, and MRI in the management of patients with gastric neoplasms. In *Gastric Cancer*. Ed. RM Gore, 120–194. Cambridge: Cambridge University Press.

14. Lee IJ, Lee JM, Kim SH et al. 2010. Diagnostic performance of 64-channel multi-detector CT in the evaluation of gastric cancer: differentiation of mucosal cancer (T1a) from submucosal involvement (T1b and T2). *Radiol*. 255:805–814.

15. Barmase M, Kang M, Wig J, Kochhar R, Gupta R, Khandelwal N. 2011. Role of multidetector CT angiography in the evaluation of suspected mesenteric ischemia. *Eur J Radiol*. 80:582–7.

16. Hara AK, Alam S, Heigh RI, Gurudu SR, Hentz JG, Leighton JA. 2008. Using CT enterography to monitor Crohn's disease activity: a preliminary study. *AJR Am J Roentgenol*. 190:1512–6.

17. Ba-Ssalamah A, Prokop M, Uffmann M, Pokieser P, Teleky B, Lechner G. 2003. Dedicated multidetector CT of the stomach: spectrum of diseases. *Radiographics*. 23:625–44.

18. Pickhardt PJ, Asher DB. 2003. Wall thickening of the gastric antrum as a normal finding: multidetector CT with cadaveric comparison. *AJR Am J Roentgenol*. 181:973–9.

19. Baker ME et al. 2009. Mural attenuation in normal small bowel and active inflammatory Crohn's disease on CT enterography: location, absolute attenuation, relative attenuation, and the effect of wall thickness. *AJR Am J Roentgenol*. 192:417–23.

20. Wittenberg J, Harisinghani MG, Jhaveri K, Varghese J, Mueller PR. 2002. Algorithmic approach to CT diagnosis of the abnormal bowel wall. *Radiographics*. 22:1093–107.

21. Tarrant AM, Ryan MF, Hamilton PA, Benjaminov O. 2008. A pictorial review of hypovolaemic shock in adults. *Br J Radiol*. 81:252–7.

22. Minordi LM, Vecchioli A, Guidi L, Mirk P, Fiorentini L, Bonomo L. 2006. Multidetector CT enteroclysis versus barium enteroclysis with methylcellulose in patients with suspected small bowel disease. *Eur Radiol*. 16:1527–36.

23. Scheirey CD, Scholz FJ, Shortsleeve MJ, Katz DS. 2011. Angiotensin-converting enzyme inhibitor-induced small-bowel angioedema: clinical and imaging findings in 20 patients. *AJR Am J Roentgenol*. 197:393–8.

24. Scholz FJ, Afnan J, Behr SC. 2011. CT findings in adult celiac disease. *Radiographics*. 31:977–92.

25. Harisinghani MG, Wittenberg J, Lee W, Chen S, Gutierrez AL, Mueller PR. 2003. Bowel wall fat halo sign in patients without intestinal disease. *AJR Am J Roentgenol*. 181:781–4.

26. Kernagis LY, Levine MS, Jacobs JE. 2003. Pneumatosis intestinalis in patients with ischemia: correlation of CT findings with viability of the bowel. *AJR Am J Roentgenol*. 180:733–6.

27. Ho LM, Paulson EK, Thompson WM. 2007. Pneumatosis intestinalis in the adult: benign to life-threatening causes. *AJR Am J Roentgenol*. 188:1604–13.

28. Meyers MA, McGuire PV. 1995. Spiral CT demonstration of hypervascularity in Crohn disease: "vascular jejunization of the ileum" or the "comb sign." *Abdom Imaging*. 20:327–32.

29. Pereira JM, Sirlin CB, Pinto PS, Jeffrey RB, Stella DL, Casola G. 2004. Disproportionate fat stranding: a helpful CT sign in patients with acute abdominal pain. *Radiographics*. 24:703–15.

30. Gore RM, Masselli G, Caroline D. 2008. Crohn's disease of the small bowel. In *Textbook of Gastrointestinal Radiology*, 3rd ed. Ed. RM Gore, MS Levine, 781–806. Philadelphia, PA: Saunders Elsevier.

31. Gore RM, Mehta UK, Berlin JW, Rao V, Newmark GM. 2006. Small bowel cancer. *Cancer Imaging*. 6:209–12.

32. Gore RM, Meyers MA. 2008. Pathways of abdominal and pelvic disease spread. In *Textbook of Gastrointestinal Radiology*, 3rd ed. Ed. RM Gore, MS Levine, 2099–2118. Philadelphia, PA: Saunders Elsevier.

33. Kul S et al. 2008. Effect of subclinical Helicobacter pylori infection on gastric wall thickness: multislice CT evaluation. *Diagn Interv Radiol*. 14:138–42.

34. Insko EK, Levine MS, Birnbaum BA, Jacobs JE. 2003. Benign and malignant lesions of the stomach: evaluation of CT criteria for differentiation. *Radiology.* 228:166–71.

35. Chen CY et al. 2009. Differentiation between malignant and benign gastric ulcers: CT virtual gastroscopy versus optical gastroendoscopy. *Radiology.* 252:410–7.

36. Levine MS. 2008. Benign tumors of the stomach and duodenum. In *Textbook of Gastrointestinal Radiology*, 3rd ed. Ed. RM Gore, MS Levine, 619–644. Philadelphia, PA: Saunders Elsevier.

37. Levine MS. 2008. Inflammatory conditions of the stomach and duodenum. In *Textbook of Gastrointestinal Radiology, 3rd ed.* Ed. RM Gore, MS Levine, 563–592. Philadelphia, PA: Saunders Elsevier.

38. Hatzaras I et al. 2007. Small-bowel tumors: epidemiologic and clinical characteristics of 1260 cases from the Connecticut tumor registry. *Arch Surg.* 142:229–35.

39. Minordi LM, Vecchioli A, Mirk P, Filigrana E, Poloni G, Bonomo L. 2007. Multidetector CT in small-bowel neoplasms. *Radiol Med.* 112:1013–25.

40. Lockhart ME, Chanon CL. 2010. Epidemiology of gastric cancer. In *Gastric Cancer*, ed. RM Gore, 1–21. Cambridge: Cambridge Univ. Press.

41. Shen YL et al. 2011. Evaluation of early gastric cancer at multidetector CT with multiplanar reformation and virtual endoscopy. *Radiographics.* 31:189–99.

42. Ogata I, Komohara Y, Yamashita Y, Mitsuzaki K, Takahashi M, Ogawa M. 1999. CT evaluation of gastric lesions with three-dimensional display and interactive virtual endoscopy: comparison with conventional barium study and endoscopy. *AJR Am J Roentgenol.* 172:1263–70.

43. Park HS et al. 2010. Three-dimensional MDCT for preoperative local staging of gastric cancer using gas and water distention methods: a retrospective cohort study. *AJR Am J Roentgenol.* 195:1316–23.

44. Lee IJ et al. 2009. Helical CT evaluation of the preoperative staging of gastric cancer in the remnant stomach. *AJR Am J Roentgenol.* 192:902–8.

45. Mahadevan D, Sudirman A, Kandasami P, Ramesh G. 2010. Laparoscopic staging in gastric cancer: an essential step in its management. *J Minim Access Surg.* 6:111–3.

46. Levine MS, Megibow AJ, Kochman ML. 2008. Carcinoma of the stomach and duodenum. In *Textbook of Gastrointestinal Radiology*, 3rd ed. Ed. RM Gore, MS Levine, 619–644. Philadelphia, PA: Saunders Elsevier.

47. Morpurgo E, Vitale GC, Galandiuk S, Kimberling J, Ziegler C, Polk HC Jr. 2004. Clinical characteristics of familial adenomatous polyposis and management of duodenal adenomas. *J Gastrointest Surg.* 8:559–64.

48. Parc Y, Mabrut JY, Shields C, Mallorca Group. 2011. Surgical management of the duodenal manifestations of familial adenomatous polyposis. *Br J Surg.* 98:480–4.

49. Aubé C, Ridereau-Zins C, Croquet V, Pessaux P. 2004. Imaging of the stomach and the duodenum. *J Radiol.* 85(4 Pt 2):503–14.

50. Anzidei M, Napoli A, Zini C, Kirchin MA, Catalano C, Passariello R. 2011. Malignant tumours of the small intestine: a review of histopathology, multidetector CT and MRI aspects. *Br J Radiol.* 84:677–90.

51. Boot H. Diagnosis and staging in gastrointestinal lymphoma. 2010. *Best Pract Res Clin Gastroenterol.* 24:3–12.

52. Gossios K, Katsimbri P, Tsianos E. 2000. CT features of gastric lymphoma. *Eur Radiol.* 10:425–30.

53. Byun JH et al. 2003. CT findings in peripheral T-cell lymphoma involving the gastrointestinal tract. *Radiology.* 227(1):59–67.

54. Choi D et al. 2002. Gastric mucosa-associated lymphoid tissue lymphoma: helical CT findings and pathologic correlation. *AJR Am J Roentgenol.* 178:1117–22.

55. Kim HJ et al. 2010. Gastrointestinal dissemination of mucosa-associated lymphoid tissue lymphoma: computed tomographic findings. *J Comput Assist Tomogr.* 34:187–92.

56. Gollub MJ. Imaging of gastrointestinal lymphoma. 2008. *Radiol Clin North Am.* 42:287–312.

57. Mendelson RM, Fermoyle S. 2005. Primary gastrointestinal lymphomas: a radiological-pathological review. Part 1: Stomach, oesophagus and colon. *Australas Radiol.* 49:353–64.

58. Karaosmanoglu D, Karcaaltincaba M, Oguz B, Akata D, Ozmen M, Akhan O. 2009. CT findings of lymphoma with peritoneal, omental and mesenteric involvement: peritoneal lymphomatosis. *Eur J Radiol.* 71:313–7.

59. Yen PP, Stevenson G. 2010. Two- and three-dimensional examination of the stomach (virtual gastroscopy): technical note. *Can Assoc Radiol J.* 61:41–3.

60. Ghimire P, Wu GY, Zhu L. 2011. Primary gastrointestinal lymphoma. *World J Gastroenterol.* 17:697–707.

61. Maglinte DDT, Lappas JC, Sandrasegaran K. 2008. Malignant tumors of the small bowel. In *Textbook of Gastrointestinal Radiology*, 3rd ed. Ed. RM Gore, MS Levine, 853–870. Philadelphia, PA: Saunders Elsevier.

62. Mendelson RM, Fermoyle S. 2006. Primary gastrointestinal lymphomas: a radiological-pathological review. Part 2: Small intestine. *Australas Radiol.* 50:102–13.

63. Sailer J, Zacherl J, Schima W. 2007. MDCT of small bowel tumours. *Cancer Imaging.* 7:224–33.

64. Ulusan S, Koc Z, Kayaselcuk F. 2008. Gastrointestinal stromal tumours: CT findings. *Br J Radiol.* 81:618–23.

65. Kim HC et al. 2004. Gastrointestinal stromal tumors of the stomach: CT findings and prediction of malignancy. *AJR Am J Roentgenol.* 184:893–8.

66. Corless CL, Barnett CM, Heinrich MC. 2011. Gastrointestinal stromal tumours: origin and molecular oncology. *Nat Rev Cancer.* 11:865–78.

67. Caram MV, Schuetze SM. 2011. Advanced or metastatic gastrointestinal stromal tumors: systemic treatment options. *J Surg Oncol.* 104:888–95.

68. Kim HC et al. 2005. Small gastrointestinal stromal tumours with focal areas of low attenuation on CT: pathological correlation. *Clin Radiol.* 60:384–8.

69. Kochhar R, Manoharan P, Leahy M, Taylor MB. 2010. Imaging in gastrointestinal stromal tumours: current status and future directions. *Clin Radiol.* 65:584–92.

70. Choi H. 2011. Imaging modalities of gastrointestinal stromal tumors. *J Surg Oncol.* 104:907–14.

71. Apfaltrer P et al. 2012. Contrast-enhanced dual-energy CT of gastrointestinal stromal tumors: is iodine-related attenuation a potential indicator of tumor response? *Invest Radiol.* 47:65–70.

72. Horton KM, Fishman EK. 2004. Multidetector-row computed tomography and 3-dimensional computed tomography imaging of small bowel neoplasms: current concept in diagnosis. *J Comput Assist Tomogr.* 28:106–16.
73. Dudeck O, Zeile M, Reichardt P, Pink D. 2011. Comparison of RECIST and Choi criteria for computed tomographic response evaluation in patients with advanced gastrointestinal stromal tumor treated with sunitinib. *Ann Oncol.* 22:1828–33.
74. Wong CS, Gong N, Chu YC et al. 2012. Correlation measurements from diffusion weighted MR imaging and FDG PET/CT in GIST patients: ADC vs. SUV. *Eur J Radiol.* 81:2122–2126.
75. Levy AD, Sobin LH. 2007. From the archives of the AFIP: Gastrointestinal carcinoids: imaging features with clinicopathologic comparison. *Radiographics.* 27:237–57.
76. Fendrich V, Bartsch DK. 2011. Surgical treatment of gastrointestinal neuroendocrine tumors. *Langenbecks Arch Surg.* 396:299–311.
77. Levy AD. 2007. Mesenteric ischemia. *Radiol Clin North Am.* 45:93–9.
78. Bushnell DL, Baum RP. 2011. Standard imaging techniques for neuroendocrine tumors. *Endocrinol Metab Clin North Am.* 40:153–62.
79. Zhang L, Ozao J, Warner R, Divino C. 2011. Review of the pathogenesis, diagnosis, and management of type I gastric carcinoid tumor. *World J Surg.* 35:1879–86.
80. Elsayes KM, Menias CO, Bowerson M, Osman OM, Alkharouby AM, Hillen TJ. 2011. Imaging of carcinoid tumors: spectrum of findings with pathologic and clinical correlation. *J Comput Assist Tomogr.* 35:72–80.
81. Akerström G, Stålberg P. 2009. Surgical management of MEN-1 and -2: state of the art. *Surg Clin North Am.* 89:1047–68.
82. Nikou GC et al. 2005. Gastrinomas associated with MEN-1 syndrome: new insights for the diagnosis and management in a series of 11 patients. *Hepatogastroenterology.* 52:1668–76.
83. Tamm EP, Kim EE, Ng CS. 2007. Imaging of neuroendocrine tumors. *Hematol Oncol Clin North Am.* 21:409–32.
84. Deschamps L, Dokmak S, Guedj N, Ruszniewski P, Sauvanet A, Couvelard A. 2010. Mixed endocrine somatostatinoma of the ampulla of vater associated with a neurofibromatosis type 1: a case report and review of the literature. *JOP.* 11:1–12.
85. Heller MT, Shah AB. 2011. Imaging of neuroendocrine tumors. *Radiol Clin North Am.* 49:529–48.
86. Wong M et al. 2009. Radiopathologic review of small bowel carcinoid tumors. *J Med Imaging Radiat Oncol.* 53:1–12.
87. Ghevariya V, Malieckal A, Ghevariya N, Mazumder M, Anand S. 2009. Carcinoid tumors of the gastrointestinal tract. *South Med J.* 102:1032–40.
88. Hakim FA, Alexander JA, Huprich JE, Grover M, Enders FT. 2011. CT-enterography may identify small bowel tumors not detected by capsule endoscopy: eight years experience at Mayo Clinic Rochester. *Dig Dis Sci.* 56:2914–9.
89. Pasieka JL. 2009. Carcinoid tumors. *Surg Clin North Am.* 89:1123–37.
90. Pera M, Riera E, Lopez R, Viñolas N, Romagosa C, Miquel R. 2001. Metastatic carcinoma of the breast resembling early gastric carcinoma. *Mayo Clin Proc.* 76:205–7.
91. Sheth S, Horton KM, Garland MR, Fishman EK. 2003. Mesenteric neoplasms: CT appearances of primary and secondary tumors and differential diagnosis. *Radiographics.* 23:457–73.
92. Desser TS, Gross M. 2008. Multidetector row computed tomography of small bowel obstruction. *Semin Ultrasound CT MR.* 29:308–21.
93. Rubesin SM, Gore RM. 2008. Small bowel obstruction. In *Textbook of Gastrointestinal Radiology,* 3rd *ed.* Ed. RM Gore, MS Levine, 871–900. Philadelphia, PA: Saunders Elsevier.
94. Shah ZK, Uppot RN, Wargo JA, Hahn PF, Sahani DV. 2008. Small bowel obstruction: the value of coronal reformatted images from 16-multidetector computed tomography—a clinicoradiological perspective. *J Comput Assist Tomogr.* 32:23–31.
95. Lazarus DE, Slywotsky C, Bennett GL, Megibow AJ, Macari M. 2004. Frequency and relevance of the "small-bowel feces" sign on CT in patients with small-bowel obstruction. *AJR Am J Roentgenol.* 183(5):1361–6.
96. Yaghmai V, Nikolaidis P, Hammond NA, Petrovic B, Gore RM, Miller FH. 2006. Multidetector-row computed tomography diagnosis of small bowel obstruction: can coronal reformations replace axial images? *Emerg Radiol.* 13:69–72.
97. Saba L, Mallarini G. 2008. Computed tomographic imaging findings of bowel ischemia. *J Comput Assist Tomogr.* 32:329–40.
98. Colon MJ, Telem DA, Wong D, Divino CM. 2010. The relevance of transition zones on computed tomography in the management of small bowel obstruction. *Surgery.* 147:373–7.
99. Maglinte DD. 2013. Fluoroscopic and CT enteroclysis: evidence-based clinical update. *Radiol Clin North Am.* 51:149–176.
100. Maglinte DD, Howard TJ, Lillemoe KD, Sandrasegaran K, Rex DK. 2008. Small-bowel obstruction: state-of-the-art imaging and its role in clinical management. *Clin Gastroenterol Hepatol.* 6:130–9.
101. Lepage-Saucier M, Tang A, Billiard JS, Murphy-Lavallée J, Lepanto L. 2010. Small and large bowel volvulus: clues to early recognition and complications. *Eur J Radiol.* 74:60–6.
102. Jang KM et al. 2010. Diagnostic performance of CT in the detection of intestinal ischemia associated with small-bowel obstruction using maximal attenuation of region of interest. *AJR Am J Roentgenol.* 194:957–63.
103. Hongo N, Mori H, Matsumoto S, Okino Y, Takaji R, Komatsu E. 2011. Internal hernias after abdominal surgeries: MDCT features. *Abdom Imaging.* 36:349–62.
104. Sheedy SP, Earnest F 4th, Fletcher JG, Fidler JL, Hoskin TL. 2006. CT of small-bowel ischemia associated with obstruction in emergency department patients: diagnostic performance evaluation. *Radiology.* 241:729–36.
105. Elsayes KM, Menias CO, Smullen TL, Platt JF. 2007. Closed-loop small-bowel obstruction: diagnostic patterns by multidetector computed tomography. *J Comput Assist Tomogr.* 31:697–701.

106. Qalbani A, Paushter D, Dachman AH. 2007. Multidetector row CT of small bowel obstruction. *Radiol Clin North Am.* 45:499–512.
107. Sarwani N, Tappouni R, Tice J. 2011. Pathophysiology of acute small bowel disease with CT correlation. *Clin Radiol.* 66:73–82.
108. Gore RM, Ghahremani GG, Marn CS. 2008. Hernias and abdominal wall pathology. In *Textbook of Gastrointestinal Radiology*, 3rd ed. Ed. RM Gore, MS Levine, 2149–2178. Philadelphia, PA: Saunders Elsevier.
109. Gore RM, Berlin JW, Mehta UK, Newmark GM, Yaghmai V. 2005. GI carcinoid tumours: appearance of the primary and detecting metastases. *Best Pract Res Clin Endocrinol Metab.* 19:245–63.
110. Maglinte DD, Howard TJ, Lillemoe KD, Sandrasegaran K, Rex DK. 2009. Small-bowel obstruction: state-of-the-art imaging and its role in clinical management. *Clin Gastroenterol Hepatol.* 6:130–9.
111. Jacobs JE, Balthazar EJ. 2008. Diseases of the appendix. In *Textbook of Gastrointestinal Radiology*, 3rd ed. Ed. RM Gore, MS Levine, 2149–2178. Philadelphia, PA: Saunders Elsevier.
112. Gore RM, Yaghmai V, Balthazar EJ CS. 2008. Diverticular disease of the colon. In *Textbook of Gastrointestinal Radiology*, 3rd ed. Ed. RM Gore, MS Levine, 2149–2178. Philadelphia, PA: Saunders Elsevier.
113. Zissin R, Osadchy A, Gayer G. 2009. Abdominal CT findings in small bowel perforation. *Br J Radiol.* 82:162–71.
114. Bennett GL, Birnbaum BA, Balthazar EJ. 2004. CT of Meckel's diverticulitis in 11 patients. *AJR Am J Roentgenol.* 182:625–9.
115. Sundaram B, Miller CN, Cohan RH, Schipper MJ, Francis IR. 2009. Can CT features be used to diagnose surgical adult bowel intussusceptions? *AJR Am J Roentgenol.* 193:471–8.
116. Segatto E, Mortelé KJ, Ji H, Wiesner W, Ros PR. 2003. Acute small bowel ischemia: CT imaging findings. *Semin Ultrasound CT MR.* 24:364–76.
117. Huprich JE, Fletcher JG. 2009. CT enterography: principles, technique and utility in Crohn's disease. *Eur J Radiol.* 69:393–7.
118. Hong SS et al. 2006. MDCT of small-bowel disease: value of 3D imaging. *AJR Am J Roentgenol.* 187:1212–21.
119. Higgins PD et al. 2007. Computed tomographic enterography adds information to clinical management in small bowel Crohn's disease. *Inflamm Bowel Dis.* 13:262–8.
120. Maglinte DD, Romano S. 2009. Diagnostic imaging of the inflammatory bowel diseases. *Eur J Radiol.* 69(2):369–370.
121. Kohli MD, Maglinte DD. 2009. CT enteroclysis in small bowel Crohn's disease. *Eur J Radiol.* 69:398–403.
122. Lee IJ et al. 2009. Multidetector row computed tomographic gastrography findings after endoscopic submucosal dissection for early gastric cancer: emphasis on time evolution and factors for predicting residual tumor. *J Comput Assist Tomogr.* 33:273–9.
123. Huprich JE. 2009. Multi-phase CT enterography in obscure GI bleeding. *Abdom Imaging.* 34:303–9.
124. Maglinte DD, Gourtsoyiannis N, Rex D, Howard TJ, Kelvin FM. 2003. Classification of small bowel Crohn's subtypes based on multimodality imaging. *Radiol Clin North Am.* 41:285–303.
125. Siddiki HA et al. 2009. Prospective comparison of state-of-the-art MR enterography and CT enterography in small-bowel Crohn's disease. *AJR Am J Roentgenol.* 193:113–21.
126. Romano S, Russo A, Daniele S, Tortora G, Maisto F, Romano L. 2009. Acute inflammatory bowel disease of the small intestine in adult: MDCT findings and criteria for differential diagnosis. *Eur J Radiol.* 69:381–7.
127. Bartone G, Severino BU, Armellino MF, Maglio MN, Castriconi M. 2008. Clinical symptoms of intestinal vascular disorders. *Radiol Clin North Am.* 46:887–9.
128. Gore RM et al. 2008. Imaging in intestinal ischemic disorders. *Radiol Clin North Am.* 2008. 46:845–75.
129. Umphrey H, Canon CL, Lockhart ME. 2008. Differential diagnosis of small bowel ischemia. *Radiol Clin North Am.* 46:943–52.
130. Gore RM, Thakrar KH, Mehta UK, Berlin J, Yaghmai V, Newmark GM. 2008. Imaging of intestinal ischemic disorders. *Clin Gastroenterol Hepatol.* 6:849–58.
131. Paterno F, Longo WE. 2008. The etiology and pathogenesis of vascular disorders of the intestine. *Radiol Clin North Am.* 46:877–85.
132. Macari M, Chandarana H, Balthazar E, Babb J. 2003. Intestinal ischemia versus intramural hemorrhage: CT evaluation. *AJR Am J Roentgenol.* 180:177–84.
133. Ofer A et al. 2009. Multidetector CT angiography in the evaluation of acute mesenteric ischemia. *Eur Radiol.* 19:624–30.
134. Furukawa A et al. 2009. CT diagnosis of acute mesenteric ischemia from various causes. *AJR Am J Roentgenol.* 192:408–16.
135. Romano S, Niola R, Maglione F, Romano L. 2008. Small bowel vascular disorders from arterial etiology and impaired venous drainage. *Radiol Clin North Am.* 46:891–908.
136. Romano S, Bartone G, Romano L. 2008a. Ischemia and infarction of the intestine related to obstruction. *Radiol Clin North Am.* 46:925–42.
137. Horton KM, Fishman EK. 2010. CT angiography of the mesenteric circulation. *Radiol Clin North Am.* 48:331–45.
138. Wiesner W, Khurana B, Ji H, Ros PR. 2003. CT of acute bowel ischemia. *Radiology.* 226:635–50.
139. Duron VP, Rutigliano S, Machan JT, Dupuy DE, Mazzaglia PJ. 2011. Computed tomographic diagnosis of pneumatosis intestinalis: clinical measures predictive of the need for surgical intervention. *Arch Surg.* 146:506–10.
140. Huprich JE et al. 2011. Prospective blinded comparison of wireless capsule endoscopy and multiphase CT enterography in obscure gastrointestinal bleeding. *Radiology.* 260:744–51.

7

Imaging of the Retroperitoneum

Ajit H. Goenka, Prabhakar Rajiah, Shetal N. Shah, and Erick M. Remer

CONTENTS

7.1 Imaging Anatomy of the Abdominal Retroperitoneum

The abdominal retroperitoneum is divided by fascial planes into the anterior and posterior pararenal spaces and the perirenal (or perinephric) space.

7.2 Compartments

7.2.1 Anterior Pararenal Space

The anterior pararenal space is confined by the posterior parietal peritoneum anteriorly, the anterior renal fascia posteriorly, and the lateroconal fascia laterally. It contains the ascending and the descending colon (pericolonic component), the duodenum, and pancreas (pancreaticoduodenal component).

7.2.2 Perirenal Space

The perirenal space is confined by the anterior renal fascia (Gerota's fascia) and posterior renal fascia (Zuckerkandl's fascia) that together comprise the renal fascia. It contains the kidneys, renal vessels, adrenal glands, renal pelves, proximal ureters, perirenal lymphatics, and perirenal fat.

7.2.3 Posterior Pararenal Space

The posterior pararenal space is confined by the posterior renal fascia anteriorly, by the transversalis fascia posteriorly, and by the psoas muscle medially. It continues laterally external to the lateroconal fascia as the properitoneal fat of the abdominal wall. Inferiorly, the posterior pararenal space is open to the pelvis [1,2], and superiorly, it continues as a thin subdiaphragmatic layer of extraperitoneal fat. It almost always contains only fat.

7.2.4 Interfascial Planes

The traditional tricompartmental anatomy described in the preceding discussion does not completely explain the spread of fluid collections or tumors in the retroperitoneum. It is now believed that the perirenal fasciae are multilaminated structures with potentially expandable interfascial planes. These are represented by the retromesenteric, retrorenal, lateroconal, and combined interfascial planes [3]. Knowledge of the anatomy and interconnections of these interfascial planes can facilitate understanding of the extent and pathways of retroperitoneal disease spread. On computed tomography (CT) and magnetic resonance imaging (MRI), retroperitoneal fascial planes are usually detected when there is an abundance of retroperitoneal fat. Fascia measuring greater than 3 mm is considered thickened and is a sensitive, though nonspecific, sign of a retroperitoneal pathologic process [4–6].

7.3 CT of the Retroperitoneum with MRI and Functional Imaging Correlation

In general, CT is the "workhorse" for evaluating retroperitoneal pathologies while MRI is more often used as a problem-solving tool. A standard CT examination includes anatomical structures from the lung bases to the symphysis pubis following the use of both oral and intravenous contrast media, with 3–5-mm slice thickness sections acquired during the portal venous phase of enhancement. MRI protocols typically contain T1-weighted images (to assess high-signal-intensity fat or hemorrhage, lymphadenopathy, and tumoral vascular invasion) and fat-suppressed T2-weighted images (to assess lymphadenopathy, muscle invasion by a disease process, cystic change or necrosis, fluid collections, and bone marrow edema). Venous-phase contrast-enhanced T1-weighted images are particularly useful for differentiating solid from nonenhancing cystic or necrotic lesions, the extent of disease, and the presence and nature of vascular thrombosis or encasement [7–11]. Functional imaging with positron emission tomography (PET) fused with CT (PET-CT) is a complementary tool for detecting, characterizing, and localizing primary and secondary retroperitoneal pathophysiological processes by demonstrating both metabolic and anatomic abnormalities. 18-F fluorodeoxyglucose (FDG) is the most commonly used radiopharmaceutical for PET-CT imaging and is the cornerstone of oncologic imaging. Intravenously injected FDG, an analog of glucose, accumulates in greater concentration within cancerous (and inflamed) cells that overexpress glucose transporter cellular receptors, and undergoes decay with emission of gamma rays that helps form the PET image [12].

7.4 Pathologic Conditions

7.4.1 Neoplastic Processes

Neoplasms in the retroperitoneum can be further categorized into four groups: (1) mesodermal tumors; (2) germ cell, sex cord, and stromal tumors; (3) neurogenic tumors; and (4) lymphoid tumors. Diagnosis of these tumors begins with affirmation of their retroperitoneal location and then determination of whether the lesion is primarily retroperitoneal or is arising secondarily from a retroperitoneal organ. Anterior displacement of retroperitoneal organs or vessels strongly suggests that a lesion is retroperitoneal (Figure 7.1). Additionally, rounded rather than "beaked" edges of an adjacent organ (negative "beak" sign) with a crescentic deformation (negative embedded organ sign) by the tumor suggest a primary retroperitoneal location [13,14].

7.4.1.1 Mesodermal Neoplasms

Soft tissue sarcomas are rare mesenchymal neoplasms that account for less than 1% of adult malignancies. However, about 15% of them originate in the retroperitoneum [15,16]. Most retroperitoneal neoplasms are malignant, and one-third of malignant retroperitoneal

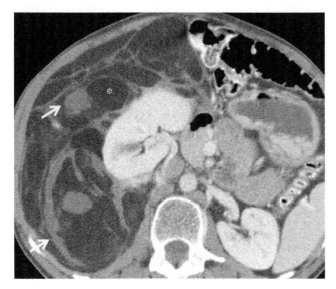

FIGURE 7.1

Well-differentiated liposarcoma in a 53-year-old woman: CECT shows large heterogeneous mass with macroscopic fat (asterisk) and enhancing, soft tissue components (arrows). Notice the anterior rotational displacement of kidney, a sign of retroperitoneal location, and negative organ embedded sign, an indication of primary retroperitoneal location.

neoplasms are sarcomas [17,18]. They typically present in the sixth and seventh decades of life and are often very large at the time of presentation since the loose connective tissue in the retroperitoneum provides little resistance to their growth [19]. Sarcomas typically develop de novo with the exception of malignant peripheral nerve sheath tumors (MPNST) that can arise from neurofibromas [20].

CT plays an important role in defining the extent of the primary tumor, evaluating direct involvement of adjacent organs and vessels, and detection of distant metastases. In general, extensive vascular involvement, peritoneal implants, and distant metastatic disease indicate unresectability [18]. Moreover, imaging evidence of tumor necrosis suggests high-grade component and portends a poor prognosis [21]. It is possible to narrow the differential diagnosis of a retroperitoneal mass based on certain imaging characteristics (Table 7.1) in combination with the pattern of involvement and patient demographics. FDG-PET has a high sensitivity in both detecting and differentiating low from intermediate and high-grade primary retorperitoneal sarcoma and can predict agressive tumor biology and disease-free survival [22]. Nevertheless, percutaneous histological sampling using imaging guidance is largely necessary to establish a definite diagnosis. Imaging is also a component of the GTNM (G-histologic grade, T-size, N-nodes, and M-metastases) system that is often used for staging retroperitoneal sarcomas [20].

Complete surgical resection is the treatment of choice for primary and recurrent retroperitoneal sarcomas. It is also the single most important independent prognostic

TABLE 7.1

Imaging Features of Sarcomas

Well-differentiated liposarcoma	Macroscopic fat; fat–fluid level
IVC leiomyosarcoma	Necrotic mass with caval and extracaval components with or without metastases
MFH	Extensive hemorrhage, absence of fat or central necrosis; "bowl of fruit sign"
Myxoid liposarcoma, MFH	Myxoid stroma
Dedifferentiated liposarcoma	Calcification, ossification, macroscopic fat

Source: Reprinted from *Radiol Clin North Am.*, Mar;50(2), Goenka AH et al., Imaging of the retroperitoneum, 333-55, vii; Copyright 2012, with permission from Elsevier.

TABLE 7.2

Features of Liposarcoma Subtypes

Well-differentiated	Low metastatic potential; low-grade histology; high local recurrence (~100%); 10% eventually dedifferentiate
Dedifferentiated	Worst prognosis; calcification or ossification may be seen (30%)
Myxoid	25% may not contain fat; "pseudocystic" appearance on unenhanced images from the myxoid component; MFH has similar appearance
Pleomorphic and round cell	Least common subtype, aggressive with little or no macroscopic fat

Source: Reprinted from *Radiol Clin North Am.*, Mar;50(2), Goenka AH et al., Imaging of the retroperitoneum, 333-55, vii; Copyright 2012, with permission from Elsevier.

factor for survival followed only by histological tumor grade [18,23–25]. Regional lymphadenopathy is found in less than 4% of soft tissue sarcomas at presentation, and less than one-third of patients have metastases at presentation [25].

7.4.1.1.1 Liposarcoma

Liposarcoma is the most common retroperitoneal sarcoma and comprises 40% of retroperitoneal sarcomas [18,26]. It originates from primitive mesenchymal cells and not from adipocytes [27]. The World Health Organization divides liposarcomas into five subtypes—well-differentiated, myxoid, dedifferentiated, round cell, and pleomorphic (Table 7.2) [20]. The most important cause of morbidity and mortality in patients with retroperitoneal liposarcoma is local disease recurrence whereas the rate of distant metastases, usually to liver and lungs, is less than 10% [16,18,28,29].

7.4.1.1.1.1 Well-Differentiated Liposarcoma Well-differentiated liposarcoma is the most common subtype

TABLE 7.3

Features That Favor Well-Differentiated Liposarcoma over Lipoma

Large size (>10 cm)
Nodular or globular components
Thick septa (>2 mm)
Soft tissue components
Low proportion of fat in mass (<75%)

Source: Reprinted from *Radiol Clin North Am.*, Mar;50(2), Goenka AH et al., Imaging of the retroperitoneum, 333-55, vii; Copyright 2012, with permission from Elsevier.

of liposarcoma. On cross-sectional imaging, it contains components that are similar in attenuation or signal intensity to macroscopic fat. Due to a paucity of intratumoral vessels, there is usually little or no contrast enhancement of the fatty component of this tumor [30]. However, streaky zones of enhancing fibrous or sclerotic components are usually seen (Figure 7.1) [31]. Areas of necrosis and calcification tend to be uncommon in all liposarcomas [28]. The main differential diagnoses on imaging studies include a lipoma (Table 7.3) or a large exophytic renal angiomyolipoma. Features that suggest an angiomyolipoma are the presence of a renal parenchymal defect from which the mass arises, enlarged intratumoral arteries, and other angiomyolipomas [32].

7.4.1.1.1.2 Other Liposarcomas Myxoid liposarcoma is the second most common subtype [27]. It is described as "pseudocystic" because the myxoid component has water attenuation or fluid signal intensity on noncontrast images. However, it tends to demonstrate a characteristic gradual, heterogeneous, and often incomplete pattern of internal enhancement on delayed contrast-enhanced images due to slow, progressive accumulation of contrast in the extracellular space [13,33]. Dedifferentiated liposarcoma contains a well-differentiated lipogenic component and a nonlipogenic (dedifferentiated) component. Therefore, it can appear as a nonlipomatous mass within, adjacent to, or encompassing a fatty mass (Figures 7.2 and 7.3) [31]. The nonlipomatous component has a similar appearance to a high-grade fibrosarcoma or a malignant fibrous histiocytoma (MFH). Pleomorphic and round cell liposarcoma are the least common subtypes and tend to present as heterogeneous tumors with little or no detectable fat and are often indistinguishable from other malignant soft tissue masses [34]. They are aggressive tumors with high tendency toward local recurrence and metastasis [27].

7.4.1.1.2 Leiomyosarcoma

Leiomyosarcoma is the second most common retroperitoneal sarcoma (30%) and two-thirds of all retroperitoneal leiomyosarcomas occur in women [18,28]. It is also the most common intraluminal venous neoplasm and the

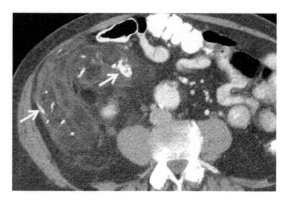

FIGURE 7.2

Axial CECT shows a heterogeneous mass with soft tissue swirls encompassing macroscopic fat in an 81-year-old woman with history of well-differentiated liposarcoma. Note the foci of calcification (arrows); this was histologically a dedifferentiated liposarcoma.

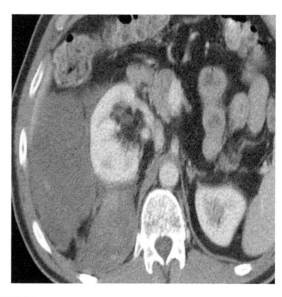

FIGURE 7.3

Axial CECT shows predominantly soft tissue attenuation posterior pararenal mass in an 85-year-old woman that was found to be a dedifferentiated liposarcoma on histopathology.

most common primary tumor of the inferior vena cava (IVC). Tumors involving the IVC may be completely external to the IVC lumen (two-thirds) (Figure 7.4); have both intraluminal and extraluminal components (one-third) (Figure 7.5); or may be purely intraluminal (5%). Purely intraluminal types occur primarily in women (80%–90% of patients) and present at a younger age (mean age, 50 years) [35]. Presenting symptoms and resectability of IVC leiomyosarcoma are variable and often depend on the segment of IVC involved. Tumors involving the upper segment (intrahepatic IVC and above) can present with Budd–Chiari syndrome; mid-segment tumors may present with right upper quadrant colic or renal insufficiency due to tumor extension into renal veins; and lower segment tumors may present with lower extremity edema.

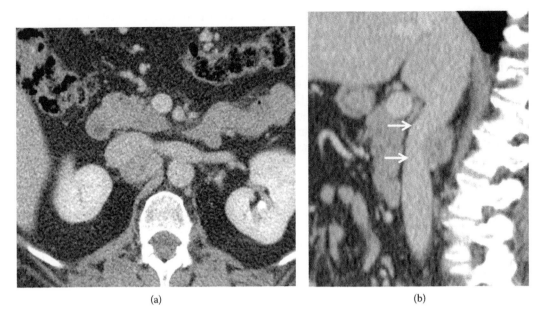

(a) (b)

FIGURE 7.4
(a) Axial and sagittal CECT shows a heterogeneous retrocaval leiomyosarcoma in a 66-year-old woman. IVC (arrows, b) is draped along the anterior surface of the lesion.

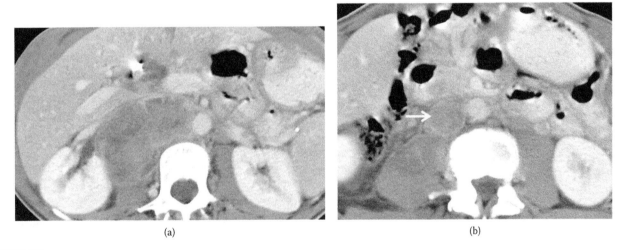

(a) (b)

FIGURE 7.5
(a) A 64-year-old man with necrotic, infiltrating mass on CECT with both intraluminal (arrow, b) and large extraluminal components—features that are pathognomonic for IVC leiomyosarcoma.

Mid-segment and lower segment tumors may be resectable but upper segment tumors are often unresectable [36,37].

Leiomyosarcomas are typically well-circumscribed masses that often contain necrosis and hemorrhage [38]. Smaller tumors may lack necrosis. Initially, adjacent organs are displaced without direct invasion, but eventually they become involved. Intracaval leiomyosarcomas are seen as polypoid or nodular masses that are firmly attached to the vessel wall and are most frequently located between the diaphragm and the renal veins. They are soft tissue masses with low to intermediate T1-signal intensity and heterogeneous intermediate to high T2-signal intensity. Fat and calcification are not typically seen. The degree of enhancement depends on the amount of muscular and fibrous components and it is usually delayed compared to the enhancement of the surrounding skeletal muscle [31,35,38,39]. Slow growth often results in formation of extensive retroperitoneal collaterals [14]. Often, it is difficult to differentiate bland tumefactive thrombus from a neoplasm. However, expansion of the vascular lumen, demonstration of feeding vessels during arterial phase, and enhancing component are the signs that favor a neoplastic etiology [31].

7.4.1.1.3 Malignant Fibrous Histiocytoma

MFH is the third most common retroperitoneal sarcoma (15%) [28] and has a male predominance (two-thirds) [40]. There are four histological subtypes of MFH—storiform-pleomorphic (most common), myxoid (second most common), giant cell, and inflammatory [20]. On CT, MFH is a large, relatively well-circumscribed soft tissue mass that spreads along fascial planes and between muscle fibers. It has low to intermediate T1-signal intensity and heterogeneously increased T2-signal intensity relative to muscle [28,29,31]. The "bowl of fruit" sign describes a mosaic of mixed low, intermediate, and high T2-signal intensity that correlates with the presence of intratumoral solid components, cystic degeneration, hemorrhage, myxoid stroma, and fibrous tissue [41]. Extensive intratumoral hemorrhage and intratumoral calcifications (20%) may also be seen [31,41,42].

7.4.1.1.4 Perivascular Epithelioid Cell Tumor

Perivascular epithelioid cell tumors (PEComas) are benign mesenchymal tumors, but have variable malignant potential. They are composed of distinctive perivascular epithelioid cells (Figure 7.6) [43]. The cells express melanocytic markers (melan-A, microphthalmia transcription factor) and smooth muscle markers (HMB-45, actin). Angiomyolipomas, lymphangioleiomyomatosis, clear cell "sugar" tumors, clear cell myomelanocytic tumors, sarcoma of perivascular cells, and pigmented melanotic tumors are included in this group [19].

7.4.1.1.5 Desmoid Tumor

Desmoid tumor (also known as deep fibromatosis, aggressive fibromatosis, or well-differentiated fibrosarcoma) accounts for less than 1% of retroperitoneal tumors [44]. It is an estrogen-dependent tumor that is more common in young women with a peak occurrence in the third decade [45,46]. It is associated with familial polyposis coli and Gardner's syndrome. Desmoids may be single or multiple. They generally have well-defined borders, but may be infiltrative. On CT, they have attenuation equivalent to muscle or greater after contrast administration [47]. On MRI, early-stage lesions are cellular and have high T2-signal intensity; but with loss of cellularity and collagen deposition, the lesion becomes hypointense. Moderate to marked enhancement is demonstrated on contrast-enhanced images [19]. They are locally aggressive lesions with high recurrence rate (50%) even after wide surgical excision [48].

7.4.1.2 Germ Cell, Sex Cord, and Stromal Tumors

7.4.1.2.1 Primary Retroperitoneal Extragonadal Germ Cell Tumor

Primary retroperitoneal extragonadal germ cell tumors (EGCTs) are hypothesized to arise from primordial midline germ cell remnants of the genital ridge that fail to migrate properly [28,49,50]. However, in general, majority of retroperitoneal EGCTs are metastases from a gonadal primary [49,51,52]. Therefore, every man with a potential primary retroperitoneal EGCT should be evaluated to exclude a coexistent testicular neoplasm (Figure 7.7). Retroperitoneal EGCTs may be seminomatous or nonseminomatous (Table 7.4). On CT and MRI, primary EGCTs are typically large, midline, enhancing masses that are of low to intermediate T1-signal intensity and intermediate to high T2-signal intensity relative to skeletal muscle. The midline location favors primary EGCT over that of metastatic lymphadenopathy from a primary testicular neoplasm [28,49,50]. The prognosis

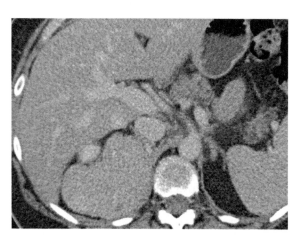

FIGURE 7.6
Axial CECT shows a mildly heterogeneous posterior pararenal space soft tissue mass in a 44-year-old woman that was found to be a PEComa.

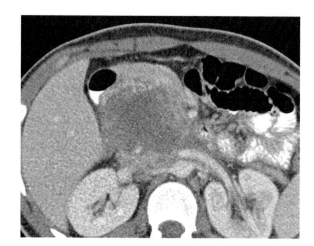

FIGURE 7.7
CECT shows a necrotic para-midline retroperitoneal mass in a 21-year-old man. Scrotal ultrasound demonstrated a "burned-out" primary tumor in the right testis, and biopsy from the mass showed metastatic mixed germ cell tumor.

TABLE 7.4

Features of Primary Extragonadal Germ Cell Tumors

Seminomatous Germ Cell Tumors	Nonseminomatous Germ Cell Tumors
Usually no elevation of tumor markers	Elevated tumor markers
Better survival (88%)	Lower survival (63%)
Homogeneous attenuation and signal intensity	Heterogeneous with areas of cystic necrosis or hemorrhage

Source: Reprinted from *Radiol Clin North Am.*, Mar;50(2), Goenka AH et al., Imaging of the retroperitoneum, 333-55, vii; Copyright 2012, with permission from Elsevier.

for and treatment of primary EGCT is equivalent to primary testicular neoplasms with retroperitoneal metastases [53]. Nonseminomatous histology, presence of nonpulmonary visceral metastases, and elevated human chorionic gonadotropin (HCG) are independent prognostic factors for shorter survival [54].

7.4.1.2.2 Growing Teratoma Syndrome

Growing teratoma syndrome is a clinical term for a retroperitoneal mass consisting of chemorefractory teratomatous elements that is defined by the following criteria: a metastatic lesion that increases in size during chemotherapy in a patient with a nonseminomatous germ cell tumor, normalization of tumor markers (AFP and/or HCG), and a predominant composition of mature teratoma at the time of resection [55]. It is a rare phenomenon with reported rates of 1.9%–7.6% in nonseminomatous germ cell tumor patients during treatment [55–57]. However, it should be considered in the differential diagnosis of a retroperitoneal metastatic lesion that shows increasing size on serial images in the setting of normal or decreasing tumor markers in a patient with a nonseminomatous germ cell tumor (Figure 7.8). Complete surgical excision is the treatment of choice and carries low risk of subsequent progression [58].

7.4.1.2.3 Primary Retroperitoneal Teratoma

Primary retroperitoneal teratomas are rare lesions that represent 6%–11% of primary retroperitoneal tumors [59,60]. Although less than 20% occur in adults, they have a greater chance of being malignant in adults than in children (14%–26% vs. 6%–7%, respectively) [20]. Alpha-fetoprotein [59,60] levels may be elevated with malignant teratomas [59]. The imaging appearance is similar to teratomas in other locations. In the retroperitoneum, they tend to be located near the upper poles of the kidneys, with preponderance on the left side [59,61] and may be solid or cystic. Solid teratomas are more frequently malignant and contain immature embryonic tissue in addition to the mature components [60,62]. Calcification can be seen in both benign and malignant tumors [62]. The presence of an internal fat–fluid level

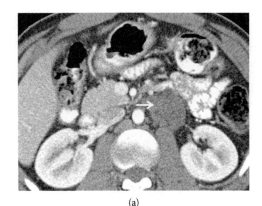

(a)

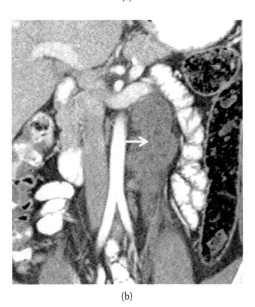

(b)

FIGURE 7.8
Residual left para-aortic mass (arrow, a—axial CECT; arrow, b—coronal CECT) in a 20-year-old man after induction chemotherapy for left testicular mixed germ cell tumor who had normalization of tumor markers. Mass was surgically resected and histopathology revealed teratoma without any evidence of malignancy—findings consistent with growing teratoma syndrome.

is almost pathognomonic of a mature cystic teratoma (Figure 7.9) [60,63]. However, this finding has also been reported in retroperitoneal liposarcoma [64]. An intraperitoneal fat–fluid level may be a sign of intraperitoneal rupture [65]. Surgical excision is recommended even for benign lesions as significant morbidity may result from continued growth [66,67].

7.4.1.3 Neurogenic Tumors

Retroperitoneal neurogenic tumors can originate from the nerve sheath (schwannoma, neurofibroma, and MPNST) (Table 7.5); ganglionic cells (ganglioneuroma, ganglioneuroblastoma, and neuroblastoma); or paraganglionic cells (paraganglioma). In toto, they constitute 10%–20% of primary retroperitoneal tumors in adults [19].

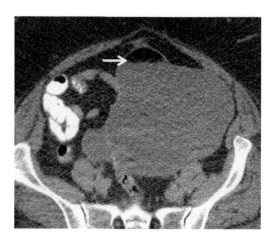

FIGURE 7.9

A 58-year-old man with a large lower retroperitoneal mass that has internal fat–fluid level (arrow) indicative of mature cystic teratoma. (Reprinted from *Radiol Clin North Am.*, Mar;50(2), Goenka AH et al., Imaging of the retroperitoneum, 333-55, vii; Copyright 2012, with permission from Elsevier.)

TABLE 7.5

Features of Benign Nerve Sheath Tumors

Schwannoma	Neurofibroma
Heterogeneous attenuation and signal intensity	Relatively homogenous
Eccentric position in relation to the parent nerve	Centered on and contiguous with the parent nerve
Low-signal-intensity capsule on MRI	Nonencapsulated
Composed of Antoni A (cellular) and Antoni B (myxoid) components	Composed of nerve sheath cells, collagenous bundles, and myxoid component
Nerve sparing surgery is possible	Resection involves excision of the parent nerve
Malignant degeneration is rare	Plexiform neurofibroma may degenerate into MPNST

Source: Reprinted from *Radiol Clin North Am.*, Mar;50(2), Goenka AH et al., Imaging of the retroperitoneum, 333-55, vii; Copyright 2012, with permission from Elsevier.

7.4.1.3.1 Schwannoma

Schwannomas are benign nerve sheath tumors of Schwann cell origin that account for up to 4% of all retroperitoneal tumors [20]. They tend to present as asymptomatic, slow growing, painless soft tissue masses [68,69]. On CT and MRI, schwannomas are sharply circumscribed masses and are usually located in the paravertebral or presacral retroperitoneum. They are of low to intermediate T1-signal intensity and high T2-signal intensity with solid enhancing components. A "target sign" consisting of a central low to intermediate T2-signal intensity fibrous tissue surrounded by peripheral high-signal-intensity myxoid tissue may be seen in both schwannomas and neurofibromas. Targetlike central enhancement may also be seen

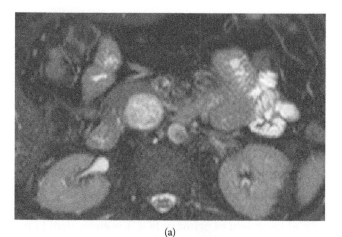

(a)

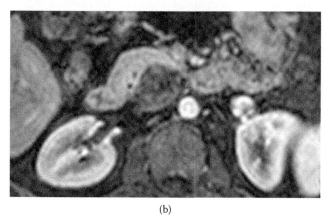

(b)

FIGURE 7.10

Relatively homogenous, well-circumscribed mass interposed between the aorta and the IVC in a 56-year-old man. On T2W MRI image (a), lesion shows targetoid pattern of hyperintensity and there is heterogeneous postgadolinium enhancement on T1WI (b). Histopathology was schwannoma. Small schwannomas tend to be homogenous but larger lesions can show a spectrum of degenerative changes.

[70]. Larger schwannomas are more likely to undergo degenerative changes, including cyst formation (in up to 66%), calcification, hemorrhage, and hyalinization (Figure 7.10) [20,71]. "Ancient schwannoma" describes a long-standing lesion with advanced degeneration [72,73]. Schwannomas are treated by surgical excision or enucleation, particularly if large or symptomatic.

7.4.1.3.2 Neurofibroma

Neurofibromas are benign nerve sheath tumors that represent 5% of all benign soft tissue neoplasms [73]. Approximately one-third of patients with a solitary neurofibroma have neurofibromatosis type 1 (NF-1), and almost every patient with multiple or plexiform neurofibromas has NF-1 [70]. Neurofibromas associated with NF-1 present in a younger age group (first two decades) are multifocal, larger (>5 cm) and are more likely to be associated with neurological symptoms than those in unaffected patients.

Neurofibromas usually have a fusiform shape that is oriented longitudinally along the course of the parent nerve. Associated muscle atrophy in the particular nerve distribution may be seen. A "split-fat sign" may be seen as a rim of fat that surrounds the tumor that originates from an intramuscular nerve [73]. As with other spinal nerve or nerve sheath tumors, a dumbbell shape is seen with spinal nerve root neurofibromas that extend through and enlarge a neural foramen [31,41,74]. In NF-1, a characteristic "bag of worms" appearance may be seen when a large conglomerate of infiltrative masses of innumerable neurofibromas diffusely thicken a parent nerve and extend into multiple nerve branches [20]. These plexiform neurofibromas in the retroperitoneum are typically bilateral and symmetrical in a parapsoas or presacral location and follow the distribution of the lumbosacral plexus (Figure 7.11) [75].

Neurofibromas have soft tissue attenuation masses on CT and demonstrate low T1-signal intensity but variably high T2-signal intensity. A "target sign," myxoid degeneration, or a whorled appearance consisting of linear or curvilinear low-signal intensity due to Schwann cell bundles and collagen fibers in a background of high signal intensity may also be seen on T2-weighted images [41,73]. Contrast enhancement is variable. Targetlike central enhancement may be encountered on CT or MRI [70].

Plexiform neurofibromas, symptomatic neurofibromas, and neurofibromas that are suspected having malignant degeneration are surgically resected along with underlying parent nerves [73].

7.4.1.3.3 Malignant Peripheral Nerve Sheath Tumor

MPNSTs include malignant schwannoma, neurogenic sarcoma, and neurofibrosarcoma [76] and represent 5%–10% of soft tissue sarcomas. About 50% of patients with MPNST have NF-1. Conversely, around 2%–5% of NF-1 patients develop MPNST, typically from preexisting neurofibromas [73,77,78]. MPNSTs in patients with NF-1 tend to present early (third decade) and have a higher histological grade and larger size than those that develop de novo [20]. Radiation exposure is another risk factor for the development of MPNST [73,78]. MPNSTs tend to be large, heterogeneous masses with central necrosis or calcification (Figure 7.12). They may exhibit poorly defined margins, associated edema, or may expand neural foramina. These features, however, may also be seen with benign neural tumors. Therefore, imaging differentiation from benign tumors is not always reliable [20]. The most important finding that should raise suspicion of MPNST is rapid enlargement of a tumor mass, particularly if associated with spontaneous and unremitting pain [79,80]. FDG-PET-CT can help distinguish benign neurogenic tumors from those that have undergone sarcomatous degeneration into MPNST in NF-1 patients [81]. Complete surgical resection is the treatment of choice and is the most important factor influencing patient survival. Local recurrence and distant metastatic disease are common. In NF-1 patients, MPNSTs have a particularly aggressive course and poor prognosis (15% survival at 5 years) [73,78].

7.4.1.3.4 Ganglioneuroma

Ganglioneuromas are benign tumors that arise from the sympathetic ganglia in the 20–40-year age group and represent 5%–10% of primary retroperitoneal tumors [76,82]. They often are asymptomatic, but approximately 57% of ganglioneuromas may be functional and produce catecholamines or androgenic hormones [83]. They typically are well-defined, longitudinally oriented, paravertebral soft tissue masses that tend to surround major blood vessels but cause little or no luminal narrowing, usually do not result in osseous changes, and only infrequently

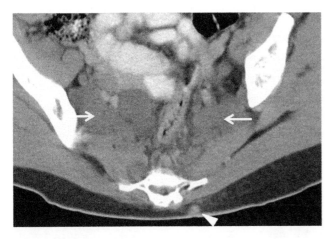

FIGURE 7.11
A 30-year-old woman with NF-1: Bilateral, plexiform, infiltrating soft tissue masses in the retroperitoneum with extension along the spinal nerve roots (arrows)—pathognomonic for plexiform neurofibroma. Note the subcutaneous neurofibroma (arrowhead).

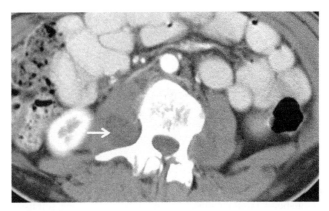

FIGURE 7.12
A 30-year-old woman with NF-1 (same patient as in Figure 7.11) developed unremitting pain in the right lower back. CECT demonstrated new heterogeneity in a preexisting plexiform neurofibroma and biopsy revealed malignant peripheral nerve sheath tumor (MPNST) (arrow).

extend into the neural foramina (Figure 7.13) [19]. Discrete punctate calcifications (20%–30%) may be present and contrast enhancement is variable [84]. On MRI, ganglioneuromas have homogeneous T1-hypointensity and variable T2-signal intensity. Like nerve sheath tumors, a whorled appearance may be seen on T2-weighted images. Imaging differentiation from the malignant ganglionic tumors

may be challenging. Metastases and younger age group favor the latter. Up to 57% of ganglioneuromas are functional and accumulate I-123-metaiodobenzylguanidine (I-123-MIBG) [85].

7.4.1.3.5 Paraganglioma

Paragangliomas are hormonally active tumors that arise from the paraganglia of the sympathetic nervous system and secrete epinephrine or norepinephrine. The paraganglia are collection of specialized neural crest cells. In the abdomen, paragangliomas occur most frequently at the renal hila and in the organs of Zuckerkandl, which are located in the para-aortic region near the inferior mesenteric artery (IMA) origin [86]. Up to 40% of paragangliomas are malignant, compared with 10% of adrenal pheochromocytomas. Malignancy is recognized by locally aggressive behavior or metastatic spread to sites that do not have paraganglia such as lymph nodes, bone, lung, or liver [14,87]. Paragangliomas may be functional in up to 60% of patients and produce symptoms due to catecholamine secretion. In affected patients, detection of elevated urinary catecholamines is the most efficacious way of characterizing an abdominal mass as a paraganglioma. However, there is poor correlation between the functional activity and the degree of malignancy [88,89].

On CT, paragangliomas are typically avidly enhancing, well-circumscribed, soft tissue masses (Figure 7.14) that may contain necrosis (40%), punctate calcification (15%), or intratumoral hemorrhage [29,76,89,90]. Intravenous administration of nonionic iodinated contrast material even without α-adrenergic blockage is now considered safe in patients with paraganglioma [91]. On MRI, they demonstrate low to intermediate T1-signal intensity and moderately high T2-signal intensity relative to skeletal muscle. They are hypervascular tumors that enhance briskly [14].

I-123-MIBG scintigraphy is a molecular tool used to detect and characterize paragangliomas that express

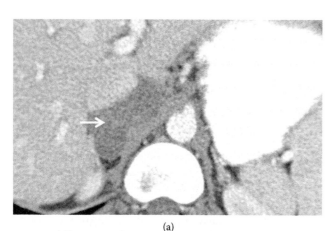

(a)

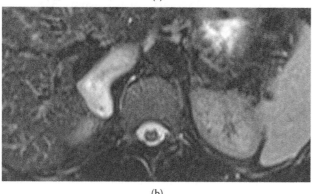

(b)

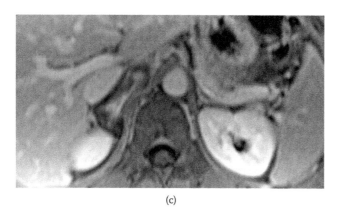

(c)

FIGURE 7.13
CECT shows a well-circumscribed, minimally enhancing, soft tissue mass in the retrocaval space (arrow, a) that displaces vessels without encasement. Lesion is hyperintense on true FISP image (b) and demonstrates minimal enhancement on postgadolinium image (c). Histopathology revealed ganglioneuroma. (Reprinted from *Radiol Clin North Am.*, Mar;50(2), Goenka AH et al., Imaging of the retroperitoneum, 333-55, vii; Copyright 2012, with permission from Elsevier.)

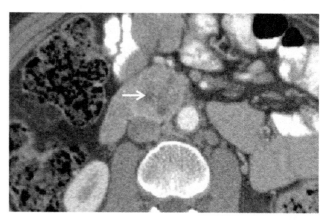

FIGURE 7.14
A 30-year-old-woman presented with heart failure with chemical evidence of hormonal secretion. CECT shows paraganglioma at the organ of Zuckerkandl (arrow).

membrane norepinephrine transporters and have a reported sensitivity of 83%–100% and specificity of 95%–100% [92,93]. It is particulary useful when there is concern for multiple primary lesions. I-123-MIBG as well as 111In-pentetreotide (Octreoscan) may be used to detect and characterize lesions in patients with hereditary syndromes, such as familial paragangliomas or multiple endocrine neoplasia. Imaging with CT or MRI is, however, performed if there is a high index of suspicion and the tumor is not found with scintigraphy since CT and MRI have a higher sensitivity [94–97]. Whenever possible, paragangliomas are treated with complete surgical resection. The limitations of histopathological criteria in predicting malignant behavior, the long natural history of the disease, and a high propensity for subsequent metastasis make extended follow-up necessary [98].

7.4.1.4 Lymphoid Neoplasms

Retroperitoneal lymph nodes are generally present in a perivascular distribution about the aorta, IVC, and iliac vessels. Lymphoma, the most common retroperitoneal malignancy, and metastatic disease are by far the most common causes of abdominopelvic lymphadenopathy [99]. Imaging differentiation between metastatic and reactive lymph nodes is based on size criteria, specifically short-axis dimension. Size criteria are location based: the upper limit of normal in the retro-crural space is 6 mm, in the retroperitoneum is 10 mm, and in the pelvis is 15 mm [100–102]. Unfortunately, relying on size criteria alone diminishes sensitivity to metastases in normal-sized lymph nodes. The presence of multiple, borderline-enlarged lymph nodes, in the 8-mm to 10-mm range, should be viewed with suspicion for an underlying pathologic process (e.g., chronic lymphocytic

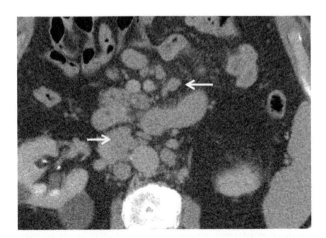

FIGURE 7.15
An 84-year-old man with incidental detection of multiple borderline-enlarged retroperitoneal (arrows) and mesenteric lymph nodes on CECT prompted investigations that led to the diagnosis of chronic lymphocytic leukemia (CLL).

leukemia) (Figure 7.15). Most normal lymph nodes have an oval shape with a preserved fatty hilum whereas malignant lymph nodes are often rounded [102,103].

7.4.1.4.1 Lymphoma

Lymphoma typically begins as local lymph node enlargement and then spreads through lymphatics to adjacent lymph nodes, commonly in the retroperitoneum, and sometimes systemically [28,104]. Conglomerate nodal masses may form and characteristically infiltrate the perinephric spaces of the retroperitoneum [28]. Whereas abdominal Hodgkin's lymphoma (HL) tends to be confined to the spleen and retroperitoneum with spread of disease to contiguous lymph nodes; non-Hodgkin's lymphoma (NHL) more commonly involves discontiguous nodal groups and extranodal sites [105,106].

On CT, nodal and extranodal lymphoma typically has homogeneous soft tissue attenuation, which is the main distinguishing factor from other neoplasms [31]. Necrosis and calcification are uncommon before therapy. Sometimes, the aorta seems to be immersed in the tumor, giving the "floating aorta" or "CT angiogram" sign (Figure 7.16). This sign is characteristic of lymphoma and is generally not seen in other retroperitoneal disorders such as sarcomas or neurogenic tumors [14]. On MRI, lymphoma typically has intermediate to slightly high T1-signal intensity and high T2-signal intensity relative to muscle. Lymphomatous nodal masses may develop low T2-signal intensity after treatment, which represents nonviable tumor or fibrosis. However, assessment of residual tumor is confounded by the presence of edema, granulation tissue, hemorrhage, or immature fibrosis, which may give rise to high T2-signal intensity up to 12 months after therapy [107]. Lymphomas are generally FDG avid on PET. The integrated interpretation of fused FDG-PET-CT performs better as compared to either modality alone in detecting and diagnosing active disease. Generally, HL and high-grade or more aggressive NHL are FDG avid. Elstrom et al. showed 100% sensitivity in disease detection for large B-cell lymphoma and mantle cell lymphoma and 98% sensitivity for Hodgkin's disease and follicular lymphoma [108]. Studies have shown that FDG-PET-CT outperforms contrast-enhanced CT by 15% in disease detection and staging, with a particular advantage in detecting extranodal disease [109]. FDG-PET-CT is also used to objectively monitor treatment repsonse: as a rule residual FDG avidity similar to or lower than mediastinal blood pool is considered complete metabolic response, irrespective of residual soft tissue on CT.

7.4.1.4.2 Metastatic Lymphadenopathy

Malignant neoplasms tend to spread initially to their regional nodal groups. However, due to complex intercommunications among regional groups of lymph

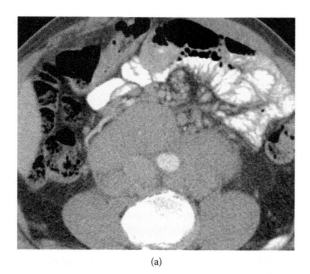

(a)

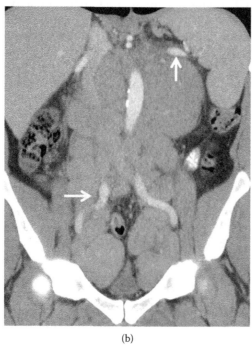

(b)

FIGURE 7.16
A 54-year-old man with homogenous, lobulated, mildly enhancing retroperitoneal masses without necrosis or calcification (a—axial and b—coronal CECT). Major vessels are encased giving positive "CT angiogram sign" (arrows). Histopathology and blood work-up showed small lymphocytic lymphoma.

nodes, lymphadenopathy may involve several contiguous or even widely separated nodal chains [20]. Most common nonlymphomatous neoplasms that lead to retroperitoneal lymphadenopathy are renal cell carcinoma, testicular carcinoma, cervical carcinoma, and prostate carcinoma. Carcinomas of the bladder, prostate, cervix, uterus, and the anorectum initially spread to the pelvic nodes (Figure 7.17). On the contrary, testicular, ovarian, and fallopian tube malignancies spread first to the retroperitoneal nodes adjacent to or near the renal hila due to

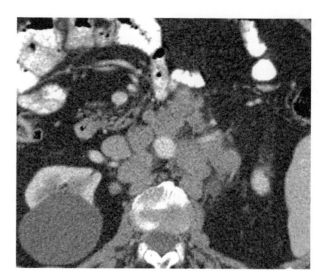

FIGURE 7.17
A 54-year-old man with multiple, discrete, enlarged, rounded retroperitoneal lymph nodes on CECT.

the spread along the gonadal vessels and may involve the pelvic nodes by retrograde spread [102]. While CT and MRI primarily detect pathological adenopathy based on abnormal size, FDG-PET-CT characterizes nodes as pathological based on active tracer uptake [110]. It often plays an important adjuvant role in helping assess therapy response. When conventional imaging is inconclusive in the postoperative patient due to extensive fibrosis, FDG can reveal hypermetabolic recurrent disease. On occasion, however, reactive or inflamed metabolically active lymph nodes may give false-positive results, while pathologic subcentimeter lymph nodes or nodes with low metabolic activity may give false-negative results.

7.4.2 Nonneoplastic Processes

7.4.2.1 Retroperitoneal Fibrosis

Retroperitoneal fibrosis (RPF) is a rare fibrotic reactive process with a prevalence of about 1 per 200,000 [111]. Most patients present during the fifth or sixth decade of life. Although a gamut of underlying etiologies may be associated with RPF, no identifiable cause may be found in two-thirds of all cases. Idiopathic RPF is also called as Ormond's disease and is more common in men (2:1) [112–114].

7.4.2.1.1 Etiology

The exact etiology of RPF is uncertain. Proposed hypotheses include either an immune-mediated reaction to a component of ruptured atherosclerotic plaque such as ceroid [113,114] or an underlying systemic autoimmune process [111]. In up to 15% of individuals, associated fibrotic processes outside the retroperitoneum may be present [115]. Other associations include autoimmune or inflammatory disease processes, asbestos exposure, and inflammatory abdominal aortic aneurysms (perianeurysmal fibrosis) [111,116]. Ergot derivatives such as methysergide (1% patients) and bromocriptine have been associated with a reversible form of RPF that tends to regress upon discontinuing these drugs [112,114]. Malignant RPF is an unusual subtype that occurs when small metastatic foci to the retroperitoneum elicit a desmoplastic response [112]. Lymphoma is the most common causal malignancy while colorectal, breast, prostate, and bladder cancers are other causes [112,114,117]. Other conditions that can lead to RPF are granulomatous infections; nonspecific gastrointestinal inflammation; retroperitoneal hemorrhage; urine extravasation; or prior irradiation or surgery [111,112,114].

7.4.2.1.2 Presentation

RPF typically originates below the aortic bifurcation at the level of the lumbosacral vertebrae. It then extends superiorly in a periaortic and pericaval distribution toward the renal hila. Typically, middle third of the ureters is encased resulting in hydroureteronephrosis [118]. However, the fibrotic process may also spread inferiorly to involve the pelvic vessels, rectosigmoid colon, urinary bladder, and other pelvic organs, or anteriorly along the celiac and superior mesenteric arteries [112,114]. Symptoms and signs are related to entrapment and compression of these retroperitoneal structures.

7.4.2.1.3 Imaging Findings

On CT, RPF has homogeneous soft tissue attenuation. On MRI, RPF has low to intermediate T1-signal intensity. The T2-weighted signal intensity and the enhancement pattern of RPF depend on the activity of the disease (Table 7.6) [112,114]. The disease progresses from chronic active inflammation to fibrous scarring [44]. The maturation process progresses laterally from the midline. Therefore, the lateral edges of the lesion tend to be T2-hyperintense and enhancing whereas the central portion tends to be more fibrotic (Figure 7.18) [113]. Factors that favor malignant RPF over idiopathic RPF on imaging are heterogeneous, enhancing soft tissue mass with poorly defined margins, adjacent osseous destruction, high T2-signal intensity in adjacent psoas muscles,

or lymphadenopathy (Figure 7.19) [28,117]. Malignant lymphadenopathy unlike RPF is lobulated and tends to displace rather than encase the aorta and the ureters [112]. Moreover, the fibrous tissue in idiopathic RPF is usually not seen between the aorta and the underlying vertebrae, in contrast to that in lymphoma or in disseminated malignancy [119]. Though there is little prospective data, FDG-PET-CT has shown promise in its ability to help differentiate active residual disease from "scar" in idiopathic RPF after treatment [120].

7.4.2.1.4 Treatment and Prognosis

Corticosteroid therapy is the mainstay of treatment. Tamoxifen has also been used successfully. Ureteral stenting or ureterolysis may be performed when medical therapy is not effective [119]. Biopsies are obtained to exclude a malignant or infectious etiology and to exclude lymphoma or metastatic lymphadenopathy, before therapy is instituted [113,114]. Idiopathic RPF carries a favorable prognosis. The mean survival of patients with malignant RPF, however, is 3–6 months after diagnosis [114,121].

7.4.2.2 Retroperitoneal Fluid Collections

Retroperitoneal fluid collections tend to be confined by the fascial planes or adhesions unless they are large, rapidly developing, or infected [4,122]. The imaging appearance of any retroperitoneal fluid collection depends on the content of collection and whether infection is present. Infected or proteinaceous collections may have high attenuation on CT, high T1-weighted signal intensity, nonenhancing internal debris, and a thick, enhancing rim.

7.4.2.2.1 Hemorrhage/Hematoma

Retroperitoneal hemorrhage may be spontaneous, posttraumatic, or secondary to other etiologies [4,28,122,123]. Spontaneous hemorrhage typically originates in the posterior pararenal space (Figure 7.20) and may extend into the properitoneal fat, pelvis, psoas muscle, or the abdominal wall musculature [122]. Traumatic hemorrhage tends to be largely confined to the retroperitoneal interfascial planes and can be clinically uncontrollable when there is extension into the subfascial plane [124]. Most bleeding

TABLE 7.6

Signal Intensity and Enhancement of RPF

RPF	T2-Signal Intensity	Enhancement	Pathophysiology
Immature, benign	Hyperintense	Present	Inflammatory edema>cellularity
Mature, benign, or after steroid therapy	Iso-hypointense	Relatively less	Decrease in edema
Malignant RPF	Heterogeneously hyperintense	Present	Hypercellularity>edema

Source: Reprinted from *Radiol Clin North Am.*, Mar;50(2), Goenka AH et al., Imaging of the retroperitoneum, 333-55, vii; Copyright 2012, with permission from Elsevier.

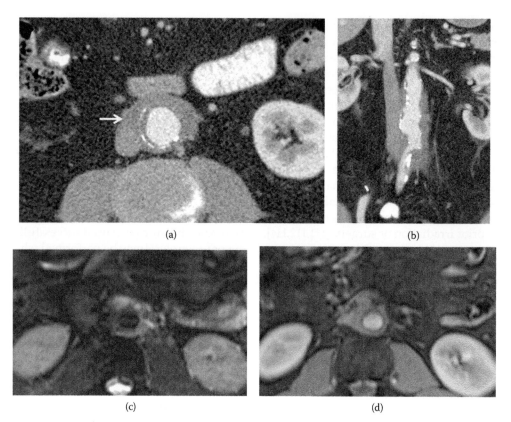

(a)   (b)

(c)   (d)

FIGURE 7.18

A 64-year-old man presented with nonspecific abdominal pain. CT scan (a, b) revealed an enhancing rim of soft tissue around the infrarenal aorta (arrow, a). Note relative sparing of retroaortic prevertebral space. Lesion is isointense on T2W image (c) and enhances on postgadolinium T1W image (d). Biopsy demonstrated benign fibrosis.

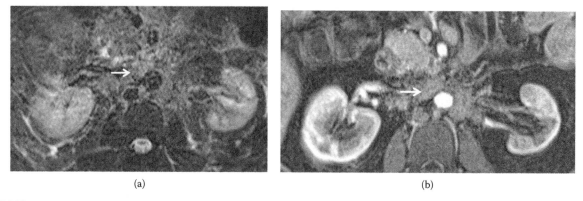

(a)   (b)

FIGURE 7.19

Malignant RP fibrosis: A 54-year-old man with heterogeneous, incomplete rind of soft tissue around the aorta. Lesion is hyperintense on STIR image (arrow, a) and shows postgadolinium enhancement (arrow, b). Biopsy showed metastatic adenocarcinoma with fibrosis. (Reprinted from *Radiol Clin North Am.*, Mar;50(2), Goenka AH et al., Imaging of the retroperitoneum, 333-55, vii; Copyright 2012, with permission from Elsevier.)

due to ruptured abdominal aortic aneursyms is confined by the psoas space.

Acute clotted hematoma typically has higher attenuation (45–80 HU) than does pure fluid (0–20 HU) or non-clotted or chronic hemorrhage (25–45 HU). This is the basis for the "sentinel clot sign," where areas of higher attenuation (acute hematoma) indicate the anatomic sites of hemorrhage origination [125]. Since MRI is typically not performed to evaluate for an acute hemorrhage, most hematomas seen on MRI are either subacute or chronic [20]. A subacute hematoma may show two outer characteristic layers of signal intensity: a thin peripheral rim with low signal intensity on all pulse sequences corresponding to hemosiderin, and an inner peripheral high T1-signal-intensity zone due to methemoglobin. This appearance of a concentric ring sign is pathognomonic

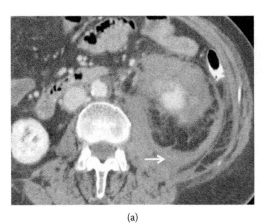
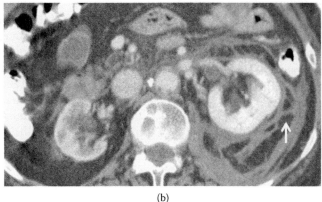

(a)   (b)

FIGURE 7.20
A 70-year-old woman developed acute drop in hemoglobin level after a cerebral angiogram. Noncontrast CT (a, b) demonstrated a retroperitoneal perinephric hematoma with extension along the retrorenal interfascial plane (arrow, a), lateral conal fascia, and the bridging septae of the perinephric space (arrow, b).

for a subacute hematoma [126]. A "hematocrit effect" (layering signal intensities or attenuations) may also be seen, especially in the setting of anticoagulation therapy or coagulopathy [127,128]. Active contrast extravasation on CT or MRI indicates ongoing arterial hemorrhage and a need for immediate supportive, angiographic, or surgical intervention [129]. The main imaging differential diagnostic consideration is a hemorrhagic tumor that typically has enhancing soft tissue components [28].

7.4.2.2.2 Lymphocele

Lymphoceles are fluid-filled cystic collections, without an epithelial lining, that usually occur at least 3–4 weeks after radical lymphadenectomy (up to 30% patients) or renal transplantation (up to 18% patients) [130–132]. They are well-circumscribed water attenuation or water signal intensity collections adjacent to surgical clips. Negative attenuation values due to lipid content, internal septa, or mural calcification may be seen [133]. Percutaneous or surgical drainage is performed for lymphoceles that are symptomatic, due to mass effect on adjacent structures, sometimes in conjunction with sclerotherapy [134].

7.4.2.2.3 Urinoma

An urinoma is an encapsulated collection of chronically extravasated urine. Urinomas are usually found in the perirenal spaces, sometimes with extension into the interfascial planes. Common causes include urinary obstruction (most common), abdominopelvic trauma, surgery, or diagnostic instrumentation [1,4,122,135]. On imaging, an urinoma is a water attenuation or water signal intensity collection. The attenuation or the signal intensity can increase progressively on contrast-enhanced studies due to leakage of the contrast-enhanced urine, thus directly confirming a urine leak (Figure 7.21) [67].

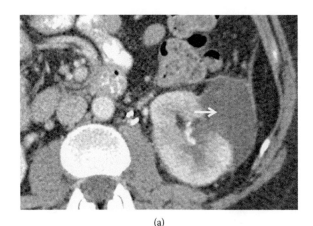

(a)

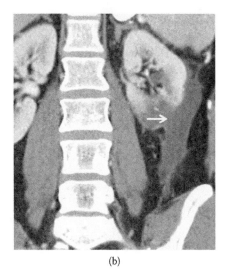

(b)

FIGURE 7.21
A 54-year-old woman underwent left laparoscopic partial nephrectomy for renal cell carcinoma. Postoperative CT scan revealed a well-circumscribed fluid pocket around the kidney (arrows, a and b) that demonstrated progressive contrast opacification on delayed images consistent with urinoma.

7.4.2.2.4 Inflammatory Collections

Infectious fluid collections in the retroperitoneum are most often due to gram-negative bacilli. Most inflammatory fluid collections originate in the anterior pararenal space from extraperitoneal portions of the gastrointestinal tract (Figure 7.22) with acute pancreatitis being one of the most common causes. Posterior pararenal space collections are usually due to extension of infection from another space. Perirenal inflammatory fluid collections are most often secondary to renal infections [136]. Inflammatory fluid collections (in particular those related to acute pancreatitis) can enter the posterior interfascial retrorenal plane, the transversalis fascia, and the abdominal wall. Fluid may also traverse the midline through the anterior interfascial retromesenteric plane, may spread inferiorly to the pelvic retroperitoneum through the combined interfascial plane, or may extend superiorly along the diaphragm to enter the mediastinum [4,124,137,138]. On imaging, inflammatory collections are localized, complex collections that show water or increased attenuation fluid, variable T1-signal intensity, intermediate to high T2-signal intensity, and thick, peripheral rim of enhancement. Layering debris, gas bubbles, or a gas–fluid level may also be seen. The presence of gas increases the specificity for the diagnosis of an abscess [28,139].

7.4.2.2.5 Psoas Muscle Fluid Collections

Fluid collections related to the psoas muscle are located in the retrofascial space posterior to the transversalis fascia [140]. Common sources of infection that may result in psoas collections include the gastrointestinal disease (most common), renal disease, or extension from lumbar osteomyelitis (Figure 7.23) [20]. Primary psoas abscesses are more likely to occur in immunocompromised patients and up to 90% are due to *Staphylococcus aureus*. In developing countries, tuberculosis is an important

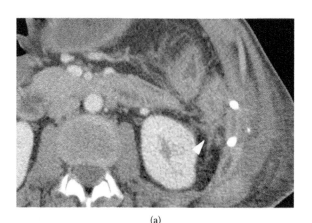

(a)

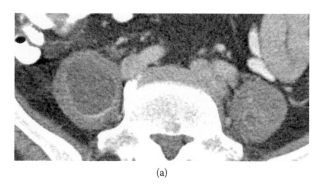

(a)

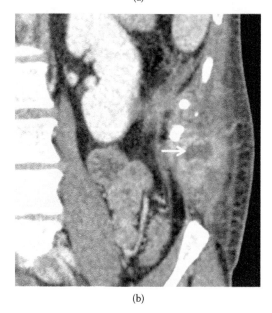

(b)

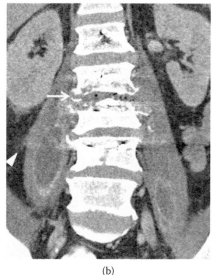

(b)

FIGURE 7.22
A 45-year-old man with Crohn's disease with colo-retroperitoneal fistula (CECT axial, a, and coronal, b) with extension of the inflammatory phlegmon along the anterior renal fascia, the lateral conal fascia (arrowhead), perinephric space, and into the lateral abdominal wall (arrow).

FIGURE 7.23
A 71-year-old male patient with multisystem organ dysfunction of unclear etiology. CECT (a, axial; b, coronal) shows bilateral psoas abscesses in contiguity with L2,3 spondylodiskitis (arrow). Note the marginal enhancement, central fluid attenuating component, and para-psoas inflammatory stranding (arrowhead).

cause of psoas abscesses [141,142]. The imaging appearance is similar to any other abscess in the retroperitoneum. Secondary findings of psoas muscle enlargement and edema; bone destruction; infiltration; and loss of surrounding fat planes may be present [142,143]. Prime differential considerations include a psoas muscle hematoma or a malignancy with cystic components. Hematomas have high attenuation on CT and a peripheral rim of high signal intensity on T1-weighted imaging secondary to methemoglobin ("concentric rim sign" described previously), may be associated with a hematocrit effect, and are typically associated with psoas muscle enlargement [126,142,143]. These findings, coupled with a history of trauma or anticoagulation therapy, are often diagnostic. Solid enhancing tissue favors a malignancy involving the psoas muscle [118].

7.4.2.3 Pneumoretroperitoneum

Retroperitoneal gas is most often the result of bowel perforation. It can originate from the duodenum (Figure 7.24) or the ascending, descending, or rectosigmoid portions of the colon. Other etiologies include superinfected necrotizing pancreatitis, necrotizing fasciitis, abscess formation, percutaneous biopsy, epidural anesthesia, extracorporeal shock-wave lithotripsy, hydrogen peroxide wound irrigation, or inferior extension of mediastinal air [118].

7.4.2.4 Miscellaneous Retroperitoneal Conditions

7.4.2.4.1 Xanthogranulomatosis/Erdheim–Chester Disease

Xanthogranulomatosis refers to the masslike accumulation of non-Langerhans lipid-laden histiocytes. It is an idiopathic process with a variable clinical course with a predisposition for the retroperitoneum. When multiple organs are involved, it is called *Erdheim–Chester disease* [144,145]. On CT and MRI, mildly enhancing infiltrative soft tissue with intermediate T1- and T2-weighted signal intensity relative to skeletal muscle is typically seen [146,147]. Circumferential periaortic involvement with associated bilateral symmetrical perirenal space involvement but with sparing of the IVC and pelvic ureters are features that differentiate it from RPF (Figure 7.25) [146]. Erdheim–Chester disease is associated with osteosclerosis, periostitis, partial epiphyseal involvement, and medullary infarction of the long bones [148].

7.4.2.4.2 Extramedullary Hematopoiesis

Extramedullary hematopoiesis (EMH) is rarely seen in the retroperitoneum. On CT and MRI, EMH appears as multiple, bilateral, homogeneous soft tissue masses with intermediate signal intensity on T1-weighted imaging, intermediate to high signal intensity on T2-weighted imaging relative to skeletal muscle, and variable

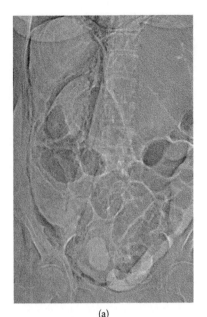

(a)

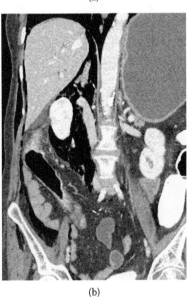

(b)

FIGURE 7.24
A 61-year-old woman who underwent endoscopic dilation of the duodenal strictures and developed abdominal pain. CT scan (a, topogram; b, coronal) revealed extensive right pneumoretroperitoneum from duodenal perforation.

enhancement [149–151]. Calcification and osseous destruction are usually not present. After blood transfusion therapy, lesions tend to shrink and develop massive iron deposition with resultant loss of enhancement [149]. Liver and splenic masses may be concurrently seen, as are skeletal changes due to chronic anemia or myelofibrosis [151].

7.4.2.4.3 Lipoma

Retroperitoneal lipomas are rare, but are the most common benign tumors of the retroperitoneum [99]. They

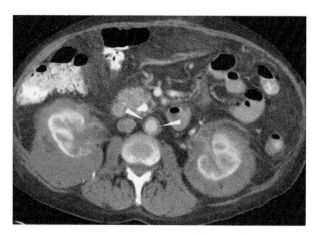

FIGURE 7.25
A 45-year-old man with Erdheim–Chester disease—note the bilateral, symmetric perinephric rind of soft tissue, periaortic involvement (arrowheads) with sparing of IVC and ureters (not seen). Patient also had histiocytic infiltration in multiple organs outside the abdomen. (Reprinted from *Radiol Clin North Am.*, Mar;50(2), Goenka AH et al., Imaging of the retroperitoneum, 333-55, vii; Copyright 2012, with permission from Elsevier.)

usually appear during periods of weight gain and are composed of large, mature adipocytes, not significantly different from the normal adult fat. They typically have homogeneous fat attenuation and signal intensity on all pulse sequences and do not enhance [152]. However, up to 31% lipomas may have enhancing nonadipose areas due to fat necrosis and associated dystrophic changes [20]. In the latter cases, a well-differentiated liposarcoma is a close imaging differential (Table 7.3).

7.4.2.4.4 Fat Necrosis

Retroperitoneal fat necrosis can present as a palpable abdominal mass, mimic other abdominal masses, including retroperitoneal liposarcoma, and rarely lead to ureteral obstruction. The most common cause of retroperitoneal fat necrosis is acute pancreatitis [153–156]. On imaging, it appears as predominantly fat attenuating or fat signal intensity lesion that may also contain foci of enhancing soft tissue or calcification. The distribution is typically peripancreatic but there may be extension into the mesenteric root, transverse mesocolon, and omentum in severe disease [157]. Fat necrosis tends to remain stable in size or shrink with time.

7.4.2.5 Retroperitoneal Nonparenchymal Cysts and Cystic Lesions

7.4.2.5.1 Lymphangioma

A retroperitoneal lymphangioma is a developmental malformation that is caused by failure of communication of retroperitoneal lymphatic tissue with the main lymphatic vessels [158]. They account for 1% of all

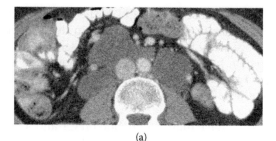

(a)

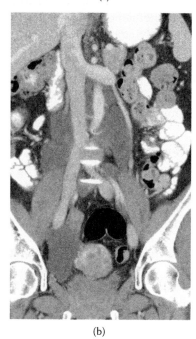

(b)

FIGURE 7.26
CECT (a, axial; b, coronal) shows a low-attenuation cystic mass that insinuates between peritoneal and retroperitoneal structures and demonstrates little enhancement—features highly suggestive of a lymphangioma.

retroperitoneal neoplasms, are more common in men, and can occur in any age group [158,159]. It characteristically appears as a fluid attenuation or fluid signal intensity, elongated, thin-walled, multiseptate cystic mass that typically insinuates between the structures (Figure 7.26). The presence of lymph fluid, chyle, may give rise to negative attenuation values or high T1- and intermediate T2-signal intensity. The presence of septa, compression of intestinal loops, and the lack of fluid in dependent recesses or mesenteric leaves are features used to differentiate lymphangiomas from ascites [67]. Surgical excision is the treatment of choice for symptomatic lesions [19,159].

7.4.2.5.2 Cystadenoma and Cystadenocarcinoma

Cystadenoma is a rare primary epithelial retroperitoneal tumor of unclear histogenesis [160] that most often occurs in women who have normal ovaries, usually in the fifth decade of life. It can be mucinous or serous and there are several clinic-pathologic subtypes. CT and MRI imaging show a well-defined unilocular homogeneous cystic mass. Internal septae, papillary projections, or soft tissue solid enhancing components may be present in cystadenocarcinoma. Surgical resection is recommended even for benign lesions due to the risk of malignant transformation [161,162].

7.4.2.5.3 Bronchogenic Cyst

Retroperitoneal bronchogenic (foregut) cysts are rare and the majority of them are found in the paramidline upper retroperitoneum adjacent to the diaphragmatic crura. They appear as sharply marginated, thin-walled, cystic lesions. However, fluid–fluid levels due to complex internal contents, mural calcification, layering milk of calcium, and rim enhancement may be seen [163–165].

7.4.2.5.4 Extralobar Pulmonary Sequestration

Subdiaphragmatic retroperitoneal localization of pulmonary sequestration can occur in up to 15% of cases [166]. On CT and MRI, a nonspecific, well-circumscribed, low-attenuation mass with low T1-weighted and high T2-weighted signal intensity is generally seen, sometimes with foci of cystic change or calcification. Contrast enhancement is variable, but is usually peripheral in distribution. Feeding systemic arterial branches to retroperitoneal extralobar pulmonary sequestrations are not usually well visualized on cross-sectional imaging, which makes a prospective diagnosis difficult [166–169].

7.4.2.5.5 Nonpancreatic Pseudocyst

Nonpancreatic pseudocysts develop due to failure of resorption of prior hematomas or abscesses. Histologically, they are similar to pancreatic pseudocysts and have no epithelial lining [170,171]. On CT and MRI, they are thin- or thick-walled cystic lesions that may demonstrate high attenuation or high T1- or T2-weighted signal intensity due to hemorrhagic, proteinaceous, or purulent contents. There may be a fluid–fluid level, internal septae, calcifications, or peripheral enhancement [170–172].

7.5 Abdominal Great Vessels

7.5.1 Aorta

7.5.1.1 Imaging Anatomy of the Aorta

The abdominal aorta is a continuation of the thoracic aorta that begins at the level of T12 vertebra. It gives visceral branches that are unpaired (celiac artery, superior mesenteric artery, and IMA) or paired (renal, adrenal, and gonadal arteries) and parietal branches that are unpaired (median sacral) or paired (subcostal, inferior phrenic, and iliolumbar arteries). The aorta bifurcates into the common iliac arteries at the level of L4. The common iliac arteries continue as external and internal iliac arteries. Anatomic variations of the abdominal aorta occur [173]. For example, accessory renal arteries are seen in up to 30% of individuals [173].

7.5.1.2 CT and MRI of the Aorta

Multi-detector CT scanners enable rapid acquisition of a large number of images of the abdominal aorta, with sub-millimeter isotropic spatial resolution, which can be reconstructed in any plane. Acquisition following contrast administration is triggered either by a bolus tracking method or by a test bolus technique. Noncontrast imaging may be helpful in patients with acute abdominal pain to evaluate for intramural aortic hematoma. In addition to noncontrast and arterial phase images, delayed venous phase images are also acquired in patients with an endovascular stent to evaluate for endoleak. Most CT protocols are acquired with 3 mm thickness, but 1 mm thickness may be required for patients being evaluated for endovascular stent planning. Radiation dose should be kept as low as reasonably achievable by using dose reduction techniques such as automatic tube-current modulation, low tube potential, high-pitch helical scanning (where possible), and iterative reconstruction algorithms. Also, virtual noncontrast images can be generated from arterial phase images using dual-source scanners [174] to diminish radiation dose. Postprocessing techniques are useful to depict anatomy and include volume rendering, shaded-surface display, maximum intensity projection (MIP), and multiplanar reconstruction (MPR). Measurements may be performed either manually or be semiautomated.

MRI of the aorta involves the use of steady-state free precession (SSFP) and T2-weighted fast-spin echo (FSE) images. The vessel wall morphology is evaluated with T2-weighted FSE images. Short-tau inversion recovery (STIR) images are used to evaluate the presence of vessel wall edema. MRI angiography is performed using T1-weighted spoiled gradient sequence following intravenous administration of gadolinium chelate. Angiographic images can also be obtained using noncontrast techniques such as navigator-gated whole-heart SSFP sequence or phase-contrast VIPR = Vastly Undersampled Isotropic PRojection technique. Noncontrast sequences are valuable in patients with severe renal dysfunction, who are at increased risk of developing nephrogenic systemic fibrosis following administration of intravenous gadolinium.

7.5.1.3 Pathologic Conditions

7.5.1.3.1 Hypoplastic Abdominal Aorta

Hypoplasia is a congenital abnormality characterized by tubular narrowing of a long segment of the aorta. Coarctation is a discrete narrowing of portion of the aorta. Congenital hypoplasia is rare in the abdominal aorta, with an incidence of 6 in 1 million [175]. It is a developmental abnormality and may be secondary to maternal infection or inflammation. It is more common in women and presents in the first to third decades of life [176]. A diagnosis of congenital hypoplasia is made after exclusion of acquired causes of aortic stenosis. Clinical symptoms include hypertension, lower extremity claudication, and absence of pulses; when all are present, it is called as mid-aortic syndrome. On CT and MRI angiography, a long segment of circumferential narrowing is seen (Figure 7.27). Occasionally, a discrete focal narrowing is seen. Extensive collateral vessel formation is often seen, indicating hemodynamically significant stenosis. Stenosis in the renal and visceral arteries is usually seen. The prognosis is generally poor and surgical bypass graft is required to prevent complications [177].

7.5.1.3.2 Atherosclerosis

Atherosclerosis is a diffuse, chronic immuno-inflammatory disease of the vascular, metabolic, and immune systems, characterized by deposition of lipid and fibrous products in the arterial wall. Atherosclerotic plaques are associated with age, high blood pressure,

and smoking [178]. On CT, atherosclerotic plaque and thrombi are seen as low-attenuation lesions in the periphery of the aortic lumen internal to mural calcifications (Figure 7.28). While plaque has irregular margins, thrombus has smooth margins with crescentic or a concentric shape with peripheral calcifications. Plaque > 4 mm, ulcers > 2 mm and mobile thrombi have higher risk of coronary artery disease [179]. Complex plaques are more prevalent in patients with myocardial infarction and are an indicator of coronary plaque instability [178]. Atherosclerotic plaques and intimal ulcers are typically asymptomatic, but may cause peripheral embolism when located in the infrarenal abdominal aorta or a proximal common iliac artery. In experimental studies, plaque has been characterized using high-resolution MRI with multicontrast sequences (T1-weighted, proton density weighted, and T2-weighted) and following contrast administration. Lipids have high signal on T1W and proton density weighted sequences, while fibrocellular components are hyperintense and calcific lesions are hypointense on T1W, T2W, and PDW sequences. Contrast enhancement is seen in unstable plaques. MRI may be used in identifying high-risk patient for cardiovascular events, serial evaluation of plaque progression and regression, and response to therapy [178].

A penetrating atherosclerotic ulcer extends through the intima into the media and is typically associated with hematoma. It is less common in the abdominal than the thoracic aorta. This process begins as an atherosclerotic intimal ulcer (stage II), evolves into an

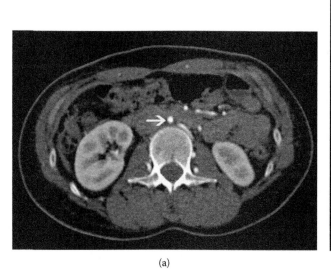

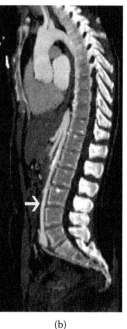

(a)   (b)

FIGURE 7.27
Abdominal aortic hypoplasia. (a) Axial contrast-enhanced CT scan in a 36-year-old female patient shows small caliber of abdominal aorta (arrow). (b) Sagittal reformatted MIP image in the same patient shows diffuse circumferential narrowing of a long segment of the abdominal aorta (arrow), with extensive collateral vessel formation. Normal caliber of the aortic bifurcation is seen.

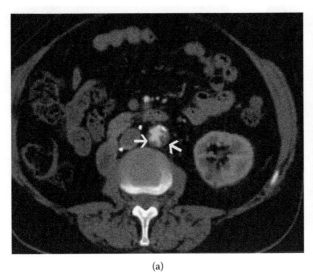 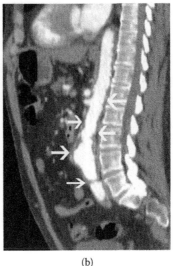

(a)   (b)

FIGURE 7.28
Atherosclerosis. (a) Axial postcontrast CT scan in a 53-year-old male shows extensive mixed, calcific, and noncalcific plaques in the abdominal aorta (arrows), causing luminal narrowing. (b) Sagittal reconstructed CT image in the same patient shows extensive atherosclerotic plaques (arrows) and intimal ulcerations of the abdominal aorta.

intimal tear (stage II), followed by hemorrhage in the media (stage III), and finally results in a full-thickness penetration of aortic wall (stage IV) [180]. It is commonly seen in elderly patients and can be either single or multiple. The clinical presentation is similar to that of aortic dissection, often presenting with acute abdominal pain. Penetrating atherosclerotic ulcer is difficult to visualize on a noncontrast CT scan. Intramural hematoma (IMH), atherosclerosis, and displaced intimal calcification can be seen. After intravenous contrast administration, a focal area of high-attenuation ulceration is seen extending through the intima into the aortic wall. A focally thick and enhancing aortic wall may be seen due to associated IMH. A penetrating ulcer should be distinguished from an intimal atherosclerotic ulcer, which is confined to the intima and is asymptomatic and without focal IMH. Saccular aneurysm formation, dissection, distal embolization, rupture, and fistula are complications of penetrating atherosclerotic ulcers. It may be challenging to distinguish a ruptured ulcer from a ruptured aneurysm. On MRI, similar appearances are seen and dislodgement of intimal calcification is difficult to visualize. A penetrating ulcer is typically managed medically, but surgery is performed if there is persistent pain, rapid enlargement, hemodynamic instability, rupture, or distal embolization. Surgery may be difficult since the aortic wall has been damaged by ulcer, resulting in higher morbidity and mortality [180].

7.5.1.3.3 Aortoiliac Occlusive Disease

Aortoiliac stenosis is a sequela of chronic atherosclerotic disease. The infrarenal abdominal aorta and the common iliac arteries are the most common locations. Stenotic lesions have been graded as four types (TransAtlantic InterSociety Consensus II), based on the lesion location, length, multiplicity, laterality, and the degree of stenosis [181]. Clinical symptoms depend on the type and location of lesion and may include intermittent hip/buttock claudication and impotence in men. CT and MRI angiography demonstrate the location and extent of the stenosis (Figure 7.29). No significant difference has been found between CT and MRI angiography in the demonstration of hemodynamically significant stenoses [182]. CT and MRI angiography are useful in treatment planning due to their ability to evaluate length, multiplicity, degree, collaterals, and coexistent femoropopliteal disease [173]. Aortoiliac occlusive disease is treated through either endovascular (balloon angioplasty and stent) or surgical procedures (aortobifemoral or axillofemoral with femoral-femoral bypass).

7.5.1.3.4 Aneurysm

An aneurysm is a focal segmental dilation of the abdominal aorta greater than 1.5 times its normal diameter, that is, >3 cm. Dilation less than 1.5 times is called ectasia. Aneurysm is more common in men than women and is seen in 4%–8% of men and 1% of women over 50 years of age [183]. The average age at diagnosis is 65–70 years [184]. There is a higher incidence of aneurysm in smokers, patients with a family history of aneursyms, and in Caucasians. Atherosclerosis is the most common cause of aneurysm. Other causes include infection, connective tissue disorders (Ehler–Danlos syndrome, Marfan syndrome,

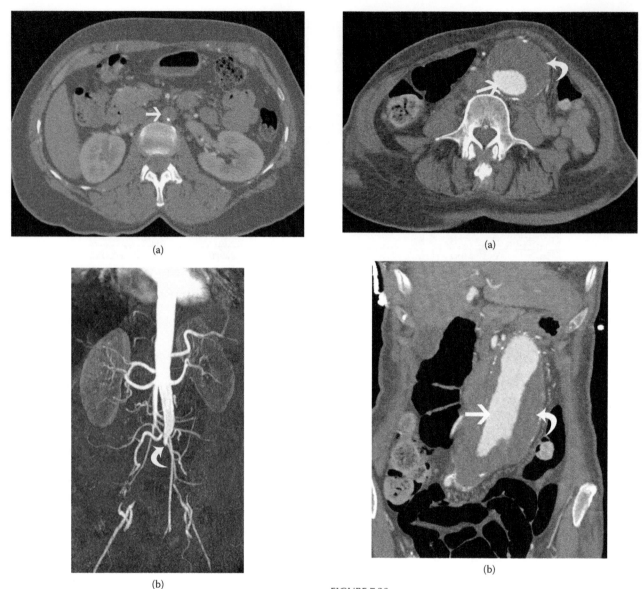

(a)

(b)

FIGURE 7.29
Aortoiliac occlusive disease. (a) Axial contrast-enhanced CT scan in a 57-year-old male shows complete occlusion of the abdominal aorta (arrow). (b) Coronal reconstructed MIP image from an MRI scan in a 59-year-old female with atherosclerotic disease shows complete occlusion of the distal abdominal aorta (arrow) and the entire length of the common iliac arteries. There is reconstruction of the external iliac arteries and the proximal internal iliac arteries through collateral vascular supply.

FIGURE 7.30
Aneurysm. (a) Axial CT angiographic image in a 72-year-old female shows a large aneurysm of the abdominal aorta measuring 6.2 cm, with a lining mural thrombus (curved arrow) and a patent contrast opacified inner lumen (straight arrow). (b) Coronal CT angiographic image in the same patient shows the fusiform nature of the aneurysm, along with the lining mural thrombus (curved arrow), calcifications, and inner patient lumen (straight arrow). There is no evidence of rupture.

homocystinuria, and pseudoxanthoma elasticum), and vasculitis (Takayasu's arteritis and giant cell arteritis) [173]. Aneurysms are believed to be caused by disruption of the extracellular matrix of the aorta, most likely secondary to the release of proinflammatory mediators.

Thoracoabdominal aneurysms can be classified (Crawford classification) as type I—proximal descending thoracic to proximal abdominal aorta; type II—proximal descending to infrarenal abdominal aorta;

type III—distal descending with abdominal aorta; and type IV—primarily abdominal aorta [185]. Aneurysms can be either fusiform or saccular in shape. A fusiform aneurysm has symmetrical dilation involving the entire circumference of aortic wall (Figure 7.30) while a saccular aneurysm is more localized with outpouching of one portion of the aortic wall. True aneurysms involve all the three aortic layers (tunica intima, media, and adventitia) without their disruption and are most commonly caused by atherosclerosis. It is more common in the infrarenal abdominal aorta. Pseudoaneurysms (false aneurysms) do not involve all the three arterial layers and are often associated with intimal and occasionally with medial disruption, with containment of blood by adventitial and periadventitial tissue. They are caused by trauma, infection, surgery, or penetrating atherosclerotic ulcers and are typically saccular. They are more common in the suprarenal abdominal aorta, due to higher likelihood of tamponade in this location due to density and rigid fixation of surrounding tissues [186]. Pseudoaneurysms are surgically treated due to risk of rupture and have high mortality rates [187].

Most of abdominal aortic aneurysms are asymptomatic and are often incidentally discovered during imaging procedures. However, they may present as a palpable pulsatile mass or with complications such as rupture, thrombotic occlusion, peripheral emboli, or fistulous communication to the bowel or IVC. Constipation, urinary retention, the urge to defecate, or syncope may also be seen due to compression of blood vessels. No symptom is seen from a contained rupture. Small aneurysms grow at the rate of 2.6–3.2 mm per year, but large aneurysms may grow faster [188].

On CT and MRI, an aneurysm is seen as focal dilation of the abdominal aorta (Figure 7.30). Mural calcification and thrombosis may also be seen. The size of the aneurysm should be measured and compared with previous scans to assess stability or growth.

7.5.1.3.5 *Ruptured Aneurysm*

Rupture is a complication of abdominal aortic aneurysm and can be either contained or free and may be acute or chronic. Rupture results from hemodynamic stress placed on the aortic wall, with a cumulative risk of rupture for aneurysms <4 cm of 1% over 6 years, 1%–3% for 4–5 cm, 6%–11% for 5–7 cm, and 20% for >7 cm [189]. The risk of rupture is also high when the aneurysm expands >0.5 cm within 6 months [190]. Rupture has a mortality of 79% when it occurs outside a hospital and 40% in the hospital [173]. The most common location of rupture is the posterolateral wall into the retroperitoneum with blood extending into the perirenal, pararenal spaces, both, or into the psoas muscle. Intraperitoneal rupture is less common and occurs from the anterior or anterolateral aortic wall. Rupture occurs rarely into the bowel (see discussion in Section 7.5.1.3.6) or into the IVC (see discussion in Section 7.5.1.3.7). The classic clinical triad of rupture is abdominal pain, pulsatile mass, and shock and is seen in 50% of patients [191]. Chronic contained ruptures are hemodynamically stable and present with pain and mass effects such as jaundice, femoral neuropathy, and inguinal hernia [191].

On CT, ruptured aneurysms are generally larger and have less thrombus and calcification than unruptured aneurysms. Focal discontinuity of the aortic wall and extravasation of contrast/blood into the retroperitoneum are specific signs of aortic rupture (Figure 7.31). Retroperitoneal hematoma adjacent to an aneurysm is the most common finding [184]. Subtle signs of impending or rupture include a new focal disruption in an otherwise circumferential aortic calcification or changes in configuration of mural calcifications since a prior study [192]. The "crescent sign" is a specific sign of impending aortic rupture [193] and indicates hemorrhage in the mural thrombus, which later penetrates the aneurismal wall and makes it weak. Well-defined crescentic areas of high attenuation that are denser than the patent lumen on an unenhanced scan and denser than psoas muscle on postcontrast scans are seen [192]. Lumen irregularity may also indicate impending rupture [193].

A chronic contained rupture is diagnosed in a patient with history of abdominal aortic aneurysm, resolved pain, stable hemodynamic status, a normal hematocrit, and CT findings of retroperitoneal hemorrhage, with pathological confirmation of an organized hematoma [194]. The "drape sign" refers to an absence of sharp posterior wall of the aorta, which drapes over the vertebral body without a distinct fat plane between aorta and vertebral body and is a sign of chronic contained rupture, even in the absence of a retroperitoneal hematoma [192]. This should be distinguished from periaortic fibrosis, lymphadenopathy, and malignant tumors of a vertebral body with soft tissue extension or of the duodenum.

Treatment of ruptured aneurysm is associated with a higher mortality (79%) than from elective surgery (5%) or endovascular repair [173,195].

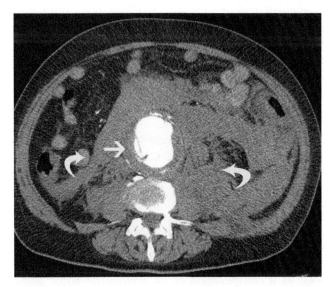

FIGURE 7.31
Ruptured aneurysm. Axial postcontrast CT image in a 73-year-old male patient with abdominal pain, syncope, hypotension, and circulatory collapse shows a large infrarenal abdominal aortic aneurysm (straight arrow) with a large retroperitoneal hematoma surrounding it (curved arrow).

7.5.1.3.6 Aortoenteric Fistula

Aortoenteric fisula is a rare, life-threatening communication between the aorta and the small bowel. It can be primary when developing from an aortic aneurysm or secondary when it is a complication of aortic surgery or endovascular stent graft repair.

The secondary type is more common than the primary (0.6–2 per million vs. 0.007 per million). A secondary fistula is more often seen following surgery than endovascular repair and can be seen between 2 weeks and 10 years following surgery. It occurs due to a combination of chronic perigraft infection and pressure on bowel from aortic pulsations [196]. Eighty percent of aortoenteric fistulas involve the duodenum, most commonly in the third and fourth portions [196]. Clinical features include gastrointestinal hemorrhage, which begins with a herald bleed before development of massive hemorrhage. Pain, pulsatile mass, and a groin mass may also be present. CT and MRI have a variable sensitivity (40%–90%) and specificity (33%–100%) in the diagnosis of aortoenteric fistula [196]. In a primary aortoenteric fistula, gas is seen adjacent to or within an aorta that has an aneurysm or a penetrating atherosclerotic ulcer. There is obliteration of fat plane between the aorta and the adjacent bowel loop. Hematoma may be seen in the retroperitoneum or within the bowel. Secondary aortoenteric fistulas are usually seen following perigraft infection. There is extensive overlap between the findings of perigraft infection and secondary aortoenteric fistula. Ectopic gas (more than 3–4 weeks after surgery) and perigraft soft tissue thickening, fluid, or hematoma (more than 2–3 months after surgery) are present in both these conditions. Disruption of the aortic wall, loss of a fat plane between aorta and bowel, and pseudoaneurysm are the other features seen in both. However, ectopic gas, focal bowel wall thickening, disruption of aortic wall, and contrast extravasation into the bowel lumen are specific features of secondary aortoenteric fistula. Extravasation of aortic contrast into the bowel lumen and leakage of enteric contrast into the aorta/paraprosthetic space are highly specific signs, but are only rarely encountered. Apart from perigraft infection, differential diagnosis for aortoenteric fistula includes mycotic aneurysm, RPF, and infectious aortitis.

7.5.1.3.7 Aortocaval Fistula

Aortocaval fistula is a communication between the abdominal aorta and the IVC. Overall, the prevalence of aortocaval fistula is 0.2%–0.9% [197]. It is most often seen as a complication of an abdominal aortic aneurysm, seen in 1% of all aneurysms and 6% of ruptured aneurysms [198]. It can also be seen following blunt or penetrating trauma [199]. It is more common in males [200]. A small fistula may be asymptomatic. A large fistula may present with a palpable mass, abdominal or back pain, a continuous machinery murmur, wide pulse-pressure, high-output cardiac failure, lower limb edema, thrombosis, claudication, or priapism [201]. A high index of clinical suspicion is essential for diagnosis, since classic imaging findings are seen in only 20%–50% of cases [202]. CT findings include early and intense opacification of the IVC and common iliac veins at the same time and with the same density as that of abdominal aorta (Figure 7.32). The IVC is distended,

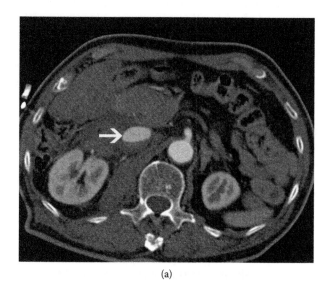

(a)

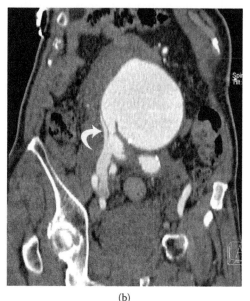

(b)

FIGURE 7.32

Aortocaval fistula. (a) Axial CT scan in a 54-year-old male patient who presented with severe abdominal pain and a pulsatile abdominal mass shows IVC opacification (arrow) at the same time as that of abdominal aorta and with similar attenuation. (b) Coronal reconstructed CT image in the same patient shows a large infrarenal abdominal aortic aneurysm, which shows a fistulous communication with the IVC (curved arrow) just above the level of bifurcation into common iliac veins, and intense and simultaneous opacification of the common iliac veins, consistent with an aortocaval fistula.

unlike aortic rupture with hypovolemia, which results in IVC collapse. The most common location of rupture is at the posterolateral wall of the abdominal aorta at or just above the aortic bifurcation. Absence of an obstructing lesion distinguishes a fistula from other causes of IVC dilation. Absence of duodenal dilation and loss of normal fat plane with intestine excludes aortoenteric fistula. Aortocaval fistula may be fatal and is treated with emergent surgery [199]. The prognosis is better than for ruptured aneurysm [203].

7.5.1.3.7.1 Imaging Before Surgical or Endovascular Graft Repair Aneurysms are repaired when they reach a diameter of 5.5 cm or when there is a size increase of >0.5 cm in 6 months or the patient is symptomatic [190]. Surgical repair is performed by opening the aorta and sewing a graft from the proximal normal aorta to the distal normal aorta or to the iliac arteries. Surgical repair is associated with more morbidity, hospital stay, and mortality (4.7% 30-day mortality) than endovascular repair [204]. An endovascular stent graft is a well-established alternative to open surgery for the treatment of abdominal aortic aneurysm, particularly in high-risk patients. The graft, which is a synthetic graft reinforced with metallic meshwork, is introduced through bilateral incisions in the femoral arteries. In addition, treatment with endovascular stent grafts is associated with faster recovery, less pain, and lower need for blood products when compared with that of open surgery [205,206].

Imaging plays an important role in the evaluation of patients undergoing endovascular or surgical grafting of abdominal aortic aneurysms. CT is the surgeons' preferred modality for evaluating an aortic aneurysm

before repair. The size of the aneurysm is measured either manually or using automated software in all the three dimensions from sections orthogonal to the axis of vessel lumen. Diameters are measured from wall to wall. The maximum antero-posterior (AP) diameter of the sac is of particular interest. The size and configuration should be compared with previous imaging studies to evaluate for growth [190]. Longitudinal measurements are useful in estimating the length of endovascular graft, but may be inaccurate in saccular or tortuous aneurysms. Three-dimensional (3D) systems are used to generate 3D models that stimulate the patient's aorta and the proposed endograft, which helps in deciding the size, shape, and position of the graft [207].

The axial length of the aneurysm neck (distance between the lowest renal artery and starting of aneurysm sac) and quality (shape and angulation) of the neck are critical factors for surgical/endovascular planning. The maximal diameters of the neck help determine device choice. Necks that are relatively straight with cylindrical shape, angulation <60% relative to long axis of aneurysm, and absence of significant thrombus or atheroma are favorable factors. Conical- or barrel-shaped neck, excessive tortuosity or angulation, and extensive atherothrombus are adverse factors. A juxtarenal aneurysm is close to or involves the renal arteries and has a higher surgical risk due to the need for suprarenal cross-clamping since it has a short neck below the renal artery (Figure 7.33a and b). It is also not suitable for the use of unfenestrated conventional endovascular stent grafts due to a higher risk of compromised renal function, type 1 endoleak, and stent migration. These aneurysms usually need a fenestrated stent graft, bridging catheters to align the fenestration with the renal artery,

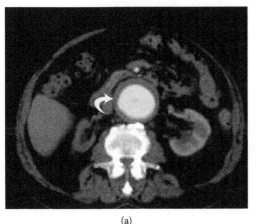
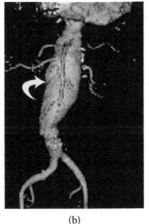
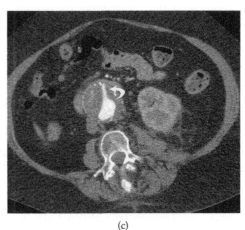

(a) (b) (c)

FIGURE 7.33
Pre-endovascular stent evaluation. (a) Axial postcontrast CT in a 63-year-old male patient shows a juxtarenal aneurysm (arrow), with occlusion of the right renal artery. Atrophic right kidney is seen. (b) Volume rendered CT image in the same patient allows exquisite demonstration of the aneurysm (arrow). (c) Axial postcontrast CT scan of a 67-year-old male patient shows a patent channel (arrow) extending through the thrombus within an aneurismal sac, which leads to a patient inferior mesenteric artery (IMA). This is a predisposing factor for a persistent type II endoleak.

and flared bridging stents to avoid endoleak. Suprarenal aneurysms extend to a level of the superior mesenteric artery or higher. Either fenestrated stent graft or surgical tube-graft placement with reimplantation of visceral branches is required. Stent migration may occur with a conical or flared aneurysm [173].

The diameter, tortuosity, and atherosclerotic burden of iliac arteries are also noted for planning device access. The main stent graft is placed through the larger and less tortuous iliac artery. Placing a friction or barbed device in a superior aneurysm neck or in iliac arteries that have extensive atherosclerotic ulceration may result in embolization, poor fixation, or endoleak [208]. The distal attachment site measurements are also essential [207]. Aortic aneurysms involve the proximal common iliac artery in 5%–46% of patients and these patients may require extension limbs [209]. Aortoiliac aneurysms extending to the iliac artery bifurcation require a bifurcated endovascular stent graft with extenders into external iliac artery and occlusion of the ipsilateral internal iliac artery. In such a situation, the contralateral common iliac aneurysm ideally should have distal margin proximal to iliac bifurcation. The common and external iliac arteries should be large enough to allow the passage of device and should have less extensive atherosclerotic calcification, tortuosity, and angulation. Common iliac artery shorter than 4 cm is also considered unfavorable [207].

The number and location of renal arteries is also important. Accessory renal arteries may be sacrificed if they are small and supply only a small portion of kidney. Accessory renal artery may limit useful length of neck and may contribute to endoleak if they communicate with aneurysm sac. Retroaortic left renal vein should be noted before surgery [208].

Patency of the mesenteric arteries should be noted. A patent IMA is seen in 10% of studies [207], usually arising from aneurysm sac and is a route for persistent endoleak following repair (Figure 7.33c). Following IMA exclusion in endovascular repair or ligation in surgical repair, colonic ischemia may develop if there is associated SMA stenosis or internal iliac stenosis or inadequate collateral supply [173].

The important parameters required for a successful endovascular stent graft repair are summarized in Table 7.7.

7.5.1.3.7.2 Evaluation of the Aorta after Graft Placement
7.5.1.3.7.2.1 Endovascular Stent Grafts CT is often used in the follow-up of patients after endovascular stent graft placement (Figure 7.34). A baseline postoperative scan is followed by scans at 1, 6, and 12 months, which are followed by annual scans for lifelong surveillance. Images are acquired before and after administration of

TABLE 7.7

Recommended Measurement for Endovascular Device Placement (AneuRx and Excluder Devices)

Proximal neck	External AP and transverse diameter <28 mm
	Length <15 mm
	Angulation with long axis of aneurysm <60°
	Not excessively conical/flared
	Atherosclerosis (involving <25% of neck circumference, <2-mm-thick thrombus)
Distal placement zone in iliac arteries	AP external diameter <13–15 mm
	Length <20 mm
	Proximal to iliac artery bifurcation
External and common iliac arteries	Size large enough to allow device access
	No focal stenosis
	Maximum tortuosity less than 120°

Source: Budovec, J.J. et al., *Radiol. Clin. N. Am.*, 48, 283–309, 2010.

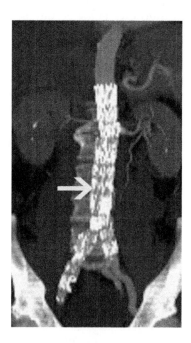

FIGURE 7.34
Normal bifurcated endovascular stent graft. Coronal reconstructed MIP image in a 66-year-old male patient shows a bifurcated endovascular stent graft (arrow) extending from the suprarenal segment of the abdominal aorta, into the common iliac arteries bilaterally and also into the right external iliac artery on the right.

contrast, both in the arterial and in the venous phases. Noncontrast scans are required to distinguish calcification and high-attenuation foci from endoleaks. MR angiography (MRA) can be used in patients who have MRI-compatible stent grafts.

Immediate complications following graft repair include rupture, ischemic, and renal complications. Other complications following EVAR: endovascular aortic repair include endoleak, thrombus, kinking, pseudoaneurysm, infection, occlusion, embolism, perforated thrombus, colonic necrosis, dissection, and hematoma [210].

Endoleak is the most common complication and refers to leakage of blood into the native aneurysml sac resulting in its expansion. Endoleak is visualized as contrast outside of the stent but within the aneurysm sac. Endoleaks are classified into five types (Table 7.8). Accurate categorization of the endoleak type is crucial, since the treatment varies with the type. Type I endoleaks occur due to a separation of the stent graft at the site of its attachment with the native aortic wall. Type 1a occurs at the proximal attachment and type 1b occurs at the distal attachment. Type 1 endoleaks occur due to complex arterial anatomy, such as short, angulated, ulcerated, trapezoidal, and thrombus-containing necks, or due to irregular, dilated, and tortuous iliac arteries. Type I endoleaks are typically seen during the graft placement. Due to the risk of rupture secondary to arterial pressure in the aneurysm sac, type I endoleaks are repaired immediately, either endovascularly with aortic cuffs or with surgical closure. On CT, acute hemorrhage or contrast leak is seen in the native aneurismal sac at the site of stent graft attachment (Figure 7.35a). Type 1C occurs due to backfilling of aneurysm sac secondary to incomplete occlusion of contralateral common iliac artery in a patient with an aorto-uniiliac stent graft with femoro-femoral artery bypass. Type IC endoleak is treated by embolization of the involved common iliac artery. Type II endoleaks are the most common type (40% of endoleaks) [211] and occur from retrograde filling of the aneurysm sac by flow through branch vessels from segments of aorta that do not have a stent or from the iliac arteries. The IMA and lumbar arteries are the common sources of type II endoleaks. On CT, type II endoleak is seen as a peripheral focus of hemorrhage or contrast leak in the aneurysm sac (Figure 7.35b) and may be identified only on a delayed scan. Due to slow leak, type II endoleaks are managed conservatively and often

undergo spontaneous resolution. In cases that show interval expansion of aneurismal sac, embolization of the lumbar or IMA or injection of hemostatic agent in the nonthrombosed part of aneurysm may be performed. Type III endoleaks occur due to structural failure of the stent graft, such as fractures, holes, or junctional separations, and are caused by stresses of arterial pulsations due to shrinking of the aneurysm sac. On CT, large collections of hemorrhage or contrast are seen centrally, away from attachment sites. Due to high risk of rupture from high pressure, type III endoleaks are repaired. Type IV endoleaks are caused by porosity of the stent graft and occur immediately following stent placement, before sealing of graft by fibrin incorporation, and are often seen in patients who are on anticoagulants. Type IV endoleak is self-healing and requires only correction of the coagulation profile. Type V endoleak or endotension refers to expansion of the native aneurysm without a visible leak. This could be either due to a small, occult leak or ultrafiltration of blood across the stent graft or an ineffective barrier to pressure transmission caused by thrombus in the native aneurysm sac [210]. Type V endoleak is a diagnosis of exclusion. It is a low-risk endoleak, but may require open repair in patients with high pressure [212].

Graft thrombosis is seen in 3%–19% of patients [213]. Thrombosis is seen as a peripheral, intraluminal, circular, or semicircular filling defect within the stent graft (Figure 7.35c and d). The thrombus may shrink spontaneously or develop into complete thrombosis [210]. Thrombosis of the graft limb is seen in 2.2%–3.9% of patients, usually due to kinking of aortic component of the stent graft within aneurysm or kinking of iliac limbs within the iliac arteries (Figure 7.35e) [173]. Stenosis of iliac graft limb has been reported in bifurcated grafts that are not fully supported by stents. Graft occlusion is, however, rare and may be seen due to thrombosis or embolus from the heart [173]. Graft kinking is seen due to shortening and decreased diameter of the aneurysm following endovascular repair, resulting in incomplete support of the stent. This is best seen on MIP or MPR images. Graft infection is rare following endovascular stent graft and is associated with high morbidity and mortality (75%) [214]. Presence of perigraft air or fluid immediately following implantation is not suggestive of infection. Fever, leukocytosis, and elevated CRP are also not specific in the early postinterventional period. Periprosthetic soft tissue thickening does not necessarily indicate infection since it may be seen as a foreign body inflammatory reaction [210]. Persistent or expanding perigraft fluid, soft tissue, or gas are features of graft infection. Pseudoaneurysm and contrast leak may also be seen (Figure 7.35f and g) [210]. Treatment is a combination of systemic antibiotics and surgical treatment.

TABLE 7.8

Types of Endoleak

Type	Description
I	Leak at the attachment side of the graft IA—Proximal attachment IB—Distal attachment IC—Backfilling of aneurysmal sac due to incomplete occlusion of contralateral common iliac artery
II	Leak by collateral vessel flow
III	Leak due to mechanical failure of the graft (junctional leak, mid graft hole, and disconnect)
IV	Leak due to graft porosity
V	Endotension

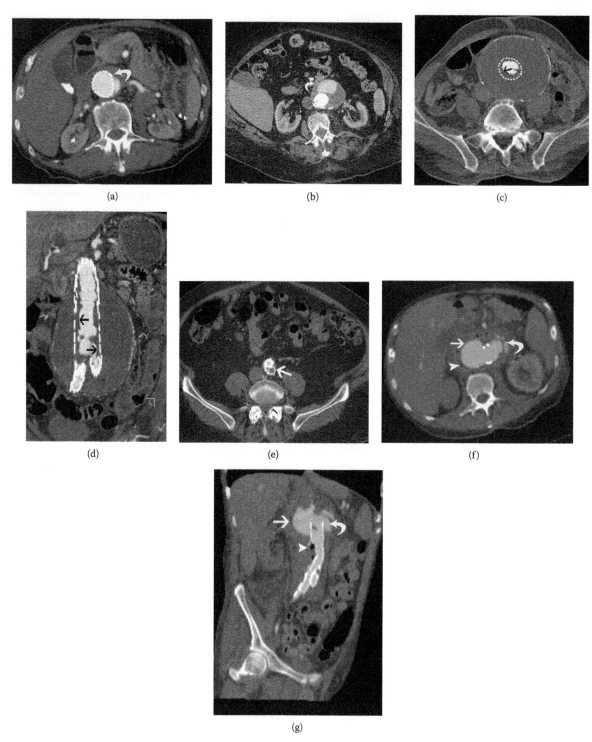

FIGURE 7.35

Complications of endovascular stent graft. (a) Axial postcontrast CT scan in a 64-year-old male shows a focal contrast leak from the proximal attachment of the stent graft with the native aorta (arrow), consistent with a type IA leak. (b) Axial postcontrast CT scan in a 56-year-old male shows an endovascular stent graft in the abdominal aorta. There is contrast opacification in the anterior part of the native aneurismal sac (arrow), which is consistent with a type 2 endoleak originating from the IMA. (c) Axial postcontrast CT scan in a 62-year-old male shows complete occlusion of the left iliac limb of EVAR (arrow). (d) Axial postcontrast CT image in a 63-year-old male patient shows circumferential thrombus (arrows) inside the endovascular stent graft. (e) Coronal reconstructed CT image in the same patient demonstrates the craniocaudal extent of the thrombus (arrows). (f) Axial postcontrast CT scan in an 89-year-old male shows extensive soft tissue with gas bubbles (arrowhead) surrounding the proximal portion of endovascular stent graft, consistent with infection. There is also a large pseudoaneurysm arising at the junction of the graft and native aorta (straight arrow). There is also contrast extravasation from the superior aspect of the stent graft on the left (curved arrow), consistent with a leak. (g) Coronal reconstructed CT image in the same patient shows the pseudoaneurysm (straight arrow), contrast leak (curved arrow), and encasing soft tissue with gas bubbles (arrowhead), consistent with infection.

Shower embolism is more common (4%–17%) following endovascular repair than in open surgery and is a serious, fatal complication [215]. This is likely caused by dispersion of mural thrombus during the procedure.

7.5.1.3.7.2.2 Surgical Grafts CT and MRI are used in the evaluation of complications following surgical graft placement. A leak is seen as extravasation of contrast from the graft, most commonly at an anastomotic site. Stenosis or occlusion of a graft is best seen on either CT or MRI angiography. Thrombus is seen as an intraluminal filling defect. Graft infection occurs in 1.3%–6% of cases and has mortality rate up to 75% [214,216]. The clinical presentation includes fever, tenderness, a pulsatile mass, and draining fistula. In the early postoperative period, graft infection might be difficult to distinguish from postoperative changes. A normal graft has a ring of fat around it and has less than 5 mm of soft tissue attenuation between the aneurysm wall and the graft (Figure 7.36). Perigraft air and fluid are suggestive of infection, but should be correlated with the length of time after surgery. While perigraft air is usually only seen up to 1 week following sugery, it may be seen beyond that and, hence, is not pathognomic of infection until 4–7 weeks after surgery [216]. Perigraft air may also be seen in aortoenteric fistula, particularly at the crossing point of transverse duodenum. Perigraft fluid is also seen normally in the early postoperative period, but is diagnostic of infection when seen beyond 3 months following surgery [216]. Any perigraft fluid present beyond 3 months following surgery should be aspirated and sent for gram stain and culture. Even if negative culture, CT or nuclear medicine scans should be done for 1 year to exclude occult infection [216]. Only rarely, fluid can be seen around a graft for up to 1 year without infection. Most of the patients with negative culture, but positive WBCs from aspirate contain *Staphylococcus epidermidis* [216]. Percutaneous drainage and placement of urokinase into the cavity are treatment options. MRI can distinguish perigraft fluid and inflammatory changes from subacute or chronic hematoma. Pseudoaneurysm may be seen at the anastomotic site and the majority is seen in patients without graft infection. However, pseudoaneurysm develops in 25% of graft infections, often presenting sooner following surgery than noninfectious causes (Figure 7.37) [217].

7.5.1.3.8 Aortic Dissection

Dissection occurs when there is a tear in the tunica intima of the aorta with resultant leak of blood into the tunica media and formation of a false lumen. Hypertension is a common cause of aortic dissection. Other causes include Marfan syndrome, connective tissue disorders, bicuspid aortic valve, Turner's syndrome, coarctation, aneurysm, aortitis, pregnancy, and cocaine use [180]. Dissection is acute when symptoms have lasted less than 2 weeks and chronic if symptoms have been present for longer than 2 weeks. The Stanford classification divides dissection into type A (75% of cases) when it involves the ascending aorta or type B when it does not involve the ascending aorta. Dissection of the abdominal aorta and iliac arteries is usually secondary to caudal extension of

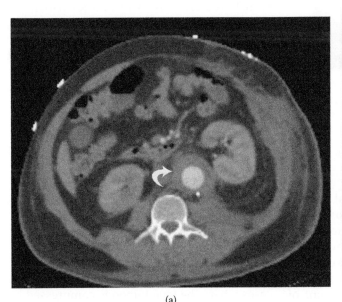
(a)

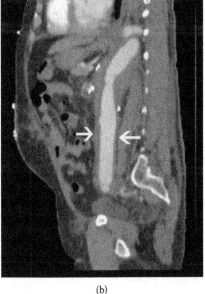
(b)

FIGURE 7.36

Normal appearances of surgical graft. Axial (a) and sagittal reconstructed (b) postcontrast CT images in a 58-year-old female patient, 2 days status postplacement of surgical aortic graft, shows smooth, soft tissue circumferentially encasing the graft (arrow), which is consistent with normal postsurgical appearances.

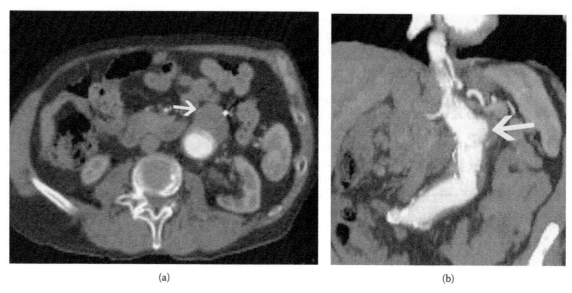

(a)   (b)

FIGURE 7.37
Surgical graft pseudoaneurysm. Axial (a) and coronal reconstructed image (b) of a 75-year-old male shows a focal pseudoaneurysm originating at the anastomosis of the surgical graft with the native abdominal aorta. The pseudoaneurysm is completely thrombosed (arrow).

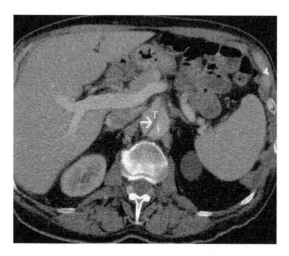

FIGURE 7.38
Aortic dissection. Contrast-enhanced axial CT image in a 54-year-old female patient with history of severe hypertension and acute chest and abdominal pain shows a dissection flap in the abdominal aorta (arrow). The smaller true lumen (T) is seen on the right and the larger false lumen (F) is seen on the left of the flap. The celiac artery (CA) is seen straddling the true and false lumens.

a thoracic aortic dissection. Occasionally, a focal abdominal aortic dissection occurs, either spontaneously or as a sequela of trauma or interventional procedures [218]. Extension to branch vessels may produce renovascular hypertension, mesenteric ischemia, or lower extremity ischemia [219].

On unenhanced CT, there may be displacement of intimal calcification toward the lumen, but no high attenuation is seen. On contrast-enhanced CT and MRI, an intimal flap is seen separating true and false lumens (Figure 7.38). Accurate identification of true and false

lumen is essential for treatment planning. The true lumen has direct continuity with the undissected proximal normal aorta at the thoracic level. The beak sign (wedge of hematoma at the leading edge of false lumen propagation) and larger size are the most useful signs to identify the false lumen [220]. The false lumen can also be identified by the presence of a cobweb sign (low-density linear areas due to residua of incompletely sheared media). Patterns of calcification and intraluminal thrombus are less reliable signs. Occlusion of branch vessels is seen in 27% of patients [221]. This may be due to either extension of the flap within the wall of the branch vessel or dynamic prolapse of the flap across branch-vessel origin [222]. A thrombus within an aneurysm should be distinguished from a dissection. Thrombus has constant circumferential relationship with aorta, irregular border, and intimal calcification deep to the thrombus, unlike a dissection that has a spiroidal configuration, smooth inner border, and intimal calcification superficial to the false lumen [180,221].

Type A dissections require surgical treatment. Uncomplicated type B dissections are treated medically and require serial follow-up CT or MRI. Type B dissections with complications, such as aneurismal enlargement, rupture, and occlusion of true lumen or visceral branches, require endovascular or surgical repair. Endovasular fenestration is performed in cases where the true lumen is compressed by the false lumen. Focal abdominal aortic dissection is usually treated with open surgical repair, although endovascular repair and conservative approaches may also be performed [219].

7.5.1.3.9 Aortic Intramural Hematoma

IMH is characterized by spontaneous hemorrhage in the tunica media of the aorta, typically due to rupture of vasa vasorum and less commonly due to a penetrating atherosclerotic ulcer or trauma that has bled into the aortic wall. Hypertension, atherosclerosis, and old age are the risk factors. Although there is no intimal tear, the media is weakened and, as a result, the clinical presentation and progression is similar to dissection. IMH is classified into Types A and B similar to aortic dissection, with 70% involving the ascending and proximal descending aorta [223]. On unenhanced CT, a crescent of high density is seen in the aortic wall, extending circumferentially in a nonspiroidal fashion that may displace the intimal calcification internally and narrow the lumen. On contrast-enhanced CT, the hematoma does not enhance. Unlike a dissection, IMH does not have an intimal tear and has a constant circumferential relationship with the aortic wall. It can extend along the aorta, rupture, or cause cerebral, mesenteric vascular, or renal insufficiency [224].

Type A IMH require emergent surgical repair, but type B IMH may be managed medically with follow-up imaging, except in the presence of aneurysm, progression, dissection, impending rupture, or end-organ ischemia, when surgery or endovascular stent is performed [225].

7.5.1.3.10 Traumatic Aortic Injury

Traumatic injury is far less common in the abdominal than in the thoracic aorta, accounting for only 4%–6% of aortic injuries. Abdominal aortic injuries account for 0.08%–0.62% of nonpenetrating abdominal traumatic injuries [173]. CT or MRI shows a focal dissection with focal flap, pseudoaneurysm, or rarely complete rupture with contrast extravasation. Traumatic pseudoaneurysm is usually seen following blunt abdominal injury, typically with the use of seat belt. It occurs due to relatively fixed location of abdominal aorta by vertebral column and lumbar vessels. Posttraumatic pseudoaneurysms are usually suprarenal [226]. Fistulous communication may be seen with the IVC or bowel.

7.5.1.3.11 Aortitis

Aortitis is inflammation of the aortic wall and can be either infectious or noninfectious in origin. A list of the several causes is given in Table 7.9 [227]. Infectious causes may be bacterial or viral. Noninfectious causes include large, medium, and small vessel vasculitis, or idiopathic inflammatory aneurysm, or RPF. Clinical presentations include abdominal pain, fever, vascular insufficiency, systemic manifestations, and elevation of acute phase reactants [228].

TABLE 7.9

Causes of Aortitis

Infectious	Bacterial	Salmonella Staphylococcus
	Mycobacterial	Mycobacterium tuberculosis
	Luetic	Syphilis
	Viral	HIV AIDS
Noninfectious	Idiopathic	Idiopathic Inflammatory aortic aneurysm Idiopathic retroperitoneal fibrosis
	Large vessel vasculitis	Takayasu's arteritis Giant cell arteritis Systemic lupus erythematosus Rheumatoid arthritis Ankylosing spondylitis Reiter's syndrome Cogan's syndrome
	Medium and small vessel vasculitis	Polyarteritis nodosa Wegener's granulomatosis Behcet's disease Relapsing polychondritis
	Radiation	

Source: Gornik, H.L., Creager, M.A., *Circulation.*, 117, 3039–51, 2008.

7.5.1.3.11.1 Takayasu's Arteritis Takayasu's arteritis (Martorell's syndrome, pulseless disease) is a chronic, progressive, granulomatous inflammatory and obliterative disease of the large vessels, particularly aorta and its branches. It is more common in women and Asians, particularly in the second and third decades [229]. It is believed to be of autoimmune origin. In the early, prepulseless phase of the disease, systemic signs (fever, malaise, weight loss, and fatigue) are present and are accompanied by elevated acute phase reactants. This is followed by vascular inflammatory phase and late quiescent phase. In the chronic occlusive phase, clinical features of stenosis, occlusion, or aneurysm are seen. The abdominal aorta is the most common segment of the aorta affected [230]. MRI can be used in the evaluation of disease activity. In the active phases of the disease, the vessel wall is thickened on T2-weighted images, and high signal intensity is seen on STIR images due to the presence of edema (Figure 7.39). Contrast enhancement may be seen on both immediate and delayed phases [231]. Occasionally, occlusion and pseudoaneurysm may be seen [230]. In the chronic phase, diffuse narrowing of the aorta and branch vessels is seen. Stenosis is seen in proximal portion of the vessels and occlusion, typically abrupt with flame-shaped termination, and collateral vessels are seen [230]. The aortic wall may be thickened, but there is no high signal edema on the STIR images

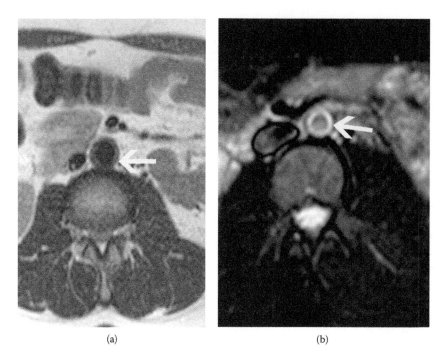

(a)   (b)

FIGURE 7.39
Takayasu's arteritis. (a) Axial T2-weighted MRI image in a 36-year-old female shows circumferential thickening of the juxta-arenal abdominal aorta (arrow). (b) Axial T2-weighted STIR image in the same patient at the same level shows high signal in the vessel wall corresponding to the area of wall thickness in T2-weighted image (arrow). The appearances are consistent with active arteritis, in this case a Takayasu's arteritis.

or contrast enhancement [232]. An aneurysm of the abdominal aorta is seen in 45% of affected patients with rupture seen in 33% of patients. Dissection and pseudoaneurysm may also be seen [230]. Similar changes to those on MRI are seen on CT, with wall thickening and contrast enhancement in the acute phase. Contrast enhancement may produce a double-ring appearance due to an outer ring of inflamed adventitia and media and an inner ring of swollen intima [233]. MRI changes of abnormal wall signal and thickening are seen earlier than that those on CT. The aim of treatment is to control active inflammation and prevent progression to vascular complications. Steroids are used in the acute phase. Vascular complications require surgical or interventional therapy [230].

7.5.1.3.11.2 Giant Cell Arteritis Giant cell arteritis is a large and medium vessel arteritis, secondary to a systemic granulomatous vasculitis that is characterized by infiltration with multinucleated giant cells and lymphocytes along with disruption of the internal elastic lamina in the acute phase and fibrosis in the chronic phase. It is more common above the age of 50 years and is associated with polymyalgia rheumatica. The aorta is involved in 15% of these patients. Involvement of the thoracic aorta, superficial temporal artery, vertebral artery, and coronary arteries is also seen. Imaging findings in the abdominal aorta are similar to those of Takayasu's arteritis [227].

7.5.1.3.11.3 Idiopathic Inflammatory Aortic Aneurysm Idiopathic inflammatory aortic aneurysm accounts for 5%–25% of abdominal aortic aneurysms [227]. Idiopathic inflammation of the aortic wall results in wall thickening and significant perianeurysmal fibrosis with adhesions to surrounding structures distinguishing it from an atherosclerotic aneurysm. It is more common in men [234]. Due to the presence of inflammation, inflammatory aneurysms are more often symptomatic than atherosclerotic aneurysms. Clinical features include abdominal pain, fever, weight loss, leukocytosis, and elevated erythrocyte sedimentation rate. CT scan shows the aneurysm, which typically has low attenuation periaortic wall thickening, affecting the anterior wall with sparing of the posterior wall. Delayed contrast enhancement of the periaortic soft tissue mass is seen. The inflammation can extend to adjacent organs such as ureter resulting in hydronephrosis or bowel resulting in a fistula and bleeding. CT can be used to delineate the craniocaudal extent and extent of adhesions to adjacent tissues, which is essential to avoid injury to adjacent organs and also for determining the operative approach, either transperitoneal or retroperitoneal [235]. MRI shows aneurysm with periaortic inflammatory wall thickening, adventitial fibrosis, and turbulent intraluminal flow (Figure 7.40). In 20%–30% of patients, hydronephrosis is seen due to ureteral involvement [236]. The risk of rupture is higher than atherosclerotic aneurysm, regardless of its size [236].

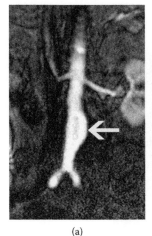 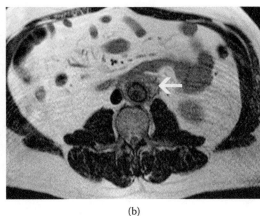 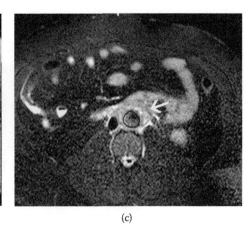

(a)   (b)   (c)

FIGURE 7.40
Inflammatory aneurysm. (a) Coronal MIP image from MRI angiography in a 55-year-old male patient shows a focal saccular aneurysm (arrow) in the infrarenal abdominal aorta. (b) Axial T2-weighted MRI image shows periaortic wall thickening (arrow), which is more prominent along the anterior than the posterior wall. (c) Axial T2-weighted STIR image at the same level shows high signal of the aortic wall thickening (arrow), consistent with an inflammatory aortic aneurysm.

Treatment is with endovascular repair or surgery, which is associated with higher mortality than for atherosclerotic aneurysm [227]. Endovascular repair has been used with success in small series and has been associated with decreased perianeurysmal soft tissue in addition to sac shrinkage [237].

7.5.1.3.11.4 Infectious Aortitis Infectious aortitis may occur in a diseased aortic wall, such as in atherosclerosis or aneurysm, or following surgery or medical device placement. Infection can be pyogenic, syphilitic, mycobacterial, or secondary to HIV. Infection spreads either through a hematogeneous route or from contiguous spread from adjacent infection or it may be directly introduced. CT shows thickening of the aortic wall with fluid and soft tissue surrounding the aorta. Occasionally, gas may be seen in the aortic wall. Complications include development of saccular aneursym or pseudoaneurysm, aneurysm rupture, dissection, and aortoenteric fistula. Treatment includes antibiotics and surgical removal. Tuberculous aneurysm is more common in HIV patients and may be associated with vertebral tuberculosis [227].

7.5.1.3.11.5 Mycotic (Infected) Aneurysm A mycotic aneurysm is an aneurysm of infectious etiology. It is a sequela of infectious aortitis that results in weakening and disruption of the aortic wall and results in a saccular aneurysm or pseudoaneurysm. Infected aneurysms account for 0.06%–2.6% of all aneurysms. Risk factors include underlying aortic disorders (atherosclerosis), immuno-compromised status, intravenous drug use, bacterial endocarditis, sepsis, and surgery or medical devices placement [228]. It is most commonly

seen in the infrarenal aorta. Clinical features include fever, leukocytosis, and features of shock in late stages. *Staphylococcus* is the most common organism isolated from infected aneurysms.

CT and MRI show a saccular aneurysm of variable size (1–11 cm) (Figure 7.41a and b) [228]. Findings suggestive of infection are the presence of perianeurysmal fluid, soft tissue stranding, and gas with an eccentric aortic aneurysm with lobular contours. Before the development of this stage, a circumferential periaortic hypodense soft tissue mass with or without rim enhancement may be seen [238]. Rapid change in the size or shape of aneurysm over a short period should raise suspicion of mycotic aneurysm [184,238]. Vertebral body destruction (Figure 7.41c and d), psoas abscess, and renal abscess may be seen. Complications of infected aneurysm include rupture, hemorrhage, sepsis, and death. Management depends on the extent of the aneurysm and associated clinical features. Prolonged systemic antibiotics may be administered in less extensive aneurysms. In extensive disease, surgical resection with debridement and abscess drainage may be necessary [228].

7.5.1.3.12 Aortic Tumors
Primary tumors of the aorta are rare, with majority of them being malignant [239]. Sarcoma is the most common primary malignant tumor of the aorta. Myxoma has also been reported in the abdominal aorta [239]. Primary tumors can originate either from the intima, which frequently result in thromboembolism, or from the media and adventitia, which form aggressive masses with intraluminal and extraluminal extension [239]. On CT and MRI, malignant aortic tumor mimics a mural

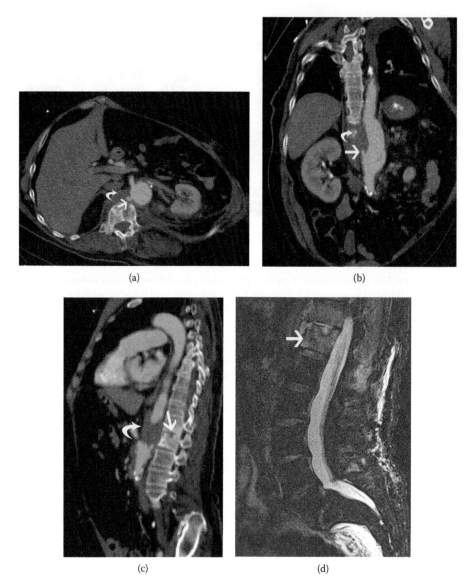

(a)

(b)

(c)

(d)

FIGURE 7.41
Mycotic aneurysm. (a) Axial and (b) coronal postcontrast CT images in a 50-year-old male presenting with abdominal pain, fever, and leukocytosis shows a saccular pseudoaneurysm (straight arrow) of the suprarenal portion of the abdominal aorta. There is a rim of soft tissue in the posterior aspect (curved arrow). (c) Sagittal CT image in the same patient shows irregular destruction of the anterior vertebral body of T12 (straight arrow), adjacent to the soft tissue (curved arrow) posterior to the pseudoaneurysm, consistent with spondylodiskitis. (d) Sagittal STIR image of the spine in the same patient shows high signal in T11 and T12 vertebral bodies (arrow) and intervertebral disk, consistent with diskitis.

thrombus. However, the presence of heterogeneity and protrusive vegetations and lack of atherosclerosis help in distinguishing a tumor from thrombus [240].

diaphragm at the level of T8 and then drains into the right atrium. Tributaries of IVC include hepatic, inferior phrenic, right gonadal, right and left renal, and suprarenal and lumbar veins. It anastomoses with the azygos vein, either directly or through the renal veins and vertebral venous plexus.

7.6 Inferior Vena Cava

7.6.1 Imaging Anatomy of the IVC

The IVC is formed by the union of the right and left common iliac veins. It courses in the retroperitoneum to the right of abdominal aorta and passes through the

7.6.2 CT and MRI of the IVC

IVC abnormalities are often discovered incidentally in scans performed for other clinical indications. If imaging is specifically performed for evaluation of the IVC, CT images are typically acquired in multiple phases following intravenous contrast administration—the portal venous phase (60–70 seconds delay) for evaluating a filling defect and arterial phase (20–30 seconds) for tumor thrombus enhancement and pre-op planning. Although the suprarenal and renal segments of IVC are visualized well in the portal venous phase, infrarenal segment may not be visualized due to admixture of noncontrast opacified blood from lower extremities. A further delayed scan (70–90 seconds) may visualize the entire IVC, but involves additional radiation [241]. MRI evaluation of the IVC can be performed using SSFP images or following contrast administration using T1-weighted spoiled gradient echo images in multiple phases.

7.6.3 Pathologic Conditions

7.6.3.1 Congenital Anamolies

Congenital anomalies of the IVC are caused by abnormal persistence of various embryonic veins. The IVC develops between the 6th and 8th weeks of gestation by the sequential union of posterior cardinal, subcardinal, and supracardinal veins. Congenital anomalies of the IVC are usually asymptomatic and are incidentally discovered during imaging studies [242].

A left-sided IVC is formed by the union of left and right common iliac veins. It extends up to the level of the left renal vein, where it passes anterior to the aorta to join normal right-sided IVC. Left-sided IVC is formed due to persistence of left supracardinal vein and regression of right supracardinal vein. It is seen in 0.2%–0.5% of the population [243]. Although a left-sided IVC does not have major clinical significance, it may pose a technical challenge in placing an infrarenal IVC filter through transjugular approach or complicate aneurym repair [244]. Double IVC is characterized by presence of both the right and left IVC below the level of the renal veins. The left IVC then drains into the left renal vein, which then drains into the right IVC. Double IVC is caused by persistence of both the right and left supracardinal veins. It is seen in 1%–3% of the population [243]. Although this anomaly also does not have a major clinical significance, undiagnosed double IVC should be considered in patients with recurrent pulmonary embolism despite IVC filter placement [244].

Interruption of IVC with azygos or hemiazygos continuation is characterized by a normal infrarenal IVC, but absent suprarenal IVC with continuation of the infrarenal IVC as an enlarged azygos vein (left IVC) or hemiazygos vein (right IVC). This is caused by absent development of right subcardinal-hepatic anastomosis and may be associated with situs abnormalities. Knowledge of the anatomy is essential before cardiac catheterization or cardiopulmonary bypass procedures [245]. Absent infrarenal IVC is likely secondary to intrauterine or periuterine IVC thrombosis [246]. In this anomaly, the lower leg veins drain through ascending lumbar veins to the azygos–hemiazygos system. These patients are prone to thrombosis and venous insufficiency [244].

In the retroaortic left renal vein, the left renal vein passes behind the aorta instead of taking the normal anterior course. This is caused by origin of left renal vein from intersupracardinal vein instead of intersubcardinal veins [243]. It is seen in 1.7%–3.4% of population [244]. In a circumaortic left renal vein, the left renal vein courses both anterior and posterior to the aorta. This is caused by origin of left renal vein from both the intersupracardinal and intersubcardinal veins and is seen in 2.4%–8.7% of population [242]. The posterior vein may be compressed by the aorta, resulting in "nutcracker phenomenon" of hypertension, hematuria, and varices [247]. Knowledge of these left renal vein anomalies is essential in planning for nephrectomy. Retrocaval ureter is characterized by location of the right ureter posterior and medial to the IVC due to development of infrarenal IVC from the right posterior cardinal vein instead of the right supracardinal vein [243]. Hydronephrosis or urinary tract infections can be caused by compression of the ureter by the IVC [248]. The abnormal course of the ureter and IVC is demonstrated on CT. Coronal images show the ureter coursing posterior and medial to the IVC, with associated hydronephrosis, producing a "fish-hook" or "reverse J" appearance [244].

7.6.3.2 IVC Thrombus and Tumors

Bland (nonmalignant) thrombus is typically seen in the IVC from extension of thrombus in the lower limb or pelvic veins. Acute thrombus expands the IVC and is seen as an intermediate attenuation filling defect within the IVC lumen that does not show contrast enhancement. Chronic thrombus does not expand the IVC.

Tumors of the IVC are more often secondary than primary. Leiomyosarcoma is the most common primary malignant tumor of the IVC (discussed in Section 7.4.1.1.2). Malignant tumors that extend into the IVC include the renal cell carcinoma, hepatocellular carcinoma, and adrenocortical carcinoma. The extent of tumor thrombus on imaging impacts the surgical approach in renal cell cancer. Benign tumors extending into the IVC include pheochromocytoma, angiomyolipoma, and intravenous leiomyomatosis [244]. Leiomyomatosis represents venous invasion of uterine fibroid in young females, seen either with a uterine fibroid or following hysterectomy.

7.7 Conclusion

In the past, the retroperitoneum has been described as a "hinterland of straggling mesenchyme, with vascular and nervous plexuses, weird embryonic rests and shadowy fascial boundarie" [20]. To date, the prospective diagnosis of a retroperitoneal pathology poses a profound clinical challenge due to the nonspecific nature of its consequent symptoms. On the contrary, cross-sectional imaging techniques have significantly contributed to our understanding of retroperitoneal anatomy and the broad spectrum of pathologies that occur. Although a precise imaging diagnosis may not be possible in every patient, the identification and accurate interpretation of a lesion's imaging characteristics can guide a reasonable line of subsequent management.

References

1. Korobkin M, Silverman PM, Quint LE et al. CT of the extraperitoneal space: normal anatomy and fluid collections. *AJR Am J Roentgenol* 1992;159(5):933–42.
2. Dodds WJ, Darweesh RM, Lawson TL et al. The retroperitoneal spaces revisited. *AJR Am J Roentgenol* 1986;147(6):1155–61.
3. Lee SL, Ku YM, Rha SE. Comprehensive reviews of the interfascial plane of the retroperitoneum: normal anatomy and pathologic entities. *Emerg Radiol* 2010;17(1):3–11.
4. Gore RM, Balfe DM, Aizenstein RI et al. The great escape: interfascial decompression planes of the retroperitoneum. *AJR Am J Roentgenol* 2000;175(2):363–70.
5. Parienty RA, Pradel J. Radiological evaluation of the peri- and pararenal spaces by computed tomography. *Crit Rev Diagn Imaging* 1983;20(1):1–26.
6. Parienty RA, Pradel J, Picard JD et al. Visibility and thickening of the renal fascia on computed tomograms. *Radiology* 1981;139(1):119–24.
7. Cyran KM, Kenney PJ. Leiomyosarcoma of abdominal veins: value of MRI with gadolinium DTPA. *Abdom Imaging* 1994;19(4):335–8.
8. Elsayes KM, Staveteig PT, Narra VR et al. Retroperitoneal masses: magnetic resonance imaging findings with pathologic correlation. *Curr Probl Diagn Radiol* 2007;36(3):97–106.
9. Low RN, Semelka RC, Worawattanakul S et al. Extrahepatic abdominal imaging in patients with malignancy: comparison of MRI imaging and helical CT in 164 patients. *J Magn Reson Imaging* 2000;12(2):269–77.
10. Low RN, Semelka RC, Worawattanakul S et al. Extrahepatic abdominal imaging in patients with malignancy: comparison of MRI imaging and helical CT, with subsequent surgical correlation. *Radiology* 1999;210(3):625–32.
11. Low RN, Sigeti JS. MRI imaging of peritoneal disease: comparison of contrast-enhanced fast multiplanar spoiled gradient-recalled and spin-echo imaging. *AJR Am J Roentgenol* 1994;163(5):1131–40.
12. Vazquez A, Liu J, Zhou Y et al. Catabolic efficiency of aerobic glycolysis: the Warburg effect revisited. *BMC Syst Biol* 2010;4:58.
13. Nishino M, Hayakawa K, Minami M et al. Primary retroperitoneal neoplasms: CT and MRI imaging findings with anatomic and pathologic diagnostic clues. *Radiographics* 2003;23(1):45–57.
14. Sanyal R, Remer EM. Radiology of the retroperitoneum: case-based review. *AJR Am J Roentgenol* 2009;192(6):S112–7; Quiz S118–21.
15. Jemal A, Siegel R, Ward E et al. Cancer statistics, 2006. *CA Cancer J Clin* 2006;56(2):106–30.
16. Shibata D, Lewis JJ, Leung DH et al. Is there a role for incomplete resection in the management of retroperitoneal liposarcomas? *J Am Coll Surg* 2001;193(4):373–9.
17. Herman K, Kusy T. Retroperitoneal sarcoma—the continued challenge for surgery and oncology. *Surg Oncol* 1998;7(1–2):77–81.
18. Lewis JJ, Leung D, Woodruff JM et al. Retroperitoneal soft-tissue sarcoma: analysis of 500 patients treated and followed at a single institution. *Ann Surg* 1998;228(3):355–65.
19. Rajiah P, Sinha R, Cuevas C et al. Imaging of uncommon retroperitoneal masses. *Radiographics* 2011;31(4):949–76.
20. Torigian DA, Ramchandani P. In: Haaga JR, Dogra VS, Forsting M et al., editors. The retroperitoneum. In *CT and MRI of the Whole Body*. Philadelphia, PA: Mosby Elsevier; 2009. pp. 1953–2040.
21. Gustafson P, Herrlin K, Biling L et al. Necrosis observed on CT enhancement is of prognostic value in soft tissue sarcoma. *Acta Radiol* 1992;33(5):474–6.
22. Brenner W, Eary JF, Hwang W et al. Risk assessment in liposarcoma patients based on FDG PET imaging. *Eur J Nucl Med Mol Imaging* 2006;33(11):1290–5.
23. Makela J, Kiviniemi H, Laitinen S. Prognostic factors predicting survival in the treatment of retroperitoneal sarcoma. *Eur J Surg Oncol* 2000;26(6):552–5.
24. Pirayesh A, Chee Y, Helliwell TR et al. The management of retroperitoneal soft tissue sarcoma: a single institution experience with a review of the literature. *Eur J Surg Oncol* 2001;27(5):491–7.
25. Swallow CJ, Catton CN. Local management of adult soft tissue sarcomas. *Semin Oncol* 2007;34(3):256–69.
26. Cormier JN, Pollock RE. Soft tissue sarcomas. *CA Cancer J Clin* 2004;54(2):94–109.
27. Sung MS, Kang HS, Suh JS et al. Myxoid liposarcoma: appearance at MRI imaging with histologic correlation. *Radiographics* 2000;20(4):1007–19.
28. Engelken JD, Ros PR. Retroperitoneal MRI imaging. *Magn Reson Imaging Clin N Am* 1997;5(1):165–78.
29. Lane RH, Stephens DH, Reiman HM. Primary retroperitoneal neoplasms: CT findings in 90 cases with clinical and pathologic correlation. *AJR Am J Roentgenol* 1989;152(1):83–9.
30. Arkun R, Memis A, Akalin T et al. Liposarcoma of soft tissue: MRI findings with pathologic correlation. *Skeletal Radiol* 1997;26(3):167–72.

31. Neville A, Herts BR. CT characteristics of primary retroperitoneal neoplasms. *Crit Rev Comput Tomogr* 2004;45(4):247–70.

32. Israel GM, Bosniak MA, Slywotzky CM et al. CT differentiation of large exophytic renal angiomyolipomas and perirenal liposarcomas. *AJR Am J Roentgenol* 2002;179(3):769–73.

33. Jelinek JS, Kransdorf MJ, Shmookler BM et al. Liposarcoma of the extremities: MRI and CT findings in the histologic subtypes. *Radiology* 1993;186(2):455–9.

34. Kim T, Murakami T, Oi H et al. CT and MRI imaging of abdominal liposarcoma. *AJR Am J Roentgenol* 1996;166(4):829–33.

35. Hartman DS, Hayes WS, Choyke PL et al. From the archives of the AFIP. Leiomyosarcoma of the retroperitoneum and inferior vena cava: radiologic-pathologic correlation. *Radiographics* 1992;12(6):1203–20.

36. Deshmukh H, Prasad SR, Patankar T et al. Internal mammary artery pseudoaneurysms complicating chest wall infection in children: diagnosis and endovascular therapy. *Clin Imaging* 2001;25(6):396–9.

37. Kieffer E, Alaoui M, Piette JC et al. Leiomyosarcoma of the inferior vena cava: experience in 22 cases. *Ann Surg* 2006;244(2):289–95.

38. McLeod AJ, Zornoza J, Shirkhoda A. Leiomyosarcoma: computed tomographic findings. *Radiology* 1984;152(1):133–6.

39. La Fianza A, Alberici E, Meloni G et al. Extraperitoneal pelvic leiomyosarcoma. MRI findings in a case. *Clin Imaging* 2000;24(4):224–6.

40. Kransdorf MJ. Malignant soft-tissue tumors in a large referral population: distribution of diagnoses by age, sex, and location. *AJR Am J Roentgenol* 1995;164(1):129–34.

41. Nishimura H, Zhang Y, Ohkuma K et al. MRI imaging of soft-tissue masses of the extraperitoneal spaces. *Radiographics* 2001;21(5):1141–54.

42. Ko SF, Wan YL, Lee TY et al. CT features of calcifications in abdominal malignant fibrous histiocytoma. *Clin Imaging* 1998;22(6):408–13.

43. Prasad SR, Sahani DV, Mino-Kenudson M et al. Neoplasms of the perivascular epithelioid cell involving the abdomen and the pelvis: cross-sectional imaging findings. *J Comput Assist Tomogr* 2007;31(5):688–96.

44. Rajiah P, Sinha R, Cuevas C et al. Imaging of uncommon retroperitoneal masses. *Radiographics* 2011;31(4):949–76.

45. Castellazzi G, Vanel D, Le Cesne A et al. Can the MRI signal of aggressive fibromatosis be used to predict its behavior? *Eur J Radiol* 2009;69(2):222–9.

46. Kreuzberg B, Koudelova J, Ferda J et al. Diagnostic problems of abdominal desmoid tumors in various locations. *Eur J Radiol* 2007;62(2):180–5.

47. Einstein DM, Tagliabue JR, Desai RK. Abdominal desmoids: CT findings in 25 patients. *AJR Am J Roentgenol* 1991;157(2):275–9.

48. Dinauer PA, Brixey CJ, Moncur JT et al. Pathologic and MRI imaging features of benign fibrous soft-tissue tumors in adults. *Radiographics* 2007;27(1):173–87.

49. Choyke PL, Hayes WS, Sesterhenn IA. Primary extragonadal germ cell tumors of the retroperitoneum: differentiation of primary and secondary tumors. *Radiographics* 1993;13(6):1365–75; Quiz 1377–8.

50. Ueno T, Tanaka YO, Nagata M et al. Spectrum of germ cell tumors: from head to toe. *Radiographics* 2004;24(2):387–404.

51. Comiter CV, Renshaw AA, Benson CB et al. Burned-out primary testicular cancer: sonographic and pathological characteristics. *J Urol* 1996;156(1):85–8.

52. Hayashi T, Mine M, Kojima S et al. Extragonadal germ cell tumor followed by metachronous testicular tumor. A case report. *Urol Int* 1996;57(3):194–6.

53. Gutierrez Delgado F, Tjulandin SA, Garin AM. Long term results of treatment in patients with extragonadal germ cell tumours. *Eur J Cancer* 1993;29A(7):1002–5.

54. Bokemeyer C, Droz JP, Horwich A et al. Extragonadal seminoma: an international multicenter analysis of prognostic factors and long term treatment outcome. *Cancer* 2001;91(7):1394–401.

55. Logothetis CJ, Samuels ML, Trindade A et al. The growing teratoma syndrome. *Cancer* 1982;50(8):1629–35.

56. Andre F, Fizazi K, Culine S et al. The growing teratoma syndrome: results of therapy and long-term follow-up of 33 patients. *Eur J Cancer* 2000;36(11):1389–94.

57. Jeffery GM, Theaker JM, Lee AH et al. The growing teratoma syndrome. *Br J Urol* 1991;67(2):195–202.

58. Spiess PE, Kassouf W, Brown GA et al. Surgical management of growing teratoma syndrome: the M.D. Anderson cancer center experience. *J Urol* 2007;177(4):1330–4; discussion 1334.

59. Wang RM, Chen CA. Primary retroperitoneal teratoma. *Acta Obstet Gynecol Scand* 2000;79(8):707–8.

60. Panageas E. General diagnosis case of the day. Primary retroperitoneal teratoma. *AJR Am J Roentgenol* 1991;156(6):1292–4.

61. Engel RM, Elkins RC, Fletcher BD. Retroperitoneal teratoma. Review of the literature and presentation of an unusual case. *Cancer* 1968;22(5):1068–73.

62. Davidson AJ, Hartman DS, Goldman SM. Mature teratoma of the retroperitoneum: radiologic, pathologic, and clinical correlation. *Radiology* 1989;172(2):421–5.

63. Engel IA, Auh YH, Rubenstein WA et al. Large posterior abdominal masses: computed tomographic localization. *Radiology* 1983;149(1):203–9.

64. Kurosaki Y, Tanaka YO, Itai Y. Well-differentiated liposarcoma of the retroperitoneum with a fat-fluid level: US, CT, and MRI appearance. *Eur Radiol* 1998;8(3):474–5.

65. Ferrero A, Cespedes M, Cantarero JM et al. Peritonitis due to rupture of retroperitoneal teratoma: computed tomography diagnosis. *Gastrointest Radiol* 1990;15(3):251–2.

66. Gatcombe HG, Assikis V, Kooby D et al. Primary retroperitoneal teratomas: a review of the literature. *J Surg Oncol* 2004;86(2):107–13.

67. Yang DM, Jung DH, Kim H et al. Retroperitoneal cystic masses: CT, clinical, and pathologic findings and literature review. *Radiographics* 2004;24(5):1353–65.

68. Hayasaka K, Tanaka Y, Soeda S et al. MRI findings in primary retroperitoneal schwannoma. *Acta Radiol* 1999;40(1):78–82.

69. Li Q, Gao C, Juzi JT et al. Analysis of 82 cases of retroperitoneal schwannoma. *ANZ J Surg* 2007;77(4):237–40.

70. Rha SE, Byun JY, Jung SE et al. Neurogenic tumors in the abdomen: tumor types and imaging characteristics. *Radiographics* 2003;23(1):29–43.

71. Takatera H, Takiuchi H, Namiki M et al. Retroperitoneal schwannoma. *Urology* 1986;28(6):529–31.

72. Loke TK, Yuen NW, Lo KK et al. Retroperitoneal ancient schwannoma: review of clinico-radiological features. *Australas Radiol* 1998;42(2):136–8.

73. Lin J, Martel W. Cross-sectional imaging of peripheral nerve sheath tumors: characteristic signs on CT, MRI imaging, and sonography. *AJR Am J Roentgenol* 2001;176(1):75–82.

74. Hughes MJ, Thomas JM, Fisher C et al. Imaging features of retroperitoneal and pelvic schwannomas. *Clin Radiol* 2005;60(8):886–93.

75. Bass JC, Korobkin M, Francis IR et al. Retroperitoneal plexiform neurofibromas: CT findings. *AJR Am J Roentgenol* 1994;163(3):617–20.

76. Rha SE, Byun JY, Jung SE et al. Neurogenic tumors in the abdomen: tumor types and imaging characteristics. *Radiographics* 2003;23(1):29–43.

77. Woodruff JM. Pathology of tumors of the peripheral nerve sheath in type 1 neurofibromatosis. *Am J Med Genet* 1999;89(1):23–30.

78. Leroy K, Dumas V, Martin-Garcia N et al. Malignant peripheral nerve sheath tumors associated with neurofibromatosis type 1: a clinicopathologic and molecular study of 17 patients. *Arch Dermatol* 2001;137(7):908–13.

79. Hrehorovich PA, Franke HR, Maximin S et al. Malignant peripheral nerve sheath tumor. *Radiographics* 2003;23(3):790–4.

80. Korf BR. Malignancy in neurofibromatosis type 1. *Oncologist* 2000;5(6):477–85.

81. Otsuka H, Graham MM, Kubo A et al. FDG-PET/CT findings of sarcomatous transformation in neurofibromatosis: a case report. *Ann Nucl Med* 2005;19(1):55–8.

82. Singh KJ, Suri A, Vijjan V et al. Retroperitoneal ganglioneuroma presenting as right renal mass. *Urology* 2006;67(5):1085. e7, e8.

83. Otal P, Mezghani S, Hassissene S et al. Imaging of retroperitoneal ganglioneuroma. *Eur Radiol* 2001;11(6):940–5.

84. Lonergan GJ, Schwab CM, Suarez ES et al. Neuroblastoma, ganglioneuroblastoma, and ganglioneuroma: radiologic-pathologic correlation. *Radiographics* 2002;22(4):911–34.

85. Miyake M, Tateishi U, Maeda T et al. A case of ganglioneuroma presenting abnormal FDG uptake. *Ann Nucl Med* 2006;20(5):357–60.

86. Remer EM, Miller FH. In: Blake MA, Boland GW, editors. Imaging of pheochromocytomas. In *Adrenal Imaging*. Totowa, NJ: Humana Press; 2009. pp. 109–27.

87. Pommier RF, Vetto JT, Billingsly K et al. Comparison of adrenal and extraadrenal pheochromocytomas. *Surgery* 1993;114(6):1160–5; discussion 1165–6.

88. Goldstein DS, Eisenhofer G, Flynn JA et al. Diagnosis and localization of pheochromocytoma. *Hypertension* 2004;43(5):907–10.

89. Hayes WS, Davidson AJ, Grimley PM et al. Extraadrenal retroperitoneal paraganglioma: clinical, pathologic, and CT findings. *AJR Am J Roentgenol* 1990;155(6):1247–50.

90. Lee KY, Oh YW, Noh HJ et al. Extraadrenal paragangliomas of the body: imaging features. *AJR Am J Roentgenol* 2006;187(2):492–504.

91. Bessell-Browne R, O'Malley ME. CT of pheochromocytoma and paraganglioma: risk of adverse events with i.v. administration of nonionic contrast material. *AJR Am J Roentgenol* 2007;188(4):970–4.

92. Shapiro B, Gross MD, Shulkin B. Radioisotope diagnosis and therapy of malignant pheochromocytoma. *Trends Endocrinol Metab* 2001;12(10):469–75.

93. Lumachi F, Tregnaghi A, Zucchetta P et al. Sensitivity and positive predictive value of CT, MRI and 123I-MIBG scintigraphy in localizing pheochromocytomas: a prospective study. *Nucl Med Commun* 2006;27(7):583–7.

94. Brink I, Hoegerle S, Klisch J et al. Imaging of pheochromocytoma and paraganglioma. *Fam Cancer* 2005;4(1):61–8.

95. Plouin PF, Gimenez-Roqueplo AP. Pheochromocytomas and secreting paragangliomas. *Orphanet J Rare Dis* 2006;1:49.

96. Rufini V, Calcagni ML, Baum RP. Imaging of neuroendocrine tumors. *Semin Nucl Med* 2006;36(3):228–47.

97. Shapiro B, Sisson JC, Shulkin BL et al. The current status of meta-iodobenzylguanidine and related agents for the diagnosis of neuro-endocrine tumors. *Q J Nucl Med* 1995;39(4 Suppl 1):3–8.

98. Hruby G, Lehman M, Barton M et al. Malignant retroperitoneal paraganglioma: case report and review of treatment options. *Australas Radiol* 2000;44(4):478–82.

99. Barker CD, Brown JJ. MRI imaging of the retroperitoneum. *Top Magn Reson Imaging* 1995;7(2):102–11.

100. Balfe DM, Mauro MA, Koehler RE et al. Gastrohepatic ligament: normal and pathologic CT anatomy. *Radiology* 1984;150(2):485–90.

101. Dorfman RE, Alpern MB, Gross BH et al. Upper abdominal lymph nodes: criteria for normal size determined with CT. *Radiology* 1991;180(2):319–22.

102. Einstein DM, Singer AA, Chilcote WA et al. Abdominal lymphadenopathy: spectrum of CT findings. *Radiographics* 1991;11(3):457–72.

103. Coakley FV, Hricak H. Imaging of peritoneal and mesenteric disease: key concepts for the clinical radiologist. *Clin Radiol* 1999;54(9):563–74.

104. Healy JC, Reznek RH. The peritoneum, mesenteries and omenta: normal anatomy and pathological processes. *Eur Radiol* 1998;8(6):886–900.

105. Blackledge G, Best JJ, Crowther D et al. Computed tomography (CT) in the staging of patients with Hodgkin's Disease: a report on 136 patients. *Clin Radiol* 1980;31(2):143–7.

106. Neumann CH, Robert NJ, Canellos G et al. Computed tomography of the abdomen and pelvis in non-Hodgkin lymphoma. *J Comput Assist Tomogr* 1983;7(5):846–50.

107. Rahmouni A, Tempany C, Jones R et al. Lymphoma: monitoring tumor size and signal intensity with MRI imaging. *Radiology* 1993;188(2):445–51.

108. Elstrom R, Guan L, Baker G et al. Utility of FDG-PET scanning in lymphoma by WHO classification. *Blood* 2003;101(10):3875–6.

109. Schiepers C, Filmont JE, Czernin J. PET for staging of Hodgkin's disease and non-Hodgkin's lymphoma. *Eur J Nucl Med Mol Imaging* 2003;30(Suppl 1):S82–8.

110. Kidd EA, Siegel BA, Dehdashti F et al. The standardized uptake value for F-18 fluorodeoxyglucose is a sensitive predictive biomarker for cervical cancer treatment response and survival. *Cancer* 2007;110(8):1738–44.

111. Vaglio A, Salvarani C, Buzio C. Retroperitoneal fibrosis. *Lancet* 2006;367(9506):241–51.

112. Amis ES Jr. Retroperitoneal fibrosis. *AJR Am J Roentgenol* 1991;157(2):321–9.

113. Gilkeson GS, Allen NB. Retroperitoneal fibrosis. A true connective tissue disease. *Rheum Dis Clin North Am* 1996;22(1):23–38.

114. Kottra JJ, Dunnick NR. Retroperitoneal fibrosis. *Radiol Clin North Am* 1996;34(6):1259–75.

115. Oguz KK, Kiratli H, Oguz O et al. Multifocal fibrosclerosis: a new case report and review of the literature. *Eur Radiol* 2002;12(5):1134–8.

116. Geoghegan T, Byrne AT, Benfayed W et al. Imaging and intervention of retroperitoneal fibrosis. *Australas Radiol* 2007;51(1):26–34.

117. Arrive L, Hricak H, Tavares NJ et al. Malignant versus nonmalignant retroperitoneal fibrosis: differentiation with MRI imaging. *Radiology* 1989;172(1):139–43.

118. Torigian DA, Ramchandani P. In: Haaga JR, Dogra VS, Forstring M et al., editors. The retroperitoneum. In *CT and MRI of the Whole Body*. New York, NY: Mosby Elsevier; 2000. pp. 484–90.

119. Geoghegan T, Byrne AT, Benfayed W et al. Imaging and intervention of retroperitoneal fibrosis. *Australas Radiol* 2007;51(1):26–34.

120. Vaglio A, Greco P, Versari A et al. Post-treatment residual tissue in idiopathic retroperitoneal fibrosis: active residual disease or silent "scar"? A study using 18F-fluorodeoxyglucose positron emission tomography. *Clin Exp Rheumatol* 2005;23(2):231–4.

121. Vivas I, Nicolas AI, Velazquez P et al. Retroperitoneal fibrosis: typical and atypical manifestations. *Br J Radiol* 2000;73(866):214–22.

122. Alexander ES, Colley DP, Clark RA. Computed tomography of retroperitoneal fluid collections. *Semin Roentgenol* 1981;16(4):268–76.

123. Danaci M, Kesici GE, Kesici H et al. Coumadin-induced renal and retroperitoneal hemorrhage. *Ren Fail* 2006;28(2):129–32.

124. Ishikawa K, Tohira H, Mizushima Y et al. Traumatic retroperitoneal hematoma spreads through the interfascial planes. *J Trauma* 2005;59(3):595–607; discussion 607–8.

125. Orwig D, Federle MP. Localized clotted blood as evidence of visceral trauma on CT: the sentinel clot sign. *AJR Am J Roentgenol* 1989;153(4):747–9.

126. Hahn PF, Saini S, Stark DD et al. Intraabdominal hematoma: the concentric-ring sign in MRI imaging. *AJR Am J Roentgenol* 1987;148(1):115–9.

127. Federle MP, Jeffrey RB Jr. Hemoperitoneum studied by computed tomography. *Radiology* 1983;148(1):187–92.

128. Federle MP, Pan KT, Pealer KM. CT criteria for differentiating abdominal hemorrhage: anticoagulation or aortic aneurysm rupture? *AJR Am J Roentgenol* 2007;188(5):1324–30.

129. Shanmuganathan K, Mirvis SE, Sover ER. Value of contrast-enhanced CT in detecting active hemorrhage in patients with blunt abdominal or pelvic trauma. *AJR Am J Roentgenol* 1993;161(1):65–9.

130. Braun WE, Banowsky LH, Straffon RA et al. Lymphoceles associated with renal transplantation: report of fifteen cases and review of the literature. *Proc Clin Dial Transplant Forum* 1973;3:185–9.

131. Petru E, Tamussino K, Lahousen M et al. Pelvic and paraaortic lymphocysts after radical surgery because of cervical and ovarian cancer. *Am J Obstet Gynecol* 1989;161(4):937–41.

132. Schweizer RT, Cho S, Koutz KOUNTZ SL et al. Lymphoceles following renal transplantation. *Arch Surg* 1972;104(1):42–5.

133. vanSonnenberg E, Wittich GR, Casola G et al. Lymphoceles: imaging characteristics and percutaneous management. *Radiology* 1986;161(3):593–6.

134. Zuckerman DA, Yeager TD. Percutaneous ethanol sclerotherapy of postoperative lymphoceles. *AJR Am J Roentgenol* 1997;169(2):433–7.

135. Titton RL, Gervais DA, Hahn PF et al. Urine leaks and urinomas: diagnosis and imaging-guided intervention. *Radiographics* 2003;23(5):1133–47.

136. Capitan Manjon C, Tejido Sanchez A, Piedra Lara JD et al. Retroperitoneal abscesses—analysis of a series of 66 cases. *Scand J Urol Nephrol* 2003;37(2):139–44.

137. Ishigami K, Khanna G, Samuel I et al. Gas-forming abdominal wall abscess: unusual manifestation of perforated retroperitoneal appendicitis extending through the superior lumbar triangle. *Emerg Radiol* 2004;10(4):207–9.

138. Ishikawa K, Idoguchi K, Tanaka H et al. Classification of acute pancreatitis based on retroperitoneal extension: application of the concept of interfascial planes. *Eur J Radiol* 2006;60(3):445–52.

139. Callen PW. Computed tomographic evaluation of abdominal and pelvic abscesses. *Radiology* 1979;131(1):171–5.

140. Simons GW, Sty JR, Starshak RJ. Retroperitoneal and retrofascial abscesses. A review. *J Bone Joint Surg Am* 1983;65(8):1041–58.

141. Muttarak M, Peh WC. CT of unusual iliopsoas compartment lesions. *Radiographics* 2000;20 Spec No:S53–66.

142. Paley M, Sidhu PS, Evans RA et al. Retroperitoneal collections—aetiology and radiological implications. *Clin Radiol* 1997;52(4):290–4.

143. Korobkin M, Silverman PM, Quint LE et al. CT of the extraperitoneal space: normal anatomy and fluid collections. *AJR Am J Roentgenol* 1992;159(5):933–42.

144. Eble JN, Rosenberg AE, Young RH. Retroperitoneal xanthogranuloma in a patient with Erdheim-Chester disease. *Am J Surg Pathol* 1994;18(8):843–8.

145. Veyssier-Belot C, Cacoub P, Caparros-Lefebvre D et al. Erdheim-Chester disease. Clinical and radiologic characteristics of 59 cases. *Medicine (Baltimore)* 1996;75(3):157–69.

146. Dion E, Graef C, Haroche J et al. Imaging of thoracoabdominal involvement in Erdheim-Chester disease. *AJR Am J Roentgenol* 2004;183(5):1253–60.

147. Fortman BJ, Beall DP. Erdheim-Chester disease of the retroperitoneum: a rare cause of ureteral obstruction. *AJR Am J Roentgenol* 2001;176(5):1330–1.

148. Dion E, Graef C, Miquel A et al. Bone involvement in Erdheim-Chester disease: imaging findings including periostitis and partial epiphyseal involvement. *Radiology* 2006;238(2):632–9.

149. Tsitouridis J, Stamos S, Hassapopoulou E et al. Extramedullary paraspinal hematopoiesis in thalassemia: CT and MRI evaluation. *Eur J Radiol* 1999;30(1):33–8.

150. Vlahos L, Trakadas S, Gouliamos A et al. Retrocrural masses of extramedullary hemopoiesis in beta-thalassemia. *Magn Reson Imaging* 1993;11(8):1227–9.

151. Mesurolle B, Sayag E, Meingan P et al. Retroperitoneal extramedullary hematopoiesis: sonographic, CT, and MRI imaging appearance. *AJR Am J Roentgenol* 1996; 167(5):1139–40.

152. Kransdorf MJ, Bancroft LW, Peterson JJ et al. Imaging of fatty tumors: distinction of lipoma and well-differentiated liposarcoma. *Radiology* 2002;224(1):99–104.

153. Andac N, Baltacioglu F, Cimsit NC et al. Fat necrosis mimicking liposarcoma in a patient with pelvic lipomatosis. CT findings. *Clin Imaging* 2003;27(2):109–11.

154. Haynes JW, Brewer WH, Walsh JW. Focal fat necrosis presenting as a palpable abdominal mass: CT evaluation. *J Comput Assist Tomogr* 1985;9(3):568–9.

155. Ross JS, Prout GR Jr. Retroperitoneal fat necrosis producing ureteral obstruction. *J Urol* 1976;115(5):524–9.

156. Takao H, Yamahira K, Watanabe T. Encapsulated fat necrosis mimicking abdominal liposarcoma: computed tomography findings. *J Comput Assist Tomogr* 2004;28(2):193–4.

157. Jeffrey RB, Federle MP, Laing FC. Computed tomography of mesenteric involvement in fulminant pancreatitis. *Radiology* 1983;147(1):185–8.

158. Davidson AJ, Hartman DS. Lymphangioma of the retroperitoneum: CT and sonographic characteristic. *Radiology* 1990;175(2):507–10.

159. Konen O, Rathaus V, Dlugy E et al. Childhood abdominal cystic lymphangioma. *Pediatr Radiol* 2002;32(2):88–94.

160. Kaku M, Ohara N, Seima Y et al. A primary retroperitoneal serous cystadenocarcinoma with clinically aggressive behavior. *Arch Gynecol Obstet* 2004;270(4):302–6.

161. Lee SA, Bae SH, Ryoo HM et al. Primary retroperitoneal mucinous cystadenocarcinoma: a case report and review of the literature. *Korean J Intern Med* 2007;22(4):287–91.

162. Pennell TC, Gusdon JP Jr. Retroperitoneal mucinous cystadenoma. *Am J Obstet Gynecol* 1989;160(5 Pt 1):1229–31.

163. Buckley JA, Siegelman ES, Birnbaum BA et al. Bronchogenic cyst appearing as a retroperitoneal mass. *AJR Am J Roentgenol* 1998;171(2):527–8.

164. McAdams HP, Kirejczyk WM, Rosado-de-Christenson ML et al. Bronchogenic cyst: imaging features with clinical and histopathologic correlation. *Radiology* 2000;217(2):441–6.

165. Liang MK, Yee HT, Song JW et al. Subdiaphragmatic bronchogenic cysts: a comprehensive review of the literature. *Am Surg* 2005;71(12):1034–41.

166. Hernanz-Schulman M, Johnson JE, Holcomb GW 3rd et al. Retroperitoneal pulmonary sequestration: imaging findings, histopathologic correlation, and relationship to cystic adenomatoid malformation. *AJR Am J Roentgenol* 1997;168(5):1277–81.

167. Furuno T, Morita K, Kakizaki H et al. Laparoscopic removal of a retroperitoneal extralobar pulmonary sequestration in an adult. *Int J Urol* 2006;13(2):165–7.

168. Kopecky KK, Bodnar A, Morphis JG et al. Subdiaphragmatic pulmonary sequestrian simulating metastatic testicular cancer. *Clin Radiol* 2000;55(10):794–6.

169. Baker EL, Gore RM, Moss AA. Retroperitoneal pulmonary sequestration: computed tomographic findings. *AJR Am J Roentgenol* 1982;138(5):956–7.

170. de Perrot M, Brundler M, Totsch M et al. Mesenteric cysts. Toward less confusion? *Dig Surg* 2000;17(4):323–8.

171. Stoupis C, Ros PR, Abbitt PL et al. Bubbles in the belly: imaging of cystic mesenteric or omental masses. *Radiographics* 1994;14(4):729–37.

172. Ros PR, Olmsted WW, Moser RP Jr et al. Mesenteric and omental cysts: histologic classification with imaging correlation. *Radiology* 1987;164(2):327–32.

173. Budovec JJ, Pollema M, Grogan M. Update on multidetector computed tomography angiography of the abdominal aorta. *Radiol Clin N Am* 2010;48:283–309.

174. Numburi UD, Schoenhagen P, Flamm SD et al. Feasibility of dual-energy CT in the arterial phase: imaging after endovascular aortic repair. *AJR Am J Roentgenol* 2010;195(2):486–93.

175. Connolly JE, Wilson SE, Lawrence PL et al. Middle aortic syndrome: distal thoracic and abdominal coarctation, a disorder with multiple etiologies. *J Am Coll Surg* 2002;194:774–81.

176. Dejardin A, Goffette P, Moulin P et al. Severe hypoplasia of the abdominal aorta and its branches in a patient and his daughter. *J Intern Med* 2004;255(1):130–6.

177. Celik T, Kursaklioglu H, Iyisoy A et al. Hypoplasia of the descending thoracic and abdominal aorta: a case report and review of literature. *J Thorac Imaging* 2006;21:296–9.

178. Momiyama Y, Fayad ZA. Plaque imaging and monitoring atherosclerotic plaque interventions. *Top Magn Reson Imaging* 2007;18:349–55.

179. Witteman JC, Kannel WB, Wolf PA et al. Aortic calcified plaques and cardiovascular disease (the Framingham study). *Am J Cardiol* 1990;66:1060–4.

180. Cataner D, Andreu M, Gallardo X et al. CT in non traumatic acute thoracic aortic disease: typical and atypical features and complications. *Radiographics* 2003; 23:S93–110.

181. Norgren L, Hiatt WR, Dormandy JA et al. Inter-Society Consensus for the management of peripheral arterial disease (TASC II). *J Vasc Surg* 2007;45(Suppl S): S5–67.

182. Heijenbrok-Kal MH, Kock MC, Hunink MG. Lower extremity arterial disease: multidetector CT angiography meta-analysis. *Radiology* 2007;245(2):433–9.

183. Pande RL, Beckman JA. Abdominal aortic aneurysm: populations at risk and how to screen. *J Vasc Interv Radiol* 2008;19(Suppl 6):S2–8.

184. Rakita D, Newatia A, Hines JJ et al. Spectrum of CT findings in rupture and impending rupture of abdominal aortic aneurysms. *Radiographics* 2007;27:497–507.

185. Svensson LG, Crawford ES, Hess KR et al. Experience with 1509 patients undergoing thoracoabdominal aortic operations. *J Vasc Surg* 1993;17(2):357–68.

186. Veith FJ, Gupta S, Daly V. Technique for occluding the supraceliac aorta through the abdomen. *Surg Gynecol Obstet* 1980;151:426–8.

187. Chase CW, Layman TS, Barker DE et al. Traumatic abdominal aortic pseudoaneurysm causing biliary obstruction: a case report and reviw of the literature. *J Vasc Surg* 1997;25(5):936–940.

188. Greehalgh RM, Forbes JF, Fowkes FG et al. Early elective open surgical repair of small abdominal aortic aneurysms is not recommended: results of the UK small aneurysm trial. Steeting committee. *Eur J Vasc Endovasc Surg* 1998;16(6):462–4.

189. Gloviczki P, Ricotta JJ II. Sabiston textbook of surgery. In: Townsend CM, Beauchamp RD, Evers BM et al., editors. *Aneurysmal Vascular Disease*. 18th edition. Philadelphia, PA: Saunders; 2007.

190. Hirsch AT, Haskal ZJ, Hertzer NR et al. ACC/AHA 2005 Practice Guidelines for the management of patients with peripheral arterial disease (lower extremity, renal, mesenteric, and abdominal aortic): AU. *Circulation* 2006; 113(11):e463.

191. Schwartz SA, Taljanovic MS, Smyth S et al. CT findings of rupture, impending rupture, and contained rupture of abdominal aortic aneurysm. *AJR Am J Roentgenol* 2007;188:W57–62.

192. Siegel CL, Cohan RH, Korobkin M et al. Abdominal aortic aneurysm morphology: CT features in patietns with ruptured and non ruptured aneurysms. *AJR Am J Roentgenol* 1994;163:1123–9.

193. Pillari G, Chang JB, Zito J et al. CT of abdominal aortic aneurysm: an in vivo pathological report with a note on dynamic predictors. *Arch Surg* 1988;123:727–32.

194. Jones CS, Reilly MK, Dalsing MC et al. Chronic contained rupture of abdominal aortic aneurysms. *Arch Surg* 1986;121:542–6.

195. Eagleton MJ, Upchurch GR. Endovascular therapy for abdominal aortic aneurysms. In *Vascular Medicine: A Companion to Braunwald's Heart Disease*. Philadelphia, PA: Elsevier; 2006.

196. Vu QDM, Menias CO, Bhalla S et al. Aortoenteric fistulas: CT features and potential mimics. *Radiographics* 2009;20:197–209.

197. Alexander JJ, Imbembo AL. Aorto-vena cava fistula. *Surgery* 1989;105:1–12.

198. Tsolakis JA, Papadoulas S, Kakkos SK et al. Aortocaval fistula in ruptured aneurysms. *Eur J Vasc Endovasc Surg* 1999;17:390–3.

199. Cinara IS, Davidovic B, Kostic DM et al. Aorto-caval fistulas: a review of eighteeen years experience. *Acta Chir Belg* 2005;105:616–20.

200. Sheward SE, Spencer RE, Hinton TR et al. Computed tomography of primary aortocaval fistula. *Comput Med Imaging Graph* 1992;16(2):121–4.

201. Hervas V, Esteban JM, García-Ferrer L. Aortocaval fistula presenting with hematuria and renal failure. *Eur J Vasc Endovasc Surg* 2007;14[extra]:33–35.

202. Gonsalez SB, Busquets JCV, Figueiras RG et al. Imaging arterivenosu fistulas. *AJR Am J Roentgenol* 2009;193(5):1425–33.

203. Mohr LL, Smith LL. Arteriovenous fistula from rupture of abdominal aortic aneurysm. *Arch Surg* 1975;110: 806–12.

204. Eliason JL, Upchurch GR Jr. Endovascular abdominal aortic aneurysm repair. *Circulation* 2008;117(13):1738–44.

205. Parodi JC, Palmaz JC, Barone HD. Transfemoral intraluminal graft implantation for abdominal aortic aneurysms. *Ann Vasc Surg* 1991;5(6):491–9.

206. Lovegrove RE, Javid M, Magee TR et al. A metaanalysis of 21,718 patients undergoing open or endovascular repair of abdominal aortic aneurysm. *Br J Surg* 2008;95(6):677–84.

207. Whitaker SC. Imaging of abdominal aortic aneurysm before and after endoluminal stent-graft repair. *Eur J Radiol* 2001;39:3–15.

208. Karkos CD, Bruce IA, Thomson GJ et al. Retroaortic left renal vein and its implications in abdominal arotic surgery. *Ann Vasc Surg* 2001;15(6):703–8.

209. Olsen PS, Schroeder T, Agerskov K et al. Surgery for abdominal aortic aneurysms. A survery of 656 patients. *J Cardiovasc Surg* 1991;32(5):636–42.

210. Mita T, Arita T, Matsunaga N et al. Complications of endovascular repair for thoracic and abdominal aortic aneurysm: an imaging spectrum. *Radiographics* 2000;20:1263–78.

211. Tolia AJ, Landis R, Lamparello P et al. Type II endoleaks after endovascular repair of abdominal aortic aneurysms: natural history. *Radiology* 2005;235(2):683–6.

212. Bashir MRI, Ferral H, Jacobs C et al. Endoleaks after endovascular abdominal aortic aneurysm repair: management strategies according to CT findings. *AJR Am J Roentgenol* 2009;192(4):W178–86.

213. Dorffner R, Thurnher S, Polterauer P et al. Treatment of abdominal aortic aneurysms with transfemoral placement of stent-grafts: complications and secondary radiologic intervention. *Radiology* 1997;204:79–86.

214. Calligaro KD, Veith FJ. Diagnosis and management of infected prosthetic aortic grafts. *Surgery* 1991; 110(5):805–13.

215. Thompson MM, Smith J, Naylor AR et al. Microembolization during endovascular and conventional aneurysm repair. *J Vasc Surg* 1997;25:179–86.

216. Orton DF, LeVeen RF, SAigh JA. Aortic prosthetic graft infections: radiologic manifestations and implications for management. *Radiographics* 2000;20:977–93.

217. Dennis JW, Littooy FN, Greisler HP et al. Anastomotic pseudoaneurysms: a continuing late complication of vascular reconstructive procedures. *Arch Surg* 1986; 121:314–7.

218. Trimarchi S, Tsai T, Eagle KA et al. Acute abdominal aortic dissection. Insight from the International Registry of Acute Aortic Dissection (IRAD). *J Vasc Surg* 2007;46(5):913–9.

219. Jonker FH, Schlosser FJ, Moll FL et al. Dissection of the abdominal aorta. Current evidence and implications for treatment strategies: a review and metanalysis of 92 patients (comment). *J Endovasc Ther* 2009;16(1):71–80.

220. McMahon MA, Squirrell CA. Multidetector CT of aortic dissection: a pictorial review. *Radiographics* 2010; 30:445–60.

221. Cambria RP, Brewster DC, Gertler J et al. Vascular complications associated with spontaneous aortic dissection. *J Vasc Surg* 1988;7:199–209.

222. Sebastia C, Pallisa E, Quiroga S et al. Aortic dissection: diagnosis and follow-up with helical CT. *Radiographics* 1999;19:45–60.

223. Litmanovich D, Bankier AA, Cantin L et al. CT and MRI in diseases of the aorta. *AJR Am J Roentgenol* 2009; 193:928–40.

224. Coady MA, Rizzo JA, Elefteriade JA. Pathologic variants of thoracic aortic dissections: penetrating atherosclerotic ulcer and intramural hematoma. *Cardiol Clin* 1999;17:637–57.

225. Blanchard DG, Sawhney NS. Aortic intramural hematoma: current diagnostic and therapeutic recommendations. *Curr Treat Options Cardiovasc Med* 2004;2(6): 99–104.

226. Miller JS, Wall MJ, Mattox KL. Ruptured aortic pseudoaneurysm 28 years after gunshot wound: case report and review of literature. *J Trauma* 1998;44:214–6.

227. Gornik HL, Creager MA. Aortitis. *Circulation* 2008; 117(23):3039–51.

228. Restrepo CS, Ocazionez D, Suri R et al. Aortitis: imaging spectrum of the infectious and inflammatory conditions of the aorta. *Radiographics* 2011;31:435–51.

229. Nastri MV, Baptista LPS, Baroni RH et al. Gadolinium-enhanced three-dimensional MRI angiography of Takayasu arteritis. *Radiographics* 2004;24:773–86.

230. Sueoshi E, Sakamoto I, Hayashi K. Aortic aneurysms in patients with Takayasu's arteritis: CT evaluation. *AJR Am J Roentgenol* 2000;175(6):1727–33.

231. Desai MY, Stone JH, Foo TKF et al. Delayed contrast-enhanced MRI of the aortic wall in Takayasu's arteritis: initial experience. *AJR Am J Roentgenol* 2005;184: 1427–31.

232. Flamm SD, White RD, Hoffman GS. The clinical application of 'edema-weighted' magnetic resonance imaging in the assessment of Takayasu's arteritis. *Int J Cardiology* 1998;66(Suppl 1):S151–9.

233. Hayashi H, Katayama N, Takagi R. CT analysis of vascular awll during the active phase of takayasu's aortitis (abstr). Eur Radiol 1991; 1 (Suppl):S239.

234. Arrive L, Correas JM, Leseche G et al. Inflammatory aneurysms of the abdominal aorta: CT findings. *AJR Am J Roentgenol* 1995;165:1481–4.

235. Cullenward MJ, Scanlan KA, Pozniak MA et al. Inflammatory aortic aneurysm: radiologic imaging. *Radiology* 1986;159(1):75–82.

236. Pennell RC, Hollier LH, Lie JT et al. Inflammatory abdominal aortic aneurysms: a thirty-year review. *J Vasc Surg* 1985;2:859–69.

237. Puechner S, Bucek RA, Loewe C et al. Endovascular repair of inflammatory aortic aneurysms: long-term results. *AJR Am J Roentgenol* 2006;186(4):1144–7.

238. Macedo TA, Stanson AW, Oderich GS et al. Infected aortic aneurysms: imaging findings. *Radiology* 2004; 231(1):250–7.

239. Daas AK, Reddy KS, Suwanjindar P et al. Primary tumors of the aorta. *Ann Thorac Surg* 1996;62:1526–8.

240. Brylka D, Demos TC, Pierce K. Primary angiosarcoma of the abdominal aorta: a case report and literature review. *Abdom Imaging* 2009;34:239–42.

241. Sheth S, Fishman EK. Imaging of the inferior vena cava with MDCT. *AJR Am J Roentgenolol* 2007;189:1243–51.

242. Minniti S, Visentini S, Procacci C. Congenital anomalies of the inferior vena cava: embryological origin, imaging features and report of three new variants. *Eur Radiol* 2002;12:2040–55.

243. Phillips E. Embryology, normal anatomy, and anomalis. In: Feeris EJ, Hipona FA, Kahn PC et al., editors. *Venography of the Inferior Vena Cava and Its Branches.* Baltimore, MD: Williams & Wilkins; 1969. pp. 1–32.

244. Kandpal H, Sharma R, Gamangatti S et al. Imaging the inferior vena cava: a road less travelled. *Radiographics* 2008;28:669–89.

245. Mazzucco A, Bortolotti U, Stellin G, Galucci V. Anomalies of the systemic venous return; a review. *J Card Surg* 1990; 5:122–133.

246. Milner LB, Marchan R. Complete absence of the inferior vena cava presenting as paraspinous mass. *Thorax* 1980; 33:798–800.

247. Gibo M, Onitsuka H. Retroaortic left renal vein with renal vein hypertension causing hematuria. *Clin Imaging* 1998; 22:422–424.

248. Bass JE, Redwine MD, Kramer LA, Huynh PT, Harris JH Jr. Spectrum of congenital anomalies of the inferior vena cava; cross-sectional imaging findings. *Radiographics* 2000; 20:639–652.

8

Abdominal Wall

Diana Tran and Damien L.Stella

CONTENTS

In the last decade, multi-detector computed tomography (CT) has facilitated fast acquisition of isotropic image data sets allowing better anatomical delineation of the abdominal wall and, combined with the improvement in CT workstations, even new clinical applications for CT. Although most abdominal wall abnormalities are usually identified on CT as incidental findings, this transformation of CT has resulted in CT becoming the primary tool for preoperative workup for planned breast reconstructive surgery where deep inferior epigastric perforator (DIEP) flap techniques are used. CT is now more reliable and accurate in characterization of inguinal region hernias and their differentiation from inguinal canal lipomas (ICLs) for which they are frequently mistaken. Ultrasound (US) is equally adequate for the evaluation of abdominal wall hernias and is preferred to CT when small inguinal region hernias are suspected. Magnetic resonance imaging (MRI) suffers with a relative lack of spatial resolution but offers the advantage of a lack of ionizing radiation and is preferred to CT in the workup of abdominal wall tumors. This chapter is divided into clinical sections (abdominal wall congenital abnormalities, hernias, hemorrhage, tumors, and CT angiography for breast free flap reconstruction) that highlight CT appearances and relevant clinical anatomy and CT techniques where appropriate.

8.1 Congenital Abnormalities of the Anterior Abdominal Wall

CT is rarely used in assessing congenital abnormalities of the anterior abdominal wall as most are usually clinically obvious at birth and CT has a limited role in their management (e.g., gastroschisis, omphalocoele, and bladder extrophy). *Urachal anomalies* are the only common abdominal wall abnormality where CT plays an important role.

The urachus is the fibrous remnant (forming the median umbilical fold) of the allantois, which drains the fetal bladder via the umbilicus. Incomplete involution of the urachal lumen gives rise to one of four forms of urachal anomaly; patent urachus, urachal sinus, urachal diverticulum, and urachal cyst. Patent urachus (persistent fistula between the bladder and umbilicus) and urachal sinus (blind-ending pouch communicating with umbilicus) usually present early in life due to continual umbilical discharge and are infrequently imaged with CT.

A urachal diverticulum (blind-ending pouch communicating with bladder) and urachal cyst (cyst without communication to bladder or umbilicus) are both

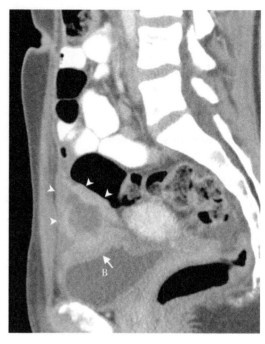

FIGURE 8.1

Sagittal multiplanar reformation showing infected urachal diverticulum (arrowheads) arising from anterior aspect of bladder dome (arrow).

usually asymptomatic and therefore present as an incidental finding on CT. They are both characterized by a midline location within the extraperitoneal fat of the anterior abdominal wall and "point" toward the umbilicus. They either directly communicate with the anterior wall of the bladder (urachal diverticulum) or are tethered to it by the urachus (urachal cyst). Both may be complicated by infection (common) or malignancy (rare). It can be difficult to differentiate between infection and tumor on CT in urachal anomalies, with needle aspiration often required to confirm diagnosis. Infection is suggested when there is mural thickening, surrounding fat stranding and a central (nonenhancing) low-density region, in keeping with abscess formation (Figure 8.1). A solid enhancing mass with calcification and/or invasion of adjacent structures suggest malignancy. The risk of malignancy increases after puberty, with 90% of cases being adenocarcinoma [1].

8.2 Abdominal Wall Hernias

An abdominal wall hernia occurs where there is a deficiency in the abdominal wall (site of the hernia neck) with resultant intra-abdominal contents (surrounded by parietal peritoneum and forming the hernia sac) bulging through for a variable distance. Abdominal wall

TABLE 8.1

CT Imaging Characteristics of Inguinal Region Fat Containing Lesions

Hernia Type	Relationship to Inferior Epigastric Vessels	Extension into Inguinal Canal	Peritoneal Lining	Femoral Vein Compression	Fat Origin
True (spermatic cord) lipoma	Anteroinferior (within the inguinal canal)	Yes	No	No	De novo
ICL	Lateral to vessels	Yes	No	No	Extraperitoneal fat
IIH	Lateral to vessels	Yes	Yes	Yes, if large	Omental or mesenteric fat
DIH	Medial to vessels	No	Yes	No	Omental or mesenteric fat
Femoral hernia	Inferior to vessels	No	Yes	Yes	Omental or mesenteric fat

hernias are classified according to their location and type. They occur in up to 5% of the population. Inguinal hernias account for about 80% of cases (2:1 ratio of indirect to direct inguinal hernias [DIH]), whereas femoral hernias make up 5%. The remaining 15% are largely made up of umbilical, epigastric, and incisional hernias [2]. Differentiation between various inguinal region fat containing lesions is outlined in Table 8.1.

8.2.1 Imaging Technique

Standard CT imaging of the abdomen and pelvis (including oral and intravenous contrast)—or targeted imaging to the region of interest—is typically sufficient to adequately show the abdominal wall defect, hernia sac and contents, identify key landmarks, and evaluate for potential complications. Although axial views provide most of the necessary information, coronal (especially for inguinal region hernias) and sagittal (especially for ventral hernias) reformats can be helpful. Postural maneuvers such as the valsalva or decubitus positions may be performed to help identify subtle hernias [3], but where there is a high suspicion and negative CT scan, US should be considered.

8.2.2 Inguinal Hernias and Inguinal Canal Lipomas

8.2.2.1 Anatomy of the Inguinal Canal

The inguinal canal is a short U-shaped canal that lies superior to the medial half of the inguinal ligament (formed by the external oblique aponeurosis folding back on itself) and courses anteroinferomedially between the aponeuroses of the external oblique, the internal oblique, and the transversus abdominis muscles. It is most easily identified on CT when there is a significant amount of fat within the canal separating the various layers and is best shown with oblique coronal reformats (Figure 8.2).

The deep (internal) ring represents the proximal opening. It corresponds to the defect in the transversalis fascia and is identified on CT by the origin of the inferior

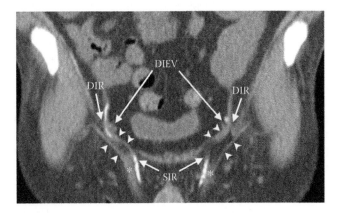

FIGURE 8.2
Oblique coronal multiplanar reformation showing normal inguinal canal (arrowheads) anatomy in a patient with calcified gonadal vessels. * = spermatic cord, DIEV = deep inferior epigastric vessels, DIR = deep inguinal ring, SIR = superficial inguinal ring.

epigastric vessels that are located inferomedially. The superficial (external) ring represents the distal opening of the inguinal canal. It corresponds to the opening in the aponeurosis of the external oblique muscle and is identified on CT superolateral to the pubic tubercle. The inguinal canal contains the spermatic cord (round ligament in females) comprising vas deferens, gonadal vessels, lymphatics, nerves, fat, and connective tissue. The normal spermatic cord contains little fat and is usually symmetrical in appearance measuring about 16 mm in diameter [4].

8.2.2.2 Inguinal Canal Lipomas

ICLs are not true lipomas of the spermatic cord (which are in fact quite rare) but represent extrusion of extraperitoneal fat (also known as properitoneal or preperitoneal fat) through the deep inguinal ring into the inguinal canal anterior to the spermatic cord [4,5]. True lipomas of the inguinal canal are circumscribed fatty masses without internal vascularity on CT (as for lipomas elsewhere) and are not a continuation of extraperitoneal fat. ICLs are present in up to 70% of

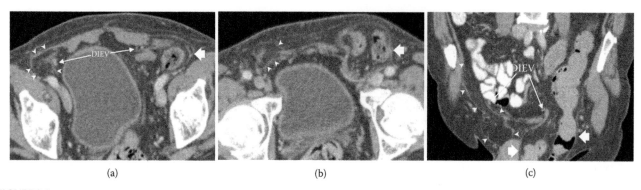

(a)   (b)   (c)

FIGURE 8.3
Axial images at the level of the deep inguinal ring (a) and superficial inguinal ring (b), and oblique coronal image (c) of the inguinal canal show a large left indirect inguinal hernia (large arrow) containing small bowel loops and a large right inguinal canal lipoma (arrowheads) with fat origin traced back to extraperitoneal fat overlying iliopsoas muscles. DIEV = deep inferior epigastric vessels.

males [5], and when large, are frequently misdiagnosed as indirect inguinal hernias (IIHs) on imaging. Their exact clinical importance is unclear, but they are associated with IIHs and have been postulated as a risk factor for both occurrence and recurrence of IIHs [6–8]. They differ from true IIHs as they do not have a peritoneal lining [5].

On axial CT, differentiation of ICLs from inguinal hernias can only be reliably achieved at the level of the deep inguinal ring, where they are seen to pass lateral to the inferior epigastric vessels into the deep inguinal ring and contain fat that can be traced back to its origin from extraperitoneal fat [4] (Figure 8.3). At and below the level of the superficial inguinal ring, it can be very difficult to differentiate between ICLs and either form of inguinal hernia on axial CT, if they only contain fat. ICLs are best appreciated on coronal imaging where the fat can be traced to its extraperitoneal origins at the deep ring, with a compressed segment passing along the inguinal canal defined by both the superior and inferior walls of the inguinal canal, expanding into a club-like bulbous mass beyond the superficial ring [4] (Figures 8.3 and 8.4).

8.2.2.3 Indirect Inguinal Hernia

IIHs are more common in men and make up most inguinal hernias in children. In boys, indirect hernias are due to a patent processus vaginalis (embryologic remnant) within the inguinal canal, and in adults, they are due to an acquired weakness of the deep inguinal ring. The hernia sac enters the deep inguinal ring lateral to the inferior epigastric artery and descends down the inguinal canal adjacent to the spermatic cord for a variable extent. Large IIHs can protrude into the scrotal sac via the superficial ring. Contents that herniate into the inguinal canal include mesenteric and/or omental

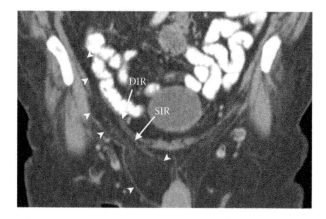

FIGURE 8.4
Oblique coronal image of a large right inguinal canal lipoma (arrowheads) arising from fat contiguous with extraperitoneal fat. Note how the fat is compressed as it passes through the deep inguinal ring (DIR) into the inguinal canal, expanding into a bulbous shape as it passes beyond the superficial inguinal ring (SIR).

fat but may also include small or large bowel and rarely bladder, ovaries, appendix, or Meckel's diverticulum.

On axial CT, IIHs are identified by their origin in the deep ring, superior and lateral to the inferior epigastric vessels (that are displaced inferiorly and medially) (Figures 8.3 and 8.5). They are differentiated from ICLs by the presence of a clearly visible peritoneal sac. They contain omental or mesenteric fat with vessels that pass posteromedially above the deep inguinal ring, as opposed to the characteristic darker fat (lower concentration of vessels) seen in the extraperitoneal fat of ICLs that arises posterolateral to the deep ring from extraperitoneal fat overlying the iliopsoas muscles [4]. The origin of omental/mesenteric fat is best appreciated on sequential coronal images, where the lack of a superior wall further helps differentiate them from ICLs [4] (Figures 8.3 and 8.5).

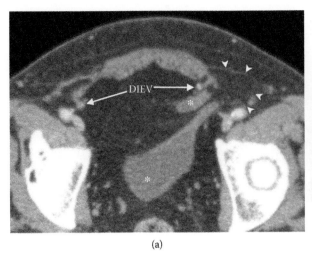
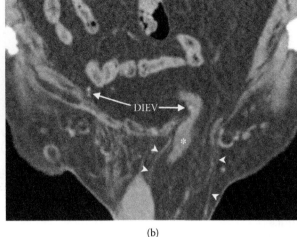

(a)   (b)

FIGURE 8.5
Axial image at the level of the deep inguinal ring (a) and oblique coronal image (b) of the inguinal canal show a large left indirect inguinal hernia (arrowheads) containing bladder (*). Note the medial displacement of the deep inferior epigastric vessels (DIEV).

8.2.2.4 Direct Inguinal Hernia

DIHs are also more common in men and occur because of acquired weakness of the transversalis fascia above the inguinal ligament and medial to the inferior epigastric vessels (Hesselbach triangle). As such, they do not enter into the inguinal canal but bulge anteroinferiorly toward or through the superficial inguinal ring, displacing the inguinal canal contents laterally. They are typically short, with a wide neck and only occasionally contain bowel, and therefore rarely obstruct or extend into the scrotum.

On axial CT, a DIH bulges the anterior abdominal wall medial to the inferior epigastric vessels, lateral to the rectus muscle (Figure 8.6). When large, DIHs compress and stretch the inguinal canal contents that are displaced laterally along with the inferior epigastric vessels, differentiating them from IIHs [2]. Like IIHs, the clearly visible peritoneal sac, lack of a superior wall, and fat contents arising from the omentum/mesentery are best appreciated on coronal imaging, differentiating them from ICLs (Figure 8.7) [4].

8.2.3 Femoral Hernias

8.2.3.1 Anatomy of the Femoral Canal

The femoral sheath is formed by the mergence of the continuation of the transversalis fascia anteriorly and the deep fascia of the thigh (fascia lata) posteriorly. It is located inferior and posterior to the inguinal ligament within the femoral triangle. The femoral sheath encircles the femoral artery and vein, with the femoral canal lying within its medial aspect. The femoral canal lies medial to the femoral vein and contains fat,

lymphatics, and the lymph gland of Cloquet. The canal is funnel shaped (wider at the abdominal end) and ends at the level of the saphenous opening. The femoral ring forms the abdominal opening of the femoral canal and is bound by the inguinal ligament (anteriorly), lacunar ligament (medially), pubic bone and pectineal ligament (posteriorly), and femoral vein (laterally).

8.2.3.2 Femoral Hernia

Femoral hernias are far less common than inguinal hernias. They are also largely confined to adults, but are more common in women, and are at much higher risk of complication than inguinal hernias. Femoral hernias occur when a hernia sac protrudes through the femoral ring into the femoral canal below the inguinal ligament. Given that all the borders of the femoral ring are rigid apart from the femoral vein, femoral hernias always compress and/or displace the femoral vein at the femoral ring.

On axial CT, the narrow femoral hernia neck emerges through the femoral ring immediately medial to the femoral vein and superolateral to the pubic tubercle. At this level, the inguinal canal lies anteromedial to the femoral hernia sac (Figure 8.8). The neck of a femoral hernia lies inferior to the origin of the inferior epigastric vessels, hence differentiating them from inguinal hernias (which emerge superolateral or superomedial to the origin of the inferior epigastric vessels) (Figure 8.9). Although the femoral vein is invariably somewhat compressed at the femoral ring in a femoral hernia, it should be noted that a large, wide-necked IIH can also compress the femoral vein (Figure 8.6). Femoral hernias do not enter the inguinal canal. They always maintain a

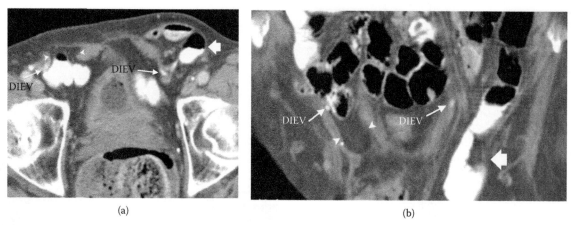

(a)   (b)

FIGURE 8.6
Axial (a) and oblique coronal (b) images showing a right direct inguinal hernia (arrowheads) containing caecum, and a large left indirect inguinal hernia (large arrow) containing small bowel loops. Note slight compression of the left femoral vein. DIEV = deep inferior epigastric vessels.

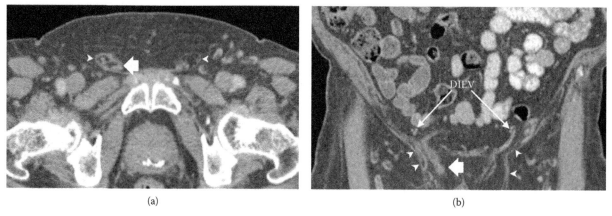

(a)   (b)

FIGURE 8.7
Axial image inferior to the superficial inguinal ring (a), and oblique coronal image (b) show a large right direct inguinal hernia (large arrow) and bilateral inguinal canal lipomas (arrowheads). Note compression and lateral displacement of the right inguinal canal lipoma. DIEV = deep inferior epigastric vessels.

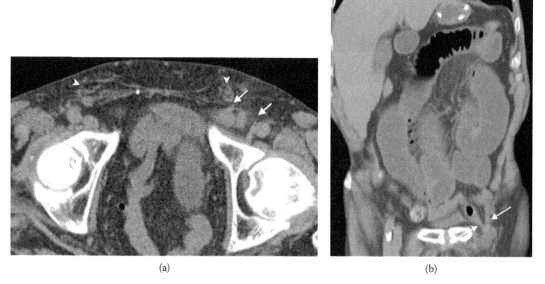

(a)   (b)

FIGURE 8.8
Axial (a) and coronal (b) images at the level of the femoral ring (defined by arrows) show an incarcerated left femoral hernia complicated by a closed loop small bowel obstruction. Note relationship to inguinal canal (arrowheads) and slit-like compression of left femoral vein.

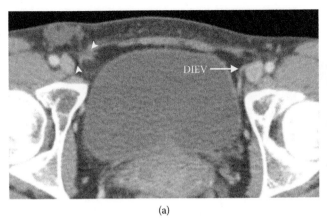 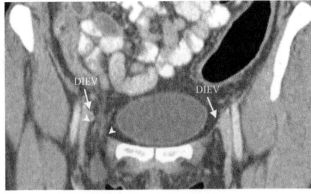

(a)   (b)

FIGURE 8.9
Axial (a) and coronal (b) images at the level of the femoral ring (defined by arrowheads) in a patient with Crohn's disease show a right sided femoral hernia containing omentum and entrapped peritoneal fluid. Note relationship to deep inferior epigastric vessels (DIEV) and slight compression of right femoral vein.

close relationship with the femoral vein as they are both contained within the femoral sheath. Their relationship to the femoral vein and inferior epigastric vessels and their differentiation from inguinal hernias are best appreciated on sequential coronal images (Figure 8.9).

8.2.4 Ventral Hernias

8.2.4.1 Midline Defects

Umbilical hernias are the most common form of midline defect. In adults, they are acquired, occurring most frequently in women (Figure 8.10). Paraumbilical hernias are a subset of umbilical hernias that do not pass through the cicatricial ring of the umbilicus but arise adjacent to the umbilicus, most commonly because of a small defect of the linea above the umbilicus. Epigastric and hypogastric hernias are uncommon and occur in the midline above and below the umbilicus, respectively, most commonly as a consequence of diastasis of the rectus abdominis muscles (Figure 8.11) or following midline laparotomy (Figure 8.12).

8.2.4.2 Paramedian Defects

Spigelian hernias occur at the lateral margin of the rectus abdominis muscle through a defect in the linea semilunaris, formed by the union of the rectus sheath and the aponeurosis of the transversus and oblique muscles. They are rare and typically occur at or below the arcuate line (where the inferior epigastric artery passes in front of the inferior border of the posterior wall of the rectus sheath) [9] (Figure 8.13). These hernias are usually interparietal, in that extruded bowel or omentum is confined between abdominal wall muscle layers (Figures 8.13 and 8.14). They typically have a narrow neck and therefore have a high frequency of incarceration [10]. Parastomal hernias are a frequent form

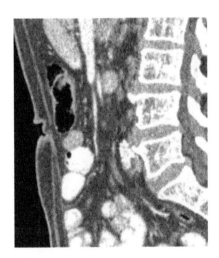

FIGURE 8.10
Sagittal image of umbilical hernia.

of incisional hernia, where the hernia sac and contents protrude through the surgical rectus defect separate from and adjacent to the stoma (Figure 8.15).

8.2.5 Lumbar Hernias

Lumbar hernias usually occur secondary to major trauma or as incisional hernias following renal surgery. Noniatrogenic lumbar hernias are rare and usually occur through relative weak areas of the thoracolumbar fascia, between muscles of the posterior abdominal wall (lumbar triangles). The superior lumber triangle is bound by erector spinae/quadratus lumborum muscles medially, the twelfth rib superiorly, and the internal oblique laterally, with the tranversalis fascia representing the floor (Figure 8.16). The inferior lumbar triangle is bound by the iliac crest inferiorly, external oblique laterally, and latissimus dorsi medially, with the internal oblique representing the floor (Figure 8.17).

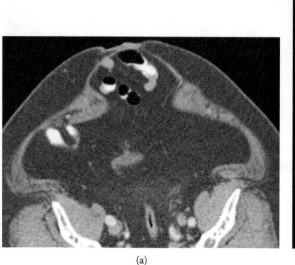

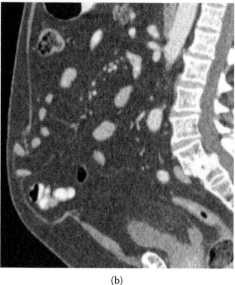

| (a) | (b) |

FIGURE 8.11
Axial (a) and sagittal (b) images showing wide-necked divarication of the recti containing small bowel loops. Note that the linea alba remains intact, and thus diastasis of the rectus abdominus muscles does not represent a true hernia.

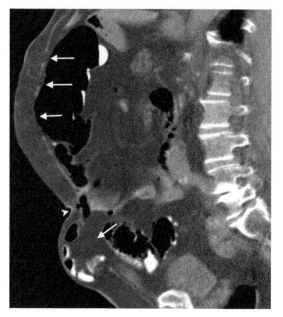

FIGURE 8.12
Sagittal image with multiple midline incisional hernias (arrows) containing omentum, colon, mesentery and small bowel. Note the small (Richter's) umbilical hernia (arrowhead) containing small bowel.

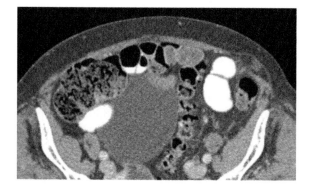

FIGURE 8.13
Axial image just below the level of the arcuate line showing a left (interparietal) Spigelian hernia containing omental fat.

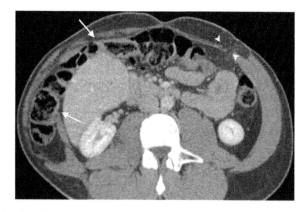

FIGURE 8.14
Axial image above the level of the arcuate line showing a narrow-necked left Spigelian hernia containing omental fat (arrowheads) and a wide-necked (interparietal) right Spigelian hernia (arrows) containing colon.

8.2.6 Other Types of Abdominal Wall Hernia

Incisional hernias occur at the site of abdominal wall weakness caused by prior surgery, particularly vertical incisions. They can occur anywhere, including at the site of laparoscopy ports, but are most frequent as ventral hernias. Hernias that occur through the abdominal wall muscles, as opposed to between them or through aponeurotic

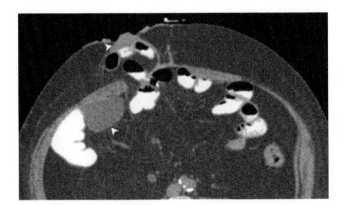

FIGURE 8.15
Parastomal hernia containing small bowel, adjacent to an ileal conduit (arrowheads).

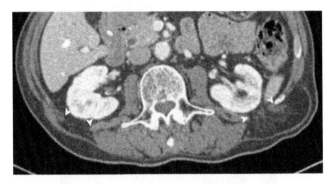

FIGURE 8.16
Small right and large left superior lumbar triangle hernias containing perirenal fat.

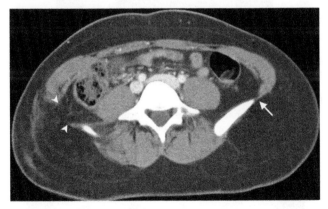

FIGURE 8.17
Acute traumatic inferior lumbar triangle hernia containing extraperitoneal fat (arrowheads). Note the normal left inferior lumbar triangle (arrow).

weaknesses, are invariably incisional or post traumatic hernias (Figure 8.18). Interparietal hernias refer to hernias where the hernia sac is located in the intermuscular plane. By definition, they do not reach the subcutaneous fat. They are uncommon and most frequently seen in lumbar and Spigelian hernias (Figures 8.13, 8.14, and 8.18). Richter's hernias occur when only a portion of the circumference of antimesenteric wall of contained bowel protrudes through

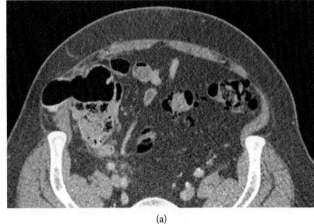

(a)

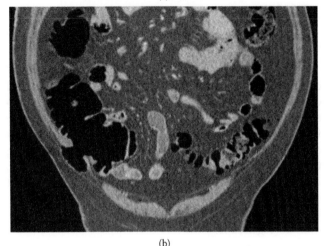

(b)

FIGURE 8.18
Axial (a) and coronal (b) images of a right lumbar (interparietal) Richter's incisional hernia containing a portion of the caecum.

the abdominal wall defect (Figures 8.12 and 8.18). They are at high risk of mural ischemia without bowel obstruction and are most frequently associated with femoral hernias [11]. Littre's and Amyand hernias refer to inguinal hernias containing a Meckel's diverticulum or appendix, (inflamed or not) respectively.

8.2.7 Abdominal Wall Hernia Complications

8.2.7.1 Incarcerated Hernias

Incarcerated hernias cannot be diagnosed on CT with certainty unless they are complicated by strangulation or bowel obstruction. They are defined by irreducibility of hernia contents on clinical examination and may be suspected on CT when a relatively narrow neck is present.

8.2.7.2 Strangulated Hernias

Strangulated hernias occur when there is vascular compromise to the hernia sac contents (whether they contain bowel or not). Signs of ischemia and venous

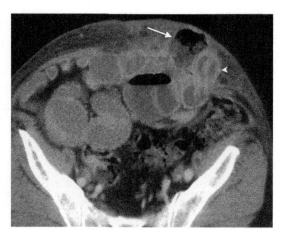

FIGURE 8.19
Incarcerated and strangulated incisional hernia containing hyperaemic small bowel (arrowhead), complicated by closed loop small bowel obstruction and local perforation (arrow).

congestion on CT include swelling, prominent increased density/haziness, and vascular engorgement of mesenteric/omental fat. Localized peritoneal fluid is also frequently seen within the sac. Strangulated hernias containing bowel loops manifest CT findings relating to closed loop bowel obstruction and venous ischemia, including mural thickening, abnormal enhancement (both hypo- or hyperenhancement), and when advanced, intramural gas and even perforation with abscess formation (Figure 8.19).

8.2.7.3 Bowel Obstruction

Bowel obstruction can occur as a complication of a hernia with or without strangulation. Small bowel obstruction is far more common than large bowel obstruction in hernias, with hernias the second most common cause of small bowel obstruction after adhesions, accounting for up to 10%–15% of cases [12]. Most bowel obstructions related to hernias are closed loop obstructions secondary to obstruction of the afferent and efferent limbs of bowel at the hernia neck. They are identified on CT by transition points at the hernial orifice, with dilation of the bowel loops within the hernia sac and proximal to the hernia, and collapsed loops of bowel distal to the hernia (Figures 8.6 and 8.20).

8.2.7.4 Abscesses

Abscess formation within abdominal wall hernias is usually a complication of strangulated hernias but may arise from direct spread of any intra-abdominal collection into a pre-existing hernia (Figure 8.21). On CT, abscesses within a hernia sac are fluid and gas containing collections demarcated by an enhancing wall, which are usually surrounded by varying degrees of

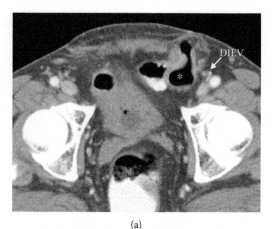

(a)

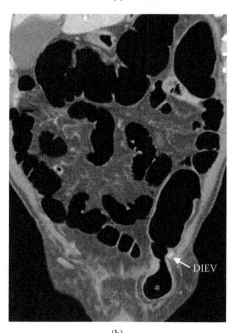

(b)

FIGURE 8.20
Axial (a) and coronal (b) images of an incarcerated left direct inguinal hernia containing sigmoid colon (*) and causing large bowel obstruction. DIEV = deep inferior epigastric vessels.

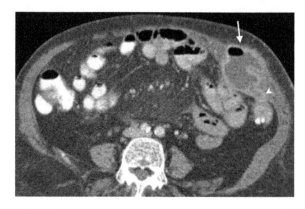

FIGURE 8.21
Abscess (arrow) secondary to perforated diverticulitis (arrowhead) within a (interparietal) spigelian hernia.

inflammatory change in adjacent abdominal wall muscles (expansion and hyperenhancement) and subcutaneous fat (haziness and vascular engorgement).

8.3 Abdominal Wall Tumors

Benign tumors of the abdominal wall are relatively common, whereas malignant tumors are uncommon. Metastases constitute the vast majority of malignant tumors. Differentiation between various benign and malignant abdominal wall tumors is not often possible on CT (with the exception of simple lipomas). Workup of abdominal wall tumors with MRI is more helpful than CT in most cases.

8.3.1 Benign Abdominal Wall Tumors

Lipomas are common benign mesenchymal fat containing tumors that frequently occur within the abdominal wall. They are well-encapsulated, homogeneous, fatty masses on CT that may contain thin internal septations. When large (greater than 10 cm), or showing contrast enhancement, or containing soft tissue nodules, or thick internal septations, liposarcomas or atypical lipomas should be suspected. Symptomatic or rapidly enlarging lesions represent clinical features suggesting malignancy. Intramuscular lipomas should be easily differentiated from interparietal hernias on CT by the lack of a hernial defect and the fact that fat within interparietal hernias can be traced back to mesenteric/omental origins (Figures 8.13, 8.14, and 8.22).

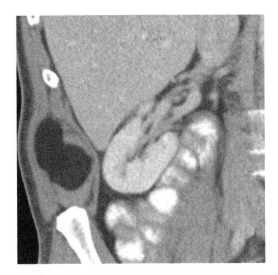

FIGURE 8.22
Coronal image of a lipoma expanding and distorting the right internal oblique muscle.

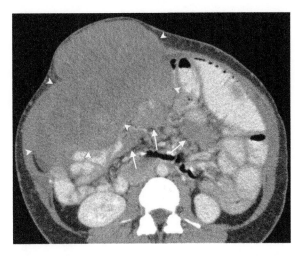

FIGURE 8.23
Patient with familial adenomatous polyposis syndrome with massive abdominal wall desmoid tumor (arrowheads), and multiple mesenteric (infiltrative) desmoid tumors (arrows).

Desmoid tumors are uncommon benign fibroblastic neoplasms that are often locally aggressive and frequently recur following surgery. They are usually solitary sporadic tumors of the anterior abdominal wall occurring most frequently in young adult females. Prior trauma, surgical incisions and pregnancy are suspected risk factors. They are also seen in 9%–18% of patients with familial adenomatous polyposis (FAP), in whom they are usually multiple and occur most commonly within the mesentery [13] (Figure 8.23). On CT, desmoid tumors have a variable homo- or heterogeneous appearance and may be hypo-, iso-, or hyperdense (more collagen) relative to muscle with well- or ill-defined margins and enhancement that ranges from minimal to marked (usually reflecting more cellular regions).

Other benign tumors of the anterior abdominal wall are uncommon and include neurofibromas. On CT, they appear as well-defined ovoid or slightly lobulated masses of (typically) low density that show variable (often heterogeneous and minimal) enhancement. Plexiform neurofibromas seen in patients with neurofibromatosis type 1 are often infiltrative, and when hypoattenuating and hypovascular, can mimic other hypodense lesions such as lymphangiomas on CT (Figure 8.24).

8.3.2 Malignant Abdominal Wall Tumors

Primary malignancy of the abdominal wall (soft tissue sarcoma or lymphoma) is rare. Common sarcomas include dermatofibrosarcoma protuberans, undifferentiated pleomorphic sarcoma (previously malignant fibrous histiocytoma), liposarcoma, and rhabdomyosarcoma.

Metastases constitute the vast majority of malignant abdominal wall tumors. Most relate to hematogenous tumor spread from melanoma, lung, breast, and

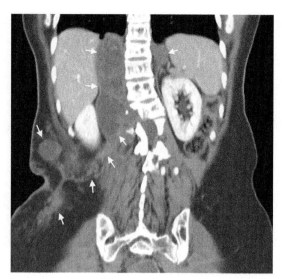

FIGURE 8.24
Patient with neurofibromatosis type 1 and an extensive plexiform neurofibroma (arrows) extending from the retroperitoneum into the right abdominal wall and subcutaneous fat.

pancreas cancers. Direct (contiguous) tumor spread from intra-abdominal primary tumors also occur and should be easily recognized as such on CT. Tumor seeding (implantation) at port sites or surgical scars is documented in renal cell carcinoma [14], colorectal cancer [15], and gynecological cancers and hepatocellular carcinoma. Lymphatic spread is mostly confined to the inguinal region where inguinal lymph nodes represent common sites of tumor spread from primary tumors arising from the lower limbs, lower rectum/anal canal, perineum, lower vagina and vulva, and penis.

8.4 Abdominal Wall Hemorrhage

Hemorrhage into the abdominal wall is usually spontaneous, often precipitated by a bleeding diathesis or anticoagulation. Secondary causes include trauma, tumors, and iatrogenic causes. They can occur anywhere in the abdominal wall but are most common within the rectus sheath. Abdominal wall hematomas may be contained within muscles or spread along fascial planes but are confined by aponeurotic attachments and muscle insertions, except in trauma where multiple bleeding sites are often involved. Rectus sheath hematomas are usually ellipse shaped but may bulge posteriorly apparently beyond the expected confines of the rectus sheath when they occur below the arcuate line (Figure 8.25).

CT is usually performed as a noncontrast study to confirm clinically suspected bleeding, when patients present with sudden onset of severe abdominal wall pain. Abdominal wall hematomas appear as heterogeneous, predominantly, hyperdense masses (relative to adjacent

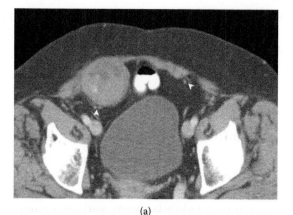

(a)

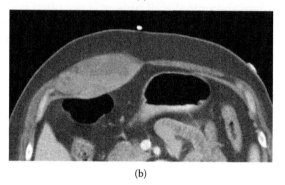

(b)

FIGURE 8.25
Two different patients with spontaneous rectus sheath hematomas while anticoagulated. The first patient (a) has a hematoma below the arcuate line, as the deep inferior epigastric vessels (arrowheads) have not yet entered in front of the posterior rectus sheath. The second patient (b) has a hematoma above the arcuate line.

muscle), often with a swirled appearance and/or areas of layering in the acute setting. They become isodense and finally hypodense as they age and are slowly resorbed. Beyond a week, granulation tissue appears at the margins, manifest as rim enhancement on CT, mimicking abscesses both clinically and radiologically at this point of temporal evolution. Hemorrhage following over anticoagulation is characterized by the appearance of a hematocrit-related fluid level. If a patient presents in a hemodynamically unstable state, CT is usually performed with intravenous contrast, timed for the arterial phase to locate the site of active bleeding (manifest as pooling of contrast) and to map the local vasculature for radiologic intervention, if required.

8.5 Abdominal Wall CT Angiography for Breast Free Flap Reconstruction

Autologous breast reconstruction using lower abdominal wall tissue as the donor site is becoming the favored form of breast reconstructive surgery following mastectomy, particularly following breast irradiation. Muscle sparing free flaps, such as the DIEP flap and superficial inferior epigastric artery (SIEA) flap, are now preferred over the transverse rectus abdominus musculocutaneous (TRAM) flap because of significantly lower donor site morbidity. The complex and highly variable anatomy of the deep inferior epigastric artery (DIEA), associated perforators, and the SIEA has created a need for preoperative vascular mapping. Since the first description of its technique in 2006 [16,17], abdominal wall CT angiography has progressively replaced color Doppler US for preoperative vascular mapping. This shift has been verified by comparative studies that have found US is less accurate, less reproducible, and more labor intensive than abdominal wall CT angiography [18–20]. Although MRI has potential in this area, it has not achieved significant popularity to date. In addition to optimizing surgical planning before attempting abdominal wall free flap autologous breast reconstruction, abdominal wall CT angiography has been shown to result in significant reduction of operating time (up to 77–100 minute reduction), improved flap outcomes, and lower morbidity [21–23]. The technique also evaluates the anterior abdominal wall for ventral hernias that may impact on planned surgery.

8.5.1 Anatomy

8.5.1.1 Deep Inferior Epigastric Artery and Vein

The DIEA arises from the external iliac artery behind the inguinal ligament and courses superomedially to enter the rectus sheath just below the arcuate line. At this point, the vessel remains as a single trunk (type I), or divides into two (type II—most common), or more (type III) trunks and continues superiorly between the posterior layer of the rectus sheath and adjacent muscle, occasionally coursing within the rectus muscle for a variable length [24]. The deep inferior epigastric vein (DIEV) forms from the venae commitantes (typically paired) that accompany the DIEA and drains into the external iliac vein. One DIEV is usually comparable in size to the adjacent DIEA.

8.5.1.2 Deep Inferior Epigastric Artery and Deep Inferior Epigastric Vein Perforators

DIEA perforators are branches of the DIEA that traverse the rectus muscle and anterior rectus sheath to supply the subcutaneous fat and skin of the overlying lower abdominal wall. Their number, caliber, location, and course are highly variable, even between sides within an individual. DIEA perforators are divided into intramuscular, subfascial (lying between the superficial margin of the rectus muscle and the anterior rectus fascia), and subcutaneous segments according to the anatomical space through which they course [24] (Figures 8.26, 8.27 and 8.28). The subfascial segment is usually absent or short. Paramedian perforators do not have a subfascial segment (instead passing medial to the rectus muscle through the linea alba) (Figure 8.28). Musculotendinous junction perforators have a muscular segment that is minimal or absent. The subcutaneous segment is variable, commonly anastomosing with the superficial inferior epigastric vessels at the level of Scarpa's fascia. The DIEV perforators accompany the perforating arteries as venae commitantes, ultimately draining into the DIEV. They also communicate with the superficial inferior epigastric vein (SIEV).

8.5.1.3 Superficial Inferior Epigastric Artery and Vein

The SIEA is absent in up to 40% of patients and when present, arises from a common origin with the superficial circumflex iliac artery (two-thirds) or as an independent vessel (one-third) [25]. The SIEA arises from the common femoral artery just below the inguinal ligament and courses superiorly anterior to the rectus sheath within the subcutaneous fat. The course, caliber, and length are highly variable. The SIEA has large accompanying venae commitantes (typically used for a SIEA adipocutaneous flap) [25]. The SIEV has a separate course to the SIEA within the subcutaneous fat of the lower anterior abdominal wall. It is usually present, complete, and of large caliber. The SIEV drains into the long saphenous vein.

8.5.2 Surgical Considerations for Breast Free Flap Reconstruction

8.5.2.1 Surgical Preferences

Some surgeons prefer to use an adipocutaneous free flap based on the SIEA as the vascular pedicle as this technique avoids dividing the anterior rectus fascia, reducing operative time and donor-site morbidity compared to using DIEP-based flaps. However, SIEA flaps are only suitable in up to 30% of patients and cannot be used when large or bilateral lower abdominal wall free flaps are required [25]. Hence, most surgeons prefer DIEP-based flaps for breast reconstruction. Given that the highly variable perforator topography determines the difficulty of the procedure and therefore the overall length of surgery, surgeons increasingly consider preoperative DIEA perforator vascular mapping with CT as an essential step in surgical planning. The desired vascular anatomical features considered favorable for breast free flap reconstruction using the lower abdominal wall are summarized in Table 8.2.

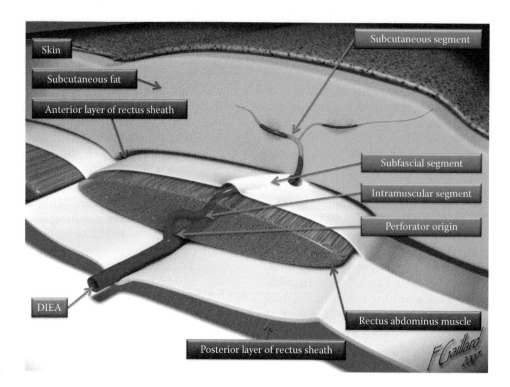

FIGURE 8.26

Three-dimensional graphic illustration of the course of a perforator (anterior musculocutaneous branch) from its origin at the deep inferior epigastric artery (DIEA) between the posterior layer of the rectus sheath and the rectus muscle, its intramuscular segment within the rectus muscle, its subfascial segment (not always present) between the anterior aspect of the rectus muscle and the anterior layer of the rectus sheath, and its end branching (subcutaneous segment) within the subcutaneous fat of the anterior abdominal wall. (Image courtesy of Francesco Gaillard MBBS, Royal Melbourne Hospital, Australia, from Phillips TJ, Stella DL, Rozen WM et al., *Radiology*, 249:32–44, 2008. With permission.)

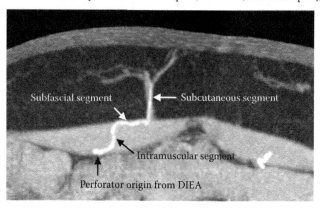

FIGURE 8.27

Axial 30 mm section MIP shows the various segments of a deep inferior epigastric artery (DIEA) perforator. Note the unopacified accompanying deep inferior epigastric vein perforator.

8.5.2.2 Desirable Superficial Inferior Epigastric Artery Features

A long length and medial course with a minimal diameter of 1.5 mm for the SIEA is preferable [25].

8.5.2.3 Desirable Deep Inferior Epigastric Artery Features

A large caliber DIEA is preferred as the vascular pedicle for a DIEP flap. Type I and II DIEAs are generally preferred in that they are more likely to supply favorable perforator vessels, including perforators with shorter intramuscular segments (type I and II DIEAs) and perforators aligned in rows along each trunk (type II DIEAs), allowing two or more smaller perforators to be used and dissected to a single trunk, if required. Medial row perforators are preferred, as dissection of lateral trunks of type II and III DIEAs risks rectus muscle denervation [24]. A lack of any intramuscular course of the DIEA is preferred, allowing for easier dissection.

8.5.2.4 Desirable Deep Inferior Epigastric Artery Perforator Features

An intramuscular segment that is short, straight, and without a substantial medial or (especially) lateral deviation is preferred, allowing for less invasive rectus-dissection [26] (Figures 8.29 and 8.30). Musculotendinous junction perforators (no intramuscular segment) are preferred by some surgeons, for similar reasons (Figure 8.31). A long subfascial segment is undesirable because of the care and time required for careful dissection [24] (Figures 8.27 and 8.28). The subcutaneous segment origin preferably lies within a 4 cm arc centered around and below the umbilicus. Vessel caliber should be at least 1 mm (better if larger) to ensure adequate adipocutaneous tissue blood supply [24] (Figure 8.29).

TABLE 8.2

Desired Arterial Anatomical Features for Abdominal Wall Free Flap Breast Reconstruction

Vessel	Origin	Length	Course	Caliber
SIEA	Direct origin from the common femoral artery	Long	Medial course	≥1.5 mm
DIEA	Not relevant (NR)	NR	Medial course and lack of intramuscular component	≥1 mm
DIEA perforators				
Intramuscular segment	Origin from type I or medial row type II/III DIEA	Short	No medial or (especially) lateral deviation	≥1 mm
Subfascial segment	Absent subfascial segment preferred	Absence preferred	Absence preferred	≥1 mm
Subcutaneous segment	Within a 4 cm arc around and below the umbilicus	NR	NR	≥1 mm

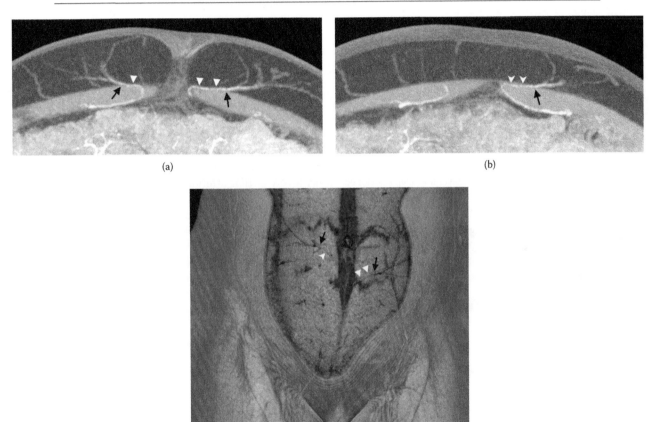

FIGURE 8.28

Sequential 20 mm axial MIP (a and b), and frontal coronal VRT with anterior clip plane (c) showing a paramedian DIEA perforator on the left and a deep inferior epigastric artery (DIEA) perforator on the right with long intramuscular course. Both perforators have a long subfascial segment (arrowheads). Arrows mark the site where the perforators penetrate the anterior rectus fascia.

8.5.2.5 Desirable Deep Inferior Epigastric Vein and Perforator, and Superficial Inferior Epigastric Vein Features

Inadequate venous drainage is the most common cause of DIEP flap failure [27]. The DIEV and the perforator vein accompanying the chosen DIEA perforator drain the DIEP flap by communicating with the SIEV. DIEV and perforator caliber should also be at least 1 mm in diameter, preferably with large communications with the SIEV. A large caliber SIEV is preferred, as are communications across the midline (especially for large flaps), not only for adequate flap drainage, but also for potential salvage surgery in cases of venous congestion. The SIEV is occasionally used as a primary venous anastomosis.

8.5.3 CT Technique

The aim of CT angiography of the abdominal wall is to capture a true arterial phase without venous contamination—particularly of the DIEV and associated

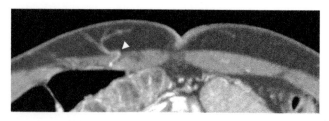

FIGURE 8.29
A 20 mm axial MIP showing favorable DIEA perforator (arrowhead) with large calibre and short, straight intramuscular segment.

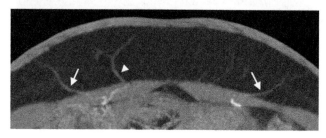

FIGURE 8.30
A 30 mm axial MIP showing surgically unfavorable deep inferior epigastric artery perforators. They have a long intramuscular segment with medial (arrowhead) or lateral deviation (arrows).

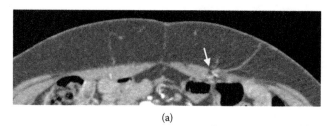

(a)

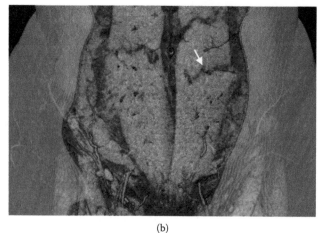

(b)

FIGURE 8.31
Thin axial MIP (A) and frontal coronal VRT with anterior clip plane (B) demonstrating a musculotendinous junction perforator (arrow). Note that the musculotendinous junctions are visible prominently on the VRT as a red color.

perforators—so as to minimize misinterpreting an isolated large venous perforator or one accompanied by a tiny arterial perforator as a large DIEA perforator (Figures 8.27 and 8.32). Given that large perforator veins (often visualized as unopacified on arterial phase CT) usually accompany large DIEA perforators, finding adequate venous drainage is rarely an issue for the surgeon [21]. The SIEV, its branches, and communications with the perforating veins are well seen on a true arterial phase study as they lie within subcutaneous fat.

Consistently achieving pure arterial phase imaging of the DIEA and its perforators is quite difficult as rapid mixing of arterial and venous blood at the vascular plexus overlying Scarpa's fascia backfills the DIEV and its tributaries early. The most robust technique proposed is that by Phillips et al. [24], which is described here (Table 8.3). As the DIEA and SIEA arise at the groin and course superiorly (flowing in a caudocranial direction), the optimal technique is to bolus trigger (100 HU threshold) the scan at the femoral artery and to scan in the caudocranial direction, thus chasing the contrast bolus. A low radiation dose technique is preferable, and therefore, it is imperative that a high iodine delivery rate (e.g., nonionic iodinated contrast 350–370 mg·mL^{-1} delivered intravenously at 4 mL·s^{-1}, equivalent to 300 mg·mL^{-1} at 5 mL·s^{-1}) be used to achieve vascular attenuation sufficient to reliably observe the intramuscular segment of DIEA perforators.

The patient should be scanned with loose clothing (to avoid distortion of the abdominal wall) in the supine position (mirroring the intraoperative position). Limiting the scan range is the most important factor in radiation dose minimization. The superior limit need not extend beyond 4 cm above the umbilicus (the superior margin of the surgical field) and the inferior limit need not extend below the mid portion of the pubic symphysis (to ensure coverage of the origin of the SIEA). This should yield an average scan range of 30 cm. Using low dose acquisition parameters tailored to the patient's body habitus (e.g., 120 kVp tube voltage and 180–200 mAs tube current), an average effective patient dose of 6 mSv can be achieved [23,28].

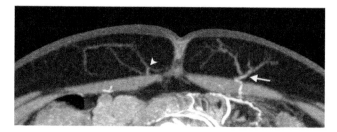

FIGURE 8.32
Axial 20 mm section maximum intensity projection shows a unopacified deep inferior epigastric vein perforator on the right (arrowhead) without accompanying artery, and a deep inferior epigastric artery perforator on the left (arrow) with accompanying unopacified deep inferior epigastric vein perforator.

TABLE 8.3

Scan Technique for CT Angiography of the Abdominal Wall

	Optimum Technique/Parameters
Collimation (mm)	Minimum possible (preferably ≤ 0.6)
Tube voltage (kV)	120
Tube current (mAs)	180–200
Rotation time (second)	Minimum possible (preferably ≤ 0.5)
Reconstruction section thickness (mm)	Minimum possible (with 20% slice overlap if image data set is not isotropic)
Bolus trigger	Trigger at the common femoral artery with 100 HU threshold
Iodine delivery rate (nonionic contrast)	350–370 mg·mL^{-1} delivered at 4 mL·s^{-1} or 300 mg·mL^{-1} at 5 mL·s^{-1}
Scanning direction	Caudal to cranial
Scan range	Pubic symphysis to 4 cm above the umbilicus (approximately 30 cm)

TABLE 8.4

Optimal Image Display Types for Vessel Characterization

Vessel	Feature	Optimal Image Display Type
SIEA	Caliber	Thin axial MIP images (10 mm) or the image data set
	Course and length	VRT or thick coronal MIP images
DIEA	Course and DIEA type	Thick coronal MIP images
	Caliber	Thick axial MIP images (20 mm)
DIEV and perforator	Caliber	Thick axial MIP images (20 and 50 mm)
SIEV	Caliber and location	VRT images
DIEA perforator		
Intramuscular segment	Origin, course, and length	Thick axial MIP images (20 and 50 mm)
Subfascial segment	Course	Thick axial MIP and VRT images
Subcutaneous segment	Origin	VRT images
	Caliber	Thick axial MIP and VRT images

8.5.4 Data Presentation to the Surgeon

Postprocessed images with annotations added by the radiologist are the most accurate and efficient way to present the data. These images should be formatted in a way that makes them usable by the surgeon as an intraoperative map. A CT workstation (thinnest possible reconstruction slice thickness image data set) is used to create axial and coronal maximum intensity projection (MIP) and volume rendered technique (VRT) images that best provide the surgeon with the information necessary to plan for breast free flap reconstruction, as detailed by Phillips et al. Their paper contains a web link (http://radiology.rsnajnls.org/cgi/content/full/249/1/32/DC1) to movies showing how these are obtained [24]. Table 8.4 summarizes which image reformats optimally display the relevant SIEA, DIEA, and perforator features.

The caliber of the SIEA is best obtained from the image data set or thin axial MIPs (10 mm). The course and length of the SIEA are best shown on VRT images (or coronal MIPs). The caliber and any intramuscular course of the DIEA are best shown on thick axial MIPs (20 mm). The course and DIEA type are best shown on coronal MIPs. The origin, course, and length of the intramuscular segment of DIEA perforators and DIEV and perforator caliber are all best appreciated on thick axial MIPs (20 mm, and 50 mm overlapping every 20 mm for vessels with a craniocaudal extent greater than 20 mm) (Figures 8.29 through 8.31). The subfascial segment and caliber of the subcutaneous segment are best viewed using a combination of thick axial MIP and VRT images (Figures 8.28 and 8.31). The origin of the subcutaneous segment (where the vessels penetrate the anterior rectus sheath) relative to the umbilicus and SIEV caliber are best displayed on VRT images (Figures 8.28, 8.31, and 8.33).

The VRT technique used is optimized for viewing the subfascial and subcutaneous segments of the DIEA perforators as a two-dimensional representation of three-dimensional information. This is best achieved using at least two colors, making the subcutaneous fat completely transparent with partly translucent skin surface [24]. Real-time manipulation of the VRT displayed volume with clip planes and/or using volume-cropping techniques, and occasional whole volume rotation is used to define any perforator subfascial segments and the subcutaneous segment origins. Using real-time anterior clip plane/volume cropping to identify where DIEA perforators penetrate the anterior rectus sheath allows each vessel to be marked on a frontal coronal VRT image (mirroring the orientation of the patient during surgery) (Figure 8.33). The location of the perforators relative to the umbilicus is best documented by superimposing a scaled grid overlay with the (0,0) point of the axis centered over the umbilicus. Thus, a "perforator map" is created that the surgeon can use perioperatively to mark suitable perforators on the patient's skin (Figure 8.33). By converting the VRT perforator map into a thick MIP volume, the relationship between the perforators' exit site through the anterior rectal fascia and the associated DIEA trunks can be identified, providing a quick overview of the degree of medial-lateral perforator intramuscular segment deviation (Figure 8.34).

If the radiologist and the referring surgeon have a close and mutual understanding of the preferences for DIEP flap reconstruction, it is possible to just mark large perforators in sequential order of likely surgical preference [26]. However, some surgeons prefer to be made aware of all identifiable perforators, particularly those near the preferred perforator. In this situation, it is necessary to differentiate large DIEA perforators (that might be used for the flap) from submillimeter vessels on the VRT perforator map by using markers of different color (Figure 8.33). Finally, it is important to teach referring surgeons on how to obtain the information they require from the various images and reformats that they are provided with, as it is very difficult to clearly and concisely convey all information required in a radiology report.

An alternative to using a CT workstation and producing MIP and VRT images is intraoperative stereotactic image-guided navigation using preoperative CT image data of perforators for DIEP flap reconstruction, first described by Rozen et al. in 2008 [29]. It is expensive and much more difficult to perform than similar techniques used for neurosurgery, given the lack of bony anatomical landmarks on the anterior abdominal wall, and is therefore not widely used at this time.

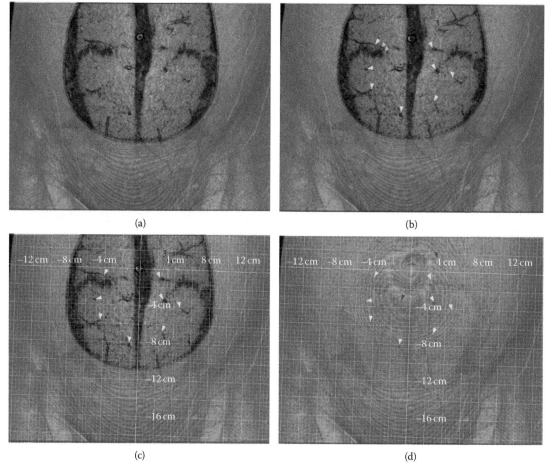

(a)

(b)

(c)

(d)

FIGURE 8.33

Steps in creation of a surgical "Perforator Map." Frontal coronal volume rendered technique with an anterior clip plane is used to remove the skin, revealing the subcutaneous and subfascial course of deep inferior epigastric artery perforators (a). Subfascial segments are identified (green arrowheads). The site where the perforators penetrate the anterior rectus sheath are marked, differentiating small (< 1mm; yellow arrowheads) from large perforators (blue arrowheads) (b). A scaled grid is overlaid, centered at the umbilicus and rotated to align with the pubic symphysis (not shown), allowing distances relative to the umbilicus to be calculated for each perforator (c). Anterior clip plane is removed, leaving the "Perforator Map" (d).

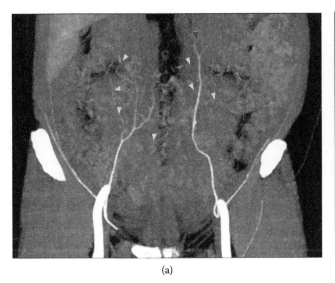
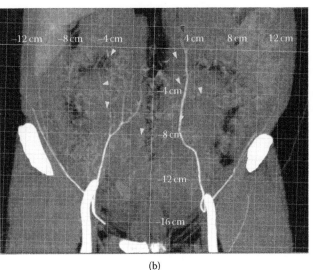

(a)   (b)

FIGURE 8.34
Same patient as for Figure 8.29. Volume rendered technique volume is now converted into a thick volume MIP, allowing identification of the deep inferior epigastric artery (DIEA) trunk(s) location within the rectus muscle and position relative to the associated perforators' exit site through the anterior rectus sheath (a). The patient has a type III DIEA on the right and a type I DIEA on the left. The scaled grid overlay is reapplied, allowing distances to be calculated (b). Note the alignment of the scaled grid with the pubic symphysis.

References

1. Yu JS, Kim KW, Lee HJ et al. (2001) Urachal remnant diseases: spectrum of CT and US findings. *Radiographics* 21:451–61.
2. Burkhardt JH, Arshanskiy Y, Munson JL et al. (2011) Diagnosis of inguinal region hernias with axial CT: the lateral crescent sign and other key findings. *Radiographics* 31:E1–12.
3. Emby DJ and Aoun G. (2003) CT technique for suspected anterior abdominal wall hernia. *AJR Am J Roentgenol* 181:431–3.
4. Fataar S. (2011) CT of inguinal canal lipomas and fat-containing inguinal hernias. *J Med Imaging Radiat Oncol* 55:485–92.
5. Heller CA, Marucci DD, Dunn T et al. (2002) Inguinal canal "lipoma". *Clin Anat* 15:280–5.
6. Carilli S, Alper A, and Emre A. (2004) Inguinal cord lipomas. *Hernia* 8:252–4.
7. Read RC and Schaefer RF. (2000) Lipoma of the spermatic cord, fatty herniation, liposarcoma. *Hernia* 4:149–54.
8. Nasr AO, Tormey S, and Walsh TN. (2005) Lipoma of the cord and round ligament: an overlooked diagnosis? *Hernia* 9:245–7.
9. Aguirre DA, Casola G, and Sirlin C. (2004) Abdominal wall hernias: MDCT findings. *AJR Am J Roentgenol* 183:681–90.
10. Zarvan NP, Lee FT, Jr., Yandow DR et al. (1995) Abdominal hernias: CT findings. *AJR Am J Roentgenol* 164:1391–5.
11. Aguirre DA, Santosa AC, Casola G et al. (2005) Abdominal wall hernias: imaging features, complications, and diagnostic pitfalls at multi-detector row CT. *Radiographics* 25:1501–20.

12. Macari M and Megibow A. (2001) Imaging of suspected acute small bowel obstruction. *Semin Roentgenol* 36:108–17.
13. Teo HE, Peh WC, and Shek TW. (2005) Case 84: desmoid tumor of the abdominal wall. *Radiology* 236:81–4.
14. Matsui Y, Ohara H, Ichioka K et al. (2004) Abdominal wall metastasis after retroperitoneoscopic assisted total nephroureterectomy for renal pelvic cancer. *J Urol* 171:793.
15. Goshen E, Davidson T, Aderka D et al. (2006) PET/CT detects abdominal wall and port site metastases of colorectal carcinoma. *Br J Radiol* 79:572–7.
16. Alonso-Burgos A, Garcia-Tutor E, Bastarrika G et al. (2006) Preoperative planning of deep inferior epigastric artery perforator flap reconstruction with multislice-CT angiography: imaging findings and initial experience. *J Plast Reconstr Aesthet Surg* 59:585–93.
17. Masia J, Clavero JA, Larranaga JR et al. (2006) Multidetector-row computed tomography in the planning of abdominal perforator flaps. *J Plast Reconstr Aesthet Surg* 59:594–9.
18. Cina A, Salgarello M, Barone-Adesi L et al. (2010) Planning breast reconstruction with deep inferior epigastric artery perforating vessels: multidetector CT angiography versus color Doppler US. *Radiology* 255:979–87.
19. Scott JR, Liu D, Said H et al. (2010) Computed tomographic angiography in planning abdomen-based microsurgical breast reconstruction: a comparison with color duplex ultrasound. *Plast Reconstr Surg* 125:446–53.
20. Rozen WM, Phillips TJ, Ashton MW et al. (2008) Preoperative imaging for DIEA perforator flaps: a comparative study of computed tomographic angiography and doppler ultrasound. *Plast Reconstr Surg* 121:1–8.

21. Clavero JA, Masia J, Larranaga J et al. (2008) MDCT in the preoperative planning of abdominal perforator surgery for postmastectomy breast reconstruction. *AJR Am J Roentgenol* 191:670–6.

22. Smit JM, Dimopoulou A, Liss AG et al. (2009) Preoperative CT angiography reduces surgery time in perforator flap reconstruction. *J Plast Reconstr Aesthet Surg* 62:1112–7.

23. Ghattaura A, Henton J, Jallali N et al. (2010) One hundred cases of abdominal-based free flaps in breast reconstruction. The impact of preoperative computed tomographic angiography. *J Plast Reconstr Aesthet Surg* 63:1597–601.

24. Phillips TJ, Stella DL, Rozen WM et al. (2008) Abdominal wall CT angiography: a detailed account of a newly established preoperative imaging technique. *Radiology* 249:32–44.

25. Spiegel AJ and Khan FN. (2007) An Intraoperative algorithm for use of the SIEA flap for breast reconstruction. *Plast Reconstr Surg* 120:1450–9.

26. Karunanithy N, Rose V, Lim AK et al. (2011) CT angiography of inferior epigastric and gluteal perforating arteries before free flap breast reconstruction. *Radiographics* 31:1307–19.

27. Cina A, Barone-Adesi L, Salgarello M et al. (2009) Multidetector CT evaluation of abdominal wall for breast reconstruction: take a look at the veins. *Radiology* 251:947–8; author reply 948.

28. Midgley SM, Einsiedel PF, Phillips TJ et al. (2011) Justifying the use of abdominal wall computed tomographic angiography in deep inferior epigastric artery perforator flap planning. *Ann Plast Surg* 67:457–9.

29. Rozen WM, Ashton MW, Stella DL et al. (2008) Stereotactic image-guided navigation in the preoperative imaging of perforators for DIEP flap breast reconstruction. *Microsurgery* 28:417–23.

9

Diseases of the Colon and Rectum

Carlo Nicola De Cecco, Davide Bellini, Giuseppe Muscogiuri, Marco Rengo,
Franco Iafrate, and Andrea Laghi

CONTENTS

9.1 Introduction

Colorectal diseases include several pathologies with a broad symptomatic spectrum. Moreover, disease overlap and dubious findings represent a frequent condition. For this reason, colorectal imaging has played since the beginning a pivotal role in disease detection and characterization.

In particular, the role of multi-detector computed tomography (MDCT) in patients with suspected colic disease has increased over time following technological innovations, and today this imaging technique plays a fundamental role in the study of the colon and rectum.

A unique feature of MDCT is its ability to accurately show the bowel wall as well as the pericolic soft tissues and adjacent structures. Therefore, abdominal CT is a highly sensitive method for the detection of intramural disease and extraluminal extension of colonic diseases.

CT examination involved different acquisition protocols related to clinical questions. In particular, an emergency condition (e.g., diverticulitis and ischemic colitis [IC]) needs a protocol that provides a fast scan of the abdomen and pelvis, without any preliminary patient preparation; on the other hand, in the identification of a suspected colon cancer or in secondary prevention (e.g., identification of an adenomatous polyp), it is required to perform a CT colonography (CTC) with accurate patient preparation.

This chapter reviews the different MDCT techniques available in colorectal evaluation and describes the imaging features of neoplastic and inflammatory conditions that affect this organ, with emphasis on distinctive imaging patterns that may help radiologists to distinguish specific disease.

9.2 Technical Aspects

9.2.1 Multi-Detector CT

MDCT is today the imaging modality of choice in the study of the abdomen. The rapid technological development has resulted in obvious benefit of the study technique. MDCT has become increasingly refined and dependent on the clinical query of the examination. However, inappropriate patient preparation and incorrect choice of the acquisition protocol are the most frequent causes of diagnostic error.

Routine abdominal CT is usually performed after oral and intravenous administration of medium contrast. If specific colonic disease is suspected, it is important to adequately opacify the entire colon. Therefore, oral medium contrast can be administered the night before the examination; this process ensures that the medium contrast has reached the colon, and it is essential for optimal organ visualization.

In urgent cases or in patients in whom limited rectosigmoid disease is suspected, positive contrast agents can be administered via the rectum (500 mL medium contrast is necessary to fill the colon).

A topogram should be obtained to confirm adequate colonic opacification before the start of the CT study. Administration of air or water through a rectal tube to distend the colon has also been reported to be helpful. Unlike positive contrast agents, air and water do not interfere with virtual colonoscopy or three-dimensional (3D) CT angiography.

Although administration of intravenous medium contrast is not essential for diagnosis of many colonic conditions, it is often helpful, especially if extracolonic extension of disease is also suspected [1].

Parenchymal enhancement is governed by the relationship of total iodine dose versus total volume of distribution (intravascular and interstitial spaces).

Several studies [2,3] showed that it is necessary to deliver an adequate amount of iodine, in the range of 500–600 mgI·kg^{-1} of total body water, to achieve an optimal parenchymal enhancement (50–60 HU).

Precontrast scan is useful to detect intraluminal bleeding, clots, and dystrophic calcification. Arterial phase should be obtained with bolus tracking technique, and it can be necessary to evaluate arterial vascularization especially in case of bowel ischemia or bleeding assessment. Portal phase must be obtained after 40 seconds from the arterial phase, and it is necessary to accurately evaluate the intestinal wall.

Equilibrium phase, about 3 minutes after intravenous injection of medium contrast, is mandatory if hepatic lesions are detected.

The abdomen should be routinely imaged from the diaphragm to the symphysis pubis.

To properly visualize the entire colon, a submillimetric collimation is suggested to perform multiplanar reconstruction. In any case, a thickness <3 mm is considered adequate.

9.2.2 CT Colonography

CTC is a colonic imaging modality based on a volumetric CT of the abdomen and pelvis where the colon, differently by a conventional CT acquisition, has been previously cleansed and distended with air or carbon dioxide. CT dataset is then edited off-line to produce multiplanar reconstructions and 3D endoscopic-like views (Figure 9.1) [4,5].

Bowel preparation represents a critical step since excessive residual stools and/or fluid may mimic or hide a colonic lesion. Current recommendations for bowel preparation require full bowel cleansing, similar to colonoscopy, in association with fecal/fluid tagging. But, ongoing research is dedicated to develop reduced bowel preparations and ultimately a preparation-free CTC, with the aim to minimize patient discomfort and to increase compliance to colorectal cancer screening; in the latter cases the use of fecal/fluid tagging is mandatory.

Patient preparation for scanning consists of air insufflation, administration of an antiperistaltic drug and, if necessary, intravenous injection of iodinated contrast medium (Tables 9.1 and 9.2).

The use of a spasmolytic agent (either hyoscine butylbromine, Buscopan®, or glucagon) is particularly useful in colonic spasm, typically in sigmoid colon, and in severe diverticular disease [6]. Buscopan® has several advantages: it is more effective than glucagon in reducing segmental collapse [7]; it has a better safety profile; it is cheaper, and it may reduce the pain associated with colonic distension.

Dual patient positioning is mandatory for standard CTC. This is required to optimize distention of all colonic segments so that solid or fluid residues will be redistributed by gravity, revealing previously obscured colonic mucosa.

Data acquisition protocols for CTC are in continuous evolution, in parallel CT scanner progress. A 16 rows MDCT scanner should now be considered as the minimum requirement.

The use of thin collimations for CTC is mandatory, since the size of detectable lesions depends fundamentally on this parameter, and should be <3 mm and >1 mm, according to the CT scan available.

Regarding scanning parameters, the kilovoltage influences image noise, contrast resolution, and dose delivered to the patient, but also density values of

TABLE 9.1

Preparation of CTC

Full Bowel Preparation	
"Wet" Colon	**"Dry" Colon**
Low-residue diet (for 3 days before the exam)	
The day before the exam	
• 4 L (34.8 g of polyethylene glycol (PEG) × 500 mL water) of PEG solution to drink at 15:00 PM OR • 2 L (34.8 g PEG × 500 mL water) of PEG solution to drink at 15:00 PM + • 5 mg bisacodyl tablets at 19:00 PM	• 5 mg bisacodyl tablets before 11:00 AM • A single dose of 45 mL sodium phosphate solution or a double dose of 296 mL magnesium citrate solution divided into two discrete doses separated by 3 hours, with the first dose taken 3–6 hours after the bisacodyl tablets

Dinner: clear liquid diet

+ Fecal/fluid tagging

Administration of positive oral contrast agent (barium or iodine):
 – Iodine: 60 mL at night on the day before the exam
 – Barium (2% w/v): 250 mL at night on the day before the exam

TABLE 9.2

Reduced Preparation of CTC

Reduced Bowel Preparation Scheme
Low-residue diet (for 3 days before the exam)
The day before the examination: • Oral intake of 80 mL diatrizoate dimeglumine/iopamidol at 15:00 PM • Oral intake of 80 mL diatrizoate dimeglumine/iopamidol at 17:00 PM • Drinking at least 2 L water during the day
Dinner: clear liquid diet

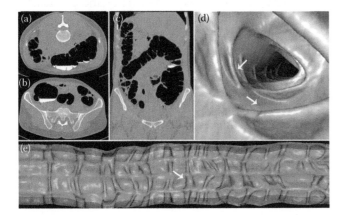

FIGURE 9.1
Computed tomography (CT) colonographic image. (a, b) Two-dimensional view in prone and supine position; tagged fluid stool are clearly visible; (c) MPR in coronal plane; (d) three-dimensional endoluminal view with colonic haustra (arrow); (e) virtual dissection of the colon.

different structures. For these reasons, it is better to keep kilovoltage at a fixed value, that is, 120 in normal-size individuals and 140 in obese patients [8]. In contrast, milliampere second (mAs) is varied according to scan protocol; in screening, CTC low mAs should be used for both prone and supine scans (50–100 mAs) (Table 9.3).

Image analysis is performed on dedicated off-line work-stations suitable for data management and reconstruction. It means powerful computers equipped with dedicated softwares, providing the radiologist with different viewing options, both two-dimensional (2D) and 3D.

Advanced visualization softwares (virtual dissection) allow the creation of a 3D model where the colon is virtually unrolled and displayed as a flat 3D rendering of the mucosal surface, similar to a gross pathologic specimen. Virtual dissection may improve reader confidence, speed-up the reading process, and increase efficiency but should be used only by readers with experience of associated distortion [9]. To improve sensitivity, especially in inexpert readers, as well as to reduce interobserver variability and perception errors, computer-aided detection (CAD) softwares are now available.

CAD is able to automatically detect the locations of suspicious polyps and masses on CTC, based on morphology, texture, density, and other math analysis.

Conventionally, CAD acts as "second reader" by pointing out abnormalities to the radiologist that otherwise might have been missed; the final diagnosis in made by radiologist.

In the end, clarification and standardization of the results in CTC reporting is mandatory to assist patients, referring physicians, and comparing examination results and reports generated in different centers.

Regarding exam indications, CTC has been addend officially on the list of methods available for screening of colorectal cancer (CRC), thanks to its several advantages: high diagnostic accuracy, similar to optical colonoscopy, high patient comfort (reduced bowel preparation, lack of sedation), and security (no complications) [10].

CTC is also considered the method of choice for the study of the colon in cases of incomplete optical colonoscopy because of dolichocolon, intolerance of the patient, intestinal spasms stenosing, or obstructing the colonic lumen. It is also recommended in elderly patients or in poor general condition and for the evaluation of diverticular disease, to provide a precise map of disease extension and severity.

9.2.3 CT Perfusion

CT perfusion (CTp) is an advanced CT technique that allows functional evaluation of tissue vascularity, measuring the temporal changes in tissue density after intravenous injection of a contrast medium bolus using a series of dynamically acquired CT images [11]. Even if it is primarily considered as a research tool, perfusion CT has found applications in oncology as well as strokes [12]. It provides quantitative data regarding perfusion parameters; might differentiate tumor tissues based on perfusion behavior; and therefore can enhance the ability to monitor chemo and radiation therapy, plan biopsies, and grade tumors.

The fundamental principle of perfusion CT is based on the temporal changes in tissue attenuation after intravenous administration of iodinated contrast medium.

In rectal cancer, perfusion CT enables the assessment of tumor vascularity. Several studies reported, in rectal cancer, a significant increment in blood flow (BF), blood volume (BV), mean transit time (MTT) and permeability compared to normal rectal wall. Moreover, tumor permeability surface and BV correlate positively with micro-vessel density and may reflect the microvascularity of colorectal tumors [13]. For these reasons, CTp has a potential role in monitoring the effects neoadjuvant chemoradiotherapy and predicting the response of rectal cancer.

For example, several studies reported that tumor with initial high BF and short MTT values tended to respond poorly to neoadjuvant therapy [14,15]. However, further studies are mandatory before the introduction of this technique in routine clinical practice.

9.2.4 Dual-Energy CT

Basic principle of dual-energy CT (DECT) is the application of two distinct energy settings making able to distinguish materials with different molecular

TABLE 9.3

Scanning Parameters of CTC

Scanning Parameters	
Asymptomatic Patient	**Symptomatic Patient**
1. Scout view	
Essential to assess bowel distension	
2. Prone scan	
Collimation: >0.625 mm, <3 mm	Collimation: >0.625 mm, <3 mm
Pitch: 1–1.5	Pitch: 1–1.5
Reconstruction thickness: 1.25 mm	Reconstruction thickness: 1.25 mm
kV: 120 (140 in obese subjects)	kV: 120
mAs: <50	mAs: <50
3. Supine scan	
Collimation: >0.625 mm, <3 mm	Post contrast scan: Portal phase, equilibrium phase (only for the liver, if necessary)
Pitch: 1–1.5	Use automated tube current modulation (ACTM) and scanning parameters as in conventional CT scan
Reconstruction thickness: 1.25 mm	
kV: 120 (140 in obese subjects)	
mAs: <50	

composition on the basis of their attenuation profiles. The result is the transition from CT density-based imaging to material-specific or spectral imaging. Several articles have investigated the role of DECT imaging in solid abdominal organs, especially in liver lesion detection and characterization [16–18].

Recently, a possible role of DECT in small bowel ischemia detection has also been described [19]. Iodine map can easily depict the absence of iodinated contrast medium in the bowel wall that can be useful in detecting ischemia before the onset of wall modifications. The same approach could also be applied to the identification of another risky and life-threatening vascular condition represented by colonic ischemia.

9.3 Colonic Diseases

9.3.1 Colorectal Cancer

CRC is the third most common type of nonskin cancer in men and women. In United States, the rate of new cases and deaths is decreasing; however, it is estimated that there are nearly 1.2 million men and women living in the United States with a previous diagnosis of CRC [20]. Age is a well-known risk factor. The median age at diagnosis is 68 for males and 72 for females. Numerous lines of epidemiologic evidence support the role of dietary factors. Lifestyle factors such as physical activity, alcohol intake, and tobacco are also positively correlated with the risk of colorectal carcinoma [21].

Genetically, CRC represents a complex disease, and genetic alterations are often associated with progression from premalignant lesion (adenomatous polyps) to invasive adenocarcinoma. The early event is a mutation of *adenomatous polyposis coli* gene, which was first discovered in individuals with familial adenomatous polyposis (FAP), a rare hereditary syndrome accounting for only about 1% of cases of colon cancer (FAP).

Colonic polyps are slow-growing overgrowths of the colonic mucosa that carry a small risk of becoming malignant. They are highly prevalent in the general population, greater than 10% in most areas [22,23].

Several studies indicate that Afro-American subjects have a higher incidence and an earlier onset of colorectal carcinoma. Males appear to have a moderately higher colonic polyp incidence than females.

Patients with isolated colonic polyps are usually asymptomatic but can experience overt or occult colonic bleeding. Colonic polyps can progress to carcinoma over several years. Morbidity from colonic polyps is related to complications, such as intestinal obstruction, bleeding, and diarrhea. Bleeding can be frank hematochezia but is often chronic and goes unnoticed by the patient.

Colon cancer can have many symptoms (changes in bowel habits, constipation, diarrhea, blood in stools, abdominal discomfort, and cramps). However, in the early stages, people with colon cancer often have no symptoms at all. Early detection through widely applied screening programs is the most important factor in the recent decline of CRC in developed countries.

In CRC screening and polyps detection, CTC has two roles: one present and the other potential. The present role is the integration into established screening programs as a replacement for barium enema in incomplete colonoscopy [24–26]. The potential role is the use of CTC as a first-line screening method together with fecal occult blood test, sigmoidoscopy, and colonoscopy. However, although CTC has been officially endorsed for CRC screening of average-risk individuals by different scientific societies including the American Cancer Society, the American College of Radiology, and the U.S. Multisociety Task Force on Colorectal Cancer, other entities, such as the U.S. Preventive Services Task Force, have considered the evidence insufficient to justify its use as a mass screening method. Nevertheless, multiple advantages exist for using CTC as a CRC screening test: high accuracy, full evaluation of the colon in virtually all patients, noninvasiveness, safety, patient comfort, and detection of extracolonic findings.

Moreover, despite the good results, there are still some open issues under debate. These are the significance of diminutive (<6 mm) polyps and the management of intermediate (6–9 mm) lesions.

The frequency of advanced lesions among patients whose largest polyp was ≤5 mm, 6–9 mm, <10 mm, and >10 mm in size was 0.9%, 4.9%, 1.7%, and 73.5%, respectively.

From a cost-effectiveness point of view, detection and removal of all polyps including those <5 mm, would be very inefficient, with a cost per year of life gained >$460,000 [27,28], absolutely unacceptable in terms of cost-effectiveness.

It is also true that this approach, not removing diminutive polyps, necessitates an extensive education of patients and physicians. In fact, according to a recently published survey [29], the majority of patients, physicians, and gastroenterologists would not choose to follow up small polyps identified by CTC with conventional colonoscopy because of the fear of missing precancerous lesions.

In case of suspected or confirmed CRC, CTC should be performed with intravenous administration of medium contrast. MDCT is valuable in planning surgery for colon cancer because it can show regional extension of tumor as well as adenopathy and distant metastases. Moreover, MDCT enables the accurate representation of the abdominal vascular anatomy that can be helpful in preoperative planning [30,31]. Radiology should report the tumor staging according to tumor node metastasis classification (Table 9.4).

9.3.1.1 CT Findings

9.3.1.1.1 Polyps

In CTC, there are two primary techniques for data interpretation: a primary 2D approach and a primary 3D approach. In 2D view, it is necessary to evaluate a lesion with multiple window width and level settings during CTC, thereby facilitating the identification of gas, high-attenuation material, and adipose tissue of polypoid lesions.

In 3D approach, including virtual dissection, sessile and flat polyps appear flame- or pea-shaped, whereas pedunculated polyps are more varied and may be flame-, club-, or bizarre-shaped.

Colonic or pedunculated polyp mobility can change the morphology of polyps with all display techniques, including virtual dissection. This change in appearance can lead to mischaracterization of the polyp as mobile stool (Figure 9.2).

9.3.1.1.2 Cancer

CT typically shows a discrete soft-tissue mass that narrows the colonic lumen. Large masses may undergo central necrosis and thus appear as a soft-tissue mass with central low attenuation or rarely air attenuation.

Local extension of tumor appears as an extracolic mass or simply as thickening and infiltration of pericolic fat. In addition, the loss of fat planes between the colon and adjacent organs is suggestive of extracolic spread. Complications of primary colonic malignancies such as obstruction, perforation, and fistula can be readily visualized with CT (Figure 9.3).

9.3.2 Diverticular Disease

9.3.2.1 Clinical Aspects and CT Indications

Diverticular disease is an increasingly common condition. There is a strong relationship between prevalence of disease and age (5% at 40 years, 30% at 60 years, and 65% at 85 years); longstanding low dietary fiber; increased consumption of red meat, salt, fat, and some hereditary disease (Marfan's and Ehler–Danlos syndromes). Diverticulosis can involve the entire gastrointestinal tract but in "westernized" population, often occurs in distal colon with involved of sigmoid colon as much as 95%; in contrast, in Asian countries, is more common the right colon involvement. In most patients, diverticular disease is asymptomatic; however, diverticulitis is developed in the 10%–30% of cases. Population with diverticulitis can be divided in two groups: simple (75%; generally responsive to medical therapy) and complicated diverticulitis (25%; associated with development of hemorrhage, abscess, perforation, obstruction, or fistula) [32]. In the setting of acute abdomen, CT is indicated when diverticulitis is suspected.

TABLE 9.4

American Joint Committee on Cancer Staging for Colon Cancer

Primary Tumors (T)	Regional Lymph Nodes (N)	Distant Metastasis (M)
Tx: Tumor cannot be assessed	Nx: Lymph nodes cannot be assessed	M0: No distant metastasis
T0: No evidence of primary tumor	N0: No regional lymph nodes metastasis	M1 Distant metastasis
T1s: Carcinoma in situ: intraepithelial or invasion of lamina proprial	N1a: 1 metastatic lymph node	M1a Metastasis confined to one organ or site (for example, liver, lung, ovary, nonregional node)
T1: Tumor invades submucosa	N1b: Metastasis in 2–3 regional lymph nodes	M1b Metastases in more than one organ/site or the peritoneum
	N1c: Tumor deposit(s) in the subserosa, mesentery, or nonperitonealized pericolic or perirectal tissues without regional nodal metastasis	
T2: Tumor invades muscularis propria	N2: Metastasis in 4 or more regional lymph nodes	
T3: Tumor invades through the muscularis propria into pericolorectal tissues	N2a: Metastasis in 4–6 regional lymph nodes	
	N2b: Metastasis in 7 or more regional lymph nodes	
T4a: Tumor penetrates to the surface of the visceral peritoneum		
T4b: Tumor directly invades or is adherent to other organs or structures		

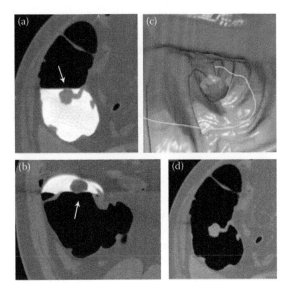

FIGURE 9.2

(a) Scan with patient in the prone position shows the presence of a pedunculated polyp in the ascending colon (arrow), covered by luminal fluid opacified by the oral iodinated contrast medium. (b) Scan with patient in the supine position. The large pedunculated polyp (arrow) is still completely covered by the luminal fluid and is visible only thanks to the opacification of the fluid itself by the oral contrast medium. (c) Coronal multiplanar reformation image obtained after electronic cleansing: the application of electronic removal of the opacified fluid, which enables the virtual cleansing of the colon by electronically subtracting the opacified fluid, shows the polypoid lesion with the peduncle. (d) Intraluminal volume rendering reconstruction after electronic cleansing: the polypoid lesions is well visualized within the lumen of the colon.

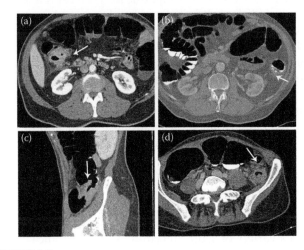

FIGURE 9.3

CT images of colon tumors. (a, b, d) On axial images, the tumor and its extramural extension is clearly visualized (arrows). Enlarged lymph nodes can also be seen. (c) Sagittal reconstruction image shows a lesion (arrow) with stenosis of the lumen.

CT has a sensitivity of 97% and specificity of 100%, with an accuracy of 98% [33] in patients with suspect acute diverticulitis.

Abdominal CT usually is performed after administration of both oral (water-soluble agent suspension) and

TABLE 9.5

CT Staging of Diverticulitis

Radiologic Characteristic	
Stage 0	Inflamed diverticulum contain within the serosa and wall thickening
Stage I	Inflamed diverticulum associated with phlegmon or abscess (<3 mm) confined in mesentery
Stage II	Inflamed diverticulum associated with abscess that invades pelvic structures
Stage III	Inflamed diverticulum associated with abscess extended to retroperitoneum or peritoneal cavity
Stage IV	Diverticulitis complicated with perforation and widespread of feces in peritoneum

intravenous of contrast agent. Good opacification of the colon permits an optimal evaluation of wall thickening, intraluminal or extraluminal air, and other signs of diverticulitis, whereas the opacification of small bowel loops decreases the possibility to confuse adjacent loop for an abscess. Intravenous administration of contrast agent can help in the individuation of inflamed diverticula.

CT scanning should include the whole abdomen, and a collimation <2.5 mm is suggested to obtain multiplanar reconstructions. Diverticular disease stage should be reported by the radiologist to properly address the treatment (Table 9.5) [34].

9.3.2.2 CT Findings

[35] identified two types of findings in diverticular disease using CTC (Figure 9.4):

1. Unequivocal findings
   a. Prediverticulosis: It represents the early stage of disease (diverticular disease without diverticula) and it is caused by myochosis. Mild regular thickening of colonic wall with minimal luminal distortion may be present.
   b. Global wall thickening: Alteration of caliber and haustral abnormalities becomes more significant with progression of myochosis. CT shows thickening >4 mm of colonic segments with short interhaustral segments. CTC shows shrinkage and distortion of lumen.
   c. Diverticulum: Herniation of mucosa and submucosa, where the vasa recta penetrate the circular muscle layer, through muscle layer covered only by serosa. CT images show an air-filled outpouching of the colonic wall. CTC shows diverticular orificium like a dark circumferential ring.
   d. Diverticular Fecalith: Fecal material remains into diverticulum and changes into fecalith

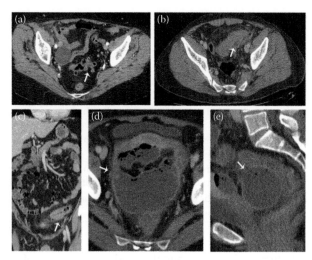

FIGURE 9.4
(a) Diverticula of sigmoid colon (arrow); (b) perisigmoid abscess (arrow) in patient with diverticulitis; (c) circumferential thickening (arrow) in patient with diverticulitis; (d, e) large peridiverticular abscess (arrow).

that looks like a pseudopolypoid lesion. On the axial images, diverticular fecalith show a hyperdense ring with hypodense center. Diverticular fecalith appears on CTC like a polypoid lesion that could be confused with polyps.

e. Inverted diverticulum: Sometimes diverticulum can invert into the lumen of colon and causes bleeding. On axial images, inverted diverticulum looks like a polypoid lesions with aerial part because of umbilication of the inverted part of diverticulum. On CTC, inverted diverticulum appears like a polypoid lesions.

f. Typical findings of diverticulitis: increased attenuation, haziness, and indistinctness of fat around diverticula usually are signs of inflamed diverticula, often associated with arrowhead signs caused by contrast funneled toward the orifice edematous of inflamed diverticulum. In 74%–90% of patients with diverticulitis, a colonic wall thickening is observed (>5 mm; focal or circumferential), whereas 98%–100% of patients present signs of pericolonic inflammation with fluid collections at the root of sigmoid mesentery. Extraluminal air in pericolonic fat can be observed, resulting from microperforation of diverticulum or in abscess.

2. Equivocal findings

a. Polyp-simulating mucosal prolapse syndrome: Sometimes in progression of diverticular disease, the thickening, shortening, and contraction of muscular layer could cause an excess of mucosa prolapsing into lumen of colon; these lesions can cause recurrent bleeding. Axial images and CTC show a polypoid lesions. Sometimes, also conventional colonoscopy has difficulties to distinguish mucosal prolapse from polyps and only histology is diagnostic.

b. Focal thickening: It is caused by fibrosis, inflammation, or tumoral process. Axial images show symmetric or asymmetric wall thickening with pericolonic lymph nodes. CTC is useful to distinguish thickened wall from polyps but not to differentiate inflammation or fibrosis from tumoral lesions.

9.3.3 Intussusception

9.3.3.1 Clinical Aspects and CT Indications

Intussusception is a process in which a segment of intestine invaginates into the adjoining intestinal lumen, causing bowel obstruction. Its estimated incidence is approximately 1 case per 2000 live births and the male-to-female ratio is approximately 3:1.

Adult intussusception is the cause of 1% of all bowel obstructions. The vast majority (95%) of intussusceptions occur in children, whereas only 5% occur in adults.

The pathogenesis of idiopathic intussusception is not well established. It is believed to be secondary to an imbalance in the longitudinal forces along the intestinal wall, frequently caused by a mass acting as a lead point or by a disorganized pattern of peristalsis. There are a lot of leading points to be considered: Meckel diverticulum, enlarged mesenteric lymph node, tumors of the mesentery or of the intestine, lymphoma, polyps, hamartomas, mesenteric or duplication cysts [36], submucosal hematomas, inverted appendiceal stumps, sutures and staples along an anastomosis, and foreign body.

In pediatric patients, signs and symptoms are based on a classic triad: vomiting, abdominal pain, and passage of blood per rectum. Adult patients usually present with a variety of acute, intermittent, and chronic symptoms that make presurgical diagnosis difficult.

The hallmark physical findings in intussusception are a right hypochondrium, sausage-shaped mass and emptiness in the right lower quadrant. Abdominal distention frequently is found if obstruction is complete.

Plain radiographs of the abdomen with the patient in the supine and upright positions are often the first diagnostic step after physical examination. However, plain abdominal radiography reveals signs that suggest intussusception in only 60% of cases [37].

Ultrasonography should be used as a first-line examination for the assessment of possible pediatric intussusception [38].

It has a high diagnostic accuracy with values of sensitivity and specificity, respectively of 97.9% and 97.8%.

CT has also been proposed as a useful tool to diagnose intussusception; the best contribution of CT is related to the possibility of differentiating between lead point and non–lead point intussusception, extremely important in determining the appropriate treatment and potentially able to reduce the prevalence of unnecessary surgery.

9.3.3.2 CT Findings

At CT, intussusception is seen as a soft-tissue mass with a target or ring-shaped appearance on face, or a sausage-like appearance in profile. A variable amount of fat attenuation material can be identified within the mass. Complete versus partial obstruction of the small bowel is determined by the degree of collapse and the amount of the residual contents in the portion of the bowel distal to the obstructed site. Passage of the contrast material through the transition zone to the collapsed distal bowel always indicates incomplete obstruction. Reported CT findings indicating strangulation include thickening and increased attenuation of the affected bowel wall, the "target" or "halo" sign, serrated beak-like narrowing at the site of obstruction, pneumatosis intestinalis, and gas in the portal veins (Figures 9.5 and 9.6).

9.3.4 Volvulus

9.3.4.1 Clinical Aspects and CT Indications

A large-bowel volvulus (LBV) is a twist of the bowel along its own mesentery, often resulting in a closed-loop obstruction. LBV accounts for 5% of all organic large-bowel obstructions and are most common among patients aged between 50 and 60 [39,40].

Genesis of an LBV requires the twist of a mobile loop around a fulcrum point. Mobile segments that can be involved include the sigmoid (60%–75%), transverse colon (5%–10%), and even cecum (25%–40%) [41].

Predisposing factors include congenital or acquired anatomical variations such as a mobile cecum, a long sigma, a history of abdominal surgery, high-fiber diet, and chronic constipation.

During LBV, strangulation of the vascular supply within the twisted mesentery leads to a decreased BF and ischemia of the bowel wall. The consequences of ischemia include mesenteric hemorrhage, intramural hematoma, lack of peristalsis, and distension, finally leading to infarction with perforation.

Clinically, this is an emergency condition. Symptoms are abdominal pain, distention, constipation, and obstipation, often accompanied by nausea, vomiting, and abdominal tenderness. Physical examination shows tympanitic percussion tones and no bowel sounds.

The differential diagnosis of acute abdominal obstruction includes small bowel volvulus, intussusception, Ogilvie's syndrome, diverticulitis, and others. CT is now a first line examination in patients with acute abdomen, and radiologists should be able to recognize the CT appearance of LBV so that the correct diagnosis can be made and catastrophic consequences can be avoided. Moreover, MDCT helps radiologists to assess the severity of the condition by analyzing the twisted loop wall and the mesentery.

9.3.4.2 CT Findings

The diagnostic criteria of an LBV is an abrupt transition between a normal and dilated bowel combined with the

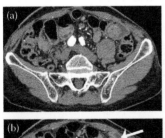
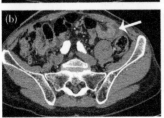
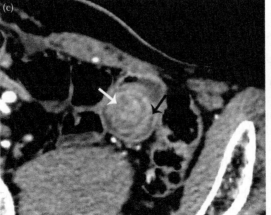
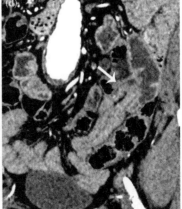

FIGURE 9.5
Small bowel intussusception in a 51-year-old man with recurrent left lower quadrant pain. (a, b, d) Cross-sectional and longitudinal diagrams show a transient intussusception; (c) typical multilayered appearance observed in the invagination of a segment of the gastrointestinal tract (intussusceptum) (white arrows) into an adjacent segment (intussuscipiens) (black arrows).

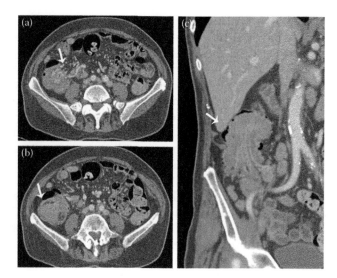

FIGURE 9.6
Large bowel intussusception in patients with intestinal lymphoma. (a, b, c) CT images show invagination of the small bowel distal loop into ascending colon (arrows).

observation of convergence of both ends of the dilated loop toward the fulcrum point. An important sign to look for is the "whirl sign," a whirlpool pattern of concentric structures (twisted intestinal loops, vessels, and mesenteric fat) that represent a torsion mechanism.

When administered, the contrast enema does not go beyond the obstruction site showing an abrupt interruption called "beak sign."

Spontaneous increased attenuation of the large bowel wall is related to transmural hemorrhagic necrosis; the absence or decreased enhancement of the large bowel wall, pneumatosis intestinalis, or thickening of the large bowel wall suggest ischemia.

Prompt recognition of these findings and quick diagnosis of LBV is mandatory, given the high rate of potentially lethal complications.

9.3.5 Inflammatory Bowel Disease

9.3.5.1 Clinical Aspects and CT Indications

Inflammatory bowel disease (IBD) is an idiopathic disease caused by a dysregulated immune response to host intestinal microflora. The two major types of IBD are ulcerative colitis (UC), which is limited to the colon, and Crohn's disease (CD), which can involve any segment of the gastrointestinal tract from the mouth to the anus, with a transmural involvement. There is a genetic predisposition for IBD, and patients with this condition are more prone to the development of malignancy.

The age distribution of newly diagnosed IBD cases is bell-shaped; the peak incidence occurs in people in the early part of the second decade of life. A second, smaller

peak in incidence occurs in patients aged 55–65 and is increasing. Approximately 10% of IBD patients are younger than 18 years.

In UC, inflammation begins in the rectum and extends proximally in an uninterrupted fashion to the proximal colon and could eventually involve the entire length of the large intestine; only mucosa and the submucosa are involved and the rectum is always affected in UC.

CD can affect any portion of the gastrointestinal tract and causes three patterns of involvement: inflammatory disease, strictures, and fistulas. The most important pathologic feature of CD is the transmural involvement.

IBD is a chronic, intermittent disease. Symptoms range from mild to severe during relapses and may disappear or decrease during remissions. In general, symptoms depend on the segment of the intestinal tract involved.

The diagnosis requires a comprehensive physical examination and a review of the patient's history. Various tests, including blood tests, stool examination, endoscopy, biopsies, and imaging studies, help exclude other causes and confirm the diagnosis.

The management of patients with IBD requires evaluation with objective tools, both at the time of diagnosis and throughout the course of the disease, to determine the location, extension, activity, and severity of inflammatory lesions, as well as the potential existence of complications. This information is crucial to select appropriate therapeutic strategies.

Magnetic resonance imaging (MRI), CT, and ultrasound (US) imaging are an adjunct to endoscopy for diagnosis of colonic IBD. MRI and CT have higher sensitivity than US, especially in analyzing deep bowel loops.

Few studies have investigated the role of CT in the UC assessment, finding an overall sensitivity of 74% [42,43]. Other preliminary studies in small samples report good correlation between disease extent by colonoscopy and positron emission tomography (PET)/CT [44,45]. However, the limited available data using CT or CTC in UC does not show adequate diagnostic performance, and colonoscopy remains the reference standard. Indications for CT are currently restricted to patients with impassable stenoses or severe comorbidities where colonoscopy is contraindicated [46].

The diagnostic utility of CT in CD colitis was investigated in several studies [47–50].

Sensitivity and specificity for Crohn's activity ranged from 60% to 90% and from 90% to 100%, respectively. However, no correlation was found between CD activity index and any specific CT finding [47].

A role for CTC has been proposed to assess postoperative recurrence, although the observed false negative rate supports continued use of colonoscopy [51], unless severe strictures.

9.3.5.2 CT Findings

At CT, the most frequent finding in both CD and UC is wall thickening. The mean wall thickness in CD (11–13 mm) is usually greater than in UC (7.8 mm). Wall thickening in UC may be diffuse and symmetric, whereas wall thickening in CD may be eccentric and segmental with skip regions.

CD has a variety of appearances at CT, depending on whether the activity is acute or chronic and whether there are complications such as obstruction, fistulas, or abscesses. CT imaging features of active small bowel CD include bowel wall thickening, mural hyperenhancement, mural stratification, the comb sign, and increased density in the perienteric fat. Chronic changes of CD include fibrotic strictures and submucosal fatty deposition in the bowel wall. Another important finding is luminal narrowing that can be reversible (when because of edema or spasm in active disease) or fixed (fibrotic strictures) (Figure 9.7).

Main common finding in UC are loss of haustration, rigid bowel wall, and bowel thickness.

Mesenteric lymphadenopathy suggests CD rather than UC, although this finding is certainly not specific for IBD (Figure 9.8).

9.3.6 Ischemic Colitis

9.3.6.1 Clinical Aspects and CT Indications

IC is an inadequate perfusion leading to colonic inflammation and is the most common form of ischemic injury to the gastrointestinal tract. It has an incidence of 4.5 per 100.000 person-years, and approximately 90% of cases

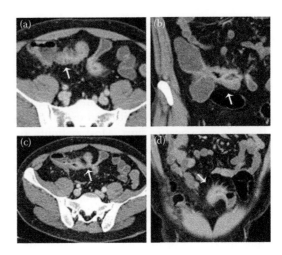

FIGURE 9.8
Active Crohn's disease. (a, b) CT scan shows mural thickening and hyperenhancement (arrows) of terminal ileum; (c) adherences with small bowel loop; (d) comb sign.

occur in patients over 60 years (mortality is over 50% in severe cases). Nevertheless, the incidence of IC is underestimated because of its frequent, mild, and transient nature.

The underlying pathophysiology is represented by an acute compromise in intestinal BF that is inadequate to ensure the metabolic demands of a region of the colon. Both arterial and venous occlusion can result in colonic ischemia.

Many conditions may predispose to IC, such as a state of increased coagulability, mesenteric artery emboli, thrombosis, trauma, congestive heart failure, transient hypotension, hypovolemia or sepsis, tumors, volvuli, adhesions, hernias, and diverticulitis. IC can also follow aortic reconstruction; it may be a complication of coronary artery bypass surgery, colonic surgery, or colonoscopy and can be idiopathic.

The colon is protected from ischemia by a collateral blood supply via a system of arcades connecting the two major arteries (superior mesenteric artery [SMA] and inferior mesenteric artery).

Segments commonly affected by IC are the junction between these two vessels (so-called watershed areas), near the splenic flexure (Griffith point) and the rectosigmoid junction, between the inferior mesenteric artery distribution and the hypogastric vascular supply (point of Sudeck).

The ischemic process, which leads to mucosal congestion, hemorrhage and edema, patchy areas of mucosal necrosis and ulcerations, tends to initially affect the mucosa and, only when severe and prolonged, the muscularis propria. Mucosal damage is reversible, occurring as a self-limiting condition, whereas necrosis of the muscle layer can lead to the development of

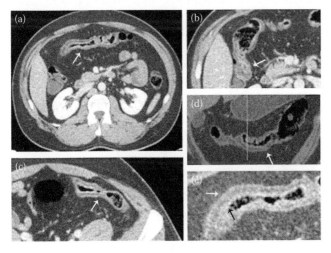

FIGURE 9.7
A 55-year-old woman with endoscopic and pathologic diagnosis of active Crohn's disease. (a–d) CT scan shows mural thickening and hyperenhancement (arrows) of trasverse colon. (e) CT enterography image shows mural hyperenhancement, mural stratification (white arrow for sierosa; asterisk for muscular layer; black arrow for mucosa), and wall thickening.

a fibrotic stricture or to necrosis with severe sepsis and perforation.

Clinically, IC may be classified into gangrenous and nongangrenous forms (80%–85% of cases). The latter can also be subdivided into transient and chronic forms.

The presentation of colon ischemia is highly variable and depends on the severity and extent of the disease. There is no specific sign. Most patients present with crampy abdominal pain, diarrhea, and an urge to defecate. The pain is mild, located over the affected part of bowel, followed by mild rectal bleeding within 24 hours. The blood can be maroon or bright red, frequently mixed with the stool. An associated ileus may be manifested by anorexia, nausea, and vomiting. Clinical examination of the abdomen reveals moderate tenderness over the affected area of the colon. Fever is unusual, but the white cell count is generally increased. In cases of severe ischemia with transmural infarction and necrosis, marked tenderness with peritoneal signs may be present on physical examination associated with metabolic acidosis and septic shock.

Diagnosis requires a high index of clinical suspicion. Attention must be paid to the presence of conditions that predispose to the disease. The differential diagnosis includes infectious colitis, IBD, pseudomembranous colitis, diverticulitis, and colon carcinoma.

Radiologic assessment of potential ischemia traditionally consisted of plain radiography of the abdomen, barium studies, and angiography. However, with continued technologic advancement, CT is being used with increasing frequency in evaluation of patients with suspected colonic ischemia.

9.3.6.2 CT Findings

CT typically shows circumferential, symmetric wall thickening with fold enlargement.

Mild thickening of the wall is considered <15 mm, marked >15–30 mm.

In the first stage immediately after occlusion, thrombus can be seen in SMA or superior mesenteric vein (SMV), but wall changes are not developed.

If there is total vascular occlusion without reperfusion (infarction), the colonic wall remains thin (paper thin wall) and unenhancing, associated with dilatation of the lumen (Figure 9.9).

In case of SMV thrombosis, the wall may show mural thickening, low attenuation because of edema, or high attenuation, which indicates intramural hemorrhage. Inflammatory changes in the pericolic fat may also be present.

Pneumatosis may be seen in advanced disease. Complications include infarction, perforation, and stricture. Occasionally, a toxic megacolon develops.

When present, the ascites is usually located mainly in the paracolic gutters and adjacent to the liver, with only a small amount of fluid in the pelvis.

9.3.7 Infectious Colitis

9.3.7.1 Clinical Aspects and CT Indications

In general, the infectious colities are typically diagnosed clinically and do not require CT for detection or differential diagnosis. However, they may be identified at CT incidentally or in cases in which the clinical symptoms are not straightforward.

There are many causes of infectious colitis. Bacterial causes include *Shigella, Salmonella, Yersinia, Campylobacter, Staphylococcus*, and *Chlamydia trachomatis*. Fungal infections such as histoplasmosis, mucormycosis, and actinomycosis can involve the colon. Viral causes of colitis include herpesvirus, cytomegalovirus, and rotavirus. Amebiasis and tuberculosis can also cause a colitis, which can resemble IBD.

A life-threatening and common type of infectious colitis is pseudomembranous colitis. It results from toxins produced by an overgrowth of the organism

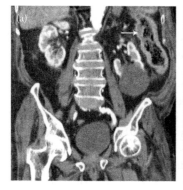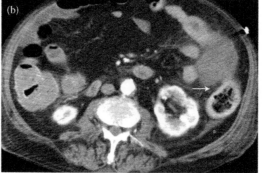

FIGURE 9.9
Ischemic colitis. (a, b) Circumferential wall thickening of descending colon (with arrow) that shows homogenous enhancement after intravenous administration of medium contrast. Ascites in paracolic gutter (asterisk).

Clostridium difficile and results in a profuse watery diarrhea with abdominal pain and fever [52].

It is now recognized to be an important nosocomial pathogen that may be associated with considerable morbidity and attributable mortality.

Pseudomembranous colitis has been associated with hypotensive episodes, chemotherapeutic agents, abdominal surgery, and complication of antibiotic therapy.

It is characterized by the presence of elevated, yellow-white plaques forming pseudomembranes on the colonic mucosa, well detected by endoscopy. The diagnosis is typically made with stool assay for the *Clostridium difficile* toxin, but the clinical presentation is often nonspecific and radiologists should be familiar with the CT findings to evaluate the extent and severity of the disease and detect potential complications.

9.3.7.2 CT Findings

There is considerable overlap of the appearances of infectious colitis at CT imaging, thus laboratory studies are necessary for definitive diagnosis (Figure 9.10). The portion of colon affected may suggest a specific organism. Gonorrhea, herpesvirus, and *Chlamydia trachomatis* typically involve the rectosigmoid. *Shigella* and *Salmonella* are usually limited to the right colon; diffuse involvement occurs in *Cytomegalovirus* and *Escherichia coli* infections [53]. Typical signs are wall thickening, low attenuation representing edema, and homogeneous enhancement of the wall. Ascites or inflammation of the pericolic fat may also be present [54]. Multiple air-fluid levels may also be observed in the colon because of increased fluid and stools.

In pseudomembranous colitis, the most common, but nonspecific, CT finding is circumferential or eccentric thickening of the colonic wall, greater than in any other inflammatory or infectious disease of the colon except CD (Figure 9.11).

The bowel wall is often irregular and shaggy, may have low attenuation because of edema, or may enhance significantly after intravenous administration of contrast material secondary to hyperemia. The target sign, originally described in UC and CD, has also been reported in pseudomembranous colitis.

9.3.8 Angiodysplasia

9.3.8.1 Clinical Aspects and CT Indications

First described by Galdabini in 1974, angiodysplasia is considered a rare condition characterized by abnormal, dilated, and tortuous small vessels with a diameter <1 cm within the mucosal and submucosal layer of the large bowel [55]. The abnormal vessels' wall is thin and fragile, consisting of endothelium or thin smooth muscle layer, and frequently bleeds resulting in blood loss from the lower gastrointestinal (LGI) tract [56]. These lesions are frequently multiple and located, in 77% of the cases, in the right colon [57].

Angiodysplasia of the gastrointestinal tract was an underestimated pathological entity for many decades. The improvement of diagnostic techniques made evident that these vascular malformations were not as rare as it was previously believed.

The prevalence of angiodysplasia of the entire gastrointestinal tract in the general population is 0.82% [58] and account for 2%–8% of all patients presenting with gastrointestinal bleeding [59]. In the general population, are usually detected in patients older than 60 years old [60] and several studies reported a strong correlation between angiodysplasia and chronic renal disease, accounting for 19%–32% of all LGI bleedings [61].

The etiology of angiodysplastic lesions is not well known. It seems to be degenerative in nature, secondary to intermittent obstruction of the submucosal veins and hypoxemia because of intestinal motility. Another hypothesis is related to altered calcium metabolism and presence of constipation, hemostatic disorders, or atherosclerotic peripheral vascular disease.

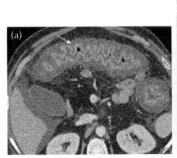
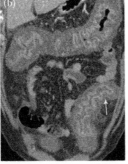

FIGURE 9.10
Pseudomembranous colitis. (a) CT enterography shows extensive luminal narrowing of the entire colon with wall thickness (asterisk) and mucosa hyperenhancement (arrow).

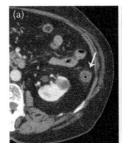
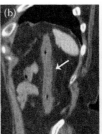
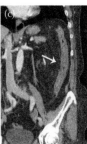

FIGURE 9.11
Infectious colitis. (a–c) Thickening of descending colon because of edema with homogeneous enhancement after intravenous administration of medium contrast (white arrow) and pericolonic fat stranding.

Angiodysplasia may be observed incidentally at colonoscopy, or patients may present with LGI bleeding. Multiple hemorrhagic episodes are common and mostly occult and intermittent in nature. In a high percentage of about 90%, bleeding stops spontaneously, and patients may present with iron deficiency anemia secondary to recurrent bleeding.

There is controversy regarding the best modality for the initial diagnosis of the cause of low gastrointestinal bleeding. Radiological tests that can be used include radionuclide scans, CT, and transcatheter arteriography. Colonoscopy possesses an eminent position in the diagnostic and also therapeutic armamentarium; however, it very challenging in the face of major active bleeding that can obscure the endoscopist's view. For these reasons, the recent guidelines suggest to use colonoscopy or radiologic testing for initial diagnosis according to local expertise and availability.

CT scanning has recently been shown to have the ability to detect bleeding as low as 0.3 mL·min^{-1}. Moreover, it has many other advantages as an initial test to localize LGI bleeding. It can often yield a diagnosis of the pathologic cause of the bleeding. In one study, CT identified the pathology, preoperatively, in 50% of cases. Defining the cause of bleeding can help determine prognosis as well as the best options for treatment. This allows patients who have lesions that are unfavorable for embolization to be triaged directly to surgery. CT can also provide information about the arterial anatomy. It can identify variant anatomy or vessel occlusions that would influence subsequent transcatheter arteriography/intervention.

9.3.8.2 CT Findings

When digestive hemorrhage is suspected, MDCT study protocol should be multiphasic to evaluate arterial and venous mesenteric vessels, to detect the bleeding source or vascular alterations of the intestinal wall, and to evaluate the amount of active endoluminal bleeding.

Typical CT findings are vascular hyperdensity in the wall of sigmoid colon; hyperdense wall thickening, when multiple vascular ectasia are present; and hemorrhage in arterial phase, resulting in contrast medium extravasation into bowel lumen.

9.3.9 Toxic Megacolon

9.3.9.1 Clinical Aspects and CT Indications

Toxic megacolon is a rare, life-threatening condition caused by worsening of colitis (10% of patients with UC, 2.3% patients with Crohn's disease, and 0.4%–3% patients with pseudomembranous colitis). The majority of toxic megacolon is caused by IBD (UC and CD), but nowadays an increase of toxic megacolon caused by pseudomembranous colitis has been established [62].

Clinical signs of disease include diarrhea or bloody diarrhea, constipation, obstipation, abdominal pain, abdominal distension, and decreased bowel sound.

CT is not routinely used for the diagnosis of toxic megacolon but could be useful especially in evaluation of complications (perforation, peritonitis, abscess, and phlebitis).

9.3.9.2 CT Findings

Dilatation of bowel >60 mm is suggestive for diagnosis of toxic megacolon.

[63] in a study of 18 patients found in the majority of cases, fat or mesenteric stranding, thickening of colonic wall between 2 and 17 mm, thickening of colonic lumen between 60 and 100 mm, abnormal haustral pattern (distorted, nodular, or asymmetrical configuration 100%), and edematous submucosal changes with multilayer aspect (target sign). Ascites were observed in 72% of patients and pleural effusions in 39%.

9.3.10 Appendicitis

9.3.10.1 Clinical Aspects and CT Indications

The appendix is a blind-ending, tubular structure (1–25 cm) arising 1.7–2.5 cm caudal to the ileocecal valve and that could lie in pelvic, preileal, postileal, or paracecal position.

Acute appendicitis are the most common surgical emergency, with a mortality of 0.2%–0.8% [64], and often patients present abdominal pain and fever. Symptoms of acute appendicitis may be similar to other abdominal pathologies such as mesenteric adenitis, cecal diverticulum, epiploic appendagitis, omental infarction, CD, terminal ileitis, cecal perforated, and appendiceal carcinoma.

Usually, obstruction of lumen causes stasis of fluid that, associated with inefficacy drainage of venous and lymphatic system, promotes development of infection. Complications of acute appendicitis include phlegmon, abscess, perforation, peritonitis, bowel obstruction, and septic seeding of mesenteric vessels [65].

CT is more sensitive than US for the diagnosis of acute appendicitis; in fact, unenhanced CT shows a sensitivity of 95%, specificity of 98%, positive predict value of 97%, and negative predict value of 98% [65–67]. CT with intravenous administration of medium contrast can be useful especially in complication detection and in patients with a small amount of intra-abdominal fat, in which the enhancement of the appendix wall can represent an inflammation sign.

9.3.10.2 CT Findings

[65] divided CT findings of acute appendicitis into appendiceal, cecal, and periappendiceal changes (Figure 9.12).

- Appendiceal changes
  - Diameter of appendix >10 mm
  - Thickening of appendiceal wall ≥3 mm
  - Hyperenhancement of appendiceal wall
  - Mural stratification of appendiceal wall
  - Appendicolith (presence in about 30% of acute appendicitis)
- Cecal changes
  - Involved of cecum show cecal apical thickening
  - "Arrowhead sign" is focal cecal thickening centered on the appendiceal orifice
  - "Cecal bar sign" because of inflammatory tissue situated at base of appendix and that divides contrast- filled cecum from appendix
- The two last signs are applicable only if cecum is filled with contrast agent.
- Periappendiceal signs:
  - Periappendiceal fat stranding
  - Extraluminal fluid
  - Lymph node enlargement
  - Phlegmon or abscess

These findings can be summarized in the classification reported in Table 9.6 [68].

Sometimes, in acute appendicitis, wall could become ischemic, necrotic, and then perforates. CT signs of perforation include extraluminal air, extraluminal appendicolith, abscess, phlegmon, and defect in enhancing of appendiceal wall (sensitivity 95% and specificity 95%). CT characteristic sign of periappendiceal abscess is a rim-enhancing fluid collection with effect mass on the bowel. Peritonitis is usually more frequent in child and is caused by early appendicular rupture before generation of adhesions, generally is associated with free-fluid in abdomen. CT with contrast is useful to distinguish ascites from peritonitis; indeed in the second situation, thickening and enhancement of peritoneal reflections are observed in association with inflammatory changes of peritoneum and omentum and hyperemic change of bowel segments. Gangrenous appendicitis represents a complication of acute appendicitis with arterial and intramural thrombosis. Usually pneumatosis, focal areas of hypoperfusion, and shaggy appendiceal wall are suggestive for diagnosis of gangrenous appendicitis.

9.3.11 Neoplasms of the Appendix

9.3.11.1 Clinical Aspects and CT Findings

Primary appendix neoplasms are uncommon and represent about 0.5%–1% of appendectomy at pathological evaluation; they are usually seen in middle-aged or older patients. Carcinoid represents the first tumor for incidence followed by epithelial neoplasms, which can be malignant or benign. About 30%–50% of patients

TABLE 9.6

Classification on CT Findings of Acute Appendicitis

Category	Imaging Findings
I	Simple acute appendicitis with imaging features (wall thickening and appendiceal enhancement) limited to appendix
II	Acute appendicitis associated with periappendiceal signs
III	Appendicitis with phlegmon or abscess
IV	Appendicitis with distal events of inflammation

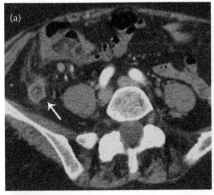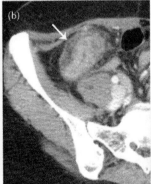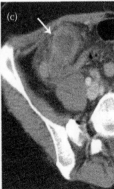

FIGURE 9.12

Appendicitis. (a, b) Enlarged appendix with marked enhancement of appendiceal wall (arrow) and adjacent fat stranding (asterisk). (c) Periappendicular abscess (arrow).

with appendiceal neoplasms manifest signs of acute appendicitis; other symptoms are: asymptomatic palpable mass, intussusception, gastrointestinal bleeding, ureteral obstruction or hematuria, or pseudomyxoma peritonei.

CT imaging could be useful for therapeutic assessment and evaluation of surgical approach.

- Appendiceal carcinoid:
  - Appendiceal carcinoid is the most common tumor of appendix, with an incidence of 15%–85%. Usually, it involves the distal appendix and rarely can cause mucocele; it generally represents an incidental finding, and it is frequently diagnosed with liver metastasis [64].
- Appendiceal adenocarcinoma:
  - Appendiceal adenocarcinoma is subdivided in two types: mucinous and nonmucinous adenocarcinoma. Mucinous tumors are characterized by slow growth, late metastases, tendency to locoregional extension, mesoappendix involvement, and lymph nodes of cecal valve.
  - Wall thickening, soft-tissue mass with periappendiceal fat stranding, and appendiceal diameter >15 mm are suggestive for diagnosis of appendiceal adenocarcinoma.
  - Mucinous epithelial tumors generally present circumferential mucosal involvement and tendency to development mucoceles (Figure 9.13).
- Mucocele and pseudomyxoma peritonei:
  - Mucocele represent dilatation of appendix caused by intraluminal accumulation of fluids and could be neoplastic

(cystoadenoma and cystoadenocarcinoma) or postinflammatory (appendicitis or endometriosis). Mucocele is a circumscribed cystic mass with calcification (highly suggestive for diagnosis of mucocele but present about in 50%).

  - Pseudomixoma peritonei is mucinous ascite arising from epithelial implants secreting extracellular mucina, and CT feature show fluid collection in peritoneum with associated calcifications.
  - Mucinous ascites on the contrary of serous ascites cause scalloping of liver and visceral surface.
- Appendiceal lymphoma:
  - Appendiceal lymphoma represents about 1.3%–2.6% of all gastrointestinal tract lymphomas, and CT features include appendiceal thickening with conserved appendix vermiform shape.

9.4 Rectum Pathologies

9.4.1 Rectal Cancer

9.4.1.1 Clinical Aspects and CT Indications

CRC is the third most common cancer worldwide [69]. Generally, it is associated with a poor prognosis because of local relapse and development of distal metastases.

Rectal cancer usually is a palpable mass in 40%–80% of patients, and rectal exploration may be useful in lesion evaluation, flexibility, and distance from anal verge [70].

Correct staging of rectal cancer (Table 9.7) is fundamental for patient management; indeed in locally

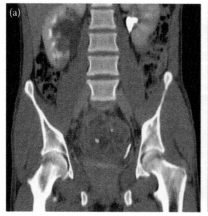
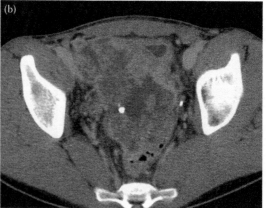

FIGURE 9.13
Cystoadenocarcinoma of the appendix. (a, b) Large cystic mass (asterisk) with heterogeneous contrast enhancement and calcifications (arrow).

TABLE 9.7

American Joint Committee on Cancer Staging for Rectal Cancer

Primary Tumors (T)	Regional Lymph Nodes (N)	Distant Metastasis (M)
Tx: Tumor cannot be assessed	Nx: Lymph nodes cannot be assessed	M0: No distant metastasis
T0: No evidence of primary tumor	N0: No regional lymph nodes metastasis	M1 Distant metastasis
T1s: Carcinoma in situ: intraepithelial or invasion of lamina proprial	N1: Metastasis in 1–3 regional lymph nodes	
T1: Tumor invades submucosa		
T2: Tumor invades muscularis propria	N2: Metastasis in 4 or more perirectal lymph nodes	
T3: Tumor invades through the muscularis propria into the subserosa or into non-peritonealized perirectal tissues		
T3a: Tumor extends <1 mm beyond muscularis propria		
T3b: Tumor extends 1–5 mm beyond muscularis propria		
T3c: Tumor extends 5–15 mm beyond muscularis propria		
T3d: Tumor extends >15 mm beyond muscularis propria		
T4: Tumor directly invades into other organs or structures and/or perforate visceral peritoneum		

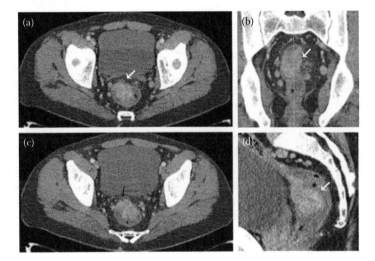

FIGURE 9.14
Rectal cancer. (a, b, d) Thickening of the rectal wall (white arrow) with hemicircunferential involvement and enlarged lymph nodes (asterisk). (c) Tumoral infiltration of the mesorectum (black arrow).

advanced cancer, surgical approach can be combined with neoadjuvant chemoradiotherapy (Figure 9.14).

CT staging of rectal cancer is not as accurate as MR, especially for the evaluation of rectal wall. In T1 and T2 stage, CT shows a diagnostic accuracy of 84% on multiplanar reformation (MPR) images versus 67% on axial images. T3 stage usually is characterized by invasion of tumor in mesorectum with evidence of strand in pericolic fat tissue; often, desmoplastic reaction can be confused with fat stranding, and T2 stage can be overstaged as T3 [71]. In T3 evaluation, CT shows an accuracy of 81% on MPR images versus 60% on axial images. T4 stage is

characterized from tumor extension in adjacent organs, and MPR images show an accuracy of 96% versus 89% of axial images.

Regarding lymph node evaluation, CT shows an accuracy on MPR images of about 84.8% versus 70.7 on axial images.

Clearly, the use of MPR images for evaluation of rectal tumor significantly increase the accuracy of cancer staging [69].

CT scan of abdomen and chest usually is sufficient for evaluation of liver and lungs that are the most common sites of rectal cancer metastases [72].

CTC is useful in evaluation of CRC and allow also the evaluation of distant metastases or synchronous colonic tumor [70].

9.4.1.2 CT Findings

CT features of rectal cancer includes the following:

1. Thickening of rectal wall
2. Presence of soft-tissue densities arising from rectum in perirectal space
3. Obliteration of presacral fat plane
4. Lymph nodes greater than 1 cm in perirectal region
5. After abdominoperineal resection, most frequent site of recurrence is the presacrococcygeal area

9.4.2 Rectal Syphilis

9.4.2.1 Clinical Aspects and CT Indications

Rectal syphilis or inflammatory pseudotumor was first described by Brunn in 1939. The name was given by Umiker et al. in 1954 because of its propensity to clinically and radiologically mimic a malignant process [73]. Inflammatory pseudotumor is a bulging lesion consisting of inflammatory cells and myofibroblastic spindle cells [74]. Inflammatory pseudotumor most commonly involves the lung and the orbit, but it has been reported to occur in nearly every site in the body, from the central nervous system to the gastrointestinal tract. Gastrointestinal tract involvement is rare, with ileocecal and gastric tumors in young girls being the most frequently described type. The causes of inflammatory pseudotumor are unknown. Some authors believe this

tumor is a low-grade fibrosarcoma with inflammatory cells [75]. The propensity of inflammatory pseudotumors to be locally aggressive, to frequently be multifocal, and to progress occasionally to a true malignant tumor supports this idea. Organisms found in association with inflammatory pseudotumor include mycobacteria associated with spindle cell tumor; Epstein–Barr virus found in splenic and nodal pseudotumors; actinomycetes and nocardiae found in hepatic and pulmonary pseudotumors, respectively; and mycoplasma in pulmonary pseudotumors [76]. There have been case reports of inflammatory pseudotumor associated with infections caused by other organisms, including *Mycobacterium avium–intracellulare* complex, *Corynebacterium equi*, *E. coli*, *Klebsiella*, *Bacillus sphaericus*, *Pseudomonas*, *Helicobacter pylori*, and *Coxiella Burnetii* [77].

9.4.2.2 CT Findings

Inflammatory condition affecting rectum usually resemble neoplastic lesions. Most common signs are diffuse thickening of the rectal wall, with circumferential involvement, and fat stranding of the mesorectum with multiple enlarged lymph nodes. Moreover, ulcerations of the wall can be present (Figure 9.15). Rectal syphilis can mimic a tumoral condition, and imaging is not able to operate a reliable distinction. For this reason, histological confirmation is mandatory in all patients presenting with anomalous symptoms or history.

9.4.3 Fistula

Fistula is an anomalous communication between two organs, structures, or organ with skin.

Perianal fistulas are subdivided into intersphinteric, trans-sphinteric, suprasphinteric, and extrasphinteric

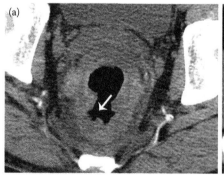 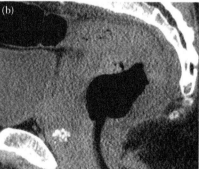 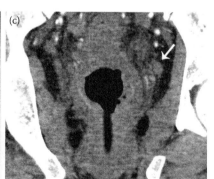

FIGURE 9.15
Rectal syphilis. (a) Contrast-enhanced axial CT image following air distention of the rectum. Severe and diffuse thickening of the rectal wall with circumferential involvement; a large ulceration is visible on the posterior wall (arrow) associated with severe fat stranding of the mesorectum and multiple enlarged lymphnodes. (b) Contrast-enhanced sagittal multiplanar reformation (MPR) CT image showing the entire involvement of the rectum. Multiple aorto-iliac lymphnodes are also evident. (c) Coronal MPR image demonstrating the presence of mesorectal lymph nodes and stranding of mesorectal fat.

and could be caused by CD, tubercolosis, pelvic infections, tumors, or radiotherapy. Most common symptom is discharge but also pain if inflammation is there.

Idiopathic fistulas are rare and generally caused by chronic anal infections. Males are affected by of perianal fistulas more than females (2:1).

Identification of fistulas with CT could be accomplished with medium contrast administration in the rectum or through fistolous orifice. However, CT is less accurate in evaluation of secondary branches of fistulas than MR [78].

Rare complication of CD could be enterovescical fistula; patients with this disease present pain, fecaluria, ematuria, dysuria, weight loss, fever, diarrhea, and rectal bleeding.

CT is useful in evaluation of enterovescical fistulas with evidence of air in bladder [79].

9.4.4 Proctitis

Proctitis could be caused from different pathologies such UC and radiation proctitis.

Usually radiation proctitis occurs in 5%–20% of patients following radiotherapy. Symptoms include urgency and rectal bleeding, diarrhea, tenesmus, and rectal pain [80]. CT is not used for evaluation of proctitis. Common findings are diffuse thickening of rectal wall and stenosis [81].

9.5 Summary

MDCT permits a complete and reliable evaluation of colorectal disease. The possibility to assess in a single fast examination the colonic lumen, extracolonic structures, and other abdominal organs allows an accurate detection of several pathological conditions. Moreover, MDCT enables a subtle disease characterization discriminating between different pathologies with similar symptoms onset.

References

1. Horton KM, Corl FM, Fishman EK. CT evaluation of the colon: inflammatory disease. *Radiographics* 2000;20(2):399–418.
2. Rengo M, Bellini D, De Cecco CN et al. The optimal contrast media policy in CT of the liver. Part I: technical notes. *Acta Radiol* 2011a;52(5):467–72.
3. Rengo M, Bellini D, De Cecco CN et al. The optimal contrast media policy in CT of the liver. Part II: clinical protocols. *Acta Radiol* 2011b;52(5):473–80.
4. Johnson CD, Hara AK, Reed JE. Computed tomographic colonography (Virtual colonoscopy): a new method for detecting colorectal neoplasms. *Endoscopy* 1997;29:454–61.
5. McFarland EG, Brink JA. Helical CT colonography (Virtual colonoscopy): the challenge that exists between advancing technology and generalizability. *Am J Roentgenol* 1999;173: 549–59.
6. Behrens C, Stevenson G, Eddy R, Mathieson J. Effect of intravenous Buscopan on colonic distention during computed tomography colonography. *Can Assoc Radiol J* 2008;59:183–90.
7. Rogalla P, Lembcke A, Ruckert JC et al. Spasmolysis at CT colonography: butyl scopolamine versus glucagon. *Radiology* 2005;236:184–8.
8. Taylor SA, Laghi A, Lefere P, Halligan S, Stoker J. European Society of Gastrointestinal and Abdominal Radiology (ESGAR): consensus statement on CT colonography. *Eur Radiol* 2007;17:575–9.
9. Burling D. CT colonography standards. *Clin Radiol* 2010;65: 474–80.
10. Neri E, Halligan S, Hellström M et al. The second ESGAR consensus statement on CT colonography. *Eur Radiol* 2012 Sep 15. [Epub ahead of print] PMID 22983280.
11. Kambadakone AR, Sahani DV. Body perfusion CT: technique, clinical applications, and advances. *Radiologic Clinics of NA* 2009;47:161–78.
12. Miles KA. Perfusion CT for the assessment of tumour vascularity: which protocol? *Br J Radiol* 2003;76:36–42.
13. Goh V, Halligan S, Daley F, Wellsted DM, Guenther T, Bartram CI. Colorectal tumor vascularity: quantitative assessment with multidetector CT—do tumor perfusion measurements reflect angiogenesis? *Radiology* 2008;249(2):510–7.
14. Bellomi M, Petralia G, Sonzogni A, Zampino MG, Rocca A. CT perfusion for the monitoring of neoadjuvant chemotherapy and radiation therapy in rectal carcinoma: initial experience. *Radiology* 2007;244(2):486–93.
15. Sahani DV, Kalva SP, Hamberg LM et al. Assessing tumor perfusion and treatment response in rectal cancer with multisection CT: initial observations. *Radiology* 2005; 234(3):785–92.
16. De Cecco CN, Buffa V, Fedeli S et al. Dual Energy CT (DECT) of the liver: conventional versus virtual unenhanced images. *Eur Radiol* 2010;20(12):2870–5.
17. De Cecco CN, Buffa V, Fedeli S et al. Preliminary experience with Dual Energy CT (DECT) of the abdomen: real versus virtual non-enhanced Images of the liver. *Radiol Med* 2010;115(8):1258–66.
18. De Cecco CN, Darnell A, Macías N et al. Virtual unenhanced images of the abdomen with second-generation dual-source dual-energy computed tomography: image quality and liver lesion detection. *Invest Radiol* 2013; 48(1):1–9.
19. De Cecco CN, Darnell A, Rengo M et al. Dual-Energy CT: oncologic applications. *Am J Roentgenol* 2012;199(Suppl 5): S98–105.
20. Howlader N, Noone AM, Krapcho M et al, eds. *SEER Cancer Statistics Review, 1975-2008*. Bethesda, MD: National Cancer Institute, 2011.

21. Hill LB, O'Connell JB, Ko CY. Colorectal cancer: epidemiology and health services research. *Surg Oncol Clin N Am* 2006;15(1):21–37.

22. Ferlitsch M, Reinhart K, Pramhas S et al. Sex-specific prevalence of adenomas, advanced adenomas, and colorectal cancer in individuals undergoing screening colonoscopy. *JAMA* 2011;306(12):1352–8.

23. Stryker SJ, Wolff BG, Culp CE, Libbe SD, Ilstrup DM, MacCarty RL. Natural history of untreated colonic polyps. *Gastroenterology* 1987 Nov;93(5):1009–13.

24. Johnson CD, MacCarty RL, Welch TJ et al. Comparison of the relative sensitivity of CT colonography and double-contrast barium enema for screen detection of colorectal polyps. *Clin Gastroenterol Hepatol* 2004;2:314–21.

25. Rockey DC, Paulson E, Niedzwiecki D et al. Analysis of air contrast barium en- ema, computed tomographic colonography, and colonoscopy: prospective comparison. *Lancet* 2005;365:305–11.

26. Sosna J, Sella T, Sy O et al. Critical analysis of the performance of double-contrast barium enema for detecting colorectal polyps > or = 6 mm in the era of CT colonography. *Am J Roentgenol* 2008;190:374–85.

27. Hassan C, Pickhardt PJ, Kim DH et al. Systematic review: distribution of advanced neoplasia according to polyp size at screening colonoscopy. *Aliment Pharmacol Ther* 2010;31:210–7.

28. Pickhardt PJ, Hassan C, Laghi A et al. Small and diminutive polyps detected at screening CT colonography: a decision analysis for referral to colonoscopy. *Am J Roentgenol* 2008;190:136–44.

29. Shah JP, Hynan LS, Rockey DC. Management of small polyps detected by screening CT colonography: patient and physician preferences. *Am J Med* 2009;122:687.e1–9.

30. Ferrari R, De Cecco CN, Iafrate F, Paolantonio P, Rengo M, Laghi A. Anatomic variations of the celiac trunk and the mesenteric arteries evaluated with 64-row CT-Angiography. *Radiologia Medica* 2007;112(7):988–98.

31. Mari FS, Nigri G, Pancaldi A et al. Role of CT angiography with three-dimensional reconstruction of mesenteric vessels in laparoscopic colorectal resections: a randomized controlled trial. *Surg Endosc* 2013 Jan 5. [Epub ahead of print].

32. Young-Fadok TM, Roberts PL, Spencer MP, Wolff BG. Colonic diverticular disease. *Curr Probl Surg* 2000;37(7):457–514.

33. Rao PM, Rhea JT, Novelline RA et al. Helical CT with only colonic contrast material for diagnosing diverticulitis: prospective evaluation of 150 patients. *Am J Roentgenol* 1998;170(6):1445–9.

34. Neff CC, vanSonnenberg E. CT of diverticulitis: diagnosis and treatment. *Radiol Clin North Am* 1989;27:743–52.

35. Lefere P, Gryspeerdt S, Baekelandt M, Dewyspelaere J, van Holsbeeck B. Diverticular disease in CT colonography. *Eur Radiol* 2003;13(Suppl 4):L62–74.

36. Gollub MJ. Colonic intussusception: clinical and radiographic features. *Am J Roentgenol* 2011;196(5):W580–5.

37. Morrison J, Lucas N, Gravel J. The role of abdominal radiography in the diagnosis of intussusception when interpreted by pediatric emergency physicians. *J Pediatr* 2009;155(4):556–9.

38. Hryhorczuk AL, Strouse PJ. Validation of US as a first-line diagnostic test for assessment of pediatric ileocolic intussusception. *Pediatr Radiol* 2009;39(10):1075–9.

39. Jones DJ. ABC of colorectal diseases. Large bowel volvulus. *BMJ* 1992;305:358–60.

40. Lau KC, Miller BJ, Schache DJ, Cohen JR. A study of large- bowel volvulus in urban Australia. *Can J Surg* 2006;49:203–7.

41. Peterson CM, Anderson JS, Hara AK, Carenza JW, Menias CO. Volvulus of the gastrointestinal tract: appearances at multimodality imaging. *Radiographics* 2009;29(5):1281–93.

42. Fletcher JG, Fidler JL, Bruining DH, Huprich JE. New concepts in intestinal imaging for inflammatory bowel diseases. *Gastroenterology* 2011;140:1795–806.

43. Johnson KT, Hara AK, Johnson CD. Evaluation of colitis: usefulness of CT enterography technique. *Emerg Radiol* 2009;16:277–82.

44. Das CJ, Makharia GK, Kumar R et al. PET/CT colonography: a novel non-invasive technique for assessment of extent and activity of ulcerative colitis. *Eur J Nucl Med Mol Imaging* 2009;37:714–21.

45. Meisner RS, Spier BJ, Einarsson S et al. Pilot study using PET/CT as a novel, noninvasive assessment of disease activity in inflammatory bowel disease. *Inflamm Bowel Dis* 2007;13:993–1000.

46. Stange EF, Travis SP, Vermeire S et al. European evidence-based Consensus on the diagnosis and management of ulcerative colitis: definitions and diagnosis. *J Crohns Colitis* 2008;2:1–23.

47. Andersen K, Vogt C, Blondin D et al. Multi-detector CT-colonography in inflammatory bowel disease: prospective analysis of CT-findings to high-resolution video colonoscopy. *Eur J Radiol* 2006;58:140–6.

48. Fiorino G, Bonifacio C, Peyrin-Biroulet L et al. Prospective comparison of computed tomography enterography and magnetic resonance enterography for assessment of disease activity and complications in ileocolonic Crohn's disease. *Inflamm Bowel Dis* 2010;17:1073–80.

49. Low RN, Francis IR, Politoske D, Bennett M. Crohn's disease evaluation: comparison of contrast-enhanced MR imaging and single-phase helical CT scanning. *J Magn Reson Imaging* 2000;11:127–35.

50. Low RN, Sebrechts CP, Politoske DA et al. Crohn's disease with endoscopic correlation: single-shot fast spin-echo and gadolinium-enhanced fat-suppressed spoiled gradient-echo MR imaging. *Radiology* 2002;222:652–60.

51. Biancone L, Fiori R, Tosti C et al. Virtual colonoscopy compared with conventional colonoscopy for stricturing postoperative recurrence in Crohn's disease. *Inflamm Bowel Dis* 2003;9:343–50.

52. Kelly CP, Pothoulakis C, LaMont JT. Clostridium difficile colitis. *N Engl J Med* 1994;330:257–62.

53. Wall SD, Jones B. Gastrointestinal tract in the immunocompromised host: opportunistic infections and other complications. *Radiology* 1992;185:327–35.

54. Philpotts LE, Heiken JP, Westcott MA, Gore RM. Colitis: use of CT findings in differential diagnosis. *Radiology* 1994;190:445–9.

55. Galdabini JJ, Waitman AC, Norellio PA, Greenfield AJ, Ezreleta M. Angiodysplasia of the colon: a cause of rectal bleeding. *J Cardiovasc Radiol* 1978;1:3–13.

56. Poralla T. Angiodysplasia in the renal patient: how to diagnose and how to treat? *Nephrol Dial Transplant* 1998;13:2188–91.

57. Meyer CT, Troncale LJ, Galloway S, Sheahan DG. Arteriovenous malformations of the bowel: an analysis of 22 cases and a review of the literature. *Medicine* 1981;60:36–48.

58. Foutch PG. Angiodysplasia of the gastrointestinal tract. *Am J Gastroenterol* 1993;88:807–18.

59. Hemingway AP. Angiodysplasia: current concepts. *Postgrad Med J* 1988;64:259–63.

60. Dodda G, Trotman BW. Gastrointestinal angiodysplasia. *J Assoc Acad Minor Phys* 1997;8:16–9.

61. Jesudason SR, Devasia A, Mathen VI, Bhaktaviziam A, Khanduri P. The pattern of angiodysplasia of the gastrointestinal tract in a tropical country. *Surg Gynecol Obstet* 1985;161:525–31.

62. Gan SI, Beck PL. A new look at toxic megacolon: an update and review of incidence, etiology, pathogenesis, and management. *Am J Gastroenterol* 2003;98(11):2363–71.

63. Imbriaco M, Balthazar EJ. Toxic megacolon: role of CT in evaluation and detection of complications. *Clin Imaging* 2001;25(5):349–54.

64. Whitley S, Sookur P, McLean A, Power N. The appendix on CT. *Clin Radiol* 2009 Feb;64(2):190–9.

65. PintoLeite N, Pereira JM, Cunha R, Pinto P, Sirlin C. CT evaluation of appendicitis and its complications: imaging techniques and key diagnostic findings. *Am J Roentgenol* 2005;185(2):406–17.

66. Ege G, Akman H, Sahin A, Bugra D, Kuzucu K. Diagnostic value of unenhanced helical CT in adult patients with suspected acute appendicitis. *Br J Radiol* 2002;75:721–5.

67. Rao PM, Rhea JT, Novelline RA, Mostafavi AA, Lawrason JN, McCabe CJ. Helical CT combined with contrast material administered only through the colon for imaging of suspected appendicitis. *Am J Roentgenol* 1997;169(5):1275–80.

68. Chalazonitis AN, Tzovara I, Sammouti E et al. CT in appendicitis. *Diagn Interv Radiol* 2008;14(1):19–25.

69. Sinha R, Verma R, Rajesh A, Richards CJ. Diagnostic value of multidetector row CT in rectal cancer staging: comparison of multiplanar and axial images with histopathology. *Clin Radiol* 2006;61(11):924–31.

70. Samee A, Selvasekar CR. Current trends in staging rectal cancer. *J Gastroenterol* 2011;17(7):828–34.

71. Shin SS, Jeong YY, Min JJ, Kim HR, Chung TW, Kang HK. Preoperative staging of colorectal cancer: CT vs. integrated FDG PET/CT. *Abdom Imaging* 2008;33(3):270–7.

72. Kosinski L, Habr-Gama A, Ludwig K, Perez R. Shifting concepts in rectal cancer management: a review of contemporary primary rectal cancer treatment strategies. *Cancer J Clin* 2012;62(3):173–202.

73. Umiker WO, Iverson LC. Post inflammatory tumor of the lung: report of four cases simulating xanthoma, fibroma or plasma cell granuloma. *J Thorac Surg* 1954; 28:55–62.

74. Dehner LP. The enigmatic inflammatory pseudotumors: the current state of our understanding, or misunderstanding (editorial). *J Pathol* 2000;192:277–9.

75. Hedlund GL, Navoy JF, Galliani CA, Johnson WH. Aggressive manifestations of inflammatory pulmonary pseudotumor in children. *Pediatr Radiol* 1999;29:112–6.

76. Wood C, Nickoloff BJ, Todes-Taylor NR. Pseudotumor resulting from atypical mycobacterial infection: a "histoid" variety of Mycobacterium avium-intracellulare complex infection. *Am J Clin Pathol* 1985;83:524–7.

77. Das Narla L, Newman B, Spottswood SS, Narla S, Kolli R. Inflammatory pseudotumor. *Radiographics* 2003;23: 719–29.

78. Sofic A, Beslic S, Sehovic N, Caluk J, Sofic D. MRI in evaluation of perianal fistulae. *Radiol Oncol* 2010;44(4):220–7.

79. Goldman SM, Fishman EK, Gatewood OM, Jones B, Siegelman SS. CT in the diagnosis of enterovesical fistulae. *Am J Roentgenol* 1985;144(6):1229–33.

80. Rustagi T, Mashimo H. Endoscopic management of chronic radiation proctitis. *World J Gastroenterol* 2011;17(41):4554–62.

81. Kennedy GD, Heise CP. Radiation colitis and proctitis. *Clin Colon Rectal Surg* 2007;20(1):64–72.

10

Posttraumatic and Postsurgical Abdomen

Matthew T. Heller and Amar B. Shah

CONTENTS

10.1 Introduction

The prompt diagnosis and treatment of patients presenting to a trauma center with possible abdominal injury remain a challenging undertaking for emergency and trauma physicians. As the abdomen is an intricate anatomic region, consisting of various compartments and complex organ systems, its evaluation can be clinically confusing and time consuming because of frequent nonspecific signs, symptoms, and physical examination findings. Although a patient's initial triage largely depends on hemodynamic stability and clinical expertise, computed tomography (CT) has evolved to play a pivotal role in the evaluation of patients presenting with abdominal trauma. The development of helical technique and multi-detector technology has allowed CT to move to the forefront of trauma imaging because of its rapid scan acquisition and volumetric imaging. This evolution has allowed more rapid and accurate diagnosis of abdominal injury, has been a major factor in the trend for nonoperative management, and has helped to guide follow-up for abdominal visceral injuries. The high temporal and spatial resolution of multi-detector CT (MDCT) have facilitated diagnosis of acute visceral and vascular injuries by allowing rapid, dynamic image acquisition during multiple phases following infusion of intravenous contrast material, allowing multiplanar and three-dimensional reconstructed images for treatment planning, and aiding in the selection of trauma patients for transcatheter embolization. In addition, although many trauma patients are routinely admitted for observation, the negative predictive value of CT has shown that hospitalization for possible abdominal injury following a normal abdominal CT examination is unnecessary in most cases, making use of trauma CT a central component of outcomes and cost containment analyses [1,2].

There are numerous mechanisms of abdominal trauma, with some of the more common presentations occurring after falls, penetrating injury, assault, and motor vehicle accidents. Motor vehicle accidents continue to be a leading cause of abdominal trauma and death for people worldwide; in the United States, injuries resulting from motor vehicle crashes are the leading cause of death for people between 11 and 33 years. In 2009, there were over 5.5 million police-reported motor vehicle crashes, resulting in 33,808 deaths and over 2.2 million injuries [3]. The clinical significance of these statistics is that most patients undergoing evaluation at a trauma center present with blunt trauma. In contrast to penetrating injury, blunt trauma adds to the complexity of the initial evaluation in several ways. First, blunt trauma is associated with multisystem injury that may act to redirect attention from the abdomen to more obvious injuries, and thereby delay diagnosis and triage of significant abdominal injury. In addition, the number and degree of abdominal viscera injured during blunt trauma is often underappreciated during the initial clinical survey because of limitations of clinical history and physical examination in patients who may be intoxicated, intubated, or in distress in the acute setting.

Therefore, a rapid, noninvasive evaluation of internal abdominal injury is paramount for prompt, accurate diagnosis, patient triage, and initiation of treatment. Diagnostic methods have evolved over the past three decades, as abdominal radiography, intravenous pyelography, nuclear medicine examinations, and diagnostic peritoneal lavage (DPL) have given way to body CT as the imaging modality of choice because of its higher sensitivity, specificity, rapidity, and universality in diagnosing acute abdominal injury [4,5].

10.2 Methods of Diagnosis in Abdominal Trauma

10.2.1 Diagnostic Peritoneal Lavage

DPL is used to diagnose hemoperitoneum in the hemodynamically stable trauma patient. There are various methods for performing DPL, ranging from open to closed technique with sensitivities ranging from 87% to 100% [6,7]. Diagnosis is based on aspiration of gross blood; however, if the initial aspiration is negative or indeterminate, sterile crystalloid is infused into the peritoneal cavity, aspirated, and sent to the laboratory for analysis. Table 10.1 lists several typical parameters that constitute a positive DPL. Despite its relatively high sensitivity, DPL suffers from lack of specificity in the evaluation of acute abdominal injury. Specifically, a positive DPL result does not quantify the volume of hemoperitoneum, the site or sites of injury, or the degree of injury. Therefore, the major disadvantage of DPL is that even low-grade injuries can produce a positive result and may prompt a nontherapeutic laparotomy. In addition, a false-positive DPL result may occur in the setting of poor technique, incisional hemorrhage, intraperitoneal extension of pelvic or retroperitoneal hemorrhage, and contamination by an anterior abdominal wall hematoma [8,9]. False-negative results have been reported in patients with diaphragmatic rupture, hematomas contained within the organ parenchyma or capsule, erroneous placement of the catheter into the extraperitoneal compartment, recovery of an insufficient volume of lavage fluid, and in cases where DPL was delayed for several hours after injury. In addition, DPL cannot detect abdominal hemorrhage because of injury of retroperitoneal organs such as the kidneys, adrenals, pancreas, and duodenum [10,11]. Therefore, the combination of cross-sectional imaging and suboptimal specificity has decreased the role of DPL in most

TABLE 10.1

Parameters Constituting a Positive DPL

1. Aspiration of blood
2. Red blood cell count >100,000
3. White blood cell count >500
4. Aspiration of bile
5. Aspiration of fecal material
6. Aspiration of gastric or intestinal contents

trauma centers. However, DPL continues to play a role in the setting of hemodynamically unstable patients and in those requiring immediate intervention for neurological injuries [12].

10.2.2 Ultrasound

Ultrasound (US) has evolved to play an important role in the evaluation of patients suspected of sustaining abdominal trauma. The portability of US allows rapid image acquisition in the trauma bay during periods of treatment and resuscitation, whereas its lack of ionizing radiation and significant cost allow performance of serial examinations. A 3.5–5 MHz probe is typically used during the transabdominopelvic examination during which the hepatorenal fossa, right subphrenic space, left subphrenic space, splenorenal recess, and pelvis (rectouterine space [pouch of Douglas] in females

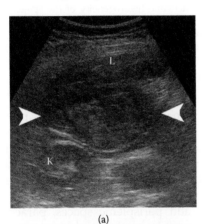

(a)

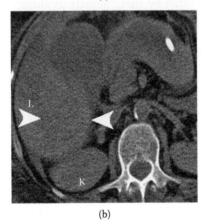

(b)

FIGURE 10.1
Hemoperitoneum. A 25-year-old male presented with abdominal pain following a motor vehicle accident. (a) Transverse ultrasound image shows heterogeneous material (arrowheads) in the hepatorenal fossa (Morrison's pouch), consistent with hematoma from liver lacerations (not shown). (b) Noncontrast computed tomography (CT) at the same anatomic level shows the hematoma (arrowheads) as mixed attenuation material in the hepatorenal fossa. L = liver, K = kidney.

and rectovesicle space in males) are scanned. The US examination is considered to be positive if free intraperitoneal fluid or hematoma is identified in any of these spaces (Figure 10.1). The examination is considered to be negative if no free fluid is identified. In some cases, the examination may be indeterminate from a technical standpoint because of poor acoustic windows from an obese body habitus, intervening bowel gas, subcutaneous emphysema, extensive soft-tissue injury, patient compliance, or a poorly distended urinary bladder.

Many trauma centers use US as a screening tool to identify free intraperitoneal fluid or hemoperitoneum. A few studies have evaluated the sensitivity of US for detection of peritoneal fluid using CT or DPL as the reference standard; in these studies, the sensitivity ranged from 63% to 86% [13,14]. The premise behind using US in the setting of abdominal trauma is similar to that of DPL; namely, there is an assumption that clinically significant abdominal injuries are associated with peritoneal fluid or hemoperitoneum. However, studies have shown that significant abdominal visceral injuries occur in the absence of hemoperitoneum, and the absence of free fluid cannot be used to exclude significant visceral injuries in stable patients [15] In addition, studies focused on abdominal CT have shown that up to 34% of patients with abdominal visceral injury following blunt abdominal trauma have no free intraperitoneal fluid on initial CT; moreover, surgery or angiographic intervention was required in up to 17% of the patients presenting without hemoperitoneum [16]. Other drawbacks of US in assessing acute abdominal injury include operator dependence, inability to reliably differentiate intraperitoneal from retroperitoneal hemorrhage, inability to identify the source of hemorrhage, and low sensitivity in diagnosing gastrointestinal (GI) injuries (Table 10.2) [13,16–18]. For evaluation of parenchymal injuries, US was shown to have the highest sensitivity for splenic injuries and lowest sensitivity for bowel injuries [13,19]. The appearance of parenchymal injuries has been reported to be quite variable and often subtle at US evaluation, with diffuse parenchymal heterogeneity being the most common abnormality [19].

TABLE 10.2

Factors Contributing to Decreased Sensitivity of US in Detecting Abdominal Injury

1. Poor acoustic window
2. Injuries occurring in absence of free fluid or hemoperitoneum
3. Inability to differentiate peritoneal from retroperitoneal fluid
4. Gastrointestinal injuries
5. Variable appearance of solid visceral injury
6. Operator experience

TABLE 10.3

Advantages of CT over DPL and US in Assessment of Abdominal Trauma

1. Ability to detect minute volumes of free fluid or blood
2. Assesses retroperitoneum in addition to peritoneum
3. Ability to identify specific site of injury
4. Increased detection of solid visceral and bowel injuries
5. Ability to identify active hemorrhage and traumatic vascular injuries
6. Nonoperator dependent
7. Less dependent on body habitus

10.2.3 Computed Tomography

Through numerous iterations of its technology, CT has evolved to become the imaging modality of choice in the evaluation of hemodynamically stable trauma patients (Table 10.3) [20]. Scanning time has drastically decreased from the early models that were limited by incremental, contiguous image acquisition to the current generations of CT that use helical technique and multi-detector technology. Multi-detector technology has allowed thinner collimation, improved spatial resolution, and decreased frequency of artifacts. Development of nonionic, low-osmolal, intravenous contrast and improvements of injector technology have allowed more widespread and efficient use of contrast material to more accurately diagnose acute vascular injuries, foci of active hemorrhage, and treatment planning.

CT technique varies somewhat between trauma centers but generally consists of acquisition of thin-section images (5 mm or thinner) through the abdomen and pelvis using helical technique. Images are most commonly acquired after the use of intravenous contrast during the portal venous phase, as this represents the time of peak parenchymal enhancement during which visceral lacerations and adjacent hematomas are most conspicuous. Some institutions use biphasic scanning of the upper abdomen when combined with chest CT so that the chest through liver and spleen are scanned during the arterial phase, followed by portal phase imaging through the entire abdomen and pelvis. This technique is felt to increase sensitivity for detection of hepatic and splenic vascular injuries, such as pseudoaneurysms and foci of active hemorrhage; by use of a biphasic protocol, active hemorrhage can be more easily identified because of its differing shape, location, and volume between the arterial and portal venous phases of the examination. In cases of suspected urinary system injury, delayed imaging after approximately 10 minutes will provide opacification of the renal collecting systems through bladder and allow identification of contrast leakage. Alternatively, diluted contrast may be instilled via a Foley catheter into the bladder, followed by scanning of the pelvis during CT cystography. Multiplanar

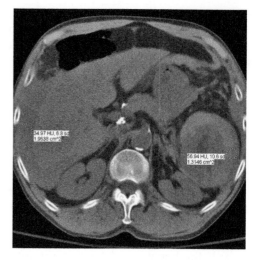

FIGURE 10.2

Sentinel clot sign because of splenic rupture. A 66-year-old female presented with diffuse abdominal pain after falling. Noncontrast CT shows parenchymal heterogeneity of the spleen and a rind of surrounding high-attenuation hemorrhage; the attenuation of the perisplenic hemorrhage measures 57 HU, whereas the attenuation of the hemoperitoneum in the perihepatic space measures 35 HU. The sentinel clot sign indicated the injured organ and guided laparotomy resulting in splenectomy.

reformatted images are can be rapidly provided with most modern CT platforms.

In addition to its speed and reproducibility, CT is extremely sensitive to small volumes of hemoperitoneum. In the supine position, the most dependent portions of the peritoneum, such as the hepatorenal fossa, perihepatic and perisplenic spaces, paracolic gutters, and pelvis, must be meticulously evaluated as a small amount of fluid or blood may be the only finding of an occult visceral or mesenteric injury. However, in cases of free intraperitoneal fluid, the location of the fluid, volume of fluid, and gender of the patient must be considered. Although both DPL and CT can detect small amounts of hemoperitoneum, CT is often able to determine a source of the hemorrhage, allow estimation of the relative amount of hemorrhage, and evaluate the retroperitoneum for acute injury. Identification of the source of hemorrhage may be made by demonstration of a visceral laceration with active contrast extravasation or by demonstration of the sentinel clot sign. The sentinel clot sign indicates that the region of highest density blood occurs adjacent to the injured organ in the setting of hemoperitoneum [21]. Identification of the sentinel clot sign may be the only finding indicating the source of hemorrhage and is especially important in patients unable to receive intravenous contrast material (Figure 10.2). Use of density measurements allows CT to differentiate between simple fluid (bile, ascites, etc), hematoma, and active bleeding. Generally, simple fluid measures near-water attenuation (0–15 HU), unclotted blood measures ~20–40 HU, hematoma measures ~40–70 HU, and active hemorrhage measures within 10 HU of contrast in the aorta [22–24]. Controversy remains of how to manage the trauma patient with free intraperitoneal fluid as the only finding on initial CT [25,26]. However, studies have indicated that immediate laparotomy is not usually required [27]. The CT finding of small volumes of free intraperitoneal fluid is a nonspecific finding that may be related to occult visceral or mesenteric injury, but may be unrelated to trauma, as in physiologic pelvic fluid during menstruation [28]. In males, recent studies have indicated that small amounts of isolated low-attenuation, free pelvic fluid is not likely to reflect occult bowel or mesenteric injury and may carry no significant clinical implication [29,30]. Regardless, the finding of free intraperitoneal fluid should be promptly communicated to the trauma team, especially when there is moderate volume of fluid or fluid in multiple sites so that appropriate follow-up can be scheduled.

10.2.4 Spleen Trauma

The spleen is the most frequently injured abdominal viscera [31,32]. The evolution of CT technology has allowed CT to play a central role in diagnosing splenic injuries and guiding their management. Contrast-enhanced helical CT has been shown to have a sensitivity of 81% and specificity of 84% in predicting the need for treatment of splenic injury and aids in the selection of hemodynamically stable patients who may be treated nonsurgically with transcatheter embolization [33]. Although the ability of CT to diagnose splenic vascular injuries has greatly improved over the past few decades, conventional angiography for high-grade splenic injuries is still indicated as not all splenic vascular injuries are detected by CT; a study evaluating the performance of postcontrast MDCT in diagnosing splenic vascular injuries revealed sensitivity and specificity of 76% and 90%, respectively [34].

The various CT findings reflect the four main types of acute splenic injury: laceration, hematoma, active hemorrhage, and vascular injuries (Table 10.4). Splenic lacerations typically appear as one or more irregularly marginated, linear, or stellate parenchymal defects (Figure 10.3). Care must be taken to differentiate a laceration from a splenic cleft that is more smoothly marginated with rounded contours; differentiation is also aided by the usual coexistence of perisplenic, subcapsular, or intraparenchymal hematomas with lacerations. Artifacts from high-density external devices, gastric contrast material, or beam hardening from adjacent ribs may also mimic splenic lacerations. In these cases, the abnormal attenuation is often extremely linear and can usually be seen to traverse multiple structures across a large section of the image. Also, the heterogeneous appearance of the splenic parenchyma during the arterial phase may

TABLE 10.4

Key Imaging Findings of Acute Splenic Injury

Injury	CT Finding
1. Laceration	Irregular linear parenchymal defect
2. Hematoma	Low or mixed attenuation collection in the parenchyma, subcapsular space, or perisplenic peritoneal spaces
3. Active hemorrhage	Ill-defined foci of extraluminal contrast that increase in volume and change shape/location on later phases of imaging
4. Vascular injuries	Round or lobulated foci of arterial enhancement that fade and become isoattenuating to splenic parenchyma on later phases

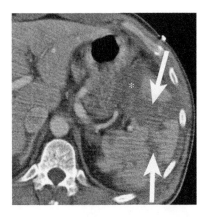

FIGURE 10.3
Splenic lacerations. A 36-year-old male presented with abdominal pain following a high-speed motor vehicle accident. Portal venous phase CT shows several linear, hypoattenuating defects (arrows) within the splenic parenchyma consistent with lacerations. There is a small amount of perisplenic hematoma (asterisk).

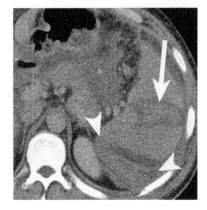

FIGURE 10.4
Splenic laceration and hematomas. A 32-year-old male presented with left upper quadrant pain after falling while mountain climbing. Portal venous phase CT shows a linear defect (arrow) consistent with laceration traversing the mid spleen. High attenuation filling the laceration is consistent with intraparenchmal hematoma. Encapsulated hematoma (arrowheads) along the posterior margin of the spleen is within the subcapsular space. Note hemoperitoneum (asterisk).

mimic lacerations or contusions; however, evaluation of the portal venous phase of imaging will show homogeneity of the parenchyma in the absence of focal injury.

Splenic hematomas may be located within the parenchyma or subcapsular space (Figure 10.4). Subcapsular hematomas typically appear as smoothly marginated, elliptical collections along the splenic margin that result in variable degrees of parenchymal compression. At noncontrast CT, the hematomas are hyperattenuating relative to the parenchyma, and appear as hypoattenuating, intermediate, density (approximately 30–60 HU) collections on postcontrast CT. Intraparenchymal hematomas manifest as irregularly marginated, linear, or stellate defects that expand the parenchyma. Over time, splenic hematomas will decrease in size and decrease in attenuation as the hemorrhage is broken down and resorbed. Splenic hematomas typically resolve over a span of 6–8 weeks after initial injury, often resulting in a small region of scarring or contour deformity; development of

a posttraumatic cyst is a rare occurrence. Although the clotted blood in hematomas has intermediate to high density (ranging from approximately 40 to 70 HU with an average of 51 HU), the attenuation of active hemorrhage is much higher (ranging from 84 to 350 HU with an average of 132 HU) (Figure 10.5) [23]. Active hemorrhage appears as linear or ill-defined foci of contrast extravasation that can occur in the splenic parenchyma, subcapsular space, or perisplenic space. Active arterial hemorrhage can be identified by an increase in the amount of contrast extravasation on images obtained during the arterial and portal venous phases of the CT examination; in addition, there is a change in the location or morphology of the extravasated contrast between the two phases of imaging (Figure 10.6).

Active splenic hemorrhage can be differentiated from a traumatic vascular injury (pseudoaneurysm or arteriovenous fistula) by evaluating the site of injury on the arterial and portal phases of the CT examination.

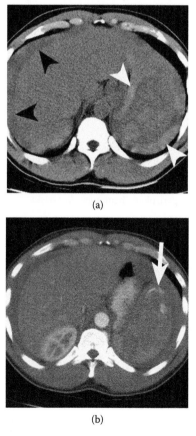

(a)

(b)

FIGURE 10.5
Active splenic hemorrhage and sentinel clot sign. A 41-year-old female presented with abdominal pain and tachycardia following a motorcycle accident. (a) Noncontrast CT shows blood in the perisplenic space (white arrowheads) to be of higher attenuation than blood in the perihepatic space (black arrowheads), consistent with the sentinel clot sign. (b) At a slightly inferior level, arterial phase CT shows extensive splenic lacerations and active extravasation (arrow) at the anterior pole.

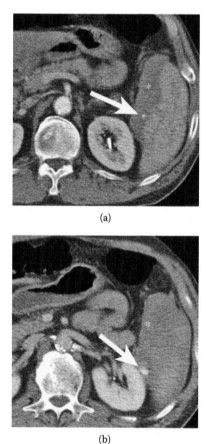

(a)

(b)

FIGURE 10.6
Subcapsular splenic hematoma with active hemorrhage. A 53-year-old male presented with abdominal pain following motor vehicle accident. (a) Arterial phase CT shows a subcapsular splenic hematoma (asterisk) and a small focus of arterial contrast extravasation (arrow). (b) Portal venous phase CT shows an increase in the amount of extravasated contrast (arrow) with changed position and location in the subcapsular hematoma (asterisk).

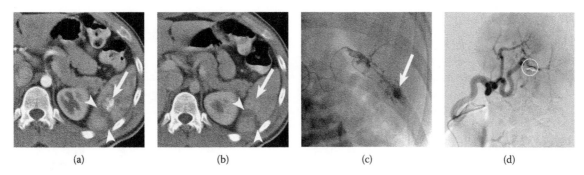

FIGURE 10.7
Splenic pseudoaneurysm. A 24-year-old male presented with left upper quadrant pain after sustaining a collision during skiing. (a) Arterial phase CT shows a marginated, round collection of contrast in the splenic parenchyma (arrow) and a laceration traversing the posterior pole of the spleen (arrowheads). (b) On the portal venous phase, the pseudoaneurysm (arrow) is barely conspicuous because of its near isoattenuation to the adjacent parenchyma, whereas the laceration (arrowheads) is well depicted. (c) Angiographic image during injection of the distal aspect of the splenic artery shows the pseudoaneurysm (arrow) as a focal round collection of contrast. (d) Following transcatheter embolization, there is no filling of the pseudoaneurysm because of coils (circle) within the supplying artery.

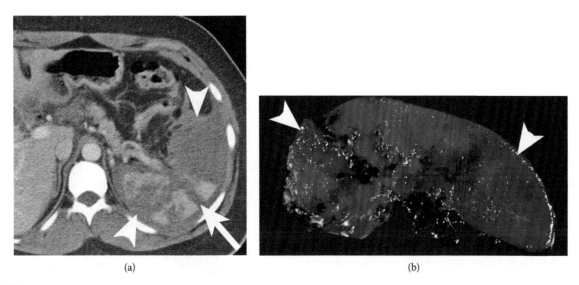

FIGURE 10.8
Splenic devascularization. A 24-year-old male presented with abdominal pain following a motor vehicle accident. (a) Portal venous phase CT shows a splenic laceration (arrow) and avascular, geographic regions (arrowheads) consistent with traumatic devascularization and regions of infarction. (b) Gross pathology specimen shows the corresponding dusky, geographic regions consistent with traumatic infarcts (arrowheads).

Traumatic vascular injuries are typically identified as well-marginated foci of abnormal contrast enhancement on the arterial phase, which then wash out or become minimally hyperdense to nearly isodense with respect to the normal splenic parenchyma on the portal venous phase of imaging (Figure 10.7). On the arterial phase, traumatic vascular injuries typically measure within 10 HU of a nearby artery [23]. In the absence of an adequate arterial phase, poor bolus timing, suboptimal contrast volume, and morbid obesity, small traumatic vascular injuries may be missed because of their near isoattenuation to adjacent splenic parenchyma [33]. Uncommonly, traumatic injury to the intima of the splenic artery can result in occlusion and subsequent infarct of the region of parenchyma

distal to the site of injury. At CT, infarcts appear as peripheral, wedge-shaped regions of hypoattenuating parenchyma because of decreased or absent enhancement (Figure 10.8). Isolated infarcts are usually not associated with perisplenic fluid or hemorrhage but may coexist with other types of splenic injury. Small splenic infarcts are often self-limited but can occasionally become superinfected or lead to splenic rupture.

The management of traumatic splenic injuries is strongly influenced by the findings at CT evaluation. A commonly used grading system based on the anatomic extent of injury at surgery has been established by the American Association for the Surgery of Trauma (AAST) (Table 10.5) [35]. It is often helpful for the interpreting radiologist to be familiar with this grading system to

TABLE 10.5

Summary of AAST Splenic Injury Grading System

Grade	Description
I	Subcapsular hematoma or laceration <1 cm
II	Subcapsular hematoma or laceration 1–3 cm
III	Capsular disruption, hematoma >3 cm, parenchymal hematoma >3 cm
IVA	Active parenchymal or subcapsular hemorrhage, pseudoaneursym or AV fistula, shattered spleen
IVB	Active intraperitoneal hemorrhage

Source: Marmery H et al., *J Am Coll Surg*, 2008, 206, 685–93.

facilitate communication with the trauma team. However, the radiologist should realize that there may be discrepancies between the clinical grade found at surgery and the CT findings and that the patient's clinical status and hemodynamic stability also play a significant role in management decisions. From an imaging standpoint, the most important finding on contrast-enhanced CT is the presence of active arterial extravasation or traumatic vascular injuries, since several studies have shown a strong correlation between CT findings of active splenic hemorrhage or traumatic vascular injury and the need for surgical or angiographic treatment [23,33,36,37] Because of the spleen's central role in immunity, nonoperative management has become the standard of care for hemodynamically stable patients with isolated splenic injury [38]. Use of transcatheter splenic artery embolization has been proven to be a useful adjunct to nonoperative management strategies, having a much lower treatment failure rate than observational management alone [39]. In patients receiving nonoperative management for traumatic splenic injuries, there has been some controversy regarding the role of follow-up CT, with some studies indicating low yield while others reporting significant progression of acute splenic injury at early follow-up CT [40,41]. Many trauma centers obtain follow-up CT in approximately 2–3 days to evaluate for increasing hematoma, extension of lacerations, development of new vascular lesions, and to assess recurrent bleeding following angioembolization or surgery. In patients with prior active hemorrhage or angiographic intervention, inclusion of noncontrast images before obtaining the contrast-enhanced series will allow easier differentiation of previously extravasated contrast from foci of persistent active hemorrhage.

10.2.5 Liver Trauma

The CT findings of acute liver injury are similar to those described for splenic injury. Hepatic lacerations are identified as irregular, linear, or stellate hypoattenuating defects (Figure 10.9). Uncomplicated lacerations evolve over the course of a few weeks and become smaller and less conspicuous on follow-up CT (Figure 10.10). Deep

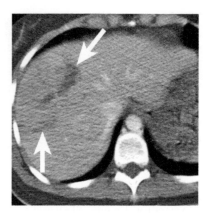

FIGURE 10.9

Liver laceration. A 33-year-old female presented after sustaining blunt abdominal trauma during a jet ski accident. Portal venous phase CT shows irregular, linear, hypoattenuating defects (arrows) within the anterior segment of the right hepatic lobe, consistent with lacerations.

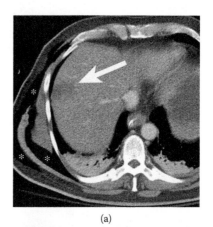

(a)

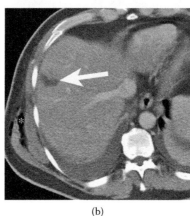

(b)

FIGURE 10.10

Evolution of liver laceration. A 47-year-old female presented with diffuse pain after sustaining blunt abdominal trauma during a motor vehicle accident. (a) Portal venous phase CT reveals an ill-defined, hypoattenuating defect (arrow) consistent with a laceration in the anterior segment of the right hepatic lobe. There is gas (asterisks) in the body wall because of trauma. (b) On follow-up CT obtained 10 days later, the laceration (arrow) is smaller and more well defined. Note the decreasing amount of gas (asterisk) in the body wall on the follow-up examination also.

lacerations (>3 cm), and those extending centrally to the level of the porta hepatis, are associated with increased risk of bile duct injury and biloma. Lacerations traversing the hepatic capsule can result in variable amount of hematoma in the perihepatic spaces and hemoperitoneum. However, not all lacerations result in hemoperitoneum; bleeding lacerations can tamponade because of accumulation of intraparenchymal hematoma (Figure 10.11), whereas others may extend to the bare area of the liver and cause hemorrhage into the retroperitoneum. Hematomas can also occur in the subcapsular space, resulting in a well-marginated elliptical collection with deformation of the adjacent parenchyma. In addition to intraparenchymal hematomas, contusions can result in regions of ill-defined heterogeneous attenuation and altered enhancement.

In contrast to the typical low to intermediate attenuation of intraparenchymal hematoma, foci of active hemorrhage are identified as a jet of high attenuation because of contrast extravasation. In cases of arterial bleeding, the active hemorrhage is typically isoattenuating to an adjacent artery. If active hemorrhage is pooling in the subcapsular or perihepatic spaces, differentiation from clotted hematoma can be made by measuring the attenuation, since active arterial extravasation was found to have much higher attenuation (ranging from 91 to 274 HU with a mean of 155 HU) compared to clotted blood within a hematoma (ranging from 28 to 82 HU with a mean of 54 HU) (Figure 10.12) [42]. In cases of active arterial extravasation, treatment is typically initiated immediately with surgical repair or angiographic intervention because of the high likelihood of developing hemodynamic instability and failure of conservative management [43,44]. Other CT findings associated with frequent urgent need for surgical or percutaneous intervention are pseudoaneurysm and laceration of a major

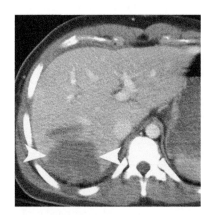

FIGURE 10.11
Hepatic intraparenchymal hematoma. An 18-year-old female presented with right-sided abdominal pain following a motorcycle crash. Portal venous phase CT shows a round, hypoattenuating region (arrowheads) in the posterior segment of the right lobe, consistent with intraparenchymal hematoma.

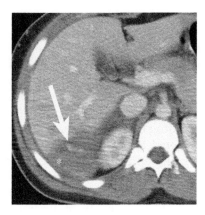

FIGURE 10.12
Active hemorrhage into hematoma. A 24-year-old female presented with pain following a motor vehicle accident. Portal venous phase CT shows a linear, high-attenuation (150 HU) focus (arrow) consistent with active contrast extravasation within the lower attenuation (60 HU) hematoma (asterisk).

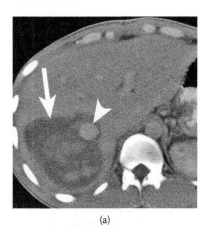

(a)

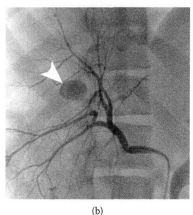

(b)

FIGURE 10.13
Hepatic intraparenchymal hematoma and pseudoaneurysm. A 23-year-old male presented with right upper quadrant pain and hypotension following a gunshot wound to the back. (a) Portal venous phase CT shows a large heterogeneous collection in the parenchyma consistent with hematoma (arrow). Within the hematoma, there is a round enhancing lesion (arrowhead). (b) Angiographic image during injection of the hepatic artery shows contrast filling an ovoid pseudoaneurysm (arrowhead). The pseudoaneurysm was successfully treated with coil embolization.

hepatic vein or the inferior vena cava (IVC) [45]. Similar to the spleen, pseudoaneurysm in the liver appear as a marginated collection of contrast that enhances on the arterial phase and generally fades or washes out on the portal phase. Pseudoaneurysms are at the risk for spontaneous rupture (Figure 10.13) and are typically treated with percutaneous catheter embolization in the acute setting. The finding of a major hepatic venous injury at CT has been noted to be an indirect finding of occult arterial injury. In addition to evaluation of the hepatic veins, the portal veins should be thoroughly evaluated for focal injury. In addition, identification of periportal low attenuation in the vicinity of a parenchymal laceration is a sign of hemorrhage dissecting along the periportal tissues. In contrast, diffuse periportal low attenuation often occurs in the setting of aggressive resuscitation because of distension of the periportal lymphatics.

There have been several proposed grading systems for blunt hepatic injury, and the most widely used classification was established by the AAST (Table 10.6). However, the AAST liver injury classification contains various criteria that cannot be assessed by CT evaluation, resulting in reports of significant discrepancies between operative and CT findings. Therefore, injury grading systems should not be the sole criterion used for clinical decision making. Rather, as with splenic injuries, the patient's clinical status and hemodynamic stability have

been found to play a more central role in the need for immediate surgery of angiographic intervention [46]. Injury grading systems are useful in facilitating communication of injury patterns between the trauma team and radiologists. A CT-based grading scheme for liver injury has been shown to assist in selecting patients for angiography and those at risk for continued bleeding or posttraumatic complications (Table 10.7) [45].

Several types of delayed complications can contribute to the morbidity and mortality following the initial liver trauma (Table 10.8). Because of the trend toward nonoperative management of liver injuries, the incidence of these delayed complications has increased over the past two decades. The most common delayed complication is hemorrhage, occurring in up to 5.9% of patients sustaining liver trauma [47]. Patients typically present with new or persistent pain, decreasing hematocrit, and ongoing transfusion requirements. CT will show findings of new or increasing hematoma, hemoperitoneum, or active contrast extravasation. Abscess may develop in regions of contaminated liver because of penetrating trauma or in regions subjected to infarction. CT findings of abscess include a well-defined fluid collection with a thick rind of enhancement and a variable degree of internal septa and gas locules. In contrast, posttraumatic bilomas are

TABLE 10.6

Summary of AAST Liver Injury Grading System

Grade	Description
I	Hematoma: subcapsular, <10% surface area
	Laceration: capsular tear, <1 cm in parenchymal depth
II	Hematoma: subcapsular, 10%–50% surface area; intraparenchymal, <10 cm in diameter
	Laceration: 1–3 cm in parenchymal depth, <10 cm long
III	Hematoma: subcapsular, >50% surface area or expanding or ruptured subcapsular hematoma with active bleeding; intraparenchymal, >10 cm or expanding or ruptured
	Laceration: >3 cm in parenchymal depth
IV	Hematoma: ruptured intraparenchymal hematoma with active bleeding
	Laceration: parenchymal disruption involving 25%–75% of a hepatic lobe or one to three Couinaud segments within a single lobe
V	Laceration: parenchymal disruption involving >75% of a hepatic lobe or more than three Couinaud segments within a single lobe
	Vascular: juxtahepatic venous injuries (i.e., retrohepatic vena cava or central hepatic veins)
VI	Vascular: hepatic avulsion

Source: Marmery H et al., *J Am Coll Surg*, 2008, 206, 685–93.

TABLE 10.7

Summary of CT-Based Grading of Liver Injury

Grade	Criteria
1	Capsular avulsion, superficial laceration(s) <1 cm deep, subcapsular hematoma <1 cm in maximum thickness, periportal blood tracking only
2	Laceration(s) 1–3 cm deep, central-subcapsular hematoma(s) 1–3 cm in diameter
3	Laceration >3 cm deep, central-subcapsular hematoma(s) >3 cm in diameter
4	Massive central-subcapsular hematoma >10 cm, lobar tissue destruction (maceration) or devascularization
5	Bilobar tissue destruction (maceration) or devascularization

Source: Wong YC et al., *J Trauma*, 2003, 54, 164–70.

TABLE 10.8

Summary of Delayed Complications of Liver Trauma

Complication	Finding
1. Hemorrhage	New or increased size of heterogeneous collection (hematoma) or active contrast extravasation within parenchyma, subcapsular space and perihepatic spaces
2. Biloma	Homogeneous, near-water attenuation fluid collection
3. Abscess	Fluid collection with irregular rind of rim enhancement and variable internal attenuation and gas

usually more homogeneous, near-water attenuation fluid collections. Other biliary complications include biliary fistula and biliary leak with resultant peritonitis. In cases of biliary fistula or leak, further evaluation with endoscopic retrograde cholangiopancreatography (ERCP), magnetic resonance cholangiopancreatography (MRCP), or hepatobiliary scintigraphy is needed to identify the site of the abnormality and guide further endoscopic or surgical treatment. In cases of bile peritonitis, CT findings include persistent or increasing volume of near-water attenuation ascites, peritoneal thickening, and hyperemia. Finally, hepatic pseudoaneurysm appears as a round or ovoid lesion that is contiguous and isoattenuating with the hepatic artery; if not urgently treated, spontaneous rupture can lead to significant hemorrhage (Figure 10.14). CT characterization of the pseudoaneurysm's size, location, and neck caliber will facilitate treatment with percutaneous embolization or surgery. The development of delayed complications

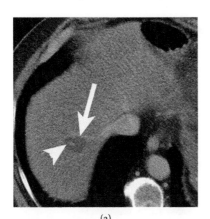

(a)

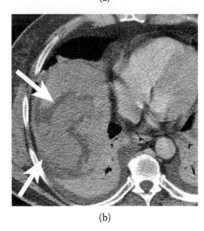

(b)

FIGURE 10.14
Hepatic pseudoaneurysm and hemorrhage. A 58-year-old male presented with abdominal pain after sustaining blunt trauma during a motor vehicle accident. (a) Portal venous phase CT shows an ovoid intraparenchymal hematoma (arrow) and a small focus on internal enhancement (arrowhead) most suggestive of a pseudoaneurysm. (b) Follow-up CT obtained because of sudden onset of increasing pain reveals extensive intraparenchymal hemorrhage (arrows) extending from the site of pseudoaneurysm.

occurs more frequently in more severe liver injuries and should be suspected in patients with persistent or increasing abdominal pain, fever, and jaundice. Although the timing of follow-up CT largely depends on the patient's clinical status, studies have suggested that the optimal time frame is between 7 and 10 days [48].

10.2.6 Gallbladder Trauma

Gallbladder injury following abdominal trauma is a rare occurrence, with the incidence reported ranging from 2% to 8% [49]. The low incidence can be accounted for by the anatomic shielding of the gallbladder by the liver and inferior ribs. Most gallbladder injuries coexist with other visceral injuries in over 90% of patients, making isolated gallbladder injury an extremely rare occurrence: coexisting abdominal injuries are most commonly observed in the liver, but can also affect the duodenum, pancreas, spleen, and kidneys [50]. The association of gallbladder injury with other visceral injuries is important clinically, as the clinical presentation and symptoms are usually dominated by injuries to the adjacent organs. Therefore, most gallbladder injuries are diagnosed at laparotomy that was prompted by signs and symptoms of associated visceral injuries. In the rare case of isolated gallbladder injury, the initial symptoms are often mild and vague, with the more fulminant clinical presentation often delayed until the onset of peritonitis.

Gallbladder injuries can be generally classified as contusion, laceration, perforation, and avulsion. Gallbladder contusions and perforations can occur following a sudden compressive blow. Pathologically, gallbladder contusions consist of intramural hematoma and are often clinically self-limited. However, lacerations and perforations consist of transmural defects that may result in leakage of bile, following penetrating or blunt trauma (Figure 10.15). Some reports have suggested that recent alcohol ingestion is contributory to gallbladder rupture because of its potential to increase tone of the sphincter of Oddi and result in gallbladder distension [51]. In contrast, the fibrosis and wall thickening associated with chronic gallbladder disease is felt to be somewhat protective against gallbladder rupture during blunt abdominal trauma [52]. Avulsion injuries are due to shear and torsion forces incurred during rapid deceleration and are subclassified as partial, complete, or total. Partial and complete avulsion injuries differ in the degree of separation of the gallbladder from the liver surface; total avulsion ("traumatic cholecystectomy") is extremely rare and occurs when there is the combination of complete separation of the gallbladder from the liver surface and disruption of the cystic artery and duct so that all anatomic attachments of the gallbladder to the liver are severed.

Although no combination of CT findings has been proven to be specific for the types of gallbladder injury,

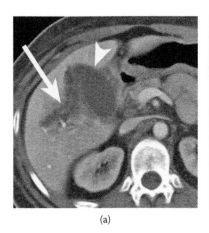
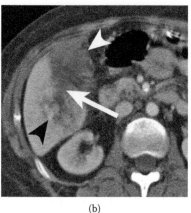

(a)   (b)

FIGURE 10.15
Gallbladder perforation. A 47-year-old male presented with right upper quadrant pain following a motorcycle crash. (a) Portal venous phase CT shows a long, linear, hypoattenuating defect (arrow) consistent with laceration extending from the level of the gallbladder fossa into the right hepatic lobe. There is an irregular margin (white arrowhead) to the gallbladder fundus at a site of wall laceration. (b) More inferiorly, there is extension of the laceration (arrow) and a focus of lobular enhancement (black arrowhead) consistent with pseudoaneurysm. The gallbladder (white arrowhead) is ill-defined and surrounded by bile and hemorrhage. A traumatic gallbladder perforation and liver lacerations were confirmed during laparotomy.

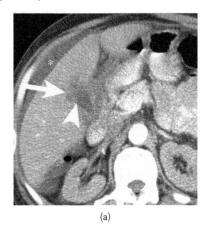
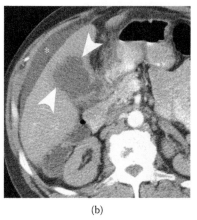

(a)   (b)

FIGURE 10.16
Gallbladder perforation. A 50-year-old male presented with right upper quadrant pain following blunt impact sustained during a motor vehicle accident. (a) Arterial phase CT shows an ill-defined hepatic contusion (arrow) along the interlobar fissure. The ventral margin of the gallbladder (arrowhead) is irregular and there is a small volume of low-attenuation fluid (asterisk) in the perihepatic spaces because of bile. (b) More inferiorly, the gallbladder fundus (arrowheads) is irregular and lobulated because of focal perforation. Note extension of low-attenuation bile (asterisk) in the perihepatic space. The patient was treated with cholecystectomy.

there are numerous findings associated with primary gallbladder injury because of blunt trauma [53,54]. Most of the CT findings of traumatic gallbladder injury involve the gallbladder wall. The CT findings of gallbladder wall irregularity and asymmetric wall thickening may be subtle but may be the only findings indicative of a mural injury ranging from contusion to perforation (Figure 10.16); in some cases, a site of microperforation may seal without intervention, and the resultant mural abnormality cannot be reliably differentiated from contusion in the absence of ancillary findings [53]. More obvious CT findings of a primary gallbladder injury include a focal mural contour defect, intraluminal mucosal flap, and a site of mucosal disruption or nonenhancement (Figure 10.17). In addition,

although the CT findings of a collapsed gallbladder lumen, subserosal fluid, pericholecystic fluid, and intraperitoneal fluid isoattenuating to bile are nonspecific in and of themselves, they are secondary signs that increase suspicion for the presence of a transmural gallbladder injury with bile leakage (Table 10.9). Although intraluminal high attenuation from acute hemorrhage into the gallbladder lumen can be due to hepatobiliary injury (hemobilia), it can also result from primary gallbladder injury [55]; however, high-attenuation material in the gallbladder lumen is a nonspecific finding and differential considerations include acute hemorrhage, vicarious excretion of intravenous contrast material, residual contrast from a recent hepatobiliary procedure, biliary sludge, and cholelithiasis. Herniation of

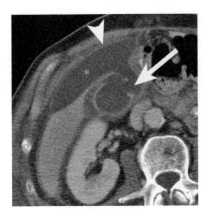

FIGURE 10.17

Gallbladder perforation. A 56-year-old male presented with right upper quadrant pain approximately three days after sustaining blunt abdominal trauma. Portal venous phase CT shows disruption of the gallbladder wall (arrow) because of perforation. Note perihepatic fluid (asterisk) and hyperemia of the adjacent peritoneal reflection (arrowhead) consistent with bile peritonitis.

TABLE 10.9

Summary of CT Findings of Traumatic Gallbladder Injury

specific
1. Focal mural contour abnormality
2. Intraluminal mucosal flap
3. Focal mural disruption or nonenhancement

Nonspecific
4. Mural edema or thickening
5. Collapsed lumen
6. Pericholecystic fluid
7. Intraluminal high attenuation

mesenteric fat through a site of gallbladder perforation has also been reported as a diagnostic CT finding, although this is quite rare [56]. Although cases of partial gallbladder avulsion may be difficult to diagnose at CT, displacement of the gallbladder may be due to complete or total avulsion or formation of a traumatic biloma.

US can also be effectively used to evaluate the gallbladder in the acute setting because of its ability to detect focal mural defects, intraluminal mucosal flaps, and foci of intramural hemorrhage. US can also be used to differentiate anechoic biliary fluid from echogenic hemorrhage in the perihepatic space. Likewise, although magnetic resonance imaging (MRI) is not typically used in diagnosing acute gallbladder injury, it has a role in differentiating intraperitoneal fluid as either bilious or hemorrhagic [57]. Hepatobiliary scintigraphy should be strongly considered as a follow-up examination in cases of suspected gallbladder perforation or laceration; in such cases, acquisition of delayed images is often crucial to prevent misinterpretation and delay in diagnosis.

Patients who have sustained a contusion or partial avulsion may be managed conservatively. In these situations, it has been suggested that a baseline hepatobiliary scan with delayed images is obtained to exclude bile extravasation followed by a repeated CT or US in approximately 3–4 weeks to assure resolution of the injury and to exclude development of a pericholecystic fluid collection [53]. Complications reported with a conservative approach include fistula formation and delayed perforation in patients who are immunocompromised [58,59]. Cholecystectomy is the preferred treatment in patients sustaining gallbladder perforation or complete or total avulsion [50].

10.2.7 Biliary Trauma

Traumatic injury to the intrahepatic and extrahepatic bile ducts is uncommon but has been reported to occur in up to 9% of patients sustaining severe liver injury [60]. Biliary injury involving the extrahepatic ducts or central intrahepatic ducts usually leads to development of significant complications, such as bile peritonitis, biloma, and biliary fistula formation [61]. There are typically no initial specific clinical signs or symptoms to suggest a biliary injury, often resulting in delayed diagnosis and treatment unless there is high clinical suspicion. In patients undergoing laparotomy for severe liver trauma, a biliary injury can be detected if there is bile staining along the hepatoduodenal ligament or lesser sac. Although no definitive correlation between the type of liver injury and presence of intrahepatic bile duct injury has been shown, intrahepatic bile duct injuries most commonly occur adjacent to the liver hilum in the setting of high-grade liver injury, with lacerations extending to the porta hepatis and caudate lobe (Figure 10.18). Although CT and US cannot resolve the focal injury to the intrahepatic bile duct, the combination of deep hepatic lacerations extending toward the hilum and low-attenuation perihepatic fluid are suggestive of intrahepatic biliary injury. In such cases, further evaluation with hepatobiliary scintigraphy, ERCP, or percutaneous cholangiography are nonsurgical methods that can diagnose biliary injury by showing extravasation of the injected material into the perihepatic spaces. MRI has also been used in some cases to secondarily diagnose biliary injury by differentiating bilious from hematogenous fluid in the peritoneal cavity [57]. In addition, persistence of simple-appearing peritoneal fluid on follow-up CT or US should raise suspicion for a biliary leak. In the uncommon complication of bile peritonitis, CT will show peritoneal fluid in conjunction with thickening and hyperemia of the peritoneal reflections. In such cases, the most likely cause of a bile leak is injury to the intrahepatic ducts, as traumatic disruption of the extrahepatic bile ducts and

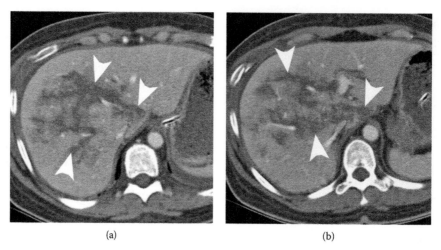

(a)   (b)

FIGURE 10.18
Intrahepatic bile duct disruption. A 43-year-old male presented abdominal pain following a motor vehicle accident. (a and b) Portal venous phase CT images show extensive lacerations (arrowheads) extending centrally into the porta hepatis and caudate lobe. During laparotomy, an intraoperative cholangiogram (not available) showed laceration of the right bile duct and bile leak requiring biliary reconstruction.

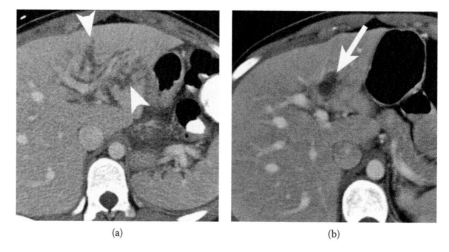

(a)   (b)

FIGURE 10.19
Biloma. A 43-year-old female presented with abdominal pain following a motor vehicle accident. (a) Portal venous phase CT shows a stellate laceration (arrowheads) in the left hepatic lobe. (b) Follow-up imaging approximately 3 weeks later shows resolution of the laceration but development of an ovoid fluid collection (arrow) consistent with biloma. The patient was treated with percutaneous drainage.

gallbladder are relatively uncommon injuries. If there is a traumatic injury involving the extrahepatic bile ducts, the ductal disruption most commonly occurs distally, as the common bile duct becomes fixated as it enters the pancreatic head; in most cases, the adjacent hepatic artery and portal vein are more tortuous and pliable and are rarely injured [62]. Similar to intrahepatic biliary injury, visualization of the site of ductal disruption is usually not possible with CT or US; secondary findings include fluid in the subhepatic and anterior pararenal spaces and possible coexistent trauma to the adjacent viscera. MRCP, ERCP, and hepatobiliary scintigraphy can diagnose an injury to the extrahepatic bile ducts and act to guide treatment.

Treatment options for acute biliary injury include placement of a stent during ERCP or surgical reconstruction of the biliary system. Bilomas and biliary fistula are delayed complications that often have an insidious course because of a slow bile leak. Most bilomas and fistula are asymptomatic and may not be diagnosed until months after the initial trauma. If sufficiently large, some bilomas may cause abdominal distension, pain, or jaundice from mass effect. CT findings consist of a well-marginated, intrahepatic or extrahepatic fluid collection measuring near-water attenuation with a thin rim of peripheral enhancement (Figure 10.19). US will reveal an avascular, loculated collection that is predominantly anechoic; some bilomas may contain thin septa and internal debris manifesting as layering low-level echoes, and differentiation of biloma from resolving hematoma or abscess may be difficult. Definitive diagnosis and treatment primarily consist of CT- or US-guided aspiration and drainage, with surgery reserved for complicated or recurrent cases. Treatment of biliary fistula is more challenging, often requiring complex surgical biliary reconstruction. However, several cases of biliary fistula have been successfully treated nonsurgically with endoscopic sphincterotomy and biliary stenting [63].

10.2.8 Pancreas Trauma

Traumatic injury of the pancreas is uncommon, occurring between 2% and 12% of patients sustaining blunt abdominal trauma [64]. The pancreas is susceptible to crush injury because of compression against the lumbar spine during rapid deceleration. Most pancreatic injuries are due to motor vehicle accidents and occur in the body, whereas the remainder are relatively evenly distributed within the remaining portions of the parenchyma. Isolated pancreatic injury is uncommon, as associated injuries to the liver, spleen, stomach, and duodenum occur in more than 90% of cases [65]. Pancreatic injuries are challenging to diagnose clinically, since symptoms and physical examination findings are nonspecific and variable. Serum amylase levels are neither sensitive nor specific in diagnosing pancreatic injury, and the reported triad of leukocytosis, fever, and elevated serum amylase is infrequently present [66,67]; in addition, amylase and lipase levels are often falsely negative during DPL because of the retroperitoneal location of the pancreas and associated fluid collections. Early diagnosis of pancreatic injury is critical since delayed complications such as abscess, sepsis, hemorrhage, and fistula develop in up to 20% of cases and may contribute to mortality [66]. In the acute setting, mortality is most common because of massive hemorrhage, whereas delayed morbidity and mortality are usual because of pancreatic duct disruption, sepsis, and multiorgan failure [68]. The mortality rate also increases when the injury involves the pancreatic head because of higher association with acute vascular injury to the IVC, splenic vein, and superior mesenteric vein [66].

Although there has been some controversy regarding the accuracy of CT for diagnosing pancreatic injuries, CT has emerged as the preferred imaging modality in the diagnosis of acute pancreatic injury [66,69]. However, diagnosis of acute pancreatic injuries can be subtle on the initial CT examination, especially in thin patients with minimal retroperitoneal fat and close apposition of retroperitoneal structures. Pancreatic injuries can be detected by identification of either direct or indirect findings. Direct signs of acute pancreatic injury include pancreatic enlargement, heterogeneity, parenchymal hemorrhage, parenchymal laceration, and transection. Pancreatic enlargement and focal or diffuse heterogeneous enhancement are findings suggestive of parenchymal contusion (Figure 10.20). Pancreatic

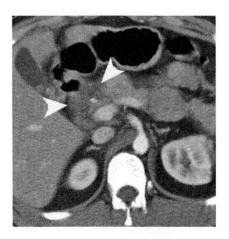

FIGURE 10.20
Pancreatic contusion. A 25-year-old male presented with mid abdominal pain following a motor vehicle accident. Portal venous phase CT shows ill-defined hypoattenuation (arrowheads) of the pancreatic neck and head because of contusion. The patient also had a laceration (not shown) of the left hepatic lobe.

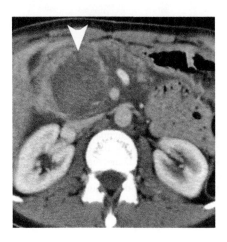

FIGURE 10.21
Pancreatic hematoma. A 27-year-old presented with epigastric pain following blunt abdominal trauma after falling from 20 ft. Portal venous phase CT shows a round, heterogeneous collection (arrowhead) within the pancreatic head (p). Hemorrhage (asterisks) dissects along the vessels in the root of the small bowel mesentery.

parenchymal hemorrhage appears as diffuse or focal increased attenuation, often with mass effect resulting in distortion of the parenchyma (Figure 10.21). Lacerations are shown as linear, hypoattenuating irregular defects in the pancreatic parenchyma. Their width is variable, depending on the amount of hemorrhage insinuating within the laceration defect (Figure 10.22). The depth of the laceration is important, as deeper lacerations (>50% pancreatic thickness in the anteroposterior diameter) have been shown to be more closely associated with pancreatic ductal injury than more superficial lacerations (<50% of the anteroposterior diameter of the pancreas) [66]. Transection occurs when a laceration extends through the entirety of the parenchyma and disrupts the pancreatic duct; determination of a full-thickness injury may be difficult unless the disrupted edges of the parenchyma are separated by hematoma (Figure 10.23). Grading schemes for pancreatic injury have been proposed that aid in predicting the severity of injury and guiding management (Table 10.10) [70].

There are several secondary findings of acute pancreatic injury that mostly hinge on the evaluation of

TABLE 10.10

Summary of CT Findings of Pancreatic Injury

Direct
1. Edema/heterogeneity
2. Parenchymal hemorrhage
3. Laceration
4. Transection

Indirect
5. Infiltration of peripancreatic fat
6. Fluid between pancreas and splenic vein
7. Fluid/hemorrhage within anterior pararenal space, lesser sac and along root of small bowel mesentery

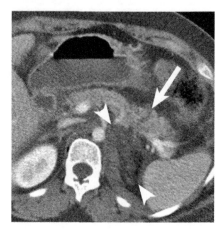

FIGURE 10.22
Pancreatic laceration. A 25-year-old male presented with left upper quadrant pain following a high-speed motor vehicle accident. Postcontrast CT shows a linear hypoattenuating defect (arrow) consistent with laceration traversing the distal body of the pancreas. There is also retroperitoneal hemorrhage (arrowheads) adjacent to the pancreas. Endoscopic retrograde cholangiopancreatography (ERCP) showed no pancreatic duct injury and the patient was managed conservatively.

TABLE 10.11

Summary of AAST Pancreas Injury Grading System

Grade	Description
I	Hematoma: Minor contusion without ductal injury
	Laceration: Superficial laceration without ductal injury
II	Hematoma: Major contusion without ductal injury or tissue loss
	Laceration: Major laceration without ductal injury or tissue loss
III	Laceration: Distal transection or pancreatic parenchymal injury with ductal injury
IV	Laceration: Proximal transection or pancreatic parenchymal injury involving the ampulla
V	Massive disruption of the pancreatic head

Source: Akhrass R et al., *Am Surg,* 1996, 62, 647–51.

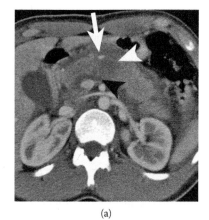

(a)

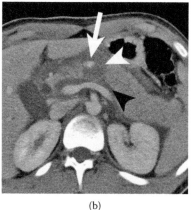

(b)

FIGURE 10.23
Pancreatic transection. A 16-year-old male presented with pain and tachycardia following a motor vehicle accident. (a) Arterial phase CT followed by (b) portal venous phase CT shows an increasing amount of active contrast extravasation (arrow) within a hypoattenuating defect (white arrowhead) in the pancreatic body, consistent with pancreatic transection. Note fluid (black arrowhead) insinuating between the dorsal margin of the pancreas and splenic and portal veins. CT findings were confirmed during surgery and the patient underwent extended distal pancreatectomy.

the peripancreatic tissue planes and adjacent viscera (Table 10.11). In patients with sufficient retroperitoneal fat, infiltration of the peripancreatic fat may be seen in cases of acute pancreatitis or extension of a small volume of hemorrhage from a parenchymal laceration. Similarly, subtle thickening of the left anterior renal fascia may be the only finding in an occult, low-grade pancreatic injury. In cases of more extensive laceration, fluid or hemorrhage can be identified in the anterior pararenal space, lesser sac, and extending along the root of the small bowel mesentery. A helpful CT finding of acute pancreatic injury is the identification of fluid between the pancreas and splenic vein, which has been reported to be present in 90% of patients with pancreatic injury following blunt abdominal trauma [71]. Since most pancreatic injuries are not isolated findings, identification of an adjacent visceral injury and correlation to the mechanism of injury are useful adjuncts in identifying an acute pancreatic trauma. For example, if the epicenter of trauma affected the right aspect of the abdomen, the pancreatic head should be thoroughly evaluated for focal injury, especially in the setting of coexisting injury to the duodenum, liver, common bile duct, and right and middle colic vessels. Midline impact typically causes a fulcrum effect of the pancreatic neck over the lumbar spine and is associated with injuries to the left hepatic lobe, transverse mesocolon, and middle colic vessels. In the setting of left-sided blunt abdominal trauma, the pancreatic tail should be thoroughly inspected, especially when there is injury to the spleen, left kidney, and distal transverse colon.

CT plays a central role in the triage of patients with acute pancreatic trauma, since treatment depends on the severity and location of the trauma and the integrity of the pancreatic duct. In cases of suspected occult ductal injury, further evaluation with MRCP or ERCP is often useful [72]. Many cases of acute pancreatic injury can be managed conservatively; examples include superficial lacerations and traumatic pancreatitis, for which supportive treatment generally consists of bowel rest and nasogastric suction. However, active hemorrhage, significant or increasing hematoma, and disruption of the pancreatic duct require laparotomy or percutaneous intervention. Pancreatic ductal disruption is treated by either surgical treatment or endoscopic stent placement. Complications from pancreatic trauma may occur weeks to years after the initial injury and are usually because of strictures or disruption of the main pancreatic duct. Complications include pancreatitis, sepsis, fistula, abscess, and pseudocyst. The timing of follow-up CT after the initial pancreatic injury is quite variable and dependent on the extent of the injury, laboratory analysis, and the patient's clinical status. Common indications for follow-up CT include persistent abdominal pain, fever, leukocytosis, increasing serial serum amylase levels, and reassessment of hematoma or fluid collections.

10.2.9 Gastrointestinal and Mesenteric Trauma

Acute GI and mesenteric injuries are less common than solid visceral injuries, occurring in only approximately 5% of patients sustaining abdominal trauma [73]. Despite their rarity, GI injuries are associated with significant morbidity and mortality if unrecognized. Patients with unrecognized bowel perforation can experience significant hemorrhage, peritonitis, and sepsis. Clinical diagnosis of GI tract, mesenteric, and omental injury is challenging because of the nonspecific signs, symptoms, and physical examination findings. Although abdominal pain and guarding are the most common symptoms associated with GI injury, symptoms may be masked in patients with distracting injuries or absent in intubated patients. Although DPL has been used to diagnose hemoperitoneum, it provides nonspecific information and does not evaluate hemorrhage because of injury of retroperitoneal structures; therefore, DPL is being used with decreasing frequency in most trauma centers. Therefore, CT has evolved over the past three decades to become the imaging modality of choice for the initial evaluation of patients with suspected GI or mesenteric injury because of its ability to provide a rapid, global view of the bowel, omentum, mesentery, and adjacent viscera. Use of thin-section (5 mm or less) MDCT performed during the portal venous phase is a common approach for abdominal trauma CT. Display of images in multiple planes and multiple window settings helps to detect subtle abnormalities, such as small amounts of pneumoperitoneum when viewed in a lung window setting. In most institutions, scanning of the trauma patient is performed without the use of oral contrast material because of its low sensitivity, as extravasation of oral contrast has been reported to occur in up to only 15% of patients with significant GI or mesenteric injury [74,75]. The trend toward omission of oral contrast in the trauma setting is based on the theoretical potential for aspiration, delay in diagnosis and treatment, and lack of proven significant additional information in the detection of substantial GI and mesenteric injury [76,77].

Acute GI injuries can result from crush injuries, shear forces incurred during rapid deceleration, and viscus rupture because of rapid increases in intraluminal pressure. The proximal jejunum and distal ileum are the most commonly injured sites of the GI tract, accounting for over 50% of all GI tract injuries, because of their relative fixation by the ligament of Treitz and the ileocolic junction, respectively (Figure 10.24) [78,79]. These sites of injury are followed by the duodenum, colon, and stomach in decreasing order of frequency (Figures 10.25 and 10.26). Historically, the sensitivity and specificity of

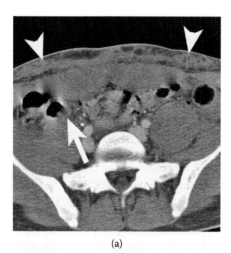

(a)

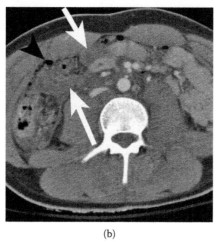

(b)

FIGURE 10.24
Laceration, ischemia and perforation of the distal ileum. A 21-year-old male presented with abdominal pain following a high-speed motor vehicle accident. (a) Portal venous phase CT shows a transverse band of subcutaneous fat infiltration (white arrowheads), consistent with "seat belt" ecchymosis. Although not well distended, a segment of ileum shows wall thickening (arrow) out of proportion to bowel elsewhere. (b) More inferiorly, there is mild wall thickening and poor perfusion of a segment of ileum (arrows), a small amount of adjacent pneumoperitoneum (black arrowhead), and a small amount of hemorrhage in the right paracolic gutter. At laparotomy, there was perforation, deserosalization and ischemia of a 20 cm segment of ileum that was resected.

CT for the detection of bowel and mesenteric injuries is reported to be 70%–95% and 92%–100%, respectively, before the advent of MDCT [80–82]. Specific CT findings of acute GI injury include full thickness laceration resulting in mural discontinuity and extravastation of oral contrast material (Table 10.12). However, these findings are relatively uncommon and have low sensitivity; for example, bowel transection with mural discontinuity has been reported to be detectable in only 7% of examinations [83]. Several more sensitive, but nonspecific, CT findings include focal mural thickening, irregular mural enhancement, infiltration of the

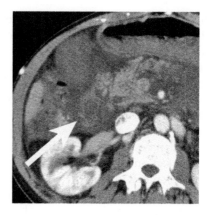

FIGURE 10.25
Duodenal perforation. A 55-year-old female presented with right-sided pain after a motor vehicle accident. Portal phase CT shows thickening and focal mural irregularity (arrow) of the descending duodenum at the site of perforation. Note fluid surrounding the duodenum and within the retroperitoneum. The perforation was repaired surgically.

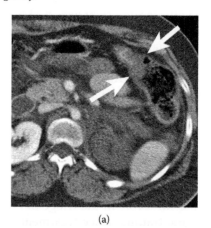

(a)

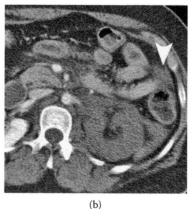

(b)

FIGURE 10.26
Colonic laceration. A 26-year-old female presented with left-sided abdominal pain after a high-speed motor vehicle accident. (a) Post-contrast CT shows focal mural thickening (arrow) of the splenic flexure of the colon. Note devascularization of the left kidney (K) because of traumatic dissection of the renal artery and a small amount of retroperitoneal hemorrhage (b) More inferiorly, there is infiltration of the pericolonic fat (arrowhead) because of hemorrhage. (c) The splayed resection specimen shows the segment of mural injury (arrows) corresponding to the segment of thickening on CT.

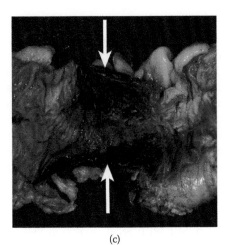

(c)

FIGURE 10.26 (*Continued*)

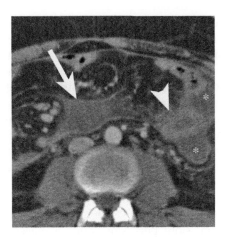

FIGURE 10.28
Small bowel laceration and mesenteric hematoma. A 33-year-old male presented with abdominal pain following blunt trauma sustained during a motor vehicle accident. Portal venous phase CT reveals a mesenteric hematoma (arrow) and a thickened segment of small bowel (arrowhead) with adjacent fluid (asterisks). An enterotomy was repaired during surgery.

TABLE 10.12

Summary of CT Findings of Bowel Injury

1. Wall thickening
2. Heterogeneous wall enhancement
3. Wall discontinuity
4. Extraluminal gas
5. Mesenteric fat infiltration
6. Mesenteric fluid/hematoma

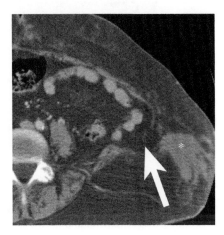

FIGURE 10.29
Traumatic hernia. A 74-year-old male presented with left side pain following a motor vehicle accident. Portal venous phase CT shows superficial hematoma (asterisk) and a defect (arrow) containing a small amount of fat in the lateral aspect of the left body wall consistent with a traumatic lumbar hernia.

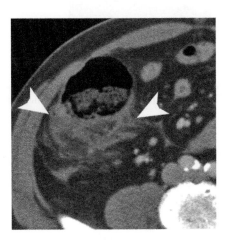

FIGURE 10.27
Colonic serosal injury. A 42-year-old male presented with right lower quadrant pain after blunt force trauma to the right aspect of the abdomen. Portal venous phase CT shows hemorrhage (arrowheads) extending from the posterior wall of the cecum into the adjacent fat. A cecal serosal injury was repaired at surgery.

mesentery adjacent to the injured segment of bowel, and free intraperitoneal fluid or hemorrhage (Figures 10.27 and 10.28). Focal bowel wall thickening or abnormal enhancement may be because of hematoma, contusion, perforation, or ischemia secondary to mesenteric vessel occlusion. Injuries of the GI tract usually occur

in the setting of multivisceral injury; for example, pancreatic head injuries and flexion/distraction fractures of L1-L2 often accompany duodenal injuries. Additionally, the body wall should be evaluated for traumatic injuries such as hematomas and traumatic hernias (Figure 10.29).

There are several pitfalls regarding GI injury with which the emergency radiologist should be aware. Although extraluminal gas should raise concern for GI perforation, there are several other etiologies to consider. For example, recent instrumentation, an indwelling peritoneal dialysis catheter, dissection of gas from pneumothorax, or extension of gas from intraperitoneal bladder rupture are all potential causes of extraluminal gas on CT. Gas dissecting between the parietal peritoneum and inner aspect of the abdominal wall also result in a false positive diagnosis of pneumoperitoneum; differentiation can be made by identification of free air elsewhere in the abdomen or by decubitus imaging. In contrast to focal mural thickening, diffuse mural thickening of the small bowel is not usually because of direct trauma, but can be due to aggressive resuscitation and subsequent fluid overload. When diffuse mural thickening occurs in the setting of diffuse mucosal hyperemia, the findings are secondary to the so-called hypoperfusion complex ("shock bowel") from severe hypotension, slow perfusion, and increased vascular permeability (Figure 10.30). Coexisting CT findings include a decompressed IVC, adrenal hyperemia, and pancreatic hyperemia and edema (Figure 10.31).

Treatment of traumatic GI injuries depends on their severity. Mural contusions are typically treated conservatively but may require resection in some cases. A focal laceration can usually be treated by enterorrhaphy with suture close of the defect. However, multifocal lacerations typically require resection of the affected bowel segment with primary anastomosis. Rectal injuries are managed by their location. Since the anterolateral aspects of the superior two-thirds of the rectum are invested by peritoneum, injuries occurring here are considered to be intraperitoneal and are managed by primary repair with fecal diversion [84]. Injuries to the inferior third and the posterosuperior aspect of the

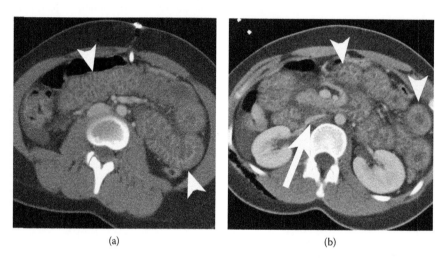

(a)   (b)

FIGURE 10.30
Shock bowel. A 39-year-old female presented with hypotension following a motor vehicle accident. (a and b) Portal venous phase CT shows diffuse wall thickening and mucosal hyperemia of the small bowel (arrowheads). The inferior vena cava (arrow in b) is collapsed because of volume loss from hemorrhage from liver and splenic lacerations (not shown).

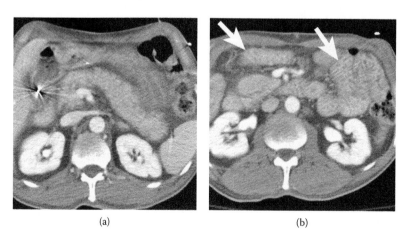

(a)   (b)

FIGURE 10.31
Shock bowel and pancreas. A 48-year-old female presented with hypotension following a motorcycle collision. (a) Portal phase CT shows pancreatic hyperemia and loss of the normal acinar architecture because of edema. (b) There is diffuse hyperemia and thickening of the small bowel (arrows) because of posttraumatic hypoperfusion complex. The inferior vena cava was not collapsed as the patient was undergoing aggressive volume resuscitation at the time of the CT.

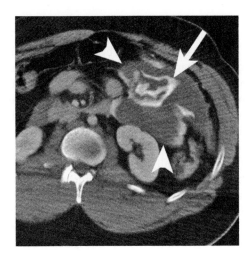

FIGURE 10.32
Mesenteric hemorrhage. A 26-year-old male presented with hypotension following a high-speed motor vehicle accident. Postcontrast CT shows a large mesenteric hematoma (arrowheads) containing regions of active contrast extravasation (arrow). Lacerations of the common hepatic artery a jejunal branch of the mesenteric artery were repaired at surgery.

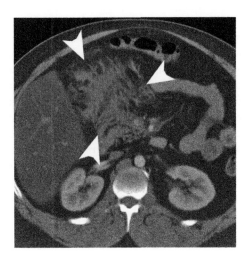

FIGURE 10.33
Transverse mesocolon hemorrhage. A 40-year-old male presented with pain following an abdominal stab wound. Portal phase CT shows an ill-defined, high-attenuation hematoma (arrowheads) along the transverse mesocolon. The skin entry site of the stab wound was located more inferiorly (not shown). At surgery, a laceration of the middle colic vein was repaired.

rectum are considered to be extraperitoneal and can be managed more conservatively, although surgery is still often required.

Mesenteric and omental injuries can occur in isolation or may accompany GI tract trauma. Although the CT finding of free intraperitoneal fluid or hemoperitoneum in the absence of an identifiable solid visceral injury should prompt meticulous search for an occult GI tract or mesenteric injury, the finding of interloop fluid or hemorrhage is a more specific finding because of its location [85]. In solid visceral trauma, resultant fluid or hemorrhage usually collects around the injured organ, in Morrison's pouch, or along the paracolic gutters. In contrast, fluid or hemorrhage secondary to bowel or mesenteric injury typically accumulates within the mesenteric leaves and assumes a triangular appearance. Other specific findings of traumatic mesenteric injury include active hemorrhage (Figure 10.32) manifested by extravasation of intravenous contrast material, hematoma, infiltration of the mesenteric fat, occlusion or luminal irregularity of mesenteric vessels, and potential internal herniation of bowel through a mesenteric defect. Omental hematoma typically appears as infiltration of the fat or formation of a heterogeneous collection within the fat or along adjoining ligaments (Figures 10.33 and 10.34). The treatment of mesenteric and omental injuries is variable, based on the degree of injury and the presence of coexisting injuries. Most small, isolated hematomas can be managed conservatively, whereas larger hematomas, mesenteric vascular injury, and active hemorrhage usually prompt laparotomy or angiographic embolization.

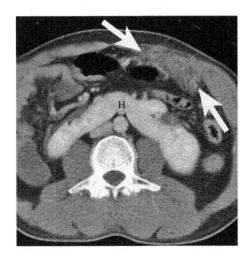

FIGURE 10.34
Omental hematoma. A 24-year-old male presented with focal pain after a bicycle accident during which his handlebars struck his left lower quadrant. Portal venous phase CT reveals a heterogeneous collection (arrows) along the left aspect of the greater omentum, consistent with hematoma. Incidental note is made of a horseshoe kidney (H).

10.2.10 Gynecologic Trauma

Although penetrating injuries to the pelvis may result in laceration and hemorrhage of the gynecologic organs, most cases of pelvic trauma involve blunt forces. Most of the blunt forces are absorbed by the pelvic bony ring and series of tightly woven ligaments that encircle and protect the uterus, ovaries, and Fallopian tubes. In addition, the lack of firm fixation of the gynecologic organs allows relative mobility during impact, thereby decreasing the likelihood of parenchymal injury during blunt trauma. Therefore, pelvic fractures occur much more frequently than do injuries to the gynecologic organs. Pelvic fractures secondary to significant compression and shear forces can result in complex fractures and fracture fragments that damage adjacent vessels. Severe hemorrhage is the leading cause of death in patients sustaining a pelvic fracture, with the vascular injury often secondary to laceration from a sharp fracture fragment. Similarly, the fracture fragments and shear forces can result in laceration of the gynecologic organs. In such cases, CT will show a variable amount of hematoma within the pelvis and will occasionally show the site of active hemorrhage as foci of contrast extravasation. Overt uterine rupture is extremely rare but the risk is increased in the gravid uterus [86]. In cases of uterine mural injury, CT will show a low-attenuation linear defect and variable mural thickening at the site of laceration. In some cases of uterine laceration, hemorrhage can fill the endometrial canal or Fallopian tube, resulting in expansion of the cavities with intermediate attenuation because of hematoma. Otherwise, involvement of the fallopian tube and ovary during blunt pelvic trauma is extremely rare but has been reported to following traumatic herniation through a defect in the broad ligament [87].

10.3 Acute Vascular Injury

10.3.1 Abdominal Aortic Aneurysm Rupture

Abdominal aortic aneurysms (AAA) are increasingly being diagnosed as older patients are screened more frequently. Risk factors associated with AA include smoking, age, hypertension, hyperlipidemia, atherosclerosis, male gender, and family history [88]. Although smoking is the risk factor believed to have a strong associating with the development of AAA, these other factors share a key role in the development of AAA. Age is an important risk factor in the development of AAA. The risk of AAA rises rapidly after the age of 55 in men and the age of 70 in wemen with a reported prevalence of 5% amongst men screened with US [89]. Family history of AAA not only have an increased risk of developing an AAA, but also a greater likelihood of aneurysms arising at a younger age with a higher risk of rupture [90].

The aortic wall is composed of three layers (intima, media, and adventitia) and derives its strength from elastin and collagen, which comprise the extracellular matrix. The weakening of these structures is believed to be the underlying cause of AAA that stems from a combination of atherosclerosis, environmental, hemodynamic, and immunologic factors [91]. Inflammatory cells within

the aortic wall, such as matrix metalloproteinases, are thought to contribute to aneurysm formation. In most cases, AAA are asymptomatic, being discovered incidentally or during imaging studies for other indications. The infrarenal aorta is the most common site of AAA formation. When symptomatic, the most common presentation is pain and tenderness; however, patients may also have a pulsatile or palpable abdominal mass and hypotension.

Most aneurysms are true aneurysms, involving all three layers of the aortic wall, rather than false or pseudoaneurysms that only involve the adventitia and the surrounding tissues. An AAA is defined as an aorta that measures greater than 3 cm. Given that most AAA are asymptomatic, the size of the aneurysm is predictive of aortic rupture. Patients with AAA measuring greater than 4 cm or larger are at increased risk for rupture, with repair suggested at 5.5 cm [92]. However, rupture can occur when the AAA measures less than 5 cm suggesting that other factors including comorbidities, aneurysm morphology, and changes to the connective tissue matrix may play a role in rupture. In addition, though aneurysms are more common in men, women are more prone to rupture than men.

Rapid diagnosis of a ruptured aortic aneurysm or an impending rupture is essential for prompt treatment (Table 10.13) (Figure 10.35). CT is the modality of choice to evaluate the aorta in patients diagnosed with acute aortic syndrome. MDCT has evolved as the modality of choice because of the speed of the examination, availability in emergent settings, and rapid interpretation time compared with MRI and US. Emergent CT AAA protocols use a combination of unenhanced and enhanced data sets. The unenhanced CT may detect AAA rupture by identifying acute (hyperdense) clot surrounding the aneurysm or displaced calcifications. The contrast-enhanced CT provides a more accurate estimation of aortic size, presence of contrast extravasation, and the relationship of the aorta to its major divisions. Impending rupture can be diagnosed when the atheromatous calcifications are displaced and a crescent of increased attenuation is within the aortic wall [93–95]. This is indicative of acute clot within the aortic wall and suggests that the aorta is unstable. A contained or impending rupture can also be suggested when the posterior aortic wall is not identifiable from the adjacent structures or if it follows the contour of the adjacent vertebral body [94,96,97].

TABLE 10.13

Features of Aortic Aneurysm Rupture

Periaortic stranding
Retroperitoneal hematoma
Extravasation of intravenous contrast
Hyperdense crescent
Discontinuity of intimal aortic calcifications or tangential calcification
Draped aorta

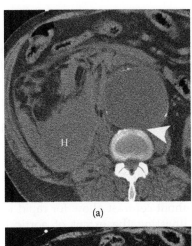

(a)

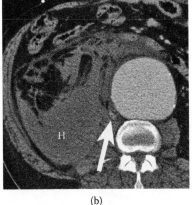

(b)

FIGURE 10.35
Ruptured abdominal aortic aneurysm. (a) Noncontrast CT shows a large infrarenal abdominal aortic aneurysm and extensive right retroperitoneal hematoma (H) of high density (40 HU), suggesting acute hemorrhage. The posterior margin of the aorta (arrowhead) is flattened and drapes along the anterior margin of the vertebral body. The calcifications of the aortic wall are laterally displaced along the right and posterolateral aspect of the aorta, suggesting the site of the potential rupture. (b) Arterial phase CT shows extravasation (arrow) of intravenous contrast adjacent to the right posterolateral edge of the aneurysm at the site of rupture. The patient was taken immediately for emergent surgery.

10.3.2 Acute Aortic Dissection

Acute aortic dissection (AAD) is most commonly caused by hypertension; however, it can also be caused by connective tissue disease, (Marfan's disease or Ehlers–Danlos syndrome), genetic syndrome (Turner's syndrome), vasculitis (Bechet's disease), or aortic root disease (bicupsid valve or other aortic valve disease) (Table 10.14). Symptomatic AAD will present with severe chest pain or back pain that is stabbing or sharp and can radiate to the back and the abdomen. Less commonly, AAD can present with syncope, neurological symptoms, abdominal pain, or syncope.

AAD involves an insult to the aortic wall, with a histologic injury to the intima, allowing blood to split the intima and media [98]. Once blood enters between these layers, the aortic flap is created that divides the aorta

TABLE 10.14

Causes of Aortic Dissection

Hypertension
Connective tissue disease
Aortic root abnormalities
Medication
Vasculitis

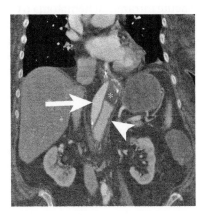

FIGURE 10.36
Aortic dissection. Coronal reformatted image from an arterial phase CT shows an aortic dissection with higher attenuation in the true lumen (arrow). The false lumen has lower attenuation, partial thrombus (asterisk), and subtle fronds (arrowhead) arising from the aortic wall because of residual nondisplaced aortic media following the dissection.

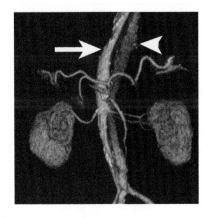

FIGURE 10.37
Aortic dissection. Three-dimensional volume rendered image shows the true lumen (arrow) giving rise to the celiac artery, superior mesenteric artery, right renal artery, and the superior left renal artery. The inferior left renal artery is less bright because of slower flow as it arises from the false lumen (arrowhead).

into a true and false lumen (Figures 10.36 and 10.37). The flap of tissue dividing the aorta is mainly composed of displaced medial tissue from the aortic wall and displaced intimal tissue. This flap will frequently contain small perforations (fenestrations) from re-entry type tears. AADs are classified by MDCT according to either the DeBakey or the Stanford classification systems

(Tables 10.15 and 10.16) [99,100]. Aortic dissections most commonly involve ascending and descending aorta (60%; DeBakey I/Stanford A), descending thoracoabdominal aorta, distal to the aortic isthmus (25%–30%; DeBakey III, Stanford B), and least commonly isolated involvement of the ascending aorta (10%–15%; DeBakey II/Stanford A) [99,100].

AAD can have symptoms and imaging features that overlap with acute intramural hematoma (AIH) and penetrating aortic ulcer (PAU) disease, which makes differentiation between these entities challenging both clinically and with MDCT. In the setting of AIH (Figure 10.38), the hemorrhage is within the vasa vasorum, and there is no clear extension through the intima; however, the hemorrhage may propagate along the aortic wall and extend through the intima. Histologically, a PAU (Figure 10.39) results in ulceration of the elastic lamina of the aortic wall, and focal hemorrhage is contained within the media; however, this too can extend along the media and lead to a dissection [101–104].

MDCT is the principal diagnostic modality used in evaluating aortic dissection. Although MRI is able to provide similar diagnostic information, the accessibility, reproducibility, and rapid acquisition time of MDCT make it the preferred modality. MDCT protocols with and without contrast allow for rapid identification of AAD, delineating the extent of aortic involvement (including the aortic root); identifying true and false lumen (Table 10.17); identifying thrombosed false lumen; and identifying potential complications including aortic rupture, extension into visceral segmental divisions, and end organ injury involving both solid and hollow viscera.

TABLE 10.15

Stanford Classification System for Aortic Dissection

Type A dissection	Ascending thoracic aorta involvement or ascending thoracic and descending thoracic and abdominal aortic involvement
Type B dissection	Descending thoracic and abdominal aorta involvement. The dissection is distal to the aortic isthmus

TABLE 10.16

DeBakey Classification System for Aortic Dissection

Type I	Ascending and descending thoracic aorta and abdominal aorta involvement
Type II	Ascending thoracic aorta involvement
Type III	descending thoracic and abdominal aorta involvement. The dissection is distal to the aortic isthmus

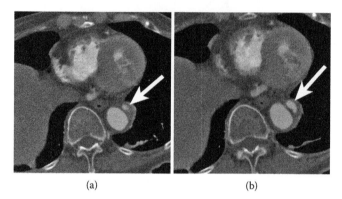

(a)   (b)

FIGURE 10.39

Penetrating aortic ulcer. (a and b) Arterial phase CT images show a focal outpouching of contrast (arrows in a and b) along the ventral margin of the aorta, consistent with a penetrating ulcer. Penetrating aortic ulcers can result in rupture, dissection, or development of a saccular aneurysm.

TABLE 10.17

Aortic Dissection: Differentiation of True from False Lumen

True Lumen	False Lumen
Smaller lumen size than false lumen	Larger lumen size than true lumen
Ovoid shape	circular shape
Higher in density on postcontrast phase	Lower in density on postcontrast phase ("delay in enhancement") or may be occluded because of slow flow with thrombus
Gives rise to celiac trunk, SMA, and right renal artery	Gives rise to the left renal artery
	Wedges around the true lumen (beak-like configuration)
	Ridge-like tissue because of residua of the media

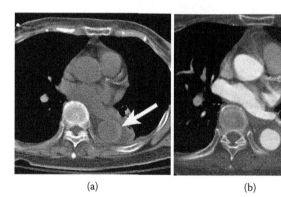

(a)   (b)

FIGURE 10.38

Acute intramural hematoma. (a) Noncontrast CT shows hyperdense intramural hematoma (arrow) that is crescentic in shape. (b) On the arterial phase CT, the crescentic hematoma (arrow) becomes less conspicuous but no discrete dissection flap was shown, most consistent with acute intramural hematoma. An alternative consideration was a thrombosed dissection flap; however, this was felt to be less likely.

Moreover, MDCT can be helpful in distinguishing AAD from AIH or PAU that can be precursors to aortic dissection and mimic AAD symptoms [104–111]. On MDCT, PAU will appear more focal than AAD and can cause focal dilation of the affected aortic segment with thrombus. Serial MDCT scans can reveal whether the insult resolves or extends into the aortic wall evolving into a dissection or causes focal dilation of the affected segment resulting in a saccular aneurysm [104]. AIH can similarly be identified by MDCT in cases where no definite flap is shown, and noncontrast images show a hyperdense crescent within the aortic wall; AIH may be suggested as the likely diagnosis, although distinguishing AIH from AAD can be difficult and aggressive management is encouraged in these settings [110].

10.3.3 Acute Thromboembolism

10.3.3.1 Normal Arterial Anatomy

The aorta gives rise to three unpaired visceral branches: the celiac artery, superior mesenteric artery (SMA), and inferior mesenteric artery (IMA). The celiac artery arises from the aorta anteriorly with a nearly 90 degree angle and a subtle superior orientation. The celiac artery supplies oxygenated blood to the distal esophagus, first and second segments of the duodenum, liver, spleen, pancreas and gallbladder. The SMA arises 1 cm distal to the celiac artery at the level of the L1 vertebral body and is inferiorly oriented with an acute angle at its origin. The SMA supplies the viscera from the duodenum (second segment) to the distal third of the transverse colon. The IMA arises at the level of the L4 vertebral body, just proximal to the aortic bifurcation, and supplies the remainder of the bowel, from the distal transverse colon to the rectum. Extensive collateral flow between visceral branches exists involving the celiac artery and SMA (pancreaticoduodenal) and SMA and IMA (Marginal artery of Drummond and Arc of Riolan) [112,113].

10.3.3.2 Normal Venous Anatomy

The small and large bowel, pancreas, and spleen venous tributaries drain into the portal vein. The hepatic and renal venous tributaries drain into the portal vein. The systemic and portal blood flow do not communicate unless there is venous obstruction [112,113].

10.3.3.3 Pathology

Vascular ischemia can occur via four mechanisms: (1) arterial thrombosis, (2) arterial embolism, (3) venous thrombosis, or (4) nonocclusive mesenteric ishchemia. Acute thrombus and embolus involving the vascular abdominal system are an uncommon set of entities that require rapid diagnosis. Thromboembolism can involve both the arterial and venous system and can involve the main arterial and venous conduits (the aorta and IVC) or their tributaries (visceral divisions). Although radiographs, Doppler US, MDCT, and MRI can all be used in the diagnostic workup, MDCT with a combination or oral, rectal, and intravenous contrast remains the primary diagnostic modality in evaluating the vessels for a cause of the symptoms.

10.3.4 Acute Mesenteric Arterial Occlusion

Acute arterial occlusion is usually secondary to a thromboembolic event and less likely caused by arterial thrombus. Risk factors include arrhythmia, myocardial infarction, low cardiac output, atherosclerosis, vasculitis, and prolonged hypotension. MDCT can distinguish between these entities as thrombus is typically located at origin of the SMA and IMA while emboli are usually located within the more distal segments of SMA and IMA [114,115]. Both emboli and thrombi appear as filling defects within the mesenteric arteries and its divisions. In the setting of arterial occlusion, the affected bowel wall segments will be thinner than the reference normal segments. Bowel wall thickening will occur in the setting of reperfusion of the affected segments. The affected segment of the bowel will have diminished enhancement or a rim of hyperenhancement (target-like appearance) following reperfusion. The adjacent mesentery will be normal unless infracted after that it is increased in attenuation [116].

10.3.5 Acute Venous Occlusion

Mesenteric vein thrombosis can be secondary to infection, portal hypertension, or hypercoaguable states. Unlike arterial occlusion, venous occlusion does not cause bowel ischemia, but rather mesenteric venous occlusion can result in bowel infarction. In contrast to arterial occlusion, venous occlusion leads to bowel wall dilatation of the affected segment, bowel wall thickening, mesenteric congestion, and ascites (Table 10.18). The impairment in venous drainage can cause a decrease in arterial blood flow that can lead to ischemia and infarction [116]. MDCT allows for the assessment of the mesenteric vessels and to assess perfusion of the bowel wall. In addition, it allows for the detection of bowel wall infarction, pneumatosis, and portal venous gas.

10.4 Postoperative Abdomen

10.4.1 Postembolization Appearance of the Spleen

The treatment of splenic injury has dramatically evolved from surgical to nonsurgical intervention with the goal of preserving splenic tissue in both the pediatric and

TABLE 10.18

MDCT Features of Mesenteric Ischemia

	Arterial Occlusion	Venous Occlusion
Bowel wall	Wall thinning or no change	Wall thickening
Bowel wall attenuation	No characteristic changes	Low density if edematous; high density if hemorrhage
Enhancement of bowel wall	Diminished; once reperfused will have a target or high-density appearance	Diminished; once reperfused will have a target or high-density appearance
Bowel dilatation	None	Moderate to marked increase
Mesenteric vessels	Defect in arteries; arterial occlusion	Venous enlargement or occlusion
Mesentery	Normal until infarct (increased attenuation)	Haziness (because of edema) and ascites

Source: Furukawa A et al., *AJR Am J Roentgenol*, 2009, 192, 408–16.

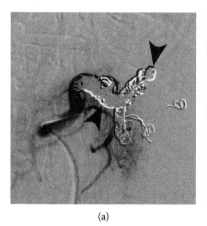 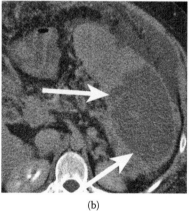 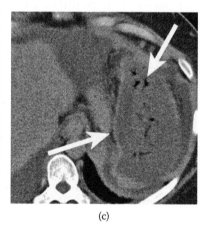

(a)   (b)   (c)

FIGURE 10.40

Splenic abscess postembolization. A patient presented with a small amount of perisplenic hematoma (not shown) following blunt abdominal trauma. (a) Because of persistent hemodynamic instability, the splenic artery was embolized with metallic coils (black arrowheads) after repeated transfusions and unsuccessful conservative management. (b) The patient experienced postoperative fevers and leukocytosis. The images show the expected splenic infarct (arrows) and upper abdominal simple ascites (c) However, more superiorly, there is a rim-enhancing gas and fluid collection (arrows) that was sampled percutaneously and was shown to be a splenic abscess.

adult populations. When conservative treatment failures or active bleeding is identified on MDCT, treatment via splenic artery emboliatization has been shown to reduce the risk of nonsurgical management. When arterial bleeding is suspected, coils are placed as distally as possible to preserve the vascular supply to the remainder of the organ [117]. In selected clinical scenarios where secondary rupture of the spleen is of high clinical concern, the splenic artery will be embolized in a proximal segment to reduce vascular pressure to the spleen and allow the spleen to heal [117].

Following embolization, splenic lesions imaged by MDCT will typically show a wedge-shaped hypodense lesion that extends to the periphery of the spleen compatible with an infarction [118]. Infarction is expected in both cases of distal splenic embolization and in up to 63% of proximal splenic embolizations [118]. Following embolization, patients may experience low-grade fevers and left upper quadrant pain secondary to embolization syndrome. The treatment site may also initially show a small amount of intrasplenic gas following treatment.

However, should the gas increase within the splenic bed, air fluid levels develop, or perisplenic pneumoperitoneum occur, splenic necrosis or abscess formation would be of greater concern (Figure 10.40) [119]. Less commonly embolization may result in further hemorrhage coil migration or iatrogenic vascular injury [120].

10.4.2 Postembolization Appearance of the Liver

The treatment of acute liver injury has also evolved to have a greater emphasis placed on nonsurgical treatment. Angiographic embolization is safe in treating acute hepatic arterial hemorrhage in patients following trauma to treat suspected sites of arterial bleeding [121]. Angioembolization can lead to abscess formation, biliary leaks, hepatic necrosis, gallbladder necrosis or ischemia (when right hepatic artery treatment is performed), biloma, transient intra-abdominal hypertension, hepatic compartment syndrome, or inflammatory syndromes [122,123]. MDCT will normally show round or irregular shaped hyopdensities at the site of vascular extravasation with no residual pooling of contrast. As the injury resolves, a large discrete subcapsular or inraparenchymal hematoma, characterized by a wall with rim enhancement can develop. However, foci of gas or air-fluid levels within the parenchyma or perihepatic space or within the evolving hematoma will be indicative of abscess though is usually only seen in severe liver injury [124].

10.4.3 Bowel Dehiscence

Segmental small and large bowel resection, either secondary to trauma, ischemia, perforation, or obstruction, requires reconstruction of the normal bowel circuit. Dehiscence can occur secondary to surgical technique, underlying sepsis, tissue hypoxia, and advanced patient age. Clinical signs that are suggestive of anastomotic dehiscence include fever, adynamic ileus, increased output in abdominal drains, leukocytosis, renal dysfunction, or cardiac dysfunction [125–129]. Identification of dehiscence at the earliest point in the postoperative setting, however, remains a diagnostic challenge, given the low specificity of clinical markers [126]. As a result, MDCT with water-soluble contrast and intravenous contrast has a key role in identifying dehiscence of the surgical anastomosis.

MDCT studies will reveal free intraperitoneal air, extravasation of water-soluble contrast, or rim-enhancing collections immediately adjacent to the surgical margins. These findings, however, may be preceded by infiltration of the fat and soft tissues at the anastomotic site that can serve as an indicator of dehiscence [130]. MDCT provides higher special resolution compared with conventional radiography, allowing for greater accuracy in identifying sites of leak [131]. Identification of dehiscence, however, is challenging in the early postoperative period, particularly if the size of the leak is not large enough to allow for extravasation of contrast and if no abscess are formed at the site of the leak [127].

10.5 Abscess and Fluid Collections

Although intrabdominal abscesses can develop in the setting of embolizaiton of the liver and spleen, abscesses can also develop in patients who have undergone laparotomy to control bleeding or for treatment of bowel, visceral, or mesenteric injury. Patients at risk for developing abscess will present with fever, leukocytosis, wound infection or dehiscence, increased drainage, or purulent material at the drainage site or unilateral pleural effusions [132].

MDCT with oral and intravenous contrast allows for rapid evaluation of the entire abdomen and pelvis for rim enhancing collections with or without air. The sensitivity of MDCT is increased compared with US because of operator variability and patient condition and the time consuming nature of MRI. Abscess and sterile collections are typically intraperitoneal in either the right or left upper quadrants (subdiaphragmatic). These occur at the site of perihepatic or perisplenic hematoma, where the hematoma has organized or in cases where bleeding was severe within the hepatectomy or splenectomy beds. Percutaneous drainage via MDCT or US is successful not only in decompressing the collection, but also in determining whether the collection is infected once the material is sent for assessment [132].

10.6 Conclusion

Abdominal trauma continues to be a significant source of morbidity and mortality, especially in young patients. The triage of abdominal trauma patients and diagnosis of their visceral injuries can be challenging for even experienced, emergency, and trauma physicians. The overlap of nonspecific signs and symptoms, variable physical examination findings, presence of distracting injuries, and potential inability of a patient to communicate, all contribute to the difficulty of clinical evaluation of the trauma patient. Therefore, diagnostic imaging has greatly evolved over the past several decades to aid in the diagnosis and management of the trauma patient. Specifically, the advent of MDCT has allowed a rapid, noninvasive means of accurately diagnosing acute abdominal injuries, judging their severity and assessing treatment response during follow-up. The refinements of intravenous contrast material and injection protocols and development of thin-section, multislice technology has allowed display of high-resolution images in multiple planes that aid in surgical planning and selecting patients for transcatheter embolization. Fast and accurate interpretation of the abdominal CT examination allows the radiologist to play a central role in the trauma center. Recognition of the key imaging findings of abdominal trauma will provide prompt diagnosis and initiation of treatment and thereby improve patient care by decreasing morbidity and mortality.

References

1. Holmes JF, McGahan JP, Wisner DH. Rate of intra-abdominal injury after a normal abdominal computed tomographic scan in adults with blunt trauma. *Am J Emerg Med* 2012;30(4):574–79.

2. Livingston DH, Lavery RF, Passannante MR et al. Admission or observation is not necessary after a negative abdominal computed tomographic scan in patients with suspected blunt abdominal trauma: results of a prospective, multi-institutional trial. *J Trauma* 1998;44:273–80; discussion 80–2.

3. U.S. Department of Transportation National Highway Traffic Safety Administration. Traffic Safety Facts. 2009 Available on-line at: http://www-nrd.nhtsa.dot.gov/Pubs/811402.pdf.

4. Federle MP. Computed tomography of blunt abdominal trauma. *Radiol Clin North Am* 1983;21:461–75.

5. Kearney PA Jr, Vahey T, Burney RE, Glazer G. Computed tomography and diagnostic peritoneal lavage in blunt abdominal trauma. Their combined role. *Arch Surg* 1989;124:344–7.

6. Henneman PL, Marx JA, Moore EE, Cantrill SV, Ammons LA. Diagnostic peritoneal lavage: accuracy in predicting necessary laparotomy following blunt and penetrating trauma. *J Trauma* 1990;30:1345–55.

7. Velmahos GC, Demetriades D, Stewart M et al. Open versus closed diagnostic peritoneal lavage: a comparison on safety, rapidity, efficacy. *J R Coll Surg Edinb* 1998; 43:235–8.

8. Powell DC, Bivins BA, Bell RM. Diagnostic peritoneal lavage. *Surg Gynecol Obstet* 1982;155:257–64.

9. Hubbard SG, Bivins BA, Sachatello CR, Griffen WO Jr. Diagnostic errors with peritoneal lavage in patients with pelvic fractures. *Arch Surg* 1979;114:844–6.

10. Kane NM, Dorfman GS, Cronan JJ. Efficacy of CT following peritoneal lavage in abdominal trauma. *J Comput Assist Tomogr* 1987;11:998–1002.

11. Hawkins ML, Bailey RL Jr, Carraway RP. Is diagnostic peritoneal lavage for blunt trauma obsolete? *Am Surg* 1990;56:96–9.

12. Nagy KK, Roberts RR, Joseph KT et al. Experience with over 2500 diagnostic peritoneal lavages. *Injury* 2000;31:479–82.

13. McGahan JP, Rose J, Coates TL, Wisner DH, Newberry P. Use of ultrasonography in the patient with acute abdominal trauma. *J Ultrasound Med* 1997;16:653–62; quiz 63–4.

14. McKenney KL, Nunez DB Jr, McKenney MG, Asher J, Zelnick K, Shipshak D. Sonography as the primary screening technique for blunt abdominal trauma: experience with 899 patients. *AJR Am J Roentgenol* 1998;170:979–85.

15. Ochsner MG, Knudson MM, Pachter HL et al. Significance of minimal or no intraperitoneal fluid visible on CT scan associated with blunt liver and splenic injuries: a multicenter analysis. *J Trauma* 2000;49:505–10.

16. Shanmuganathan K, Mirvis SE, Sherbourne CD, Chiu WC, Rodriguez A. Hemoperitoneum as the sole indicator of abdominal visceral injuries: a potential limitation of screening abdominal US for trauma. *Radiology* 1999;212:423–30.

17. Chiu WC, Cushing BM, Rodriguez A et al. Abdominal injuries without hemoperitoneum: a potential limitation of focused abdominal sonography for trauma (FAST). *J Trauma* 1997;42:617–23; discussion 623–25.

18. Yoshii H, Sato M, Yamamoto S et al. Usefulness and limitations of ultrasonography in the initial evaluation of blunt abdominal trauma. *J Trauma* 1998;45:45–50; discussion 50–51.

19. Richards JR, McGahan JP, Jones CD, Zhan S, Gerscovich EO. Ultrasound detection of blunt splenic injury. *Injury* 2001;32:95–103.

20. van der Vlies CH, Olthof DC, Gaakeer M, Ponsen KJ, van Delden OM, Goslings JC. Changing patterns in diagnostic strategies and the treatment of blunt injury to solid abdominal organs. *Int J Emerg Med* 2011;4:47.

21. Orwig D, Federle MP. Localized clotted blood as evidence of visceral trauma on CT: the sentinel clot sign. *AJR Am J Roentgenol* 1989;153:747–9.

22. Mirvis SE, Whitley NO, Vainwright JR, Gens DR. Blunt hepatic trauma in adults: CT-based classification and correlation with prognosis and treatment. *Radiology* 1989;171:27–32.

23. Shanmuganathan K, Mirvis SE, Sover ER. Value of contrast-enhanced CT in detecting active hemorrhage in patients with blunt abdominal or pelvic trauma. *AJR Am J Roentgenol* 1993;161:65–9.

24. Shanmuganathan K, Mirvis SE, Reaney SM. Pictorial review: CT appearances of contrast medium extravasations associated with injury sustained from blunt abdominal trauma. *Clin Radiol* 1995;50:182–7.

25. Harris HW, Morabito DJ, Mackersie RC, Halvorsen RA, Schecter WP. Leukocytosis and free fluid are important indicators of isolated intestinal injury after blunt trauma. *J Trauma* 1999;46:656–9.

26. Livingston DH, Lavery RF, Passannante MR et al. Free fluid on abdominal computed tomography without solid organ injury after blunt abdominal injury does not mandate celiotomy. *Am J Surg* 2001;182:6–9.

27. Rodriguez C, Barone JE, Wilbanks TO, Rha CK, Miller K. Isolated free fluid on computed tomographic scan in blunt abdominal trauma: a systematic review of incidence and management. *J Trauma* 2002;53:79–85.

28. Levine CD, Patel UJ, Wachsberg RH, Simmons MZ, Baker SR, Cho KC. CT in patients with blunt abdominal trauma: clinical significance of intraperitoneal fluid detected on a scan with otherwise normal findings. *AJR Am J Roentgenol* 1995;164:1381–5.

29. Yu J, Fulcher AS, Wang DB et al. Frequency and importance of small amount of isolated pelvic free fluid detected with multidetector CT in male patients with blunt trauma. *Radiology* 2010;256:799–805.

30. Drasin TE, Anderson SW, Asandra A, Rhea JT, Soto JA. MDCT evaluation of blunt abdominal trauma: clinical significance of free intraperitoneal fluid in males with absence of identifiable injury. *AJR Am J Roentgenol* 2008;191:1821–6.

31. Stivelman RL, Glaubitz JP, Crampton RS. Laceration of the Spleen due to nonpenetrating trauma. one hundred cases. *Am J Surg* 1963;106:888–91.

32. Federle MP, Goldberg HI, Kaiser JA, Moss AA, Jeffrey RB Jr, Mall JC. Evaluation of abdominal trauma by computed tomography. *Radiology* 1981;138:637–44.

33. Shanmuganathan K, Mirvis SE, Boyd-Kranis R, Takada T, Scalea TM. Nonsurgical management of blunt splenic injury: use of CT criteria to select patients for splenic arteriography and potential endovascular therapy. *Radiology* 2000;217:75–82.

34. Marmery H, Shanmuganathan K, Mirvis SE et al. Correlation of multidetector CT findings with splenic arteriography and surgery: prospective study in 392 patients. *J Am Coll Surg* 2008;206:685–93.

35. Moore EE, Cogbill TH, Jurkovich GJ, Shackford SR, Malangoni MA, Champion HR. Organ injury scaling: spleen and liver (1994 revision). *J Trauma* 1995;38: 323–4.

36. Federle MP, Courcoulas AP, Powell M, Ferris JV, Peitzman AB. Blunt splenic injury in adults: clinical and CT criteria for management, with emphasis on active extravasation. *Radiology* 1998;206:137–42.

37. Omert LA, Salyer D, Dunham CM, Porter J, Silva A, Protetch J. Implications of the "contrast blush" finding on computed tomographic scan of the spleen in trauma. *J Trauma* 2001;51:272–7; discussion 7–8.

38. Cocanour CS. Blunt splenic injury. *Curr Opin Crit Care* 2010;16(6):575–81.

39. Requarth JA, D'Agostino RB Jr, Miller PR. Nonoperative management of adult blunt splenic injury with and without splenic artery embolotherapy: a meta-analysis. *J Trauma* 2011;71:898–903; discussion 903.

40. Gomez D, Haas B, Al-Ali K, Monneuse O, Nathens AB, Ahmed N. Controversies in the management of splenic trauma. *Injury* 2012;43(1):55–6.

41. Federle MP. Splenic trauma: is follow-up CT of value? *Radiology* 1995;194:23–4.

42. Willmann JK, Roos JE, Platz A et al. Multidetector CT: detection of active hemorrhage in patients with blunt abdominal trauma. *AJR Am J Roentgenol* 2002;179:437–44.

43. Fang JF, Chen RJ, Wong YC et al. Pooling of contrast material on computed tomography mandates aggressive management of blunt hepatic injury. *Am J Surg* 1998;176:315–9.

44. Wong YC, Wang LJ, See LC, Fang JF, Ng CJ, Chen CJ. Contrast material extravasation on contrast-enhanced helical computed tomographic scan of blunt abdominal trauma: its significance on the choice, time, and outcome of treatment. *J Trauma* 2003;54:164–70.

45. Poletti PA, Mirvis SE, Shanmuganathan K, Killeen KL, Coldwell D. CT criteria for management of blunt liver trauma: correlation with angiographic and surgical findings. *Radiology* 2000;216:418–27.

46. Poletti PA, Wintermark M, Schnyder P, Becker CD. Traumatic injuries: role of imaging in the management of the polytrauma victim (conservative expectation). *Eur Radiol* 2002;12:969–78.

47. Griffen M, Ochoa J, Boulanger BR. A minimally invasive approach to bile peritonitis after blunt liver injury. *Am Surg* 2000;66:309–12.

48. Pachter HL, Knudson MM, Esrig B et al. Status of nonoperative management of blunt hepatic injuries in 1995: a multicenter experience with 404 patients. *J Trauma* 1996;40:31–8.

49. Soderstrom CA, Maekawa K, DuPriest RW Jr, Cowley RA. Gallbladder injuries resulting from blunt abdominal trauma: an experience and review. *Ann Surg* 1981;193:60–6.

50. Jaggard MK, Johal NS, Choudhry M. Blunt abdominal trauma resulting in gallbladder injury: a review with emphasis on pediatrics. *J Trauma* 2011;70:1005–10.

51. Pirola RC, Davis AE. Effects of ethyl alcohol on sphincteric resistance at the choledocho-duodenal junction in man. *Gut* 1968;9:557–60.

52. Hall ER Jr, Howard JM, Jordan GL, Mikesky WE. Traumatic injuries of the gall bladder. *AMA Arch Surg* 1956;72:520–4.

53. Erb RE, Mirvis SE, Shanmuganathan K. Gallbladder injury secondary to blunt trauma: CT findings. *J Comput Assist Tomogr* 1994;18:778–84.

54. Scaglione M, Rossi G, Pinto F et al. [Gallbladder blunt trauma: comparison between radiologic and anatomosurgical findings]. *Radiol Med* 1998;96:592–5.

55. Berland LL, Doust BD, Foley WD. Acute hemorrhage into the gallbladder diagnosed by computed tomography and ultrasonography. *J Comput Assist Tomogr* 1980;4:260–2.

56. Ajlan AM, Alqahtani A, Kellow Z. Intracholecystic fat herniation in traumatic gallbladder perforation: a case report. *J Comput Assist Tomogr* 2009;33:408–9.

57. Baumgartner FJ, Barnett MJ, Velez M, Chiu LC. Traumatic disruption of the gallbladder evaluated by computerized tomography and magnetic resonance imaging. *Br J Surg* 1988;75:386–7.

58. Fawaz F, Kim SK. Traumatic cholecystitis. *W V Med J* 1985;81:32–4.

59. Grimes OF, Steinbach HL. Traumatic cholecystocutaneous fistula. *AMA Arch Surg* 1955;71:68–70.

60. Sugimoto K, Asari Y, Sakaguchi T, Owada T, Maekawa K. Endoscopic retrograde cholangiography in the nonsurgical management of blunt liver injury. *J Trauma* 1993;35:192–9.

61. D'Amours SK, Simons RK, Scudamore CH, Nagy AG, Brown DR. Major intrahepatic bile duct injuries detected after laparotomy: selective nonoperative management. *J Trauma* 2001;50:480–4.

62. Rydell WB Jr. Complete transection of the common bile duct due to blunt abdominal trauma. *Arch Surg* 1970;100:724–8.

63. Sugiyama M, Abe N, Masaki T, Mori T, Atomi Y. Endoscopic biliary stent placement for treatment of gallbladder perforation due to blunt abdominal injury. *Gastrointest Endosc* 2000;52:275–7.

64. Ilahi O, Bochicchio GV, Scalea TM. Efficacy of computed tomography in the diagnosis of pancreatic injury in adult blunt trauma patients: a single-institutional study. *Am Surg* 2002;68:704–7; discussion 7–8.

65. Madiba TE, Mokoena TR. Favourable prognosis after surgical drainage of gunshot, stab or blunt trauma of the pancreas. *Br J Surg* 1995;82:1236–9.

66. Wong YC, Wang LJ, Lin BC, Chen CJ, Lim KE, Chen RJ. CT grading of blunt pancreatic injuries: prediction of ductal disruption and surgical correlation. *J Comput Assist Tomogr* 1997;21:246–50.

67. Bouwman DL, Weaver DW, Walt AJ. Serum amylase and its isoenzymes: a clarification of their implications in trauma. *J Trauma* 1984;24:573–8.

68. Bradley EL 3rd, Young PR Jr, Chang MC et al. Diagnosis and initial management of blunt pancreatic trauma: guidelines from a multiinstitutional review. *Ann Surg* 1998;227:861–9.

69. Akhrass R, Kim K, Brandt C. Computed tomography: an unreliable indicator of pancreatic trauma. *Am Surg* 1996;62:647–51.

70. Oniscu GC, Parks RW, Garden OJ. Classification of liver and pancreatic trauma. *HPB (Oxford)* 2006;8:4–9.

71. Lane MJ, Mindelzun RE, Sandhu JS, McCormick VD, Jeffrey RB. CT diagnosis of blunt pancreatic trauma: importance of detecting fluid between the pancreas and the splenic vein. *AJR Am J Roentgenol* 1994;163: 833–5.

72. Soto JA, Alvarez O, Munera F, Yepes NL, Sepulveda ME, Perez JM. Traumatic disruption of the pancreatic duct: diagnosis with MR pancreatography. *AJR Am J Roentgenol* 2001;176:175–8.

73. Rizzo MJ, Federle MP, Griffiths BG. Bowel and mesenteric injury following blunt abdominal trauma: evaluation with CT. *Radiology* 1989;173:143–8.

74. Hanks PW, Brody JM. Blunt injury to mesentery and small bowel: CT evaluation. *Radiol Clin North Am* 2003;41:1171–82.

75. Butela ST, Federle MP, Chang PJ et al. Performance of CT in detection of bowel injury. *AJR Am J Roentgenol* 2001;176:129–35.

76. Stafford RE, McGonigal MD, Weigelt JA, Johnson TJ. Oral contrast solution and computed tomography for blunt abdominal trauma: a randomized study. *Arch Surg* 1999;134:622–6; discussion 6–7.

77. Clancy TV, Ragozzino MW, Ramshaw D, Churchill MP, Covington DL, Maxwell JG. Oral contrast is not necessary in the evaluation of blunt abdominal trauma by computed tomography. *Am J Surg* 1993;166:680–4; discussion 4–5.

78. Kim HC, Shin HC, Park SJ et al. Traumatic bowel perforation: analysis of CT findings according to the perforation site and the elapsed time since accident. *Clin Imaging* 2004;28:334–9.

79. Hawkins AE, Mirvis SE. Evaluation of bowel and mesenteric injury: role of multidetector CT. *Abdom Imaging* 2003;28:505–14.

80. Multicentre Aneurysm Screening Study Group. Atri M, Hanson JM, Grinblat L, Brofman N, Chughtai T, Tomlinson G. Surgically important bowel and/or mesenteric injury in blunt trauma: accuracy of multidetector CT for evaluation. *Radiology* 2008;249:524–33.

81. Stuhlfaut JW, Soto JA, Lucey BC et al. Blunt abdominal trauma: performance of CT without oral contrast material. *Radiology* 2004;233:689–94.

82. Hamilton P, Rizoli S, McLellan B, Murphy J. Significance of intra-abdominal extraluminal air detected by CT scan in blunt abdominal trauma. *J Trauma* 1995;39:331–3.

83. Brofman N, Atri M, Hanson JM, Grinblat L, Chughtai T, Brenneman F. Evaluation of bowel and mesenteric blunt trauma with multidetector CT. *Radiographics* 2006;26:1119–31.

84. Cleary RK, Pomerantz RA, Lampman RM. Colon and rectal injuries. *Dis Colon Rectum* 2006;49:1203–22.

85. Levine CD, Gonzales RN, Wachsberg RH, Ghanekar D. CT findings of bowel and mesenteric injury. *J Comput Assist Tomogr* 1997;21:974–9.

86. Dash N, Lupetin AR. Uterine rupture secondary to trauma: CT findings. *J Comput Assist Tomogr* 1991;15:329–31.

87. Karcaaltincaba D, Avsar F, Iskender C, Korukluoglu B. Unusual mechanism of isolated torsion of fallopian tube following minor trauma. Herniation through a broad ligament tear. *Saudi Med J* 2007;28:637–8.

88. Lederle FA, Johnson GR, Wilson SE et al. Prevalence and associations of abdominal aortic aneurysm detected through screening. Aneurysm Detection and Management (ADAM) Veterans Affairs Cooperative Study Group. *Ann Intern Med* 1997;126:441–9.

89. Multicentre Aneurysm Screening Study Group (MASS): cost effectiveness analysis of screening for abdominal aortic aneurysms based on four year results from randomised controlled trial. *BMJ* 2002;325:1135.

90. Frydman G, Walker PJ, Summers K et al. The value of screening in siblings of patients with abdominal aortic aneurysm. *Eur J Vasc Endovasc Surg* 2003;26:396–400.

91. Isselbacher EM. Thoracic and abdominal aortic aneurysms. *Circulation* 2005;111:816–28.

92. Brewster DC, Cronenwett JL, Hallett JW Jr, Johnston KW, Krupski WC, Matsumura JS. Guidelines for the treatment of abdominal aortic aneurysms. Report of a subcommittee of the Joint Council of the American Association for Vascular Surgery and Society for Vascular Surgery. *J Vasc Surg* 2003;37:1106–17.

93. Gonsalves CF. The hyperattenuating crescent sign. *Radiology* 1999;211:37–8.

94. Mehard WB, Heiken JP, Sicard GA. High-attenuating crescent in abdominal aortic aneurysm wall at CT: a sign of acute or impending rupture. *Radiology* 1994;92:359–62.

95. Arita T, Matsunaga N, Takano K et al. Abdominal aortic aneurysm: rupture associated with the high-attenuating crescent sign. *Radiology* 1997;204:765–8.

96. Halliday KE, al-Kutoubi A. Draped aorta: CT sign of contained leak of aortic aneurysms. *Radiology* 1996;199:41–3.

97. Siegel CL, Cohan RH, Korobkin M, Alpern MB, Courneya DL, Leder RA. Abdominal aortic aneurysm morphology: CT features in patients with ruptured and nonruptured aneurysms. *AJR Am J Roentgenol* 1994;163:1123–9.

98. Rakita D, Newatia A, Hines JJ, Siegel DN, Friedman B. Spectrum of CT findings in rupture and impending rupture of abdominal aortic aneurysms. *Radiographics* 2007;27:497–507.

99. Debakey ME, Henly WS, Cooley DA, Morris GC Jr, Crawford ES, Beall AC Jr. Surgical management of dissecting aneurysms of the aorta. *J Thorac Cardiovasc Surg* 1965;49:130–49.

100. Daily PO, Trueblood HW, Stinson EB, Wuerflein RD, Shumway NE. Management of acute aortic dissections. *Ann Thorac Surg* 1970;10:237–47.

101. Stanson AW, Kazmier FJ, Hollier LH et al. Penetrating atherosclerotic ulcers of the thoracic aorta: natural history and clinicopathologic correlations. *Ann Vasc Surg* 1986;1:15–23.

102. Welch TJ, Stanson AW, Sheedy PF 2nd, Johnson CM, McKusick MA. Radiologic evaluation of penetrating aortic atherosclerotic ulcer. *Radiographics* 1990;10:675–85.

103. Cooke JP, Kazmier FJ, Orszulak TA. The penetrating aortic ulcer: pathologic manifestations, diagnosis, and management. *Mayo Clin Proc* 1988;63:718–25.

104. Hayashi H, Matsuoka Y, Sakamoto I et al. Penetrating atherosclerotic ulcer of the aorta: imaging features and disease concept. *Radiographics* 2000;20:995–1005.

105. Tsai TT, Nienaber CA, Eagle KA. Acute aortic syndromes. *Circulation* 2005;112:3802–13.

106. Mukherjee D, Eagle KA. Aortic dissection—an update. *Curr Probl Cardiol* 2005;30:287–325.

107. Cho KR, Stanson AW, Potter DD, Cherry KJ, Schaff HV, Sundt TM 3rd. Penetrating atherosclerotic ulcer of the descending thoracic aorta and arch. *J Thorac Cardiovasc Surg* 2004;127:1393–9; discussion 9–401.

108. Ganaha F, Miller DC, Sugimoto K et al. Prognosis of aortic intramural hematoma with and without penetrating atherosclerotic ulcer: a clinical and radiological analysis. *Circulation* 2002;106:342–8.

109. von Kodolitsch Y, Csosz SK, Koschyk DH et al. Intramural hematoma of the aorta: predictors of progression to dissection and rupture. *Circulation* 2003;107:1158–63.

110. Evangelista A, Mukherjee D, Mehta RH et al. Acute intramural hematoma of the aorta: a mystery in evolution. *Circulation* 2005;111:1063–70.

111. Manghat NE, Morgan-Hughes GJ, Roobottom CA. Multi-detector row computed tomography: imaging in acute aortic syndrome. *Clin Radiol* 2005;60:1256–67.

112. Martinez JP, Hogan GJ. Mesenteric ischemia. *Emerg Med Clin North Am* 2004;22:909–28.

113. Lewiss RE, Egan DJ, Shreves A. Vascular abdominal emergencies. *Emerg Med Clin North Am* 2011;29:253–72, viii.

114. Wiesner W, Khurana B, Ji H, Ros PR. CT of acute bowel ischemia. *Radiology* 2003;226:635–50.

115. Oldenburg WA, Lau LL, Rodenberg TJ, Edmonds HJ, Burger CD. Acute mesenteric ischemia: a clinical review. *Arch Intern Med* 2004;164:1054–62.

116. Furukawa A, Kanasaki S, Kono N et al. CT diagnosis of acute mesenteric ischemia from various causes. *AJR Am J Roentgenol* 2009;192:408–16.

117. Madoff DC, Denys A, Wallace MJ et al. Splenic arterial interventions: anatomy, indications, technical considerations, and potential complications. *Radiographics* 2005;25 Suppl 1:S191–211.

118. Killeen KL, Shanmuganathan K, Boyd-Kranis R, Scalea TM, Mirvis SE. CT findings after embolization for blunt splenic trauma. *J Vasc Interv Radiol* 2001;12:209–14.

119. Boscak A, Shanmuganathan K. Splenic trauma: what is new? *Radiol Clin North Am* 2012;50:105–22.

120. Haan JM, Biffl W, Knudson MM et al. Splenic embolization revisited: a multicenter review. *J Trauma* 2004;56:542–7.

121. Yoon W, Jeong YY, Kim JK et al. CT in blunt liver trauma. *Radiographics* 2005;25:87–104.

122. Letoublon C, Morra I, Chen Y, Monnin V, Voirin D, Arvieux C. Hepatic arterial embolization in the management of blunt hepatic trauma: indications and complications. *J Trauma* 2011;70:1032–6; discussion 6–7.

123. Misselbeck TS, Teicher EJ, Cipolle MD et al. Hepatic angioembolization in trauma patients: indications and complications. *J Trauma* 2009;67:769–73.

124. Hsieh CH, Chen RJ, Fang JF et al. Liver abscess after nonoperative management of blunt liver injury. *Langenbecks Arch Surg* 2003;387:343–7.

125. Herlinger H MD, Birnbaum BA, eds. Post-Surgical Small Bowel. In Lappas and William L. Campbell. "*Clinical Imaging of the Small Intestine*" New york: springer; 2001: 507–525.

126. Alves A, Panis Y, Pocard M, Regimbeau JM, Valleur P. Management of anastomotic leakage after nondiverted large bowel resection. *J Am Coll Surg* 1999;189:554–9.

127. Doeksen A, Tanis PJ, Wust AF, Vrouenraets BC, van Lanschot JJ, van Tets WF. Radiological evaluation of colorectal anastomoses. *Int J Colorectal Dis* 2008;23:863–8.

128. Lim M, Akhtar S, Sasapu K et al. Clinical and subclinical leaks after low colorectal anastomosis: a clinical and radiologic study. *Dis Colon Rectum* 2006;49:1611–9.

129. Sutton CD, Marshall LJ, Williams N, Berry DP, Thomas WM, Kelly MJ. Colo-rectal anastomotic leakage often masquerades as a cardiac complication. *Colorectal Dis* 2004;6:21–2.

130. Herlinger H, Maglinte DDT, Birnbaum BA, eds. In Lappas and William L. Campbell. *Clinical Imaging of the Small Intestine*. New york: springer; 2001: 507–525.

131. Scardapane A, Brindicci D, Fracella MR, Angelelli G. Post colon surgery complications: imaging findings. *Eur J Radiol* 2005;53:397–409.

132. Goins WA, Rodriguez A, Joshi M, Jacobs D. Intra-abdominal abscess after blunt abdominal trauma. *Ann Surg* 1990;212:60–5.

Section II

Urogenital

11

Kidney and Ureters

Pedram Rezai, Rita Agarwala, and Mark Pisaneschi

CONTENTS

11.1 Introduction

Multi-detector row computed tomography (MDCT) plays an indispensable role in the evaluation of kidneys and ureters. Recent advances in CT technology have allowed expansion and improvement of the armamentarium of diagnostic tools in the evaluation of genitourinary tract. For example, dual-energy CT acquisition is a recent and promising technique that provides energy- and material-specific data in addition to anatomic information [1]. Application of dual-energy acquisition has several applications in the evaluation of genitourinary system with CT such as improved determination of stone type in urolithiasis [2,3] and superior characterization of enhancement in renal lesions [4]. This chapter will provide an overview of the more common disorders of kidneys and ureters with emphasis on CT findings.

Depending on the clinical indication and patient-specific variables, MDCT is usually performed as a multistage examination. Thorough knowledge of patient's medical history and the clinical scenario in question is crucial. An understanding of different protocols and rationale behind them helps the radiologist choose the protocol that is optimized for each patient, yields the necessary information and keeps radiation and contrast exposure in check. Nonenhanced images are usually obtained for the evaluation of urinary stones, calcifications, hemorrhage, and determination of baseline attenuation values for quantification of enhancement in suspicious renal masses [5,6]. Of note, water density images reconstructed from contrast-enhanced images obtained by dual-energy CT acquisition can serve as virtual nonenhanced images by removing the iodine content and may eliminate the need to obtain a conventional nonenhanced scan [4].

The timing of contrast-enhanced phases varies with the speed of intravenous (IV) contrast material injection. Arterial phase images obtained 25–80 seconds after administration of IV contrast yield the characteristic "corticomedullary phase" appearance and facilitate evaluation of hypervascular tumors, aneurysms, arteriovenous malformations, and fistulas. Because of incomplete opacification of the medulla during this phase, small medullary lesions might remain obscured. Uniform opacification of renal cortex and medulla is achieved when scan is performed 85–120 seconds after administration of IV contrast, which is known as the "nephrogram phase." Filling of collecting system and ureters by contrast may be depicted on delayed images obtained 3–5 minutes after administration of IV contrast, which is known as the delayed, "pyelogram or equilibrium phase." Delayed scan through the full length of ureters has widely replaced the traditional methods such as intravenous pyelogram (IVP) and retrograde ureterography. Nonenhanced CT of the abdomen combined with arterial phase images of the kidney and delayed images of the abdomen and pelvis yield CT urogram or CT-IVP and provides the most comprehensive evaluation of the urinary tract in the setting of hematuria [5,7].

11.2 Kidney

11.2.1 Anatomy

11.2.1.1 Normal Anatomy

The superior urinary organs, kidneys and ureters, and their vessels are the original, native structures of the retroperitoneum. The retroperitoneum is located posterior to the peritoneal cavity and is bounded anteriorly by the posterior parietal peritoneum and posteriorly by the transversalis fascia (TF).

Renal parenchyma is surrounded by the renal capsule, which sharply delineates the border between parenchyma and perinephric fat. Subcapsular accumulation of blood or other fluids may have mass effect on the underlying parenchyma usually with little extension into the perirenal fat. This phenomenon can lead to hypertension secondary to renal parenchymal compression, which is

known as Page kidney and represents a rare cause of secondary hypertension [8]. Renal parenchyma is composed of 5–11 lobes consisting of the inner pyramid-shaped medulla (pyramids of Malpighi) surrounded by the outer cortex. Renal cortex extends between pyramids as renal columns of Bertin. A prominent column of Bertin may mimic a renal mass [9]. Tips of the renal pyramids terminate as 5–11 renal papillae. Each renal papilla is surrounded by a cup-shaped minor calyx. Fusion of minor calyces results in formation of 2 or 3 major calyces (infundibula), which drain into the renal pelvis.

Kidneys and their pedicles are surrounded by the perinephric fat. The space occupied by the kidneys and perinephric fat, proximal renal collecting system, hilar vessels, and adrenal glands is known as the "perirenal space (PRS)." PRS is limited anteriorly by the thinner anterior renal fascia (ARF) (Gerota fascia) and posteriorly by the thicker posterior renal fascia (PRF) (Zuckerkandl fascia) (Figure 11.1). During embryologic development, kidneys ascend from the pelvis to the retroperitoneum. Consequently, the ARF and PRF narrow as they extend inferiorly, explaining the inverted cone appearance of the PRS (Figure 11.2). Ureters pass through the apex of the cone. During ascent, kidneys rotate 90° medially, which explains the medial orientation of the renal hilum [10–13].

Collections in the right PRS can extend superiorly into the bare area of the liver and vice versa. Similarly, collections in the left PRS can extend to the subphrenic space.

It has been shown that the inferior aspect of the renal cone communicated with the retroperitoneal space of the lower abdomen and pelvis. This explains inferior extension of perirenal fluid into the retroperitoneal space of the lower abdomen and pelvis and vice versa.

There is no connection between the medial aspects of the PRSs above the level of renal hila, which has been

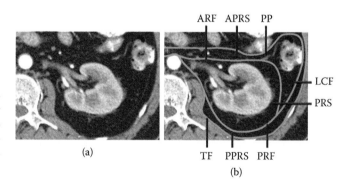

FIGURE 11.1

Axial corticomedullary phase CT image of the left kidney without (a) and with (b) highlighted fascial planes showing anterior renal fascia (ARF), posterior renal fascia (PRF), and lateroconal fascia (LCF) dividing retroperitoneum into the anterior pararenal space (APRS), perirenal space (PRS), and posterior pararenal space (PPRS). The asterisk shows communication between the medial aspects of PRSs. TF = transversalis fascia, PP = posterior peritoneum.

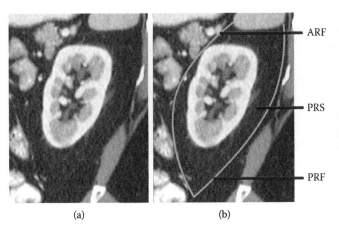

(a)   (b)

FIGURE 11.2
Sagittal corticomedullary phase CT image of the left kidney without (a) and with (b) highlighted ARF and PRF showing the inverted cone appearance of the PRS.

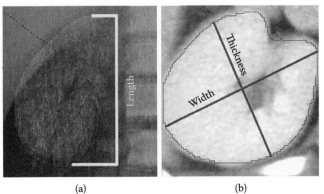

(a)   (b)

FIGURE 11.3
Volume-rendered image (a) and axial CT image of the right kidney at the level of maximum transaxial diameter (b) show the reproducible technique for quantification of renal length, width, and thickness. Note that maximum transaxial diameter and its perpendicular diameter commonly lie in an oblique plane, and not necessarily in anteroposterior and mediolateral planes.

attributed to the presence of celiac truck and superior mesenteric artery. However, communication between the medial aspects of PRSs exists below this level (Figure 11.1) [12].

Anterior pararenal space (APRS) is located anterior to the PRS and is anteriorly bounded by the peritoneum, posteriorly by the ARF, and laterally by the lateroconal fascia (LCF), which is the anterior projection of the PRF. APRS contains ascending and descending colon, pancreas, and duodenum (Figures 11.1 and 11.2). PPRS, located posterior to the PRS, is bounded anteriorly by the PRF and posteriorly by the TF. PPRS is a potential space and contains a small amount of adipose tissue (Figures 11.1 and 11.2) [10–13].

Ultrasonography has traditionally been the preferred imaging modality for evaluation of renal size. However, quantification of renal volume on CT by voxel count method has been regarded as the most accurate method for determination of renal volume. Unfortunately, voxel count method requires a dedicated workstation with three-dimensional (3D) image processing capabilities and is currently not widely available. On the other hand, determination of unidimensional diameters of kidney may be performed on almost every Picture Archiving and Communication System (PACS) workstation and is widely available. For reproducible measurements on CT, standardized renal unidimensional diameters may be defined as follows (Figure 11.3): width (cm) defined as the longest transaxial renal diameter; thickness (cm) defined as the longest diameter perpendicular to width on the same axial image; length (cm) defined as vertical distance between upper and lower poles. It has been shown that by incorporation of the product (P) of standardized unidimensional diameters (width, thickness, and length) into the formula: $V = 0.4 \times P + 30$, renal volume in milliliter can be measured with comparable

accuracy to voxel count method. In 177 consecutive Northern American patients who underwent abdominal CT mean values for left and right renal volume (voxel count), width, thickness, and length were 192 mL, 185 mL, 7 cm, 5 cm, and 10 cm, respectively [14].

11.2.1.2 Congenital Anomalies

11.2.1.2.1 Renal Ectopia

Renal ectopia is a general term used to define any displacement of the kidneys caused by abnormal migration from their origin in the true pelvis to their normal retroperitoneal position. Simple ectopia refers to malposition of a kidney that is normally lateralized. During normal development, kidneys rotate 90° medially by the time they have reached their normal retroperitoneal position. With simple ectopia, failure to complete ascent and medial rotation occurs. Most simple ectopias are clinically asymptomatic. Patients with pelvic kidneys, an extreme form of simple ectopia, are more prone to incomplete ureteral drainage because of abnormal ureteral angulation. Horseshoe kidney (Figure 11.4) is considered a bilateral simple ectopia associated with fusion of lower (more common), upper, or both poles across the midline and is usually located anterior to the great vessels. Similar to other forms of ectopia, horseshoe kidneys are usually positioned caudally, which has been attributed to extension of isthmus across the aorta at the level of inferior mesenteric artery origin. Occasionally, the isthmus is drained by a third ureter. Because of malrotation and passage of ureters over the isthmus, horseshoe kidneys are more prone to insufficient ureteral drainage and consequent infection and stone formation. It has been shown that transitional cell carcinoma (TCC) is up to four times more common in patients with horseshoe

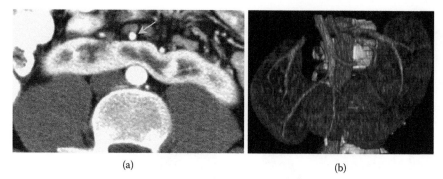

(a)   (b)

FIGURE 11.4
Axial corticomedullary phase CT image (a) and corresponding 3D volume-rendered image (b) showing a horseshoe kidney with isthmus crossing the midline anterior to the inferior vena cava and aorta and posterior to inferior mesenteric artery (arrow). Note that isthmus is composed of enhancing, functional renal tissue.

kidney compared to general population. Furthermore, horseshoe kidneys are more susceptible to injury during blunt abdominal trauma [15,16].

11.2.1.2.2 Persistent Fetal Lobulation

As mentioned before, renal lobe is considered the functional unit of the kidney and is composed of cortex, medulla, and papilla. In the neonatal kidney, functional units are separated by surface grooves. By the age of 4–5 years, these surface grooves normally disappear and adjacent lobes fuse. Incomplete fusion of lobes is seen in 5% of population and results in persistent fetal lobulation that appears as discrete cortical grooves. Kidneys have a scalloped appearance with smooth indentations and normal cortical thickness (10 mm). As opposed to reflux nephropathy in which indentations overlie the calyces, in persistent fetal lobulation calyces are centered between indentations. Persistent fetal lobulation does not have any clinical significance but may be mistaken for other entities such as tumors or renal scarring [15].

11.2.1.2.3 Hypertrophied Column of Bertin

As mentioned before, column of Bertin represents hypertrophy of the renal cortex. Hypertrophied column of Bertin does not have any clinical significance but may be confused with a renal mass [9].

11.2.2 Renal Masses

Most renal masses are currently discovered incidentally on cross-sectional imaging examinations performed for a complaint not related to the urinary system. It has been estimated that more than half of patients over the age of 50 years have at least one renal mass [17]. Renal masses are best characterized with nonenhanced phase followed by nephrographic and excretory phase, all performed with thin sections. Coronal and sagittal images may provide better characterization of lesions that are elusive on axial images and should

be routinely reviewed [18–20]. Conditions that mimic a renal mass such as hypertrophied column of Bertin, hypertrophied parenchyma adjacent to parenchymal scar, vascular abnormalities, infarction, trauma, infection, and hemorrhage should be excluded. Ipsilateral perinephric fat stranding should raise the suspicion for an inflammatory process. Contributory clinical information should be taken into account in the radiological evaluation of renal masses. Renal masses are subdivided into cystic and solid masses and will be further discussed [9,21].

11.2.2.1 Cystic Renal Masses

Cystic renal masses range in biological behavior from non-neoplastic to neoplastic, which determines whether they may be left alone, followed or excised. A cystic renal mass is defined as any mass predominantly composed of fluid filled spaces. On CT, attenuation values between 0 and 20 HU represent simple fluid and any mass predominantly composed of fluid density material can be categorized as a cystic mass [22]. Another fundamental imaging characteristic of cystic renal mass on CT is lack of enhancement. An attenuation difference of 10 HU or less is usually applied to define lack of enhancement. Attenuation difference values of 10–20 HU and more than 20 HU represent equivocal and unequivocal enhancement, respectively and require further investigation [9,23]. However, it is important to keep in mind that factors including but not limited to size of the cystic mass, CT technique, volume averaging, and pseudoenhancement can affect attenuation values [24].

The Bosniak classification has remained the main guideline for classification and management of cystic renal masses. Size is not a fundamental feature of Bosniak classification [22,25–27]. However, it has been suggested that smaller masses are more likely to be benign and probability of malignancy in cysts smaller than 1 cm is extremely low [28].

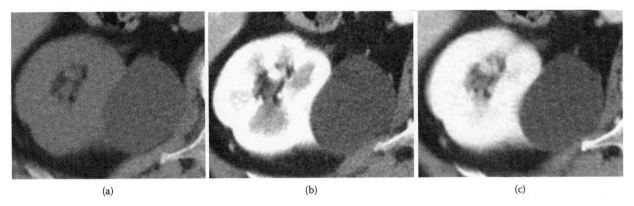

(a)   (b)   (c)

FIGURE 11.5
Nonenhanced (a), corticomedullary (b), and nephrographic (c) phase axial CT images of the right kidney in a 61-year-old male shows well-marginated, nonenhancing cysts that contain homogenous low-attenuating fluid (0–20 HU) with no calcifications, septations, or enhancing nodular soft tissue consistent with Bosniak category I renal cyst.

Bosniak category I masses (Figure 11.5) are simple renal cysts and represent the most common renal mass detected by imaging modalities. Simple cysts are well-marginated, nonenhancing cysts that contain homogenous low-attenuating fluid (0–20 HU) with no calcifications, septations, or enhancing nodular soft tissue and have a barely perceptible, hairline-thin wall. Category I cystic lesions are always benign and do not require any additional workup [9].

Minimally complicated cysts fall into Bosniak category II masses (Figure 11.6) and usually contain a few thin septations that do not show any enhancement. Fine border-forming calcification or small areas of thickened calcification may be observed in the cyst wall or septa. Hyperattenuating cysts are defined as homogeneous cysts that contain fluid with higher attenuation than water (>20 HU) on nonenhanced images that do not enhance after administration of IV contrast. Hyperattenuating cysts are also classified as Bosniak category II. Of note, attenuation values of 20–40 HU and >40 HU represent proteinaceous and hemorrhagic content, respectively. Absence of de-enhancement on delayed CT is another feature of hyperattenuating cysts that correspond to lack of vascularity and may help differentiate a hyperattenuating cyst from a vascular lesion. This principle is particularly helpful in cases with no prior nonenhanced images. Category II cystic lesions may be reliably considered benign and do not warrant any additional workup. Category IIF ("F" stands for follow) represent a group of slightly more complicated cystic masses than group II that cannot be reliably considered benign and require follow-up. Multiple (more than a few) thin septa with perceived enhancement, minimal smooth wall/septal thickening and harboring thick, irregular/nodular calcification qualify a cystic lesion to be classified as category IIF. Hyperattenuating renal masses larger than 3 cm are also classified in this category. The recommended follow-up interval is at

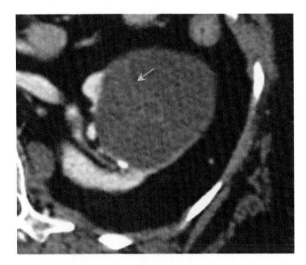

FIGURE 11.6
Nephrographic-phase axial CT image in a 56-year-old man showing a cystic left renal mass that contains a small area of thickened calcification in the medial cyst wall and a few hairline-thin septa (arrow) with no measurable enhancement consistent with benign but complicated renal cyst, which is classified as Bosniak category II renal cyst.

6 months, followed by yearly studies for a minimum of 5 years. Size and morphologic stability (no increase in septal thickening or nodularity) in a category IIF mass after 5 years is consistent with benign biological behavior and does not require additional follow-up [9,27].

Bosniak category III masses (Figure 11.7) are complicated indeterminate cystic masses characterized by: thick, irregular wall, multiple, thick septa with measurable enhancement and thick or nodular calcification. Category III cystic renal masses have a reasonable chance of being malignant (30%–100%), which justifies surgical resection despite the fact that up to two-third of patients might undergo unnecessary surgery. Differential diagnoses of category III lesions include benign etiologies such as hemorrhagic or infected cysts and malignant etiologies such as multilocular cystic nephroma, mixed epithelial and stromal tumor of the kidney and cystic renal cell carcinoma (RCC). Approximately 15% of RCCs are cystic due either to extensive necrosis or cystic growth pattern [9,29].

Bosniak category IV masses (Figure 11.8) not only have all the characteristics of category III masses, but also contain enhancing soft-tissue and/or nodular components adjacent to or separate from the wall or septa. Cystic renal lesions in this category are almost always malignant unless proven otherwise and should be surgically removed [9].

11.2.2.2 Solid Renal Masses

Solid renal masses are mainly composed of enhancing tissue with little or no fluid components. An enhancing renal mass should be considered neoplastic after excluding inflammatory and vascular abnormalities

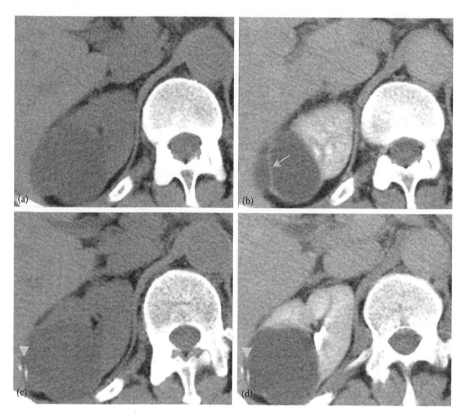

FIGURE 11.7
Axial nonenhanced (a and c) and delayed (b and d) phase CT images in a 53-year-old male show a cystic left renal mass with thick septa showing measurable enhancement (arrow) (b) and peripheral calcification (arrowheads) (c and d) corresponding to Bosniak category III cystic mass. Benign and malignant causes of category III cystic renal masses cannot be distinguished by cyst features. A benign, septated cyst was diagnosed at surgical pathologic evaluation.

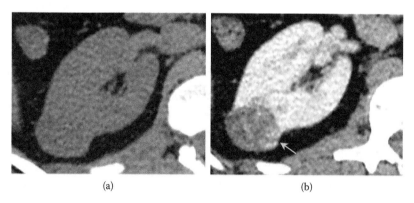

(a)   (b)

FIGURE 11.8
Nonenhanced (a) and nephrographic (b) phase axial CT images in a 26-year-old male show a cystic right renal mass with solid enhancing nodules (arrow), which was classified as Bosniak category IV cystic mass. RCC was diagnosed at surgical pathologic evaluation.

and pseudotumors. Taking into account relevant clinical information such as age, gender, personal history of malignancy, family history of and genetic predisposition to RCC may help in diagnosing the etiology of a renal mass. Although the majority of solid masses are solitary, multiple renal masses are most likely because of multifocal RCC and multiple oncocytomas, both as part of hereditary syndromes, or rarely lymphoma [9,21].

11.2.2.2.1 Renal Cell Carcinoma

RCC is a heterogeneous group of tumors with distinct histopathologic features arising from proximal convoluted tubules of renal cortex. RCC accounts for up to 90% of renal solid masses and is more frequently seen in elderly males [30,31]. Multifocal and bilateral tumors are seen in around 4% of RCC cases and could be hereditary. Multiple conventional RCCs are associated with von Hippel–Lindau disease [32]. Currently, most RCCs are discovered incidentally and the classic triad of hematuria, flank pain, and a palpable abdominal mass is seen in a very small minority of patients and heralds a poor prognosis [30,33]. This trend has resulted in earlier detection of RCCs, which can translate into improved outcomes achieved with less invasive interventions [33]. Patients with renal failure are at higher risk of developing RCC against the background of acquired cystic disease of dialysis and require ongoing surveillance [21].

RCC has been referred to as the prototypic ball-type mass (Figures 11.9 and 11.10) [31,34]. Ball-type masses enlarge by means of additive expansion responsible for their spherical shape and exophytic growth that can deform renal contour. After administration of IV contrast, a distinct interface between the mass and the surrounding renal parenchyma is typically seen. Because of high vascularity, some masses may be obscured during the corticomedullary phase. However, vascular lesions become more conspicuous against the background of enhanced renal parenchyma during the nephrographic phase. Excretory phase CT images may be helpful in demonstration of distortion and displacement of the pyelocaliceal system by the adjacent mass and should be routinely performed in the evaluation of all solid renal masses [21,31,34].

Clear cell RCC is the conventional, most common histologic subtype and accounts for up to 80% of cases [35]. High vascularity of conventional RCC produces strong enhancement on corticomedullary phase images (change in attenuation of as much as 100 HU) (Figure 11.9) and de-enhancement on delayed images [36]. Strong enhancement on corticomedullary phase makes small or peripherally located RCCs difficult to identify against the background of normal cortical enhancement. Consequently, nephrographic-phase images are usually most sensitive for detection of RCC [18,23,37].

De-enhancement on delayed CT images may serve as a useful tool for differentiation of RCC from high-density cyst in the evaluation of a well-demarcated, homogenous, high-attenuating renal mass (>30 HU) [38]. It has been shown that fast kilovoltage-switching dual-energy CT is highly specific in excluding enhancement and moderately to highly sensitive in detecting enhancement of renal lesions without the need to perform a dedicated nonenhanced phase [4]. Enhancement is usually homogenous in small RCCs but may be heterogeneous in larger RCCs because of the areas of necrosis (Figure 11.11). It has been shown that quantification of degree and heterogeneity of enhancement may be useful in differentiation of different subtypes of small RCCs [39]. Calcification may be seen on nonenhanced CT in up to 30% of RCCs and is characteristically central as opposed to thin, peripheral calcification associated with benign cysts [19].

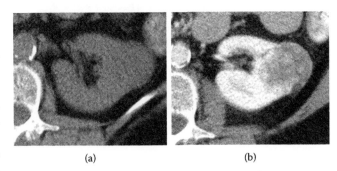

(a)   (b)

FIGURE 11.9
Nonenhanced (a) and nephrographic (b) phase axial CT images in a 62-year-old female showing an exophytic, ball-type left renal mass with strong heterogeneous enhancement. Conventional RCC with focal extension into the perinephric fat was diagnosed at surgical pathologic evaluation.

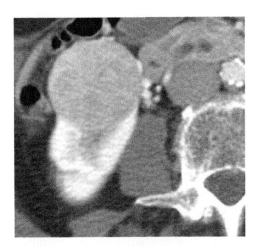

FIGURE 11.10
Nephrographic-phase axial CT image in an 82-year-old female showing a solid, exophytic, ball-type right renal mass with homogenous enhancement. Papillary RCC was diagnosed at surgical pathologic evaluation.

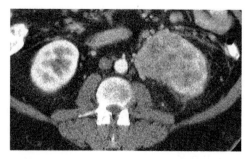

FIGURE 11.11
Contrast-enhanced axial CT image in a 72-year-old male shows a solid, ill-defined, necrotic left renal mass with heterogeneous enhancement and extracapsular spread. RCC was diagnosed at surgical pathologic evaluation. Note the exophytic and associated renal contour deformity.

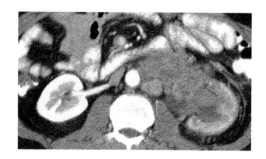

FIGURE 11.12
Axial contrast-enhanced corticomedullary phase CT image in 46-year-old male with bilateral lower extremity swelling reveals a large, infiltrative, heterogeneous, necrotic left renal mass with abnormal retroperitoneal soft-tissue attenuation representing retroperitoneal extension of tumor into the left renal vein. An enlarged, retroperitoneal lymph node (arrow) is noted adjacent to the aorta. Diagnosis of high-grade conventional RCC was made at surgical pathologic evaluation.

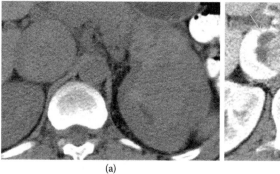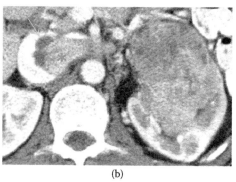

(a)   (b)

FIGURE 11.13
Nonenhanced (a) and corticomedullary (b) axial CT images in a 43-year-old male show a large, heterogeneously enhancing left renal mass extending into the left renal vein and inferior vena cava. Surgical pathologic evaluation revealed a grade 3 clear renal carcinoma with minimal invasion into the perinephric fat. Tumor fragments were identified in the tumor thrombus compatible with CT finding of enhancing soft-tissue density (asterisk) within the left renal vein and inferior vena cava adjacent to the nonenhancing thrombus (arrow).

Papillary (10%–15%) and chromophobe-type (5%) RCC are the second and third most common tumor subtypes (Figure 11.10) [40]. It is worth mentioning that some papillary RCCs exhibit less enhancement (10–20 HU increase), which may render differentiation from a cystic lesion difficult [41].

Extension of the disease into perinephric fat, vascular structures, lymph nodes, and adjacent or distant organs should be evaluated in every case for proper tumor staging (Figures 11.12 and 11.13). Of note, invasion of the perinephric fat by the tumor might not be depicted on CT; nevertheless, this differentiation does not usually affect the surgical approach. Venous invasion typically presents as tissue plug with the renal veins (Figure 11.12) or inferior vena cava (Figure 11.13) and is usually associated with presence of tumor thrombus within the vein. Lymph nodes smaller than 1 cm are usually benign, those between 1 and 2 cm are indeterminate (metastatic versus reactive) and those larger than 2 cm are almost always metastatic. Stage I (T1, N0, M0) tumors are 7 cm or smaller and are confined to the kidneys with those

smaller than 4 cm being classified as T1a and those between 4 and 7 cm as T1b. Stage II (T2, N0, M0) are also confined to the kidneys but are larger than 7 cm. It should be noted that nephron-sparing surgery may be considered for tumors smaller than 7 cm. Any extension of tumor or tumor thrombus into the adjacent structures such as perinephric fat, renal vein, or inferior vena cava but not beyond the anterior or PRF with or without involvement of one regional lymph node is classified as stage III (Figures 11.12 and 11.13). Stage IV is defined as any extension of the tumor beyond the ARF or PRF, involvement of more than one regional lymph node or presence of distant metastasis (Figure 11.14) [13,42].

Surgical resection remains the mainstay of treatment for all stages of RCC. CT is highly accurate for surveillance for recurrence after surgical resection. Local recurrence may manifest as an irregular, enhancing lesion displacing adjacent structures and frequently involving the psoas and quadratus muscles. Lymphatic recurrence is less common and usually takes place adjacent to renal vascular pedicle. Distant metastasis is the

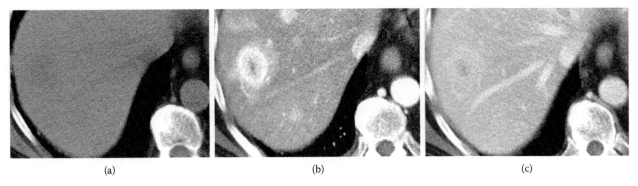

(a)   (b)   (c)

FIGURE 11.14
Nonenhanced (a), arterial (b), and portal venous (c) phase axial CT images in a 61-year-old male 1 year after he was diagnosed with invasive clear cell carcinoma of the left kidney and subsequently underwent left radical nephrectomy show multiple hypervascular liver lesion best depicted on the arterial phase images. Note de-enhancement of the lesions on the portal venous phase images.

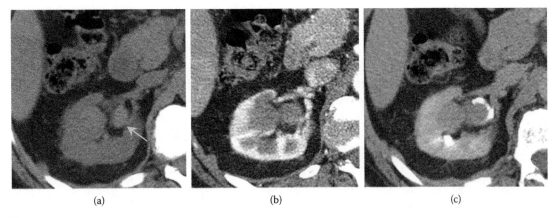

(a)   (b)   (c)

FIGURE 11.15
Nonenhanced (a), corticomedullary (b), and delayed (c) phase axial CT images of the right kidney in a 53-year-old male who presented with hematuria showing increased attenuation in right renal pelvis (arrow) on nonenhanced phase CT image (a). With administration of IV contrast, faint enhancement of the soft-tissue mass invading the sinus structures is depicted (b). Delayed image (c) further characterizes the renal pelvis mass infiltrating renal parenchyma and encasing the native collecting system, which is most consistent with advanced TCC that was confirmed by surgical pathologic evaluation. Note how TCC uses renal parenchyma as scaffolding for its infiltrative growth and how kidney's native bean-shaped morphology is preserved with little distortion of its contour. Also note how differentiation of TCC from nonenhanced medulla can be challenging on corticomedullary phase, rendering nephrographic phase necessary for optimal radiological evaluation.

most common form of recurrence; is typically hypervascular; and is observed in lungs, mediastinum, bones, liver, contralateral kidney, and adrenal gland and brain (Figure 11.14) [9,42].

11.2.2.2.2 Transitional Cell Carcinoma

TCC accounts for approximately 10% of renal malignancies [21]. Renal TCC arises from transitional urothelium and is seen in the renal pelvis, infundibulum, and caliceal regions in decreasing frequency [43]. TCCs are typically low-grade, superficial, and papillary (projecting intraluminally) producing focal intraluminal mass in the collecting system [44]. Aggressive TCC is characterized by either local, mucosal extension manifested by mural thickening and luminal narrowing or systemic spread via hematogenous or lymphatic invasion and is seen in up to 15% of cases [44,45]. Upper-tract TCCs are more common in elderly males [46]. Smoking, chemical carcinogens, and drugs (cyclophosphamide, analgesics)

have been associated with TCC. Since carcinogens bathe the entire urothelium, TCCs are often multifocal with synchronous and metachronous tumors, emphasizing the necessity for vigilant surveillance [46,47].

Early tumors are confined to the muscularis layer and are separated from the renal parenchyma by renal sinus fat. Advanced TCCs extend centrifugally into the renal parenchyma in an infiltrating pattern that distorts normal architecture but typically preserve the reniform shape of the affected kidney (Figure 11.15). Consequently, TCC has been referred to as the prototypic bean-type mass. Instead of spherical enlargement seen in ball-type masses, bean-type lesions use renal parenchyma as scaffolding for their infiltrative growth leading to the typical ill-defined borders. Infiltrative growth usually results in preservation of kidney's native bean-shaped morphology with little distortion of kidney contour. As a result, bean-type lesions may be invisible on nonenhanced CT. On nonenhanced CT, the intraluminal portion is usually hyperattenuating compared to the surrounding urine. Subtle invasion of sinus structures or dilatation of collecting system may be the only indicators of TCC on nonenhanced CT. With administration of IV contrast, differentiation of TCC from nonenhanced medulla can be impossible on corticomedullary phase. Best seen on nephrographic phase, the infiltrative, parenchymal element of TCC enhances less than normal renal parenchyma and characteristically less than RCC. Encasement or obliteration of the native collecting system by an intraluminal element is best depicted on the excretory phase especially when combined with multiplanar reformatting. The parenchymal infiltration may replace significant portions or even the entire kidney with subsequent incomplete or complete alteration of renal enhancement [13,21].

11.2.2.2.3 Angiomyolipoma

Angiomyolipoma are benign neoplasms that should be excluded in the evaluation of incidental solid renal masses. Most angiomyolipomas are characterized by the presence of areas of fat within a noncalcified renal mass on nonenhanced CT. Diagnostic feature of angiomyolipoma

on CT is presence of well-marginated fat (<−20 HU) arising from cortex (Figure 11.16) [48]. Up to 5% of small angiomyolipomas contain little or no fat and appear as a hyperattenuating mass on nonenhanced CT that enhance homogeneously and are thus, indistinguishable from small RCC. Presence of small, discrete pockets of fat might contribute to establishing the correct diagnosis [13,49,50].

Vascular component of angiomyolipoma is unusually weak predisposing to aneurysm formation and making hemorrhage into PRS the most common complication. Tumors larger than 4 cm are at increased risk for hemorrhage and warrant therapeutic intervention (Figure 11.17) [51,52]. Most angiomyolipomas (up to 90%) are solitary and more common among middle-aged women. Multifocal, usually bilateral, angiomyolipoma is seen in association with tuberous sclerosis [53].

11.2.2.2.4 Oncocytoma

Oncocytoma is another benign renal tumor arising from proximal renal tubules. Oncocytomas are characterized with homogeneous enhancement and central, stellate, low-attenuating scar on CT. Similar to RCC, oncocytoma

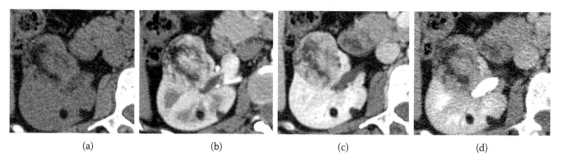

(a)　　　　　　　(b)　　　　　　　(c)　　　　　　　(d)

FIGURE 11.16
Nonenhanced (a), corticomedullary (b), nephrographic (c), and delayed (d) phase axial CT images of the right kidney in a 43-year-old female showing a solid, well-marginated, fat-containing enhancing mass consistent with angiomyolipoma. Note the additional two lesions in the posterior aspect of the right kidney.

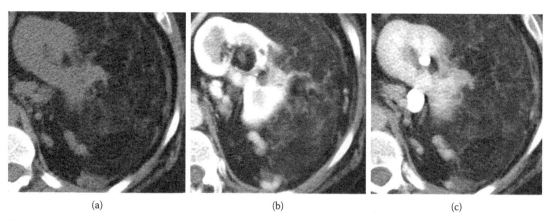

(a)　　　　　　　　　　(b)　　　　　　　　　　(c)

FIGURE 11.17
Nonenhanced (a), corticomedullary (b), and delayed (c) phase axial CT images in a 48-year-old female showing a large solid mass, mainly composed of fat, arising from the lower pole of the left kidney with minimal enhancement. Consequently, tumor was resected and a diagnosis of angiomyolipoma extending into the perinephric fat with no evidence of hemorrhage was made at surgical pathology evaluation.

is a ball-type mass and occurs more often in elderly male patients. In addition, imaging characteristics are not sufficiently diagnostic and histopathological diagnosis is warranted. As a result, oncocytomas remain the most frequently excised benign solid renal mass [21,54].

11.2.2.2.5 Renal Medullary Carcinoma

Renal medullary carcinoma (RMC) is a rare histologic subtype of RCC that arises from caliceal epithelium in or near the renal papilla and follows an infiltrative (bean-type) growth pattern. Most RMCs are located deep in the medulla, which results in caliectasis without pelviectasis. RMCs usually have ill-defined margins and encase or interrupt adjacent collecting system structures. Seen almost exclusively in patients with sickle cell trait, RMC develops in a younger population and has a predilection for right kidney. RMC usually present with hematuria, flank/abdominal pain and palpable mass and are extremely aggressive with very poor survival due to disseminated disease at the time of diagnosis [55,56].

11.2.2.2.6 Renal Lymphoma

Since kidney does not have any native lymphoid tissue, primary involvement by a lymphoproliferative process is extremely rare. On the other hand, evidence of kidney involvement has been documented in 34%–68% of patients with lymphoma at autopsy studies. Nevertheless, renal involvement has been reported on CT in up to 8% of patients with lymphoma. Renal involvement typically occurs in the setting of disseminated disease and is more frequent with non-Hodgkin's lymphoma. Although presentation of lymphoma on CT

is diverse, multiple bilateral renal masses associated with retroperitoneal lymphadenopathy is the most common presentation and is seen in up to 60% of patients with lymphoma (Figure 11.18). Contiguous spread from adjacent involved lymph nodes into the kidney, usually through an infiltrative process, is another presentation of renal lymphoma and is seen in up to 25% of patients (Figure 11.19). Encasement of renal artery or vein characteristically does not result in obstruction or thrombosis in renal lymphoma (Figure 11.18). Seen in 20% of patients, diffuse infiltration of kidneys by affected lymphocytes is usually bilateral and manifests as smooth generalized renal enlargement (Figure 11.20). A solitary mass is the least common form of renal involvement in lymphoma and is seen in fewer than 10% of patients. On CT, renal lymphoma presents as a mass with soft-tissue attenuation and homogeneous enhancement, which is

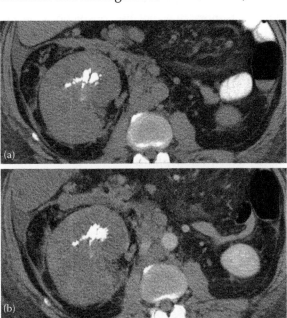

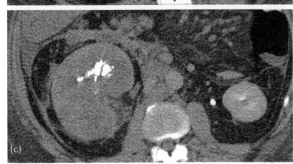

FIGURE 11.19
Nonenhanced (a), corticomedullary (b), and delayed (c) phase axial CT images in a 55-year-old male with lymphoma showing extensive retroperitoneal lymphadenopathy with contiguous spread to the right kidney. Note the necrotic appearance of the mass and impaired right renal function as a result of neoplastic infiltration. Central calcification observed in this case is not a typical manifestation of lymphoma and may be the result of spontaneous bleeding or prior treatment.

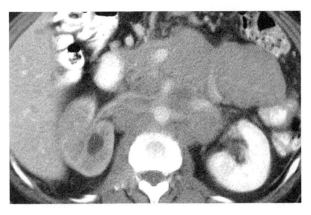

FIGURE 11.18
Nephrographic-phase axial CT image in a 52-year-old female with diffuse lymphocytic lymphoma showing a large, homogeneous retroperitoneal mass invading the right kidney through hilum and enveloping hilar vessels. Note the replacement of right renal parenchyma by neoplastic cells and that patency of the encased vessels are maintained despite the massive tumor burden.

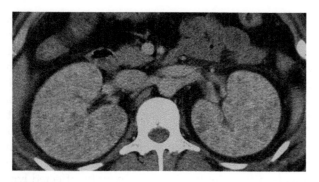

FIGURE 11.20
Nephrographic-phase axial CT image in a 41-year-old male with infiltrative renal lymphoma showing diffuse, bilateral enlargement of the kidneys and patchy deposition of neoplastic cell within the parenchyma. Note that both kidneys have retained their normal contours and reniform configurations.

commonly less intense than normal parenchyma. Small medullary tumors may not be conspicuous on corticomedullary phase and require nephrographic-phase images. Calcification may be seen in a subset of cases but is not a typical manifestation of lymphoma on CT and may be the result of spontaneous hemorrhage or prior treatment (Figure 11.19) [9,13,21,57].

11.2.3 Infections

11.2.3.1 Acute Pyelonephritis

Pyelitis refers to an ascending urinary tract infection, usually in the setting of vesicoureteral reflux, which has reached the renal pelvis without involvement of renal parenchyma. Further progression of infection from renal pelvis to parenchyma, known as nephritis, initially results in lobar parenchymal inflammation as opposed to multifocal and peripheral inflammation associated with the less common hematogenous spread. Eventually, regardless of origin, most inflammatory foci become confluent, yielding a similar appearance. The Society of Uroradiology has recommended that the term "acute pyelonephritis" be adopted to describe all of the above-mentioned levels of infectious involvement. Patients with acute pyelonephritis typically present with pyuria, flank pain, and fever with chills. Imaging has a limited role in the diagnosis of acute pyelonephritis in adults and diagnosis is usually made clinically. However, imaging may yield valuable information regarding potential underlying congenital abnormalities that predispose to infection and complications. CT usually does not show any specific findings in mild acute pyelonephritis. More severe involvement results in focal swelling or enlargement of the entire kidney. Focal swelling is usually associated with decreased enhancement as a result of under-perfusion and associated necrosis (Figure 11.21). Swelling may persist for months and if severe enough, may cause permanent

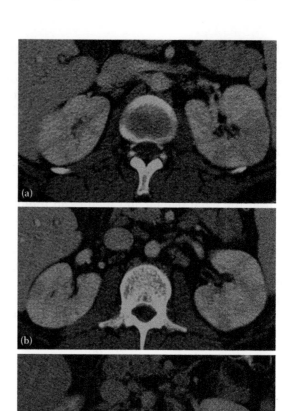

FIGURE 11.21
Nephrographic (a and b) and delayed (c) phase axial CT images in a 31-year-old male with acute flank pain, dysuria, and chills show bilateral, multifocal wedge-shaped areas of heterogeneous attenuation that extends from papillae to cortex. Effacement of renal sinus and loss of corticomedullary differentiation are also noted. These findings are highly suggestive of acute pyelonephritis. Also note hyperenhancement of the left collecting system, which is consistent with left-sided pyelitis.

scarring of the affected lobes (Figure 11.22). Focal swelling may present as areas of decreased and increased attenuation compared to normal parenchyma on non-enhanced images, representing areas of necrosis and focal hemorrhage, respectively. Parenchymal perfusion defects associated with ascending and hematogenous infection usually manifest as wedge-shaped and multiple, rounded low-attenuation defects, respectively. Perfusion defects correlates with severity of infection and is seen on contrast-enhanced CT in up to two thirds of patients. Interestingly, involved segments may show enhancement on delayed images. Additional CT findings may include perinephric inflammation manifested as thickening of Gerota's fascia and perinephric fat stranding. Renal infection confined to a single lobe is called focal pyelonephritis and may mimic renal neoplasms on CT (Figure 11.22). Lack of a well-defined,

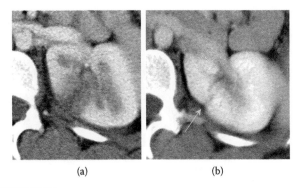

(a)   (b)

FIGURE 11.22

Corticomedullary phase axial CT image (a) in a 17-year-old female with dysuria, fever, and chills showing focal swelling and decreased focal enhancement consistent with acute, mild, focal pyelonephritis of the left kidney, which was successfully treated with IV antibiotics. Follow-up nephrographic-phase axial CT image (b) after 6 months show complete resolution of swelling, normal enhancement with no perfusion defect and smooth focal indentation (arrow) representing scarring of the affected lobe.

perceptible capsule and absence of impression on renal contour helps distinguish focal pyelonephritis from RCC. Patients with suspected uncomplicated acute pyelonephritis are treated medically with antibiotics. Poor response after 72 hours of antibiotic treatment and high-risk patients such as immunocompromised and diabetic patients require radiological examination for evaluation of complications, which is preferably accomplished with CT. Abscess refers to any intraparenchymal or extraparenchymal collection of purulent material that may extend to PRS. Up to 75% of all renal abscesses occur in diabetics. Abscesses typically present as round or geographic, nonenhancing, low-attenuation collections that may show rim enhancement (Figure 11.23). The abscess rims are not true capsules and are frequently nodular. Extraparenchymal abscess collections may occasionally extend into adjacent structures, such as the psoas muscles [13,15,58].

11.2.3.2 Chronic Pyelonephritis

Chronic pyelonephritis is a common descriptor for active chronic infection and multiple recurrent infections, which have similar radiological appearance. Vesicoureteral reflux is characterized by thickening and dilatation of the caliceal system. Reflux into collecting tubules is more common in compound papillae located in the renal poles, which results in the typical loss of renal parenchyma at these locations, manifested as renal scarring on imaging. Scarring results in inhomogeneous contrast enhancement and may cause caliceal clubbing secondary to retraction of papilla and cortical thinning. With progression, scarring eventually results in small, lobulated kidneys usually associated with distorted and clubbed calyces. Compensatory hypertrophy of the noninvolved,

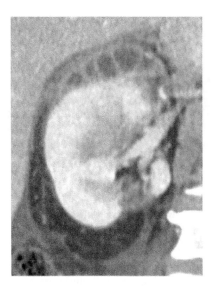

FIGURE 11.23

Corticomedullary phase coronal CT image in a 36-year-old diabetic female with acute pyelonephritis and poor response to antibiotic treatment show a loculated, rim-enhancing, extraparenchymal collection of nonenhancing, low-attenuation material consistent with multiloculated renal abscess.

contralateral kidney and ipsilateral residual normal renal parenchyma may be observed. The latter may present as a pseudotumor. Quantification of residual renal parenchymal volume on CT or magnetic resonance imaging may provide prognostic data on the expected renal function [13,58,59].

11.2.3.3 Emphysematous Pyelonephritis

Emphysematous pyelonephritis is a life-threatening, rapidly progressive necrotizing infection of the kidneys characterized by formation of gas within renal parenchyma or in its surroundings. Emphysematous pyelonephritis is highly associated with poorly controlled diabetes (up to 90% of cases), immunocompromised status, and urinary tract obstruction usually secondary to calculi, neoplasm, or sloughed papilla. Emphysematous pyelonephritis can rapidly become systemic and progress to fulminant sepsis, which carries a high-mortality rate. CT is the imaging modality of choice in the evaluation of emphysematous pyelonephritis. CT findings include enlargement and destruction of parenchyma, with or without necrosis, associated with presence of gas (small bubbles or linear streaks), fluid, and air-fluid levels (Figure 11.24). Distribution of the gas follows two distinct patterns that have been found to correlate with prognosis: type 1 is characterized by presence of streaky or mottled areas of gas with characteristic absence of intrarenal or extrarenal fluid collections; type 2 is characterized by gas in direct association with fluid collection (intraparenchymal or perirenal) or gas within the

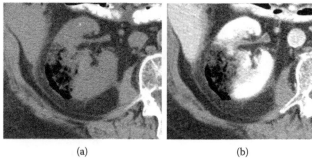

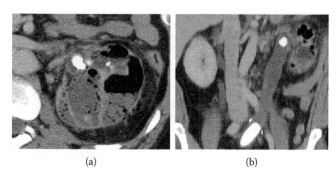

FIGURE 11.24
Nonenhanced (a) and nephrographic (b) phase axial CT images in an 80-year-old female with poorly controlled diabetes showing enlargement of the right kidney, destruction of renal parenchyma associated with presence of intraparenchymal gas consistent with emphysematous pyelonephritis. Note perinephric fat stranding and thickening of the adjacent posterior renal fascia. Also note hyperenhancement and slight wall thickening of the collecting system that signifies the ascending nature of the infectious process.

FIGURE 11.25
Corticomedullary phase axial (a) and coronal (b) CT images in a 59-year-old male with obstructive uropathy as a result of large, left ureteral and renal pelvis calculi showing destruction of renal parenchyma associated with presence of air-fluid level, which is most consistent with type 2 emphysematous pyelonephritis.

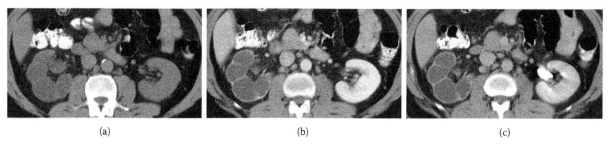

FIGURE 11.26
Nonenhanced (a), nephrographic (b), and delayed (c) phase axial CT images in a 45-year-old male with medical history of recurrent, right-sided urinary tract infections show relative enlargement and nonenhancement of the right kidney, which is consistent with XGP. Although a large staghorn calculus is seen in most cases, it could be absent in a subset of cases similar to the present case.

collecting system (Figure 11.25). Type 1 is associated with a more aggressive clinical course and significant mortality (69% for type 1 versus 18% for type 2) [13,58–60].

11.2.3.4 Xanthogranulomatous Pyelonephritis

Xanthogranulomatous pyelonephritis (XGP) is a chronic, granulomatous inflammatory process that often leads to renal parenchymal destruction. XGP is most commonly associated with renal pelvic calculus, hydronephrosis or superimposed recurrent bacterial infections. Destruction of the renal parenchyma is mainly a consequence of inflammatory response rather than obstruction per se, and results in loss of renal function. CT is the imaging modality of choice for the evaluation of XGP. The main characteristics of XGP on CT include kidney enlargement associated with impaired function (Figure 11.26), contracted renal pelvis associated with presence of central calculus, expansion of calices (Figure 11.27), and inflammatory changes in the perinephric fat. The central branching, low-attenuating areas within the collecting system correspond to the extensive inflammatory infiltrates that fill and expand the collecting system and

should not be mistaken for hydronephrosis. The central branching inflammatory process commonly shows rim enhancement on CT. Fistula formation and psoas muscle abscess are among the most significant extrarenal manifestations of XGP [13,57,59,61–63].

11.2.3.5 Tuberculosis

Prevalence of tuberculosis in developed countries has been rising mainly because of the spread of human immunodeficiency virus infection and the emergence of multidrug-resistant mycobacterial strains. Urinary tract is the most common site of extrapulmonary tuberculosis. Although renal involvement always results from hematogenous seeding from the lungs, less than 50% of patients with urinary tract tuberculosis have radiographic evidence of prior pulmonary tuberculosis. Bilateral, cortical granulomas develop following hematogenous seeding in patients with intact cellular immunity and remain dormant until reactivation occurs. High perfusion rate of renal cortex and favorable oxygen tension favor bacilli implantation in this location. Despite bilateral hematogenous seeding, clinically significant disease

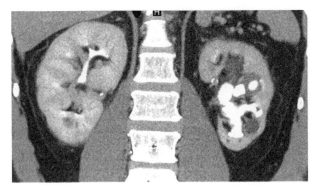

FIGURE 11.27
Delayed phase coronal CT image in a 58-year-old male show a central staghorn calculus in the left renal pelvis associated with expansion of calices and impaired renal function consistent with XGP.

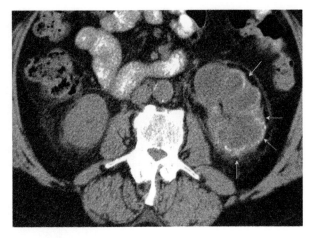

FIGURE 11.28
Nonenhanced phase axial CT image in a 65-year-old male with known history of pulmonary tuberculosis show calcification of left kidney (arrows), complete destruction of renal parenchyma (autonephrectomy) and replacement of renal parenchyma with inflammatory debris and caseous necrotic tissue.

is usually unilateral upon reactivation. Reactivation is characterized with enlargement and coalescence of cortical granulomas. Capillary rupture results in delivery of organisms to the medulla that follows stepwise stages of granuloma formation and enlargement, caseous necrosis, and cavitation that eventually leads to complete destruction of renal parenchyma (autonephrectomy) if left untreated (Figure 11.28). Communication of the granulomas with the collecting system can lead to further extension of the infection into the urothelium. The host's immune response triggers fibrosis and calcium deposition that further contributes to obstruction and renal dysfunction. Retroperitoneal extension commonly associated with involvement of adjacent organs may occur in untreated patients. CT is helpful in the evaluation of renal and extrarenal extent of tuberculosis. CT is the most sensitive imaging modality for detection of renal calcifications, which is seen in the majority of patients and is considered the hallmark of genitourinary tuberculosis (Figure 11.28). Knowledge of CT attenuation values may facilitate evaluation of genitourinary tuberculosis. Fluid-filled calices and calculi have attenuation values of 0–10 HU and greater than 120 HU, respectively. Inflammatory debris and tissue with caseous necrosis have attenuation value of 10–30 HU (Figure 11.29). Diffuse calcification of renal parenchyma, forming a cast of the kidney with autonephrectomy, is known as putty-like calcification and has an attenuation value of 50–120 HU. Tuberculosis-related papillary necrosis leaves cavitary defects within the medulla after sloughing off. A cavity that communicates with the collecting system is readily seen on CT. A sloughed-off papilla is seen as a triangular caliceal filling defect on CT and may cause ureteral obstruction. Additional CT findings of genitourinary tuberculosis include cortical thinning (focal or global), parenchymal scarring, and fibrotic urothelial strictures (highly suggestive of tuberculosis). CT urography is helpful in the evaluation of urothelial mucosal abnormalities [58,59,64,65].

11.2.3.6 Malakoplakia

Malakoplakia is a rare, inflammatory process characterized by abnormal host response to chronic infection as a result of altered, abnormal intracellular processing of ingested organisms. Although any urothelial-lined location may be involved, the condition is most commonly seen in the urinary bladder. Malakoplakia is associated with recurrent urinary tract infection, HIV infection, renal transplant, and autoimmune disorders. Since malakoplakia most commonly presents as urothelial mucosal mass, the most frequent renal finding is obstruction. Direct involvement of the kidney typically manifests as an infiltrative multifocal process that might coalesce into a large dominant mass that distorts renal contour. The classic appearance of malakoplakia is an enlarged kidney with multiple, minimally enhancing masses. Imaging findings can usually suggest malakoplakia in the appropriate clinical context [59,66,67].

11.3 Ureters

11.3.1 Anatomy

11.3.1.1 Normal Anatomy

The ureters are retroperitoneal tubes approximately 25–30 cm in length that consist of an outer fibrous, a middle muscular, and an inner mucosal layer. The outer fibrous layer, adventitia, is continuous with the renal capsule and adventitia of the urinary bladder. The muscularis layer consists of outer circular and inner longitudinal

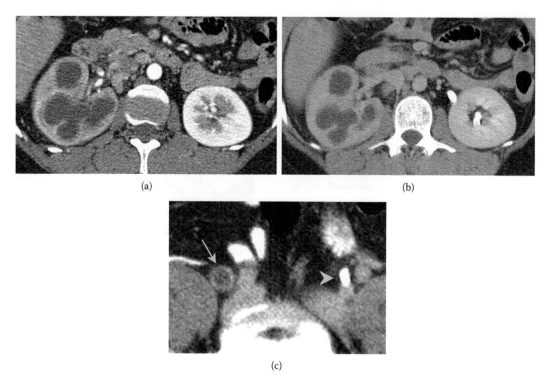

FIGURE 11.29
Corticomedullary (a) and delayed (b) phase axial CT images in a 35-year-old female with documented pulmonary tuberculosis show dilated, fluid-filled calices, cortical thinning and replacement of renal parenchyma with inflammatory debris, and caseous necrosis, which represent renal tuberculosis. Magnified view from delayed phase axial CT image (c) shows lack of filling of right ureter (arrow) with contrast and circumferential right ureteral wall thickening. The left ureter (arrowhead) is filled with contrast and appears normal.

muscular layers. Mucosal layer is lined with transitional epithelium supported by the submucosal connective tissue of the lamina propria. The ureters begin at the ureteropelvic junction and descend inferomedially along the psoas major muscles projecting over the transverse processes of the lumbar vertebrae until they reach the true pelvis. Ureters cross anterior to the common iliac or proximal external iliac vessels before they cross the pelvic inlet to enter the true pelvis where they may be compromised by an aneurysm. Ureters course medially at the pelvic brim (edge of the pelvic inlet) to sacroiliac joint and then laterally near the ischial spine before they finally turn medially at the level of inferior greater sciatic foramen to enter the bladder trigone through the ureterovesical junction. Three normal constrictions of the ureter include ureteropelvic junction, pelvic brim, and ureterovesical junction [15,68].

11.3.1.2 Congenital Anomalies

11.3.1.2.1 Ureteral Duplication

Duplication of the ureters is the most common anomaly of the urinary tract. Duplication is more common in women and is familial in many cases. Most duplication anomalies are unilateral and those that are bilateral tend to be asymmetrical. A duplication anomaly in which the two ureters join before inserting into the bladder

is considered incomplete as opposed to separate insertions in complete duplication. According to the Weigert–Meyer rule, in a duplicated renal collecting system the upper pole moiety ureter inserts inferior and medial to the ureter, draining the lower pole moiety. Consequently, the ureter, draining the upper pole moiety is more likely to be ectopic, obstructed, and to end in an ureterocele. Ectopic upper pole moiety is more common in females and unlike males, always ends below the continence mechanism of the bladder. This can result in incontinence because of insertion of ureter distal to the external sphincter, uterus, or vagina (associated with vaginal infection and interlabial mass). Although ectopic ureter is not associated with incontinence in males because of insertion of ureter proximal to the external sphincter, ureteral ectopia within the vas deferens may cause epididymo-orchitis. The lower pole ureter usually inserts at or near the normal location; however, it is prone to reflux as a result of short intravesicular segment or distortion of its ureterovesical junction by an upper pole ectopic ureterocele. Duplications may be difficult to detect on nonenhanced axial CT images. However, contrast-enhanced visualization of two ureters provides sufficient evidence to establish the diagnosis (Figure 11.30). Detection of an occult ectopic ureter associated with a small and poorly functioning renal segment can be difficult to diagnose with imaging [7,15,68].

11.3.1.2.2 *Ureteral Obstruction*

Congenital narrowing at the ureteropelvic junction is the most common cause of antenatal hydronephrosis and is bilateral in up to 30% of cases. Varying degrees of hydronephrosis without accompanying ureterectasis is seen depending on the severity of stenosis. Anomalous formation of inferior vena cava from a persistent right posterior cardinal vein rather than the right supracardinal vein results in retrocaval (circumcaval) positioning of the right ureter. Retrocaval ureter is usually asymptomatic and is discovered incidentally in most instances. Compression of the retrocaval right ureter can cause varying degrees of proximal ureteral obstruction and hydronephrosis and abrupt medial deviation of the normal-caliber, poststenotic distal ureter that result in the "J" or fishhook appearance of the ureter [7,15].

11.3.2 Neoplasms

TCC accounts for approximately 90% of ureteral malignancies and is associated with exposure to tobacco, industrial dyes, and chemicals, and drugs such as phenacetin and cyclophosphamide. Approximately 75% of ureteral TCCs occur in the distal third of the ureter. Bathing of the entire collecting system with concentrated amounts

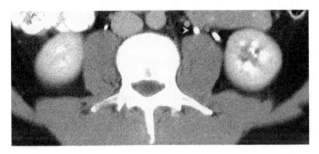

FIGURE 11.30
Delayed phase axial CT image in a 37-year-old asymptomatic female shows duplicated left ureter (arrowhead) with normal size opacified with excreted contrast.

of carcinogens leads to the development of synchronous and metachronous lesions. Close urologic surveillance and frequent radiological evaluation is therefore mandatory, especially in the first 2 years after the diagnosis of TCC has been established [15,43,46].

Traditionally, ureteral disease has been evaluated with IV urogram and retrograde ureterography, which only allow evaluation of the ureteral lumen. Instead, CT urogram allows visualization of intraluminal, mural, and extraluminal abnormalities and has widely replaced the traditional methods. One potential disadvantage of CT urography over the traditional methods is acquisition of images over a very short period of time during which all segments of the collecting system might not be in a distended and opacified state. This shortcoming may be addressed by augmentation of urinary flow rate by administration of IV furosemide or saline. It is important to remember that absence of obstruction does not rule out presence of tumors in the collecting system. As a result, opacification combined with distention of the collecting system is the key to optimal evaluation and detection of small lesions. CT urography is indicated in the evaluation of patients with hematuria and suspected collecting system neoplasms, surveillance of those with prior urothelial malignancies and evaluation of disease progression and treatment response. Nonenhanced images are necessary to determine attenuation values for nonenhancing filling defects. Ureteral TCC most typically presents as wall thickening of varying degrees that may become obstructive or as a mass that manifests itself as a filling defect in an opacified collecting system (Figure 11.31). Slow growth of the TCC may lead to pre- and postobstructive dilatation of the affected ureter, which is usually seen in more advanced stages. TCC is typically hyperattenuating (5–30 HU) to urine but has lower density than filling defects caused by clot (40–80 HU) or calculus (>100 HU) on nonenhanced images. Contrast-enhanced images further aid in confirming location and extent of the lesion (Figure 11.32). TCC can show early enhancement and

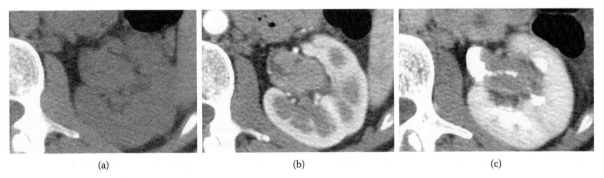

(a) (b) (c)

FIGURE 11.31
Nonenhanced (a), corticomedullary (b), and delayed (c) phase axial CT images in a 39-year-old female with hematuria show a hyperattenuating left proximal collecting system fullness on nonenhanced image (a). Corticomedullary phase image (b) shows irregular wall thickening hyperattenuating to urine but with lower density than the renal cortex. Delayed phase image (c) best depicts the renal pelvis intraluminal mass with encasement of the collecting system consistent with TCC. Note de-enhancement of the tumor on the delayed image.

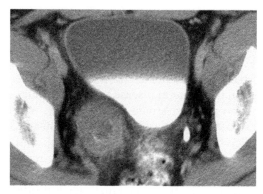

FIGURE 11.32
Delayed phase axial CT image in a 76-year-old male with right-sided hydronephrosis shows ill-defined, obstructive wall thickening of the right ureter. Diagnosis of high-grade TCC was made at surgical pathologic evaluation.

de-enhancement on contrast-enhanced images. TCC metastasizes via lymphatics and hematogenously to the liver, lungs, and bones [7,69–73].

Leukoplakia is squamous metaplasia of the urothelium, secondary to chronic irritation by factors such as calculi, chronic infection, and schistosomiasis infection. Leukoplakia is a premalignant condition associated with development of squamous cell carcinoma and may manifests as mural filling defects. Squamous cell carcinoma of the ureter is less frequent than TCC and manifests as an infiltrative process with superficial spread. Like other urothelial neoplasms, manifestations of urothelial squamous cell carcinoma on CT urography range from a mild circumferential focal wall thickening to a large obstructive mass [15].

11.3.3 Infections

11.3.3.1 Ureteritis

Ureteritis is usually associated with ipsilateral pyelonephritis. Diagnosis is usually made clinically and imaging is performed for the evaluation of complications. Diffuse enhancement and circumferential wall thickening of the urothelium is depicted on CT, often associated with periureteric and perinephric stranding (Figure 11.24) [74].

11.3.3.2 Emphysematous Pyelitis

Emphysematous pyelitis is a less aggressive form of emphysematous infection of the upper urinary tract characterized by isolated presence of gas in the collecting system. Emphysematous pyelitis is also associated with diabetes and urinary obstruction and is more common among females and carries significantly less mortality compared to emphysematous pyelonephritis. Other etiologies of air within the collecting

system such as recent instrumentation and fistula should be excluded. On CT, emphysematous pyelitis presents with gas within a dilated collecting system in the absence of parenchymal gas and can be accurately differentiated from emphysematous pyelonephritis (Figure 11.33) [59].

11.3.3.3 Pyonephrosis

Pyonephrosis is acute infection with formation of pus within an obstructed collecting system. Rapid intervention is crucial in the management of pyonephrosis, which if left untreated, may result in rapid, often permanent, decline in renal function and septic shock. Pyonephrosis should be suspected in any patient with urinary tract obstruction who presents with fever and flank pain. Ultrasound findings, particularly presence of echogenic debris, provide high accuracy in diagnosis of pyonephrosis versus simple hydronephrosis. CT shows dilatation and obstruction of the collecting system, wall thickening of the renal pelvis, inflammatory changes in the parenchyma or perinephric space and high-attenuation values of the fluid within collecting system. Distinguishing simple hydronephrosis from pyonephrosis on the basis of fluid attenuation measurements may be difficult on CT and remains a diagnostic challenge [59].

11.3.4 Urolithiasis

Etiologies of urinary tract obstruction range from benign to malignant and from intrinsic to the urinary tract to extrinsic. Urolithiasis is the most common cause of ureteral obstruction and results from migration of renal calculi into the ureter in the vast majority of cases and will be discussed in more detail. Other etiologies of ureteral obstruction include intrinsic or extrinsic tumors, ischemia, trauma, adjacent Crohn's disease, infection, retrocaval ureter, ovarian vein syndrome, endometriosis, and retroperitoneal fibrosis. Retroperitoneal fibrosis is a progressive fibrotic process that can be idiopathic or caused by inflammatory aortic aneurysm, medications (hydralazine, ergot alkaloids) or retroperitoneal metastasis, abscess, or hematoma. On CT, retroperitoneal fibrosis appears as a confluent mass centered at the level of L4 vertebral body, with or without encasement of ureters [15,74,75].

It has been shown that nonenhanced CT has a high sensitivity (95%–98%) and specificity (96%–100%) in the diagnosis of urolithiasis. Evaluation of number, size, and location of calculi and presence of hydronephrosis are routinely performed on CT. Recent CT innovations has allowed for new applications such as quantification of stone burden, assessment of fragility, and differentiation between different types of stones. IV contrast

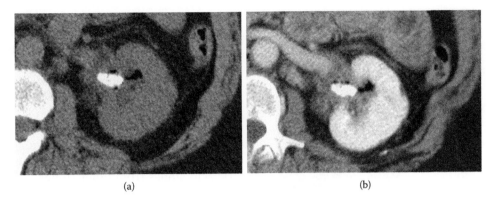

FIGURE 11.33
Nonenhanced (a) and nephrographic (b) phase axial CT images in a 55-year-old female show an ureteropelvic junction stone, periureteral inflammation, and presence of gas in the collecting system consistent with emphysematous pyelitis. Note the absence of parenchymal gas.

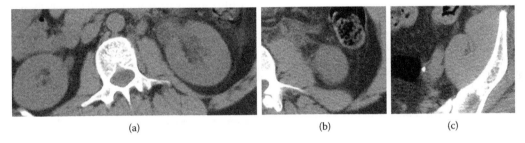

FIGURE 11.34
Nonenhanced phase axial CT images (a–c) in a 52-year-old male with acute left flank pain show hydronephrosis, hydroureter, perinephric fat stranding, periureteral edema, left-sided kidney enlargement with lower attenuation value, thickening of the lateroconal fascia and a stone within the left ureteral lumen.

material administration is not routinely required for the diagnosis of urolithiasis on CT. However, administration of contrast may be indicated for differentiation of distal ureteral stones from phleboliths and vascular calcifications or further evaluation of incidental findings. Because of the craniocaudal orientation of the collecting system, coronal reformation has been shown to be a useful adjunct to axial images in the evaluation of urolithiasis and improves detection of urinary stones that may remain unrecognized on axial images. Most stones have a greater attenuation value than the surrounding soft tissue (>200 HU) and may be radiolucent on conventional radiographs. All stones with an attenuation value of 200 HU or more are visible on nonenhanced CT. Stones with soft-tissue attenuation (15–30 HU) include pure matrix stones and stones made of indinavir, are difficult to visualize and are more likely to be missed on nonenhanced CT. Contrast-enhanced images in equivocal circumstances depicts stones as filling defects on delayed phase images. The most direct sign for ureterolithiasis on CT is depiction of stone within the ureteral lumen associated with ureteral dilatation proximal to obstruction and normal ureteral caliber distal to obstruction (Figure 11.34). It should be noted that ureteral dilatation may be absent in a minority of

cases. Nevertheless, the diagnosis of ureterolithiasis can be supported by the following secondary signs on CT: hydroureter, hydronephrosis, perinephric fat stranding or edema, periureteral edema, kidney enlargement with lower attenuation value on the affected side, and thickening of the LCF (Figure 11.34). The "soft-tissue rim sign" and "comet tail sign," have been shown to be useful in the differentiation of ureteral stones from extraluminal calcifications such as phleboliths. The soft-tissue rim sign represents the edematous ureteral wall around the calculus that manifests as a halo of soft-tissue attenuation around a calcific focus and is very specific for ureteral calculi (Figure 11.35). On the other hand, depiction of an eccentric, tapering soft-tissue area adjacent to the calcification is a reliable feature in the diagnosis of phleboliths and is referred to as the comet tail sign. Another helpful feature for differentiation is the presence of central lucent area seen in phleboliths as opposed to the opacified centers seen in calculi. Depiction of unilateral ureteral dilatation and perinephric stranding and failure to depict a stone on CT could be due to recent passage of stone or stones with insufficient size or attenuation. In the absence of ureteral dilatation or perinephric stranding, the likelihood of renal stone is very low [3,76,77].

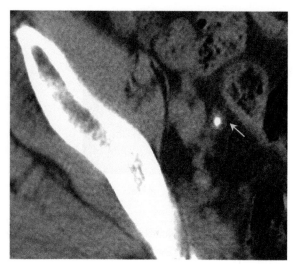

FIGURE 11.35

Magnified, nonenhanced phase axial CT image in a 54-year-old male with acute right flank pain shows a halo of soft-tissue attenuation around a calcific focus representing an edematous right ureteral wall around the calculus (arrow), which is referred to as "soft-tissue rim sign" and is highly specific for ureteral calculi.

Assessment of stone burden on CT is one of the most important aspects of radiological evaluation in patients with urolithiasis and commands treatment strategies and management options. Assessment of stone burden is usually performed by measurement of greatest dimension of the stone to the closest millimeter on CT. Bone window settings may be more accurate than soft-tissue window settings in quantification of stone diameter. Quantification of stone volume provides a more accurate assessment of stone burden but is not currently widely available [3,78].

Stone fragility can be assessed by evaluation of internal structure of a stone on CT. Evaluation of stone fragility may optimize selection of treatment modality. Internal structure of stones, best appreciated with thin-slice CT viewed with bone window settings, is classified as either homogeneous or heterogeneous. Although homogeneous stones have a uniform internal structure, heterogeneous stones contain areas with low-attenuation values. It has been shown that the irregularities in heterogeneous stones may serve as focal points for absorption of shock wave energy that results in stone disintegration and fragmentation. Conversely, homogeneous stones tend to be less susceptible to shock wave and often require more comminution and more extensive treatment [3,79–81].

Determination of stone composition on CT has been traditionally based on measurement of stone's attenuation values. The following attenuation values have been proposed for different types of urinary calculi: uric acid: (200–450) HU; struvite: (600–900) HU; cystine: (600–1100) HU; calcium phosphate: (1200–1600) HU;

and calcium oxalate: (1700–2800) HU. Unfortunately, in vivo differentiation between different types of stones is complicated and less reliable because of variation in size of stone and subsequent inconsistency in placement of the region of interest. More importantly, the majority of stones (up to 65%) have mixed composition and overlapping attenuation ranges, which further complicates differentiation of stone types based on attenuation values. As a result, quantification of CT attenuation values is most valuable in differentiating uric acid stones from other stones. It has been shown that dual-energy CT is a more robust method in determination of stone composition. Inherent variation in chemical composition of different stones allows characterization of different tissues and elements through dual-energy postprocessing algorithm. Dual-energy CT may allow differentiation of uric acid, cystine, struvite, and calcium oxalate stones. However, application of dual-energy CT in the evaluation of stone composition is still under investigation and is not widely available [3,79,82–87].

References

1. Vrtiska, T. J. et al. 2010. Genitourinary applications of dual-energy CT. *AJR Am J Roentgenol* 194(6):1434–42.
2. Grosjean, R. et al. 2008. Characterization of human renal stones with MDCT: advantage of dual energy and limitations due to respiratory motion. *AJR Am J Roentgenol* 190(3):720–8.
3. Kambadakone, A. R. et al. 2010. New and evolving concepts in the imaging and management of urolithiasis: urologists' perspective. *Radiographics* 30(3):603–23.
4. Kaza, R. K. et al. 2011. Distinguishing enhancing from nonenhancing renal lesions with fast kilovoltage-switching dual-energy CT. *AJR Am J Roentgenol* 197(6):1375–81.
5. Johnson, P. T., K. M. Horton, and E. K. Fishman. 2010. Optimizing detectability of renal pathology with MDCT: protocols, pearls, and pitfalls. *AJR Am J Roentgenol* 194(4):1001–12.
6. Yuh, B. I., and R. H. Cohan. 1999. Different phases of renal enhancement: role in detecting and characterizing renal masses during helical CT. *AJR Am J Roentgenol* 173(3):747–55.
7. Silverman, S. G., J. R. Leyendecker, and E. S. Amis, Jr. 2009. What is the current role of CT urography and MR urography in the evaluation of the urinary tract? *Radiology* 250(2):309–23.
8. Oliveira, G. H., and A. Schirger. 2003. Images in clinical medicine. Page kidney. *N Engl J Med* 348(2):129.
9. Silverman, S. G. et al. 2008. Management of the incidental renal mass. *Radiology* 249(1):16–31.
10. Bechtold, R. E. et al. 1996. The perirenal space: relationship of pathologic processes to normal retroperitoneal anatomy. *Radiographics* 16(4):841–54.

11. DeMeo, J. H., A. S. Fulcher, and R. F. Austin, Jr. 1995. Anatomic CT demonstration of the peritoneal spaces, ligaments, and mesenteries: normal and pathologic processes. *Radiographics* 15(4):755–70.

12. Lim, J. H., B. Kim, and Y. H. Auh. 1998. Anatomical communications of the perirenal space. *Br J Radiol* 71(844):450–6.

13. Surabhi, V. R. et al. 2008. Neoplastic and non-neoplastic proliferative disorders of the perirenal space: cross-sectional imaging findings. *Radiographics* 28(4):1005–17.

14. Rezai, P. et al. 2010. A best fit model for estimation of renal volume at MDCT. In *American Roentgen Ray Society (ARRS)*. San Diego.

15. Cannon, C. L. 2009. *McGraw-Hill Specialty Board Review Radiology*. New York, NY: McGraw-Hill.

16. Turkvatan, A., T. Olcer, and T. Cumhur 2009. Multidetector CT urography of renal fusion anomalies. *Diagn Interv Radiol* 15(2):127–34.

17. Tada, S. et al. 1983. The incidence of simple renal cyst by computed tomography. *Clin Radiol* 34(4):437–9.

18. Cohan, R. H. et al. 1995. Renal masses: assessment of corticomedullary-phase and nephrographic-phase CT scans. *Radiology* 196(2):445–51.

19. Sheth, S. et al. 2001. Current concepts in the diagnosis and management of renal cell carcinoma: role of multidetector CT and three-dimensional CT. *Radiographics* 21 Spec No:S237–54.

20. Zagoria, R. J. 2000. Imaging of small renal masses: a medical success story. *AJR Am J Roentgenol* 175(4):945–55.

21. Dyer, R., D. J. DiSantis, and B. L. McClennan. 2008. Simplified imaging approach for evaluation of the solid renal mass in adults. *Radiology* 247(2):331–43.

22. Bosniak, M. A. 1986. The current radiological approach to renal cysts. *Radiology* 158(1):1–10.

23. Israel, G. M., and M. A. Bosniak. 2005. How I do it: evaluating renal masses. *Radiology* 236(2):441–50.

24. Tappouni, R. et al. 2012. Pseudoenhancement of renal cysts: influence of lesion size, lesion location, slice thickness, and number of MDCT detectors. *AJR Am J Roentgenol* 198(1):133–7.

25. Bosniak, M. A. 1991. The small (less than or equal to 3.0 cm) renal parenchymal tumor: detection, diagnosis, and controversies. *Radiology* 179(2):307–17.

26. Bosniak, M. A. 1997. Diagnosis and management of patients with complicated cystic lesions of the kidney. *AJR Am J Roentgenol* 169(3):819–21.

27. Israel, G. M., and M. A. Bosniak. 2003. Follow-up CT of moderately complex cystic lesions of the kidney (Bosniak category IIF). *AJR Am J Roentgenol* 181(3):627–33.

28. Bosniak, M. A., and N. M. Rofsky. 1996. Problems in the detection and characterization of small renal masses. *Radiology* 198(3):638–41.

29. Bosniak, M. A. 2003. Should we biopsy complex cystic renal masses (Bosniak category III)? *AJR Am J Roentgenol* 181(5):1425–6; author reply 1426.

30. Cohen, H. T., and F. J. McGovern. 2005. Renal-cell carcinoma. *N Engl J Med* 353(23):2477–90.

31. Pickhardt, P. J. et al. 2000. From the archives of the AFIP. Infiltrative renal lesions: radiologic-pathologic correlation. Armed Forces Institute of Pathology. *Radiographics* 20(1):215–43.

32. Choyke, P. L. 2003. Imaging of hereditary renal cancer. *Radiol Clin North Am* 41(5):1037–51.

33. Leslie, J. A., T. Prihoda, and I. M. Thompson. 2003. Serendipitous renal cell carcinoma in the post-CT era: continued evidence in improved outcomes. *Urol Oncol* 21(1):39–44.

34. Hartman, D. S. et al. 1988. Infiltrative renal lesions: CT-sonographic-pathologic correlation. *AJR Am J Roentgenol* 150(5):1061–4.

35. Bostwick, D. G., and J. N. Eble. 1999. Diagnosis and classification of renal cell carcinoma. *Urol Clin North Am* 26(3):627–35.

36. Kim, J. K. et al. 2002. Differentiation of subtypes of renal cell carcinoma on helical CT scans. *AJR Am J Roentgenol* 178(6):1499–506.

37. Birnbaum, B. A., J. E. Jacobs, and P. Ramchandani. 1996. Multiphasic renal CT: comparison of renal mass enhancement during the corticomedullary and nephrographic phases. *Radiology* 200(3):753–8.

38. Macari, M., and M. A. Bosniak. 1999. Delayed CT to evaluate renal masses incidentally discovered at contrast-enhanced CT: demonstration of vascularity with deenhancement. *Radiology* 213(3):674–80.

39. Jung, S. C., J. Y. Cho, and S. H. Kim. 2012. Subtype differentiation of small renal cell carcinomas on three-phase MDCT: usefulness of the measurement of degree and heterogeneity of enhancement. *Acta Radiol* 53(1):112–8.

40. Paspulati, R. M., and S. Bhatt. 2006. Sonography in benign and malignant renal masses. *Radiol Clin North Am* 44(6):787–803.

41. Ruppert-Kohlmayr, A. J. et al. 2004. Differentiation of renal clear cell carcinoma and renal papillary carcinoma using quantitative CT enhancement parameters. *AJR Am J Roentgenol* 183(5):1387–91.

42. Ng, C. S. et al. 2008. Renal cell carcinoma: diagnosis, staging, and surveillance. *AJR Am J Roentgenol* 191(4):1220–32.

43. Wong-You-Cheong, J. J., B. J. Wagner, and C. J. Davis, Jr. 1998. Transitional cell carcinoma of the urinary tract: radiologic-pathologic correlation. *Radiographics* 18(1):123–42; quiz 148.

44. Urban, B. A. et al. 1997a. CT appearance of transitional cell carcinoma of the renal pelvis: Part 1. Early-stage disease. *AJR Am J Roentgenol* 169(1):157–61.

45. Urban, B. A. et al. 1997b. CT appearance of transitional cell carcinoma of the renal pelvis: Part 2. Advanced-stage disease. *AJR Am J Roentgenol* 169(1):163–8.

46. Browne, R. F. et al. 2005. Transitional cell carcinoma of the upper urinary tract: spectrum of imaging findings. *Radiographics* 25(6):1609–27.

47. Yousem, D. M. et al. 1988. Synchronous and metachronous transitional cell carcinoma of the urinary tract: prevalence, incidence, and radiographic detection. *Radiology* 167(3):613–8.

48. Bosniak, M. A. 1981. Angiomyolipoma (hamartoma) of the kidney: a preoperative diagnosis is possible in virtually every case. *Urol Radiol* 3(3):135–42.

49. Jinzaki, M. et al. 1997. Angiomyolipoma: imaging findings in lesions with minimal fat. *Radiology* 205(2):497–502.

50. Takahashi, K. et al. 1993. CT pixel mapping in the diagnosis of small angiomyolipomas of the kidneys. *J Comput Assist Tomogr* 17(1):98–101.

51. Oesterling, J. E. et al. 1986. The management of renal angiomyolipoma. *J Urol* 135(6):1121–4.

52. Rimon, U. et al. 2006. Ethanol and polyvinyl alcohol mixture for transcatheter embolization of renal angiomyolipoma. *AJR Am J Roentgenol* 187(3):762–8.

53. Logue, L. G., R. E. Acker, and A. E. Sienko. 2003. Best cases from the AFIP: angiomyolipomas in tuberous sclerosis. *Radiographics* 23(1):241–6.

54. Davidson, A. J. et al. 1993. Renal oncocytoma and carcinoma: failure of differentiation with CT. *Radiology* 186(3):693–6.

55. Davidson, A. J. et al. 1995. Renal medullary carcinoma associated with sickle cell trait: radiologic findings. *Radiology* 195(1):83–5.

56. Davis, C. J. Jr., F. K. Mostofi, and I. A. Sesterhenn. 1995. Renal medullary carcinoma. The seventh sickle cell nephropathy. *Am J Surg Pathol* 19(1):1–11.

57. Urban, B. A., and E. K. Fishman. 2000. Renal lymphoma: CT patterns with emphasis on helical CT. *Radiographics* 20(1):197–212.

58. Kawashima, A. et al. 1997. CT of renal inflammatory disease. *Radiographics* 17(4):851–66; discussion 867–8.

59. Craig, W. D., B. J. Wagner, and M. D. Travis. 2008. Pyelonephritis: radiologic-pathologic review. *Radiographics* 28(1):255–77; quiz 327–8.

60. Wan, Y. L. et al. 1996. Acute gas-producing bacterial renal infection: correlation between imaging findings and clinical outcome. *Radiology* 198(2):433–8.

61. Goldman, S. M. et al. 1984. CT of xanthogranulomatous pyelonephritis: radiologic-pathologic correlation. *AJR Am J Roentgenol* 142(5):963–9.

62. Hayes, W. S., D. S. Hartman, and I. A. Sesterbenn. 1991. From the archives of the AFIP. Xanthogranulomatous pyelonephritis. *Radiographics* 11(3):485–98.

63. Loffroy, R. et al. 2007. Xanthogranulomatous pyelonephritis in adults: clinical and radiological findings in diffuse and focal forms. *Clin Radiol* 62(9):884–90.

64. Kenney, P. J. 1990. Imaging of chronic renal infections. *AJR Am J Roentgenol* 155(3):485–94.

65. Muttarak, M., W. N. ChiangMai, and B. Lojanapiwat. 2005. Tuberculosis of the genitourinary tract: imaging features with pathological correlation. *Singapore Med J* 46(10):568–74; quiz 575.

66. Dobyan, D. C., L. D. Truong, and G. Eknoyan. 1993. Renal malacoplakia reappraised. *Am J Kidney Dis* 22(2):243–52.

67. Hartman, D. S. et al. 1980. Renal parenchymal malacoplakia. *Radiology* 136(1):33–42.

68. Raman, S. S. et al. 2007. Surgically relevant normal and variant renal parenchymal and vascular anatomy in preoperative 16-MDCT evaluation of potential laparoscopic renal donors. *AJR Am J Roentgenol* 188(1):105–14.

69. Caoili, E. M. et al. 2002. Urinary tract abnormalities: initial experience with multi-detector row CT urography. *Radiology* 222(2):353–60.

70. Joffe, S. A. et al. 2003. Multi-detector row CT urography in the evaluation of hematuria. *Radiographics* 23(6):1441–55; discussion 1455–6.

71. Kawashima, A. et al. 2004. CT urography. *Radiographics* 24 Suppl 1:S35–54; discussion S55–8.

72. Silverman, S. G. et al. 2006. Multi-detector row CT urography of normal urinary collecting system: furosemide versus saline as adjunct to contrast medium. *Radiology* 240(3):749–55.

73. Xu, A. D. et al. 2010. Significance of upper urinary tract urothelial thickening and filling defect seen on MDCT urography in patients with a history of urothelial neoplasms. *AJR Am J Roentgenol* 195(4):959–65.

74. Wasnik, A. P. et al. 2011. Multimodality imaging in ureteric and periureteric pathologic abnormalities. *AJR Am J Roentgenol* 197(6):W1083–92.

75. Moe, O. W. 2006. Kidney stones: pathophysiology and medical management. *Lancet* 367(9507):333–44.

76. Boulay, I. et al. 1999. Ureteral calculi: diagnostic efficacy of helical CT and implications for treatment of patients. *AJR Am J Roentgenol* 172(6):1485–90.

77. Smith, R. C. et al. 1996. Diagnosis of acute flank pain: value of unenhanced helical CT. *AJR Am J Roentgenol* 166(1):97–101.

78. Preminger, G. M. et al. 2007. 2007 Guideline for the management of ureteral calculi. *Eur Urol* 52(6):1610–31.

79. Kim, S. C. et al. 2007. Cystine calculi: correlation of CT-visible structure, CT number, and stone morphology with fragmentation by shock wave lithotripsy. *Urol Res* 35(6):319–24.

80. Williams, J. C., Jr. et al. 2002. High resolution detection of internal structure of renal calculi by helical computerized tomography. *J Urol* 167(1):322–6.

81. Zarse, C. A. et al. 2007. CT visible internal stone structure, but not Hounsfield unit value, of calcium oxalate monohydrate (COM) calculi predicts lithotripsy fragility in vitro. *Urol Res* 35(4):201–6.

82. Bellin, M. F. et al. 2004. Helical CT evaluation of the chemical composition of urinary tract calculi with a discriminant analysis of CT-attenuation values and density. *Eur Radiol* 14(11):2134–40.

83. Deveci, S. et al. 2004. Spiral computed tomography: role in determination of chemical compositions of pure and mixed urinary stones—an in vitro study. *Urology* 64(2):237–40.

84. Fletcher, J. G. et al. 2009. Dual-energy and dual-source CT: is there a role in the abdomen and pelvis? *Radiol Clin North Am* 47(1):41–57.

85. Johnson, T. R. et al. 2007. Material differentiation by dual energy CT: initial experience. *Eur Radiol* 17(6):1510–7.

86. Primak, A. N. et al. 2007. Noninvasive differentiation of uric acid versus non-uric acid kidney stones using dual-energy CT. *Acad Radiol* 14(12):1441–7.

87. Sheir, K. Z. et al. 2005. Determination of the chemical composition of urinary calculi by noncontrast spiral computerized tomography. *Urol Res* 33(2):99–104.

12

Bladder

Masahiro Jinzaki, Hirotaka Akita, and Eiji Kikuchi

CONTENTS

12.1 Introduction

Bladder disease consists of a wide spectrum of conditions including neoplasms, nonneoplastic masses and inflammatory change, similar to diseases of other organs. Although significant overlap in the clinical features and radiologic findings exists among bladder diseases, some have specific radiologic features that may dictate subsequent clinical management or that may change the treatment strategy.

Of the various modalities used to image the urinary bladder, ultrasonography and cystoscopy have been widely used mainly for the detection of bladder tumors, whereas computed tomography (CT) and magnetic resonance imaging (MRI) have been used for tumor staging. Both ultrasonography and cystoscopy have disadvantages such as operator dependence and invasiveness respectively. The introduction of multi-detector-row CT (MDCT) has enabled the easy acquisition of thin slice section images with any plane of the reformatted images. This advancement has helped CT to become a useful tool not only for staging, but also for detection [1–3]. MRI continues to possess superior soft-tissue contrast over CT and can further contribute to the evaluation of bladder disease.

12.2 Normal Anatomy

The urinary bladder is situated within an extraperitoneal structure behind the symphysis, with the peritoneum covering only the superior surface of the bladder dome. The space anterior to the bladder and behind the abdominal wall is called the retropubic space (space of Retzius). Posterior to the urinary bladder, the seminal vesicles or lower uterine segment lies within the perivesical space. At the apex, the dorsal and ventral walls meet and the urachus starts and runs to the umbilicus. Unlike the bladder neck which is fixed, the rest of the bladder moves relatively freely within the fat, thus, its shape and position changes, depending on the volume of urine that it contains. The trigone of the bladder, a trianglular region on the dorsal wall, is marked by the two ureteric orifices and the internal urethral orifice. Between the ureteric orifices is a muscular ridge, known as the interureteral ridge, which is produced by the intravesical extension of the longitudinal muscles of the ureters. This ridge is usually thickened and should not be mistaken for focal bladder thickening.

The bladder wall consists of four layers: (1) the urothelium that lines the bladder lumen, (2) the lamina propria (submucosa), (3) the muscularis propria, and (4) the outermost serosa. The urothelium is composed of three to seven layers of stratified flat cells. The lamina propria is very vascular, and its thickness varies with the degree of bladder. The muscular layer is the detrusor muscle that consists of three layers: an inner longitudinal, a middle circular, and an outer longitudinal. A loose layer of connective tissue forms the outermost serosa.

12.3 CT Scanning Protocol

During the era of helical CT, an oral contrast agent was routinely administered to opacify the gastrointestinal tract. With the introduction of MDCT, thin slice section images or reformatted images has simplified the identification of the bowel and other organs, making contrast opacification of the gastrointestinal tract not as essential as it was previously, although it remains useful for the evaluation of enterovesical fistula. For MDCT, only the

oral intake of water at least 10–15 minutes before scanning is recommended to keep the bladder distended.

For pelvis imaging, the most widely used protocol is a single-phase injection of 100mL of 300–350 mgI/mL administered at a rate of 2 mL/s or less following a 90–120-second delay. This protocol is adequate in most cases. For further refinement targeting the urinary bladder, early enhanced image acquisition is recommended, consisting of a single-phase injection of 100mL of 300–350 mgI/mL administered at a rate of 3 mL/s or higher following a 60–70-second delay [1–3]. Bladder cancer is best enhanced using this timing. Further delay causes the decreased enhancement of the bladder cancer and also causes the contrast material to fill the bladder. A typical examination of the pelvis usually also includes an abdominal study. In abdominal studies, this timing corresponds to the portal phase of the liver.

For four-detector systems, a 2.5 mm slice thickness reconstructed at 5–7 mm intervals and a pitch of 0.75–1.5 is used [1,2]. A 2.5 mm thickness and 50% overlap reconstruction is recommended. For 16-row detector CT or higher, 1–1.25 mm or smaller collimation and reconstruction at 1–1.25 mm or less is recommended to improve the detection rate as well as to improve the quality of the reformatted image [3]. A gantry rotation speed of 0.5–0.8 seconds is used. The use of some sort of dose modulation system that varies the mA per slice is optimal. Sagittal and coronal reformats can be easily performed and are useful for anatomic delineation.

In selected cases, additional excretory-phase CT images obtained after a delay of approximately 7–10 minutes may be useful for outlining bladder tumors or upper urinary tract tumors [4–7]. Thus, when including surveillance for synchronic multifocal upper urinary tract tumors in patients with bladder cancer, one recommendation is to take the first image of the bladder after a 60–70-second delay, then to obtain a nephrographic phase image of the kidney after a 90–100-second delay, followed by excretory-phase images. When reading excretory-phase images, a wider window and a higher level should be selected.

12.4 Bladder Neoplasms

Bladder neoplasms can arise from any of the bladder layers. Such neoplasms are broadly classified as either epithelial that account for approximately 95% of all bladder neoplasms, or nonepithelial (mesenchymal) that account for 5% [8]. Most bladder neoplasms are malignant, and only approximately 1% of all bladder neoplasms are benign.

12.4.1 Bladder Cancer

Urothelial malignancy may arise from any part of the urinary tract but occurs in the bladder in more than 90% of cases. Bladder cancer is a malignancy that is relatively common in the elderly. The median age of diagnosis is around 70 years. It is also more common in men, with a male to female ratio of 3:1 [9]. Histologically, 90% of all bladder cancers are urothelial carcinoma (UC), 5% are squamous cell carcinoma (SCC), and less than 2% are adenocarcinoma or other variants [10]. The most common form of presentation (~80% of cases) is hematuria that is typically painless, intermittent, and gross. The prognosis depends on the pathologic stage, which is most often determined using the TNM system [11] (Figure 12.1 and Table 12.1). The cellular grading of bladder cancer is also a predictor of prognosis and usually correlate well with the staging. Lymphatic spread occurs to the regional lymph nodes in the perivesical, sacral, presacral, hypogastric, obturator, external, and internal iliac groups and the common iliac chain [12]. Spread to the paraaortic lymph nodes is considered distant metastasis. Hematogenous metastasis most commonly occurs to the lung, bones, liver, and adrenal glands [13]. Direct extension into the prostatic urethra, seminal vesicle, or vagina can also occur.

12.4.1.1 Urothelial Carcinoma

UC is characterized by multifocality with synchronous and metachronous lesions in the bladder and upper tract [8]. Multicentric bladder lesions occur in up to 30%–40% of cases. Upper tract lesions occur in 2%–4% of UC cases and are seen most frequently when multiple bladder lesions are present [14]. Approximately 75%–85% of UC may present as a nonmuscle invasive tumor (Ta, T1, or carcinoma in situ), and approximately 20% is muscle invasive tumors extending into the detrusor muscle or deeper (T2≤) or metastatic malignancy [15]. In nonmuscle invasive tumors, treatment by cystoscopic resection with or without intravesical immunotherapy or chemotherapy have a good prognosis. However, tumor recurrence rate is high and occurs even after a 5-year tumor-free period, suggesting the need for longer follow-up [16]. Nonmetastatic muscle invasive bladder tumors are treated aggressively with radical cystectomy and lymph node dissection. However, approximately 30% of patients eventually develop local or distant recurrences, most appearing within 1 year [17]. Metastatic UC are treated with current cisplatin-based combination chemotherapy, and progressive disease after frontline chemotherapy is characterized by a short survival [18].

With CT imaging, UC may be detected either as focal masses or asymmetric wall thickening (Figures 12.2 and 12.3). In rare cases, bladder cancers may produce

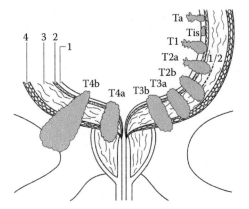

1. Mucosa, 2. Submucosa, 3. Muscle, 4. Perivesical fat

FIGURE 12.1
TNM classification.

TABLE 12.1

TNM Staging of Bladder Cancer

Primary Tumor (T)

Tx Primary tumor cannot be assessed.

T0 No evidence of primary tumor.

Ta Noninvasive papillary carcinoma.

Tis Carcinoma in situ: "flat tumor."

T1 Tumor invades subepithelial connective tissue.

T2 Tumor invades muscularis propria.

T2a Tumor invades superficial muscularis propria (inner half).

T2b Tumor invades deep muscularis propria (outer half).

T3 Tumor invades perivesical tissue.

T3a Microscopically.

T3b Macroscopically (extravesical mass).

T4 Tumor invades any of the following: prostatic stroma, seminal vesicles, uterus, vagina, pelvic wall, and abdominal wall.

T4a Tumor invades prostatic stroma, uterus, and vagina.

T4b Tumor invades pelvic wall, and abdominal wall.

Regional Lymph Nodes (N)

NX Lymph nodes cannot be assessed.

N0 No lymph node metastasis.

N1 Single regional lymph node metastasis in the true pelvis (hypogastric, obturator, external iliac, or presacral lymph node).

N2 Multiple regional lymph node metastases in the true pelvis (hypogastric, obturator, external iliac, or presacral lymph node).

N3 Lymph node metastases to the common iliac lymph nodes.

*Regional lymph nodes include both primary and secondary drainage regions. All other nodes above the aortic bifurcation are considered distant lymph nodes.

Distant Metastasis (M)

M0 No distant metastasis

M1 Distant metastases

diffuse symmetric bladder wall thickening. Intraluminal tumors may occasionally show fine calcifications (Figure 12.4). To evaluate bladder tumors, a cystoscopy or ultrasonography is typically performed as the initial examination. The main advantage of conventional CT over cystoscopy or ultrasonography is the better definition of perivesical invasion and lymph node involvement or distant metastases. Macroscopic extravesical

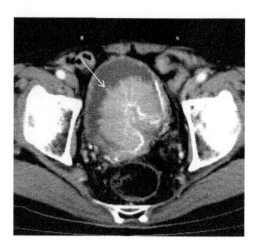

FIGURE 12.2
Urothelial carcinoma. Axial enhanced CT image shows a large, lobular mass (arrows) within the bladder.

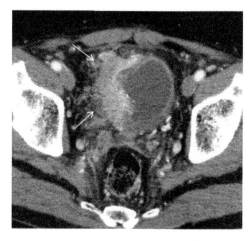

FIGURE 12.3
Urothelial carcinoma. Axial enhanced CT image of the bladder shows an enhancing area of asymmetric wall thickening (arrows).

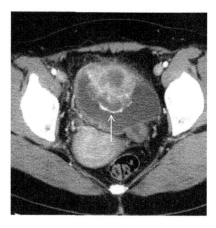

FIGURE 12.4
Urothelial carcinoma with calcification. Axial enhanced CT image of the bladder shows a large mass with peripheral calcification (arrow) that represents urothelial carcinoma with sarcomatoid change.

extension (T3b) is seen on CT as an irregular, ill-defined, outer bladder wall and by the presence of soft-tissue nodules or fat stranding in the surrounding perivesical fat (Figure 12.5). The diagnostic accuracy for perivesical invasion is reportedly 83%; however, since it cannot discriminate the extent of invasion into the muscular wall of the bladder, the overall accuracy of conventional CT for the staging of bladder cancer has been as low as 55% [19,20]. In comparison, MRI has a higher accuracy of 93% for the diagnosis of perivesical invasion and is also superior at detecting muscle invasion [19]. Thus, in terms of the tumor penetration of the bladder wall, MRI provides more reliable information than conventional CT. Lymph node metastases are mainly assessed by size: lymph nodes with a short axis greater than 1 cm in size are considered suspicious [21] (Figure 12.6). However, the presence of enlarged lymph nodes does not always indicate metastasis and may instead represent reactive alterations. Thus, the reported diagnostic

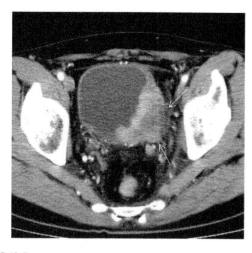

FIGURE 12.5
Urothelial carcinoma with perivesical invasion. Axial enhanced CT image of the bladder shows a large urothelial carcinoma with irregular soft-tissue stranding (arrows) from tumor invasion into the perivesical fat.

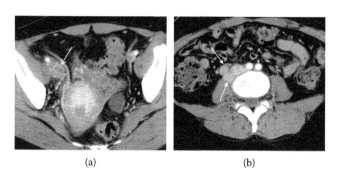

(a)   (b)

FIGURE 12.6
Lymph node metastases. Axial enhanced CT image shows LN metastases in right external iliac groups (a: arrow) and right common iliac lymph nodes (b: arrows).

accuracy for LN staging is equally low for CT and MRI and is reported to be 5% and 60%, respectively [22,23]. With the introduction of MDCT, the acquisition of thinner slice images has paved the way to increasing the role of CT in detection and also has helped overcome limitations of conventional CT in the diagnostic accuracy for detecting perivesical fat invasion. Furthermore, MDCT urography has been found to be superior to excretory urography for the evaluation of upper urinary tract lesions [6,7].

Thin-section, early enhanced CT and thin-section, excretory-phase CT have increased the detection rate for bladder cancers. When obtaining early enhanced images at 60–80 seconds after contrast injection, most bladder cancers show an early enhancement that is more pronounced than that of the normal bladder wall [2]. As a result, bladder cancers can be nicely outlined by the surrounding unenhanced urine. Thin-section, early enhanced CT with multiplanar reformation (MPR) detects 89%–97% of all bladder cancers [1–3] (Figure 12.7). Reviewing the bladder in at least two planes (usually axial and coronal) helps detect small bladder lesions that were not seen in a single orientation [1] (Figure 12.8). Also, MPR further enhances the role of CT in detecting bladder lesions located at the bladder base (near the prostate and urethra) are often difficult to detect and can be difficult to distinguish from prostatic enlargement or periurethral tissue (Figure 12.9). For this approach to be successful, adequate bladder distention must be ensured. This can be accomplished by asking the patient not to void his or her bladder for at least an hour before imaging [1]. Thin-section, excretory-phase CT also has relatively high sensitivities in the range of 79%–89.7%. Thus, if CT shows a definite bladder lesion, a flexible cystoscopy can be omitted and the patient can proceed directly to a rigid cystoscopy, biopsy, and transurethral resection [24,25]. However, neither early enhanced nor excretory-phase images have a sufficient sensitivity to allow this modality to replace flexible cystoscopy in a diagnostic pathway. Even with MDCT, various possible causes of false-negative or false-positive diagnoses of bladder cancer exist. Some small lesions ≤5 mm in diameter can be missed, especially since overdistension of the bladder can flatten some lesions. Also, the bladder wall is often asymmetrically thickened in patients who have undergone transurethral resections or intravesical immunotherapy or chemotherapy (Figure 12.10) [26]. Furthermore, some inflamed posttreatment bladders show areas of abnormal enhancement that mimic tumor hyperenhancement; such appearances not only result in false-positive diagnoses, but also make any cancers that may be present more difficult to detect.

MDCT has also improved the diagnosis of perivesical invasion: from 83% using conventional CT to 93%

using thin-section, early enhanced CT [2]. This accuracy is almost equal to that of MRI. Perivesical invasion is the most critical factor among the degrees of tumor penetration of the bladder wall for deciding the management strategy. Thus, in most cases, MDCT alone may be sufficient for the diagnosis of tumor staging. The false diagnosis of perivesical invasion is caused by false-negative findings arising from microscopic fat invasion

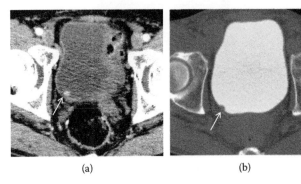

(a)   (b)

FIGURE 12.7
Small urothelial carcinoma. (a) Early enhanced axial CT image shows a small enhancing mass (arrow) within the bladder. (b) Excretory-phase axial CT image shows the masses as a small filling defect (arrow) within the bladder.

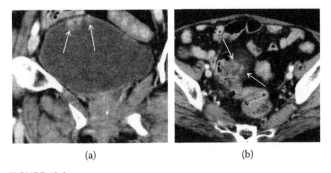

(a)   (b)

FIGURE 12.8
Small urothelial carcinoma located in the dome of the bladder. (a) Oblique coronal enhanced CT image shows small masses (arrows) in the bladder dome. (b) These tumors (arrows) are difficult to detect on axial image.

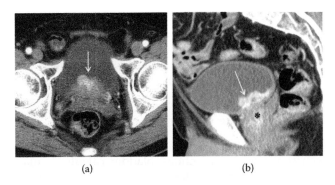

(a)   (b)

FIGURE 12.9
Urothelial carcinoma located at the bladder base. (a) Axial enhanced CT image shows enhanced lesion (arrow) in part of enlarged prostate gland. (b) Sagittal enhanced CT image clearly shows that the lesion (arrow) is separate from prostate gland (*).

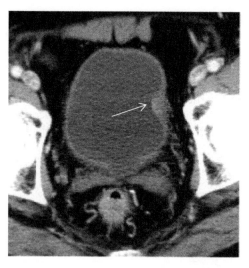

FIGURE 12.10
Bladder wall asymmetrically thickened in patients with a history of transurethral resection. Axial enhanced CT image shows focal wall thickening (arrow) in the left side wall of the bladder. Histological examination showed only focal inflammation and fibrosis.

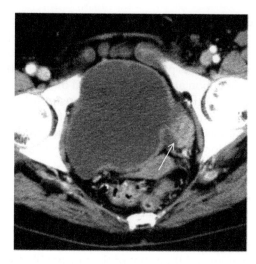

FIGURE 12.11
Bladder cancer in bladder diverticulum. Axial enhanced CT image shows a large left-sided diverticulum with an enhancing mass (arrow).

or false-positive findings arising from perivesical soft-tissue stranding as a result of edema or inflammation caused by factors such as posttransurethral resection performed within a week before the CT examination [2]. Regarding the differentiation of nonmuscle-invasive bladder cancer from muscle-invasive bladder cancer, MRI is still superior to MDCT.

Excretory urography has been used in patients with suspected bladder cancer for its ability to show small upper urinary tract lesions. Recently, excretory-phase CT images have begun to replace excretory urography for the evaluation of the upper urinary tract because of their superiority for the detection and localization of upper urinary tract cancers [6,7].

CT is valuable for detecting bladder cancers originating in the bladder diverticulum (Figure 12.11), especially when the lesions are inaccessible by cystoscopy. Although these patients often develop SCCs, most of these lesions are UCs. The prognosis of bladder cancers originating in the diverticulum is poorer than those of cancers originating elsewhere in the lumen of the bladder because of the difficulty in their diagnosis and the occurrence of early invasion because of the lack of a muscular layer in the diverticulum.

12.4.1.2 Squamous Cell Carcinoma

Patients with SCC usually have a history of chronic or recurrent bladder infections, bladder calculi, or bladder diverticula or schistomisasis. Even in the absence of distant metastasis, the prognosis of SCC remains dismal because of high rate of locoregional recurrence [27]. Aggressive local treatment with radical cystectomy is the treatment of choice. Unfortunately, SCC is a

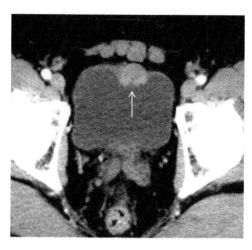

FIGURE 12.12
Squamous cell carcinoma. Axial enhanced CT image of the bladder shows focal wall thickening (arrow) protruding into the perivesical fat. The tumor showed microscopic fat invasion on pathological specimen.

chemo-resistant tumor, and currently no chemotherapy regimen has yet been found.

Upon CT examination, the imaging findings show either focal or diffuse bladder wall thickening or a single bulky enhancing mass, and the lesions are typically sessile, rather than papillary (Figure 12.12) [28,29]. These findings are nonspecific and difficult to differentiate from other bladder neoplasms. SCC originating from the diverticulum is sometimes accompanied by surface calcification [30].

12.4.1.3 Adenocarcinoma

Adenocarcinoma is classically associated with bladder exstrophy, persistent urachus, and a malignant transformation in patients with cystitis glandularis. It can be classified as primary adenocarcinoma, urachal carcinoma (urachal carcinoma is described in the following section of this chapter), or secondary (metastatic) adenocarcinoma. The mean age at the time of presentation for primary adenocarcinoma is 60 years, with urachal cancer occurring approximately 10 years earlier. Primary adenocarcinoma is three times more predominant in men. The histological subtype of primary adenocarcinoma includes enteric, mucinous, and signet ring cell types, etc., among which the signet ring cell type is associated with the worst prognosis [31]. Adenocarcinoma is virtually always invasive and the prognosis is poor with a 5-year survival rates range from 0% to 31% [32]. Primary adenocarcinoma is poorly responsive to radiation and chemotherapy, and thus, patients should be treated with radical cystectomy. Metastatic adenocarcinoma to the bladder is more common than primary adenocarcinoma. Distinguishing primary disease from metastases on imaging findings is important because of the different treatment options.

Tumors may be exophytic, papillary, sessile, ulcerating, or infiltrating. According to one study evaluating primary nonurachal adenocarcinoma, diffuse bladder wall thickening visible upon CT examination was seen in three-fourths of the patients (mean thickness, 1.8 cm), and most patients had perivesical fat stranding [33]. Lymphadenopathy and the direct invasion of the rectus muscle are seen in one-fourth of all patients. A propensity to peritoneal metastases has also been noted.

12.4.2 Urachal Carcinoma

The urachus is a midline musculofibrous band that extends from the umbilicus to the anterior dome of the bladder. The normal urachus is most commonly lined by transitional epithelium. Urachal carcinomas represent less than 0.5% of all bladder cancers [34]. Urachal adenocarcinoma occurs equally often in men and women and predominantly manifests as adenocarcinoma, of which 75% are mucin-producing adenocarcinoma and 15% are non-mucin-producing adenocarcinoma. This situation is probably due to the metaplasia of the urachal mucosa into columnar epithelium followed by malignant transformation. Urachal adenocarcinoma may be associated with cystitis cystica and cystitis glandularis. The remaining 10% of urachal carcinomas are classified as urothelium, squamous cell, or anaplastic cell types [35]. While the majority, or approximately 90%, of urachal carcinomas arise in the juxtavesical portion of the urachus, a few arise in the middle of the urachus (6% of cases) or near the umbilical end (4%) [35].

Urachal carcinoma is diagnosed when patients present with an enteric-type adenocarcinoma of the bladder, at the bladder dome or elsewhere in the midline as having an urachal tumor unless proven otherwise [36].

Because the tumor growth occurs in an area that is relatively silent clinically, patients with urachal carcinoma generally present late in the disease course. At the time of the initial diagnosis of the primary lesion, 64% of all patients have pathologically proven local perivesical fat invasion, and distant metastases are present in approximately 30% of all patients [37]. Thus, the prognosis of patients with urachal carcinoma is poor, and the 5-year survival rate is 6.5%–15% [38]. In the absence of metastatic disease, surgically resectable tumors are treated with either total or partial cystectomy with en bloc resection of the urachal ligament and umbilicus. The roles of chemotherapy and radiotherapy are unclear, although some reports showed that chemotherapy had a potential to induce an objective response in some case [39,40].

The CT demonstration of a midline mass with calcification above or anterior to the bladder is highly suspicious of urachal carcinoma. A component with low-attenuation, reflecting the mucin content, is seen in the majority of cases, while a minority of lesions (16%) are purely solid (Figures 12.13 and 12.14) [37,41]. Calcification occurs in 50%–72% of cases and may be punctate, stippled, or curvilinear and peripheral [37,41–43]. Since this tumor has a tendency to involve the bladder wall and to grow in the perivesical space toward the umbilicus, the multiplanar images obtained using MDCT are more useful for clarifying the location and the extension of the tumor than conventional CT [44]. A discrete spiculation or fat stranding is suggestive of tumor infiltration [41]. However, CT is not accurate for identifying the microscopic invasion of extravesical fat tissue. Metastases occur initially in the pelvic lymph nodes, followed by systemic metastases to the lung, brain, liver, and bone.

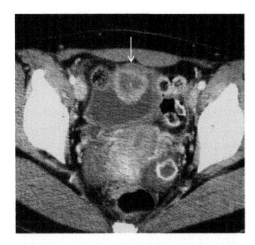

FIGURE 12.13
Urachal carcinoma with low-attenuation component. Axial enhanced CT image shows a midline enhancing mass (arrow) with central low attenuation and a punctuate calcification in the anterior aspect of the bladder.

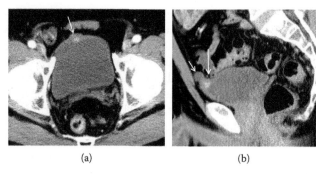

                    (a)   (b)

FIGURE 12.14
Urachal carcinoma. (a) Axial enhanced CT image shows a midline solid enhancing mass (arrow) contiguous with the anterior aspect of the bladder. (b) Sagittal enhanced CT image shows the tumor (long arrow) located near the small, anterosuperior outpouching (short arrow) representing a urachal diverticulum.

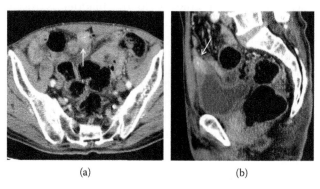

                    (a)   (b)

FIGURE 12.15
Infectious urachal remnant. (a) Axial enhanced CT image shows an enhancing mass (arrow) with puncture calcification just beneath the abdominal wall in the midline. (b) Sagittal enhanced CT image clearly shows the mass (arrow) is extending toward the umbilicus.

The differentiation of juxtavesical urachal carcinomas and primary tumors of the bladder dome can be difficult; however, unlike vesical tumors, urachal tumors are judged based on the location of an extravesical component of the lesion. Furthermore, infected urachal remnants are often difficult to distinguish from urachal carcinoma (Figure 12.15). Many cases of infection exhibit inflammatory spread to the adjacent fat tissue, mimicking invasive urachal carcinoma. The presence of hematuria, mural nodularity, and calcification on CT images is more suggestive of carcinoma than of infected urachal remnants [45,46].

12.4.3 Mesenchymal Tumors

The most common mesenchymal tumor of the bladder is leiomyoma [31]. Leiomyosarcoma is the most common malignant mesenchymal bladder tumor in adults. Rhabdomyosarcoma is the most common bladder tumor in patients under the age of 10 years. Other mesenchymal tumors include paraganglioma, lymphoma, hemangioma, neurofibroma, granular cell tumors,

angiosarcoma, osteosarcoma and malignant fibrous histiocytoma.

12.4.3.1 Leiomyosarcoma

Leiomyosarcoma arises from bladder smooth muscle. An increased prevalence is seen after pelvic radiation therapy or prior systemic cyclophosphamide chemotherapy. The age range is relatively wide at 25–88 years with a male to female ratio of 2–3:1 [31,47]. Urinary bladder leiomyosarcomas have always been considered highly aggressive tumors that require aggressive surgical extirpation, and a radical cystectomy with wide margins should be performed whenever possible.

Leiomyosarcoma tends to be present as an irregular, ulcerating mural mass with a mean size of 7 cm [31,47]. It can be difficult to distinguish leiomyoma from leiomyosarcoma based on imaging alone. However, necrosis is common in leiomyosarcomas, which tend to be poorly circumscribed invasive masses.

12.4.3.2 Rhabdomyosarcoma

Rhabdomyosarcoma is a sarcoma that recapitulates the morphologic and molecular features of skeletal muscle. It is rarely seen in adults and is most commonly observed in children, with a mean patient age of 4 years, affecting boys more than girls at a ratio of 3:1 [8]. Almost all bladder rhabdomyosarcomas are of embryonal subtype, and the genetically distinct alveolar subtype is extremely rare in the bladder [31]. In adults, rhabdomyosarcomas are usually the pleomorphic subtype. Over the last 40 years, the management of patients with rhabdomyosarcoma has changed radically from surgical resection to chemotherapy [48].

CT typically shows large, nodular masses [49]. The growth pattern for embryonal rhabdomyosarcoma is classified into two groups: polypoid type, involving mostly intraluminal tumors and associated with a favorable prognosis; and invasive type, involving the entire bladder wall and usually adjacent organs and associated with a poor prognosis [31]. The botryoid subtype is found at the end of the spectrum of polypoid types and has a lobulated appearance resembling a cluster of grapes.

12.4.3.3 Leiomyoma

Leiomyomas are noninfiltrative smooth muscle tumors arising in the submucosa, but their growth may be submucosal (7%), intravesical (63%), or extravesical (30%) [50]. Most are small with a mean size of less than 2 cm [8], asymptomatic, and discovered incidentally. Leiomyomas are considered to occur equally in men and women with a wide age range of 22–78 years [47].

However, some studies have reported a preponderance in women [51,52]. Leiomyomas are benign tumors without malignant potential. Thus, local excision is the treatment of choice. A preoperative suspicion of a leiomyoma is important for preventing unnecessary radical surgery. Previous reports have suggested that asymptomatic patients with a high probability of leiomyoma based on imaging, biopsy, and cystoscopy evaluations can be followed up without invasive surgery [53,54]. However, partial surgical resection is currently the standard procedure for confirming the diagnosis and for definitive treatment.

CT features include either a smooth, homogeneous mass protruding into the bladder lumen (intravesical type) or an extrinsic mass (extravesical type) [55] (Figure 12.16). Degenerated leiomyomas have more heterogeneous signal characteristics. Leiomyoma can be difficult to distinguish from leiomyosarcoma in larger, extravesical types. Although few studies have evaluated the enhancement pattern on CT images, one study reported that the tumors show a variable pattern of enhancement on MRI findings, with some enhancing homogeneously and others showing little enhancement [56]. Typically, leiomyomas exhibit a low-signal intensity on T2-weighted images [57]; thus, in this regard, MR imaging is superior to CT for characterization and demonstrating the submucosal origin and muscular preservation [58].

12.4.3.4 Paraganglioma

Paraganglioma arises in the chromaffin cells of the sympathetic chain in the detrusor muscle layer. It can occur anywhere in the bladder, but is typically found near the trigone. The age range at the time of onset is relatively wide at 10–78 years, and a female preponderance has been observed [8]. A characteristic clinical syndrome consisting of palpitations, sweating, headache, and syncope with hypertension during micturition, occurs in 50% of patients [58]. Hematuria is common. Nonfunctioning pheochromocytomas have also been reported. Most lesions are sporadic; however, they can also be associated with familial syndromes, including neurofibromatosis, von Hippel-Lindau syndrome, Sturge-Weber syndrome, tuberous sclerosis, and multiple endocrine neoplasia [59]. Treatment involves local excision under adrenergic blockade. Long-term follow-up is necessary, because the histology is not predictive of malignancy.

Bladder paraganglioma is usually a solid, homogeneous, lobulated, well-marginated mass (Figure 12.17). An intramural or submucosal location and marked enhancement after contrast administration are key characteristics [56]. Ring calcification around the circumference of the mass is highly suggestive of a bladder paraganglioma [60]. Occasionally, cystic areas can occur

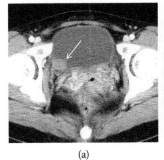 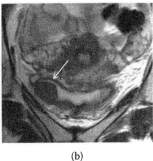

(a)　　　　　　　　　　　　(b)

FIGURE 12.16
Leiomyoma. (a) Axial enhanced CT image shows a well-marginated intramural mass (arrow) within the right posterior side of the bladder. b) Coronal T2-weighted MR image shows the intramural low-intensity mass (arrow).

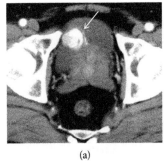 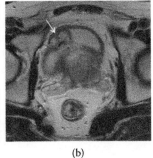

(a)　　　　　　　　　　　　(b)

FIGURE 12.17
Paraganglioma. (a) Axial enhanced CT image of the bladder shows a well-marginated marked enhancing mass (arrow). (b) Axial T2-weighted MR image shows the intramural high-intensity mass (arrow).

as a result of necrosis or hemorrhage. Bladder paraganglioma is also characterized by a high-signal intensity on T2-weighted images [59]. MR imaging also has an advantage over CT for demonstrating the submucosal origin of the tumor.

12.4.3.5 Lymphoma

Primary bladder lymphoma is rare, as there is no lymphoid tissue in the bladder, but secondary involvement of the bladder may be present in 10%–25% of patients with lymphoma and leukemia [61]. Most lesions are low-grade MALT lymphoma [31] and have a good prognosis. High-grade primary lymphomas are less common, constituting approximately 20% of all cases, and are mostly diffuse large B-cell type [62]. If a pathological examination reveals high-grade lymphoma of the bladder, the possibility of systemic lymphoma should be excluded. Treatment may consist of chemotherapy, local radiation therapy, or surgery, or a various combinations of these therapies.

CT findings are nonspecific but may consist of a mural-based nodular mass, usually in the region of the bladder base (Figure 12.18). The tumors may result in solitary (70%), multiple (20%), or diffuse wall thickening (10%) of the bladder wall [31]. One study reported a large homogeneously enhanced solitary mass with no paravesical fat infiltration [63]. Although the radiological findings for bladder lymphoma and the more common UC cannot be differentiated, the presence of a large mass without extravesical spreading should raise the possibility of lymphoma or rhabdomyosarcoma, and the mass should not be assumed to be a UC [63].

12.4.4 Secondary Bladder Tumors

Secondary bladder tumors or metastases to the bladder are rare, constituting only approximately 1% of all malignant bladder lesions. The most common secondary tumor is melanoma, followed by metastases from the stomach, colon, pancreas, and ovary. Direct invasion by tumors in the adjacent pelvic organs, such as prostate, sigmoid, and cervical cancers, is more common than hematogenous metastases.

Radiographically, secondary bladder tumors are seen as one or more mural masses projecting into bladder

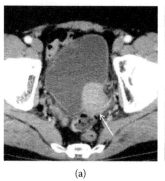 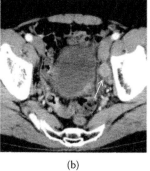

| (a) | (b) |

FIGURE 12.18
Lymphoma. (a) Axial enhanced CT image of the bladder shows a large homogeneously enhancing solitary mass (arrow) in the posterolateral bladder wall on the left. (b) Lymph node involvement is also seen (arrow).

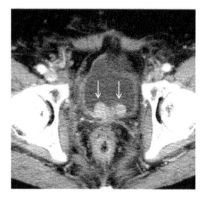

FIGURE 12.19
Metastases to the bladder in a patient with history of prostate carcinoma. Axial enhanced CT image shows multiple masses (arrows) protruding into the bladder lumen on the bladder trigone.

lumen (Figure 12.19). One study reported that secondary bladder tumors were almost always solitary, and 54% were located in the bladder neck or trigone [64].

12.5 Nonneoplastic Bladder Masses

Most bladder masses are neoplastic, but other masses with nonneoplastic origins can develop secondary to infiltrative diseases, such as endometriosis and proliferative diseases. The clinical and radiologic findings for nonneoplastic masses may overlap with those for bladder neoplasms; thus, histologic evaluations are necessary.

12.5.1 Endometriosis

Although the urinary tract is not usually involved in patients with endometriosis, the bladder is the most frequently affected site [65,66]. Bladder endometriosis affects premenopausal women and occurs in about 6% of patients with endometriosis [8]. Bladder endometriosis can occur spontaneously after the direct implantation of endometrium, typically at the vesicouterine pouch, or following pelvic surgery. Often, these masses penetrate the muscle into the submucosa, producing an obtuse bulge (mural mass) into the bladder lumen. Less frequently, endometriosis can grow through the mucosa and produce a polypoid mass [67]. Cyclic hematuria is highly suggestive of bladder endometriosis, but it occurs in only 20% of cases [66]. The treatment for symptomatic bladder endometriosis consists of a partial cystectomy.

The main CT feature of endometriotic bladder masses is localized bladder wall thickening with occasional protrusion inside the bladder lumen, mimicking bladder cancer. The CT findings can be nonspecific; thus, the location of the lesions is helpful in diagnosing this disease [68] (Figure 12.20). The masses are usually located anterior to the vesicouterine pouch and can come in contact with an adenomyotic nodule of the anterior aspect of the uterus [69]. MRI, on the other hand, has specific findings, showing a lesion with a heterogeneous T2-lowintense irregular marginated wall thickness and occasional T1 hyperintense spots.

12.5.2 Inflammatory Pseudotumor (Myofibroblastic Tumor)

An inflammatory pseudotumor is a nonneoplastic proliferation of myofibroblastic spindle cells and inflammatory cells with myxoid components. The bladder is a common site of inflammatory pseudotumor in the genitourinary tract. It can occur at any age but typically appears in

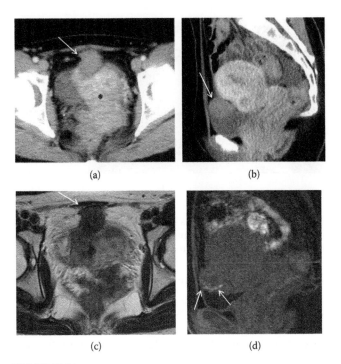

(a)　　　　(b)

(c)　　　　(d)

FIGURE 12.20
Endometoriosis. (a) Axial enhanced CT image shows localized lesion (arrow) in the anterior aspect of the bladder wall. * = uterus (b) Sagittal enhanced CT image shows protrusion (arrow) inside the bladder lumen. (c) Axial T2-weighted MR image shows the lesion (arrow) is predominantly low-signal intensity. (d) Fat-suppressed T1-weighted MR images show hemorrhagic foci with high-signal intensity within a soft-tissue mass (arrows).

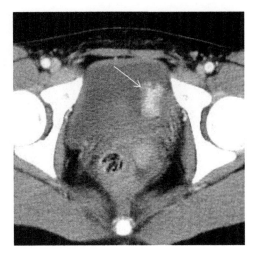

FIGURE 12.21
Inflammatory pseudotumor. Axial enhanced CT image shows an enhancing intraluminal mass without extension into the perivesical fat (arrow).

young adults, with an average age of onset of 28 years. It is two times more common in women than in men [70]. This disease has come to be known by several different names, such as inflammatory myofibroblastic tumor, plasma cell granuloma or pseudotumor, xanthomatous pseudo tumor, pseudosarcomatous myofibroblastic proliferation, inflammatory myofibroblastic proliferation, and myofibroblastoma. Inflammatory pseudotumor of the urinary tract mimics malignant tumors and can potentially be misdiagnosed as rhabdomyosarcoma. The preoperative recognition of this benign lesion using an imaging-guided biopsy is critical to avoid unnecessary surgery.

On CT images, inflammatory pseudotumor usually appears as a polypoid intraluminal mass or a submucosal mass with or without extension into the perivesical fat [71]. Intramural solid and cystic variants may also occur. A pattern of ring-like enhancement is often observed on CT and MRI findings because the central region is composed of necrotic tissue while the periphery is composed of fascicles of spindle cells in edematous stroma with myxoid components, vessels, and inflammatory cells [72] (Figure 12.21). Inflammatory pseudotumor is suspected when an enhancing tumor is surrounded by a clot, particularly in young adults [73]. Large lesions invading through the bladder and having

a substantial extravesical component make differentiation from rhabdomyosarcoma and myxoid leiomyosarcoma difficult.

12.5.3 Cystitis Cystica/Glandularis

Cystitis cystica and cystitis glandularis are common chronic reactive inflammatory disorders secondary to *Escherichia coli* infection, calculi, or tumors and are most commonly found in women [74]. Chronic irritation results in metaplasia of the urothelium, which proliferates into buds (nests of von Brunn). The urothelium grows downward into the connective tissue beneath the epithelium in the lamina propria [75] and then differentiates into cystic deposits of cystitis cystica or into intestinal columnar mucin-secreting glands (goblet cells), resulting in cystitis glandularis. Cystitis glandularis occasionally transforms into adenocarcinoma [75]. Treatment usually involves the removal of the source of irritation and surgical excision of the area of inflammation. Careful monitoring is needed because of the possible association with adenocarcinoma.

Masses from cystitis cystica and cystitis glandularis vary in number and size (Figure 12.22). They consist of multiple small 2- to 5-mm smooth walled rounded lucent masses or, in rare cases, be up to 2–3 cm in size. Cystitis glandularis may develop into a papillary or polypoid mass making it difficult to differentiate from cancer. However, the distinguishing feature of cystitis cystica and cystitis glandularis is that the muscle layer should be intact [68].

12.5.4 Nephrogenic Adenoma

Nephrogenic adenoma is not a neoplastic mass but rather a benign proliferative response of the bladder urothelium to chronic irritation by calculi, infection,

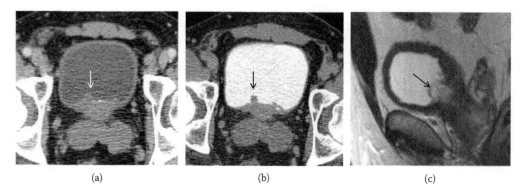

(a)   (b)   (c)

FIGURE 12.22
Cystitis cystica (Courtesy to Takehiko Gokan in Showa University). (a) Axial enhanced CT image shows a smooth walled rounded lucent mass (arrow) projecting into the bladder lumen. (b) Excretory-phase axial CT image shows the masses as s a small-sized filling defect (arrow) within the bladder. c) T2-weighted MR image clearly shows the tumor as a high-intensity lesion (arrow), which reflects the cystic nature of this lesion.

injury, or previous surgery; a typical patient may have a history of repeated biopsies for UC. This process results in papillary and tubular growths, which have a similar histologic appearance to the proximal tubules of a nephron, thus its name. Nephrogenic adenomas involve the lamina propria but not the muscle layer and are three times more common in men than in women [76]. Although this condition is not considered to be premalignant, nephrogenic adenomas can recur in up to 63% of all cases [76]. These lesions can occur in diverticula or at sites of previous surgery. Varying amounts of stromal calcification can be found histologically [77]. The optimal treatment is endoscopic resection.

Very few reports have described CT findings for nephrogenic adenoma. One study reported that CT revealed diffuse wall thickening or an irregular mass [78]. Another reported that the mass consisted of moderately enhanced soft tissue with coarse curvilinear calcification in the luminal aspect [79]. No distinctive radiographic features of nephrogenic adenoma exist that enable it to be differentiated from tumors or other inflammatory lesions. When examined using a cystoscopy, nephrogenic adenoma also resembles UC or chronic cystitis with multiple polypoid or single sessile growths [80]. Thus, a diagnosis can only be made with a histologic evaluation, since imaging and cystoscopic findings are nonspecific.

12.5.5 Malacoplakia

Malacoplakia is a chronic granulomatous condition consisting of rare yellow–gray plaques that are strongly associated with *E. coli* infection [81]. Although this disease can affect any organ, the urinary tract is the most common system to be involved, and the bladder is the most frequently affected organ (40% of patients with malacoplakia have bladder involvement and 16% have renal involvement) [81]. The disease is more common in patients with diabetes mellitus or in

immunocompromised individuals. The pathogenesis of malacoplakia is mainly thought to involve impaired host defenses and defective phagocytosis. The disease is four times more frequent in women than in men [81]. Presenting symptoms include gross hematuria and signs of urinary tract infection such as hesitancy, dysuria, and frequency. Patients may have variable proteinuria as well as leukocytes and erythrocytes in their urine. Treatment regimens include antibiotics, ascorbic acid, and a cholinergic agonist.

The imaging characteristics of malacoplakia vary. Multiple, polypoid, vascular, solid masses, or circumferential wall thickening may be present. Compression of the orifice of the ureter may cause dilatation of the upper urinary tract, and invasion of the perivesical space may cause bone destruction [82,83]. Less commonly, the condition may also involve the uterus or an extravesical anterior mass [84]. Because the imaging appearances of malacoplakia are often similar to those of neoplasms, a biopsy is essential for diagnosis.

12.6 Infection and Inflammation

12.6.1 Emphysematous Cystitis

Emphysematous urinary tract infection is considered to result from necrotizing inflammation with gas formation caused by *E. coli*, *Klebsiella* species, or mixed infections and less commonly by *Proteus*, *Citrobacter*, streptococci, or *Candida*. [85]. This disease is a rare condition and is always found in patients with diabetes mellitus. The clinical course can vary from asymptomatic infection to fulminant sepsis [86]. The mortality rate is reported to be approximately 20%. Treatment includes appropriate antimicrobial agents and control of the underlying disease.

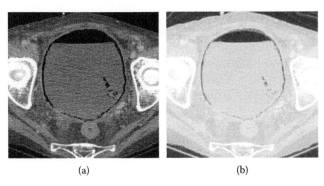

(a)   (b)

FIGURE 12.23
Emphysematous cystitis. (a) Axial enhanced CT image shows distension of the urinary bladder. (b) Image with a wider window and a higher level clearly shows the distribution of the gas.

The gas is initially formed in the bladder wall and subsequently passes through the mucosa into the lumen of the bladder (Figure 12.23). Plain films typically show gas within the bladder and irregular streak radiolucencies within the bladder wall. The best diagnostic modality is CT that clearly shows the mural and luminal location of the gas.

12.6.2 Radiation- and Cyclophosphamide-Induced Cystitis

Hemorrhagic cystitis may occur after cyclophosphamide chemotherapy or irradiation of the bladder. Radiation injury is a dose-dependent complication of radiation therapy performed for the treatment of bladder or other pelvic malignancies [87]. Lower doses of radiation (30 Gy external beam therapy over a 4-week period) can cause mild cystitis, with higher doses of up to 70 Gy causing longer-term effects. Acute radiation cystitis occurs during or soon after radiation treatment. Late radiation cystitis can develop from 6 months to 20 years after radiation therapy. Cyclophosphamide-related cystitis occurs from systemic or local chemotherapy with a frequency of 2%–40% [88]. The excretion of hepatic metabolites of cyclophosphamide in the urine produces edema, ulceration, hemorrhage, and necrosis of the urothelium. The main presenting symptom during the acute phase is hematuria, which may vary from mild to severe, life-threatening hemorrhage. Symptoms during the chronic phase are mostly related to the contraction of the bladder and consist of frequency, urgency, dysuria, hematuria, and incontinence.

The CT appearance is an abnormal bladder wall with focal or diffuse irregular thickening (Figure 12.24). Hypervascularity in the wall and bleeding vessels result in intraluminal clotting (Figure 12.25) [89]. In the chronic phase, the bladder has a small volume and cannot be fully distended because of fibrosis. Calcification may be seen in rare cases. Perforation of the bladder is a rare late complication of radiation therapy but is life-threatening.

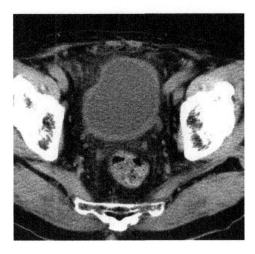

FIGURE 12.24
Radiation cystitis post radiation therapy for bladder cancer. Axial unenhanced CT image shows diffuse thickening of bladder wall.

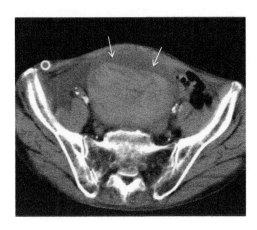

FIGURE 12.25
Cyclophosphamide cystitis. Axial unenhanced CT image shows the bladder occupied by high-density lesion (arrows) consistent with a hematoma.

12.6.3 Eosinophilic Cystitis

Eosinophilic cystitis, a rare chronic inflammatory disease of the bladder, is characterized by an infiltrate of eosinophils into the bladder wall and is associated with variable degrees of fibrosis and muscle necrosis [90]. It can occur in patients with atopy, with peripheral eosinophilia, or after bladder surgery, but it may also be idiopathic. Whether the disease represents a distinct entity is controversial, since eosinophilic infiltrates are also seen in other conditions and disorders, such as adverse reactions to drugs and food, parasitic or bacterial infections, UC, autoimmune disorders, and eosinophilic enteritis. Hematuria (macroscopic or microscopic) and frequency are the most common presenting symptoms, but other symptoms include irritative voiding symptoms, and a few patients may be asymptomatic. Treatment is relatively conservative, since eosinophilic cystitis typically runs a benign, self-limiting course following the

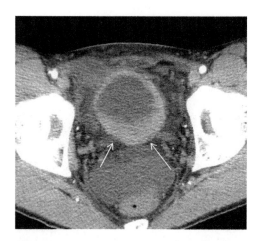

FIGURE 12.26
Eosinophilic cystitis. Axial enhanced CT image shows asymmetric thickening (arrows) of bladder wall.

removal of the etiologic factor, if known. When an intercurrent infection is present, local transurethral resection can be supplemented with the administration of antihistamines and various anti-inflammatory drugs.

At radiologic evaluation, single masses are observed more frequently than multiple bladder masses and may be sessile [90,91]. The bladder wall may appear normal or thickened (Figure 12.26) [92]. A cystic variant with an enhanced wall may be seen. In the fibrotic stage, the bladder is small and contracted, possibly resulting in hydronephrosis. Since the clinical and imaging features overlap with those of other disorders, particularly neoplasms that may coexist with eosinophilic cystitis, a biopsy is needed in both children and adults [91].

12.6.4 Schistosomiasis

Bladder schistosomiasis is one of the most common parasitic infections in the world, and is most prevalent in Africa [93]. Genitourinary tract infection is caused by the *Schistosoma haematobium* species. Eggs that enter the urine are trapped in the bladder walls and produce a granulomatous response that often causes linear streaks of calcium in the bladder or masses of large conglomerations of eggs. The chronic inflammatory response of schistosomiasis is a well-known predisposing factor for squamous carcinoma. Symptoms are nonspecific and are most commonly dysuria, suprapubic pain, microscopic hematuria, and frequency. Praziquantel may be administered to patients to destroy the adult worms and to incite the eggs to hatch. It has no effect on the chronic fibrotic changes in the bladder wall and ureters.

During the acute phase, nodular bladder wall thickening can be observed using CT [68]. Ureteral dilatation may be present because of the partial obstruction of the ureterovesical junction. The chronic phase is characterized by a contracted, fibrotic, thick-walled bladder with typically curvilinear calcifications [68]. A nodular lesion may

develop secondary to the granulomatous response, or secondary carcinoma, typically squamous carcinoma. In a follow-up examination, the absence of wall calcification in an area that was previously calcified may indicate a bladder tumor. A definitive diagnosis is made when eggs are found in the urine during a microscopic examination.

12.7 Fistulae

Bladder fistulae may involve the intestine (enterovesical fistula), colon (colovesical fistulae), skin (vesicocutaneous fistula), urethra (vesicourethral fistula), or female reproductive tract (vesicovaginal or vesicouterine fistulae) [94]. Enterovesical and colorectal fistulae are the most prevalent. Other fistulae usually occur secondary to surgical procedures or trauma.

Enterovesical and colorectal fistulae are diagnosed primarily based on the clinical features of pneumaturia, fecaluria, and recurrent urinary tract infections. Enterovesical fistulae are most frequently caused by Crohn's disease. Enterovesical fistulae occur in 1.7%–7.7% of patients with Crohn's disease and most often arise from the ileum (64% of cases) or colon (21%) [95]. Colovesical fistulae most frequently involve the rectosigmoid colon. The most frequent cause is diverticulitis followed by colon cancer. Treatment consists of surgery, with resection of the abnormal bowel segment and closure of the bladder defect, when Crohn's disease or diverticulitis is the cause.

CT is the primary imaging modality for suspected cases of enterovesical fistulae. Although CT often fails to show the fistulous tract, air within the bladder, focal irregularities of the wall, and the tethering of focal bladder wall thickening with focal thickening of a loop of bowel adjacent to the bladder are typical findings (Figures 12.27 and 12.28) [94,95]. These findings are suggestive of this disease. The presence of orally administered contrast material in the bladder is diagnostic of a fistula between the bowel and the bladder. Initial scanning should also be performed after the oral administration of contrast material but before the intravenous administration of contrast material to show bladder enhancement. A cystoscopy is accepted as a routine component of the work-up, but it fails to actually show the fistula in more than half of all cases [96]. The advantages of CT are its noninvasive nature and its ability to show any associated intra-abdominal processes. Intravesical air, in particular, is a key finding. The diagnosis of a fistula may also be made using fluoroscopic studies of enterography, barium enema, or cystography. However, these modalities are less sensitive from a diagnostic perspective [94].

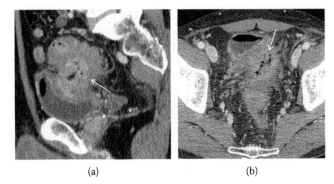

(a)   (b)

FIGURE 12.27
Enterovesical fistulas because of diverticulitis. (a) Sagittal enhanced CT image shows wall thickening of the sigmoid colon and the adjacent bladder, and soft-tissue mass (arrow) enveloped in between. Fistula is not detected within the soft-tissue mass; however, intravesical air suggests the existence of enterovesical fistula. (b) Axial enhanced CT image shows the soft-tissue mass (arrow) contains air, resulting from abscess formation.

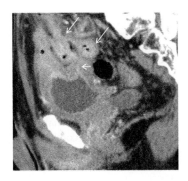

FIGURE 12.28
Enterovesical fistulas because of Crohn's disease. Sagittal enhanced CT image shows wall thickening of the ileum (long arrows) and the adjacent bladder with linear structure suggesting fistula (short arrow). The inflammatory process also extends to urachal remnant (*).

References

1. Jinzaki M, Tanimoto A, Shinmoto H et al. Detection of bladder tumors with dynamic contrast-enhanced MDCT. *AJR Am J Roentgenol* 2007;188:913–918.
2. Kim JK, Park SY, Ahn HJ, Kim CS, Cho SK. Bladder cancer: analysis of multi-detector row helical CT enhancement pattern and accuracy in tumor detection and perivesical staging. *Radiology* 2004;231:725–731.
3. Park SB, Kim JK, Lee HJ, Choi HJ, Cho KS. Hematuria: portal venous phase multi-detector row CT of the bladder: a prospective study. *Radiology* 2007;245:798–805.
4. Mc Tavish JD, Jinzaki M, Zou KH, Nawfel RD, Silverman SG. Multi-detector row CT urography: comparison of strategies for depicting the normal urinary collecting system. *Radiology* 2002;225:783–790.
5. Caoili EM, Cohan RH, Korobkin M et al. Urinary tract abnormalities: initial experience with multi-detector row CT urography. *Radiology* 2002;222:353–360.
6. Jinzaki M, Matsumoto K, Kikuchi E et al. Comparison of CT urography and excretory urography in the detection and localization of urothelial carcinoma of the upper urinary tract. *AJR Am J Roentgenol* 2011;196:1102–1109.
7. Wang LJ, Wong YC, Huang CC et al. Multidetector computerized tomography urography is more accurate than excretory urography for diagnosing transitional cell carcinoma of the upper urinary tract in adults with hematuria. *J Urol* 2010;183:48–55.
8. Murphy WM, Grignon DJ, Perlman EJ. *Tumors of the kidney, bladder, and related urinary structures.* Washington, DC: American Registry of Pathology, 2004;241–361.
9. Scosyrev E, Noyes K, Feng C, Messing E. Sex and racial differences in bladder cancer presentation and mortality in the US. *Cancer* 2009;115:68–74.
10. Lopez-Beltran A. Bladder cancer: clinical and pathological profile. *Scand J Urol Nephrol Suppl* 2008;218:95–109.
11. Edge SB, Byrd DR, Compton CC, eds. Urinary bladder. In: *AJCC cancer staging manual.* 7th ed. New York, NY: Springer, 2010;367–374.
12. Dorin RP, Daneshmand S, Eisenberg MS et al. Lymph node dissection technique is more important than lymph node count in identifying nodal metastases in radical cystectomy patients: a comparative mapping study. *Eur Urol* 2011;60:946–952.
13. Shinagare AB, Ramaiya NH, Jagannathan JP et al. Metastatic pattern of bladder cancer: correlation with the characteristics of the primary tumor. *AJR Am J Roentgenol* 2011;196:117–122.
14. Millan-Rodriguez F, Chechile-Toniolo G, Salvador-Bayarri J, Huguet-Pérez J, Vicente-Rodríguez J. Upper urinary tract tumors after primary superficial bladder tumors: prognostic factors and risk groups. *J Urol* 2000;164:1183–1187.
15. Babjuk M, Oosterlinck W, Sylvester R et al. EAU guidelines on non-muscle-invasive urothelial carcinoma of the bladder, the 2011 update. *Eur Urol* 2011;59:997–1008.
16. Matsumoto K, Kikuchi E, Horiguchi Y et al. Late recurrence and progression in non-muscle-invasive bladder cancers after 5-year tumor-free periods. *Urology* 2010;75:1385–1390.
17. Hautmann RE, Gschwend JE, de Petriconi RC, Kron M, Volkmer BG. Cystectomy for transitional cell carcinoma of the bladder: results of a surgery only series in the neobladder era. *J Urol* 2006;176:486–492.
18. von der Maase H, Sengelov L, Roberts JT et al. Long-term survival results of a randomized trial comparing gemcitabine plus cisplatin, with methotrexate, vinblastine, doxorubicin, plus cisplatin in patients with bladder cancer. *J Clin Oncol* 2005;23:4602–4608.
19. Kim B, Semelka RC, Ascher SM, Chalpin DB, Carroll PR, Hricak H. Bladder tumor staging: comparison of contrast-enhanced CT, T1- and T2-weighted MR imaging, dynamic gadolinium-enhanced imaging, and late gadolinium-enhanced imaging. *Radiology* 1994;193:239–245.
20. Tanimoto A, Yuasa Y, Imai Y et al. Bladder tumor staging: comparison of conventional and gadolinium-enhanced dynamic MR imaging and CT. *Radiology* 1992;185:741–747.

21. Vinnicombe SJ, Norman AR, Nicolson V, Husband JE. Normal pelvic lymph nodes: evaluation by CT scanning after bipedal lymphangiography. *Radiology* 1995;194:349–355.

22. Paik ML, Scolieri MJ, Brown SL, Spirnak JP, Resnick MI. Limitations of computerized tomography in staging invasive bladder cancer before radical cystectomy. *J Urol* 2000;163:1693–1696.

23. Husband JE. Computer tomography and magnetic resonance imaging in the evaluation of bladder cancer. *J Belge Radiol* 1995;78:350–355.

24. Turney BW, Willatt JM, Nixon D, Crew JP, Cowan NC. Computed tomography urography for diagnosing bladder cancer. *BJU Int* 2006;98:345–348.

25. Knox MK, Cowan NC, Rivers-Bowerman MD, Turney BW. Evaluation of multidetector computed tomography urography and ultrasonography for diagnosing bladder cancer. *Clin Radiol* 2008;63:1317–1325.

26. Cohan RH, Caoili EM, Cowan NC, Weizer AZ, Ellis JH. MDCT urography: exploring a new paradigm for imaging of bladder cancer. *AJR Am J Roentgenol* 2009;192:1501–1508.

27. Kassouf W, Spiess PE, Siefker-Radtke A et al. Outcome and patterns of recurrence of nonbilharzial pure squamous cell carcinoma of the bladder: a contemporary review of The University of Texas M D Anderson Cancer Center experience. *Cancer* 2007;110:764–769.

28. Narumi Y, Sato T, Hori S et al. Squamous cell carcinoma of the uroepithelium: CT evaluation. *Radiology* 1989;173:853–836.

29. Wong JT, Wasserman NF, Padurean AM. Bladder squamous cell carcinoma. *Radiographics* 2004;24:855–860.

30. Dondalski M, White EM, Ghahremani GG, Patel SK. Carcinoma arising in urinary bladder diverticula: imaging findings in six patients. *AJR Am J Roentgenol* 1993;161:817–820.

31. Eble JN, Sauter G, Epstein JI, Sesterhenn IA, eds. *Pathology and genetics of tumours of the urinary system and male genital organs.* World Health Organization Classification of Tumours. Lyon, France: IARC Press, 2004:89–149.

32. Abol-Enein H, Kava BR, Carmack AJ. Nonurothelial cancer of the bladder. *Urology* 2007;69:93–104.

33. Hughes MJ, Fisher C, Sohaib SA. Imaging features of primary nonurachal adenocarcinoma of the bladder. *AJR Am J Roentgenol* 2004;183:1397–1401.

34. Henly DR, Farrow GM, Zincke H. Urachal cancer: role of conservative surgery. *Urology* 1993;42:635–639.

35. Beck AD, Gaudin JH, Bonham DG. Carcinoma of the urachus. *Br J Urol* 1970;42:555–562.

36. Molina JR, Quevedo JF, Furth AF et al. Predictors of survival from urachal cancer: a Mayo Clinic study of 49 cases. *Cancer* 2007;110:2434–2340.

37. Thali-Schwab CM, Woodward PJ, Wagner BJ. Computed tomographic appearance of urachal adenocarcinomas: review of 25 cases. *Eur Radiol* 2005;15:79–84.

38. Kwok-Liu JP, Zikman JM, Cockshott WP. Carcinoma of the urachus: the role of computed tomography. *Radiology* 1980;137:731–734.

39. Siefker-Radtke AO, Gee J, Shen Y et al. Multimodality management of urachal carcinoma: the M. D. Anderson Cancer Center experience. *J Urol* 2003;169:1295–1298.

40. Yazawa S, Kikuchi E, Takeda T et al. Surgical and chemotherapeutic options for urachal carcinoma: report of ten cases and literature review. *Urol Int* 2012;88:209–214.

41. Brick SH, Friedman AC, Pollack HM et al. Urachal carcinoma: CT findings. *Radiology* 1988;169:377–381.

42. Narumi Y, Sato T, Kuriyama K et al. Vesical dome tumors: significance of extravesical extension on CT. *Radiology* 1988;196:383–385.

43. Lee SH, Kitchens HH, Kim BS. Adenocarcinoma of the urachus: CT features. *J Comput Assist Tomogr* 1990;14:232–235.

44. Machida H, Ueno E, Nakazawa H, Fujimura M, Kihara T. Computed tomographic appearance of urachal carcinoma associated with urachal diverticulum is diagnosed by cystoscopy. *Abdom Imaging* 2008;33:363–366.

45. Candamio MJD, Pombo F, Arnal F, Busto L. Xanthogranulomatous urachitis: CT findings. *J Comput Assist Tomogr* 1998;22:93–95.

46. Chen WJ, Hsieh HH, Wan YL. Abscess of urachal remnant mimicking urinary bladder neoplasm. *Br J Urol* 1992;69:510–512.

47. Martin SA, Sears DL, Sebo TJ, Lohse CM, Cheville JC. Smooth muscle neoplasms of the urinary bladder: a clinicopathologic comparison of leiomyoma and leiomyosarcoma. *Am J Surg Pathol* 2002;26:292–300.

48. Seitz G, Dantonello TM, Int-Veen C et al. Treatment efficiency, outcome and surgical treatment problems in patients suffering from localized embryonal bladder/prostate rhabdomyosarcoma: a report from the Cooperative Soft Tissue Sarcoma trial CWS-96. *Pediatr Blood Cancer* 2011;56:718–724.

49. Agrons GA, Wagner BJ, Lonergan GJ, Dickey GE, Kaufman MS. Genitourinary rhabdomyosarcoma in children: radiologic-pathologic correlation. *RadioGraphics* 1997;17:919–937.

50. Knoll LD, Segura JW, Scheithauer BW. Leiomyoma of the bladder. *J Urol* 1986;136:906–908.

51. Goluboff ET, O'Toole K, Sawczuk IS. Leiomyoma of bladder: report of case and review of literature. *Urology* 1994;43:238–241.

52. Park JW, Jeong BC, Seo SI et al. Leiomyoma of the urinary bladder: a series of nine cases and review of the literature. *Urology* 2010;76:1425–1429.

53. Cornella JL, Larson TR, Lee RA, Magrina JF, Kammerer-Doak D. Leiomyoma of the female urethra and bladder: report of twenty-three patients and review of the literature. *Am J Obstet Gynecol* 1997;176:1278–1285.

54. Bai SW, Jung HJ, Jeon MJ et al. Leiomyoma of the female urethra and bladder: a report of five cases and review of the literature. *Int Urogynecol J Pelvic Floor Dysfunct* 2007;18:913–917.

55. Dighe MK, Bhargava P, Wright J. Urinary bladder masses: techniques, imaging spectrum, and staging. *J Comput Assist Tomogr* 2011;35:411–424.

56. Chen M, Lipson SA, Hricak H. MR imaging evaluation of benign mesenchymal tumors of the urinary bladder. *AJR Am J Roentgenol* 1997;168: 399–403.

57. Sundaram CP, Rawal A, Saltzman B. Characteristics of bladder leiomyoma as noted on magnetic resonance imaging. *Urology* 1998;52:1142–1143.

58. Wong-You-Cheong JJ, Woodward PJ, Manning MA, Sesterhenn IA. From the archives of the AFIP: neoplasms of the urinary bladder: radiologic-pathologic correlation. *Radiographics* 2006;26:553–580.

59. Crecelius SA, Bellah R. Pheochromocytoma of the bladder in an adolescent: sonographic and MR imaging findings. *AJR Am J Roentgenol* 1995;165:101–103.

60. Asbury WL Jr, Hatcher PA, Gould HR, Reeves WA, Wilson DD. Bladder pheochromocytoma with ring calcification. *Abdom Imaging* 1996;21:275–277.

61. Bates AW, Norton AJ, Baithun SI. Malignant lymphoma of the urinary bladder: a clinicopathological study of 11 cases. *J Clin Pathol* 2000;53:458–461.

62. Horasanli K, Kadihasanoglu M, Aksakal OT, Ozagari A, Miroglu C. A case of primary lymphoma of the bladder managed with multimodal therapy. *Nat Clin Pract Urol* 2008;5:167–170.

63. Maninderpal KG, Amir FH, Azad HA, Mun KS. Imaging findings of a primary bladder maltoma. *Br J Radiol* 2011;84:e186–e190.

64. Bates AW, Baithun SI. Secondary neoplasms of the bladder are histological mimics of nontransitional cell primary tumours: clinicopathological and histological features of 282 cases. *Histopathology* 2000;36:32–40.

65. Chapron C, Chopin N, Borghese B et al. Deeply infiltrating endometriosis: pathogenetic implications of the anatomical distribution. *Hum Reprod* 2006;21:1839–1845.

66. Batler RA, Kim SC, Nadler RB. Bladder endometriosis: pertinent clinical images. *Urology* 2001;57:798–799.

67. Bazot M, Darai E, Hourani R et al. Deep pelvic endometriosis: MR imaging for diagnosis and prediction of extension of disease. *Radiology* 2004;232:379–389.

68. Wong-You-Cheong JJ, Woodward PJ, Manning MA, Davis CJ. From the archives of the AFIP: inflammatory and nonneoplastic bladder masses: radiologic-pathologic correlation. *Radiographics* 2006;26:1847–1868.

69. Kinkel K, Frei KA, Balleyguier C, Chapron C. Diagnosis of endometriosis with imaging: a review. *Eur Radiol* 2006;16:285–298.

70. Young RH. Pseudoneoplastic lesions of the urinary bladder and urethra: a selective review with emphasis on recent information. *Semin Diagn Pathol* 1997;14:133–146.

71. Fujiwara T, Sugimura K, Imaoka I, Igawa M. Inflammatory pseudotumor of the bladder: MR findings. *J Comput Assist Tomogr* 1999;23:558–561.

72. Sugita R, Saito M, Miura M, Yuda F. Inflammatory pseudotumour of the bladder: CT and MRI findings. *Br J Radiol* 1999;72:809–811.

73. Narla LD, Newman B, Spottswood SS, Narla S, Kolli R. Inflammatory pseudotumor. *RadioGraphics* 2003;23:719–729.

74. Grignon DJ, Sakr W. Inflammatory and other conditions that can mimic carcinoma in the urinary bladder. *Pathol Annu* 1995;30:95–122.

75. Thrasher JB, Rajan RR, Perez LM, Humphrey PA, Anderson EE. Cystitis glandularis: transition to adenocarcinoma of the urinary bladder. *N C Med J* 1994;55:562–564.

76. Porcaro AB, D'Amico A, Ficarra V et al. Nephrogenic adenoma of the urinary bladder: our experience and review of the literature. *Urol Int* 2001;66:152–155.

77. O'Shea PA, Callaghan JF, Lawlor JB, Aeddy VC. "Nephrogenic adenoma": an unusual metaplastic change of urothelium. *Urology* 1981:125:249–252.

78. Zingas AP, Kling GA, Crotte E, Shumaker E, Vazquez PM. Computed tomography of nephrogenic adenoma of the urinary bladder. *J Comput Assist Tomogr* 1986;10:979–982.

79. Patel PS, Wilbur AC. Nephrogenic adenoma presenting as a calcified mass. *AJR Am J Roentgenol* 1988;150:1071–1072.

80. Peeker R, Aldenborg F, Fall M. Nephrogenic adenoma: a study with special reference to clinical presentation. *Br J Urol* 1997;80:539–542.

81. Stanton MJ, Maxted W. Malacoplakia: a study of the literature and current concepts of pathogenesis, diagnosis and treatment. *J Urol* 1981;125:139–146.

82. Steele B, Vade A, Lim-Dunham J. Sonographic appearance of bladder malacoplakia. *Pediatr Radiol* 2003;33:253–255.

83. Bidwell JK, Dunne MG. Computed tomography of bladder malakoplakia. *J Comput Assist Tomogr* 1987;11:909–910.

84. Baumgartner BR, Alagappian R. Malakoplakia of the ureter and bladder. *Urol Radiol* 1990;12:157–159.

85. Mokabberi R, Ravakhah K. Emphysematous urinary tract infections: diagnosis, treatment and survival (case review series). *Am J Med Sci* 2007;333:111–116.

86. Perlmutter AE, Mastromichaelis M, Zaslau S. Emphysematous cystitis: a case report and literature review. *W V Med J* 2004;100:232–233.

87. Iyer RB, Jhingran A, Sawaf H, Libshitz HI. Imaging findings after radiotherapy to the pelvis. *AJR Am J Roentgenol* 2001;177:1083–1089.

88. Bennett AH. Cyclophosphamide and haemorrhagic cystitis. *J Urol* 1974;111:603–606.

89. McCarville MB, Hoffer FA, Gingrich JR, Jenkins JJ 3rd. Imaging findings of hemorrhagic cystitis in pediatric oncology patients. *Pediatr Radiol* 2000;30:131–138.

90. Teegavarapu PS, Sahai A, Chandra A, Dasgupta P, Khan MS. Eosinophilic cystitis and its management. *Int J Clin Pract* 2005;59:356–360.

91. Itano NM, Malek RS. Eosinophilic cystitis in adults. *J Urol* 2001;165:805–807.

92. Verhagen PC, Nikkels PG, de Jong TP. Eosinophilic cystitis. *Arch Dis Child* 2001;84:344–346.

93. Neal PM. Schistosomiasis—an unusual cause of ureteral obstruction: a case history and perspective. *Clin Med Res* 2004;2:216–227.

94. Yu NC, Raman SS, Patel M, Barbaric Z. Fistulas of the genitourinary tract: a radiologic review. *RadioGraphics* 2004;24:1331–1352.

95. Solem CA, Loftus EV Jr, Tremaine WJ, Pemberton JH, Wolff BG, Sandborn WJ. Fistulas to the urinary system in Crohn's disease: clinical features and outcomes. *Am J Gastroenterol* 2002;97:2300–2305.

96. Woods RJ, Lavery IC, Fazio VW, Jagelman DG, Weakley FL. Internal fistulas in diverticular disease. *Dis Colon Rectum* 1988;31:591–596.

13

Male Pelvis

Jurgen J. Fütterer

CONTENTS

13.1 Introduction

13.1.1 Bladder

The urinary bladder is a muscular sac and elastic-walled organ in the pelvis. The bladder is part of the urinary system. The produced and excreted urine is transported from the kidneys, passing through the ureters, to the bladder. The functions of the bladder are to store and to allow the urine to exit via the urethra.

Diseases of the bladder can be divided into a number of categories: cystitis, bladder stones, urine incontinence, and bladder cancer. Bladder cancer is the third most common cancer in males and the tenth most common cancer in females [1]. It is estimated that 73,510 men and women (55,600 men and 17,910 women) will be diagnosed and 14,880 men and women will die of cancer of the urinary bladder in 2012 [2]. In women, the disease is diagnosed at a more advanced stage, and women have a higher mortality rate than men. Early diagnosis of bladder cancer is essential if it is assumed that this confers a better prognosis. Urinary bladder cancer has a high recurrence rate, necessitating long-term surveillance after initial therapy.

13.1.2 Anatomy of the Urinary Bladder

The urinary bladder is an extraperitoneal organ surrounded by fat, with peritoneum covering only the superior surface of the bladder. The orifices of the ureters at the ureterovesical junction are joined by an elevated ridge covered by mucosa [3]. The bladder trigone is a triangular region on the inferior wall, marked at its corners by the ureterovesical junction and urethra [4].

The wall of the urinary bladder is composed of four layers. The most inner layer, the urothelium, has varying thickness depending on the degree of bladder distension. The uroepithelium consists of three to seven layers of transitional cells. The underlying lamina propria is highly vascularized and is composed of blood vessels, loose connective tissue, nerves, adipose tissue, and a variable amount of smooth muscle fibers (muscularis mucosae). The third layer, the muscularis propria (detrusor) is composed of large bundles of muscle. The outermost serosa, including perivesical adipose tissue, is the fourth layer (Figure 13.1.) [5,6].

13.1.3 Pathology

Bladder cancer can arise from any of the four layers and can be classified as epithelial and nonepithelial. About 90% of bladder tumors are urothelial in origin. Urothelial tumors exhibit a spectrum of neoplasia ranging from a benign papilloma through carcinoma in situ to invasive carcinoma [4]. Squamous cell carcinomas account for 6%–8% of all bladder cancers. Adenocarcinomas are rare and typically represent urachal cancer [7].

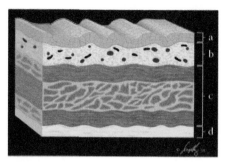

FIGURE 13.1
Normal bladder wall. Diagram shows (a) urothelium, (b) lamina propria, (c) muscularis propria (detrusor muscle), and (d) adventitia. (Reprinted from Siegel R, Naishadham D, Jemal A., *CA Cancer J Clin.*, 62(1), 10, 2012. With permission.)

TABLE 13.1

TNM Classification Bladder Cancer

Primary Tumor (T)	
TX	Primary tumor cannot be assessed
T0	No evidence of primary tumor
Ta	Noninvasive papillary carcinoma
Tis	Carcinoma in situ: "flat tumor"
T1	Tumor invades subepithelial connective tissue
T2	Tumor invades muscularis propria
pT2a	Tumor invades superficial muscularis propria (inner half)
pT2b	Tumor invades deep muscularis propria (outer half)
T3	Tumor invades perivesical tissue
pT3a	Microscopically
pT3b	Macroscopically (extravesical mass)
T4	Tumor invades any of the following: prostatic stroma, seminal vesicles, uterus, vagina, pelvic wall, abdominal wall
T4a	Tumor invades prostatic stroma, uterus, vagina
T4b	Tumor invades pelvic wall, abdominal wall
Regional Lymph Nodes (N)	
NX	Lymph nodes cannot be assessed
N0	No lymph node metastasis
N1	Single regional lymph node metastasis in the true pelvis (hypogastric, obturator, external iliac, or presacral lymph node)
N2	Multiple regional lymph node metastases in the true pelvis (hypogastric, obturator, external iliac, or presacral lymph node)
N3	Lymph node metastases to the common iliac lymph nodes
Distant Metastasis (M)	
M0	No distant metastasis
M1	Distant metastasis

Bladder cancer is staged using the tumor-node-metastasis (TNM) staging system (Table 13.1) [8]. In this system, T stage is based on the degree of invasion of the bladder wall. Urothelial cancer can be divided into

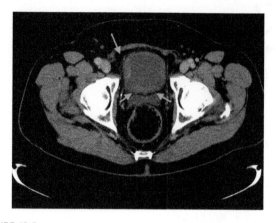

FIGURE 13.2
Multifocal urothelial bladder cancer stage 2a (cystectomy was performed).

nonmuscle-invasive or muscle-invasive disease. In approximately 70% of the cases, the cancer is confined to the mucosa (noninvasive papillary carcinoma or carcinoma in situ) or submucosa (pathology stage T1). Malignant urothelial tumors confined to the bladder mucosa are termed nonmuscle invasive tumors. Carcinoma in situ is a high-grade and aggressive manifestation of transitional cell carcinoma of the bladder that has a highly variable course, and, therefore, difficult to manage [9]. Carcinoma in situ represents 5%–10% of the nonmuscle-invasive bladder cancers [10]. One-third of the patients with urothelial cancer of the bladder will be diagnosed with a muscle-invasive tumor (pathology stage ≥T2) or metastatic disease at the time of diagnosis. In addition, approximately 30% of patients who initially diagnosed with nonmuscle-invasive tumor will develop muscle-invasive tumors in the course of the follow-up after bladder-sparing treatment.

Approximately 30% of bladder cancers are already multifocal at the time of initial diagnosis (Figure 13.2). Nearly 15% of urothelial carcinoma in the upper urinary tract lead to the subsequent development of bladder tumors.

The most common etiologic factors for urothelial tumors are cigarette smoking and occupational exposure to chemical carcinogens [11,12]. Cigarette smokers have a substantial increase in risk of cancer of the urinary tract. They have an approximately threefold higher risk of urinary tract cancer than nonsmokers [13]. Bladder diverticula have an increased risk (2%–10%) of developing cancer as a result of urine stasis. Tumors occurring in diverticula have a propensity to invade perivesical fat early because of the lack of muscle in their wall [4].

13.1.4 Bladder Cancer Clinical Staging and Management

Patient classically presents with painless gross hematuria occurring in about 80%–90% of the cases. The workup of these patients depends on the local situation.

As a result, there remains wide variation in the imaging methods. This may consist of renal and bladder ultrasound examination and urine cytology for triage prior to cystoscopy. Other institutions perform computed tomographic (CT) urography, whereas others use cystoscopy as the first line of investigation. Nevertheless, cystoscopy and CT urography are complementary and have a definite management role in patients who present with hematuria. Urinalysis has a high specificity (94%) for the detection of bladder cancer [14].

Cystoscopy to evaluate the urinary bladder wall and urethral mucosa is an important part of pretreatment planning. Cystoscopic-guided biopsy of bladder lesions is performed to assess the pathology, grade, and penetration depth of these malignant-looking tumors. Transurethral resection of bladder tumor is performed for complete resection of superficial bladder tumors.

Irritative bladder symptoms such as dysuria, urgency, or frequency of urination occur in 20%–30% of patients with bladder cancer. Although irritative symptoms may be related to more advanced muscle-invasive disease, carcinoma in situ is especially likely to cause such symptoms (Figure 13.3).

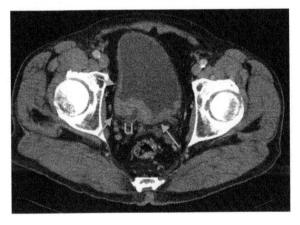

FIGURE 13.3
Carcinoma in situ with involvement of the dorsal bladder wall and right urethra.

After the diagnosis of a solid bladder cancer, imaging is usually performed to stage the disease in these patients. Treatment decisions and prognosis for bladder cancer are based on the depth of muscle invasion by the tumor, degree of differentiation of the tumor, and presence or absence of metastatic disease.

13.1.5 Diagnosis

Distinguishing patients with muscle invasion from those with noninvasive muscle growth is critical for the care of patients with bladder cancer. Radical cystectomy with meticulous lymph node dissection is the treatment of choice for patients with invasion of the muscular layer, whereas bladder-sparing treatment options are available for superficial tumors [15].

Epithelial masses derive from the most superficial layer of the bladder wall. They often appear as irregular, intraluminal filling defects. This filling defect can be detected on the intravenous urogram (IVU). However, IVU is a not sensitive imaging modality, because small tumors can be missed. In less than 67% of the cases, a filling defect is visible on the IVU [14,16]. A filling defect can also be explained by a clot, fungus ball, radiolucent stone, and so on.

Multi-detector CT (MDCT), with its isotropic high-quality multiplanar image reconstruction capability, is used as a routine procedure for the assessment of the depth of tumor invasion, lymph node involvement and presence of organ metastases [17]. CT urography is emerging as a "one-stop" diagnostic imaging technique that offers a thorough evaluation of the urinary tract for stones, renal masses, and urothelial neoplasms in a single examination [18,19]. CT urography is defined as MDCT examination of the kidneys, ureters, and bladder with at least one imaging series acquired during the excretory phase after IV contrast administration [20].

Tumors can be papillary (Figure 13.4), sessile, or nodular. Most urothelial tumors are located at the bladder base. Tumors that cause ureteral obstruction are 92%

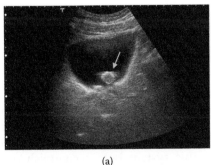

(a)

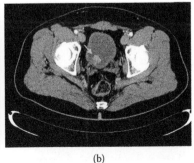

(b)

FIGURE 13.4
(a) Trans abdominal ultrasound in a patient with macroscopic hematuria shows a papillary lesion in the dorsal bladder wall. (b) Multi-detector computed tomography (CT) shows highly vascular lesion.

muscle-invasive [21,22]. Tumor may appear as an intra-luminal mass or focal wall thickening. Identification of the primary lesion may be difficult in areas of the bladder neck and dome [23]. Lesions may be missed without adequate bladder distention, especially small, flat tumors. Oral hydration with water (1000 mL) prior to the examination is a patient preparation strategy to prevent this. Turning the patients several times before the excretory phase imaging may improve homogeneous contrast distribution on the bladder (Figure 13.5). CT shows calcification within the lesion in about 5% of cases (Figure 13.6). Differentiation of cancerous tissue from nonspecific wall edema, blood clots, or tissue debris (that mimic the appearance of a tumor) may be difficult. Transurethral biopsy or resection decreases the diagnostic accuracy as a result of blood, edema (focal wall thickening), and perivesical fat stranding. To further improve in the differentiation, IV contrast material is used. Bladder cancer tends to show peak enhancement with the 60-second scanning delay and may be readily

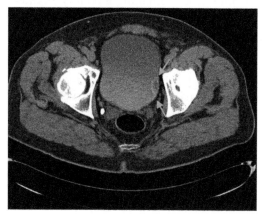

FIGURE 13.5
Urothelial bladder cancer in the bladder wall (stage T1 after TURT). Poor opacification of the bladder lumen this may be improved by turning the patient.

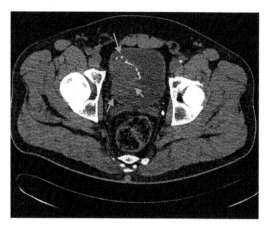

FIGURE 13.6
Calcifications in the large bulky lesion expanding into the bladder lumen.

detected with CT [24]. Once the tumor has extended into the perivesical fat, increased attenuation or infiltration is noted in the fat.

Results of CT urography depends on the specific population studied. In a patient population with microscopic hematuria, a sensitivity of 40% was achieved compared to cystoscopy [25]. In a high-risk group (i.e., gross hematuria), unequivocal results for CT urography were found compared to cystoscopy. A sensitivity of 93% and specificity of 99% was achieved in the detection of bladder cancer [26]. An advantage of CT urography is that it avoids any morbidity associated with cystoscopy [27]. Carcinoma in situ tumors rather than organ-confined tumors are associated with CT urography undetectability [28]. A system for investigating patients with hematuria according to predetermined risk factors is suggested by Nolte-Ernsting and Cowan (Table 13.2) [29].

Overall accuracy for local bladder cancer staging in clinical studies is approximately 55% [23,30–35]. In most studies, the disease is overstaged. CT urography cannot accurately distinguish nonmuscle-invasive from muscle-invasive bladder cancer and cannot detect microscopic perivesical spread of tumor (stage T3a disease). The use of contrast agent improved the detection and staging performance, however, until there is little evidence to confirm these initial findings [23].

Lymph node metastases in noninvasive muscle tumors are infrequent. Lymphogenic metastases occur mainly to the perivesical lymph nodes. The lymphatic drainage is to the nodes along the external iliac vein, next to the obturator lymph nodes followed by the presacral and retroperitoneal lymph nodes. Deep muscle layer infiltration or extravesical invasion increases the likelihood of lymph node metastases to 20%–30% and 50%–60%, respectively [36]. Size and shape criteria are used for detecting lymph node metastases. The accuracy of CT for staging of lymph nodes is between 70% and 98% with 20%–40% false negatives [37]. Hematogenous spread of bladder cancer is a late event that occurs predominantly to the liver, lung, bone, and brain.

13.2 Prostate

13.2.1 Introduction

The male reproductive system encompasses a number of organs including the testes, ejaculatory ducts, the seminal vesicles, prostate, and penis. The function of this system is to accomplish reproduction. The main role of the prostate gland is to produce and secrete an alkaline fluid. This helps to energize and protect the sperm during intercourse in the vaginal canal.

TABLE 13.2

Differentiated Workup of (Painless) Hematuria

Lowest Risk	Low Risk	Medium Risk	High Risk
Microscopic hematuria age <40 years	Macroscopic hematuria age <40 years	Microscopic hematuria age >40 years	Macroscopic hematuria age >40 years
Cystsocopy + ultrasound	Cystsocopy + ultrasound	Cystsocopy + ultrasound	Cystsocopy + CT urography
If negative:	If negative and symptoms continue:	If negative and symptoms continue:	Clinical referral
Watch and wait	Conventional urography	Conventional urography or CT urography	

Source: Adapted from Clayman RV et al. *J Urol.*, 131:715–6, 1984.

The prostate changes and commonly enlarges with age. The most frequent types of benign prostate diseases are prostatitis and benign prostatic hyperplasia (BPH). Prostate cancer is the most common noncutaneous malignancy in males [1]. In an early stage, prostate cancer is commonly asymptomatic because most cancers are located in the peripheral zone. Few patients have symptoms of the lower urinary tract because of obstruction. Prostate cancer patients rarely present with symptoms of hematuria or hematospermia. Prostate cancer is suspected in patients with elevated prostate-specific antigen (PSA) value. The urologic workup in patients with elevated PSA consists of a digital rectal examination and systematic 10–12 core Transrectal ultrasound (TRUS)-guided biopsy session. The latter is done to diagnose the cancer; unfortunately, TRUS understages the Gleason score in about 40% of the patients. Imaging plays a central role in the detection, localization, staging, and local recurrence detection in prostate cancer patients.

13.2.2 Anatomy of the Prostate

The prostate is a small gland and situated directly caudal to the bladder. On the basis of embryological origins, the prostate is anatomically divided into three zones that are eccentrically located around the urethra: the innermost transition zone, the central zone, and the outermost peripheral zone. Knowledge of the zonal anatomy of the prostate is very useful, considering that many prostatic diseases have a zonal distribution. The prostate gland envelops the prostatic urethra and the ejaculatory ducts. The seminal vesicles are paired grapelike pouches filled with fluid that are located caudolateral to the corresponding deferent duct, between the bladder and rectum. The prostate is divided into apex and base (directed upward to the inferior border of the bladder).

In the elderly patient, the transition and central zone is difficult to discern because of compression of the central zone by BPH in the transition zone. Seventy percent of all prostate cancers are located in the peripheral zone, whereas 20% emerge from the transition zone, and 10% from the central zone. The neurovascular bundle

courses bilaterally along the posterolateral aspect of the prostate and is a preferential pathway of tumor spread.

13.2.3 Prostatitis and Prostate Abscess

The prevalence of prostatitis ranges between 2% and 16%, depending on the definition used by the evaluating physician [38]. Prostatitis may occur at any age and race, however, its incidence increases with age. Prostatitis is a diffuse disease and inflammatory condition that is not well understood. There are several classes in prostatitis: acute, chronic, and asymptomatic [39]. Perineal pain and increased frequency of (painful) voiding are the most common symptoms in chronic prostatitis, whereas in acute prostatitis, symptoms of acute onset of fever and severely tender prostate are on the foreground.

The most common type of infectious agent granulomatous prostatitis is bacillus Calmette-Guérin (BCG). After transurethral resection, intravesical instillation of BCG is administered in patients with nonmuscle-invasive urothelial cell carcinoma [40]. BCG prostatic reflux can be extensive such that the peripheral zone as well as the central and transition zones of the prostate are involved by the inflammatory response [41].

Inadequate treatment of acute prostatitis may result in the transformation into a prostatic abscess. Other causes for abscess include bladder outlet obstruction such as benign prostatic hypertrophy, indwelling urethral catheters, lower urinary tract instrumentation such as cystoscopy, and more invasive procedures such as prostate biopsy [42]. The most common organism causing prostatic abscess is *Escherichia coli*, followed closely by *S. aureus* [43]. With CT, prostatic abscesses appear as a single or multilocular area of low attenuation [44,45]. TRUS and CT of the prostate should only be performed in cases where laboratory analysis is equivocal, when no improvement is observed following medical therapy, and development of urosepsis. Ruling out a prostatic abscess in these patients is a strong indication to proceed to imaging studies. Small abscesses are easier to detect with high-resolution TRUS than with CT. CT can be applied to detect spread beyond the prostate capsule and to plan drainage route.

13.2.4 Benign Prostate Hyperplasia

Worldwide, 30 million men have symptoms related to BPH. This disease occurs normally at the age of 30 or above and also is associated with sexual dysfunction and lower urinary tract symptoms. According to the National Institute of Health, BPH affects more than 50% of men over age 60 and as many as 90% of men over the age of 70.

Benign prostate hyperplasia refers to a regional nodular growth of varying combinations of glandular and stromal proliferation that occurs in almost all men who have testes and who live long enough [46]. BPH is a benign disease of the prostate gland and consists of nodular hypertrophy of the fibrous, muscular, and glandular tissue within the periurethral and transition zones. The exact pathophysiology of BPH in the prostate is unknown. It is probably associated with hormonal changes that occur as men age.

Generally, TRUS of the prostate is performed to assess prostate volume and to rule out prostate cancer. However, TRUS is not indicated for the evaluation of BPH. MDCT has no place in the evaluation of BPH.

13.2.4.1 Prostate Cancer

From autopsy studies, it is known that prostate cancer can be found in 55% of men in their fifth and 64% in their seventh decade of life, respectively. Prostate cancer is very common in elderly males, and it occurs with a lifetime risk of one in ten. MDCT of the prostate has little soft-tissue contrast resolution to discern the different zones within the prostate. Intraprostatic detection of prostate cancer is only possible in advanced stages (i.e., gross capsule invasion; Figure 13.7). The TNM classification system for prostate cancer is presented in Table 13.3. Two studies revealed low sensitivity (26%–29%) with reasonably high specificity (80%–89%) in local staging prostate cancer [47,48]. As a result, MDCT has limited additional value for local staging and detection of prostate cancer.

MDCT pelvis can be performed in high-risk patients (PSA >20, biopsy Gleason score 8–10, or clinical stage T3 disease) for lymph node metastases detection. This patient group has an increased pretest probability for lymph node metastases. Patients with low-risk prostate cancer are unlikely to have metastatic disease documented by bone scan or CT [49]. Size and shape criteria are used to define a lymph node as potentially bearing metastasis [50]. Jager et al. [50] recommended a threshold of 10 mm in the short-axis diameter for oval lymph node and 8 mm for round lymph node as criteria for the diagnosis of lymph node metastases (Figure 13.8). The diagnostic sensitivity and specificity of CT in staging of pelvic lymph nodes in patients with prostate cancer is 0.42 (95% CI 0.26–0.56) and 0.82 (95% CI 0.80–0.83), respectively [51].

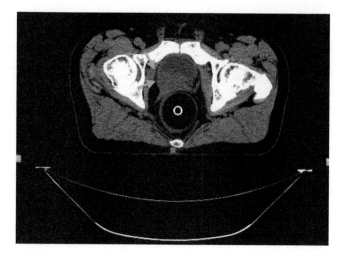

FIGURE 13.7
Stage T4 prostate cancer with invasion in the bladder neck and wall.

TABLE 13.3

Tumor-Node-Metastasis Classification of Prostate Cancer

T—Primary Tumor	
TX	Primary tumor cannot be assessed
T0	No evidence of primary tumor
T1	Clinically inapparent tumor not palpable or visible by imaging
T1a	Tumor incidental histological finding in 5% or less of tissue resected
T1b	Tumor incidental histological finding in more than 5% of tissue resected
T1c	Tumor identified by needle biopsy (e.g., because of elevated PSA-level)
T2	Tumor confined within the prostate
T2a	Tumor involves one half of one lobe or less
T2b	Tumor involves more than half of one lobe, but not both lobes
T2c	Tumor involves both lobes
T3	Tumor extends through the prostatic capsule
T3a	Extracapsular extension (unilateral or bilateral) including microscopic bladder neck involvement
T3b	Tumor invades seminal vesicle(s)
T4	Tumor is fixed or invades adjacent structures other than seminal vesicles: external sphincter, rectum, levator muscles, and/or pelvic wall
N—Regional Lymph Nodes	
NX	Regional lymph nodes cannot be assessed
N0	No regional lymph node metastasis
N1	Regional lymph node metastasis
M—Distant Metastasis	
MX	Distant metastasis cannot be assessed
M0	No distant metastasis
M1	Distant metastasis
M1a	Nonregional lymph node(s)
M1b	Bone(s)
M1c	Other site(s)

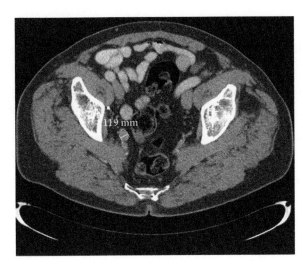

FIGURE 13.8
Pathologic lymph node of 12 mm next to the right internal iliac artery in a patient with stage T3 prostate cancer.

References

1. Siegel R, Naishadham D, Jemal A. Cancer statistics, 2012. *CA Cancer J Clin.* 2012;62(1):10–29.

2. National Cancer Institute. Estimated new cancer cases and deaths for 2012. http://seer.cancer.gov/csr/1975_2009_pops09/results_single/sect_01_table.01.pdf. Accessed June 20, 2013.

3. Verma S, Rajesh A, Prasad SR et al. Urinary bladder cancer: role of MR imaging. *Radiographics.* 2012;32(2):371–87.

4. Wong-You-Cheong JJ, Woodward PJ, Manning MA, Sesterhenn IA. Neoplasms of the urinary bladder: radiologic-pathologic correlation. *Radiographics.* 2006;26(2):553–80.

5. Mills SE, ed. *Histology for Pathologists,* 2nd ed. Philadelphia, PA: Lippincott Williams … Wilkins, 2007.

6. Humphrey PA, Dehner LP, Pfeifer JD. *The Washington Manual of Surgical Pathology.* Philadelphia, PA: Lippincott Williams & Wilkins, 2012.

7. Skinner DG, Lieskovsky G, eds. *Diagnosis and Management of Genitourinary Cancer.* Philadelphia, PA: Saunders, 1988.

8. Edge SB, Byrd DR, Compton CC et al. *Urinary Bladder. AJCC Cancer Staging Manual.* 7th ed. New York, NY: Springer, 2010:497–505.

9. Lamm DL. Carcinoma in situ. *Urol Clin N Am.* 1992;19:499–508.

10. Lamm DL, Herr HW, Jakse G et al. Updated concepts and treatment of carcinoma in situ. *Urol Oncol.* 1998;4:130–8.

11. Murta-Nascimento C, Schmitz-Dräger BJ, Zeegers MP et al. Epidemiology of urinary bladder cancer: from tumor development to patient's death. *World J Urol.* 2007;25(3):285–95.

12. Murphy WM, Grignon DJ, Perlman EJ. *Tumors of the Kidney, Bladder, and Related Urinary Structures.* Washington, DC: American Registry of Pathology, 2004:394.

13. Glas AS, Roos D, Deutekom M, Zwinderman AH, Bossuyt PM, Kurth KH. Tumor markers in the diagnosis of primary bladder cancer. A systematic review. *J Urol.* 2003;169:1975–82.

14. Zeegers MP, Tan FE, Dorant E, van Den Brandt PA. The impact of characteristics of cigarette smoking on urinary tract cancer risk: a meta-analysis of epidemiologic studies. *Cancer.* 2000;89(3):630–9.

15. Kaufman DS, Shipley WU, Feldman AS. Bladder cancer. *Lancet.* 2009;374(9685):239–49.

16. DeFelippo NP, Fortunato RP, Mellins HZ, Richie JP. Intravenous urography: important adjunct for diagnosis of bladder tumours. *Br J Urol.* 1984;56:502–5.

17. Stenzl A, Cowan NC, De Santis M et al. Treatment of muscle-invasive and metastatic bladder cancer: update of the EAU guidelines. *Eur Urol.* 2011;59:1009–18.

18. O'Connor OJ, Fitzgerald E, Maher MM. Imaging of Hematuria. *AJR Am J Roentgenol.* 2010;195:W263–7.

19. Blick CG, Nazir SA, Mallett S et al. Evaluation of diagnostic strategies for bladder cancer using computed tomography (CT) urography, flexible cystoscopy and voided urine cytology: results for 778 patients from a hospital haematuria clinic. *BJU Int.* 2012;110(1):84–94.

20. Van Der Molen AJ, Cowan NC, Mueller-Lisse UG et al. CT urography: definition, indications and techniques. A guideline for clinical practice. *Eur Radiol.* 2008;18(1):4–17.

21. Hillman BJ, Silvert M, Cook G et al. Recognition of bladder tumors by excretory urography. *Radiology.* 1981;138:319–23.

22. Hatch TR, Barry JM. The value of excretory urography in staging bladder cancer. *J Urol.* 1986;135:49.

23. Paik ML, Scolieri MJ, Brown SL, Spirnak JP, Resnick MI. Limitations of computerized tomography in staging invasive bladder cancer before radical cystectomy. *J Urol.* 2000;163:1693–6.

24. Kim JK, Park SY, Ahn HJ, Kim CS, Cho KS. Bladder cancer: analysis of multi-detector row helical CT enhancement pattern and accuracy in tumor detection and perivesical staging. *Radiology.* 2004;231:725–31.

25. Albani JM, Ciaschini MW, Streem SB, Herts BR, Angermeier MW. The role of computerized tomographic urography in the initial evaluation of hematuria. *J Urol.* 2007;177:644–8.

26. Turney BW, Willatt JMC, Nixon D, Crew JP, Cowan NC. Computed tomography for diagnosing bladder cancer. *BJU Int.* 2006;98:345–8.

27. Clayman RV, Reddy P, Lange PH. Flexible fiberoptic and rigid-rod lens endoscopy of the lower urinary tract: a prospective controlled comparison. *J Urol.* 1984;131:715–6.

28. Wang LJ, Wong YC, Ng KF, Chuang CK, Lee SY, Wan YL. Tumor characteristics of urothelial carcinoma on multidetector computerized tomography urography. *J Urol.* 2010;183:2154–60.

29. Nolte-Ernsting C, Cowan NC. Understanding multislice CT urography techniques: many roads lead to Rome. *Eur Radiol.* 2006;16:2670–86.

30. Ficarra V, Dalpiaz O, Alrabi N, Novara G, Galfano A, Artibani W. Correlation between clinical and pathological

staging in a series of radical cystectomies for bladder carcinoma. *BJU Int*. 2005;95:786–90.

31. Barentsz JO, Jager GJ, Witjes JA, Ruijs SHJ. Primary staging of urinary bladder carcinoma: the role of MR imaging and a comparison with CT. *Eur Radiol*. 1996;6:134–9.

32. MacVicar AD. Bladder cancer staging. *BJ Int*. 2000;86 Suppl 1:111–22.

33. Husband JE, Olliff JF, Williams MP, Heron CW, Cherryman GR. Bladder cancer: staging with CT and MR imaging. *Radiology*. 1989;173:435–40.

34. Baltaci S, Resorlu B, Yagci C, Turkolmez K, Gogus C, Beduk Y. Computerized tomography for detecting perivesical infiltration and lymph node metastasis in invasive bladder carcinoma. *Urol Int*. 2008;81:399–402.

35. Tritschler S, Mosler C, Straub J et al. Staging of muscle-invasive bladder cancer: can computerized tomography help us to decide on local treatment? *World J Urol*. 2011;30(6):827–31.

36. Barentsz JO, Witjes JA, Ruijs SHJ. What is new in bladder cancer imaging. *Urol Clin North Am*. 1997;24:583–602.

37. Dhar NB, Klein EA, Reuther AM, Thalmann GN, Madersbacher S, Studer UE. Outcome after radical cystectomy with limited or extended pelvic lymph node dissection. *J Urol*. 2008;179(3):873–8; discussion 878.

38. Dighe MK, Bhargava P, Wright J. Urinary bladder masses: techniques, imaging spectrum, and staging. *J Comput Assist Tomogr*. 2011;35(4):411–24.

39. Krieger JN, Riley DE, Cheah PY, Liong ML, Yuen KH. Epidemiology of prostatitis: new evidence for a worldwide problem. *World J Urol*. 2003;21:70–4.

40. Krieger JN, Nyberg L, Nickel JC. NIH consensus definition and classification of prostatitis. *JAMA*. 1999;282(3):236–7.

41. Lamm DL, van der Meijden PM, Morales A et al. Incidence and treatment of complication of bacillus Calmette-Guérin intravesical therapy in superficial bladder cancer. *J Urol*. 1992;147:596–600.

42. Humphrey PA. BCG prostatitis. *J Urol*. 2012;188(3): 961–2.

43. Dattilo WR, Shiber J. Prostatitis or prostatic abscess. J Emerg Med. 2013;44(1):e121-2.

44. Weinberger M, Cytron S, Servadio C, Block C, Rosenfeld JB, Pitlik SD. Prostatic abscess in the antibiotic era. *Rev Infect Dis*. 1998;10:239–49.

45. Davidson KC, Garlow WB, Brewer J. Computerized tomography of prostatic and periurethral abscess: 2 case reports. *J Urol*. 1986;135:1257–8.

46. Hanno PM, Malkowicz SB, Win AJ. *Chapter 14, Penn Clinical Manual of Urology*, 1st ed. Philadelphia, PA: Saunders-Elsevier, 2007.

47. Tarcan T, Turkeri L, Biren T, Küllü S, Gürmen N, Akdaş A. The effectiveness of imaging modalities in clinical staging of localized prostatic carcinoma. *Int Urol Nephrol*. 1996;28:773–9.

48. Barbieri A, Monica B, Sebastio N, Incarbone GP, Di Stefano C. Value and limitations of transrectal ultrasonography and computer tomography in preoperative staging of prostate carcinoma. *Acta Biomed Ateneo Parmense*. 1997;68:23–6.

49. Abuzallouf S, Dayes I, Lukka H. Baseline staging of newly diagnosed prostate cancer: a summary of the literature. *J Urol*. 2004;171:2122–7.

50. Jager GJ, Barentsz JO, Oosterhof GO, Witjes JA, Ruijs SJ. Pelvic adenopathy in prostatic and urinary bladder carcinoma: MR imaging with a three-dimensional TI-weighted magnetization-prepared-rapid gradient-echo sequence. *AJR Am J Roentgenol*. 1996;167:1503–7.

51. Hövels AM, Heesakkers RA, Adang EM. The diagnostic accuracy of CT and MRI in the staging of pelvic lymph nodes in patients with prostate cancer: a meta-analysis. *Clin Radiol*. 2008;63:387–95.

14

Female Pelvis: Uterus, Ovaries, Fallopian Tubes, and Vagina

Valdair Muglia, Jorge Elias Jr., and Fabiano Lucchesi

CONTENTS

14.1 Introduction

Although ultrasonography (US) remains the method of choice for evaluation of female pelvic abnormalities because of its great availability, lack of contralateral effects and good accuracy, with a few authors claiming that magnetic resonance imaging (MRI) should be the "next step" or problem-solving method, considering its higher specificity, the use of computed tomography (CT) imaging in pelvic diseases has steadily increased in the last years. The introduction of multi-detector CT (MDCT) significantly improved accuracy of CT, allowing high-resolution images in several planes, facilitating the diagnosis.

This chapter will focus on the CT techniques employed to evaluate the most frequent female pelvic affections as well as the most frequent indications and respective tomographic findings.

14.2 Normal Anatomy of Female Pelvis

The detailed approach of the anatomical structures that constitute the female pelvis is beyond the scope of this chapter. Here, only those aspects of normal radiologic anatomy essential for better understanding of the diseases included in the text, especially those details more relevant for tomographic images, have been described.

14.2.1 Uterus

The normal uterus shows pyriform shape and central or lateral position in the pelvis. It has been described, roughly, as three different parts, namely fundus, body, and cervix (Figure 14.1). During pregnancy, it is still possible to individualize the isthmus, located between the body and cervix. The uterus varies in appearance depending on the phase of menstrual and reproductive cycle of women. The orientation of the major axis of the body and cervix may be different, assuming importance in the planning and interpretation of imaging studies, depending on their clinical indication. The uterus is considered anteflexed or retroflexed when the major axis of the body of the uterus is anterior or posterior in relation to the cervix, respectively. Uterus is called anteverted or retroverted when the major axis of the cervix in relation into the major axis of the vagina assumes a posterior or anterior position [1].

There are three distinct zones in the body of the uterus: endometrium, junctional zone, and myometrium [2]. The endometrium comprises the inner portion of the uterine corpus, usually presenting as low-density tubular image, dividing the corpus. It varies in thickness in accordance with the menstrual cycle and female hormone level [3].

The junctional zone lies between the endometrium and myometrium; however, it is not often seen on CT images. Its thickness is variable according to the patient's age and hormonal changes. The upper limit of normal range described in the medical literature is 8 mm [4]. The myometrium is slightly darker than endometrium on CT images.

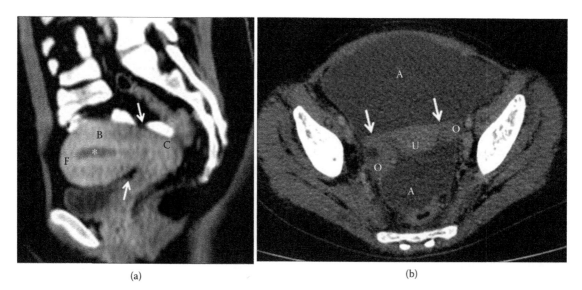

(a)   (b)

FIGURE 14.1
(a) Sagittal reformatation showing uterine anatomy. C: cervix; B: body; F: fundus. Asterisk indicates the endometrial cavity and arrows anterior and posterior cul-de sac. (b) Axial—Patient with severe ascites that improves visualization of broad ligament (arrows), ovaries (O) and uterus (U).

14.2.2 Cervix

The cervix usually shows a cylindrical appearance, starting in the lower body portion and protruding into vaginal lumen. It communicates the uterine cavity through the vagina by endocervical canal. The portion that projects into the vagina is named ectocervix, and the remaining portion corresponds to the supravaginal cervix. It consists predominantly of muscle and fibrous component while the endocervical canal is outlined by columnar epithelium. On CT images, one can distinguish only the endocervical canal and the muscular mass of the cervix [3,5].

14.2.3 Vagina

The vagina is a fibromuscular tubular structure, with walls showing a hypodense appearance on CT images. It is divided into three segments, using the bladder as reference [2]. The proximal portion contains the fornix surrounding the cervix [1] and the distal opens in the vulva.

14.2.4 Parametrium

The parametrium is a band of fibrous tissue between the layers of broad ligament, formed by the cardinal and uterosacral ligaments, extending laterally to the cervix [6]. The parametrium contains ovarian ligament, uterine and ovarian blood vessels, nerves, lymphatic vessels, mesonephric remnants, and the distal portion of the ureter. Although the broad ligament is rarely

seen, when ascites is present, it is possible to detect all these anatomic details (Figure 14.2) [5]. It also represents an important anatomical reference in the staging of cancer of the cervix [6].

14.2.5 Vaginal Recesses

The peritoneal reflections in the pelvis create two virtual spaces around the uterus. Peritoneum covers the vesical roof, descends to cover almost the entire posterior bladder surface until the level of the uterine cervix, and then goes upside in the whole anterior uterine wall. The space formed on this route is called anterior cul-de-sac. After covering the uterine fundus, the peritoneal membrane descends along its posterior wall, until the rectovaginal septum, when bends to describe an ascending trajectory on the anterior rectal surface. This space is called posterior cul-de-sac, extensively known by the eponym, Douglas' cul-de-sac (Figure 14.1a).

14.2.6 Ovaries

The ovaries can be detected by CT images since prepuberal ages. They are better visualized during the reproductive phase when they are usually identified on CT images by oval images with homogeneous low density, except when functional cysts and/or follicles are seen as more hypodense structures (Figure 14.1b). Usually, the amount of hemorrhage created by follicle disruption in ovulation is not enough to be detected by tomographic images.

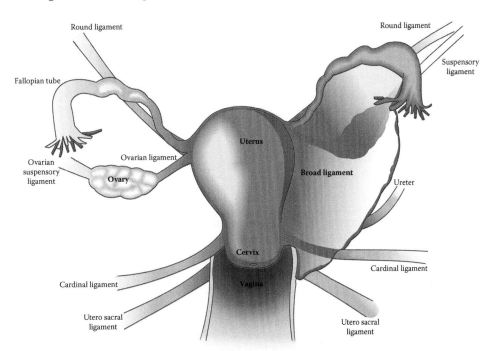

FIGURE 14.2
Drawing showing the main ligaments involving uterus and ovaries.

14.2.7 Pelvic Ligaments

As mentioned earlier, the broad ligament is a large peritoneal fold formed by two layers of peritoneum, draped over the uterus with lateral extension to pelvic wall. The superior limit is given by the fallopian tube medially and the suspensory ligament of the ovary more laterally, and the inferior edge of the broad ligament ends at the cardinal ligament (Figure 14.2).

The round ligament is a sheet of fibroconnective tissue attached to the anterolateral uterine fundus, inferior and anterior to the fallopian tube and anterior to the ovarian ligament. It has an oblique course within the broad ligament to enter the internal inguinal ring ending in the labia majora. The round ligament is seen on CT images as a thin soft-tissue band extending laterally from the fundus and gradually tapering from its relatively broad uterine base.

14.3 Protocols and Techniques

When a female pelvic CT is ordered, patients usually have been evaluated previously with transvaginal ultrasound (TVUS) or other imaging method. It is very important to know what indication was for CT scanning and ask patients to bring all the previous examination reports. Patients are instructed to fast for about 4–6 hours. It is not necessary to scan with a full distended bladder; however, a good degree of vesical filling improves bladder and uterine evaluation since uterine anteversion may be (partially) corrected. The use of antiperistaltic drugs, such as hyoscine butylbromide, intravenously or intramuscularly, is not recommended since MDCT scanning times is too short. In our daily clinical practice, we use gel to distend the vaginal lumen, allowing better assessment of the cervix and vagina [7,8], especially when assessing uterine neoplasias. The examination is performed with the patient in supine position only, except when questions about bladder wall status arise and prone position may add information [8].

The pelvis should be imaged using thin sections of 1–2 mm width and high-resolution matrix (512 × 512, at least). Although frequently used in the past, we have not performed noncontrast pelvic CT imaging, except when urinary lithiasis is suspected. There is no need for dynamic contrast-enhanced series in the pelvis. Sometimes, when secondary involvement of bladder wall is suspected, a delayed series, with full bladder distension may be necessary. Contrast-enhanced images are obtained after injection of 80–200 mL iodinated contrast, depending on patient's weight, usually 1.5–2.0 mL·kg^{-1} [9,10].

An important issue when using CT imaging is radiation dose control. This has been detailed in Chapter 2 of the first book in this series, but is always valuable to remind that imaging should be made the less harmful as possible.

14.4 Uterine Diseases

14.4.1 Congenital Malformations

Congenital uterine malformations result from altered development of the Müllerian ducts during fetal life. The prevalence rates vary greatly, with reports ranging from 0.06% to 38%, which can be partially explained by the lack of a standardized classification system. Nonetheless, once a Müllerian duct anomaly (MDA) is identified, it is important to correctly classify the anomaly as women with history of miscarriage and infertility have higher prevalence of congenital uterine anomalies compared with unselected population [11].

Because of the intrinsic uterine anatomy, composed mainly by muscular tissue, CT findings of congenital uterine malformations are often inconspicuous. Most of the cases will show an enlarged uterus only. However, in particular cases, mainly in those with complications related to partial uterine obstruction in duplicated anomalies, it is possible to have findings that can simulate parauterine thick-wall cystic-like lesions.

Many consider the combination of laparoscopy or laparotomy with hysteroscopy or hysterosalpingography to be the best evaluation to classify these anomalies; however, all these methods are invasive. Three-dimensional ultrasound and dedicate pelvic MRI are noninvasive methods that can play an important role in this setting, allowing to classify the anomaly. A modified Buttram and Gibbons classification is widely used and should be known (Table 14.1).

14.4.2 Leiomyomas and Other Benign Tumors

Uterine leiomyomas, or fibroids, are benign neoplasm of smooth-muscle cell origin interspersed with fibrous connective tissue. It is the most common pelvic tumor found in women, reportedly present in greater than 20% of women over the age of 30. Although US is the modality of choice to evaluate uterine leiomyomas, the high prevalence of this benign tumor makes it a frequently encountered finding in CT exams performed for other clinical indications [13,14].

Most women with leiomyomas are asymptomatic, presenting as incidental findings in imaging exams. Symptoms that may relate to leiomyomas are palpable pelvic mass and/or pelvic pain, and increased and

TABLE 14.1

Modified Buttram and Gibbons Classification of MDA

Class I	Segmental agenesis or hypoplasia	It may occur as part of a congenital syndrome or as a result of chromosomal defects.
Class II	Unicornuate uterus	This anomaly is the result of non- or rudimentary development of one Müllerian duct.
Class III	Uterus didelphys	Result of nearly complete failure of fusion of the Müllerian ducts. No communication is present between the duplicated endometrial cavities. Nonobstructive uterus didelphys is usually asymptomatic. Unilateral vaginal obstruction may become symptomatic at menarche and manifest as dysmenorrhea.
Class IV	Bicornuate uterus	Incomplete fusion of the uterovaginal horns at the level of the fundus. Accounts for approximately 10% of MDA. Consists of two symmetric cornua that are fused caudal, with communication of the endometrial cavities.
Class V	Septate uterus	Failure of resorption of the final fibrous septum between the two Müllerian ducts results in a septate uterus. It is the most common MDA (55%) and has a high association with infertility.
Class VI	Arcuate uterus	Characterized by a mild indentation of the endometrium at the uterine fundus as a result of near complete resorption of the uterovaginal septum.
Class VII	Diethylstilbesterol (DES) exposure	DES, a synthetic estrogen agent, was frequently used until the 1970s in pregnant women with vaginal bleeding, in an attempt to prevent miscarriage.

Source: Buttram VC, Gibbons WE. *Fertil Steril* 1979; 32:40–46.

disproportionate vaginal bleeding. All of these can be associated with compressive symptoms (bladder, uterus, and rectum). The clinical findings of uterine leiomyomas can often be correlated to the location and size of the lesion, that is, subserosal, intramural, or submucosal, as well as fundic, cornual, cervical, or uterine body. Uterine leiomyomas may grow in response to an estrogenic stimulus, increasing in size during pregnancy or with oral contraceptive treatment. They do not appear until after menarche and usually reduce in size after menopause.

Most of leiomyomas have the same CT attenuation of myometrium and can be overlooked. When detected by CT, most leiomyomas without any kind of degeneration cause uterine enlargement and/or lobulated uterine contour (Figure 14.3) [14,15]. Diverse degenerative changes may occur in leiomyomas resulting in several CT features correlating with pathological changes as cystic degeneration, calcification, infection, necrosis, or fatty degeneration (Figure 14.4). The presence of calcification, usually a coarse dystrophic type, is the most specific sign of leiomyoma (Figure 14.5) [14]. Enhancement of leiomyoma varies on CT, and areas of low attenuation within a leiomyoma after contrast administration may suggest the possibility of degeneration or infarction [13,15]. There are many reports describing unusual CT features in rare manifestations of leiomyoma or in complications [16–18]. CT was proved accurate in detecting twisted subserosal leiomyoma, although being able to depict the torsion of the vascular pedicle [17].

Uterine artery embolization (UAE) has been increasingly used to treat patients with symptomatic uterine fibroids. CT following UAE may be requested because

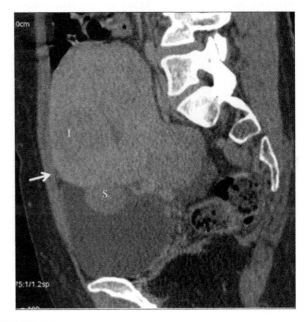

FIGURE 14.3
Sagittal reformation. An enlarged uterus exhibits intramural (I) and subserosal (S) leiomyomas causing focal bulging of uterine contours (arrow).

of acute pelvic pain, chest discomfort, or pyrexia, and/or for complications that may require treatment in acute phase [19]. Visualization of gas in uterus and uterine vessels following UAE is an expected finding that should not be misinterpreted as a sign of infection [19]. A branching serpiginous linear distribution of gas may be seen in uterine vessels up to 1 month after UAE without associated clinical signs to suggest infection [19]. The differentiation between postembolization syndrome

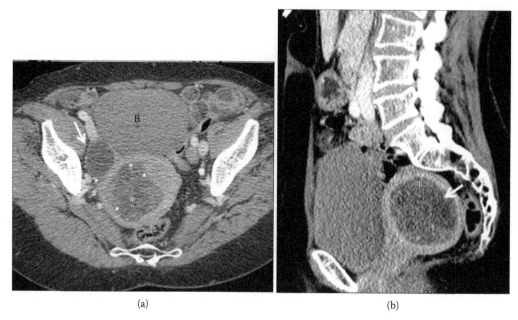

(a)   (b)

FIGURE 14.4
Leiomyoma with fat degeneration. (a) Axial image showing a distended bladder (B) and a very hypodense leiomyoma (*). A functional cyst is seen in the right ovary (arrow). (b) Sagittal reformation showing areas of very low density compatible with fat (arrow). (Courtesy of Prof. Antonio Westphalen, University of California, San Francisco.)

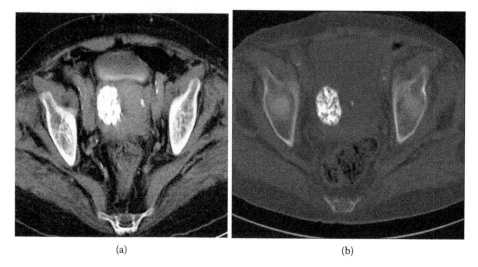

(a)   (b)

FIGURE 14.5
Heavily calcified leiomyoma. (a) and (b) Axial images with soft-tissue and bone settings showing an irregular and coarse calcium deposit in a subserosal leiomyoma, the most typical appearance.

and infection is of paramount importance and must be accomplished through clinic–laboratory correlation and good communication between the gynecologist and the radiologist.

Rarely, myometrium neoplasia may be malignant, a leiomyosarcoma. The incidence of malignant neoplasia is less than 1.0% and has been estimated to be as low as 0.2%. Differentiation between leiomyoma and leiomyosarcoma is not possible by imaging alone and we must rely on histopathological exams in cases where a rapid

enlargement of a uterine fibroid-like lesion is documented [13].

14.4.3 Endometrial Polyps and Hyperplasia

The endometrial cavity of the uterus is central, flat, and triangular [20]. The endometrium in premenopausal women appears as a hypodense, hypovascular stripe relative to myometrium, with variable thickness, according to the menstrual cycle. In postmenopausal women, the endometrium is frequently atrophic and not seen at CT, although it can be confidently seen in approximately one-half of asymptomatic postmenopausal women on routine contrast-enhanced CT examinations [21]. Sagittal reconstruction images are helpful to further evaluate the endometrium on CT [20]. Homogenous fluid-attenuation endometrial cavity content may occur in elderly with substenotic cervix because of mucus accumulation (Figure 14.6). However, a thickened endometrium or the presence of fluid within the endometrial canal in postmenopausal women who are complaining of vaginal bleeding is suspicious for malignancy. In this setting, it is important to apply the correct upper limit of the short-axis endometrial thickness of 12 mm, as reported by Lim et al., to prevent overdiagnosis of endometrial fluid or thickening in asymptomatic women [21]. Endometrial thickness above 12 mm requires further work up diagnosis and possible etiologies would be endometrial hyperplasia and neoplasm. However, the sensitivity of CT for diagnosing a thickened endometrium previously identified by TVUS was reported as low as 53.1% [20].

Endometrial hyperplasia is an abnormal proliferation of endometrial stroma and glands and represents a spectrum of endometrial changes ranging from glandular atypia to frank neoplasia [22]. A definitive diagnosis can be made only with biopsy, and imaging cannot reliably allow differentiation between hyperplasia and carcinoma. Up to one-third of endometrial carcinoma is believed to be preceded by hyperplasia [22].

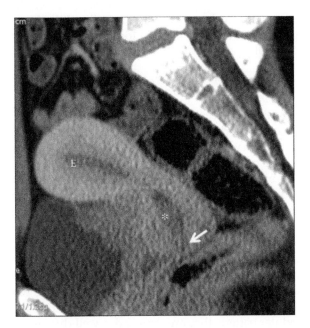

FIGURE 14.6
Endocervix stenosis. The endocervical canal (*) and the endometrium (E) are distended by mucous accumulation secondary to a substenotic exocervix (arrow).

Endometrial polyp is a benign nodular protrusion of the endometrial surface that consists of irregularly distributed endometrial glands and stroma. It is composed of a stroma of focally or diffusely dense fibrous or smooth muscle tissue, thick-walled vessels, and endometrial glands. Endometrial polyps represent a common cause of postmenopausal bleeding and are most frequently seen in patients receiving unopposed estrogens, such as tamoxifen [22]. CT may show a thickened endometrium stripe in cases of endometrial polyps; however, diagnosis cannot be established by CT only. To date, there are no reports in the literature of endometrial polyp findings on CT, although it is possible to anticipate that polyps would be hyperdense after injection of contrast because of their hypervascularization. Newer CT techniques as virtual hysteroscopy have been reported and may improve the evaluation of endometrial cavity by CT [23].

14.4.4 Uterine Neoplasms

14.4.4.1 Cervical

Cervical cancer is the third most common gynecologic malignancy. Worldwide, there are an estimated 529,000 new cases of cervical cancer and 275,000 deaths per year [24]. About 85% of cancers and 80% of deaths from cervical cancer occur in developing countries [24]. Approximately 85% of the cases are squamous cell carcinoma and most of the remaining cases correspond to adenocarcinoma. Uncommon subtypes include adenosquamous carcinoma, lymphoma, adenoma malignum, and small-cell carcinoma, the latter tending to be locally invasive, as well to have distant metastases [25]. Cervical carcinoma arises from a precursor lesion of dysplasia affecting the cervical epithelium and it is typically related to prior infection with human papillomavirus (HPV). The HPV vaccine has been shown to prevent potentially precancerous lesions of the cervix, and a reduction in incidence is projected in the near future.

The prognosis for patients with cervical cancer is markedly affected by the extent of disease at the time of diagnosis. The prognosis is based on the stage (Table 14.2 and Figure 14.7), volume, and grade of tumor; histologic type; status of the lymph nodes; and vascular invasion. Assessment of the stage of disease is important in determining whether the patient may benefit from surgery or will receive radiation therapy.

CT can be used for staging advanced disease, planning radiation therapy, and monitoring recurrence, although because of inferior contrast resolution, it has been replaced by MRI. More recently, MDCT technology has improved CT staging for cervical cancer because of thinner slices, better spatial resolution, and the availability of multiplanar reconstructions, allowing better detection of parametrial extension, pelvic sidewall invasion, local organ involvement, adenopathy, local tumor recurrence,

TABLE 14.2

FIGO Cervical Cancer Staging

Stage 0	Carcinoma in situ (preinvasive)
Stage I	Tumor confined to uterus
IA	Microscopic invasion only
IA1	Stromal invasion not more than 3 mm deep and 7 mm wide
IA2	Stromal invasion more than 3 mm but not more than 5 mm deep, and not more than 7 mm wide
IB	Clinically visible lesion or lesion greater in size than IA2
IB1	More than 5 mm deep, and more than 7 mm wide
IB2	Larger than 4 cm in greatest dimension
Stage II	Tumor invasion beyond cervix but not to pelvic wall or lower third of vagina
IIA	No parametrial invasion
IIB	Parametrial invasion
Stage III	Tumor extension to pelvic wall and/or lower third of vagina and/or tumor causing hydronephrosis or nonfunctioning kidney
IIIA	Tumor involvement of the lower third of the vagina without pelvic sidewall involvement
IIIB	Tumor involvement of the pelvic sidewall and/or hydronephrosis or a nonfunctioning kidney
Stage IV	
IVA	Tumor invasion of bladder or rectum and/or extension beyond true pelvis
IVB	Distant metastasis

Source: Data from Pecorelli S, *Int J Gynaecol Obstet,*105(2):103–104, 2009.

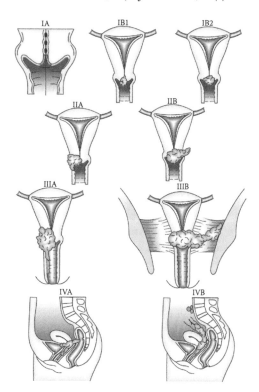

FIGURE 14.7
Drawing depicting FIGO staging for cervical uterine cancer. (Adapted from Narayan K, Mckenzie AF, Hicks RJ, Fisher R, Bernshaw D, Bau S. *Int J Gynecol Cancer* 2003; 13:657–663.)

and distant metastatic disease [15]. Nonetheless, a recent ACRIN® trial reported that CT had sensitivity of only 42% for detecting advanced disease, with sensitivity and specificity for detecting parametrial invasion ranging from 14% to 38% and 84% to 100%, respectively [27,28].

The primary tumor CT features include heterogeneous mass that is hypoattenuating relative to normal stroma after injection of contrast agent (Figure 14.8). Areas of low attenuation secondary to necrosis, ulceration, or reduced vascularity may occur [29]. Up to 50% of stage IB cervical cancers still are described as undetectable because they are isodense to normal cervical parenchyma [30]. Microscopic and small-volume cervical tumors cannot be identified by CT.

CT staging of cervical carcinoma comprises the evaluation of periureteral fat plane for direct parametrial extension, evaluation distance of tumor from pelvic muscles and vessels, and evaluation of lymph nodes. Encasement of the ureter and parametrial soft-tissue mass is considered specific sign of parametrial invasion on CT (Figure 14.9). Other signs of parametrial disease are perivascular invasion and thickening of the uterosacral ligaments. When stranding of the parametrial fat is present, it must be greater than 3–4 mm thick to be considered as parametrial invasion, as inflammatory tissue (or even normal parametrial structures) may also appear as soft-tissue strands [4].

Diagnosis of pelvic wall invasion can be made if there is a gap less than 3 mm between the tumor and pelvic muscles or if there is vascular encasement [30]. Cervical cancer can spread along the external iliac vessels, internal iliac vessels, and presacral tissues [30]. All three routes of spread lead to the common iliac lymph nodes (Figure 14.10) and, eventually, to the para-aortic lymph nodes [30].

14.4.4.2 Endometrial Cancer

Endometrial cancer is the most common gynecologic malignancy in developed countries, accounting for 6% of all cancers in women, with approximately 40,000 new cases reported in the United States each year [31]. Typically, it occurs in perimenopausal women and has risk factors associated with increased estrogen exposure such as nulliparity, chronic anovulation, and obesity [25]. Postmenopausal uterine bleeding is the main symptom and lead to early detection in majority of cases. Endometrial cancer has the best prognosis of the gynecologic cancers, with a 5-year relative survival rate of 86% [15,32]. The most prevalent histologic subtype is endometrioid adenocarcinoma, which account for 75% to 80% of all cases [33]. Depending on the glandular pattern, they are classified as well-differentiated (grade 1) to anaplastic (grade 3) tumors [32].

The role of imaging in endometrial cancer comprises the evaluation of symptomatic patients for a possible

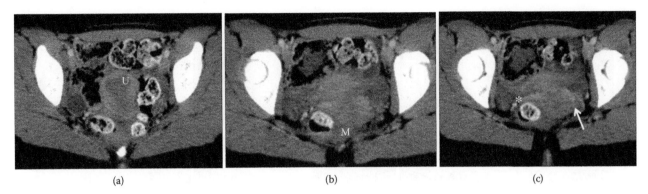

FIGURE 14.8
(a), (b), and (c) Uterine cervix cancer. Axial postcontrast images. (a) The endometrial space (U) is distended because of cervical obstruction caused by a mass (M) seen on (b) and (c) images. The mass shows heterogeneous enhancement with several hypovascular areas (arrow in [c]) and invades the parametrium, asterisk in (c).

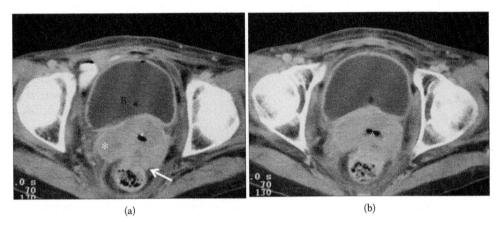

FIGURE 14.9
Invasive cervical uterine neoplasia. (a) and (b) An invasive lesion is seen extending from the cervix to the rectum (arrow). Laterally, the lesion involves the parametrium (*), but there is no pelvic wall extension. A small amount of gas (^) is seen within the cervical canal on (b). (B = bladder).

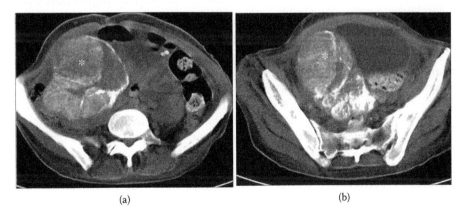

FIGURE 14.10
Metastatic uterine cervical cancer. (a) and (b) Axial images of the pelvis showing a large mass (*), partially calcified (hyperdense areas) in the projection of right iliac lymphatic chain in a patient with nodal recurrence.

endometrial abnormality, which is best accomplished by TVUS, characterization, and staging of disease in those with known pathology, which was previously detected by CT, MRI, or PET-CT [25].

As mentioned, the sensitivity of CT to detect a thickened endometrium is as low as 53.1% [20], thus CT is not useful to diagnose endometrial cancer. However, endometrial cancer cases may appear on CT as an enlarged uterus, and, occasionally, a mass, usually hypodense to the normal uterine tissue, will be displayed causing heterogeneous attenuation in the endometrium and/or myometrium (Figure 14.11) [15]. CT images after contrast

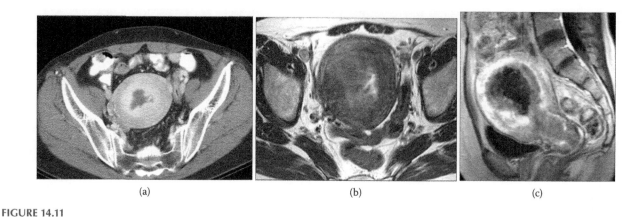

(a)   (b)   (c)

FIGURE 14.11
Endometrial carcinoma. (a) Computed tomography (CT) postcontrast image. An infiltrative lesion is seen extending to the inner myometrium (arrow) in an enlarged uterus. (b) and (c) Axial T2 and Sagittal T1-weighted postcontrast magnetic resonance (MR) images. The invasive nature of the lesion is clearly seen on axial T2 (arrow) and also the hypovascular pattern of tumor is reinforced on MR images. The lesion extends inferiorly until the cervix (arrow in [c]).

TABLE 14.3

FIGO Endometrial Carcinoma Staging

	Primary tumor cannot be assessed
	No evidence of primary tumor
0	Carcinoma in situ (preinvasive carcinoma)
I	Tumor confined to corpus uteri
IA	Tumor limited to endometrium or invades less than one-half of the myometrium
IB	Tumor invades one-half or more of the myometrium
II	Tumor invades stromal connective tissue of the cervix but does not extend beyond the uterus
IIIA	Tumor involves serosa and/or adnexa (direct extension or metastasis)
IIIB	Vaginal involvement (direct extension or metastasis) or parametrial involvement
IVA	Tumor invades bladder mucosa and/or bowel mucosa (bullous edema is not sufficient to classify a tumor as T4)

injection may show an enhancing lesion in the myometrium. A fluid-filled endometrial cavity may signify an obstructing tumor or may be secondary to surgery or radiation.

Staging of endometrial cancer is based on surgico-pathologic International Federation of Gynecology and Obstetrics (FIGO) criteria, as shown in Table 14.3.

CT is valuable for staging endometrial cancer with reported sensitivity of 83% and specificity of 42% for the assessment of depth of myometrial invasion, and a sensitivity of 25% and a specificity of 70% for the depiction of cervical invasion [34]. A more recent study using a 16-row CT scanner has shown sensitivity, specificity, and accuracy for evaluating myometrial invasion of 100%, 80%, and 95%, respectively, and for assessing cervical infiltration of 78%, 83%, and 81%, respectively [35]. So, although MRI remains as the preferred imaging method to stage endometrial cancer, CT can be considered an alternative to MRI examination [35].

For detection of extrauterine disease, accuracy of CT is approximately 86% [15]. CT can demonstrate invasion to the adjacent organs, such as bladder and rectum [32]. Distant metastases from endometrial cancer are most often seen in extrapelvic lymph nodes and peritoneum (Figure 14.12) [32]. Nodal metastases from endometrial cancer involve pelvic and para-aortic nodes, similarly to cervical cancer (Figure 14.10) [25]. Middle and inferior uterine tumors drain to the parametrial and obturatory nodes, whereas proximal body and fundus tumors drain to the common iliac and para-aortic nodes. Endometrial cancer can also spread via the round ligament to inguinal nodes [25]. The likelihood of nodal spread increases in the presence of greater than 50% invasion of the myometrium and also with higher tumor histologic grade [25].

14.4.4.3 Gestational Trophoblastic Neoplasms

Gestational trophoblastic neoplasms (GTNs) encompass a spectrum of placental lesions from the premalignant hydatidiform mole (complete and partial) through malignant invasive mole, choriocarcinoma, and the rare placental site trophoblastic tumor [36]. Despite treatment, up to 20% of hydatidiform mole can develop malignant disease. All these patients must be followed with serial blood tests for beta human chorionic gonadotropin (beta-HCG). If beta-HCG increases or maintain high serum levels, patients must be assessed for possible metastases [37].

Ultrasound remains the method of choice for initial diagnosis, and can also predict invasive and recurrent disease. MRI has an increasing use in assessing extrauterine tumor spread, tumor vascularity, and overall staging. The role of CT in GTN is essentially in the detection of metastatic disease. Even so, Sanders and Rubin (1987) reported three different types of CT appearance of GTN: (1) uterus of normal size containing irregular central or eccentric areas of hypodensity (Figure 14.13), (2) uniformly enlarged

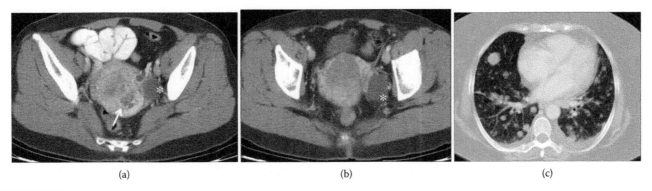

FIGURE 14.12
Metastatic endometrial carcinoma. (a) and (b) CT postcontrast images showing an enlarged uterus with an ill-defined mass (M) that is seen invading myometrium and abutting uterine contours with fat stranding (arrows in [a] and [b]). There is an enlarged lymph node on left iliac chain (N). (c) Axial image of chest with lung settings. Several soft-tissue nodules throughout both lungs. Small amount of bilateral pleural effusion.

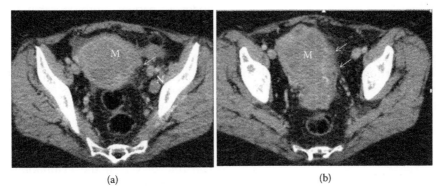

FIGURE 14.13
Gestational trophoblastic neoplasia. (a) and (b) Axial, postcontrast images demonstrating an infiltrative lesion within the endometrium, involving the myometrium of posterior wall of the uterine body. Small vesicles, giving the aspect of "grapefruit," are seen in (a) (arrow). Theca-lutein cysts are seen in the left ovary (asterisk in [a] and [b]). (Courtesy of Prof. Antonio Westphalen, University of California San Francisco.)

uterus with areas of hypodensity, and (3) lobular uterus with focal uterine or cervical enlargement [38]. They also described that 50% of the third type had irregular areas of hypodensity. Extrauterine pelvic disease may appear on CT exams as bilateral ovarian enlargement with multilocular theca lutein cysts (Figure 14.13). Enhancing parametrial soft tissue is characteristic of local spread.

Metastatic disease occurs in up to 19% of all GTN, mainly in choriocarcinoma [37]. The route of spread is hematogenous, and most commonly metastases occur in the lungs, in up to 87% [37].

14.5 Vulva, Vagina, and Urethra

14.5.1 Normal Variants and Congenital Diseases

The vagina is seen as a rectangular soft-tissue structure inferior to the cervix (Figure 14.1). The vulva is seen as a triangular soft-tissue structure. Vaginal congenital anomalies as atresia, vaginal duplication, and abnormalities of

gonadal differentiation and ambiguous genitalia can occur, but CT resolution is suboptimal to depict these anomalies. Eventually, Gartner's duct cysts can be seen on CT.

14.5.2 Benign and Malignant Masses

Benign tumors of the vagina are rare. Some reported tumors include neurofibromas, hemangiomas, fibroepithelial polyps, leiomyomas, rhabdomyomas, and Müllerian mixed tumors. They typically present as mobile rounded submucosal or polypoid masses. Simple excision is both diagnostic and therapeutic in these cases.

14.5.3 Carcinoma of the Vagina

Vaginal cancer is a rare gynecologic malignancy representing only 1%–2% of all gynecologic neoplasms [39]. According to the FIGO, cases should be classified as vaginal carcinomas only after the exclusion of cervical, urethral, or vulvar origins [39]. Carcinoma of the vagina occurs mainly in postmenopausal females, 85%–90%

above 50 years [40]. Eighty to ninety percent of primary vaginal malignancies are squamous cell carcinomas and approximately 5%–10% are adenocarcinomas. The leading risk factor for vaginal intraepithelial neoplasia and subsequent squamous cell vaginal carcinoma is long-lasting infection with HPV type 16 [40].

Prognosis of the disease depends on age, histologic type, and tumor stage (Table 14.4).

Five-year survival rates are about 95% for stage 0, 75% for stage I, 60% for stage II, 35% for stage III, and 20% for stage IVA [39]. CT can provide information about the size, shape, and position of the tumor, and is used to evaluate direct spreading to paravaginal tissues, other organs, or pelvic wall, as well as to evaluate regional and distant lymph nodes (Figure 14.14).

14.5.4 Vulvar Cancer

Vulvar cancer is a rare malignancy in women accounting for 4%–5% of the genital malignancies [41]. It occurs in elderly women with peak of incidence in eighth decade of age, although the proportion of young patients has risen fourfold because of its association with HPV infections [41]. It is most commonly squamous cell carcinoma

TABLE 14.4

FIGO Vaginal Cancer Staging

	Primary tumor cannot be assessed
	No evidence of primary tumor
0	Carcinoma in situ
I	Tumor confined to vagina
II	Tumor invades paravaginal tissues but not to pelvic wall
III	Tumor extends to pelvic wall[a]
IVA	Tumor invades mucosa of the bladder or rectum and/ or extends beyond the true pelvis (Bullous edema is not sufficient evidence to classify a tumor as T4.)

[a]*Note:* Pelvic wall is defined as muscle, fascia, neurovascular structures, or skeletal portions of the bony pelvis.

in type, though other histologic types do occur. The labia majora is the most common site of involvement and accounts for about 50% of cases. The labia minora accounts for 15%–20% of cases. The clitoris and Bartholin glands are less frequently involved [42].

Dissemination of vulvar cancer usually leads to infiltration of the vagina, urethra, perineum, and anus [41]. The pattern of spread is influenced by the histology. Well-differentiated lesions tend to spread along the surface with minimal invasion, whereas anaplastic lesions are more likely to be deeply invasive. Also, it can disseminate to inguinal and femoral lymph nodes, which has direct correlation to the depth of invasion and diameter of the tumor. Hematogenous spread appears to be uncommon, but distant metastases to lung, liver, and bone may occur.

Survival is most dependent on the staging (Table 14.5) and mainly on the pathologic status of the inguinal nodes. In patients with operable disease without nodal involvement, the overall survival (OS) rate is 90%; however, in patients with nodal involvement, the 5-year OS rate is approximately 50%–60% [43]. Although not routinely needed, CT is useful in advanced cases to evaluate involved lymph nodes and/or organ infiltration to help planning the therapeutic options [41].

14.5.5 Female Urethra

The role of CT in the evaluation of the female urethra is limited, although newer techniques have been described as CT voiding cystourethrography [44]. CT can reliably demonstrate urethral calculi as it can depict certain urethral abnormalities incidentally discovered at CT performed for other abdominopelvic indications. Contrast-enhanced CT can help characterize urethral diverticulum as a cystic mass with wall thickening and enhancement at the level of the pubic symphysis [45]. CT can reliably show urethral calculi in the dependent portion of diverticula as well as diagnose inflammatory process in urethral diverticula [45]. An enhancing solid

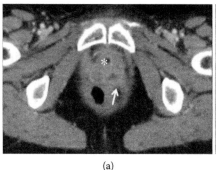
(a)

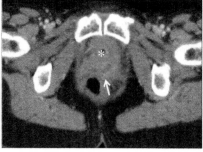
(b)

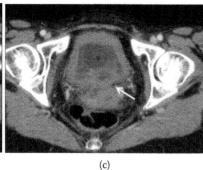
(c)

FIGURE 14.14
Vaginal cancer. (a), (b), and (c) Axial postcontrast CT images showing an ill-defined lesion in the vaginal vault (arrows in [a] and [b]) invading the vesical trigonum (arrow in [c]). A small, round, hypodense structure represents vesical catheter through the urethra (asterisk in [a] and [b]).

TABLE 14.5

FIGO Vulvar Cancer Staging

	Primary tumor cannot be assessed
	No evidence of primary tumor
0	Carcinoma in situ (preinvasive carcinoma)
I	Tumor confined to the vulva or vulva and perineum, 2 cm or less in greatest dimension
IA	Tumor confined to the vulva or vulva and perineum, 2 cm or less in greatest dimension, and with stromal invasion no greater than 1 mm
IB	Tumor confined to the vulva or vulva and perineum, 2 cm or less in greatest dimension, and with stromal invasion greater than 1 mm
II	Tumor confined to the vulva or vulva and perineum, more than 2 cm in greatest dimension
III	Tumor of any size with contiguous spread to the lower urethra and/or vagina or anus
IVA	Tumor invades any of the following: upper urethra, bladder mucosa, rectal mucosa, or is fixed to the pubic bone

mass within a diverticular cavity suggests a neoplasm. CT can also be used for regional staging of urethral neoplasm prior to surgery.

14.6 Adnexal

14.6.1 Normal Appearance

As previously described, ovaries are best seen on CT during the reproductive phase when they are identified on tomographic images by oval structures with homogeneous low density, except for the presence of small cysts that represent follicles. The volume of ovary can be variable, but an intact parenchymal appearance and volume as high as 15–18 cm^3 can be normal. Several conditions, inflammatory/infectious and neoplastic, may alter the adnexa and will be discussed in Sections 14.6.2 and 14.6.3.

14.6.2 Inflammatory Diseases

Pelvic inflammatory disease (PID) is an important cause of pelvic pain and morbidity. Most affected women are those in reproductive ages. Usually, this is a chronic and indolent infection, with most of the patients complaining of chronic and refractory pelvic pain. Rarely, this infection will have an acute and more severe presentation with pelvic [46].

Ultrasound is the first choice to approach patients with suspected PID. CT is reserved for cases suspicious for complications such as hydro/pyosalpinx and tuboovarian abscess (TOA) [46,47].

Hydrosalpinx results from tubal obstruction and will appear as tubular, hypodense structures, in close relation with the uterine fundus (Figure 14.15). If obstruction

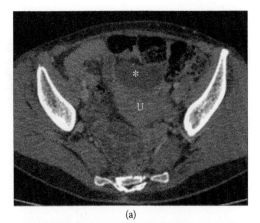

(a)

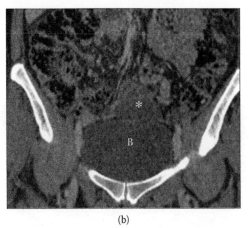

(b)

FIGURE 14.15

Hydrosalpinx. Axial (a) and coronal (b) images demonstrate an elongated, tubular structure (*) extending from right adnexal region to anterior and superior to the uterus (U). B (bladder) in coronal reformattation.

persists, hydrosalpinx may be complicated by infection of its contents. Pyosalpinx will share a similar appearance, although one may expect more heterogeneous content in the lumen. The most typical appearance for dilated tubes, either hydro-or pyosalpinx, is the ultrasonographic features of "spoke-wheel" appearance given by the mucosal folds within the tube lumen (Figure 14.16). This sign will be scarcely seen on tomographic images. TOA is the more worrisome complication of inflammatory pelvic disease. Clinically, patients will present with severe pelvic pain; on gynecological examination, usually there will be a palpable, tender, mass on cul-de-sac or adnexal region. US will show a complex mass, with ill-defined borders and heterogeneous echogenicity, sometimes with mixed, cystic-solid components [48]. CT will show a heterogeneous mass on adnexal region with hypodense, nonenhancing areas that correspond to necrosis (Figure 14.17). Ancillary findings include a small amount of fluid around the mass and in posterior cul-de-sac, as well as diffuse increase in density of fat. Postcontrast images demonstrate areas of heterogeneous enhancement with rim-pattern around necrotic areas [47,49].

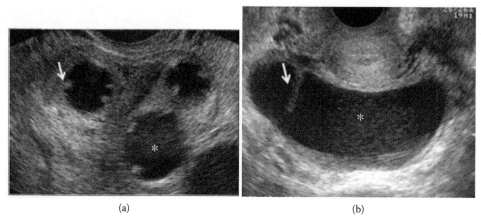

(a)   (b)

FIGURE 14.16
Hydrosalpinx on US. (a) and (b) Two different cases of hydrosalpinx showing the most typical appearance of this condition. The "spoke-wheel" appearance (asterisk) is seen as small dots representing mucosal folds protrude to lumen (arrow). (b) The same finding in the longest axis of the tube.

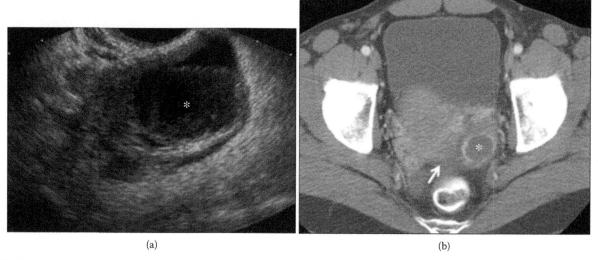

(a)   (b)

FIGURE 14.17
Tubo-ovarian abscess. (a) US showing a complex mass (*) with several irregular echoes. (b) CT scan, postcontrast showing a left adnexal lesion, with rim-like enhancement (asterisk) and a small amount of fluid adjacent (arrow).

14.6.3 Adnexal Lesions

Adnexal masses are common lesions in general population. The term adnexal encompasses lesions from ovaries, fallopian tubes, parametrium and adjacent peritoneum, bowel, and also uterine lesions with exophytic growth [50,51]. Benign lesions are the most common adnexal masses seen on premenopausal women. In elderly, postmenopausal women, benign lesions are still more common. In recent studies observing high-risk, postmenopausal population, the prevalence of ovarian cancer was estimated in 0.1% against 0.8% to 1.8% of benign lesions [52]. However, the risk of developing a malignant (ovarian) lesion in this group (post menopausal women) is up to 12 times higher than premenopausal ones [51,52].

In this scenario, preoperative workup of adnexal masses is crucial for a correct management of this lesion. US has been the first choice, because of wide availability, lack of ionizing radiation, and good sensitivity and specificity [53]. CT and MRI have been reserved for workup of indeterminate lesion seen on US. Tomographic imaging has several papers when evaluating adnexal lesions: (1) define if ovarian or from other adnexal origin; (2) if it is clearly benign or potentially malignant, to determine if a safe follow-up is recommended or surgery is indicated when really necessary and; (3) when possible, to determine preoperative diagnosis (mature teratoma for example). To determine if a lesion is from ovaries or not, one may rely on some anatomical landmarks: (1) the ovarian space is just beneath the iliac vessels bifurcation; and (2) ovaries lie anterior or antero-medial to the ureters. However, the most specific sign for defining an ovarian lesion is the relation between the mass and gonadal vein. Volumetric images allow reconstruction depicting the gonadal vein (usually enlarged, when a tumor is present) originating from the mass, confirming the ovarian origin and the laterality (Figure 14.18).

In addition, CT has been extensively used in various clinical conditions, mainly for evaluation of abdominal/pelvic pain in emergency settings, which has resulted in frequent detection of adnexal masses as incidental findings [54]. The addition of MDCT has improved detection and characterization of adnexal lesions [53,55].

14.6.4 Benign Adnexal Lesions

Functional cysts represent the most common lesions in the ovaries. Usually, they appear on CT images as homogeneous, hypodense lesions, with no enhancement after intravenous contrast media, especially in women during the reproductive ages (Figure 14.19). The mean diameter of functional cysts is about 3.0 cm, but cysts up to 6.0–7.0 cm may be found. Functional cysts may occur in postmenopausal women, although they are much less frequent in this group [55].

Care should be taken when interpreting hypodense/cystic lesions in the adnexal. Depending on the scanner, technique, and protocols used in acquisition, internal components such as septa and/or vegetations may be missed. As a result, a complex lesion may be mistaken as a simple cyst delaying correct diagnosis and the appropriate assessment (Figure 14.20).

Theca-lutein cysts are frequent in early pregnancy or when hormonal disturbs result in elevation of serum levels of progesterone. Their tomographic appearance is indistinguishable from simple/functional cysts (Figure 14.13a). Differentiation must rely on clinical history [54,56].

Peritoneal inclusion cysts (PICs) are not true cysts; rather, they represent a nonneoplastic reactive mesothelial proliferation. The development of a PIC depends on the presence of an active ovary and peritoneal adhesion. The adhesion extends to the ovarian surface, but do not invade. PICs may simulate simple cysts, hydrosalpinx, and even ovarian cancer, when they present as complex cystic lesions [57].

Ovarian torsion is not a frequent event and is more common among prepubertal girls and during pregnancy. When present, an ovarian mass predisposes to the ovary torsion [58]. Clinically, patients will present with an acute onset of pelvic pain. Imaging findings reflects the underlying pathologic events, so the more severe the ischemia, the more conspicuous the imaging features, which include increase in volume, fluid in cul-de-sac, and lack of enhancement on postcontrast images. Enlarged vessels may be seen around the ovary [59,60].

Patients suspected to have ectopic pregnancy are usually imaged by TVUS. CT will be used only when this diagnosis is not suspected and an adnexal (or abdominal) mass is detected. The most common site for ectopic pregnancy is the uterine tubes. A few reports of CT are available in literature and imaging findings may show an adnexal mass, a fallopian tube hematoma with enhancing walls, and, rarely, a gestational saclike structure [61,62].

The polycystic ovary syndrome, also known as Stein–Leventhal syndrome, may cause enlarged ovaries, but the diagnosis is usually straightforward by TVUS, and CT imaging has no role in this affection [50].

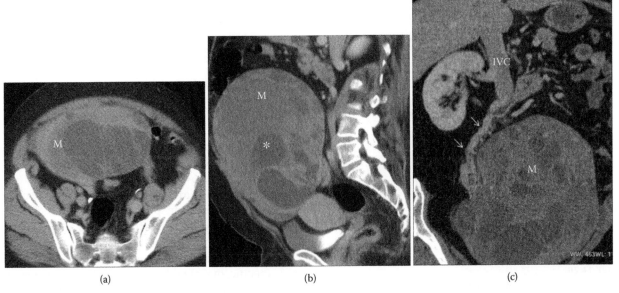

(a) (b) (c)

FIGURE 14.18

The gonadal vein sign. (a) and (b) Axial and sagittal CT images showing a huge abdominopelvic mixed lesion, with cystic components (M). Although located predominantly in the pelvis and in right hemiabdomen, no definite conclusion about its origin is possible with these images. (c) Curved reformatation following the path of right gonadal vein (arrows), undoubtedly confirm the origin of the lesion (IVC = inferior vena cava).

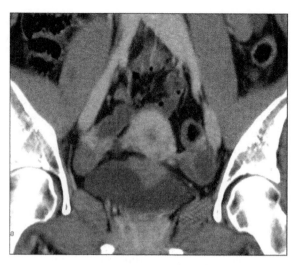

FIGURE 14.19
Functional cyst. The most common cystic lesion in premenopausal women. A hypodense, homogeneous, small cyst in the left ovary (*). B-bladder and U-uterus.

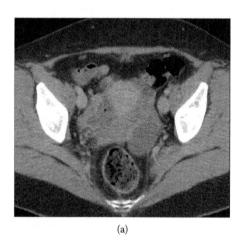

(a)

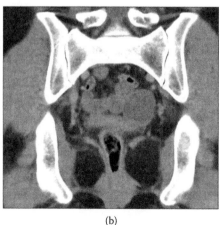

(b)

FIGURE 14.20
Complex cyst mistaken as a simple cyst. (a) and (b) Axial and coronal images demonstrate a left adnexal lesions, with an homogeneous density and no enhancement. The 34-year-old patient underwent a follow-up US (not available) 2 months later that showed a complex cystic lesion. After surgical removal, a serous adenocarcinoma was found.

Cystic lesions in adnexa may originate from other uncommon sites. Paraovarian cysts, also known as paratubal cysts, originate in broad ligaments. They are a relative common cystic lesion, representing about 10%–20% of adnexal cysts. Women in third and fourth decades are the most affected. They should be suspected when the ovary is seen separate from the cyst. Usually, they are unilocular and homogeneous [50,57].

Mesenteric cysts may occupy the adnexa, but it is an extremely uncommon lesion and adnexal is an atypical location for these cysts. Usually asymptomatic, the tomographic appearance is nonspecific, but most common appearance is a unilocular and homogeneous cystic lesion. Other benign adnexal lesions include hydro- and pyosalpinx already discussed. Endometrial cysts, an important differential diagnosis, will be discussed later in Section 14.7.

14.6.5 Ovarian Neoplasms

Primary ovarian tumors can be divided according to histologic types as epithelial, germ-cell, and sexual cord/stromal origin. Epithelial tumors are the most common histopathologic type of malignant ovarian tumor, accounting for about 85% of cases [56,63]. Besides primary tumors, ovaries may be a site of metastatic lesions.

The incidence of ovarian histologic subtypes varies intensely according to age of patients. Therefore, for a more accurate interpretation of ovarian neoplasms, one should know some important clinical aspects, summarized in Table 14.6. Tomographic imaging has several roles in ovarian neoplasms: recognize typical benign lesions impeding unnecessary exploration; detect suspect lesions and contribute for surgical planning when lesions are already diagnosed. It is also important for follow-up of treated patients.

14.6.6 Germ-Cell Neoplasms

Mature cystic teratomas derive from germ cells present in ovaries. They are the most common ovarian neoplasm in some reports and the most prevalent among young patients. The three germ-cell layer components may be present, although ectodermal ones predominate, and according to that such lesions are often referred to as dermoid cysts [63,64].

Most teratomas are asymptomatic and discovered incidentally at routine pelvic examination. However, they may predispose to ovarian torsion and, rarely, rupture causing a chemical peritonitis.

The features of mature teratomas on CT are usually very specific, mainly when a young female present with an adnexal mass with fat tissue and calcifications inside. Fat can be confirmed by measuring and obtaining densities under –20 HU [56,65]. Sometimes, even a tooth may be recognized on tomographic images (Figure 14.21).

TABLE 14.6

Ovarian Cancer: Clinical and Epidemiological Aspects According to Histologic Types

Tumor Type	Peak of Incidence (Age)	Clinical and Imaging Aspects
Germ-cell tumors		
Mature teratoma	10–20 years	Asymptomatic—fat and calcification
Stromal/sexual cord cells		
Granulosa cell tumors	1—Prepubertal	Precocious puberty
	2—Menacme	Endometrial hyperplasia/carcinoma
Fibromas	Middle age	Asymptomatic or Meigs syndrome
Epithelial		
Cystadenoma/carcinoma	40–60s	Ascites. Complex cystic mass
Endometrioid tumor	40–60s	Endometrial hyperplasia/carcinoma
Metastases		
Metastases	40–70s	Ascites, peritoneal seeding

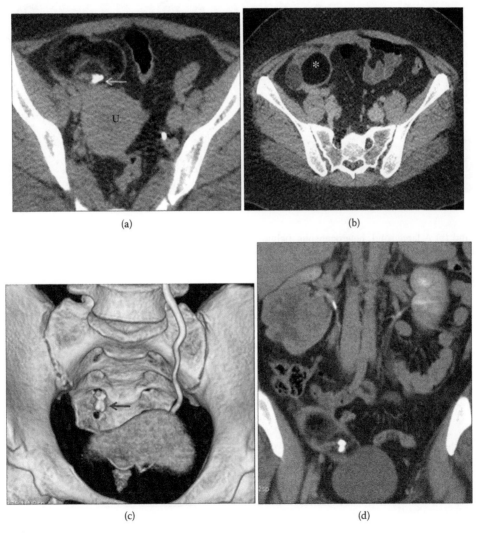

(a) (b)

(c) (d)

FIGURE 14.21

Mature teratoma in the right ovary. (a) and (b) Axial images demonstrate a complex lesion in right adnexa, with calcification (arrow in [a]) and fat (asterisk in [b]). The volume rendering reconstruction showed a well-defined tooth (red arrow in [c]). (d) Incidentally, a large renal cell carcinoma is seen in lower pole of right kidney. U=uterus.

Although the mature teratoma, the most frequent germ-cell tumor, is benign, it is not always benign. Malignant variants of teratoma may occur, as well as other histologic subtypes. Disgerminomas represent the most common malignant variant. These lesions will present on CT images, usually as large, vascularized lesions, but without specific signs (Figure 14.22) [65,66].

14.6.7 Stromal and Sexual-Cord Lesions

Tumors of gonadal stromal origin have a few histologic subtypes, including fibromas, thecomas, and fibroth-ecomas. Histologically, they are composed of fibrocon-nective tissue and theca cells with lipid-rich cytoplasm [56,67]. The theca cells may secrete estrogens that will give the clinical symptoms of early puberty (Table 14.6).

Fibromas are composed of bundles of spindle cells without theca cells and, therefore, have no hormonal effect [68]. They represent about 4% of all ovarian tumors and are more common in women in reproductive ages. Usually asymptomatic, fibromas will appear on CT images as solid adnexal masses, which make them an important differential diagnosis for malignant lesions, although, in contrast to aggressive lesions, they show only minimal and delayed enhancement on postcontrast images. Large lesions are associated with pleural effusion and ascites in a triad known as Meigs syndrome, present in about 40% of all fibromas [56,67–69]. The tomographic appearance of stromal tumors is nonspecific, but it is more characteristic on MRI, as the fibrous component show low signal on T1- and T2-weighted images (Figure 14.23).

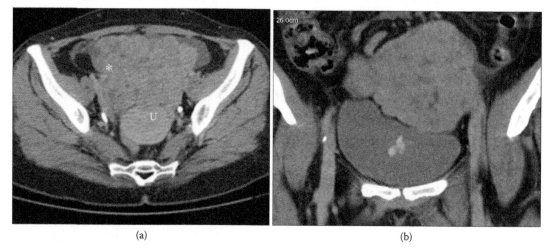

(a)   (b)

FIGURE 14.22
Disgerminoma. (a) and (b) A large solid, heterogeneous, pelvic mass (*) is seen in young female, extending superior and anterior to the uterus (U), from the left adnexa. The mass showed a heterogeneous enhancement on postcontrast images.

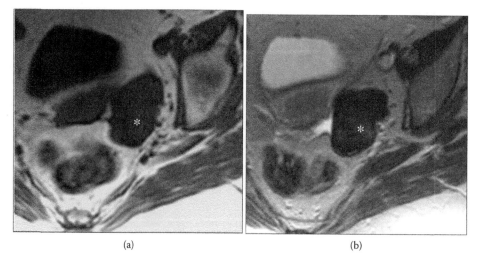

(a)   (b)

FIGURE 14.23
Left ovary fibroma. (a) and (b) Axial T1- and T2-weighted images show an oval, well-defined lesion (*) on left adnexa with marked low signal on both sequences. Along with a poor enhancement on postcontrast images (not shown here), this is the most typical appearance for ovarian fibroma. (Courtesy of Prof. Antonio Westphalen, University of California, San Francisco.)

14.6.8 Epithelial Neoplasias

Epithelial neoplasias of ovaries share a wide range of histologic types, varying from benign to frankly malignant lesions, encompassing the borderline tumors. These lesions have an increasing incidence from the third decade of life and reach their peak about sixth and seventh decade [56,65].

Epithelial tumors are usually cystic or mixed, solid-cystic lesions. Benign lesions usually are uni- or multilocular cysts without solid components. They may have septa, which are usually thin and with regular surfaces. Typical findings of malignant lesions are the following: solid or mixed (cystic-solid); large lesions, usually more than 5.0 cm in the largest axis; irregular and thick septae [70,71]. Postcontrast images may show marked enhancement, reflecting the rapid growth and marked neovascularization (Figure 14.24). Recently, some studies have shown that malignant lesions may be defined by the pattern of enhancement on dynamic contrast studies. As mentioned earlier, in the presence of cystic lesions, a complete search for internal components of the lesion should

be performed, ideally on workstation where different settings of brightness/contrast may improve the visualization of vegetations and/or thick, irregular septae.

When staging ovarian cancer, radiologists should be aware of pathways used by this neoplasia to disseminate. There are four mechanisms of spreading: intraperitoneal dissemination; direct invasion of adjacent organs; lymphatic dissemination, especially to iliac and periaortic lymph nodes; and hematogenous spread to distant organs. Malignant cells, when disseminating in peritoneal cavity, usually induce ascites formation and peritoneal seeding (Figure 14.25). The staging of ovarian cancer is shown in Table 14.7. CT and MRI have similar accuracy for staging of ovarian cancer, reported as 92% and 97%, respectively [71].

Relapsing disease is suspected when serum levels of CA-125 increase and is usually investigated by CT or MRI. The relapsing may be systemic or local (Figure 14.26). Imaging is essential in the follow-up of

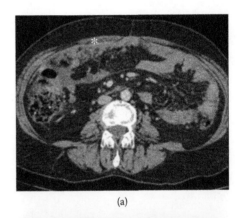

(a)

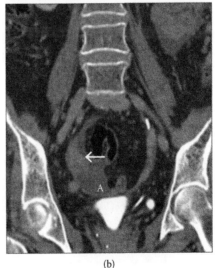

(b)

FIGURE 14.25
Signs of ovarian metastatic disease. (a) Axial scan obtained just above the iliac crest showing thickening of omentum compatible with peritoneal dissemination (*). (b) Coronal reformatation showing small amount of free fluid in the pelvis (A) and a peritoneal nodule compatible of metastatic dissemination (arrow).

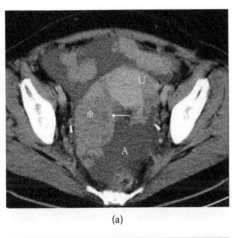

(a)

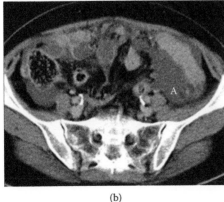

(b)

FIGURE 14.24
Serous adenocarcinoma of right ovary. (a) and (b) Axial tomographic images demonstrate a mixed lesion on right ovary (*), with a few cystic areas inside (arrow in [a]). There is a marked ascites (A) in the pelvis, an ancillary finding of ovarian epithelial tumors.

TABLE 14.7

FIGO Ovarian Cancer Staging

IA	Lesion limited to one ovary
IB	Growth extends to both ovaries
IC	IA/IB with capsular involvement, tumor rupture, positive washing/ascites
IIA	Extension or metastases to uterus and/or uterine tubes
IIB	Involvement of other pelvic organs rather than uterus
IIC	IIA/IIB with capsular involvement, tumor rupture, positive washing/ascites
IIIA	Microscopic peritoneal implants
IIIB	Peritoneal implants less than 2.0 cm
IIIC	Peritoneal implants more than 2.0 cm, retroperitoneal or pelvic adenopathy
IV	Distant metastases (liver, pleuropulmonar, brain, etc.)

patients operated for ovarian cancer since serum levels of CA-125 may not elevate in some cases of recurrence.

14.6.9 Ovarian Metastases

Metastases to ovaries are uncommon and represent only 1%–2% of all ovarian neoplasms. The most common primary sites are gastrointestinal tract, mainly stomach and colon, and breast [72].

In 1896, Friedrich Ernst Krukenberg, a German pathologist, described metastatic signet-ring cell adenocarcinomas of the ovaries, with sarcomatous stroma. He first interpreted such lesions as primary of ovaries. Later on they were recognized as secondary lesions from gastrointestinal tract, mainly from stomach and colon [73].

Ovarian metastases are bilateral in up to 30% of cases. The most typical appearance on CT is solid lesions with cystic components within and with marked enhancement on postcontrast images. In the majority of cases, the primary lesion is advanced and secondary signs as ascites and peritoneal carcinomatosis may be detected (Figure 14.27). They must be differentiated from enlarged lymph nodes, using ureters as references. The

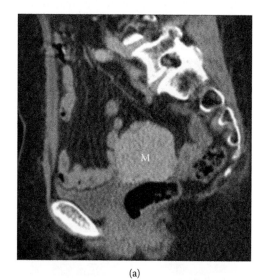

(a)

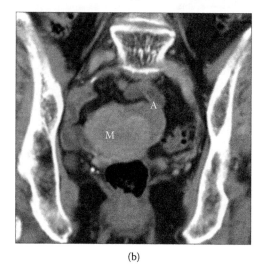

(b)

FIGURE 14.26
Ovarian cancer recurrence. In the sagittal and coronal reformatation is noticeable the postsurgical status, without uterus and ovaries. An irregular, soft-tissue mass (M) is seen surrounded by a small amount of fluid (A) in a case of recurrence of ovarian epithelial tumor.

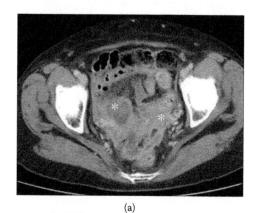

(a)

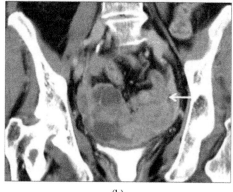

(b)

FIGURE 14.27
Krukenberg tumor. (a) Axial scan of the pelvis showing a bilateral mixed mass (*) with several cystic components. (b) Coronal reformatation showing the uterus (arrow) dislocated to the left and involved by the lesions.

ovaries are usually located anterior or medial to the ureters, meanwhile adenopathy are located lateral or posterolateral to ureters [72,74].

14.7 Adenomyosis and Endometriosis

Endometriosis may be defined as the occurrence of endometrial tissue outside the endometrium and the myometrium. Adenomyosis can be defined as the presence of endometrial glands deeper than one large field of view on microscopic pathologic specimens. In recent past, adenomyosis were called "internal endometriosis" and "external endometriosis" was the name for what we know as endometriosis [75,76].

The most common sites for endometriosis are the ovaries, uterine serosal surface, peritoneum, pelvic ligaments, and, less commonly, vagina, rectovaginal septum, rectum, and bladder. The so-called deep pelvic endometriosis is defined as the presence of invasive endometriotic lesions extending more than 5 mm from the peritoneal surface into adjacent structures and is associated with fibrosis and muscular hyperplasia. Patients' complaints will depend on the site(s) of deposition of endometriotic tissues and dysmenorrhea, deep dyspareunia, chronic pelvic pain, or infertility may occur [76].

The imaging findings will reflect the form of occurrence of endometriotic tissues. In the ovaries, the most common presentation will be a cystic lesion with huge amount of internal debris (hemosiderin and its product of degradation), the well-known endometrial cyst or endometrioma [77]. Outside the ovaries, the endometriotic tissue may be deposited on peritoneal surface of pelvic organs and that will be the most challenging presentation of endometriosis in all imaging methods, because of the flat nature of such deposits. When the endometriotic tissues invade deep portion of the pelvis, they usually induce an inflammatory response that ultimately will result in fibrotic, retractile tissues and may cause adherences between organs. This is common in the rectovaginal septum and among posterior surface of the uterus and rectum and/or sigmoid. The CT finding of rectal tethering in the direction of uterus had been described as a very specific sign for deep endometriosis (Figure 14.28).

The endometriotic implants may arise in distant sites including abdominal wall, mediastinum, and pleural space [78]. A more worrisome complication of endometriosis is the malignant transformation of endometrial implants, either in ovaries or extraovarian. Solid components or mural nodules with vivid enhancement on postcontrast images are suspicious and should be investigated [79].

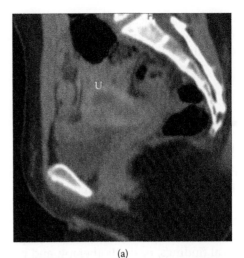

(a)

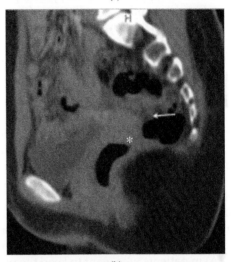

(b)

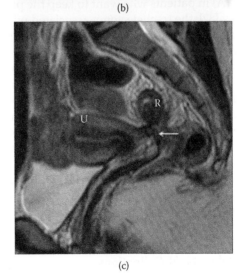

(c)

FIGURE 14.28

Deep endometriosis. (a) and (b) In sagittal tomographic images, it is possible to see the uterus (U) and thin strands (arrow in [b]) irradiating from the posterior surface of the cervix (*). (c) Same patient. A sagittal T2-weighted image clearly shows a hypoinytense thickening of rectovaginal septum (arrow) and bands of low signal intensity extending to rectal wall, in a tethered appearance. (R=rectum.)

Recently, CT colonoscopy has been described to be useful for planning surgical approach of endometriotic lesions extending to rectal/sigmoid wall [80].

14.8 Treated Pelvis

Depending on the gynecological disease, the therapeutic possibilities include surgery, chemotherapy, and radiotherapy alone or associated, determining changes in the pelvic organs that can be evaluated by imaging methods. In a didactic way, we will divide our approach in postsurgical findings, postradiotherapy, and pelvic fluid collections. Fistulas, another complication of surgical procedures and radiation therapy, are detailed in Section 14.9.

14.8.1 Postoperative Changes

The indication for pelvic surgery covers benign and malignant conditions. The choice of imaging method will depend on the clinical indication, either to evaluate the findings of a specific surgical intervention or possible associated conditions, such as hematomas, urinomas, lymphoceles, abscesses, visceral perforations, suture dehiscence, and fistulae [81].

Within the scope of uterine cancer, surgery, depending on the stage, may include trachelectomy or radical hysterectomy. For the initial cases of cancer of the cervix (FIGO—IA) in patients who want to keep the possibility of fertility [82], the trachelectomy associated with pelvic lymphadenectomy represents a conservative and curative therapeutic option [83].

In imaging studies, the postsurgical aspect will be a normal uterine body, with pyriform aspect, sitting on the vaginal dome (termino-terminal anastomosis). The other possible postsurgical aspect include isthmic stenosis, represented as secondary dilatation of the uterine cavity; diffuse vaginal thickening; and prominence of the pelvic venous plexus [83,84].

Following radical hysterectomy (FIGO IB and II) and without signs of neoplasm recurrence, a possible fibrotic scar may be seen around the vaginal dome [85].

14.8.2 Pelvic Fluid Collections

Fluid collections found in the postoperative period may correspond to hemorrhages/hematomas, lymphoceles, seromas, and abscesses.

The lymphoceles represent homogeneous accumulation of lymph in the lymphatic chains pathway, usually with spontaneous resolution [85]. The identification of a

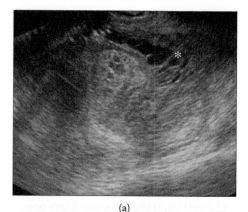

(a)

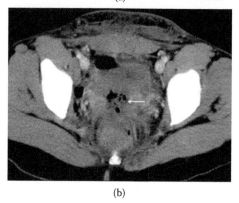

(b)

FIGURE 14.29
Postsurgical abscess. (a) Ultrasonography image of patient complaining of pelvic pain just after a hysterectomy for a cervical uterine cancer. A complex collection is seen around the vaginal vault (*). (b) Axial CT scan showing a ill-defined fluid collection containing gas bubbles.

more hyperdense content on precontrast CT (70–90 HU) in postsurgical fluid collection favors the possibility of a hematoma, especially with a hematic level identified. Collections with the presence of gas, always correlated with appropriate clinical setting, indicate the possibility of an abscess (Figure 14.29) [81].

The postoperative collections can be approached percutaneously, guided by ultrasound and CT [86–88].

14.8.3 Actinic Changes

Imaging studies after radiotherapy of the uterus aim to assess the presence of residual or recurrent neoplastic lesions. The major complications of radiation therapy are the fibrotic scars and development of fistulas.

The posttreatment fibrosis may be indistinguishable of residual tumor or recurrence, if it assumes a mass-like form. Since morphology is not a good discriminator, post contrast images may be helpful, but not in the immediate posttreatment period. Fibrotic scars may show contrast enhancement for a long and variable period, usually no less than 2–3 months, but may persist for almost a year. As tumor recurrence always enhances, differentiation may be not possible on early posttreatment period [89].

When assessing tumor response, reduction of tumor volume has been the most frequent parameter to evaluate. Recently, the degree of enhancement has been tested as a predictor of cervical cancer response after radiation therapy. If MRI is used, measurement of apparent diffuse coefficient is another predictor being investigated [90].

Other possible additional findings in imaging studies after radiation therapy include intestinal disorders, such as increased density of submucosal rectal and sigmoid colon (proctitis) and increase in density of perirectal fatty tissue; urological disorders, such as diffuse bladder wall thickening (cystitis); and bone changes, such as conversion of fatty marrow and osteitis actinic [91].

14.9 Fistulas

The pelvic fistulas have different etiologies; the most frequent causes are postoperative conditions, inflammatory and infectious disease, primary pelvic neoplasms, and complications after chemotherapy and radiation therapy. The diagnosis is suspected by the signs and symptoms, which will depend on location of fistulous pathway. The role of imaging methods is confirmation of a clinical suspected fistula: location, extent, and complexity of the fistula path [90,92].

The fistula pathway may cross the various pelvic organs and according to this route, different communications may be established. The most common ones are vesicovaginal and enterovaginal fistulas, for those of neoplastic etiology [86].

The imaging methods for approaching fistulas are MRI and CT. Both may depict the route of a fistula with much more details than fistulography, using conventional radiology. When using CT, we perform volumetric acquisition in pre- and postcontrast series, allowing multiplanar reformatation, since sagittal, coronal, and oblique planes are crucial, when fistulas are suspected (Figure 14.30). The CT scans may benefit from the additional use of oral and rectal contrast and excretory phase for better evaluation of vesical fistula. As an alternative, retrograde vesical filling with iodinated contrast media may be helpful for characterization of vesicovaginal and rectovesical fistulas.

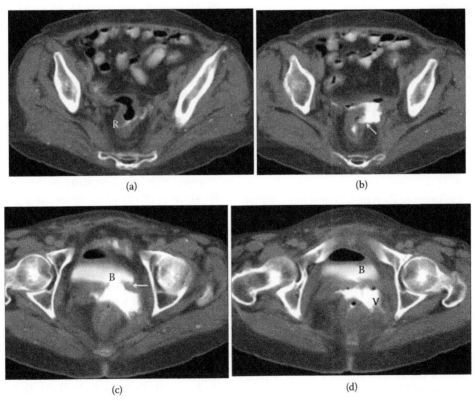

(a) (b)

(c) (d)

FIGURE 14.30
Recto-vaginal-vesical fistula. This patient had surgery and radiation therapy for a uterine cervical cancer and a complex fistula was suspected. The bladder was filled with diluted iodinated contrast media. Axial images in a craniocaudal direction—the contrast media are seen extending posteriorly to the rectum (R) and a rectovaginal fistula is clearly seen in (b) (arrow). The contrast media is seen passing through a defect on posterior bladder (B) wall to the vagina (V), arrow in (c).

References

1. Farthing A. Clinical Anatomy of the Pelvis and Reproductive Tract. Dewhurst's Textbook of Obstetrics & Gynaecology, Seventh Edition, Ed: D. Keiths Diamond. pp. 1–9. Hoboken, NJ: Wiley Online Library, 2008.

2. Fosbanger MC, Walsh JW. CT Anatomy of the female pelvis: a second look. *Radiographics* 1994; 14:51–66.

3. Wasnik AP, Mazza MB, Liu PS. Normal and variant pelvic anatomy on MRI. *Magn Reson Imaging Clin N Am* 2011; 19:547–566.

4. Vick CW, Walsh JW, Wheelock JB, Brewer WH. CT of the normal and abnormal parametria in cervical cancer. *AJR Am J Roentgenol* 1984; 143(3):597–603.

5. Foshager MC, Walsh JW. CT anatomy of the female pelvis: a second look. *Radiographics* 1994; 14:51–64.

6. Okamoto Y, Tanaka YO, Nishida M, Tsunoda H, Yoshikawa H, Itai Y. MR imaging of the uterine cervix: imaging-pathologic correlation. *Radiographics* 2003; 23:425–445.

7. Tsili AC, Tsampoulas C, Dalkalitsis N, Stefanou D, Paraskevaidis E, Efremidis SC. Local staging of endometrial carcinoma: role of multidetector CT. *Eur Radiol* 2008; 18(5):1043–1048.

8. Sala E, Wakely S, Senior E. MRI of malignant neoplasms of the uterine corpus and cervix. *AJR Am J Roentgenol* 2007; 188:1577–1587.

9. Mortelé KJ, Oliva MR, Ondategui S, Ros PR, Silverman SG. Universal use of nonionic iodinated contrast medium for CT: evaluation of safety in a large urban teaching hospital. *AJR Am J Reontgen* 2005; 184:31–34.

10. Elicker B, Coackley F, Cho K, Fong C, Hampton T, Gordon R, Mackenzie J. Guidelines on the administration of intravenous iodinated contrast media. Home page of University of California at San Francisco, Department of Radiology & Biomedical Imaging. http://www.radiology.ucsf.edu/patient-care/patient-safety/contrast/iodinated (accessed on June 12, 2012).

11. Chan YY, Jayaprakasan K, Zamora J, Thornton JG, Raine Fenning N, Coomarasamy A. The prevalence of congenital uterine anomalies in unselected and high-risk populations: a systematic review. *Hum Reprod Update* 2011; 17(6):761–771.

12. Buttram VC Jr, Gibbons WE. Müllerian anomalies: a proposed classification. (An analysis of 144 cases). *Fertil Steril* 1979; 32(1):40–46.

13. Casillas J, Joseph RC, Guerra JJ Jr. CT appearance of uterine leiomyomas. *Radiographics* 1990; 10(6):999–1007.

14. Karasick S, Lev-Toaff AS, Toaff ME. Imaging of uterine leiomyomas. *AJR Am J Roentgenol* 1992; 158:799–780.

15. Siddall KA, Rubens DJ. Multidetector CT of the female pelvis. *Radiol Clin N Am* 2005; 43:1097–1118.

16. Boni RA, Hebisch G, Huch A, Stallmach T, Krestin GP. Multiple necrotic uterine leiomyomas causing severe puerperal fever: ultrasound, CT, MR, and histological findings. *J Comput Assist Tomogr* 1994; 18:828–831.

17. Roy C, Bierry G, Ei Ghali S, Buy X, Rossini A. Acute torsion of uterine leiomyoma: CT features. *Abdom Imaging* 2005; 30(1):120–123.

18. Togashi K, Nishimura K, Nakano Y, Itoh H, Torizuka K, Ozasa H, Watanabe T. Cystic pedunculated leiomyomas of the uterus with unusual CT manifestations. *J Comput Assist Tomogr* 1986; 10(4):642–644.

19. Verma SK, Gonsalves CF, Baltarowich OH, Mitchell DG, Lev Toaff AS, Bergin D. Spectrum of imaging findings on MRI and CT after uterine artery embolization. *Abdom Imaging* 2010; 35(1):118–128.

20. Grossman J, Ricci ZJ, Rozenblit A, Freeman K, Mazzariol F, Stein MW. Efficacy of contrast-enhanced CT in assessing the endometrium. *AJR Am J Roentgenol* 2008; 191(3):664–669.

21. Lim PS, Nazarian LN, Wechsler RJ, Kurtz AB, Parker L. The endometrium on routine contrast-enhanced CT in asymptomatic postmenopausal women: avoiding errors in interpretation. *Clin Imaging* 2002; 26(5):325–329.

22. Nalaboff KM, Pellerito JS, Ben-Levi E. Imaging the endometrium: disease and normal variants. *Radiographics* 2001; 21(6):1409–1424.

23. Celik O, Karakas HM, Hascalik S, Tagluk ME. Virtual hysterosalpingography and hysteroscopy: assessment of uterine cavity and fallopian tubes using 64-detector computed tomography data sets. *Fertil Steril* 2010; 93:2383–2384.

24. Tay SK. Cervical cancer in the human papillomavirus vaccination era. *Curr Opin Obstet Gynecol* 2012; 24:3–7.

25. Narayan K, Mckenzie AF, Hicks RJ, Fisher R, Bernshaw D, Bau S. Relation between FIGO stage, primary tumor volume, and presence of lymph node metastases in cervical cancer patients referred for radiotherapy. *Int J Gynecol Cancer* 2003; 13:657–663.

26. Pecorelli S. Revised FIGO staging for carcinoma of the vulva, cervix, and endometrium. *Int J Gynaecol Obstet* 2009; 105(2):103–104.

27. Hricak H et al. Role of imaging in pretreatment evaluation of early invasive cervical cancer: results of the intergroup study American College of Radiology Imaging Network 6651-Gynecologic Oncology Group 183. *J Clin Oncol* 2005; 23(36):9329–9337.

28. Mitchell DG et al. Early invasive cervical cancer: MRI and CT predictors of lymphatic metastases in the ACRIN 6651/GOG 183 intergroup study. *Gynecol Oncol* 2009; 112(1):95–103.

29. Sawyer RW, Walsh JW. CT in gynecologic pelvic diseases. *Semin Ultrasound CT MR* 1988; 9(2):122–142.

30. Pannu HK, Fishman EK. Evaluation of cervical cancer by computed tomography: current status. *Cancer* 2003; 98(9 Suppl):2039–2043.

31. Jemal A, Bray F, Center MM, Ferlay J, Ward E, Forman D. Global cancer statistics. *CA Cancer J Clin* 2011; 61(2):69–90.

32. Akin O, Mironov S, Pandit-Taskar N, Hann LE. Imaging of uterine cancer. *Radiol Clin N Am* 2007; 45(1):167–182.

33. Zaino RJ, Kurman R, Herbold D, Gliedman J, Bundy BN, Vote R, Advani H. The significance of squamous differentiation in endometrial carcinoma. Data from a Gynecologic Oncology Group study. *Cancer* 1991; 68(10):2293–2302.

34. Hardesty LA, Sumkin JH, Hakim C, Johns C, Nath M. The ability of helical CT to preoperatively stage endometrial carcinoma. *AJR Am J Roentgenol* 2001; 176:603–606.

35. Balleyguier C et al. Staging of uterine cervical cancer with MRI: guidelines of the European Society of Urogenital Radiology. *Eur Radiol* 2011; 21:1102–1110.

36. Wagner BJ, Woodward PJ, Dickey GE. From the archives of the AFIP. Gestational trophoblastic disease: radiologic-pathologic correlation. *Radiographics* 1996; 16(1):131–148.

37. Allen SD, Lim AK, Seckl MJ, Blunt DM, Mitchell AW. Radiology of gestational trophoblastic neoplasia. *Clin Radiol* 2006; 61(4):301–313.

38. Sanders C, Rubin E. Malignant gestational trophoblastic disease: CT findings. *AJR Am J Roentgenol* 1987; 148:165–168.

39. Di Donato V, Bellati F, Fischetti M, Plotti F, Perniola G, Panici PB. Vaginal cancer. *Crit Rev Oncol Hematol* 2012; 81:286–295.

40. Lilic V, Lilic G, Filipovic S, Visnjic M, Zivadinovic R. Primary carcinoma of the vagina. *J BUON* 2010; 15(2):241–247.

41. Dittmer C, Fischer D, Diedrich K, Thill M. Diagnosis and treatment options of vulvar cancer: a review. *Arch Gynecol Obstet* 2012; 285(1):183–193.

42. Perez CA, Camel HM, Galakatos AE, Grigsby PW, Kuske RR, Buchsbaum G, Hederman MA. Definitive irradiation in carcinoma of the vagina: long-term evaluation of results. *Int J Radiat Oncol Biol Phys* 1988; 15(6):1283–1290.

43. Gallup DG, Talledo OE, Shah KJ, Hayes C. Invasive squamous cell carcinoma of the vagina: a 14-year study. *Obstet Gynecol* 1987; 69(5):782–785.

44. Kim SH, Kim SH, Park BK, Jung SY, Hwang SI, Paick JS, Kim SW. CT voiding cystourethrography using 16-MDCT for the evaluation of female urethral diverticula: initial experience. *AJR Am J Roentgenol* 2005; 184(5):1594–1596.

45. Chou CP et al. Imaging of female urethral diverticulum: an update. *Radiographics* 2008; 28(7):1917–1930.

46. Kruszka PS, Kruszka SJ. Evaluation of acute pelvic pain in women. *Am Fam Physician* 2010; 82(2):141–147.

47. Yitta S, Hecht EM, Slywotzky CM, Bennett GL. Added value of multiplanar reformation in the multidetector CT evaluation of the female pelvis: a pictorial review. *Radiographics* 2009; 29(7):1987–2003.

48. Vandermeer FQ, Wong-You-Cheong JJ. Imaging of acute pelvic pain. *Clin Obstet Gynecol* 2009; 52(1):2–20.

49. Ghiatas AA. The spectrum of pelvic inflammatory disease. *Eur Radiol* 2004; 14:E184–E192.

50. Asch E, Levine D, Kim Y, Hecht JL. Histologic, surgical, and imaging correlations of adnexal masses. *J Ultrasound Med* 2008; 27(3):327–342.

51. Dørum A, Blom GP, Ekerhovd E, Granberg S. Prevalence and histologic diagnosis of adnexal cysts in postmenopausal women: an autopsy study. *Am J Obstet Gynecol* 2005; 192:48–54.

52. McDonald JM, Modesitt SC. The incidental postmenopausal adnexal mass. *Clin Obstet Gynecol* 2006; 49:506–516.

53. van Nagell JR, DePriest PD. Management of adnexal masses in postmenopausal women. *Am J Obstet Gynecol* 2005; 193:30–35.

54. Asayama Y et al. MDCT of the gonadal veins in females with large pelvic masses: value in differentiating ovarian versus uterine origin. *AJR Am J Roentgenol* 2006 Feb; 186(2):440–448.

55. Tsili AC, Tsampoulas C, Charisiadi A, Kalef-Ezra J, Dousias V, Paraskevaidis E, Efremidis SC. Adnexal masses: accuracy of detection and differentiation with multidetector computed tomography. *Gynecol Oncol* 2008; 110(1):22–31.

56. Jeong YY, Outwater EK, Kang HK. Imaging evaluation of ovarian masses. *Radiographics* 2000; 20(5):1445–1470.

57. Kiran J. Imaging of peritoneal inclusion. *AJR Am J Roentegenol* 2000; 174:1559–1563.

58. Lee YR. CT imaging findings of ruptured ovarian endometriotic cysts: emphasis on the differential diagnosis with ruptured ovarian functional cysts. *Korean J Radiol* 2011; 12(1):59–65.

59. Roche O, Chavan N, Aquilina J, Rockall A. Radiological appearance of gynaecological emergencies. *Insight Imaging* 2012; 3:265–275.

60. Wilkinson C, Sanderson A. Adnexal torsion—a multimodality imaging review. *Clin Radiol* 2012; 67(5):476–478.

61. Coulier B, Malbecq S, Brinon PE, Ramboux A. MDCT diagnosis of ruptured tubal pregnancy with massive hemoperitoneum. *Emerg Radiol* 2008; 15(3):179–182.

62. Pham H, Lin EC. Adnexal ring of ectopic pregnancy detected by contrast-enhanced CT. *Abdom Imaging* 2007; 32(1):56–58.

63. Gostout BS, Pachman DR, Lechner R. Recognizing and treating ovarian cancer. *Minn Med* 2012; 95:40–42.

64. Koonings PP, Campbell K, Mishell DR Jr, Grimes DA. Relative frequency of primary ovarian neoplasms: a 10-year review. *Obstet Gynecol* 1989; 74:921–926.

65. Kurtz AB et al. Diagnosis and staging of ovarian cancer: comparative values of Doppler and conventional US, CT, and MR imaging correlated with surgery and histopathologic analysis—report of the Radiation Diagnostic Oncology Group. *Radiology* 1999; 212:19–27.

66. Park SB, Cho KS, Kim JK. CT findings of mature cystic teratoma with malignant transformation: comparison with mature cystic teratoma. *Clin Imaging* 2011; 35:294–300.

67. Lai CH, Chang TC, Hsueh S, Wu TI, Chao A, Chou HH, Wang PN. Outcome and prognostic factors in ovarian germ cell malignancies. *Gynecol Oncol* 2005; 96:784–791.

68. Bazot M et al. Fibrothecomas of the ovary: CT and US findings. *J Comput Assist Tomogr* 1993; 17:754–759.

69. Kawamoto S, Urban BA, Fishman EK. CT of epithelial ovarian tumors. *Radiographics* 1999; 19:S85–S102.

70. Tsili AC, Tsampoulas C, Argyropoulou M, Navrozoglou I, Alamanos Y, Paraskevaidis E, Efremidis SC. Comparative evaluation of multidetector CT and MR imaging in the differentiation of adnexal masses. *Eur Radiol* 2008; 18(5):1049–1057.

71. Asch E, Levine D, Pedrosa I, Hecht JL, Kruskal J. Patterns of misinterpretation of adnexal masses on CT and MR in an academic radiology department. *Acad Radiol* 2009; 16(8):969–980.

72. Kim SH, Kim WH, Park KJ, Lee JK, Kim JS. CT and MR findings of Krukenberg tumors: comparison with primary ovarian tumors. *J Comput Assist Tomogr* 1996; 20:393–398.

73. Krukenberg F. Ueber das Fibrosarcoma ovarii mucocellulare (Carcinomatodes). *Arch Gynecol* 1896; 50:287–321.

74. Saksouk FA, Johnson SC. Recognition of the ovaries and ovarian origin of pelvic masses with CT. *Radiographics* 2004; 24:S133–S146.

75. Jung SI, Kim YJ, Jeon HJ, Jeong KA. Deep infiltrating endometriosis: CT imaging evaluation. *J Comput Assist Tomogr* 2010; 34(3):338–342.

76. Coutinho AC Jr, Coutinho EPD, Aidar MN, Gasparetto EL, De Oliveira CMA, Ribeiro EB. Magnetic resonance imaging in deep pelvic endometriosis: iconographic essay. *Radiol Brasil* 2008; 41:129–134.

77. Chamié LP, Blasbalg R, Pereira RM, Warmbrand G, Serafini PC. Findings of pelvic endometriosis at transvaginal US, MR imaging, and laparoscopy. *Radiographics* 2011; 31:E77–E100.

78. Accetta I, Accetta P, Accetta AF, Maia FJ, Oliveira AP. Abdominal wall endometrioma. *Rev Col Bras Cir* 2011; 38(1):41–44.

79. Tsili AC, Argyropoulou MI, Koliopoulos G, Paraskevaidis E, Tsampoulas K. Malignant transformation of an endometriotic cyst: MDCT and MR findings. *J Radiol Case Rep* 2011; 5(1):9–17.

80. Vassilieff M et al. Computed tomography-based virtual colonoscopy: an examination useful for the choice of the surgical management of colorectal endometriosis. *Gynecol Obstet Fertil* 2011; 39(6):339–345.

81. Paspulati RM, Dalal TA. Imaging of complications following gynecologic surgery. *Radiographics* 2010; 30:625–642.

82. Shepherd JH, Crawford RA, Oram DH. Radical trachelectomy: a way to preserve fertility in the treatment of early cervical cancer. *Br J Obstet Gynaecol* 1998; 105:912–916.

83. Sahdev A, Jones J, Shepherd JH, Reznek RH. MR Imaging appearances of the female pelvis after trachelectomy. *Radiographics* 2005; 25:41–52.

84. Peppercorn PD et al. Role of MR imaging in the selection of patients with early cervical carcinoma for fertility-preserving surgery: initial experience. *Radiology* 1999; 212:395–399.

85. Jeong YY, Kang HK, Chung TW, Seo JJ, Park JG. Uterine cervical carcinoma after therapy: CT and MR imaging findings. *Radiographics* 2003; 23:969–981.

86. Gupta S et al. Various approaches for CT-guided percutaneous biopsy of deep pelvic lesions: anatomic and technical considerations. *Radiographics* 2004; 24:175–189.

87. Walser E, Raza S, Hernandez A, Ozkan O, Kathuria M, Akinci D. Sonographically guided transgluteal drainage of pelvic abscesses. *AJR Am J Roentegen* 2003; 181:498–500.

88. Feld R. Treatment of pelvic abscesses and other fluid collections: efficacy of transvaginal sonographically guided aspiration and drainage. *Am J Roentgen* 1994; 163:1141–1145.

89. Addley HC, Vargas HA, Moyle PL, Crawford R, Sala E. Pelvic imaging following chemotherapy and radiation therapy for gyneco logic malignancies. *Radiographics* 2010; 30:1843–1856.

90. Vincens E et al. Accuracy of magnetic resonance imaging in predicting residual disease in patients treated for stage IB2/II cervical carcinoma with chemoradiation therapy. Correlation of radiologic findings with surgicopathologic results. *Cancer* 2008; 113:2158–2165.

91. Narayanan P, Nobbenhuis M, Reynolds KM, Sahdev A, Reznek RH, Rockall AG. Fistulas in malignant gynecologic disease: etiology, imaging, and management. *Radiographics* 2009; 29:1073–1083.

92. Weber TM, Sostman HD, Spritzer CE, Ballard RL, Meyer GA, Clark Pearson DL, Soper JT. Cervical carcinoma: determination of recurrent tumor extent versus radiation changes with MR imaging. *Radiology* 1995; 194:135–139.

Section III

Muscle and Skeleton

15

Degenerative and Traumatic Diseases of the Spine

Evangelos N. Perdikakis

CONTENTS

15.1 Degenerative Diseases of the Spine

15.1.1 Introduction

Spine degeneration is among the leading causes of functional incapacity and chronic disability in both sexes. A number of different mechanical, traumatic, nutritional, and genetic factors have been implicated in the cascade of spine degeneration. Even though several causes are responsible for the physiological age-related spinal changes, the main impact of trauma, either in the forms of acute traumatism or chronic overload that leads to micro–macro instability is especially of paramount importance. The role of imaging in the degenerative pathology of the spine usually comes from the need for identifying the reason for the clinical problem of pain. However, the radiologist should always bear in mind that the presence of degenerative changes is by no means an indicator of symptoms as there is a very high prevalence of spine degeneration in asymptomatic individuals. Radicular or nonradicular pain may be because of degeneration of various anatomically involved spine portions that should be interpreted always in the relevant clinical history. Thus, symptom provocation might be the result of disc degeneration, bony endplate osteochondrosis and facet joint osteoarthrosis that may act alone or in combination. In addition, far from the morphologic or mechanical factors that may be implicated in the etiology of pain in the degenerative spine, the role of different inflammatory mediators complicates the issue even more. In this chapter, an overview of the spectrum of degenerative diseases of the spine is provided. Special emphasis is directed to multi-detector computed tomography (MDCT) imaging appearance of degenerative spine disorders, since MDCT offers several advantages with its superior spatial resolution. The image acquisition at a submillimeter scale together with the availability of multiplanar reformations can reveal the underlying etiology of symptomatology and contribute in establishing the correct diagnosis and thus in tailoring the appropriate therapy.

15.1.2 Osseous Degenerative Changes

15.1.2.1 Degenerative Changes in the Vertebral Bodies

The changes that can be observed in the vertebral bodies because of intervertebral disk degeneration can be manifested in the following two ways: (1) osteophyte formation and (2) bone marrow changes in the adjacent endplates.

15.1.2.1.1 Osteophyte Formation

They occur on the upper or lower margins of the vertebral body that is adjacent to the degenerated disk. Usually they take the form of a bony excrescence protuberance and their pathogenesis is related to chronic traction forces on Sharpey's fibers (traction osteophytes). These bony spurs typically develop where these fibers attach to the vertebral body. Osteophytes are usually anterolateral in location and extend initially in the horizontal and then in the vertical direction. Spondylosis deformans and intervertebral osteochondrosis are common terms that encompass these age-related vertebral alterations. Differential diagnosis is needed from syndesmophytes that develop in ankylosing spondylitis, from enthesophytes that are commonly seen in psoriatic arthritis and Reiter syndrome and from diffuse idiopathic skeletal hyperostosis (DISH) but this is beyond the scope of this chapter. In the thoracolumbar spine, osteophytes are located anterolaterally and do not present difficulties in recognition. In the cervical spine, however, osteophyte formation may occur in a posterior location (degenerative osteoarthritis of uncovertebral joints). During image interpretation the differentiation of disk abnormalities from posteriorly located osteophytes is extremely difficult even with MDCT and magnetic resonance imaging (MRI). Since both the disk material and the bony spurs may contribute to neural compression and symptomatology, the combination of disk degeneration, bulging, and associated posteriorly protruded bony osteophytes in the cervical spine has led in the use of the term diskovertebral or diskosteophytic complex. MDCT offers

several advantages in the evaluation of bony details and thus is an excellent imaging method for osteophyte depiction and their possible impact in spinal neural elements. (Figures 15.1 through 15.4)

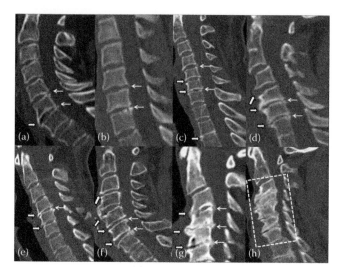

FIGURE 15.1
The sagittal MPR–MDCT images in eight patients show various degrees of osseous vertebral degenerative changes in the cervical spine. Anteriorly projecting osteophytes are shown with thick arrows and posteriorly located diskosteophytic changes are shown with thin arrows (a–h). Marked central spinal stenosis is noted in h (in dashed line).

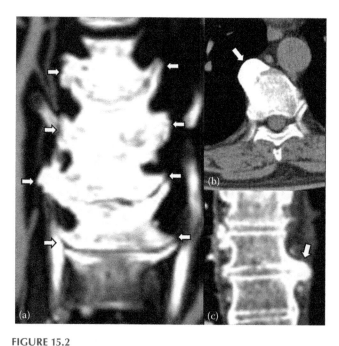

FIGURE 15.2
(a) The coronal MIP–MDCT image show laterally projecting osteophytes (arrows) in the cervical spine. (b) The axial MDCT image shows a large anterolateral osteophyte (arrow) in the thoracic spine. (c) Laterally projecting osteophytes (arrow) in the lower thoracic spine.

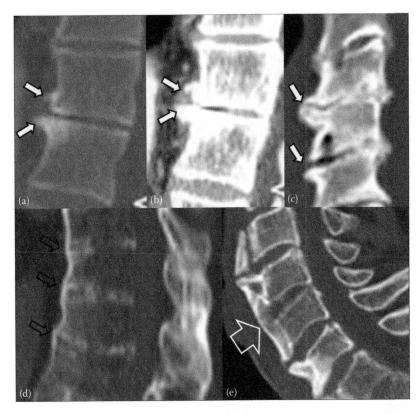

FIGURE 15.3
Differential diagnosis of osteophytosis. Sagittal MDCT images. (a–b) Degenerative osteophytic changes (arrows) in the lumbar spine. (c) Degenerative osteophytic changes (arrows) in the cervical spine. (d) Ankylosing spondylitis in the thoracolumbar spine (open black arrows). (e) DISH in the cervical spine (open white arrow).

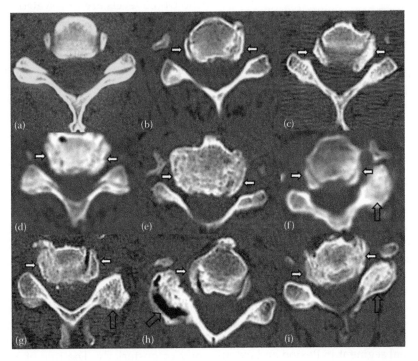

FIGURE 15.4
(a) The axial MDCT image shows the normal spinal anatomy at the level of the uncovertebral joints. (b–i) Different patients with degenerative osteophytic changes of the uncovertebral joints (arrows) and degenerative osteophytosis of the facet joints (open black arrows). Note the resulting foraminal stenoses because of the aforementioned degenerative changes in comparison to panel a.

15.1.2.1.2 Bone Marrow Changes

The role of MRI in bone marrow disorders is of paramount importance because it can evaluate marrow pathology to a better extent than MDCT. Signal intensity changes in vertebral body marrow adjacent to the endplates of degenerated disks are a common observation on MRI evaluation of the degenerated spine. Parallel bands of abnormal signal in the endplates may take three main forms that represent the response of the vertebral bone marrow to the adjacent disk degeneration. Modic type I changes show decreased signal intensity on T1-w images and increased signal intensity on T2-w images. Histopathologically, they are correlated with the associated inflammatory and vascularized fibrous changes of the bone marrow adjacent to the degenerated disk. Modic type II endplate changes are shown with increased signal intensity both on T1-w and T2-w sequences because of focal fatty replacement. Finally, Modic type III changes are depicted by a decreased signal intensity on both T1-w and T2-w MR images and correlate with extensive bony sclerosis. MDCT cannot be used in the evaluation of type I, II endplate bone marrow changes and can only depict the bony sclerosis in type III changes. For that reason, the role of MDCT is limited and MRI is definitely the modality of choice in studying the degenerative bone marrow disorders. Furthermore, MRI offers the ability to study the degenerative marrow changes in relation to time. Type I may convert to type II or reestablish a normal signal appearance. Type II changes have been shown to be more stable over time but may also convert to type I, type III, or a mixed pattern of type I and II. The clinical significance of these changes remains obscure but is postulated that type I changes are related to some degree of instability and reconversion of either type I or II to normal signal intensity may serve as an indicator of good clinical-surgical outcome (Figure 15.5).

15.1.2.2 Degenerative Changes in the Facet (Zygapophyseal) Joints

The facet joints are true diarthrodial synovium lined joints with hyaline cartilage overlying subchondral bone, a synovial membrane, and a joint capsule. They are formed by the inferior articular process of the above vertebra, which articulates with the superior articular process of the vertebra bellow. The anterior aspect of the facet joint is covered by the ligamentum flavum. Various studies have shown the important biomechanical role of facet joints in load transmission, in stabilizing the corresponding spinal segment in flexion and extension, and in restricting the axial rotation in rotational spinal kinematics. Knowledge of facet innervations is of paramount importance prior to description of the

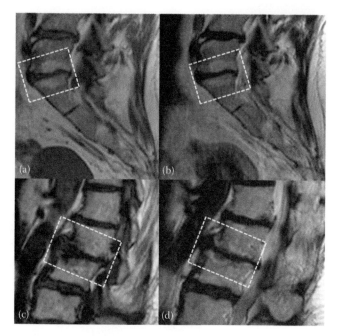

FIGURE 15.5
The sagittal (a) T1-w and (b) T2-w MR images show typical Modic type II endplate changes. The sagittal (c) T1-w and (d) T2-w MR images show mixed Modic type I–II endplate changes.

degenerative changes of the zygapophyseal joints. Each facet joint is innervated by the medial branches of the primary dorsal rami from the same level and the above spinal level. For example, the zygapophyseal joints at the L4–L5 levels are innervated by both the L4 and the L3 medial branches. Facet joint degeneration is considered a multifactorial process that is intimately tied to the intervertebral disc degeneration. From an anatomical, functional, and biomechanical point of view, each spinal segment consists of an anteriorly situated intervertebral disc and the posteriorly located paired facet joints hence the term "three-joint complex." Disk degeneration has been shown to increase the stresses on the facet joints. The sequelae and progress of micro- and macro-instability produced in conjunction with disk pathology results in facet osteroarthritis (osteoarthrosis and osteophytosis). Although MRI is considered the modality of choice in the evaluation of disc degeneration, MDCT scanning provides superior anatomic bony detail for the evaluation of facet osteoarthritic changes. The characteristic MDCT findings that can be depicted are the same as osteoarthritis elsewhere in the body: articular cartilage loss, subchondral bone irregularity and sclerosis, and subarticular cyst and osteophyte formation. Synovial cysts may also develop from degenerated zygapophyseal joints and can be found either anteriorly or posteriorly. The role of MDCT in the depiction of these degenerative synovial cysts is limited and MRI is preferred because of better soft tissue differentiation. Facet joint osteoarthrosis may be an important factor of spinal stenosis because of the resulting compression of the adjacent neural structures (central canal stenosis, lateral recess stenosis, and foraminal stenosis). Facet osteoarthritis, which may even occur independently of disk degeneration, may cause hypermobility of the facet joint and subsequently may lead to degenerative spondylolisthesis. Finally, facet joint ostearthritic changes may provoke pain independently even without neural compression because of richly innervated synovium and joint capsule. In such patients, diagnostic spinal injections under fluoroscopic or MDCT guidance allow

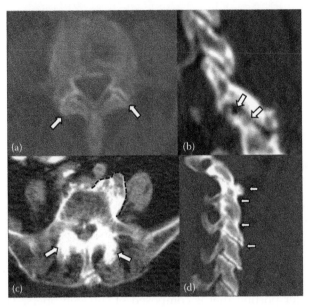

FIGURE 15.6
Facet degeneration in four patients. (a) Axial MDCT image in the lumbar spine. (b) Sagittal MDCT image in the lower cervical spine. (c) Axial MDCT image in the lumbosacral spine. (d) Sagittal MDCT image in the upper cervical spine. The arrows show characteristic osteoarthritic changes. A large anterolaterally projecting vertebral osteophyte is shown in panel c (dashed line).

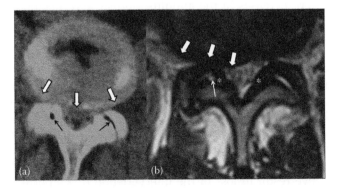

FIGURE 15.7
(a) The axial MDCT image shows central spinal stenosis because of diffuse disk bulging (large arrows), ligamentum flavum hypertrophy (asterisks), and facet joint osteoarthritis (thin black arrows). (b) The axial T2-w MR image shows right foraminal stenosis resulting from disk protrusion (large arrows), ligamentum flavum hypertrophy (asterisks), and facet osteoarthritis. A small synovial cyst is shown with thin arrow.

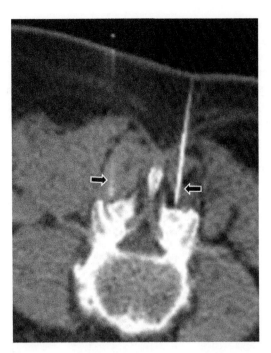

FIGURE 15.8
Diagnostic facet injections under MDCT guidance. Arrows showing the needles.

a functional assessment of these anatomic structures that are suspected to be sources of pain (Facet joint syndrome is the proposed clinical term in use) (Figures 15.4 and 15.6 through 15.8).

15.1.2.3 Degenerative Changes in the Posterior Spinal Elements

The degenerative changes of the disk and/or the zygapophyseal joints alters the local biomechanics in the posterior elements of the spine (spinous processes, supraspinatous ligament, interspinous ligaments, and paravertebral extrinsic and intrinsic muscles) and the increased chronic stress forces may result in degeneration of the aforementioned structures. This is especially evident in the lumbar spinal segments with a resulting increased hyperlordotic appearance and an associated pseudofaceted manifestation (Baastrup disease/ phenomenon). Controversy exists, however, as whether Baastrup disease is a normal finding of the aging spine or not. MDCT with sagittal reconstructions shows characteristic signs of this hyperlordotic degenerative appearance with lack of space between the adjacent spinous processes and the associated sclerotic bony changes—osteophyte formation. In advanced cases, bursae formation or true synovial joints may develop between the opposing spinous processes and MRI is the imaging modality of choice for depicting these changes that may be the cause of symptoms. The paravertebral intrinsic muscles of the lumbar spine are important for spine stabilization and mobility because they regulate the tonus and motion of the spine. In chronic stages of spine degeneration, muscular atrophy with fatty infiltration is observed in cross-sectional imaging studies. Nevertheless, the relationship between these changes and pain provocation remains controversial. (Various examples are shown in Figures 15.9 through 15.12.)

15.1.3 Disk Degeneration

The intervertebral disk together with the articulating superior and inferior vertebral bodies constitute a cartilaginous joint (amphiarthrosis). The normal disk consists of an inner portion called nucleus pulposus and is surrounded by the annulus fibrosus. The nucleus pulposus is eccentrically located and in more close relation to the posterior surface of the intervertebral disk and

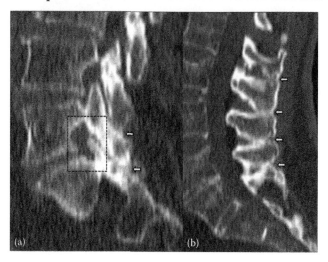

FIGURE 15.9
(a) Foraminal stenosis (in dashed line) because of facet hypertrophy and mild grade I degenerative anterolisthesis of L5 vertebra. Note degenerative changes in the posterior processes (arrows). (b) More extensive degenerative changes in the posterior processes (arrows) with a hyperlordotic lumbar spine appearance.

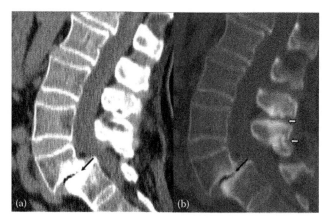

FIGURE 15.10
(a–b) Degenerative grade II spondylolisthisis. There is anterolisthesis of L5 vertebra (black arrow) and associated degenerative changes in the posterior spinal processes (white arrows).

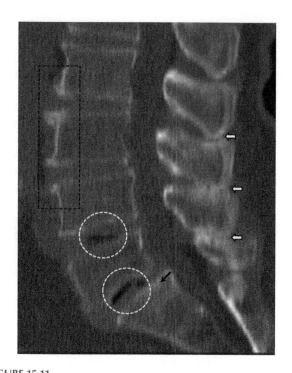

FIGURE 15.11
The sagittal MDCT image shows lumbar spinal degenerative changes with the presence of vacuum disk phenomenum in L4, L5 (dashed circles) disks, grade I degenerative spondylolisthesis of L5 vertebra in relation to S1 (black arrow), anteriorly projecting vertebral osteophytes (dashed rectangle), and degeneration of the posterior spinal processes (arrows).

is composed of water and proteoglycans. The annulus fibrosus has an inner portion of fibrocartilage and an outer portion that is composed of collagen fibers. The annulus fibrosus is anchored to the adjacent vertebral bodies by the Sharpey's fibers. With degeneration and normal aging a number of pathophysiologic changes appear both in the nucleus pulposus and the annulus fibrosus. The term "disk degeneration" may include any or all of the following underlying pathology: type II collagen increases in the annulus, fibrosis and mucinous degeneration of the annulus may occur, diffused bulging of the annulus and narrowing of the normal disk space is observed, annular tears and fissures develop, dehydration of the nucleus pulposus, and a change in its relative proteoglycan composition occurs. The water content and the integrity of the annulus appear to be important factors for the functional role of the intervertebral disk in stress absorption and load transmission in the vertebral column.

The degenerative and age-related changes mentioned above result in loss of the intervertebral disk's normal capacities, mainly loss of its elasticity, and MRI is considered the preferred imaging modality for depiction of these changes, which are manifested with loss of signal intensity in T2-w images. Furthermore, MR imaging is considered the most accurate anatomic method for the clinical assessment of the degenerated disk. A proposed classification system for lumbar disk degeneration that uses a five grading scale is currently in clinical use and is based on MR signal intensities, disk structure, the differentiation between nucleus and annulus fibrosus, and disk height. This classification system has shown good intra- and interobserver agreement and is applied in clinical practice at any level in the spinal column (cervical, thoracic, or lumbar region). The morphological disk abnormalities have been thus categorized in: (1) normal disk, (2) disk bulging, (3) disk protrusion, (4) disk extrusion, and (5) disk sequestration or free fragment. The term "disk herniation" is deliberately omitted from discussion because it encompasses a broad pathology, as the herniated material may include part of the nucleus pulposus, cartilaginous portions, fragmented apophyseal bony material, or disorganized annular tissues. In other words the term "herniation" may refer both to extrusion and protrusion and its use should be avoided in a radiologic report. However, the terms "broad-based disk herniation" (involving between 25% and 50% [90–180°] of the disc circumference) and "focal disk herniation" (involving less than 25% [90°] of the disc circumference) are still being used in the everyday clinical practice.

Analytically, the aforementioned terminology of disk degeneration is presented in Table 15.1.

Apart from the morphologic classification mentioned above, in a radiologic report the clinicians should also be informed about the location and site of the focal disk abnormalities as well as the relationship with the

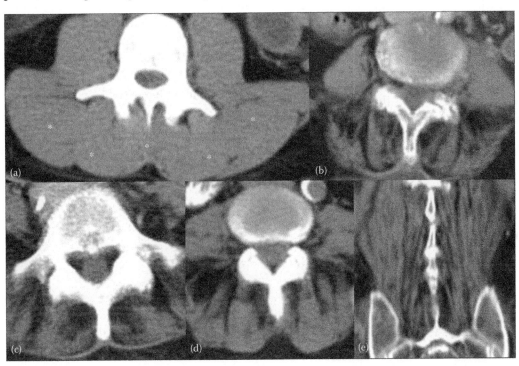

FIGURE 15.12
The axial (a) MDCT image shows the normal muscle mass (asterisks) of the paravertebral muscles in a male patient. The axial (b), (c), and (d) and the coronal (e) MDCT images in four different patients show degenerative muscle changes with muscle mass atrophy and diffuse fatty infiltration.

TABLE 15.1

Terminology of Disk Degeneration

Normal disk	The disk does not reach beyond the border margin of the adjacent vertebral bodies.
Disk bulging	The disk extends symmetrically and circumferentially beyond the margins of the adjacent vertebral bodies.
Disk protrusion	There is a focal or asymmetric extension of the disk material beyond the adjacent vertebral body margin. The disk origin (disk base) is broader than any other dimension of the protrusion.
Disk extrusion	There is more pronounced extension of the disk beyond the vertebral body margin. The disk base is usually narrower than the diameter of the extruded material (calculations should be done in all planes to determine the true dimensions). The extruded material may migrate posteriorly or upward or downward in relation to the adjacent vertebral bodies but maintains connection with the parent disk.
Disk sequestration	It is defined as an extruded disk material that loses attachment to the parent disk (hence the synonymous term free-disk fragment). The sequestered disk fragment may migrate either cranially or caudally.

neural elements. This is of principal clinical relevance because the treating physician can determine the correlation of symptoms with the reported anatomic disk abnormality and this information may influence treatment options or surgical planning. A complete imaging evaluation should thus include a description of the focal disk abnormality in the concept of location as following: (1) centrally located, (2) in left or right paracentral location, (3) in left or right foraminal location, and (4) left or right extraforaminal (otherwise called far lateral) located. A new MRI-based classification system that assesses the compromised nerve root in relation to the focal disk abnormality has recently been proposed. According to this study, the relation between the nerve root and the degenerated disk could be described as following: no contact, contact without nerve root deviation, contact with nerve root deviation, and finally, evidence of nerve root compression. Regardless of the classification proposed above, the relationship of the focal disk abnormality with the neural elements should definitely be included in an MR examination report.

In this section, an overview of the spectrum of disk degeneration is provided. Emphasis is given on MRI because MRI has become the standard of reference regarding disk abnormalities' evaluation. The superior soft tissue differentiation and characterization of MRI is a dominant significant feature in the accurate evaluation of the patient with back pain. The role of MDCT despite its superior spatial resolution is of limited value in disk degeneration. Focal disk abnormalities can be depicted and different window-level modifications together with selection of an appropriate reconstruction filter may allow correct identification of disk degeneration. The vacuum disk phenomenum (representing N_2 gas from negative pressure inside the abnormal space of the degenerated disk) can easily be manifested in MDCT exams. However, neural elements and neural compromise is better examined with MRI. Furthermore, differentiation of disk material from facet joint synovial cysts, perineural cysts, conjoined nerve roots, and tumors of the spinal canal is difficult to be carried out with MDCT. Nevertheless, in certain contraindications to MRI and in postoperative spine imaging MDCT might serve as a valuable alternative. (Illustrative cases in Figures 15.13 through 15.17.)

15.1.4 Spinal Stenosis

Spinal stenosis is defined as narrowing either of the central spinal canal or of the neural foramen or of the lateral recess or any combination of these anatomic areas.

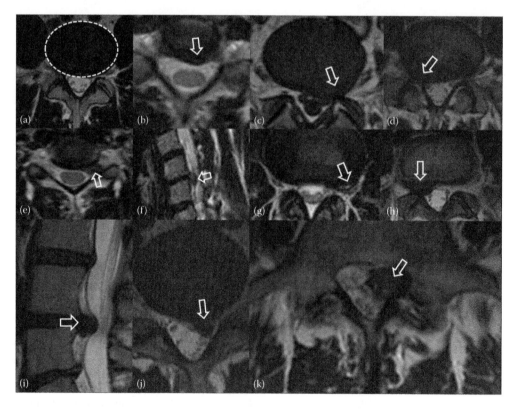

FIGURE 15.13

Disk contour abnormalities (all images are in T2-w sequence besides c and k, which are in T1-w). (a) Diffuse disk bulging, (b) left paracentral protruded disk, (c) left foraminal protruded disk, (d) right foraminal protruded disk, (e–f) left paracentral extruded disk, (g) left foraminal–extraforaminal extruded disk, (h) right foraminal extruded disk, (i) centrally extruded disk, (j) left paracentral extruded disk, and (k) sequestered disk material in the lateral recess (arrows and dashed circle point to the disk contour abnormalities).

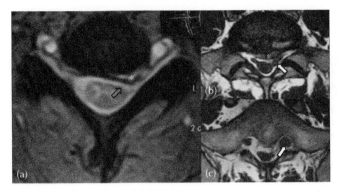

FIGURE 15.14
The axial (a) T2-w MR image shows a left paracentral protruded disk (asterisk) that causes thecal sac deformation (open arrow). The axial (b), (c) T1-w MR images show a centrally protruded disk (asterisk) that contacts the nerve root and causes diffuse nerve root edema (arrow). Compare with normal right nerve root.

According to etiology, spinal stenosis is classified as: (1) congenital-developmental (e.g., idiopathic achondroplasia, short padicle syndrome, and osteopetrosis) and (2) acquired (most commonly because of degenerative disease). Developmental and congenital stenosis can also be exacerbated by superimposed acquired degenerative changes and thus become symptomatic. The degenerative spinal changes mentioned above may contribute to spinal stenosis either alone or in combination (disk bulges–protrusions–extrusions, intervertebral osteochondrosis, facet osteoarthritic changes, ligamentum flavum hypertrophy, or inward buckling). Various other causes, besides degeneration, could be responsible for spinal stenosis and can be identified in cross-sectional imaging studies such as tumors, fractures, spondylolysis

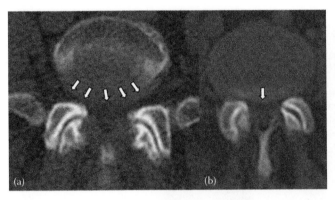

FIGURE 15.15
MDCT appearance of disk contour abnormalities. (a) Diffuse disk bulging (arrows). (b) Centrally protruded disk (arrow).

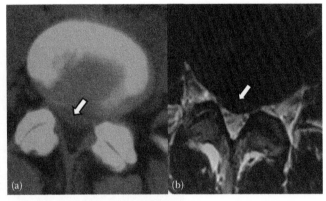

FIGURE 15.16
Correlation of MDCT and MRI in disk contour abnormalities. The axial (a) MDCT and the axial (b) T2-w MR images both nicely depict a centrally extruded disk (arrows).

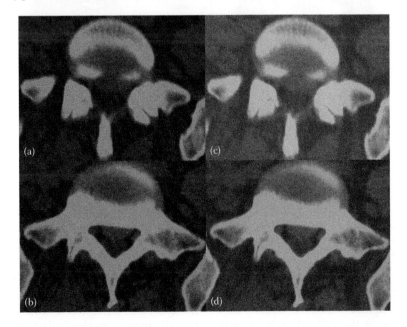

FIGURE 15.17
Role of window-level and reconstruction filter-kernel adjustment in disk contour abnormality depiction. The axial (a and b) and (c and d) MDCT images in different window-level and filter selection show a centrally extruded disk that contacts the thecal sack.

15.1.5 Focus Points in Spine Degeneration

Degenerative Diseases of the Spine

Osseous Degenerative Changes	Disk Degeneration	Spinal Stenosis

• Vertebral Bodies
  I. Osteophyte formation
  II. Bone marrow changes (Modic I, II, III)
• Facet Joint Osteoarthritis
  I. Articular cartilage loss
  II. Subchondral bone irregularity-sclerosis
  III. Subarticular cyst formation
  IV. Osteophyte formation
  V. Synovial cyst formation
  VI. (and evaluation of ligamentum flavum degenerative changes)
• Posterior Spinal Elements
  I. Baastrup Disease
  II. (and evaluation of muscle atrophy and fatty infiltration of paravertebral muscles)
	• Terminology
	  I. Disk Bulging
	  II. Disk Protrusion
	  III. Disk Extrusion
	  IV. Disk Sequestration
	• Location
	  I. Central
	  II. Paracentral
	  III. Foraminal
	  IV. Extraforaminal
	• Relation with neural elements
	  I. Evaluate thecal sac contour
	  II. Evaluate nerve roots
		• Narrowing
		  I. Central spinal canal
		  II. Neural foramen
		  III. Lateral recess
		  IV. Any combination of the above anatomic areas
		• Imaging signs of severe spinal stenosis
		  I. Swelling/edema of nerve root
		  II. Cord myelopathy-myelomalacia
		  III. Elongation of the cauda equina
		  IV. Enhancement of the nerve roots in post gadolinium MR sequences

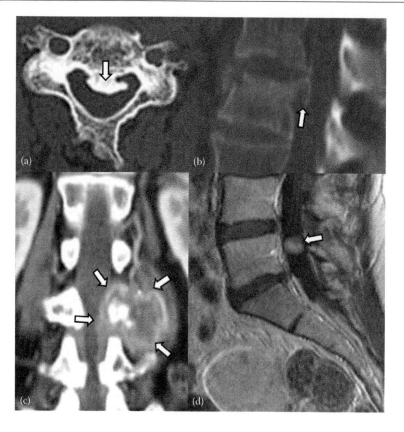

FIGURE 15.18

Spinal stenosis from various causes. (a) The axial MDCT image shows ossification of the posterior longitudinal ligament (arrow) causing central canal stenosis. (b) The sagittal MDCT image shows a seatbelt thoracic fracture with fractured material (arrow) in the central canal. (c) The coronal contrast-enhanced MDCT image depicts a breast cancer metastasis (arrows) causing central canal and foraminal stenosis. (d) The sagittal contrast enhanced T1-w MR image shows an ependymoma (arrow) occupying the central canal.

with spondylolisthisis, epidural lipomatosis, ossification of the posterior longitudinal ligament, and Paget disease.

Symptomatology from spinal stenosis is usually nonspecific and includes any of the following: back pain, neurogenic claudication, radiculopathy, and pain that is exacerbated or alleviated with postural changes. It is important to emphasize that imaging alone does not indicate that a patient is symptomatic. Physical examination, electrodiagnostic tests are additional informative diagnostic methods that should be correlated with cross-sectional imaging modalities (MRI and MDCT). In addition to that, absolute measurements of the bony spinal canal (anteroposterior diameter) provide little help in the determination of the clinical significance of the observed spinal stenosis. Measurements of the cross-sectional area of the central canal in a Picture Archiving and Communication System (PACS) station (in mm²) could be conducted, however, in the lumbar level and an area <75–100 mm² has been shown to correlate with the likelihood of symptomatic central spinal stenosis.

The superiority of MRI over MDCT in the evaluation of spinal stenosis is accentuated by the fact that we are trying to determine and report a possible impact on neural elements. The most important cross-sectional imaging finding in MRI exams that may be used as a criterion of the severity of the spinal stenosis is the shape of thecal sac and the amount of residual subarachnoid space as seen on axial T2-w images. Additional MRI findings that may indicate a severe spinal stenosis are swelling and edema of the compressed nerve root, cord myelopathy–myelomalacia, a relative elongation of the cauda equina either above or below the stenotic segment and enhancement of the nerve roots in postgadolinium sequences. The last finding has been shown to be a negative prognostic sign for complete resolution of symptoms even after successful decompression surgery. (Various cases of degenerative spinal stenosis are described in Figures 15.1, 15.4, 15.7, 15.9, 15.13, and 15.14, whereas Figure 15.18 shows examples of spinal stenosis because of other causes.)

15.2 Traumatic Diseases of the Spine

15.2.1 Introduction

Traumatic injuries of the spine represent a major cause of disability and have an increased socioeconomic cost mainly because they can result in partial or complete paralysis. They are frequently encountered in level one trauma center patients with serious high velocity/high force accidents such as motor vehicle accidents (MVA), falling, and sports injuries. Furthermore, benign or malignant diseases may predispose to traumatic spinal injuries without the presence of a high-velocity/high-intensity applied force. For that reason, in the definition of spinal fractures one item should always be firstly taken into account. "What is the bone status prior to the applied force?" Acute traumatic fractures occur as a result of increased biomechanical stress on a normal bone. Pathologic spinal fractures occur as a response to normal or slightly increased stress on a weakened bone. Fatigue and overuse injuries-fractures occur in response to a chronic repetitive biomechanical stress on a normal bone background. The correct diagnosis of spinal trauma is based on a thorough clinical examination and is tailored by the associated radiological findings. The diagnostic

imaging of spinal trauma has been revolutionized with the advent of MDCT and MRI. Plain film radiography used to be the initial imaging procedure in the evaluation of traumatic injuries of the spine but has now been replaced by MDCT. For example, anteroposterior, lateral, oblique, swimmer's, and open mouth odontoid views as well as flexion-extension radiographs of the cervical spine have been largely substituted by MDCT and its multiplanar reconstructions in both the coronal and sagittal planes. In addition, plain radiographs have shown a lower sensitivity for identifying traumatic spine lesions compared to cross-sectional imaging studies, particularly MDCT. Not only is MDCT more accurate in diagnosing spinal injury, it also has been shown to reduce imaging time and patient manipulation and this is of paramount importance in cervical spine traumatic injuries and multi-injured patients. The principal limitation of MDCT is its inability to directly evaluate the spinal cord and the supporting ligamentous structures. However, these limitations have been overcome with the use of MRI and its crucial role in patients with neurologic deficits and suspected spinal cord injury is well-established, nowadays. MRI has an inherent superior contrast resolution with higher sensitivity for soft-tissue injuries and is currently performed in any injured patient with signs of myelopathy, radiculopathy, progressive neurologic deficit, and/or an unexpected level of clinical signs above the level of the radiographically or MDCT-detected injury. The purpose of this chapter is to present characteristic radiographic features of common and uncommon traumatic disorders of the spine with emphasis on their MDCT findings.

15.2.2 Traumatic Injuries of the Normal Spine

15.2.2.1 Normal Developmental Variants That Should Not Be Interpreted as Fractures

Several developmental variants can simulate a fracture, and this is especially important in the evaluation of cervical spine injury in pediatric patients. Knowledge of the normal embryologic development and anatomy is essential to avoid misinterpretation of normal epiphyses or synchondroses as fractures (Figures 15.19 and 15.20). "Synchondroses" can be distinguished by their characteristic locations and smooth-well corticated margins whereas fractures have irregular and nonsclerotic margins. The atlas (C1) develops from three primary ossification centers and in the axon (C2) there are four ossification centers. Normal absence or delayed fusion of the ossification centers can be confused with C1 or C2 fracture. A potential source of confusion is the presence of clefts resulting from anomalous ossification centers. These clefts are more commonly encountered in the thoracic and lumbar spine but they can also be depicted in the cervical spine (Figure 15.21). Five types of vertebral

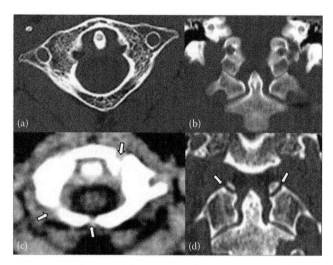

FIGURE 15.19

(a and b) Normal MDCT appearance of C1-C2. (c) Normal synchondroses (arrows) of the atlas in a 14-month-old boy. (d) Normal atlas synchondroses (arrows) in a 36-year-old male patient.

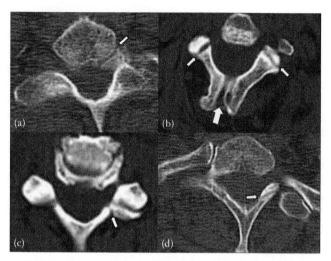

FIGURE 15.21

MDCT imaging of normal vertebral clefts. (a) Neurocentral cleft. (b) Bilateral spondylolysis clefts (small arrows) and spinal cleft (large arrow). (c and d) Retroisthmic clefts.

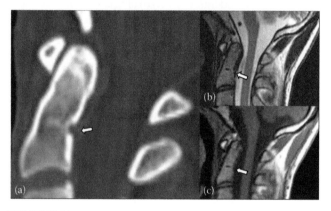

FIGURE 15.20

The sagittal (a) MDCT image and the sagittal T2-w (b), T1-w (c) MR images in a 20-year-old male show the normal synchondrosis (arrows) of the dens.

clefts have been described in the literature and are presented in Table 15.2.

Occipitalization of the atlas is a normal anatomic variation with lack of segmentation at the atlanto-occipital junction and is easily recognized with MDCT sagittal reformations. The os terminale is a secondary ossification center that appears at the tip of the odontoid process and normally fuses by the age of 12. It may persist, however, unfused and simulate a fracture of the odontoid tip. It must also be reminded that the apex of the odontoid is V-shaped before it ossifies or may persist that way and latter in adult life. Os odontoideum is considered a developmental anatomic variant and its cause is controversial. Some considered it to be an old fracture of the odontoid process that did not unite and others believe that it may be a large os terminale associated with a hypoplastic odontoid process. Limbus vertebra

TABLE 15.2

Normal Vertebral Clefts

Neurocentral synchondrosis	Location: at the posterolateral corner of the vertebral body
Retrosomatic cleft	Location: in the pedicle anterior to the transverse process
Spondylolysis involving the pars	Location: posterior to the transverse process
Retroisthmic cleft	Location: in the lamina
Spinal cleft	Location: in the spinous process

may be mistaken as fracture in the thoracolumbar spine. It is manifested as a cleft at the superior (rarely at the inferior) corner of the vertebral body. Some consider it to be an unfused ring apophysis, whereas others believe that it is the result of an intravertebral disk herniation similarly to Schmorl's nodes development. (Examples are shown in Figures 15.22 and 15.23.)

15.2.2.2 Biomechanics of Acute Traumatic Spinal Injury

Denis' three column model of spinal stability is very useful in understanding and interpreting the various patterns of traumatic spinal injury. The anterior column consists of the anterior longitudinal ligament, the anterior half of the vertebral bodies, the anterior part of the intervertebral disks, and the associated supporting soft tissues. The middle column consists of the posterior longitudinal ligament, posterior half of the vertebral bodies, and the posterior half of the annulus fibrosis (disk and supporting soft tissues). Finally, the posterior column consists of the neural arch, facet joints, and posterior soft tissue elements (mainly ligaments). Injury and disruption of only one column is considered a rather stable

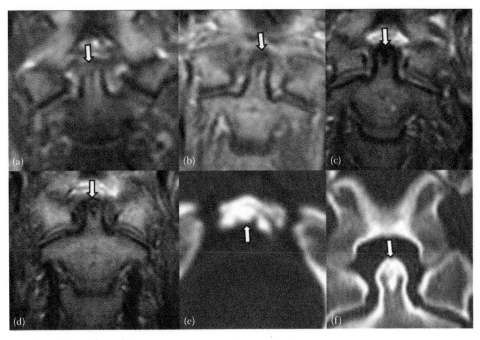

FIGURE 15.22
(a–d) The coronal T1-w MR images show different degrees of ossification and fusion of os terminale (arrows) in four patients. (e) The axial MDCT image shows an unfused os terminale (arrow). (f) The coronal MDCT image shows a fused os terminale. The characteristic V-shaped configuration of the dens can still be identified.

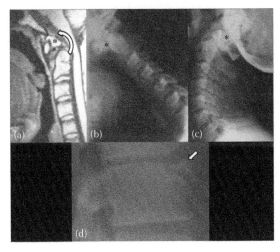

FIGURE 15.23
The sagittal (a) T1-w MR image shows an os odontoideum (asterisk) tilted anteriorly (curved arrow). The dynamic flexion (b) and extension (c) radiographs verify instability of the os. (d) The lateral radiograph shows a limbus vertebra variation (arrow).

injury and may be treated conservatively. Disruption of two or more columns is considered to result in spinal instability and mandates surgical intervention. The integrity of the middle column is considered the most crucial to spinal stability. The forces that may act alone or in combination and produce acute spinal trauma are usually in the form of flexion, extension, compression, shearing, rotation, and distraction. A complete

and detailed history of the traumatic event and mechanism of injury should be obtained, whenever possible, to tailor image interpretation. Flexion is the most common mechanism of trauma in spinal injuries and results in compressive forces in the anterior column and tension within the posterior elements. Extension forces act in the opposite way upon the spine. They increase tensile forces in the anterior column and compressive forces, posteriorly. Compression acts in an axial mode of force distribution and results in fractures that may involve all three columns as in burst fractures. Distraction forces are the opposite of compression ones and the spinal element (usually vertebra) is pulled in opposite directions in the plane of applied force. Rotational and shearing forces usually act in combination and cause ligamentous laxity and rupture resulting thus in dislocations. Last but not least, a radiologist should always bear in mind that spinal fractures may be encountered in contiguous and discontiguous levels of the spine. For that reason, once a spinal fracture is depicted, careful evaluation of adjacent vertebrae and in certain cases of the whole spine should be carried out. Fractures of C1 and C2 may be associated, for example, with fractures of the lower cervical spine. The reported incidence of second-level spinal fractures has been estimated to be 15%–17% by MDCT and 50% by MRI examinations. In addition, calcaneal fractures after fall from height (as in suicide attempts) have been associated with an increased risk of thoracolumbar spinal fractures.

15.2.2.3 Cervical Spine Injuries

Cervical spine injuries can be categorized based on the mechanism of applied force. The alignment of the vertebrae and the height of vertebral bodies should be evaluated and MDCT reformations (multiplanar reformations [MPRs]) provide the best means for that purpose. The four vertebral lines that are used in plain radiographic examinations for cervical spine trauma evaluation can be recognized in sagittal MDCT–MPRs as well (anterior vertebral line, posterior vertebral line, spinal laminar line, and posterior spinous line). Prevertebral soft tissue swelling should also be observed, although the width of prevertebral soft tissues could be quite variable. In adults, the normal measurements is less than 5 mm at the C3 and C4 level and increases up to 22 mm at the level of C6. In children, however, the prevertebral soft tissues should not exceed more than 2/3 the width of the C2 body at the level of C3 through C4 and should not measure more than 16 mm at the level of C6. In addition, the normal lordotic cervical alignment should be evaluated in every sagittal MDCT–MPR although loss of lordosis may be because of muscle spasm, patient positioning, backboard, or cervical collar use. The presence of several normal variations can make MDCT evaluation of the pediatric cervical spine difficult. These are presented in Table 15.3.

Besides identification of a cervical spine fracture and in the concept of the Denis three column model, any additional radiographic signs of instability should be evaluated and included in a MDCT report. These are the following:

1. Vertebral compression >25°
2. Widening of intervertebral disk space, facet discongruency, and widened interspinous space
3. Subluxation of one vertebral body on another >3.5 mm
4. Kyphosis or angulation >11°
5. Multiple fractures in one spinal segment

TABLE 15.3

Normal Variations in Pediatric Cervical Spine

Pseudosubluxation at C2–C3 and C3–C4 level	In children <8 years, because of physiologic laxity of the cervical spine (step-off <1.5–2 mm). May mimic Hangman's fracture.
Pseudospread of C1 upon C2	In children <7 years, because of discrepancy in the growth rate of the C1 in comparison to the C2. May mimic Jefferson's fracture.
Secondary ossification centers	May mimic fracture lines. Typical location and the smooth and corticated margins allows differentiation.
C3 vertebral body wedging	In children <7 years, normal wedging of the C3 vertebral body. Not to be mistaken with compressive fracture.

Specific types of cervical spine injuries including fractures, dislocations, and fracture–dislocations are presented in Table 15.4 and illustrated cases are shown in Figures 15.24 through 15.30.

15.2.2.4 Thoracolumbar Spine Injuries

The most common biomechanical forces of spinal injury that are implicated in the thoracolumbar trauma are in the form of compression and flexion distraction and over 90% of fractures occur at the T11–L4 level. However, complex mechanisms of injury can be encountered especially in MVA. In such cases, careful inspection of abdominal and thoracomediastinal structures needs to be carried out because of the possible concomitant presence of severe thoracoabdominal trauma. MDCT with images reconstructed in the sagittal and coronal planes clearly depicts the radiographic findings of thoracolumbar fractures. Particular attention should be given to the height and configuration of all vertebral bodies as well as in their alignment because any offset or malalignment of the vertebral bodies could help in the identification of isolated fractures or fracture-dislocations. If the injury is limited to the anterior column, it is considered stable. Once an anterior column fracture is depicted; however, special attention is needed to identify any additional radiographic features that may indicate thoracolumbar spine instability. These are presented in Table 15.5, and specific types of thoracolumbar fractures are described in Table 15.6 and illustrated in Figures 15.31 through 15.33.

15.2.2.5 Penetrating Spinal Injuries

In general, penetrating injuries can be differentiated into two types: (1) high-energy injuries or (2) low-energy injuries. Low-energy injuries are usually the result of low-velocity guns and sharp cutting objects, such as knives, arrows, glass, sharp, sticks, etc. High-energy injuries are the consequence of high-velocity projectiles, for example, those from military weapons, and typically are characterized from a widespread tissue destruction than low-energy injuries. Although traditionally penetrating injuries were described in the medical literature from military surgeons in the battlefields, the widespread use of guns and the increased criminal rates in the modern western societies has led in a significant increase of morbidity and mortality from these injuries. From a ballistic point of view, the severity of a bullet wound depends on its velocity, special type of bullet used, and the vital structures through the bullet trajectory. The result on the body structures can be either by direct impact or by kinetic energy transfer, or

TABLE 15.4

Specific Types of Cervical Spine Injuries

Craniocervical dissociation	It is a rare and often fatal injury. Most often caused by MVA and concomitant facial and intracranial injuries are often present. It can be further classified into three subtypes: anterior dislocation, posterior dislocation, and longitudinal distraction. The tectorial membrane and the alar ligaments have to be disrupted for this dislocation to occur. A variety of angles, lines, and measurements have been described and used for the imaging assessment of this fatal spine injury: (a) The Wackenheim clivus line (b) The Kaufman's method (condylar gap method) (c) The Powers' ratio (d) The basion-dens interval (e) The basion-posterior axial line method (Harris method) (f) The predental interval
"Jefferson" fracture	It actually represents a burst fracture of C1 ring. The mechanism of trauma is usually a direct impact on the top of the head (common in swimming pool-diving accidents). The axial loading forces cause the lateral masses of the atlas to slide apart disrupting thus the C1 ring, which breaks in several places but in children an isolated fracture line involving the synchondrosis may be observed.
Atlantoaxial rotatory displacement	It can be caused by minor trauma and represents a rotational injury of C1 on C2. Patients typically present with painful torticollis and limited range of motion. It has been classified into four subtypes by Fielding and Hawkins: Type I: C1 is rotated on C2 with the odontoid acting as the pivot and with no anterior displacement. Type II: C1 is rotated on C2 with the lateral mass as the pivot and there is <5 mm of anterior displacement. Type III: C1 is rotated on C2 with more than 5 mm of anterior displacement of C1 upon C2. Type IV: There is posterior displacement of C1 on C2. MDCT images in the axial plane can illustrate the relationships between the occiput, atlas, and axis and show the rotation of C1 on C2.
Odontoid (dens) fractures	They represent the most common fractures of the cervical spine in children, and they are also the most commonly missed cervical spine fractures in plain radiographs. According to the location of the fracture, three types are described: Type 1 is an avulsion of the odontoid tip. It is considered a stable injury and treated with immobilization. Type 2 (most common pattern of dens injury) is a transverse fracture at base of the dens. There is 30%–50% incidence of nonunion and is considered unstable and treated with primary fusion. Type 3 is an unstable fracture extending into the body of C2. MDCT–MPRs in the sagittal and coronal plane are invaluable in the correct diagnosis of odontoid fractures.
"Hangman's" fracture	It is an unstable fracture of the upper cervical spine that is more commonly seen at C2 level. The mechanism of trauma is hyperextension and distraction injury that results in bilateral neural arch fractures (common dashboard injury when the patient hits the head on the dashboard). Usually the cord is not damaged unless there is severe displacement and angulation.
"Clay-Shoveler's" fracture	This fracture occurs at any level of the lower cervical spine but most commonly involves the C6, C7, and T1. It is an isolated fracture of the spinous process. The mechanism of trauma is an avulsion injury of the supraspinatus ligaments upon the spinous process.
Flexion teardrop fracture	It is the result of a severe flexion force acting on the C-spine that causes disruption of the posterior ligaments and anterior wedge compression vertebral fracture. The teardrop fracture is a severe flexion injury that may result in permanent neurologic damage. MDCT sagittal and coronal MPRs images show a characteristic triangular bony fragment at the anterior–inferior border of the fractured-vertebral body and associated displacement and traumatic stenosis in the central canal.
Unilateral locked facets	It is the result of flexion, distraction, and rotation that causes facet joint dislocation. There is a characteristic locking of the facet in an overriding position. MDCT in the axial plane together with MPRs can reveal this characteristic type of injury.
Bilateral locked facets	Bilateral disarticulation of the facets. The mechanism of injury is similar to unilateral locked facets but there is a higher incidence of severe cord injury.
SCIWORA	It is defined as the presence of objective neurological signs of myelopathy because of trauma but with the absence of fracture or ligamentous instability noted on radiographs or CT. MRI can help in the correct diagnosis by revealing a number of neural and extraneural findings such as cord edema, cord hematoma, cord transaction, ligamentous disruption, edema or hematoma in the paravertebral muscles, disc edema or traumatic disk herniation, and epidural or subdural hemorrhage.

a combination of both mechanisms. For the aforementioned reason, the anatomic structures may be injured even in the absence of direct contact with a high-energy bullet. In addition, bony fractured fragments and bullet fragmentation can result in secondary projectiles that cause additional injuries. Penetrating spinal injuries can be quickly and accurately evaluated with MDCT obviating thus or guiding a surgical exploration. Sagittal and coronal reformations can reveal the trajectory course and MDCT angiographic protocols provide additional information regarding vessel damage. Therefore, a detailed evaluation regarding vertebral fractures and the distribution and location of foreign bodies and possible spinal canal involvement in the trajectory course can be achieved by MDCT in a noninvasive way (Figures 15.34 and 15.35).

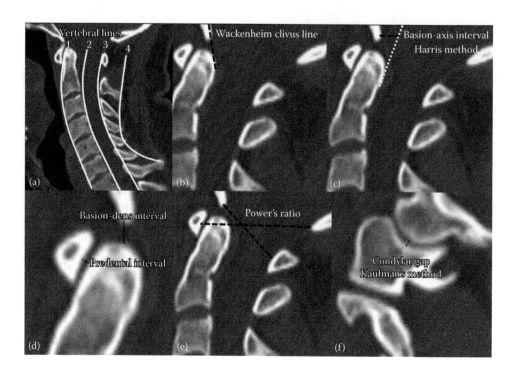

FIGURE 15.24

(a) Normal MDCT evaluation of anterior vertebral line (1), posterior vertebral line (2), spinal laminar line (3), and posterior spinous line (4). (b–f) Normal measurements and lines for evaluation of craniocervical dissociation: (b) The Wackenheim clivus baseline should lie tangentially to the posterior aspect of the dens. (c) The basion-axis interval is the distance between the basion and a line drawn along the posterior aspect of the dens and should normally be between 4 and 12 mm. (d) The predental interval is the normal space between the anterior arch of atlas and the anterior surface of the odontoid process and should normally vary between 3 and 5 mm. The basion-dens interval is the distance between the basion and the tip of the dens and should be <12 mm. (e) The Powers' ratio is calculated as the ratio of the distance between the basion and the posterior arch of atlas to the distance between the opisthion and the anterior arch of atlas and if the ratio is >1 is indicative of atlantooccipital dislocation. (f) The condylar gap should measure <5 mm.

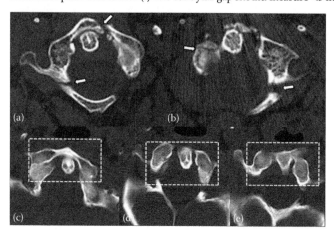

FIGURE 15.25

(a and b) Jefferson burst C1 fracture (arrows) in a 71-year-old male after fall from his house roof. (c–e) Atlantoaxial rotatory displacement (note rotation of C1-C2 in rectangle) in a 21-year-old male involved in MVA.

15.2.3 Traumatic Injuries on a Pathologic Background

15.2.3.1 Benign Vertebral Fractures

Benign vertebral lesions such as hemangiomas, aneurysmal bone cysts, osteoblastomas, and giant-cell tumors may predispose to a pathologic vertebral fracture in

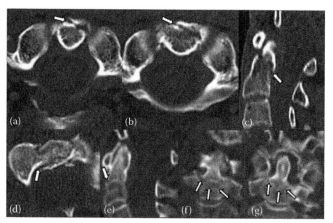

FIGURE 15.26

(a–c) Dens type II fracture. (d–g) Dens type III fracture. The arrows show the fracture lines.

the absence of any severe force applied. MDCT with its superior spatial resolution can provide the valuable information and lead to the correct diagnosis. Vertebral hemangiomas particularly constitute nearly 30% of all skeletal hemangiomas and multiplicity is observed in 1/3 of cases. They are most commonly located in the lower thoracic and upper lumbar spine and are easily depicted in MDCT images by a characteristic coarse-thickened

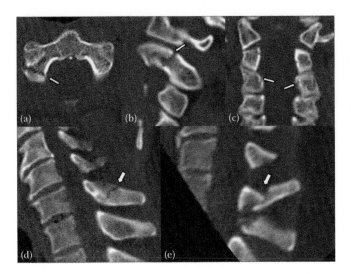

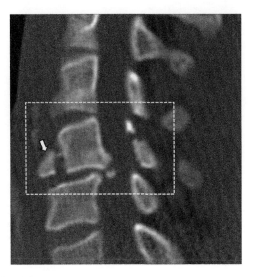

FIGURE 15.27

The axial (a), sagittal (b), and coronal (c) MDCT images show a Hangman's fracture in a 35-year-old male with a head dashboard injury in a MVA. The sagittal (d) MDCT image shows a nondisplaced "Clay-Shoveler's" fracture. The sagittal (e) MDCT image shows a displaced "Clay-Shoveler's" fracture.

FIGURE 15.28

The sagittal MDCT image shows a teardrop fracture of C5 in a 22-year-old male involved in a motorbike racing accident. Note the characteristic triangular bony fragment (arrow) and the severe associated displacement and traumatic stenosis (in rectangle).

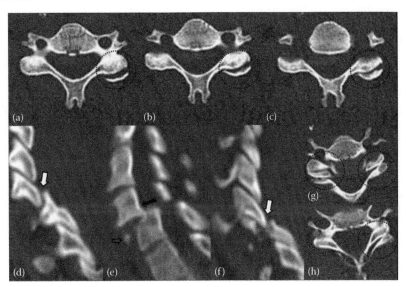

FIGURE 15.29

(a–c) The axial MDCT images show a unilateral locked facet dislocation (in dashed circle). The sagittal (d–f) and axial (g and h) MDCT images show bilateral locked facet fracture dislocation (white arrows and in dashed circles) in a 15-year-old male patient involved in MVA. There is severe anterolisthisis (black arrow) and a bony fragment of the superior border of the anteriorly wedged fractured vertebral body (open arrow).

vertical trabecular appearance. Although they are usually asymptomatic giant hemangiomas and atypical-aggressive forms may predispose to vertebral collapse (Figure 15.36).

Insufficiency spinal fractures are a leading cause for low-back pain without the presence of an acute traumatic event (normal stress exerted on a weakened bone). There are many causes that may predispose to insufficiency fractures in the spine, and Table 15.7 shows the most common ones.

Special emphasis will be given in this section in "osteoporotic fractures" as they represent a common and serious health problem. Osteoporosis is considered by far the most common metabolic disease in the western world that is reported to affect one in two women and one in five men over the age of 50 years. It is a systemic disease characterized by a reduction in bone mass (quantitative bone abnormality), and this is a distinguishing feature from osteomalacia and rickets disease, which are qualitative bone abnormalities. The

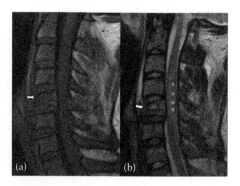

FIGURE 15.30
The (a) sagittal T1-w and (b) T2-w MR images of a SCIWORA in a 20-year-old male patient involved in an MVA. There is an occult fracture of C5 vertebral body (arrow) and severe cord edema (asterisks).

TABLE 15.5

MDCT Evidence of Thoracolumbar Instability

- Vertebral compression that exceeds 50% of vertebral body height
- Evidence of posterior vertebral body line disruption
- Widening of the facet joints, interpinous and interpediculate spaces
- Over 2 mm of noticeable vertebral body displacement
- Severe accompanying disk space narrowing

TABLE 15.6

Specific Types of Thoracolumbar Spine Injuries

Anterior wedged compression fracture	It is the result of anterior flexion forces that cause compression of the superior endplate of the vertebrae. The characteristic MDCT feature in the sagittal plane is a reduction in the anterior height of the vertebral with intact medial and posterior column.
Burst fracture	It is the result of compression forces that act in all three vertebral columns. Usually they are observed in falling accidents from height. On MDCT, fracture lines can be depicted in all three columns and this type of fracture can be associated with traumatic spinal canal stenosis.
Seatbelt injury	The mechanism of trauma is a hyperflexion injury of the waist. It commonly occurs in MVA with the body restrained in a sitting position by the automobile's belt. The injury is usually observed at the T12, L1, and L2 level. MDCT can reveal the fracture lines and the associated thoracoabdominal soft tissue changes. Different names have also been given to this type of injury depending on the spinal elements involved: for example, Chance fracture and Smith's fracture.
Lateral compression fracture	It is caused by lateral flexion. MDCT in coronal reconstructions is extremely helpful.
Spinal process fracture	These can involve the spinal process or the transverse processes. They can occur as an isolated—usually avulsion—injury but they can be an indication of a severe spinal trauma with concomitant severe life-threatening thoracoabdominal injuries.

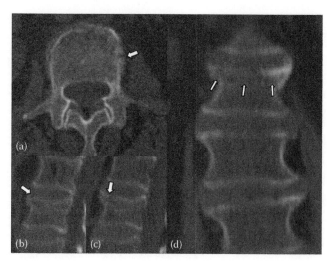

FIGURE 15.31
The axial (a), sagittal (b and c), and coronal (d) MDCT images show an anterior wedge compression fracture (arrows) in a 70-year-old male patient after fall from the stairs. The fracture is considered stable because it involves only the anterior column according to Denis classification.

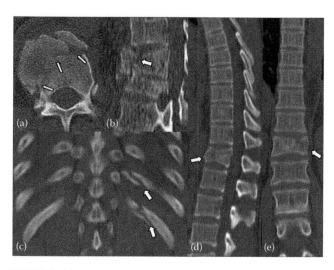

FIGURE 15.32
(a and b) The axial and sagittal MDCT images show a burst lumbar fracture (arrows) in a 69-year-old female patient after fall from height. (c–e) The coronal (c) and sagittal (d and e) MDCT images show a seatbelt injury and concomitant rib fractures in a 20-year-old male patient involved in an MVA. The fractured vertebra is considered unstable because it involves both the anterior and middle spinal column.

loss in bone mass results in an increase in bone fragility and this decreased biomechanical bone strength predisposes to fracture. The risk of fracture has been seen to increase with advancing age, and vertebral fractures are the most common ostoporotic insufficiency fractures. Recent guidelines from the International Osteoporosis Foundation and the European Society of Skeletal Radiology have shown that there is evidence that vertebral fractures are an underreported entity.

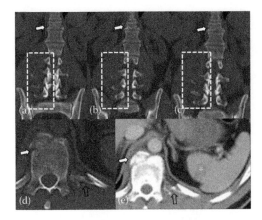

FIGURE 15.33

The coronal (a–c) MDCT images show multiple fractures of transverse processes of the lumbar vertebras (in rectangles) in 40-year-old male involved in an MVA. Note an associated anteriorly wedge compression fracture of T11 vertebra (white arrows) and a rib fracture (open arrow) with adjacent spleen laceration (asterisk) in axial (d and e) MDCT images.

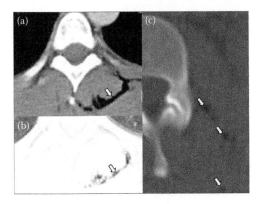

FIGURE 15.34

The axial (a–c) MDCT images show a stab wound from knife in a 19-year-old male patient involved in a bar fight. The presence of air bubbles (arrows) help in the identification of the injury and lung window levels are especially helpful in that task.

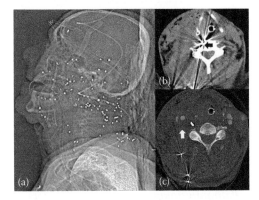

FIGURE 15.35

The CT scanogram (a) and the axial (b and c) MDCT images of an armed robbery victim show multiple pellets from a shotgun. A pellet is identified in a cervical vertebra (black arrow in b) and an associated traumatic-near total occlusion of the ipsilateral vertebral artery is identified (small arrow in c). Acute extravasation is also noted in the paravertebral soft tissues (large arrow in c).

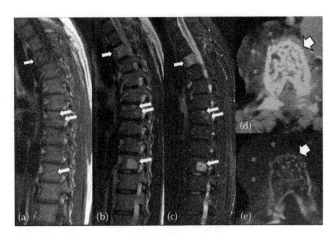

FIGURE 15.36

The sagittal (a) T1-w, (b) T2-w, and (c) STIR MR images in a 50-year-old male patient show an atypical giant vertebral thoracic hemangioma (thick arrows) and multiple small hemangiomas (thinner arrows) in lower vertebras. The axial (d and e) MDCT images in a 77-year-old female patient show an aggressive hemangioma occupying the entire thoracic vertebral body (with a characteristic "polka dot" CT appearance). There are perivertebral soft tissue changes (asterisks) attributed to recurrent episodes of fracture-hemorrhage and exraosseous hemangioma extension.

TABLE 15.7

Predisposing Factors for Insufficiency Spinal Fractures

- Postmenopausal osteoporosis
- Senile osteoporosis
- Irradiation therapy
- Corticosteroid therapy
- Osteomalacia
- Rickets disease
- Paget's disease
- Rheumatoid arthritis
- Hyperparathyroidism
- Renal osteodystrophy
- Osteogenesis imperfecta
- Fibrous dysplasia
- Organ transplant recipients
- Tabes dorsalis
- High dose fluoride therapy

However, osteoporotic vertebral fractures are considered a significant prognostic factor and a predictor of future fractures in osteoporotic patients and their accurate depiction and reporting may play a vital role in the diagnosis and proper management of osteoporosis. The spectrum of MDCT findings in insufficiency osteoporotic fractures ranges from minor severe anterior wedge compression to biconcave vertebral deformities and to the presence of an intravertebral gas cleft that is considered indicative of osteonecrosis, also referred to as "Kümmell disease" (Figure 15.37). Certain indexes such as spinal fracture index and the spine deformity index can be calculated but these scores are not frequently used in clinical practice. MRI, on the other hand, is the preferred imaging technique for defining

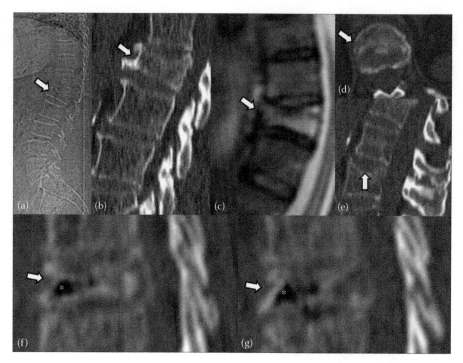

FIGURE 15.37
(a and b) The CT scanogram and the sagittal MDCT image show an incidentally depicted wedge-shaped osteoporotic fracture (arrows) of L1 in an 87-year-old female patient. (c) The sagittal STIR MR image shows bone edema and vertebral deformity indicative of an acute osteoporotic fracture (arrow) of T10 in an 82-year-old female patient presented with low-back pain. (d and e) The axial and sagittal MDCT images show an acute concave osteoporotic fracture (arrows) of L3 in 97-year-old female patient. (f and g) The sagittal MDCT images show Kummell disease (vertebral osteonecrosis) of T10 vertebra (arrow) in a 72-year-old male patient. Note the characteristic intravertebral vacuum cleft (asterisks).

the age of the fracture, by showing bone marrow edema in the acute and subacute phases. Nevertheless, correct identification of vertebral osteoporotic fractures in MDCT exams can have a tremendous impact on the quality of life of the patient with, or at risk of, osteoporosis. The radiologist may be the first to suggest the diagnosis and guide the patient and treating physician to more precise and accurate methods of mineral bone density assessment (dual-energy x-ray absorptiometry and quantitative CT).

15.2.3.2 Malignant Vertebral Fractures

Malignant vertebral fractures can result from metastases, multiple myeloma, primary malignant bone tumors, primary or secondary lymphoma, diffuse marrow diseases such as leukemia, and myeloproliferative diseases (Figure 15.38). The neoplastic infiltration can be either focal or diffuse and in the last the differential diagnosis between osteoporotic and malignant pathologic fractures may be difficult. MDCT can assist in the differential diagnosis of a benign from a malignant vertebral fracture mostly based on morphological criteria. A convex posterior border of the vertebra, the presence of additional lesions, or an accompanying soft tissue mass in the epidural or para-prevertebral space

are signs of a malignant fracture. In addition, MDCT may provide additional information on tumor matrix and may guide to a specific tumor diagnosis especially in primary bone tumors (e.g., "rings and arcs" internal tumor matrix in chondrosarcoma). MRI is undoubtedly more useful in visualizing bone marrow pathology but MDCT is definitely preferred in the assessment of the stability of a malignant fracture since it directly visualizes the bony structures and shows the fracture lines in a more detailed fashion. The continuous development of new imaging techniques that are currently in clinical practice such as positron emission tomography-computed tomography and MR diffusion and perfusion of the spine may assist in the difficult task of the differential diagnosis of benign from malignant vertebral fractures.

15.2.4 Overuse-Stress Injuries of the Spine

15.2.4.1 Pathophysiology and Imaging Strategy

Overuse and stress-related injuries of the spine are common in athletes of all levels and in military recruits. Despite their prevalence in high-elite and semiprofessional athletic endeavors, osseous stress injuries are increasingly been seen in amateur athletes-"weekend

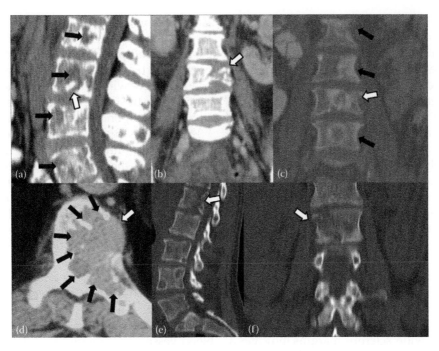

FIGURE 15.38
Malignant pathologic fractures. (a) Sagittal MDCT image: multiple lumbar metastases (black arrows) from breast Ca in a 69-year-old female patient. Note an endplate fracture (white arrow). (b) Coronal MDCT image: Lateral compressive malignant fracture (arrow) of L2 in 56-year-old female patient with GI AdenoCa. (c) Coronal MDCT image: biconcave compressive malignant fracture of L3 (white arrow) in a 70-year-old female patient with multiple metastases (black arrows) from breast Ca. (d) Axial MDCT image: plasmocytoma (black arrows) occupying the entire thoracic vertebral body in a 67-year-old male patient and causing pathologic fracture (white arrow). (e and f) Sagittal and coronal MDCT images showing a pathologic fracture of L1 (arrow) in a 37-year-old female patient with AdenoCa of unknown primary and multiple bone metastases.

warriors" and the radiologist may play a key role in the detection of subtle bone abnormalities and identify the stress injuries at an earlier stage. This is of paramount importance because early detection can result in reduced recovery time and minimize the risk of the injury or the evolution into a complete stress–fatigue fracture. Proper communication between the treating physician and the radiologist as well as a thorough history regarding the sports activity (e.g., recent change in an existing training program, participation in a new sport, or using a new sports equipment) may increase the radiologists' awareness in identifying these stress injuries.

In general, osseous stress injuries are the result of an imbalance between loads applied to bone and the ability of bone to respond to these changes. They could be described as a form of subacute trauma that is typically caused by repetitive movements—forces. The aforementioned repetitive application of force may result in bone weakening (imbalance between resorption and new bone formation because of overwhelming activity of osteoclasts over the osteoblasts). If the inciting sports-overuse activity is not discontinued, then stress injury develops to microfracture and finally may result to complete fracture.

Plain radiographs have a low sensitivity for detection of stress injuries at initial stage. Once the healing process proceeds then sclerosis, periostitis, and callus formation can be identified on radiographic exams. MDCT with multiplanar reformats is a more accurate modality for detecting an incomplete fracture line and may also be used for assessment of osseous healing. In the past, bone scans were used for the diagnosis of these occult injuries but nowadays MRI is considered the imaging modality of choice for early detection, proper characterization, and staging. It is important, however, to use an appropriate MR protocol that includes both anatomic (T1-weighted) sequences and fluid-sensitive sequences (short tau inversion recovery [STIR]) to establish the correct diagnosis.

15.2.4.2 Common Overuse-Stress Injuries of the Spine

Spondylolysis is a fracture-defect in the pars interarticularis of the lamina. Its cause is controversial and the osseous defect of the pars interarticularis is thought to be a developmental or acquired stress fracture secondary to chronic low-grade trauma. It has been postulated that it may be an overuse-related injury during infancy that results from repeated falls of the toddlers when they try to walk. The excess continuous stress on the lower lumbar spine during these falls may result in pars fracture defect. Various reports of acute symptomatic spondylolysis in pediatric or adolescent patients have been described and are associated with a strenuous or sports-related activity. The most probable pathogenetic mechanism of lumbar spondylolysis is most likely multifactorial with a stress fracture occurring through a congenitally weak or dysplastic pars interarticularis. However, spondylolysis is reported in nearly 10% of the asymptomatic population and correlation of imaging findings with the clinical scenario is of outmost importance. The role of imaging is to detect spondylolysis, to differentiate acute and active lesions from chronic inactive nonunion, to grade the defect and guide treatment, and to assess bony healing. Traditionally, the pars defect was detected on oblique lateral radiographs (Scottie dog sign) but MDCT with its multiplanar reformations may provide additional information with prognostic treatment value. The MDCT demonstration of a pars defect with wide, sclerotic margins indicates a chronic nonunion that has no potential for healing with conservative treatment. On the contrary, a pars defect with incomplete fracture line or narrow, sharp, noncorticated margins indicative of an acute fracture could benefit from immobilization using a spinal brace with a thoraco–lumbo–sacral orthosis. Plain radiography and MDCT are not sensitive for detection of the early

stress response without a fracture line and MRI is considered the primary investigation for adolescents with back pain and presumed stress reactions of the lumbar pars interarticularis. In MR examinations, bone marrow edema with or without a fracture line in the pars interarticularis are the imaging characteristics of stress-related symptomatic spondylolysis (Figures 15.39 and 15.40).

Intraosseous disk herniations (Schmorl's nodes) are herniations of nucleus pulposus into the trabecular bone through the vertebral endplate. The classification of Schmorl's nodes in overuse-stress-related injuries of the spine could be criticized, because they represent a common abnormality detected in MRI exams of asymptomatic population. Their incidence has been estimated in nearly up to 20% on MRI exams in people without low-back pain and in human cadaver studies, the prevalence of Schmorl's nodes is reported to be even higher. It has been postulated that intraosseous disk herniations develop through congenitally weak points in the cartilaginous disc plates, which may have been left by small blood vessesl or through small defects from notochord remnants. Nevertheless, symptomatic Schmorl's nodes have been reported in the literature and MRI can help distinguish these cases by showing the adjacent bone marrow edema. Vascularity may develop as a secondary process surrounding an intraosseous disk hernia and is considered a normal response of the vertebra that should not be confused with tumor or diskitis (Figure 15.41).

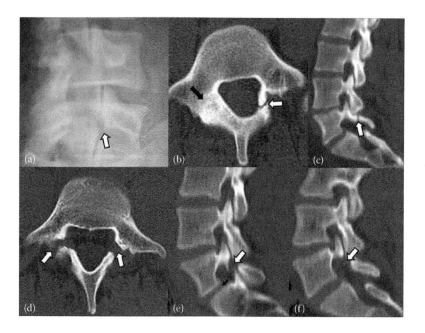

FIGURE 15.39
(a) The lateral oblique radiograph shows the characteristic "Scotty dog sign" of spondylolysis (arrow) in a 25-year-old military recruit. (b and c) The axial and sagittal MDCT images show spondylolysis (white arrow) and a contralateral healed pars defect (black arrow) of L5 in a 30-year-old male football player. (d–f) Bilateral painful spondylolysis (arrows) with grade I spondylolisthisis (small arrow) in an 8-year-old male basketball player.

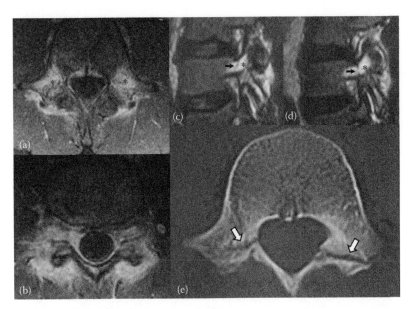

FIGURE 15.40
The axial contrast enhanced fat saturated (a and b) T1-w and the sagittal (c and d) STIR MR images in a 15-year-old male presented with low-back pain after a skateboarding competition show edema (asterisks) and occult fracture lines (black arrows) in bilateral L4 pedicles, consistent with acute spondylolysis. The axial (e) MDCT image verified the fracture lines. Associated soft tissue reactive changes are identified in panels a and b.

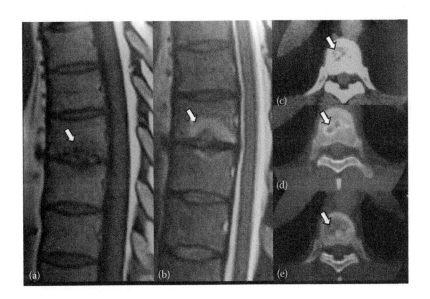

FIGURE 15.41
The sagittal (a) T1-w and (b) T2-w MR images show a symptomatic Schmorl's hernia (arrows) with surrounding bone edema in a 31-year-old male military officer that presented with back pain after 2-months training in parachute jumps. The axial (c–e) MDCT images verify the intraosseous disk herniation (arrows).

Finally, bone marrow changes can be depicted in asymptomatic high-elite athletes and the differentiation of normal stress-related changes from stress-related injuries could be a difficult task. The pattern and distribution of bone marrow changes together with other associated imaging findings (e.g., occult fracture lines, periosteal reactions, and avulsion injures) may contribute in the correct assessment and classification of these findings. In conclusion, close collaboration between the radiologist, sports physician, orthopedic surgeon, physical therapist, and the patient is mandatory for the early detection and subsequent correct management of stress-related spinal injuries (Figures 15.42 and 15.43).

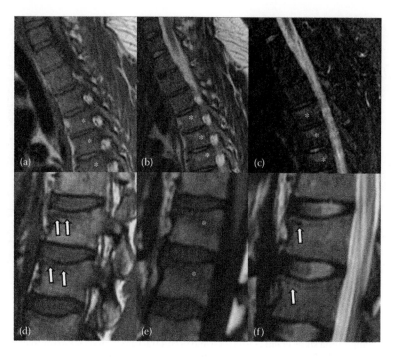

FIGURE 15.42
The sagittal (a) T1-w, (b) T2-w, and (c) STIR MR images show mild stress reaction bone edema (asterisks) in the thoracic vertebrae of a 21-year-old basketball player. The sagittal (d and e) T1-w and (f) T2-w MR images show bone marrow edema (asterisks) and occult fracture lines in the L1, L2 vertebrae of a 21-year-old male military recruit after 2 months intense and strenuous athletic training.

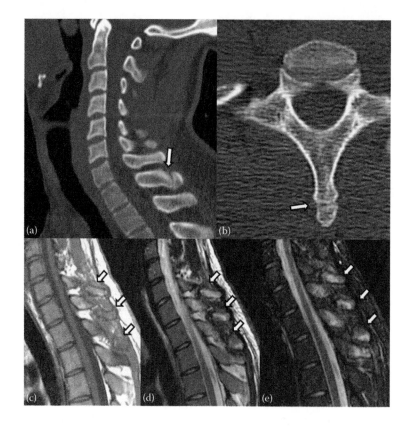

FIGURE 15.43
The sagittal (a) and axial (b) MDCT images in a 17-year-old male gymnastics athlete show a nonunion (arrows) of an avulsed injury of the T1 spinous process tip. The sagittal (c) T1-w, (d) T2-w, and (e) STIR MR images show multiple avulsed fractures (arrows) of the thoracocervical spinous processes in a 22-year-old military recruit after intense and strenuous training in a special armed forces unit.

15.2.5 Focus Points in Spinal Trauma

Traumatic Diseases of the Spine

Acute Traumatic Injuries of the Normal Spine	Traumatic Injuries on a Pathologic Background	Overuse-Stress Injuries of the Spine

• Knowledge of normal anatomic and developmental variants that should not be interpreted as fractures
• Denis' three column model to assess spinal stability
• Specific types of cervical spine trauma
  I. Craniocervical dissociation
  II. "Jefferson's" fracture
  III. Atlantoaxial rotatory displacement
  IV. Odontoid (Dens) fractures
  V. "Hangman's" fracture
  VI. "Clay-Shoveler's" fracture
  VII. Flexion teardrop fracture
  VIII. Unilateral locked facets
  IX. Bilateral locked facets
  X. SCIWORA
• Specific types of thoracolumbar spine trauma
  I. Anterior wedged compression fracture
  II. Burst fracture
  III. Seatbelt injury
  IV. Lateral compression fracture
  V. Spinal process fracture
• Penetrating spinal injuries
  I. High-energy injuries
  II. Low-energy injuries
	• Benign factors predisposing to spinal trauma
	  I. Benign vertebral lesions (for example, hemangiomas, aneurysmal bone cysts)
	  II. Diseases that predispose to insufficiency fractures (for example, osteoporosis)
	  III. Inflammatory arthropathies that alter spinal biomechanics (e.g. ankylosing spondylitis, rheumatoid arthritis)
	• Malignant fractures
	  I. Metastases
	  II. Primary malignant bone tumors
	  III. Multiple myeloma
	  IV. Primary or secondary lymphoma
	  V. Diffuse marrow diseases (leukemia and myeloproliferative diseases)
		• Pathophysiology and imaging strategy
		  I. Common in athletes of all levels (elite athletes and "weekend warriors") and in military recruits
		  II. Caused by repetitive microtrauma
		  III. Thorough history regarding the sports-overuse activity should be obtained
		  IV. MRI for early detection
		  V. Use of appropriate MR protocol: anatomic sequences (T1-weighted) and fluid-sensitive sequences (STIR or T2-w with fat saturation)
		  VI. Close collaboration between the radiologist, sports physician, orthopedic surgeon, physical therapist and the patient helps depiction and correct management

Acknowledgments

The author thanks Apostolos Karantanas, Associate Professor of Radiology from the University of Crete, Argyro Voloudaki, Head of MDCT Department from the University Hospital of Heraklion-Crete, and Stefanos Lahanis, Head of MRI Unit from the 401 Military Hospital of Athens for their valuable guidelines and advices in medical imaging.

Bibliography

1. Leone A, Cassar-Pullicino VN, Guglielmi G, Bonomo L. 2009. Degenerative lumbar intervertebral instability: what is it and how does imaging contribute? *Skeletal Radiol* 38:529–33.
2. Rahme R, Moussa R. 2008. The modic vertebral endplate and marrow changes: pathologic significance and relation to low back pain and segmental instability of the lumbar spine. *AJNR Am J Neuroradiol* 29:838–42.
3. Rao RD, Currier BL, Albert TJ et al. 2007. Degenerative cervical spondylosis: clinical syndromes, pathogenesis, and management. *J Bone Joint Surg Am* 89:1360–78.
4. Gallucci M, Limbucci N, Paonessa A, Splendiani A. 2007. Degenerative disease of the spine. *Neuroimaging Clin N Am* 17:87–103.
5. Madigan L, Vaccaro AR, Spector LR, Milam RA. 2009. Management of symptomatic lumbar degenerative disk disease. *J Am Acad Orthop Surg* 17:102–11.
6. Hong SH, Choi JY, Lee JW, Kim NR, Choi JA, Kang HS. 2009. MR imaging assessment of the spine: infection or an imitation? *Radiographics* 29:599–612.
7. Khalatbari K, Ansari H. 2008. MRI of degenerative cysts of the lumbar spine. *Clin Radiol* 63:322–8.
8. Leone A, Guglielmi G, Cassar-Pullicino VN, Bonomo L. 2007. Lumbar intervertebral instability: a review. *Radiology* 245:62–77.
9. Modic MT, Ross JS. 2007. Lumbar degenerative disk disease. *Radiology* 245:43–61.
10. Manaster BJ, May DA, Disler DG. 2007. *Muskuloskeletal Imaging: The Requisites in Radiology.* Philadelphia, PA, Mosby-Elsevier.
11. Brant WE, Helms CA. 2006. *The Brant and Helms Solution: Fundamentals of Diagnostic Radiology.* Philadelphia, PA, Lippincott, Williams & Wilkins.
12. Kaplan PA, Helms CA, Dussault R, Major NM, Anderson MW. 2001. *Musculoskeletal MRI.* Philadelphia, PA, W.B. Saunders.
13. Kalichman L, Hunter DJ. 2007. Lumbar facet joint osteoarthritis: a review. *Semin Arthritis Rheum* 37:69–80.

14. Khan AM, Girardi F. 2006. Spinal lumbar synovial cysts. Diagnosis and management challenge. *Eur Spine J* 15:1176–82.

15. Freund M, Sartor K. 2006. Degenerative spine disorders in the context of clinical findings. *Eur J Radiol* 58:15–26.

16. Roh JS, Teng AL, Yoo JU, Davis J, Furey C, Bohlman HH. 2005. Degenerative disorders of the lumbar and cervical spine. *Orthop Clin North Am* 36:255–62.

17. Pathria M. 2005. Imaging of spine instability. *Semin Musculoskelet Radiol* 9:88–99.

18. Gallucci M, Puglielli E, Splendiani A, Pistoia F, Spacca G. 2005. Degenerative disorders of the spine. *Eur Radiol* 15:591–8.

19. Kwong Y, Rao N, Latief K. 2011. MDCT findings in Baastrup disease: disease or normal feature of the aging spine? *AJR Am J Roentgenol* 196:1156–9.

20. Bierry G, Kremer S, Kellner F, Abu Eid M, Bogorin A, Dietemann JL. 2008. Disorders of paravertebral lumbar muscles: from pathology to cross-sectional imaging. *Skeletal Radiol* 37:967–77.

21. Müller D, Bauer JS, Zeile M, Rummeny EJ, Link TM. 2008. Significance of sagittal reformations in routine thoracic and abdominal multislice CT studies for detecting osteoporotic fractures and other spine abnormalities. *Eur Radiol* 18:1696–702.

22. Ergun T, Lakadamyali H. 2010. CT and MRI in the evaluation of extraspinal sciatica. *Br J Radiol* 83:791–803.

23. Varlotta GP, Lefkowitz TR, Schweitzer M et al. 2011. The lumbar facet joint: a review of current knowledge: part 1: anatomy, biomechanics, and grading. *Skeletal Radiol* 40:13–23.

24. Varlotta GP, Lefkowitz TR, Schweitzer M et al. 2011. The lumbar facet joint: a review of current knowledge: part II: diagnosis and management. *Skeletal Radiol* 40:149–57.

25. Hurri H, Karppinen J. 2004. Discogenic pain. *Pain* 112:225–8.

26. Fritz J, Niemeyer T, Clasen S et al. 2007. Management of chronic low back pain: rationales, principles, and targets of imaging-guided spinal injections. *Radiographics* 27:1751–71.

27. Kennedy DJ, Shokat M, Visco CJ. 2010. Sacroiliac joint and lumbar zygapophysial joint corticosteroid injections. *Phys Med Rehabil Clin N Am* 21:835–42.

28. Milette PC. 2001. Reporting lumbar disk abnormalities: at last, consensus! *AJNR Am J Neuroradiol* 22:428–9.

29. Pfirrmann CW, Metzdorf A, Zanetti M, Hodler J, Boos N. 2001. Magnetic resonance classification of lumbar intervertebral disc degeneration. *Spine* 26:1873–8.

30. Fujiwara A, Lim TH, An HS et al. 2000. The effect of disc degeneration and facet joint osteoarthritis on the segmental flexibility of the lumbar spine. *Spine* 25:3036–44.

31. Kettler A, Wilke HJ. 2006. Review of existing grading systems for cervical or lumbar disc and facet joint degeneration. *Eur Spine J* 15:705–18.

32. Park YH, Taylor JA, Szollar SM, Resnick D. 1994. Imaging findings in spinal neuroarthropathy. *Spine* 19:1499–504.

33. Chen CK, Yeh L, Resnick D et al. 2004. Intraspinal posterior epidural cysts associated with Baastrup's disease: report of 10 patients. *AJR Am J Roentgenol* 182:191–4.

34. Fardon DF, Milette PC. 2001. Nomenclature and classification of lumbar disc pathology. Recommendations of the Combined task Forces of the North American Spine Society, American Society of Spine Radiology, and American Society of Neuroradiology. *Spine (Phila Pa 1976)* 26:E93–113.

35. Pfirrmann CW, Dora C, Schmid MR, Zanetti M, Hodler J, Boos N. 2004. MR image-based grading of lumbar nerve root compromise due to disk herniation: reliability study with surgical correlation. *Radiology* 230:583–8.

36. Jinkins JR. 2004. Acquired degenerative changes of the intervertebral segments at and suprajacent to the lumbosacral junction. A radioanatomic analysis of the nondiscal structures of the spinal column and perispinal soft tissues. *Eur J Radiol* 50:134–58.

37. Van Goethem JW, Maes M, Ozsarlak O, van den Hauwe L, Parizel PM. 2005. Imaging in spinal trauma. *Eur Radiol* 15:582–90.

38. Looby S, Flanders A. 2011. Spine trauma. *Radiol Clin North Am* 49:129–63.

39. Griffith JF, Guglielmi G. 2010. Vertebral fracture. *Radiol Clin North Am* 48:519–29.

40. Cassar-Pulicino V, Imhof E. 2006. *Spinal Trauma-An Imaging Approach*. New York, Stuttgart, Thieme.

41. Goldberg AL, Kershah SM. 2010. Advances in imaging of vertebral and spinal cord injury. *J Spinal Cord* 33:105–16.

42. Khanna G, El-Khoury GY. 2007. Imaging of cervical spine injuries of childhood. *Skeletal Radiol* 36:477–94.

43. Chang W, Alexander MT, Mirvis SE. 2009. Diagnostic determinants of craniocervical distraction injury in adults. *AJR Am J Roentgenol* 192:52–8.

44. Bensch FV, Kiuru MJ, Koivikko MP, Koskinen SK. 2004. Spine fractures in falling accidents: analysis of multidetector CT findings. *Eur Radiol* 14:618–24.

45. Hsu JM, Joseph T, Ellis AM. 2003. Thoracolumbar fracture in blunt trauma patients: guidelines for diagnosis and imaging. *Injury* 34:426–33.

46. Herzog C, Ahle H, Mack MG et al. 2004. Traumatic injuries of the pelvis and thoracic and lumbar spine: does thin-slice multidetector-row CT increase diagnostic accuracy? *Eur Radiol* 14:1751–60.

47. Steenburg SD, Sliker CW, Shanmuganathan K, Siegel EL. 2010. Imaging evaluation of penetrating neck injuries. *Radiographics* 30:869–86.

48. Osborn TM, Bell RB, Qaisi W, Long WB. 2008. Computed tomographic angiography as an aid to clinical decision making in the selective management of penetrating injuries to the neck: a reduction in the need for operative exploration. *J Trauma* 64:1466–71.

49. Woo K, Magner DP, Wilson MT, Margulies DR. 2005. CT angiography in penetrating neck trauma reduces the need for operative neck exploration. *Am Surg* 71: 754–8.

50. Link TM, Guglielmi G, van Kuijk C, Adams JE. 2005. Radiologic assessment of osteoporotic vertebral fractures: diagnostic and prognostic implications. *Eur Radiol* 15:1521–32.

51. Williams AL, Al-Busaidi A, Sparrow PJ, Adams JE, Whitehouse RW. 2009. Under-reporting of osteoporotic vertebral fractures on computed tomography. *Eur J Radiol* 69:179–83.

52. Libicher M, Appelt A, Berger I et al. 2007. The intravertebral vacuum phenomenon as specific sign of osteonecrosis in vertebral compression fractures: results from a radiological and histological study. *Eur Radiol* 17:2248–52.

53. Link TM. 2010. The Founder's Lecture 2009: advances in imaging of osteoporosis and osteoarthritis. *Skeletal Radiol* 39:943–55.

54. Baur-Melnyk A. 2009. Malignant versus benign vertebral collapse: are new imaging techniques useful? *Cancer Imaging* 2;9 Spec No A:S49–51.

55. Karchevsky M, Babb JS, Schweitzer ME. 2008. Can diffusion-weighted imaging be used to differentiate benign from pathologic fractures? A meta-analysis. *Skeletal Radiol* 37:791–5.

56. Tokuda O, Hayashi N, Taguchi K, Matsunaga N. 2005. Dynamic contrast-enhanced perfusion MR imaging of diseased vertebrae: analysis of three parameters and the distribution of the time intensity curve patterns. *Skeletal Radiol* 34:632–8.

57. Cho WI, Chang UK. 2011. Comparison of MR imaging and FDG-PET/CT in the differential diagnosis of benign and malignant vertebral compression fractures. *J Neurosurg Spine* 14:177–83.

58. Navas A, Kassarjian A. 2011. Bone marrow changes in stress injuries. *Semin Musculoskelet Radiol* 15:183–97.

59. Groves AM, Cheow HK, Balan KK, Housden BA, Bearcroft PW, Dixon AK. 2005. 16-Detector multislice CT in the detection of stress fractures: a comparison with skeletal scintigraphy. *Clin Radiol* 60:1100–5.

60. Leone A, Cianfoni A, Cerase A, Magarelli N, Bonomo L. 2011. Lumbar spondylolysis: a review. *Skeletal Radiol* 40:683–700.

61. Hollenberg GM, Beattie PF, Meyers SP, Weinberg EP, Adams MJ. 2002. Stress reactions of the lumbar pars interarticularis: the development of a new MRI classification system. *Spine* 27:181–6.

62. Micheli LJ, Curtis C. 2006. Stress fractures in the spine and sacrum. *Clin Sports Med* 25:75–88.

63. Niemeyer P, Weinberg A, Schmitt H, Kreuz PC, Ewerbeck V, Kasten P. 2006. Stress fractures in the juvenile skeletal system. *Int J Sports Med* 27:242–9.

64. Ferry AT, Graves T, Theodore GH, Gill TJ. 2010. Stress fractures in athletes. *Phys Sportsmed* 38:109–16.

65. Dixon S, Newton J, Teh J. 2011. Stress fractures in the young athlete: a pictorial review. *Curr Probl Diagn Radiol* 40:29–44.

66. Kornaat PR, de Jonge MC, Maas M. 2008. Bone marrow edema-like signal in the athlete. *Eur J Radiol* 67:49–53.

16

Inflammatory Diseases of the Spine

Joaquín Martín, José M. Mellado, and Laura Pérez del Palomar

CONTENTS

16.1 Introduction

Infectious diseases of the spine are rare but may associate with significant morbidity. Long-standing infections, aggressive germs, and inappropriate treatments may result in high morbidity or mortality. This chapter will mainly discuss infectious disorders of the musculoskeletal components of the spine. Consequently, intradural infections and noninfectious inflammatory conditions will be obviated.

16.2 Anatomical Review

The spine usually consists of 33 vertebrae. The upper 24 vertebrae are named cervical (7 vertebrae), thoracic (12 vertebrae), and lumbar (5 vertebrae). The lower nine vertebrae are fused to form the sacrum and coccyx. Articulations between C1 and C2 have special features, while sacral and coccygeal vertebrae are usually fused. The bodies of adjacent vertebrae are connected by specialized cartilaginous joints known as intervertebral discs. Interapophyseal joints (found throughout the whole spine) and uncovertebral joints (only present at the cervical spine) are synovial joints.

Several ligaments stabilize the spine and protect the intervertebral discs. The major ligaments are the anterior and posterior longitudinal ligaments, which extend along the anterior and posterior surfaces of the vertebras bodies, and the ligamentum flavum, which extends along the posterior surface of the spinal canal, connecting the vertebral laminae (Figure 16.1).

The arterial supply of the spine varies with age, which influences the pathophysiology of infectious conditions. The vertebral bodies are vascularized by the vertebral and ascending cervical arteries at the cervical spine, by the posterior intercostal arteries at the thoracic spine, by the lumbar and iliolumbar arteries at the lumbar spine, and by the sacral arteries at the sacrococcygeal level.

Infectious conditions predominate at the lumbar spine. At this site, several pairs of lumbar arteries originating from the abdominal aorta run through the paravertebral spaces and irrigate the vertebral bodies. Spinal arteries are distal branches of the lumbar arteries, which irrigate the spinal canal and spinal cord. The vascularization of the vertebral bodies derives from peripheral, metaphyseal, and anterolateral nutrient arteries (Figure 16.2). All of these arise directly from the lumbar artery, except the nutrient arteries that originate from the spinal artery within the spinal canal [1].

The venous drainage of the vertebral body has a tree-like configuration, with confluent vessels originating from

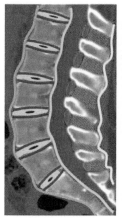
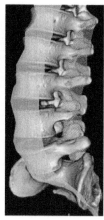
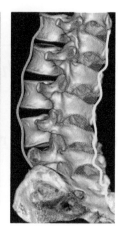

FIGURE 16.1
Ligamentous structures of the lumbar spine: anterior longitudinal ligament (orange line), posterior longitudinal ligament (green line), ligamentum flavum (purple areas), interspinous ligament (purple dotted areas), intertransverse ligament (blue dotted areas), supraspinous ligament (yellow line) and facet capsulary ligament (green areas).

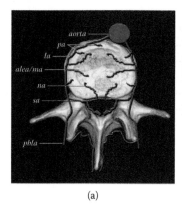
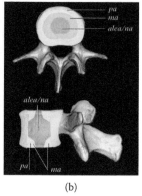

(a)   (b)

FIGURE 16.2
(a) Arterial vascularization of the lumbar vertebra: lumbar artery (la), anterolateral equatorial artery (alea), metaphyseal artery (ma), nutrient arteries (na), posterior branch of lumbar artery (pbla), spinal arteries (sa), and peripheral arteries (pa). (b) This figure shows axial and sagittal zones of arterial vascularization of the lumbar vertebral body.

the metaphysis and draining into the centre of the vertebral body to form the basivertebral vein, which drains into the internal vertebral venous plexuses through the Hahn's canal (Figure 16.3). These plexuses may look particularly prominent in some asymptomatic individuals. They run along the spinal canal and neural arcs and anastomose with veins that pierce the cortical bone of the vertebral bodies, thus originating the so-called Batson's vertebral plexus, which distally continues with the pelvic veins [2].

The discovertebral complex is formed by the nucleus pulposus, the annulus fibrosus, and the cartilaginous endplates (Figure 16.4). The vertebral endplates present a central part covered by hyaline cartilage and a peripheral elevated rim of cortical bone, not covered by cartilage, called ring apophysis. The nucleus pulposus is a mucoprotein gel located at the center of the disc. The annulus fibrosus consists of several layers of fibrocartilage, which surrounds the nucleus pulposus. The outer fibers of the annulus fibrosus are known as Sharpey's fibers and are inserted into the ring apophysis.

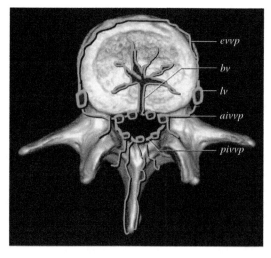

FIGURE 16.3
Perivertebral veins around the lumbar vertebra: external vertebral venous plexus (evvp), basivertebral vein (bv), lumbar vein (lv), anterior internal vertebral venous plexus (aivvp), and posterior internal vertebral venous plexus (pivvp).

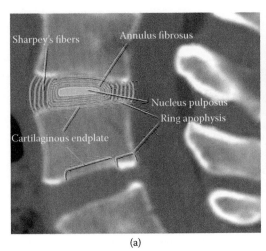 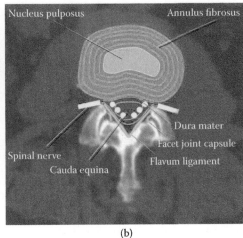

(a) (b)

FIGURE 16.4
Discovertebral complex at the lumbar spine. (a) Sagittal-reformatted multi-detector computed tomography (MDCT) image shows the disc structure, which consists of a central nucleus pulposus and a peripheral annulus fibrosus. The outer fibers of annulus fibrosus insert into the ring apophysis, which is the part of the vertebral endplate that is not covered by hyaline cartilage. (b) Axial MDCT image shows the relationship between neural structures (cauda equina and spinal nerves), intervertebral disc, and facet joint.

16.3 Spondylodiscitis

Spinal infectious diseases can be caused by bacterial, fungal, or parasitic organisms. Osteomyelitis of the vertebral body is the most common primary infectious condition of the spine, although this is typically followed by disc involvement. In fact, inflammation can affect one or more of spinal structures, causing single lesions or variable combination of spondylitis, discitis, spondylodiscitis, pyogenic facet arthritis, epidural abscess, meningitis, polyradiculopathy, and myelitis [3].

16.3.1 General Considerations

Spondylodiscitis typically derives from hematogenous seeding, owing to antegrade flow (through nutrient arterioles) or retrograde flow (through venous plexus) [4,5]. Early osteomyelitis typically involves the most anterior aspect of the subchondral region of the vertebral body (Figure 16.5), irrigated by terminal vessels. Spondylodiscitis may also follow local spread from contiguous contaminated sources (Figures 16.6 and 16.7) or be secondary to direct inoculation, in a clinical setting of trauma, surgery [6], vertebroplasty [7], spinal anesthesia, and other invasive procedures.

Progression of the germ into the vertebral body, disc, and adjacent soft tissues occurs in a gradual fashion, which directly influences imaging findings. This progression varies according to the dissemination route, patient's age and condition, and responsible germ, which can be divided into pyogenic (Figure 16.8) and tuberculous (Figure 16.9) types.

Pyogenic spondylodiscitis is the most frequent type of spondylitis, frequently caused by hematogenous spread from the genitourinary tract, skin, or upper respiratory tract. Less frequently, it may originate from direct extension by contiguous infected organs such as the oropharynx, pleural space, and thoracic or abdominal wall. More rarely, it may be secondary to invasive procedures such as surgery, discography, or vertebroplasty. The most common organism is *Staphylococcus aureus*, identified in up to 60% of cases. Main risk factors are age (more frequent in patients of 60 to 70 years old), sex (slightly more frequent in men), debilitating diseases (diabetes, renal failure, cirrhosis, cancer, and immunosuppressive states), and other conditions such as intravenous drug use or recent spinal instrumentation procedures.

Tuberculous spondylitis is caused by mycobacterium tuberculosis. Although the prevalence of tuberculosis had declined in developed countries, infections are becoming progressively common in specific populations, such as those related to third world immigration and immunosuppressed states. Tuberculosis usually involves the respiratory system, although any organ can be reached. Skeletal involvement has been reported to occur in 1%–5% of all tuberculous patients. In developing countries, skeletal tuberculosis may be more common in children, while adults are more commonly affected in developed countries [8].

Clinical presentation of both pyogenic and tuberculous spondylodiscitis is nonspecific, consisting of back pain, muscle spasm, and inconstant fever. Chills, night sweats, and weight loss may occur. Symptoms take 2–3 weeks to appear. Torpid or insidious presentations typically cause delays in diagnosis. Severe damage may lead

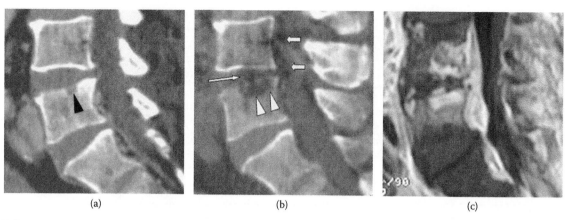

(a)   (b)   (c)

FIGURE 16.5

Sagittal MDCT image (a) in a patient suffering intestinal obstruction shows a small erosion in the upper endplate of L5 (black arrowhead), which was overlooked. Follow-up MDCT 20 days later was performed (b), which showed larger erosions of the superior vertebral endplate (white arrowhead), mild hypodensity within the adjacent disc (thin arrow), and anterior epidural fluid collection (thick arrows). Subsequent magnetic resonance imaging (MRI) (c) confirmed the suspicion of spondylodiscitis associated with epidural abscess.

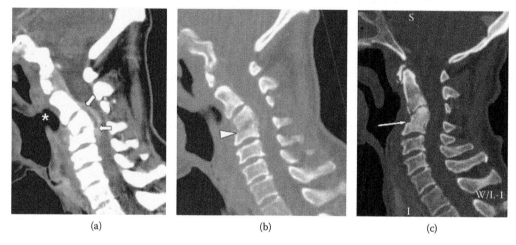

(a)   (b)   (c)

FIGURE 16.6

Sagittal MDCT image after intravenous contrast administration (a and b), performed in a patient with neck pain, following oropharyngeal biopsy. The MDCT with soft tissue algorithm reconstruction (a) shows a cavity within the prevertebral soft tissues (asterisk), associated with cervical spondylodiscitis and anterior epidural abscess (thick arrows). The MDCT image with bone algorithm (b) shows decrease in C3–C4 disc space height (arrowhead), erosion in adjacent plates, and wedging of C4. Follow-up MDCT, performed 12 months later (c), shows disappearance of the disc space (thin arrow) with fusion of the C3–C4 bodies, sclerosis, and kyphotic deformation.

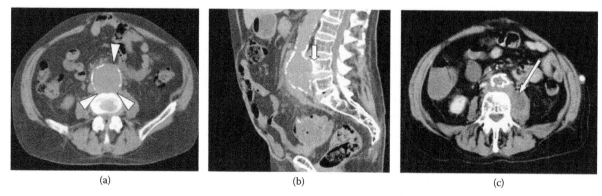

(a)   (b)   (c)

FIGURE 16.7

Asymptomatic patient monitored for lung cancer with known aortic aneurysm. Axial MDCT image (a) shows increased diameter of the aortic aneurysm and discontinuity of wall calcifications (arrowheads). Note focal sclerosis (thick arrow) on adjacent L4 vertebral body (b). Intraoperatively, infected and disrupted aortic aneurysm was found. A follow-up study (c) shows a small persistent psoas abscess (thin arrow).

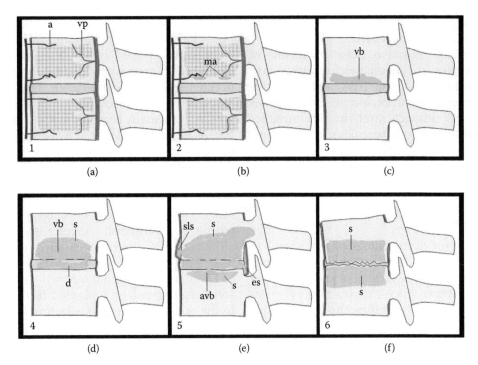

FIGURE 16.8
Patterns of pyogenic spondylitis. The germ arrives through terminal arteries (a) or venous plexuses (vp) to the vertebral metaphysis, causing microinfarcts and microabscesses (ma) that lead to bone resorption. The infection extends through the vertebral bone (vb) into the intervertebral disc (d) and to adjacent vertebral body (avb). There may also be subligamentous (sls) or epidural (es) extension. Subsequently, sclerosis may develop (s), particularly evident in the healing phase, when loss of disc height is also advanced.

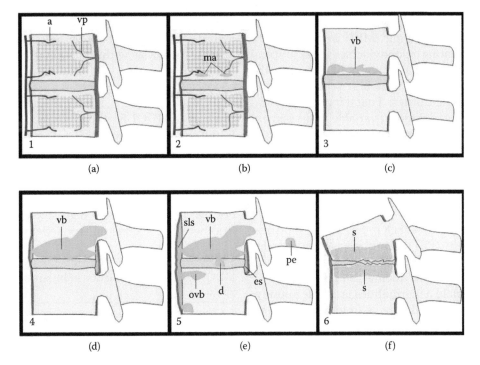

FIGURE 16.9
Patterns of tuberculous spondylitis. The germ arrives through terminal arteries (a) or venous plexuses (vp) to the vertebral metaphysis. These cause microinfarcts and microabscesses (ma) leading to bone resorption. The infection extends through the vertebral bone (vb) and to subligamentous spaces (sls). Later, infection can reach other vertebral bodies (ovb) with little or no disc involvement (d), extend to posterior elements (pe), and originate epidural (es) and paravertebral collections. Sclerosis (s) appears late in the disease. Vertebral collapse, ankylosis, and kyphosis are common.

to spinal instability and neurologic morbidity, which are uncommon in the early stages [4].

Identification of the causative factor by means of blood culture is typically difficult. Serologic tests such as erythrocyte sedimentation rate (ESR) and C-reactive protein (CRP) are sensitive but nonspecific. Leukocytosis is commonly found, although rarely in old, immuno-compromised patients or in tuberculous and parasitic infections [4]. Due to the relative unspecificity of the clinical and laboratory tests, imaging modalities are essential for the diagnosis of spinal infections.

16.3.2 Imaging Modalities

Abnormal findings on plain radiographs appear 2 to 8 weeks after the onset of disease. Significant findings include focal bone osteolysis, erosion of endplates, narrowing of intervertebral spaces, destruction of vertebral bodies, and soft tissue swelling. As degenerative disease and noninfectious inflammatory diseases can show similar changes, radiologic differential diagnosis may be particularly challenging [3].

Scintigraphy is a sensitive but nonspecific test. Technetium-99m phosphate complexes or gallium-67 citrate are the most frequently used radionuclides. Fractures, noninfectious inflammatory diseases, and tumors may show similar scintigraphic patterns [9]. High false-negative rates have been described in patients with active tuberculous infection [8].

Magnetic resonance imaging (MRI) is the modality of choice for evaluating spondylodiscitis [4]. Typical MRI findings include signal abnormalities within the involved disc and adjacent vertebral bodies, and ill-defined contiguous endplates. Following administration of intravenous gadolinium, variable enhancement of the involved disc and adjacent vertebral bodies is typically found. MRI may show abnormal thickening and enhancement of epidural space and paraspinal soft tissues. Homogeneous enhancement is consistent with phlegmon, while ring enhancement associates with abscess.

18F fluorodeoxyglucose (FDG) total-body positron emission tomography (PET) scanning has been used for evaluating spondylodiscitis. PET is more sensitive and specific than MRI and can distinguish between active Modic type 1 endplate abnormalities and true spondylodiscitis: FDG uptake will only be found in infectious conditions [10].

16.3.2.1 *Multi-Detector Computed Tomography (MDCT) Technique*

MDCT is a widely available modality that may be used when spinal infection or tumor are suspected. However, early infections and small tumors may be hard to detect, in comparison with MRI. Also, MDCT requires high doses of ionizing radiation and intravenous iodinated contrast. When MRI is not available or is contraindicated, MDCT represents a useful alternative. In the rest of cases, MRI will be used as the modality of choice for suspected spinal infection.

MDCT is usually acquired with 120 kV and automatic tube current modulation. Low-dose protocols may be used, although significantly decreased spatial resolution of bony structures can occur. The range of study should be limited to the symptomatic region. In this regard, previous x-rays may help select the optimal range of study. Full-spine imaging may be required whenever multilevel involvement is suspected, although MDCT is rarely used in this particular setting. Data sets are reconstructed with a slice width of 1 mm, reconstruction interval of 0.8 mm, bone and soft tissue kernel, and adapted field of view, targeted to the spine. Intravenous administration of iodinated contrast may help evaluate soft tissue involvement and paraspinal abscess.

Axial images are optimal for evaluating the spinal canal, the contour of the intervertebral discs, the foramina, the facet joints, and the paraspinal soft tissues. Sagittal reconstructions are used for evaluating intervertebral spaces, vertebral endplates, and regional bone density. Coronal reconstructions are useful for visualizing paraspinal soft tissues. Multiplanar and tridimensional displays, readily available on workstations, may identify early erosions of vertebral endplates or small areas of osteolysis within the cancellous bone [11].

16.3.2.2 *MDCT Role*

The role of MDCT for the evaluation of spinal infection is multiple (Table 16.1). MDCT optimally depicts the osseous structures of the spine, particularly mild erosions of vertebral endplates, and may detect soft tissue calcifications or abnormal gas bubbles. However, abnormalities of bone density as seen on MDCT images do not necessarily correlate with signal changes on MRI. In other words, bone marrow edema, an MRI feature,

TABLE 16.1

MDCT Role in the Evaluation of Inflammatory Disease of the Spine

- Number and location of affected vertebral levels
- Extent of cancellous and cortical involvement
- Evaluation of disc height
- Evaluation of paraspinal and epidural involvement
- Degree of spinal canal stenosis
- Severity of pathologic fracture
- Evaluation of local sequelae (kyphosis, ankylosis, sinus tract)
- Image-guided percutaneous aspiration of collections or biopsy
- Surgical planning
- Follow-up of disease

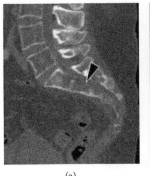
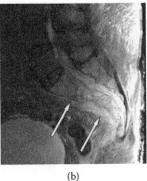
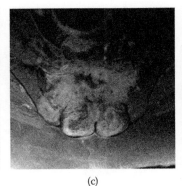
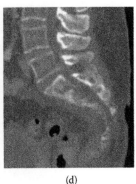

(a) (b) (c) (d)

FIGURE 16.10
Patient with severe anal pain. Initial MDCT study (a) shows mild hypodensity within sacral cancellous bone (black arrowhead). Corresponding sagittal fat–suppressed T_2-weighted MR image (b) shows bone and soft tissue edema, consistent with sacral osteomyelitis (thin arrows). Axial fat–suppressed contrast-enhanced T_1-weighted MR image (c) shows heterogeneous enhancement of involved areas. Follow-up MDCT image, performed 2 months later (d), shows a mixed pattern of osteolysis and osteosclerosis within the sacrum.

TABLE 16.2

Histopathological Features and Corresponding Imaging Appearance

	Radiography	MDCT	MRI
Bone marrow edema	Not assessed	Not assessed	Low signal on T_1 weighted, high signal on T_2 weighted
Vertebral endplate erosion	Difficult to assess	Modality of choice	Moderately difficult to assess
Bone sclerosis	High density	High density	Low signal on T_1 weighted and T_2 weighted
Discal edema	Not assessed	Difficult to assess	Low signal on T_1 weighted, high signal on T_2 weighted
Decrease in disc height	Difficult to assess	Modality of choice	Modality of choice
Soft tissue edema	Not assessed	Difficult to assess	Low signal on T_1-weighted, high signal on T_2-weighted solid homogenous enhancement
Soft tissue abscess	Difficult to assess	Hypodense, rim enhancement	Low signal on T_1-weighted, high signal on T_2-weighted rim enhancement
Paravertebral calcifications	Difficult to assess	Modality of choice	Difficult to assess
Epidural abscess	Not assessed	Difficult to assess	Low signal on T_1-weighted, high signal on T_2-weighted, rim enhancement
Cord compression	Not assessed	Not assessed	Cord deformity, myelopathy

TABLE 16.3

Local Complications of Spondylodiscitis

- Decrease in disc space height
- Fibrous or bony ankylosis
- Vertebral wedging, gibbus deformity
- Pathologic fracture
- Medullary or nerve root compression
- Chronic spondylitis
- Sinus tract

cannot be seen on MDCT studies, which is to be considered a significant handicap for early detection of spinal infection (Figure 16.10) (Table 16.2).

Soft tissue resolution of MDCT, particularly in contrast-enhanced studies, allows the evaluation of paraspinal soft tissues. However, involvement of the epidural space and intradural structures is significantly suboptimal, owing to beam-hardening artifacts, and requires additional MRI [11]. MDCT is also used for evaluating potential complications, such as cord or root compression, pathologic fractures, spinal instability, and gibbus deformity (Table 16.3). Deep venous thrombosis within regional veins may lead to septic emboli [12] (Figure 16.11).

Isolation of the causative germ by percutaneous aspiration is usually required for establishing an effective treatment. MDCT is widely used for planning biopsies and drain fluid collections. Large samples should be obtained and appropriate cultures performed, in order to maximize the sensitivity of the procedure. MDCT avoids damage to vital structures and confirms the presence of the needle tip within the inflammatory tissue (Figure 16.12). MDCT-guided aspiration may be diagnostic in 53% to 86% of cases. Histological examination of the biopsied specimen is also useful to establish differential diagnosis not only between pyogenic and tuberculous infection but also between infection and tumor [13].

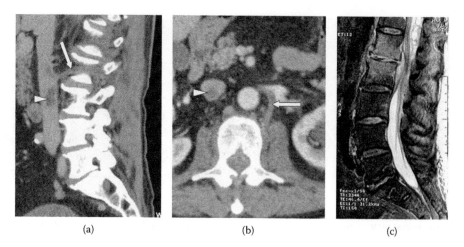

FIGURE 16.11

(a) Sagittal and (b) axial MDCT images show thrombosis of lumbar vein (arrows) and inferior vena cava (arrowheads). Corresponding sagittal fat–suppressed T_2-weighted MR image (c) shows signs of L1/2 spondylodiscitis and epidural abscess.

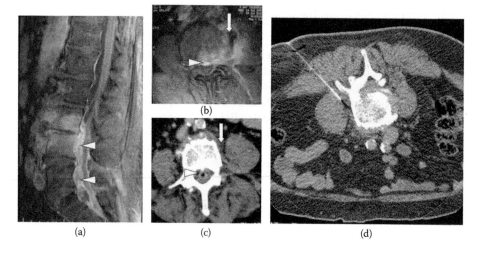

FIGURE 16.12

(a) Sagittal and (b) axial fat–suppressed contrast-enhanced T_1-weighted MR images and axial MDCT images (c and d) in a patient with L3/4 spondylodiscitis show a small paraspinal collection (arrows) and associate epidural phlegmon (arrowheads). CT-guided aspiration (d) was performed.

16.3.2.3 MDCT Features

The radiological manifestations of pyogenic and tuberculous infection slightly differ, although findings may show considerable overlap [3] (Table 16.4).

Pyogenic spondylitis predominates in the lumbar spine (48%) followed by the thoracic (35%) and cervical spine (6.5%) [9]. Pyogenic discitis in children may be a primary disorder, due to persisting vascular channels in intervertebral discs. Involvement of pedicle, laminae, and spinous process is uncommon in pyogenic infection (3%–12%). When present, tuberculous infection should be suspected [14]. Cervical spondylitis may progress anteriorly, thus leading to retropharyngeal abscess (anteriorly) and mediastinitis (inferiorly). Thoracic spondylitis may also cause mediastinitis, empyema,

TABLE 16.4

MDCT Findings in Spondylodiscitis

- Focal osteolysis of vertebral bodies
- Erosion of vertebral endplates
- Lytic fragmentation of vertebral bodies
- Bone sclerosis
- Sequestra
- Loss of disc height
- Paraspinal soft tissue swelling
- Paraspinal soft tissue fluid collection
- Paraspinal calcification
- Epidural abscess

and pericarditis, while lumbar spondylitis can cause peritonitis.

Tuberculosis predominates on the lower thoracic and upper lumbar levels [15] (Table 16.5). Reactive sclerosis and local periosteal reaction are rare [8].

TABLE 16.5

Main Features of Pyogenic and Tuberculous Spondylitis

	Pyogenic Spondylitis	Tuberculous Spondylitis
Spinal level	Lumbar	Lower thoracic, upper lumbar
Distribution	Single level	Multiple levels, skip lesions
Clinical presentation	Back pain, muscle spasm, fever	Insidious
ESR, CRP	Increased	Often normal
Disc involvement	Early	Late
Bone sclerosis	Present	Sparse or absent
Neural arc involvement	Rare	Common
Soft tissue abscess	Small, local	Large (calcifications, sinus tracts)
Extension	Through discs	Subligamentous
Sequelae	No significant deformity	Gibbus deformity

Destruction of the intervertebral disc is also a rare, late finding [16]. Tuberculous spondylitis usually propagates under the anterior or posterior longitudinal ligaments (Figure 16.13), in a multilevel fashion. Neural arc involvement is common (Figure 16.14), and paraspinal abscesses are typically large. Sinus tracts into adjacent organs or skin may occur [15]. Calcifications within paraspinal soft tissues are virtually diagnostic of tuberculosis [8,17]. Collapse of anterior vertebral body, kyphotic angulation, and discovertebral ankylosis may be particularly dramatic (Figure 16.6c). Brucellar [18] (Table 16.6) and fungal spondylitis [11,19] (Table 16.7) are similar to tuberculous spondylitis. Hydatid disease of the spine, however, shows more specific imaging features [20] (Figure 16.15) (Table 16.8).

Focal osteoporosis and cortical erosion are common in both types of spondylodiscitis, while severe bone fragmentation is more characteristic of tuberculous

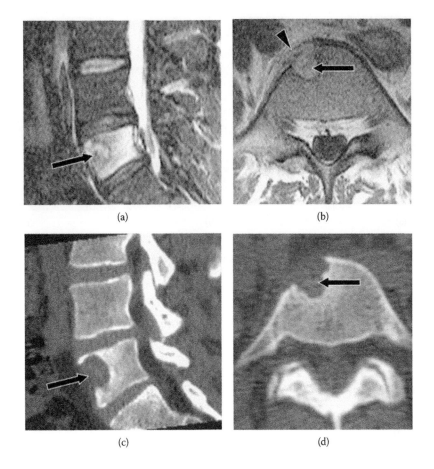

(a)

(b)

(c)

(d)

FIGURE 16.13

A 30-year-old patient with tuberculous infection of the L5 vertebral body. Sagittal STIR (Short Tau Inversion Recovery) (a) and axial contrast-enhanced T$_1$-weighted (b) MR images show L5 spondylitis, anterior lytic lesion with cortical disruption (arrows), and subligamentous extension (arrowhead). Sagittal (c) and axial (d) MDCT images with bone algorithm reconstruction accurately delimit anterior well-defined lytic lesion (arrows), unrelated to intervertebral space. (With kind permission from Springer Science+Business Media: *Eur Radiol*, MR imaging of spinal infection: Atypical features, interpretative pitfalls and potential mimickers, 14, 2004, 1980–1989, Mellado JM, Fig 1.)

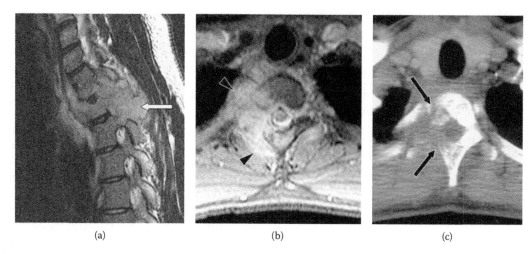

(a)	(b)	(c)

FIGURE 16.14

Young patient with cervicodorsal tuberculous spondylitis. Sagittal T_2-weighted (a) and axial gradient-echo (b) MR images show pseudotumoral involvement of vertebral body and neural arch (white arrow), with paraspinal soft tissue mass (arrowheads). Axial CT (c) shows an osteolytic lesion involving both vertebral body and neural arch (black arrows). A CT-guided biopsy revealed spinal tuberculosis. (With kind permission from Springer Science+Business Media: *Eur Radiol*, MR imaging of spinal infection: Atypical features, interpretative pitfalls and potential mimickers, 14, 2004, 1980–1989, Mellado JM, Fig 2.)

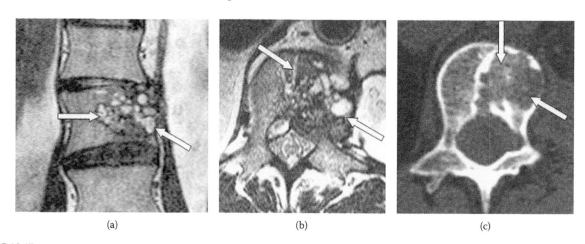

(a)	(b)	(c)

FIGURE 16.15

Spinal hydatidosis in a 65-year-old woman with a history of hydatid disease of the liver. Coronal (a) and axial (b) T_2-weighted MR images show a cystic multiloculated bone lesion (arrows) in the L2 vertebral body. Axial CT image (c) shows a well-defined lytic lesion. (With kind permission from Springer Science+Business Media: *Eur Radiol*, MR imaging of spinal infection: Atypical features, interpretative pitfalls and potential mimickers, 14, 2004, 1980–1989, Mellado JM, Fig 14.)

TABLE 16.6

Imaging Features of Brucellar Spondylodiscitis

- Involvement of lower lumbar spine
- Intact vertebral architecture
- Preserved neural arc
- Relatively preserved discs
- Minimal soft tissue involvement
- No gibbus deformity

TABLE 16.7

Imaging Features of Fungal Spondylodiscitis

- Multilevel involvement
- Involvement of neural arc
- Relatively preserved discs
- Prominent soft tissue involvement

TABLE 16.8

Imaging Features of Vertebral Hydatid Disease

- Cystic multiloculated bone lesions
- Cortical erosions
- No rim enhancement after contrast administration
- Potential extension into adjacent soft tissues

infection. Focal resorption of cancellous bone (Figures 16.5 and 16.16a) typically represents an early finding, which is usually followed by erosion of vertebral endplates. These areas of bone loss typically correlate with regional signal abnormalities on MRI, which look hypointense on T_1-weighted sequences and hyperintense on T_2-weighted sequences.

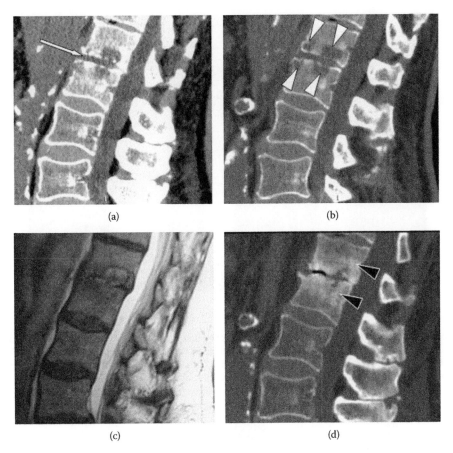

FIGURE 16.16

T12-L1 spondylodiscitis in an 80-year-old man with long-standing lumbar pain. Sagittal-reformatted MDCT with soft tissue (a) and bone (b) algorithm show disc (arrow) and bone (arrowheads) involvement. Corresponding sagittal T_2-weighted MR image (c) confirms the diagnosis. Follow-up MDCT 6 months later (d) shows typical sequelae, with loss of intervertebral space, endplate erosions, and sclerosis (black arrowheads). Note mild anterior wedging of L1.

Bony sequestrations are more common in chronic tuberculous spondylitis. On MDCT, they appear as small dense fragments within larger lytic areas (Figure 16.17). Bone sclerosis is a reparative mechanism associated to many degenerative and inflammatory processes and is more common in pyogenic infection (Figure 16.16d). It relates to Modic type 3 changes [21], which typically show low signal on T_1- and T_2-weighted sequences. This finding does not necessarily indicate absence of active infection [22]. In chronic cases, extensive sclerosis can be visualized [23] (Figure 16.18).

Disc hypodensity and loss of disc height may reflect water accumulation, which appears hypointense on T_1-weighted sequences and hyperintense on T_2-weighted sequences. However, mild hypodensity on sagittal-reformatted MDCT images is hard to appreciate. Small focal or diffuse infection-induced disc protrusion is frequently found [24], it may be bulky and cause radicular compression [25]. Loss of disc height is characteristic of advanced stages, reflecting destruction of the disc (Figures 16.5b and 16.16a). In advanced and chronic cases, discovertebral ankylosis may be found (Figure 16.6c).

Paraspinal soft tissue swelling and paraspinal fluid collections are usually adjacent to the involved disc. MDCT typically shows asymmetric enlargement of the involved muscle groups. Iodinated contrast may help differentiate phlegmonous changes from true abscesses (Figure 16.19). Fluid collections may contain gas bubbles, sequestra, or calcifications [26]. Epidural abscess may occasionally be seen on MDCT, due to loss of epidural fat and rim enhancement (Figure 16.6a). However, distinction between epidural abscess and granulation tissue is difficult, even on MRI [27].

Infection of a single vertebral body without involvement of adjacent disc and spondylodiscitis involving a single vertebral body and a single contiguous disc are considered atypical early findings [28]. Skip lesions involving noncontiguous discovertebral levels are rare in pyogenic infection [11], but rather characteristic of spinal tuberculosis. Preservation or widening of the intervertebral disc may occur. Distant epidural abscesses should be ruled out. Massive paraspinal abscesses are rare in pyogenic infection [23].

Postoperative spondylodiscitis represents a particularly difficult diagnostic challenge. Staphylococcus

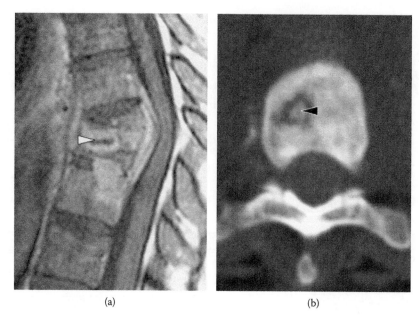

FIGURE 16.17
Sagittal contrast-enhanced T_1-weighted MR image (a) in a patient with pyogenic spondylodiscitis of T10 vertebral body shows a hypointense structure (white arrowhead) surrounded by a thick rim of intense enhancement. Note the epidural phlegmon. Axial CT image (b) through the T10 vertebral confirms the existence of a sequestration (black arrowhead). (With kind permission from Springer Science+Business Media: *Eur Radiol*, MR imaging of spinal infection: Atypical features, interpretative pitfalls and potential mimickers, 14, 2004, 1980–1989, Mellado JM, Fig 12.)

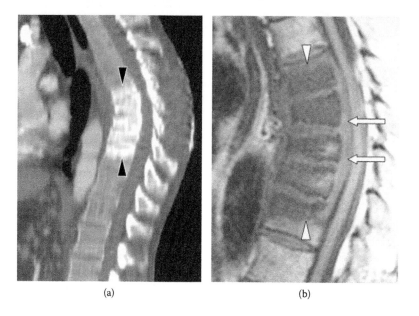

FIGURE 16.18
Sagittal-reformatted CT image (a) in a patient with long-standing dorsal pain shows sclerosis of T6 to T10 vertebral bodies (black arrowheads) and erosion of vertebral endplates. Sagittal T_1-weighted MRI image (b) shows remarkable hypointensity of involved vertebral bodies (white arrowheads) and epidural phlegmon (arrows). These atypical finding are consistent with chronic infectious spondylodiscitis. (With kind permission from Springer Science+Business Media: *Eur Radiol*, MR imaging of spinal infection: Atypical features, interpretative pitfalls and potential mimickers, 14, 2004, 1980–1989, Mellado JM, Fig 11.)

is the most common organism involved. The clinical presentation is nonspecific. Although ESR is almost always increased, it is also nonspecific in operated patients. Increased CRP may indicate an infectious complication, especially if it was known to be negative before surgery [29]. Imaging findings may take a few weeks to become evident, but show no specific patterns. The persistence of normal postoperative findings beyond 3 weeks after the intervention, the progression of findings in two imaging studies, and the clinical suspicion may help diagnose a postoperative infection [9].

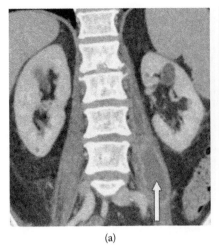 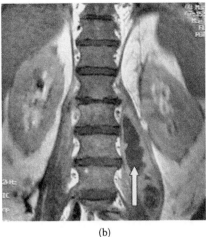 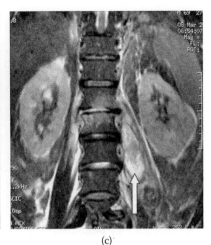

(a) (b) (c)

FIGURE 16.19
Coronal contrast-enhanced MDCT (a), contrast-enhanced T_1-weighted (b), and non-enhanced T_2-weighted (c) MR images show L2/3 spondylodiscitis with associated abscess of left psoas muscle (arrows).

16.3.3 Differential Diagnosis of Spondylodiscitis

Various spinal disorders may mimic spondylodiscitis, such as erosive intervertebral osteochondrosis, ankylosing spondylitis, destructive spondyloarthropathy, and Schmörl's nodes [30].

Modic et al. [21] described MRI changes associated to the degeneration of the discovertebral complex. Modic type 1 changes are hypointense on T_1-weighted imaging and hyperintense on T_2-weighted imaging, representing bone marrow edema. Modic type 2 changes are hyperintense on T_1-weighted imaging and isointense or slightly hyperintense on T_2-weighted imaging and represent conversion of normal red hematopoietic bone marrow into yellow fatty marrow as a result of marrow ischemia. Modic type 3 changes are described as hypointense on T_1- and T_2-weighted imaging and represent subchondral bone sclerosis. Mixed types 1/2 and 2/3 Modic changes have also been reported, suggesting that these changes can convert from one type to another and that they all present different stages of the same pathologic process. Imaging features of spondylodiscitis may present a variety of Modic changes, including type 1 in early stages, type 3 in advanced disease, or mixed types. From a differential standpoint, the presence of disc vacuum phenomenon should be considered a valuable sign of disc degeneration [31].

Erosive osteochondrosis represents an advanced stage of intervertebral osteochondrosis, and commonly presents multifocal involvement. It may associate with degenerative scoliosis of the lumbar spine and may mimic infectious disease. In these cases, MRI should be performed. Presence of disc hyperintensity, loss of nuclear cleft on T_2-weighted images, extensive bone marrow edema involving both sides of the disc, and epidural abscesses are associated with infectious spondylodiscitis. On the opposite, discal vacuum phenomenon, well-defined sclerosis, and erosions of vertebral endplates suggest erosive osteochondrosis [32] (Figure 16.20).

Early ankylosing spondylitis involves the anterior corners of the vertebral bodies, originating marginal enthesitis that are followed by syndesmophyte formation. In more advanced stages, diffuse involvement of discovertebral units and posterior elements may occur. Pseudoarthrosis may complicate ankylosing spondylitis. They are seen as areas of discovertebral destruction and adjacent sclerosis on plain films and sagittal-reformatted MDCT images. These changes, which are referred to as the Andersson lesion, may certainly resemble disc infection.

Destructive spondyloarthropathy associated with hemodialysis also presents with decreased disc height, erosions, and subchondral sclerosis. The absence of subchondral hyperintensity on T_2-weighted sequences is the main difference with infectious spondylitis.

In the acute Schmörl's node, there is focal erosion of the vertebral endplate, surrounded by edema. The absence of abnormalities on the surrounding soft tissues may help rule out an infectious process.

Vertebral tuberculosis can also mimic vertebral metastatic disease [23]. Metastatic disease often involves several contiguous or noncontiguous vertebrae, with occasional involvement of neural arcs. Prevertebral soft tissue involvement, diffuse osteolytic destruction, gas within bone and soft tissues, and intervertebral disc involvement are more characteristics of infection [33].

16.3.4 Treatment

Medical treatment is best applied after isolation of causative germ. When the agent is not identified, empiric treatment for pyogenic infection is commonly used.

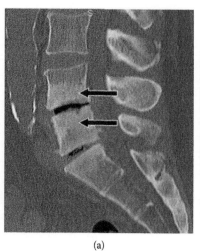
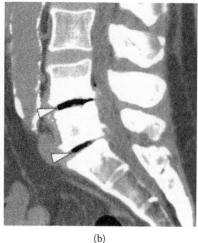
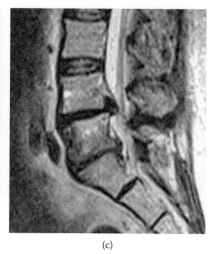

(a)   (b)   (c)

FIGURE 16.20
Sagittal-reformatted MDCT images with soft tissue (a) and bone algorithm reconstruction (b), and T$_2$-weighted MR images (c) in a patient with lumbar pain. Loss of disc height and discal vacuum phenomenon, along with sclerosis and well-defined vertebral endplates, are consistent with degenerative intervertebral osteochondrosis.

The effectiveness of conservative treatment can be estimated by reduction of pain, resolution of fever and leukocytosis, and decreased ESR. A decrease in ESR value during the first month of treatment is considered a predictor of good prognosis [34].

Indications for surgical treatment include neural compression, spinal instability, severe kyphosis, and failure of conservative treatment [35]. Most authors include intractable pain [36] and epidural abscess as surgical indications, even in the absence of neurologic deficits [37].

16.4 Septic Arthritis of the Facet Joint

Pyogenic arthritis of the facet joint is a very rare condition. Most cases are considered to be secondary to spinal osteomyelitis of the vertebral body. However, direct hematogenous dissemination has been reported [38]. Pyogenic arthritis of the facet joint may also derive from steroid injection [39] or acupuncture treatment [40]. The predominant causative bacteria are *S. aureus* and *S. epidermidis*, and both ESR and CRP are usually elevated. Characteristic symptoms include persistent back pain in 90% of patients and fever in 50% [41]. Lumbar spine is the predominant site of involvement. Epidural abscess formation complicates 25% of the cases, of which 38% develop severe neurologic deficit [38]. Systemic complications such as endocarditis [42] have been described. Uncomplicated cases, treated with percutaneous drainage and antibiotics, may do better than those treated with antibiotics alone. Cases complicated by an epidural abscess and severe neurologic deficit should undergo immediate decompressive laminectomy.

16.5 Spontaneous Epidural Abscess

Spinal epidural abscess is frequently associated with spondylodiscitis, facet infection, posterior paraspinal abscess, and retroperitoneal abscess [9]. Also, it may associate with spinal intervention or pyomyositis [43]. However, epidural abscess may also be spontaneous. Spontaneous epidural abscess is a rare, potentially devastating condition. *S. aureus* is the most frequent germ. It predominates in the thoracic spine because the epidural space and the venous plexus are larger in that region [44]. The presenting symptoms are spinal pain and fever, and neurological deficits due to cord compression and ischemia may occur. MRI is the technique of choice for evaluating the spinal canal. Contrast-enhanced MDCT has low sensibility for detecting small abscesses and may be particularly insensitive at the lower cervical and high thoracic spine. Spontaneous epidural abscesses may have a high morbidity with quick progression to paraplegia or quadriplegia [9]. An efficient treatment typically includes surgical decompression and antibiotics.

16.6 Paraspinal Abscess

Paraspinal abscesses may appear associated with discitis, spondylitis, arthritis of facet joints, or epidural abscess. They are widely described in the literature as a complication of invasive spinal procedures such as facet joint infiltration [39], epidural anesthesia [45], or vertebral surgery [46]. Psoas muscle is the most frequent location, but other paraspinal muscles may also get involved. Paraspinal abscess may derive from distant infectious pathology of skeletal, urological, or gastrointestinal origin [47]. Less frequently, it may associate with infected abdominal aortic aneurysm [48] or pregnancy [49]. On these occasions, drainage and excision of graft must be considered.

References

1. Ratcliffe JF. 1982. An evaluation of the intra-osseous arterial anastomoses in the human vertebral body at different ages. A microarteriographic study. *J Anat* 134(Pt 2):373–82.

2. Wiley AM, Trueta J. 1959. The vascular anatomy of the spine and its relationship to pyogenic vertebral osteomyelitis. *J Bone Joint Surg Br* 41-B:796–809.

3. Tali ET. 2004. Spinal infections. *Eur J Radiol* 50(2):120–33.

4. Hong SH, Choi JY, Lee JW, Kim NR, Choi JA, Kang HS. 2009. MR imaging assessment of the spine: Infection or an imitation? *Radiographics* 29:599–612.

5. Mahboubi S, Morris MC. 2001. Imaging of spinal infections in children. *Radiol Clin North Am* 39:215–22.

6. Peruzzi P, Rousseaux P, Scherpereel B et al. 1988. [Spondylodiscitis after surgery of lumbar disk hernia. Apropos of 12 cases in 1796 operations]. *Neurochirurgie* 34(6):394–400.

7. Schofer MD, Lakemeier S, Peterlein CD, Heyse TJ, Quante M. 2011. Primary pyogenic spondylitis following kyphoplasty: A case report. *J Med Case Reports* 5:101.

8. Burrill J, Williams CJ, Bain G, Conder G, Hine AL, Misra RR. 2007. Tuberculosis: A radiologic review. *Radiographics* 27:1255–73.

9. DeSanto J, Ross JS. 2011. Spine infection/inflammation. *Radiol Clin North Am* 49(1):105–27.

10. Stumpe KDM, Zanetti M, Weishaupt D, Hodler J, Boos N, Von Schulthess GK. 2002. FDG positron emission tomography for differentiation of degenerative and infectious endplate abnormalities in the lumbar spine detected on MR imaging. *AJR Am J Roentgenol* 179(5):1151–7.

11. Stäbler A, Reiser MF. 2001. Imaging of spinal infection. *Radiol Clin North Am* 39(1):115–35.

12. Lee JS, Kim KW. 2011. Disseminated septic emboli, septic thrombosis of the vena cava and the common iliac and renal veins, and retroperitoneal abscess secondary to pyogenic spondylitis of the lumbar spine: A case report. *J Bone Joint Surg Am* 93(11):e59.

13. Mondal A. 1994. Cytological diagnosis of vertebral tuberculosis with fine-needle aspiration biopsy. *J Bone Joint Surg Am* 76(2):181–4.

14. Babinchak TJ, Riley DK, Rotheram EB. 1997. Pyogenic vertebral osteomyelitis of the posterior elements. *Clin Infect Dis* 25:221–4.

15. De Backer AI, Mortelé KJ, Vanschoubroeck IJ et al. 2005. Tuberculosis of the spine: CT and MR imaging features. *JBR–BTR* 88(2):92–7.

16. Almeida A. 2005. Tuberculosis of the spine and spinal cord. *Eur J Radiol* 55(2):193–201.

17. Meyer CA, Vagal AS, Seaman D. 2011. Put your back into it: Pathologic conditions of the spine at chest CT. *Radiographics* 31(5):1425–41.

18. Lee HJ, Hur JW, Lee JW, Lee SR. 2008. Brucellar spondylitis. *J Korean Neurosurg Soc* 44(4):277–9.

19. Son JM, Jee WH, Jung CK, Kim SI, Ha KY. 2007. Aspergillus spondylitis involving the cervico-thoracolumbar spine in an immunocompromised patient: A case report. *Korean J Radiol* 8(5):448–51.

20. Tüzün M, Hekimoğlu B. 1998. Hydatid disease of the CNS: Imaging features. *AJR Am J Roentgenol* 171(6):1497–500.

21. Modic MT, Masaryk TJ, Ross JS, Carter JR. 1988. Imaging of degenerative disk disease. *Radiology* 168(1):177–86.

22. Dagirmanjian A, Schils J, McHenry M, Modic MT. 1996. MR imaging of vertebral osteomyelitis revisited. *AJR Am J Roentgenol* 167:1539–43.

23. Mellado JM, Pérez del Palomar L, Camins A, Salvadó E, Ramos A, Saurí A. 2004. MR imaging of spinal infection: Atypical features, interpretive pitfalls and potential mimickers. *Eur Radiol* 14:1980–9.

24. Jinkins JR, Bazan C 3rd, Xiong L. 1996. MR of disc protrusion engendered by infectious spondylitis. *J Comput Assist Tomogr* 20(5):715–8.

25. Yilmaz C, Akar A, Civelek E et al. 2010. Brucellar discitis as a cause of lumbar disc herniation: A case report. *Neurol Neurochir Pol* 44(5):516–9.

26. Ralls PW, Boswell W, Henderson R, Rogers W, Boger D, Halls J. 1980. CT of inflammatory disease of the psoas muscle. *AJR Am J Roentgenol* 134(4):767–70.

27. Kirzner H, Oh YK, Lee SH. 1988. Intraspinal air: A CT finding of epidural abscess. *AJR Am J Roentgenol* 151(6):1217–8.

28. Ledermann HP, Schweitzer ME, Morrison WB, Carrino JA. 2003. MR imaging findings in spinal infections: Rules or myths? *Radiology* 228(2):506–14.

29. Kulkarni AG, Hee HT. 2006. Adjacent level discitis after anterior cervical discectomy and fusion (ACDF): A case report. *Eur Spine J* 15(Suppl 5):559–63.

30. Jevtic V. 2001. Magnetic resonance imaging appearances of different discovertebral lesions. *Eur Radiol* 11(7):1123–35.

31. D'Anastasi M, Birkenmaier C, Schmidt GP, Wegener B, Reiser MF, Baur-Melnyk A. 2011. Correlation between vacuum phenomenon on CT and fluid on MRI in degenerative disks. *AJR Am J Roentgenol* 197(5):1182–9.

32. Champsaur P, Parlier-Cuau C, Juhan V et al. 2000. Differential diagnosis of infective spondylodiscitis and erosive degenerative disk disease. *J Radiol* 81(5):516–22.

33. VanLom KJ, Kellerhouse LE, Pathria MN et al. 1988. Infection versus tumor in the spine: Criteria for distinction with CT. *Radiology* 166(3):851–5.

34. Carragee EJ, Kim D, van der Vlugt T, Vittum D. 1997. The clinical use of erythrocyte sedimentation rate in pyogenic vertebral osteomyelitis. *Spine (Phila Pa 1976)* 22:2089–93.

35. Gouliouris T, Aliyu SH, Brown NM. 2010. Spondylodiscitis: Update on diagnosis and management. *J Antimicrob Chemother* 65(Suppl 3):iii11–24.

36. Chen WH, Jiang LS, Dai LY. 2007. Surgical treatment of pyogenic vertebral osteomyelitis with spinal instrumentation. *Eur Spine J* 16(9):1307–16.
37. Darouiche RO. 2006. Spinal epidural abscess. *N Engl J Med* 355(29):2012–20.
38. Muffoletto AJ, Ketonen LM, Mader JT, Crow WN, Hadjipavlou AG. 2001. Hematogenous pyogenic facet joint infection. *Spine(Phila Pa 1976)* 26(14):1570–6.
39. Park MS, Moon SH, Hahn SB, Lee HM. 2007. Paraspinal abscess communicated with epidural abscess after extra-articular facet joint injection. *Yonsei Med J* 48(4):711–4.
40. Daivajna S, Jones A, O'Malley M, Mehdian H. 2004. Unilateral septic arthritis of a lumbar facet joint secondary to acupuncture treatment—A case report. *Acupunct Med* 22(3):152–5.
41. Rhyu KW, Park SE, Ji JH, Park I, Kim YY. 2011. Pyogenic arthritis of the facet joint with concurrent epidural and paraspinal abscess: A case report. *Asian Spine J* 5(4):245–9.
42. Hoelzer BC, Weingarten TN, Hooten WM, Wright RS, Wilson WR, Wilson PR. 2008. Paraspinal abscess complicated by endocarditis following a facet joint injection. *Eur J Pain* 12(3):261–5.
43. Bowen DK, Mitchell LA, Burnett MW, Rooks VJ, Martin JE. 2010. Spinal epidural abscess due to tropical pyomyositis in immunocompetent adolescents. *J Neurosurg Pediatr* 6(1):33–7.
44. Oktenoglu T, Sasani M, Cetin B et al. 2011. Spontaneous pyogenic spinal epidural abscess. *Turk Neurosurg* 21(1):74–82.
45. Yang YW, Chen WT, Chen JY, Lee SC, Chang Y, Wen YR. 2011. Bacterial infection in deep paraspinal muscles in a parturient following epidural analgesia. *Acta Anaesthesiol Taiwan* 49(2):75–8.
46. Mückley T, Schütz T, Hierholzer C, Potulski M, Beisse R, Bühren V. 2003. [Psoas abscess after anterior spinal fusion]. *Unfallchirurg* 106(3):252–8.
47. Montero PG, Lagunadel Estal P, Gómez ML, Pastor AC, Navarro MG. 2011. Pyogenic and tuberculous abscesses of the psoas muscle. *Rev Clin Esp* 211(11):572–8.
48. Alvi AR, UrRehman Z, Nabi ZU. 2010. Pyogenic psoas abscess: Case series and literature review. *Trop Doct* 40(1):56–8.
49. Nelson DB, Manders DB, Shivvers SA. 2010. Primary iliopsoas abscess and pregnancy. *Obstet Gynecol* 116(Suppl 2):479–82.

17

Imaging of Spinal Tumors with Emphasis on MDCT

José M. Mellado, Susana Solanas, Joaquín Martín, and J. Dámaso Aquerreta

CONTENTS

17.1 Introduction

Spinal tumors may be classified as intramedullary, intradural-extramedullary, and extradural. In this review, we will focus on extradural tumors of the spine. Metastatic disease, multiple myeloma, and lymphoma are the most common malignant extradural tumors of the spine, while hemangioma is the most common benign vertebral tumor. Imaging plays a major role in the diagnosis and management of spinal tumors. However, inherent limitations of imaging modalities should be kept in mind, such as cost, availability, radiation dose, acquisition time, and diagnostic accuracy. A systematic approach is useful for characterizing tumors of the spine. The diagnosis of spinal tumors is based on patient age, topographic features,

lesion pattern, and histopathological analysis after biopsy. Among other modalities, multi-detector computed tomography (MDCT) is considered one of the most versatile tools for diagnosis and management of spinal tumors [1,2].

17.2 Anatomical Review

The spine usually consists of 33 vertebrae. The upper 24 vertebrae are grouped under the cervical (7), thoracic (12), and lumbar (5) vertebrae. The lower nine vertebrae fuse to form the sacrum and coccyx. A typical lumbar vertebra consists of a vertebral body and a neural arch (Figure 17.1). The neural arch is formed

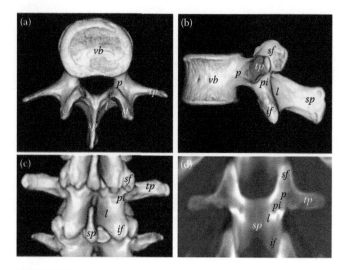

FIGURE 17.1
Normal anatomy of a lumbar vertebral (L4) as seen on axial (a), lateral (b), and posterior coronal (c, d) volume-rendered MDCT images. A typical vertebra consists of a vertebral body (vb) and a neural arch. The neural arch is formed by a pair of pedicles (p) and a pair of laminae (l), and supports two superior articular processes (sf), two inferior articular processes (if), two transverse processes (tp), and one spinous process (sp). Note the position of the pars interarticularis (pi) on the confluence of other posterior elements.

by a pair of pedicles and laminae, and it supports two superior articular processes, two inferior articular processes, two transverse processes, and one spinous process. The bodies of adjacent vertebrae are connected by specialized cartilaginous joints known as intervertebral discs. The concavities above and below the pedicles enclose the intervertebral foramina and the spinal roots. Synovial joints are formed between the inferior articular facets of one vertebra and the superior articular facets of the vertebrae below. Different ligaments reinforce the vertebral joints [3].

The thoracic vertebrae are intermediate in size between those of the cervical and lumbar regions. The upper vertebrae are much smaller than those in the lower part of the thoracic region. The thoracic vertebrae are distinguished by the presence of facets on the sides of the bodies for articulation with the heads of the ribs, and facets on the transverse processes of all, except the eleventh and twelfth, for articulation with the tubercles of the ribs [3].

The cervical vertebrae are the smallest of the true vertebrae, and their transverse processes are pierced by a foramen. The first, second, and seventh cervical

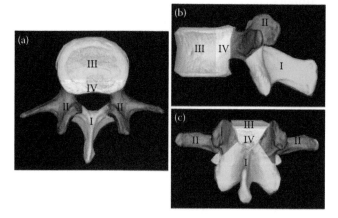

FIGURE 17.2
Diagram based on axial (a), lateral (b), and posterior coronal (c) volume-rendered MDCT images show the topographic classification of vertebral tumors as suggested by James Weinstein. Within these zones, the tumor is described as intraosseous, extraosseous, or distant metastasis.

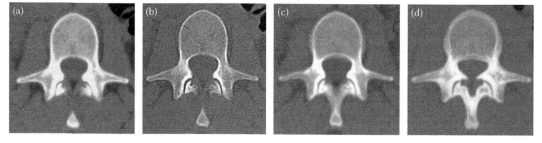

FIGURE 17.3
Axial two-dimensional reformatted and three-dimensional volume-rendered MDCT images of L3 lumbar vertebra. A 3-mm-thick image with bone window and soft-tissue reconstruction algorithm (a) offers incomplete display of neural arch and suboptimal spatial resolution. A 3-mm-thick image with bone reconstruction algorithm significantly improves spatial resolution (b). A 10-cm-thick volume-rendered image (c) offers complete display of vertebral body, neural arch, and its processes. A 10-cm-thick axial MIP image (d) offers complete vertebral display, with increased density and artefactual thickening of cortical bone.

vertebrae are slightly different. The first cervical vertebra is called the atlas, and it has anterior arch, posterior arch, and lateral masses. The second cervical vertebra is called the axis and has a vertebral body, an odontoid process, and a neural arch. The seventh cervical vertebra has a prominent spinous process [3].

In 1983, Francis Denis introduced the concept of the three spine columns. Traumatic lesions involving two columns are unstable, which means that isolated

posterior ligamentous disruption does not necessarily imply spinal instability [4]. In 1989, James Weinstein proposed a model designed for improving surgical planning of spinal tumors (Figure 17.2). In this model, the vertebra is delineated into four zones, which are used to describe the location of the primary tumors and metastatic lesions [5].

The vertebrae are composed of cortical and cancellous bone. Cortical bone is denser, stronger, and stiffer than

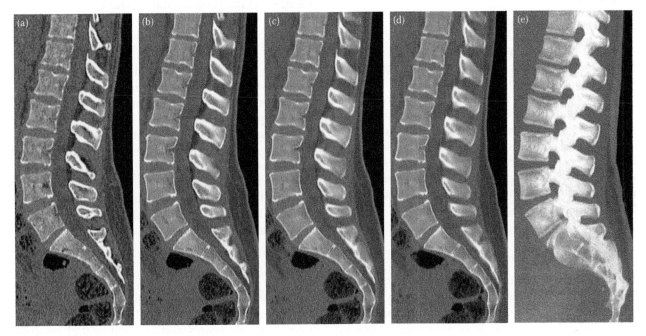

FIGURE 17.4
Sagittal reformatted MDCT images with bone window and bone reconstruction algorithm, displayed with 1 (a), 3 (b), 6 (c) and 9 (d) mm thickness, and sagittal thick-slab MIP (e).

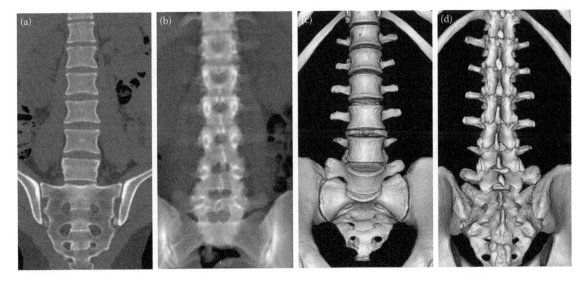

FIGURE 17.5
Coronal curved reformatted (a), coronal thick-slab MIP (b), anterior coronal volume-rendered (c), and posterior coronal volume-rendered (d) MDCT images of the lumbo-sacral spine.

cancellous bone. Cancellous bone predominates in the vertebral bodies, is highly vascular, and frequently contains red bone marrow, which partly explains the high prevalence of some tumors within that area. Conversely, cancellous bone and red bone marrow are comparatively less abundant in neural archs [6].

17.3 Imaging Modalities

Conventional radiography, radionuclide bone scan (RBS), MDCT, magnetic resonance (MR) imaging, and positron emission tomography-computed tomography (PET-CT), among other modalities, play a complementary role in the assessment of spinal tumors. At present, technical advances have made possible whole-spine imaging with virtually all modalities. Radiography and RBS used to be first-line tools for initial assessment of spinal tumors. At present, MDCT and MR imaging are extensively used in the work-up of spinal tumors, but PET-CT is also increasingly used (Table 17.1).

17.3.1 Conventional Radiography

According to the American College of Radiology (ACR) practice guidelines, spine radiographies may be useful in the clinical setting of suspected spinal tumor [7] (ACR 2012). If the patient is symptomatic, a focused

radiographic examination should be carried out. However, this modality provides minimal data on the integrity of the bone marrow and the presence of lesions due to the complex anatomy of the vertebrae. In addition, osteolytic bone lesions only become radiographically evident after more than 30% through 50% of bone mineral content is lost at the site of the disease. When a spinal tumor has caused a pathologic fracture, weight-bearing full-spine x-rays may be used to evaluate spinal balance and the need for stabilization.

17.3.2 Radionuclide Bone Scan

The RBS is a simple and cost-effective modality for whole-body screening when multifocal spine tumors are suspected. 99m Tc methylene diphosphonate is the most frequently used isotope. RBS helps detect areas of increased osteoblastic activity, which may relate to osteolytic or osteoblastic lesions. Multiple lesions suggest metastases. However, focal lesions may be hard to interpret, and multiple myeloma could not be detected. Other patterns include diffuse involvement (superscan), photopenic lesions (cold lesions), flare phenomena, and soft-tissue lesions [8].

17.3.3 Multi-Detector Computed Tomography

MDCT provides great anatomical detail of the spine [2,9]. The routine use of submillimeter collimation generates isotropic voxels and optimal spatial resolution.

TABLE 17.1

Imaging Modalities

	Advantages	Disadvantages
Radiography	Low cost Widely available	Ionizing radiation Superposition of multiple structures Low sensitivity
RBS	Fast overview of the whole skeleton High sensitivity for cortical lesions Low ionizing radiation Low cost	Low sensitivity for medullary lesions Low specificity Low spatial resolution
MDCT	Fast overview of bones and organs High sensitivity and specificity for large enough lesions Image-guided biopsy Widely available	High Ionizing radiation dose Low sensitivity for small lesions Inappropriate for routine screening
MRI	Fast whole-body survey High sensitivity and specificity Anatomical (T1+STIR) and functional (DWI) No ionizing radiation	Whole-body survey lacks anatomical detail High cost
PET	Whole-body overview High sensitivity and specificity Low ionizing radiation No undesirable effects of radiopharmaceuticals	Low spatial resolution High cost Low availability
PET-CT	Whole-body overview High sensitivity and specificity No undesirable effects of radiopharmaceuticals	High cost Low availability Ionizing radiation

Significant reductions in data acquisition times are possible with large pitches and fast gantry rotation times. MDCT of a vertebral tumor may be tailored to a specific spinal segment and are performed with a small field of view. However, large body datasets, acquired with a standard collimation of 64 × 0.5 mm, can be retrospectively reconstructed with a slice width of 0.5 mm, reconstruction interval of 0.3 mm, bone and soft-tissue kernel, and adapted field-of-view, targeted to the spine.

Modern MDCT provides tube current modulation, leading to substantial dose reduction in comparison with scans with fixed milliamperes. Axial (Figure 17.3), sagittal (Figure 17.4), and coronal (Figure 17.5) reformatted and volume-rendered images are available in real-time, interactive display. Conversely, other forms of visualization as shaded surface rendering are more rarely used. Intravenous iodinated contrast may add diagnostic value by helping to define the extent of soft-tissue involvement.

MDCT is widely used for determining the size, number, and location of already known vertebral tumors, but is not a routine modality for survey of metastatic bone involvement. It is probably the most accurate method for evaluating the extent of cancellous and cortical involvement in large lesions. It can also help determine the degree of paraspinal soft-tissue infiltration and the existence of distant-associated lesions, among other roles (Table 17.2).

On MDCT images (Figure 17.6), cortical bone has a denser appearance than cancellous bone. However, areas of relative hypodensity are commonly encountered at the posterior aspect of vertebral bodies and along lower transverse processes (Figure 17.7). Unfortunately, bone marrow evaluation cannot be reliably performed on MDCT, although an inverse relationship between fatty bone marrow and bone mineral density has been suggested [10].

TABLE 17.2

MDCT Role in the Evaluation of Spinal Tumors

Size, number, and location of vertebral lesions

Extent of cancellous and cortical involvement

Degree of paraspinal infiltration

Distant extra-spinal associated lesions

Tumor matrix

Degree of spinal canal or foraminal stenosis

Risk of pathologic fracture

Severity of pathologic fracture (height loss, angular kyphosis)

Discrimination between metastatic and non-malignant fracture

Search of unknown primary malignancy

Image-guided percutaneous biopsy

Surgical and radiotherapy planning

Oncologic follow-up

17.3.4 Magnetic Resonance Imaging

MR imaging has been considered the modality of choice for detecting areas of infiltration of bone marrow and is superior to MDCT for evaluation of the epidural space and neural structures. Sagittal, axial, and coronal sequences are commonly used for evaluation of spinal tumors. T1-weighted images are helpful for evaluation of normal bone marrow, fat content, subacute hemorrhage, and tissue enhancement. T2-weighted sequences,

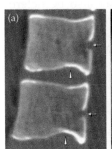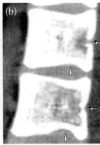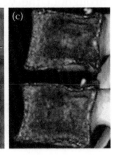

FIGURE 17.6
Sagittal-reformatted with bone (a), soft-tissue (b) windows, and trimmed volume-rendered (c) MDCT images depict the cross-sectional appearance of cortical and cancellous bone of thoracic vertebral bodies. Note heterogeneous bone density at the posterior third of vertebral bodies, particularly conspicuous around the basivertebral veins (arrows), which constitutes a normal finding. Also note mild regular depression at the posterior aspect of vertebral endplates (arrowheads), a normal finding that has been related to notochordal remnants.

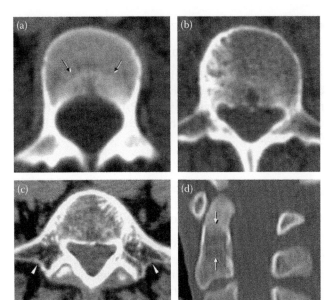

FIGURE 17.7
Examples of normal variations of bone density on MDCT images of the spine. In young individuals, an ill-defined area of increased bone density may be seen around the basivertebral vein (black arrows in a), but is rarely found in the elderly population (b). Also, ill-defined areas of normal hypodensity are seen on transverse processes of the lumbosacral junction (arrowheads in c) and at the base of the odontoid process (white arrows in d).

particularly those with fat saturation, are optimal for detection of most vertebral lesions and may help evaluate the contour of the spinal canal and the cord involvement. Full-spine and whole-body MR imaging, including diffusion-weighted sequences, have been advocated for evaluating bone metastases [11,12].

On MRI, red marrow exhibits intermediate to slightly high signal on both T1- and T2-weighted sequences, while yellow marrow shows signal similar to fat on all pulse sequences. The distribution of red bone marrow throughout the vertebral bodies may also be heterogeneous. Small areas of yellow marrow are occasionally found surrounding the basivertebral veins. In the elderly population, predominance of vertebral yellow marrow is a common finding [13–15].

17.3.5 FDG-PET and PET-CT

Uptake of 18F FDG (fludeoxyglucose) by tumor cells allows for early detection and monitoring the response to therapy within the marrow, bone, and soft tissues. The hybrid techniques, SPECT/CT (Single-Photon Emission Computed Tomography) and PET/CT, recently introduced into clinical practice, provide a better anatomic localization of scintigraphic findings and may improve the diagnostic accuracy of SPECT and PET in detecting malignant bone involvement [16].

17.4 Hystologic Types of Spinal Tumors

According to the histologic types, spinal tumors may be primary and metastatic. A wide variety of primary neoplasms can involve the spine. Primary spinal tumors can be classified according to their tissue of origin (Table 17.3).

17.5 Imaging Features of Spinal Tumors

A classification of spinal tumors according to location has been suggested (Table 17.4) [2]. When a single vertebral lesion is found, additional lesions should be systematically ruled out. Multiple lesions suggest a specific differential diagnosis (Table 17.5). Imaging features provide useful clues for tumor characterization (Table 17.6). Benign and malignant spine tumors may present with pathologic fractures, although osteoporotic compression fractures are much more common. Discriminating between both entities (Figure 17.8 and Table 17.7) and determining the severity of the fracture (Figure 17.9) may be challenging tasks [17–19].

TABLE 17.3

Classification of Primary Spinal Tumors by Tissue of Origin

Osteogenic	Enostosis (bone island)
	Osteoid osteoma
	Osteoblastoma
	Osteosarcoma
Chondrogenic	Osteochondroma
	Chondroblastoma
	Chondrosarcoma
Fibrogenic	Fibrous dysplasia
Vascular	Hemangioma
	Epithelioid hemangioendothelioma
Hematopoietic, reticuloendothelial, lymphatic	Histiocytosis
	Plasmocytoma, multiple myeloma
	Lymphoma
	Leukemia
	Ewing sarcoma
	Notochordal chordoma
Unknown	Aneurysmal bone cyst (ABC)
	Giant cell tumor (GCT)

TABLE 17.4

Spinal Tumors According to Location

Vertebral Body		Neural Arch and Its Processes	
Benign (rare, except hemangioma)	Malignant (common)	Benign (common)	Malignant (rare)
Hemangioma	Metastasis	Osteoid osteoma	Chondrosarcoma
Eosinophilic granuloma	Plasmocitoma*	Osteoblastoma†	Osteosarcoma
	Myeloma*	Osteochondroma	Ewing sarcoma
Giant cell tumor*	Lymphoma	Aneurysmal bone cyst†	
	Chordoma		

*Common extension into the neural arch.　†Common extension into the vertebral body.

TABLE 17.5

Multiple Spinal Tumors

Skip Lesions	Contiguous Levels
Metastasis	Osteosarcoma
Myeloma	Chondrosarcoma
Lymphoma	Myeloma
Enostosis	Lymphoma
Hemangioma	Ewing sarcoma
Eosinophilic granuloma	Chordoma
	Aneurysmal bone cyst
	Giant cell tumor

17.6 Primary Spinal Tumors

Primary tumors of the spine are uncommon, representing less than 5% of all bone tumors. While metastatic disease and multiple myeloma are multifocal, most primary tumors of the spine are solitary lesions. In patients

TABLE 17.6

Imaging Features of Spinal Tumors

Radiographic Pattern	Osteolytic, Osteoblastic, Mixed
Matrix	Osteoblastic tumors can display amorphous ossifications Reactive bone sclerosis is found adjacent to osteoid osteoma and osteoblastoma Cartilage-forming tumors exhibit punctate comma-shaped or annular calcifications Fibrous dysplasia manifests as ground-glass attenuation
Fluid–fluid levels	Suggestive of aneurysmal bone cyst
Vertical striations	Suggestive of hemangioma
Fat content	Suggestive of hemangioma, fibrous dysplasia, Paget disease, and Schmörl node
Margins	Benign tumors exhibit geographic bone destruction and sclerotic margins GCT, ABC, and hemangioma may be aggressive looking Malignant tumors exhibit poorly defined margins and permeative bone destruction
Soft-tissue involvement	Malignant tumors may have paraspinal or epidural soft-tissue mass Also aneurysmal bone cysts, aggressive hemangioma and eosinophilic granuloma
Growth rate	Slow-growing rate in benign tumors Fast-growing rate in malignant tumors
Loco-regional extension	Tumors of the cervical spine may involve supraaortic trunks Tumors of the thoracic spine may involve pleura, mediastinum, and ribs Tumors of the lumbar spine may involve retroperitoneum Sacral tumors may involve the sacroiliac joints and pelvis
Stenosis	Epidural infiltration or pathologic fracture may cause spinal canal and foraminal stenosis
Pathologic fracture	Benign and malignant spinal tumors may cause pathologic fracture

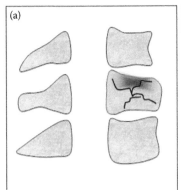 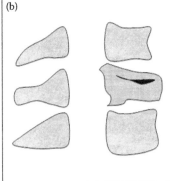 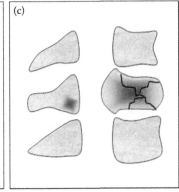

FIGURE 17.8

Diagram shows the imaging characteristics of acute osteoporotic fracture (a), chronic osteoporotic fracture (b) and acute pathologic fracture secondary to spine tumor (c). In acute osteoporotic lesions, fracture lines are visible, mild anterior wedging is common, and posterior wall may be preserved. In chronic osteoporotic fractures, mild retropulsion of the superior aspect of the posterior wall is a common finding, typically with an irregular contour and minimal canal compromise. Also, subchondral or diffuse bone sclerosis of the vertebral body, linear subchondral bands, or intraosseous air may be present. In acute pathologic fracture secondary to bone tumor, height loss of the vertebral body associates with commonly heterogenous density, convex posterior wall, and occasional abnormalities of the neural arch.

TABLE 17.7

Differential Diagnosis of Compression Fracture

Acute Osteoporotic Compression Fracture	Pathologic Fracture Secondary to Spine Tumor
Hypointense band on T1w and T2w	Convex posterior wall
Partially preserved bone marrow	Signal changes on neural arch
Retropulsed fragment	Epidural or focal paraspinal mass
Other compression fractures	Other vertebral lesions

under 30 years of age, spinal tumors are benign except for Ewing sarcoma and osteosarcoma. In patients over 30 years of age, most tumors are malignant except for vertebral hemangiomas and bone islands. Back pain is the most relevant symptom, but some lesions are incidental findings on routine imaging. The diagnosis of primary tumors of the spine is based on patient age, sex, site of the lesion, and tumor pattern as seen at radiological examinations (Table 17.8) [2,18].

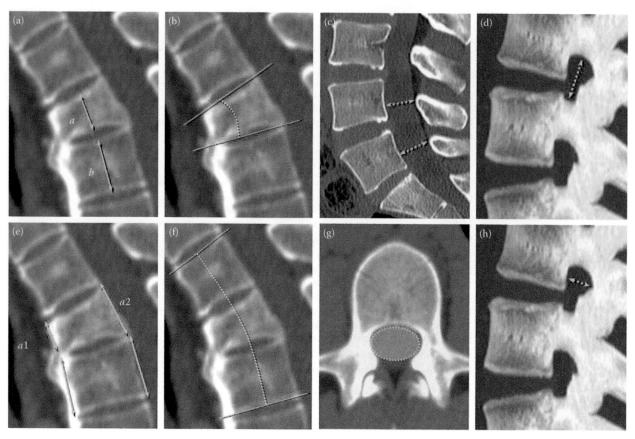

FIGURE 17.9
Measurement of vertebral body loss (a, b), wedge angle (c), kyphosis angle (d), AP diameter of the spinal canal (e), and area of spinal canal (f). In the lumbar spine, AP diameter of 10 mm indicates canal stenosis. Cross-sectional dural sac areas less than 75 mm² are correlated with stenosis. Measurement of foraminal height (g) and foraminal AP diameter (h) are also shown.

TABLE 17.8

Primary Tumors of the Spine

Lesion	Patient Age	Spinal Location	Matrix	Imaging Findings
Osteoid osteoma	2nd	Posterior elements Lumbar spine	Bone-forming tumor	Radiolucent nidus Surrounding sclerosis
Osteoblastoma	2nd–3rd	Posterior elements Thoracic and lumbar spine	Bone-forming tumor	Expansile lesion Calcifications May resemble osteoid osteoma
Osteosarcoma	2nd–4th 7th–9th	Vertebral body Thoracic and lumbar spine	Bone-forming tumor	Osteolytic and osteoblastic areas, soft-tissue mass
Osteochondroma	2nd–3rd	Posterior elements Cervical spine	Cartilage-forming tumor	Classic exostosis
Chondrosarcoma	4th–5th	Vertebral body Thoracic spine	Cartilage-forming tumor	Osteolysis lesion Punctate calcification
Ewing's sarcoma	2nd–3rd	Vertebral body Lumbo-sacral spine	Reticulo-endothelial tumor	Osteolytic lesion Soft-tissue mass
Vertebral hemangioma	Any age (peak 4th)	Vertebral body Thoracic spine	Vascular tumors Fat content	Thickened vertical trabeculae Occasional aggressive pattern
Chordoma	Middle-aged	Vertebral body Sacro-coccygeal Spheno-occipital Contiguous vertebral involvement	Notochord origin Cartilage component	Destructive midline lesion Soft-tissue mass associated
Aneurysmal bone cyst	Young patients	Posterior elements Thoracic spine	Unknown origin Fluid–fluid levels	Lytic expansive lesion Fluid–fluid levels

TABLE 17.8 (*Continued*)

Primary Tumors of the Spine

Lesion	Patient Age	Spinal Location	Matrix	Imaging Findings
Giant cell tumor	2nd–3rd	Vertebral body Sacrum	Unknown origin	Osteolytic geographic area Soft-tissue density No mineralized matrix
Myeloma Plasmocytoma	4th–8th (peak 65 years)	Vertebral body Thoracic and lumbar spine	Hematopoietic and Lymphatic tumor	Punched-out osteolytic lesions Uniform size Loss of bone mineral density
Lymphoma	5th–7th	Vertebral body Thoracic spine Contiguous vertebral involvement	Hematopoietic and Lymphatic tumor	Osteolytic, osteoblastic or mixed; aggressive appearance Soft-tissue mass

17.6.1 Bone-Forming Tumors

A bone island, also termed solitary enostosis, is a hamartoma. It appears as a solitary area of mature, lamellar bone located within an area of cancellous bone. It predominates in the thoracic and lumbar vertebral bodies. Most are 1 through 2 mm in size, but some can be up to 1 through 2 cm or more. They may be multiple, as in osteopoikilosis. Uptake on bone scan is decreased, but may be increased in less than 10% of cases. Most lesions remain stable. Radiography and MDCT demonstrate round osteoblastic lesions with peripheral "brush border" and identical density to cortical bone (Figure 17.10). The differential diagnosis includes osteosarcoma and osteoblastic metastasis [2,18].

Osteoid osteoma is a benign bone lesion with a nidus of less than 2 cm surrounded by a zone of reactive bone. It occurs most commonly in the long bones, especially the femur, but may also involve the neural arch (Figure 17.11) or the vertebral body (Figure 17.12). The tumor presents a peak age in the early twenties. It causes pain at night, which is promptly relieved with salicylates. The male to female ratio is 2:1. Classic radiological presentation includes radiolucent nidus surrounded by reactive sclerosis in the cortex of the bone. However, osteoid osteoma may involve the cortical bone, the cancellous bone, or the subperiosteal region [20,21]. Sometimes, and depending on location, it cannot be visible in the sclerotic reaction. For example, in the posterior arch, sclerosis is difficult to assess so the nidus predominates. However, this sclerosis is more evident when tumor is located in peripheral areas of the vertebral body.

Osteoblastoma is a rare benign bone tumor. The tumor may have a slow indolent course or mimic malignancy. On CT, osteoblastomas may be similar to osteoid osteomas, but grow larger than 2.0 cm in diameter. They may also appear as expansive lesions with sclerotic rim and calcifications (Figure 17.13). More rarely, osteoblastomas may have an aggressive-looking appearance. Other diagnoses that share similar clinical, radiographic, and histologic features with conventional osteoblastoma

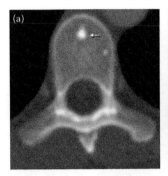
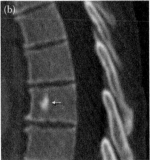

FIGURE 17.10

A 42-year-old woman who presented with abdominal pain. Axial (a) and sagittal reformatted (b) MDCT images show a small hyperdense lesion on the T7 vertebral body (arrows), consistent with a bone island.

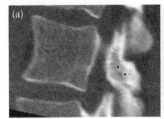
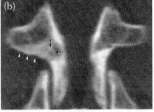

FIGURE 17.11

A 34-year-old woman with back pain. Sagittal (a) and coronal reformatted (b) MDCT images show a small osteolytic yuxta-cortical nidus within the pars interarticularis of a lumbar vertebra (arrows). Note mild reactive sclerosis around the lesion (arrowheads). The findings are consistent with osteoid osteoma.

include osteoid osteoma, giant cell tumor, and fibrous dysplasia [21].

Osteosarcoma is a high-grade malignant osteoblastic lesion that contains variable amounts of osteoid, cartilage, or fibrous tissue (Figure 17.14). Previous radiation therapy and Paget disease may associate. More frequently, the tumor arises in vertebral body, but secondary extension into posterior elements is common. CT usually demonstrates variable densely mineralized matrix, predominantly osteosclerotic pattern, but most frequently has mixed osteosclerotic–osteolytic appearance. Purely lytic pattern is also seen [22].

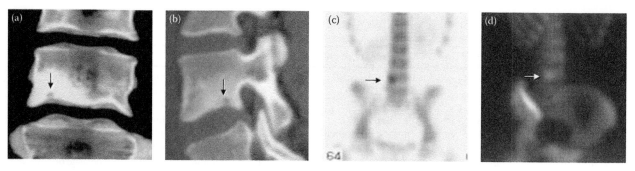

FIGURE 17.12
Subchondral osteoid osteoma of L4 vertebral body in a young man. Coronal (a) and sagittal (b) volume-rendered MDCT images show a small osteolytic nidus (arrows), surrounded by reactive sclerosis. Corresponding radionuclide bone scan (c,d) shows a small focus of increased uptake at L4 (arrows).

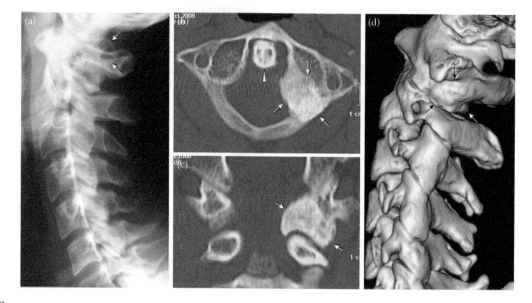

FIGURE 17.13
A 27-year-old man with neck pain. Lateral radiograph (a) shows an abnormal bony structure projected on the posterior arch of C1 (arrows). Axial (b), coronal reformatted (c) and oblique coronal volume rendered (d) MDCT images show an expansive osteblastic lesion involving the left lateral mass of C1. The lesion has well-defined margins and slight heterogeneous density, but no periosteal reaction or soft-tissue mass are seen. Mild contralateral displacement of the odontoid process is found (arrowhead). The findings are consistent with osteoblastoma, which has remained stable for an 8-year follow-up.

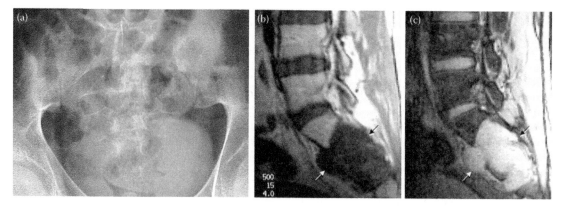

FIGURE 17.14
Sacral osteosarcoma. AP radiograph of the sacrum (a) reveals mild hyperdensity projected within the sacrum. Sagittal T1-weighted (b) and STIR (Short Tau Inversion Recovery) (c) MR images show an aggressive-looking mass of the sacrum, which is found to involve the presacral space and the spinal canal (arrows). The histopathological evaluation revealed an osteosarcoma.

17.6.2 Cartilage-Forming Tumors

Spinal osteochondroma is uncommon, representing only 1% through 4% of solitary exostosis. Hereditary multiple exostosis and previous radiation therapy may predispose. Spinal osteochondroma predominates in the cervical segment. It tends to arise from posterior elements, especially the spinous process, but may also involve the vertebral body. Osteochondromas are composed of cortical and medullary bone with an overlying hyaline cartilage cap and must demonstrate continuity with the underlying parent bone cortex and medullary canal [23,24].

Vertebral chondroblastoma is an exceedingly rare tumor. The radiological features of vertebral chondroblastomas are non-specific, showing a hypodense lesion with well-defined boundary. The differential diagnoses include aneurysmal bone cyst, osteoblastoma, giant cell tumor, eosinophilic granuloma, spondylitis (especially of tuberculous origin), chondromyxoid fibroma, and metastasis [2].

Vertebral chondrosarcomas are also very uncommon. Radiography of chondrosarcoma reveals an aggressive tumor with calcified mass with bone destruction affecting posterior elements and vertebral body. Chondroid matrix mineralization is well shown by CT, where nonmineralized portions correspond to low attenuation zones [2].

17.6.3 Hematopoietic, Reticuloendothelial, and Lymphatic Tumors

Eosinophilic granuloma of the spine is rare, especially in adults. There is a particular high prevalence of lesions in the cervical spine [2]. The radiographic characteristics of spinal eosinophilic granuloma consist of complete or incomplete collapse of the vertebral body; absence of an osteolytic area; preservation of pedicles, posterior elements, and adjacent disk spaces; absence of adjacent paravertebral soft-tissue mass; and increased opacity in the collapsed body. Neurologic deficits, angular kyphosis, and vertebra plana may occur [2].

Multiple myeloma is a malignant proliferation of plasma cells within the cancellous bone. Plasmocytoma represents focal bone involvement and may be considered the early stage of multiple myeloma. Myeloma is seen between the 4th and 8th decades of life. The thoracic and lumbar segments are most commonly affected. Radiographically, multiple myeloma may present as solitary lesion, diffuse myelomatosis, osteopenia (85%), or sclerotic lesions. CT imaging shows punched-out osteolytic lesions, with discrete margins and uniform size. Compression fractures may occur (Figure 17.15) [25]. In diagnosis of myeloma, CT is an alternative if

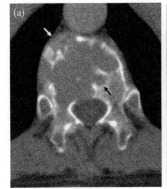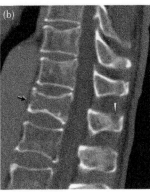

FIGURE 17.15
A 68-year-old man with back pain and constitutional syndrome. Axial (a) and sagittal reformatted (b) MDCT images show an osteolytic lesion within the T12 vertebral body (black arrow). The tumor has lobulated well-defined non-sclerotic borders, with areas of aggressive cortical destruction, and a small soft-tissue mass (white arrow). The sagittal reformation reveals a pathologic fracture with mild height loss and integrity of posterior wall. Additional osteolytic lesions are observed (note a small one at the T12 spinous process, arrowhead in b). The histopathologic analysis revealed multiple myeloma.

MRI is not available. CT provides greater sensitivity than conventional radiographies with similar radiation dose, improves detection of areas with high fracture risk, increases the appreciation of lytic and blastic lesions, and allows doing CT-guided biopsy on specific lesions with increased activity. This improves specimen's results compared with standard sternum or iliac bone marrow biopsies [26,27].

Primary lymphoma of bone is a rare disease, usually with nonspecific appearance in images studies, showing lytic bone destruction (Figure 17.16) with soft-tissue mass associates. Presence of periosteal reaction, soft-tissue mass, or pathologic fracture at initial presentation has been suggested as indicators of poor prognosis. Secondary involvement from systemic lymphoma is more frequently seen, resulting from hematogenous spread or direct invasion from adjacent lymph nodes [28].

Ewing sarcoma of the spine is an aggressive and a rare malignant tumor. It is seen in young people, with a slight male predominance. Lumbosacral vertebral is the most frequent site. Lesions arise in the vertebral body. Lesions may be lytic, sclerotic, or mixed, with associated partial or total vertebral compression. CT may show a permeative bone lesion and collapse of the vertebral body. Extraosseous extension into the spinal canal or paraspinal soft-tissue mass is uncommon. The tumor can metastasize to lungs, other bones, and lymph nodes [2].

Vertebral hemangiomas are slowly growing lesions with well-know radiologic features (Figure 17.17). They typically appear osteolytic, well-defined, with a

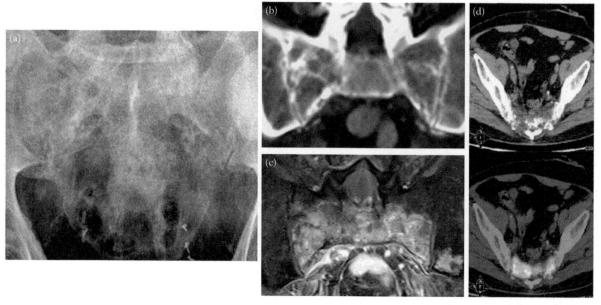

FIGURE 17.16
Primary sacral lymphoma. A 71-year-old man with history of rectal adenocarcinoma, who presented with sacral pain and gait disturbance. AP radiograph (a) and coronal reformatted MDCT image (b) show a mixed osteolytic and osteoblastic lesion involving both sacral wings. Coronal STIR image (c) shows diffuse involvement of the sacrum, but also of contiguous left iliac bone. The PET-CT (d) revealed pathologic enhancement of the involved area.

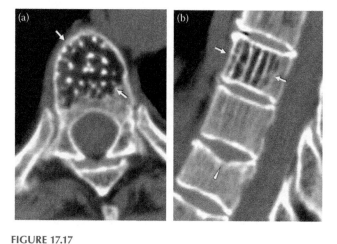

FIGURE 17.17
A 76-year-old woman with monoclonal gammopathy and severe back pain. Axial (a) and sagittal reformatted (b) MDCT images show an osteolytic lesion within the T9 vertebral body, which shows well-defined minimally sclerotic borders (arrows) and a prominent trabecular pattern with vertical striations, characteristic of vertebral hemangioma. A compression fracture of T11 (arrowhead) is also seen.

prominent trabecular pattern of vertical striations. More rarely, hemangiomas may show a soft-tissue component (Figure 17.18), or exhibit an aggressive pattern, mimicking malignant tumors and becoming symptomatic. Compression of neural elements may be secondary to extra-osseous extension, to vertebral fracture, or less frequently to enlargement of adjacent blood vessels. There may be an inverse relationship between the amount of

intraosseus fatty stroma and the aggressiveness of the hemangioma [29].

Chordoma is a rare and aggressive tumor that arises from remnants of embryonic notochord. Chordomas predominate at the spheno-occipital and sacrococcygeal regions. They are usually found at the fifth to sixth decade of life. They usually present as expansive destructive lesions within the vertebral body, typically centered in the midline. One or more contiguous vertebrae may be involved, with sparing of the discs and posterior elements. Imaging studies invariably show lytic bone destruction and extraosseous soft-tissue mass associated, sometimes with "mushroom" appearance (Figure 17.19). Amorphous calcifications are frequents, more in sacrococcygeal lesions [2,30].

Benign notochordal cell tumors, also called giant notochordal rests, are recently discovered intraosseous lesions of notochordal cell origin that are usually asymptomatic or indolent (Figure 17.20). However, pain, sometimes severe, is commonly present. Roentgenographic studies are either normal or show sclerosis within the involved vertebral body. The normal vertebral body configuration is maintained without bone expansion. Multicentric foci may occur. CT is normal, or demonstrates whatever sclerosis is present. Significantly, however, no bone destruction is evident. MRI studies invariably demonstrate a lesion that most often has a low T1- and high T2-weighted signal intensity, and which is almost always non-enhancing [31].

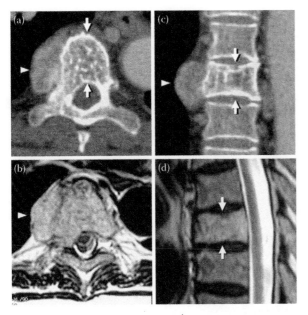

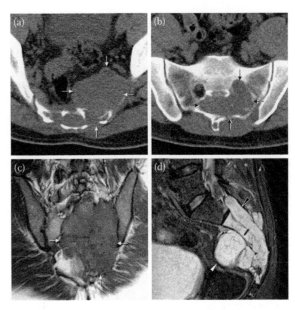

FIGURE 17.18

An 80-year-old woman with endometrioid ovarian carcinoma and a solitary vertebral lesion. Axial (a) and coronal sagittal reformatted (b) MDCT images and axial (c) and sagittal (d) T2-weighted MR images show an osteolytic lesion within the T7 vertebral body. The imaging findings are suggestive of vertebral hemangioma. The association of a right paraspinal mass (arrowhead) and the existence of an already known ovarian malignancy (data not shown) was necessary a CT-guided fine-needle aspiration, which ruled out metastatic disease.

FIGURE 17.19

Sacral chordoma. A 50-year-old man with 2-year-long sciatic pain. Axial MDCT images (a, b) show an osteolytic lesion with associated soft-tissue mass involving the sacrum (arrows). On coronal T1-weighted MR images (c), the lesion has a solid appearance and exhibits low signal intensity (arrows). On sagittal STIR sequence (d), the lesion is found to extend into both the presacral space (white arrowhead) and the spinal canal (black arrowhead).

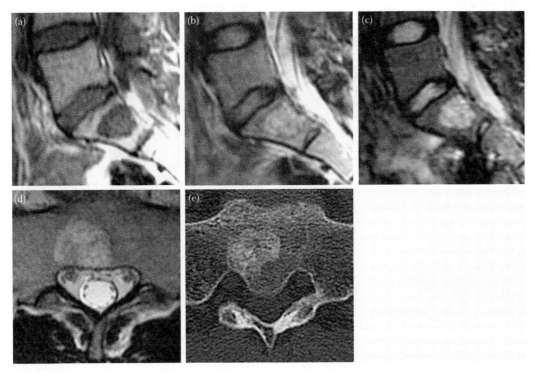

FIGURE 17.20

An 18-year-old woman who presented with non-specific lumbar pain. Sagittal T1-weighted (a), T2-weigthed (b), and STIR (c) MR images show a well-defined non expansive sacral lesion. Axial T2-weighted MR image (d) and axial MDCT image (e) reveal the lesion is near the midline. The well-defined focus of sclerosis at CT, and the absence or cortical remodelling or permeation rules out chordoma. The findings are consistent with a benign notochordal cell tumor.

Aneurysmal bone cysts are usually found in young patients, usually at the second to third decade of life. They result from trauma or tumor-induced anomalous vascular process. In one third of cases, a preexisting lesion can be identified (the giant cell tumor being the most common). The spine is involved in 12% through 30% of the cases. Aneurysmal bone cysts predominate at the posterior elements of thoracic vertebrae. On CT images, aneurysmal bone cysts appear as osteolytic lesions with expanded contour, internal septa, and fluid–fluid levels. The differential diagnosis of an expansive lesion of the posterior vertebral elements includes giant cell tumor, osteoblastoma, aneurysmal bone cyst, eosinophilic granuloma, and multiple myeloma [32].

Giant cell tumor is composed of stromal cell with uniformly distributed osteoblastic giant cell. Involvement of the spine is not usual. It is commonly benign, but its size and soft tissue component may simulate a malignant neoplasm and may be locally aggressive. Giant cell tumors also involve young patients. They appear as osteolytic and expansive lesions, without mineralized matrix. On CT images, sacral lesions have a soft tissue density with well-defined margins that may show a thin rim of sclerosis. Areas of hemorrhage and necrosis are shown like foci of low attenuation. CT imaging performed after intravenous injections of contrast material reveals enhancement of the tumor, which reflects an increase in the vascular supply (Figure 17.21) [33].

Other primary spinal tumors of another nature or origin in other structures may be seen, including fibrous dysplasia, intra-osseous schwannoma (Figure 17.22), and parosteal lipoma (Figure 17.23).

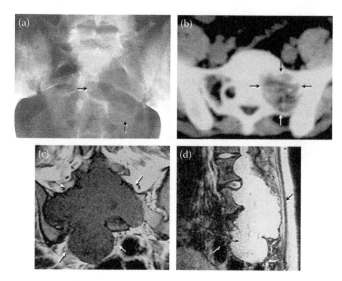

FIGURE 17.22
Sacral schwannoma. AP radiograph (a), axial CT image (b), axial T1-weighted (c), and sagittal T2-weighted (d) MR images reveal a well-defined osteolytic tumor involving the left sacral wing, the presacral space, the spinal canal, and the retrospinal soft-tissues (arrows). Histopathological evaluation was consistent with intraosseous schwannoma.

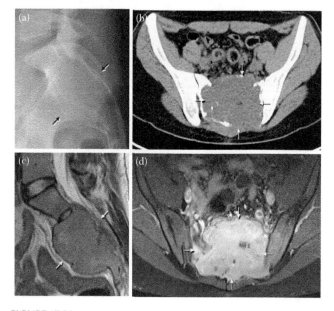

FIGURE 17.21
Sacral giant cell tumor. Lateral radiograph (a) and axial CT image (b) show an expansive osteolytic tumor involving the sacrum and the presacral space. Sagittal T2-weighted (c) and contrast-enhanced T1-weighted (d) MR images show marked enhancement of the tumor and spinal canal involvement (arrows). Histopathological evaluation was consistent with giant cell tumor.

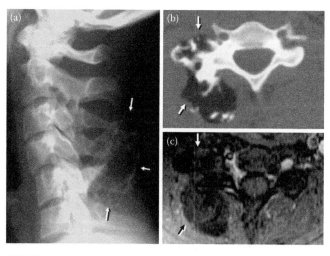

FIGURE 17.23
A 28-year-old man with palpable lump at the posterior aspect of the neck. Lateral radiograph of the cervical spine (a) reveals a round soft-tissue mass with linear calcifications near the spinous processes. Axial CT (b) and axial fat-suppressed T1-weighted MR image (c) reveal an exostosis of right lateral elements of C5, associated with a fatty soft-tissue mass (arrows). The findings are consistent with parosteal lipoma.

17.7 Vertebral Metastases

Vertebral metastases are common events in oncologic patients. Early detection is essential for optimal therapy. Imaging plays a crucial role in the work-up of bone metastases. The purpose of imaging is to identify the lesion, to determine its full extent, to characterize it, to assess accompanying complications—such as fractures and cord compression—and to monitor response to therapy. Detection of bone metastases is based on visualization of tumor infiltration or detection of bone reaction to the malignant process. A comprehensive understanding of epidemiology, physiopathology, clinical features, and prognostic indicators of vertebral metastases is required in order to design efficient diagnostic strategies and cost-effective personalized treatments [34].

17.7.1 Epidemiology

The skeletal system is the most common site for metastases in oncology patients. In fact, metastases are the most common malignant bone tumors. The prevalence of bone tumors varies considerably with the type of tumor, but is likely to increase, owing to the increased survival time of many malignant diseases. Approximately 30% to 70% of all those diagnosed with carcinoma are predicted to have metastasis to bone at the time of their death. Bone metastases are particularly prevalent in breast and prostate cancers because of the relative prevalence of these diseases (Table 17.9). Also, bone is the most common initial site of metastasis for breast and prostate cancers. Bone metastases from melanoma, kidney, thyroid, and lung cancers are also highly prevalent [34–37].

Bone metastases may be the initial manifestation of previously unknown malignancies. Twenty percent of histologically proven vertebral metastases occur as the initial manifestation of malignancy. This is particularly common in lung cancer, cancer of unknown primary site, multiple myeloma, and non-Hodgkin's lymphoma. Symptoms are non-specific in one third of these patients. The diagnosis is suggested when specific imaging features are found. This is typically followed by further imaging and imaging-guided techniques in order to confirm the diagnosis, establish the extent of the disease, and find the primary tumor [38].

Bone metastases are much more commonly found during periodical follow-ups in oncology patients. In this population, newly detected vertebral lesions are usually interpreted as metastatic disease, related to progression or recurrence. However, these may also represent metastases from a second unknown primary tumor or benign lesions, with a prevalence and probability of 2%. Despite this low prevalence, management of presumptive recurrence in the absence of biopsy proof can lead to errors such as inappropriate therapy for benign disease or incorrect management of a second malignant disease [39].

17.7.2 Pathogenesis

Bone involvement in metastases occurs by means of three main mechanisms: (1) direct extension, (2) retrograde venous flow, and (3) seeding with tumor emboli via the blood circulation.

Direct invasion of the axial skeleton may result from adjacent primary tumors. The left side of the vertebral bodies is commonly infiltrated by contiguous pathologic lymph nodes, because the left-sided nodes are closer to bone than the right (Figure 17.24). Direct skeletal invasion typically starts with cortical permeation and is usually accompanied by a detectable soft tissue mass, a feature that is unusual in metastases that arise by hematogenous spread [35,40].

TABLE 17.9

Incidence of Bone Metastases at Postmortem Examination

Primary Tumor	Prevalence of Bone Metastases (%)
Breast	65–75
Prostate	65–75
Thyroid	60
Lung	30–40
Kidney	20–25
Melanoma	15–25

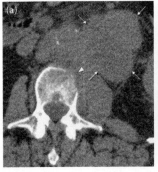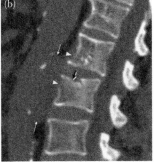

FIGURE 17.24
A 66-year-old man who presented with left sciatic pain. Axial (a) and sagittal-reformatted (b) non-enhanced MDCT images show a retroperitoneal mass (white arrows), which erodes the anterior cortical of L1 and L2 vertebral bodies (arrowheads). Note pathologic fracture on L2 (black arrow). The CT-guided biopsy revealed CD20-positive B-cell lymphoma.

Retrograde venous flow through the valveless vertebral venous plexus is probably the major mechanism when spread from intra-abdominal cancer involves the vertebrae. Antegrade seeding of tumor emboli is also possible. Both hematogenous routes initially involve the cancellous bone, which contains great amounts of red marrow, followed by secondary cortical destruction. The predominant involvement of axial skeleton in adults (over 90%) is probably due to its great amount of red marrow, and also due to its rich vascularity [35].

In bone metastases, tumor cells produce factors that directly or indirectly induce the formation of osteoclasts that stimulates bone destruction. The relationship between the osteoclastic and osteoblastic remodeling processes determines whether a predominant lytic, sclerotic, or mixed pattern is seen on radiographs [41,42].

17.7.3 Distribution

The spine is most commonly affected by bone metastasis, followed by the pelvis, proximal femur, ribs, proximal humerus, and skull. Metastatic seeding predominates in the thoracic spine (accounting for about 70% of cases), with the lumbar spine being the next most involved site (20% of cases). The cervical spine is affected in approximately 10% of cases. Multiple spinal levels are affected in about 30% of patients [35,37].

Extradural metastases of the spine account for approximately 95% of secondary spinal tumors, although lymphomas may occur in the epidural space without bone involvement. Metastatic spinal tumors seldom breach the dura. Intradural extramedullary metastases are uncommon and represent tertiary spread from cerebral secondary sites, transmitted through the cerebrospinal fluid. Intramedullary tumors are rare, arise through hematogenous spread, and comprise approximately 3.5% of spinal metastases.

Vertebral metastases predominantly involve the posterior aspect of the vertebral body (Figure 17.25). Although destruction of the pedicle was considered an early sign of vertebral metastasis (Figure 17.26), the blurring of the pedicle in the conventional radiographies occurs rather late in the metastatic process and often accompanies extensive destruction of the vertebral body. Certain carcinomas show a predilection for particular skeletal sites. Primary tumors arising from the pelvis have a predilection for the lumbosacral spine [35,43].

17.7.4 Clinical Features

Skeletal metastases cause considerable morbidity in patients with advanced cancer. Skeletal morbidity includes severe pain, pathologic fracture, spinal cord or nerve root compression, spinal instability, and hypercalcemia. Metastatic disease may remain confined to the skeleton, but causes a dramatic decline in quality of life and eventual death almost entirely due to skeletal complications and their treatment [35].

Bone metastases are the most common cause of cancer-related pain, although two thirds of vertebral metastases may remain painless. Different sites of bone metastases are associated with distinct clinical pain syndromes. Back pain with or without neurologic

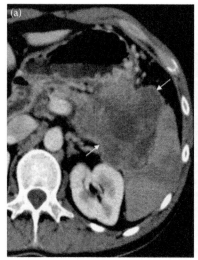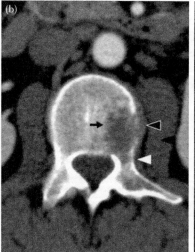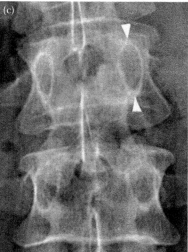

FIGURE 17.25
A 41-year-old man who presented to the emergency room with abdominal pain of 1-month duration. Axial contrast-enhanced MDCT (a) reveals a mass within the pancreatic tail (white arrows), which was found to infiltrate the gastric wall and the splenic capsule. A close-up through the upper aspect of L2 (b) shows an ill-defined osteolytic lesion of the vertebral body (black arrow), causing cortical permeation and mild soft-tissue involvement (black arrowhead). The left L2 pedicle, seen on MDCT image and AP radiograph (c) (white arrowheads), appears mostly preserved.

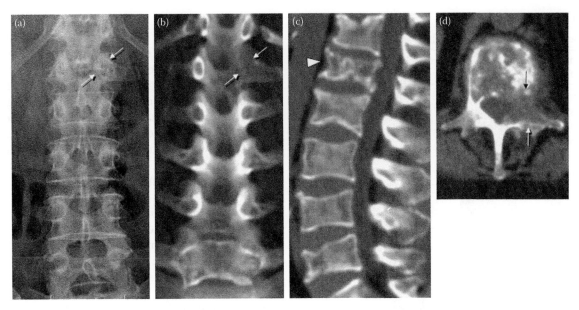

FIGURE 17.26
A 65-year-old woman who presented to the emergency room with abdominal pain. AP radiograph (a) (decubitus view) shows a missing left L1 pedicle (white arrows), which was initially overlooked. A year later, the patient presented colonic obstruction caused by sigmoid neoplasia, breast cancer, and metastatic disease. Coronal volume-rendered MDCT image (b) clearly depicts the missing pedicle, which has been termed the "winking owl sign" (white arrows). Corresponding sagittal reformatted (c) and axial (d) MDCT images further contribute to demonstrate the extent of metastatic disease.

complications may derive from bone destruction, pathologic fracture, epidural extension, or spinal instability.

Spinal cord compression is a medical emergency that reflects vertebral metastases with expansion into the epidural space through the intervertebral foramina, venous hematogenous spread, or pathologic fracture (Figure 17.27).

17.7.5 Diagnostic Imaging of Vertebral Metastases

Radiography remains useful but is considered relatively insensitive in the detection of early or small metastatic lesions. The so-called pedicle sign remains a valuable radiologic indicator of metastases on plain films, but is not considered an early sign [44,45]. As previously stated, the radiographic appearance of bone metastases is often useful in suggesting the nature of the underlying primary malignancy (Table 17.10). On radiographs and MDCT, vertebral metastases may be osteolytic, sclerotic, or mixed. Lytic lesions may be seen in almost all tumor types, but are particularly common in lung cancer. Metastases from renal cell or thyroid carcinomas are almost always osteolytic, and may be outstandingly expansile. Bone metastases of bladder cancer tend to be lytic as well, but may be osteoblastic. Blastic lesions are frequently seen in prostate (Figure 17.28) and breast cancer, occasionally in carcinoid tumors (Figure 17.29), and also in stomach, pancreas, cervix, and colorectal cancer.

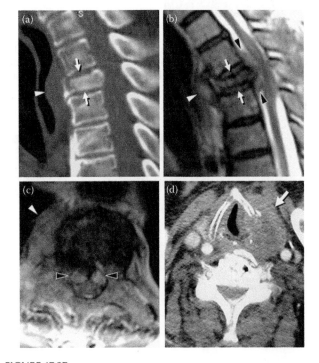

FIGURE 17.27
An 81-year-old without prior history of trauma, who presented with motor weakness and sensory loss in the extremities. Sagittal reformatted MDCT image (a), sagittal T2-weighted MR image (b), and axial T2-weighted MR image (c) show a pathologic fracture of T3 vertebral body (small arrows), with convex posterior wall, epidural mass (black arrowheads), and focal paraspinal mass (white arrowheads). Axial MDCT image through the upper neck (d) reveals a left-hemilarynx tumor (large arrow). The patient underwent radiation therapy.

TABLE 17.10

Radiologic Appearance of Vertebral Metastases

Commonly Osteolytic (75%)	Commonly Osteoblastic (15%)		Commonly Mixed (10%)
Lung	Male	Female	Breast
Kidney	Prostate	Breast	Lung
Thyroid	Bladder		Ovary
Stomach	Carcinoid		Cervix
Colon	Seminoma		Testis
Melanoma	Osteosarcoma		

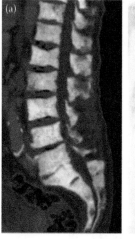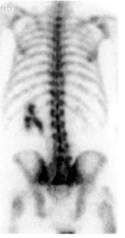

FIGURE 17.28
A 78-year-old man with prostate cancer and elevated PSA (1438). Sagittal MIP (a) shows diffuse osteoblastic metastases in the axial skeleton. Corresponding radionuclide bone scan (b) shows increased skeletal uptake.

MDCT is expected to detect vertebral metastases before many of them become radiographically obvious. Although MDCT scan is superior to radiographs, it is also relatively insensitive to small intramedullary lesions or relatively large lesions with intermediate density that do not stand out from its surrounding tissue, and has the disadvantage of limited skeletal coverage and high radiation dose. In addition, evaluation of bone marrow and soft-tissue involvement are difficult on MDCT. Conversely, MDCT is the modality of choice for image-guided percutaneous biopsy of vertebral tumors (Figure 17.30).

Although radiography and CT may have a role, the appropriateness of these modalities in such a clinical setting is considered low by the ACR. RBS, MR imaging, PET, and PET-CT are also available for the work-up of bone metastases, being the most appropriate according ACR [46]. RBS is regarded as a cost-effective whole-body screening test for assessment of bone metastases, but has low specificity. MR imaging is widely considered the modality of choice for bone marrow evaluation and soft-tissue involvement, aiding in characterization of pathologic fractures. Metastatic seeding in the bone marrow is characterized by long T1 relaxation times, whereas T2 relaxation times are variable, depending on tumor morphology. Whole-body MR imagining has been postulated as an alternative to RBS for screening of the entire skeleton. PET-TC combines the morphologic and functional approach, but cost considerations may limit a more systematic indication.

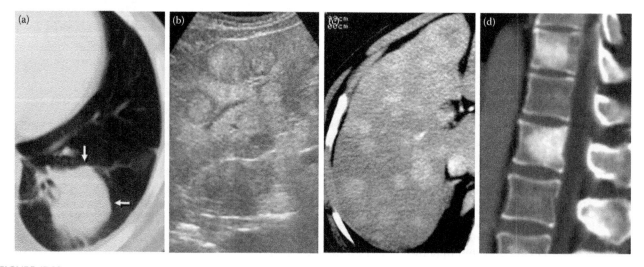

FIGURE 17.29
A 49-year-old man studied by productive cough and fever of 1 month duration, a chest CT (a) showed a left lower lobe pulmonary mass (arrowheads). A percutaneous biopsy identified a carcinoid tumor, and a left lower lobectomy was performed. Histology confirmed carcinoid tumor. Ten years later, the patient presented with right hypochondriac pain and abnormal liver function tests. An abdominal ultrasound (b) showed hyperechogenic liver metastases. The liver lesions were markedly hypervascular at portal-phase MDCT (c). Ultrasound-guided liver biopsy was consistent with carcinoid liver metastases. Osteoblastic vertebral metastases were also found on MDCT (d). On follow-ups, liver metastases have shown a slow progression, while osteoblastic metastases have remained rather stable.

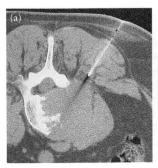

FIGURE 17.30
MDCT-guided biopsy in a 63-year-old patient with prior history of renal cell carcinoma and melanoma.

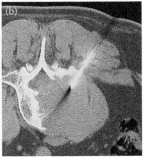

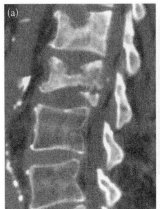

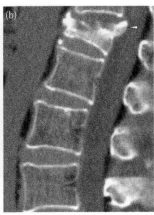

FIGURE 17.32
Sagittal reformatted MDCT images show the difficulties for discriminating pathologic fracture secondary to malignant infiltration (a), and chronic compression fracture (b) of the thoracolumbar vertebrae. Note the characteristic superior retropulsion of posterior wall in non-malignant fracture (arrowhead in b), and also the diffuse reactive sclerosis that may be confused with malignant infiltration.

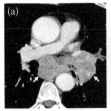

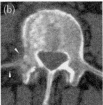

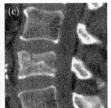

FIGURE 17.31
A 67-year-old man with microcytic lung cancer. Axial contrast-enhanced MDCT image (a) reveals mediastinal and left hilar lymphadenopathies (arrows). Axial MDCT through L4 (b) shows abnormal bone density of vertebral body, with a mixed pattern that associates cortical permeation and involvement of right pedicle and right transverse process (arrowheads). Sagittal reformatted MDCT image of the lumbar spine (c) shows a compression fracture of L4 vertebral body, which appears outstandingly heterogeneous. The findings are consistent with spinal metastases and pathologic fracture.

17.7.6 Differential Diagnosis

In a patient with known malignancy, a compression fracture may represent a pathologic fracture (Figure 17.31). However, pathologic fractures may be difficult to differentiate from chronic traumatic or osteoporotic compression fractures, which may also occur in oncologic patients (Figure 17.32). In addition, a solitary lesion of the spine in the oncologic patient may represent highly prevalent benign conditions, such as hemangioma or Paget disease (Figure 17.33). The differential diagnosis of ivory vertebra includes osteoblastic metastases, lymphoma, Paget disease, and osteosarcoma in the adult population. In children, metastases from neuroblastoma and medulloblastoma should be added to the list. Also, a number or additional benign disorders may mimic metastatic disease, which includes bone islands, eosinophilic granuloma, mastocytosis, osteopoikilia, osteomalacia and renal osteodystrophy, chronic osteomyelitis, tuberous sclerosis, Schmörl nodes, amyloidosis, or cystic angiomatosis.

17.7.7 Follow-Up

The initial manifestation of healing in an osteolytic metastatic lesion is a sclerotic rim of reactive bone. With

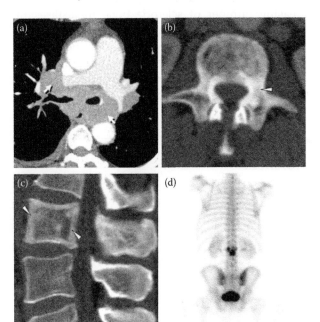

FIGURE 17.33
A 62-year-old man with microcytic lung cancer. Axial contrast-enhanced MDCT image (a) reveals extensive mediastinal and hilar lymphadenopathies (arrows). Axial (b) and sagittal reformatted (c) MDCT images show abnormal cortical thickening (arrowheads) and increased density within cancellous bone. Although a diagnosis of osteoblastic metastases may be considered, the above-described findings are consistent with Paget disease. Corresponding radionuclide bone scan reveals increased uptake of L2, and rules out multifocal disease.

progressive healing, sclerosis increases and advances from periphery of the lesion to its center (Figure 17.34). The lesion shrinks and eventually resolves. For a mixed osteolytic-sclerotic lesion, a healing response to therapy is demonstrated as uniform lesional sclerosis, whereas increasing osteolysis indicates disease progression.

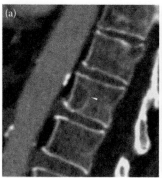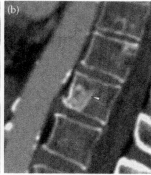

FIGURE 17.34
A 70-year-old woman, with long-standing multiple myeloma. Sagittal reformatted MDCT (a) reveals multiple osteolytic lesions within vertebral bodies. The patient received appropriate treatment (Lenalidomide and Dexamethasone). One year later, the follow-up study (b) reveals reactive peripheral sclerosis within the dominant lesion (arrowheads).

Purely sclerotic lesions are more difficult to assess. An increasing number of sclerotic bone metastases may be difficult to distinguish from the healing of sclerotic lesions that were not previously identified. From a RECIST (Response Evaluation Criteria In Solid Tumors) standpoint, bone metastases are considered non-measurable lesions [47].

References

1. Greenspan A. 2004. Radiologic evaluation of tumors and tumor-like lesions. In: *Orthopedic imaging: a practical approach.* ed. Greenspan A. 4th ed. Philadelphia, PA: Lippincott Williams & Wilkins, 529–570.
2. Rodallec MH, Feydy A, Larousserie F et al. 2008. Diagnostic imaging of solitary tumors of the spine: what to do and say. *Radiographics* 28(4):1019–41.
3. Testut L. 1932. Columna vertebral. In: *Tratado de anatomía humana,* 8th ed., ed. Testut L and Latarjet A. Barcelona: Salvat, 52–106.
4. Denis F. 1983. The three column spine and its significance in the classification of acute thoracolumbar spinal injuries. *Spine (Phila Pa 1976)* 8(8):817–31.
5. Weinstein JN. 1989. Surgical approach to spine tumors. *Orthopedics* 12:897–905.
6. Kricun ME. 1985. Red-yellow marrow conversion: its effect on the location of some solitary bone lesions. *Skeletal Radiol* 14(1):10–9.
7. ACR–ASSR–SPR–SSR practice guideline for the performance ofspine radiography, revised 2012, http://www.acr.org/~/media/ACR/Documents/PGTS/guidelines/Spine_Radiography.pdf.
8. Dickinson F, Liddicoat A, Dhingsa R, Finlay D. 2000. Magnetic resonance imaging versus radionuclide scintigraphy for screening in bone metastases. *Clin Radiol* 55(8):653.

9. Pretorius ES, Fishman EK. 1999. Volume-rendered three-dimensional spiral CT: musculoskeletal applications. *Radiographics* 19(5):1143–60.
10. Shen W, Chen J, Gantz M et al. 2012. MRI-measured pelvic bone marrow adipose tissue is inversely related to DXA-measured bone mineral in younger and older adults. *Eur J Clin Nutr* doi: 10.1038/ejcn.2012.35. [Epub ahead of print]
11. Barceló J, Vilanova JC, Riera E et al. 2007. Diffusion-weighted whole-body MRI (virtual PET) in screening for osseous metastases. *Radiologia* 49(6):407–15.
12. Vilanova JC, Barceló J. 2008. Diffusion-weighted whole-body MR screening. *Eur J Radiol* 67(3):440–7.
13. Dooms GC, Fisher MR, Hricak H, Richardson M, Crooks LE, Genant HK. 1985. Bone marrow imaging: magnetic resonance studies related to age and sex. *Radiology* 155:429–32.
14. Ricci C, Cova M, Kang YS et al. 1990. Normal age-related patterns of cellular and fatty bone marrow distribution in the axial skeleton: MR imaging study. *Radiology* 177(1):83–8.
15. Vogler JB, Murphy WA. 1988. Bone marrow imaging. *Radiology* 168(3):679–93.
16. Even-Sapir E. 2005. Imaging of malignant bone involvement by morphologic, scintigraphic and hybrid modalities. *J Nucl Med* 46(8):1356–67.
17. Jung HS, Jee WH, McCauley TR, Ha KY, Choi KH. 2003. Discrimination of metastatic from acute osteoporotic compression spinal fractures with MR imaging. *Radiographics* 23(1):179–87.
18. Murphey MD, Andrews CL, Flemming DJ, Temple HT, Smith WS, Smirniotopoulos JG. 1996. Primary tumors of the spine: radiologic pathologic correlation. *Radiographics* 16(5):1131–58.
19. Snyder BD, Cordio MA, Nazarian A et al. 2009. Noninvasive prediction of fracture risk in patients with metastatic cancer to the spine. *Clin Cancer Res* 15(24):7676–7683.
20. Kransdorf MJ, Stull MA, Gilkey FW, Moser RP. 1991. Osteoid osteoma. *Radiographics* 11:671–96.
21. Saccomanni B. 2009. Osteoid osteoma and osteoblastoma of the spine: a review of the literature. *Curr Rev Musculoskelet Med* 2(1):65–7.
22. Avcu S, Akdeniz H, Arslan H, Toprak N, Unal O. 2009. A case of primary vertebral osteosarcoma metastasizing to pancreas. *JOP* 10(4):438–40.
23. Murphey MD, Choi JJ, Kransdorf MJ, Flemming DJ, Gannon FH. 2000. Imaging of osteochondroma: variants and complications with radiologic-pathologic correlation. *Radiographics* 20(5):1407–34.
24. Tajima K, Nishida J, Yamazaki K, Shimamura T, Abe M. 1989. Case report 545: Osteochondroma (osteocartilagenous exostosis) cervical spine with spinal cord compression. *Skeletal Radiol* 18(4):306–9.
25. Angtuaco EJ, Fassas AB, Walker R, Sethi R, Barlogie B. 2004. Multiple myeloma: clinical review and diagnostic imaging. *Radiology* 231(1):11–23.
26. Avva R, Vanhemert RL, Barlogie B, Munshi N, Angtuaco EJ. 2001. CT-guided biopsy of focal lesions in patients with multiple myeloma may reveal new and more

aggressive cytogenetic abnormalities. *AJNR Am J Neuroradiol* 22(4):781–5.

27. Mahnken AH, Wildberger JE, Gehbauer G, Schmitz-Rode T et al. 2002. Multidetector CT of the spine in multiple myeloma: comparison with MR imaging and radiography. *AJR Am J Roentgenol* 178:1429–36.

28. Mulligan ME, McRae GA, Murphey MD. 1999. Imaging features of primary lymphoma of bone. *AJR Am J Roentgenol* 173(6):1691–7.

29. Friedman DP. 1996. Symptomatic vertebral hemangiomas: MR findings. *AJR Am J Roentgenol* 167:359–64.

30. Wippold FJ, Koeller KK, Smirniotopoulos JG. 1999. Clinical and imaging features of cervical chordoma. *AJR Am J Roentgenol* 172(5):1423–6.

31. Kyriakos M. 2011. Benign notochordal lesions of the axial skeleton: a review and current appraisal. *Skeletal Radiol* 40(9):1141–52.

32. Kransdorf MJ, Sweet DE. 1995. Aneurysmal bone cyst: concept, controversy, clinical presentation, and imaging. *AJR Am J Roentgenol* 164(3):573–80.

33. Junming M, Cheng Y, Dong C et al. 2008. Giant cell tumor of the cervical spine: a series of 22 cases and outcomes. *Spine (Phila Pa 1976)* 33(3):280–8.

34. Georgy BA. 2008. Metastatic spinal lesions: state-of-the-art treatment options and future trends. *AJNR Am J Neuroradiol* 29(9):1605–11.

35. Coleman RE. 2006. Clinical features of metastatic bone disease and risk of skeletal morbidity. *Clin Cancer Res* 12(20 Pt 2):6243s–6249s.

36. Patten RM, Shuman WP, Teefey S. 1990. Metastases from malignant melanoma to the axial skeleton: A CT study of frequency and appearance. *AJR Am J Roentgenol* 155(1):109–12.

37. Rybak LD, Rosenthal DI. 2001. Radiological imaging for the diagnosis of bone metastases. *Q J Nucl Med* 45(1):53–64.

38. Schiff D, O'Neill BP, Suman VJ. 1997. Spinal epidural metastasis as the initial manifestation of malignancy: clinical features and diagnostic approach. *Neurology* 49(2):452–6.

39. Cronin CG, Cashell T, Mhuircheartaigh JN et al. 2009. Bone biopsy of new suspicious bone lesions in patients with primary carcinoma: prevalence and probability of an alternative diagnosis. *AJR Am J Roentgenol* 193(5):W407–10.

40. Batson OV. 1942. The role of the vertebral veins in metastatic processes. *Ann Intern Med* 16:38–45.

41. Fidler IJ. 2003. The pathogenesis of cancer metastasis: the "seed and soil" hypothesis revisited. *Nat Rev Cancer* 3:453–8.

42. Guise TA. 2002. The vicious cycle of bone metastases. *J Musculoskelet Neuronal Interact* 2(6):570–2.

43. Cheong HW, Peh WC, Guglielmi G. 2008. Imaging of diseases of the axial and peripheral skeleton. *Radiol Clin North Am* 46(4):703–33.

44. Algra PR, Heimans JJ, Valk J, Nauta JJ, Lachniet M, Van Kooten B. 1992. Do metastases in vertebrae begin in the body or the pedicles? Imaging study in 45 patients. *AJR Am J Roentgenol* 158(6):1275–9.

45. Jacobson HG, Poppel MH, Shapiro JH, Grossberger S. 1958. The vertebral pedicle sign: a roentgen finding to differentiate metastatic carcinoma from multiple myeloma. *AJR Am J Roentgenol* 80:817–21.

46. Roberts CC, Daffner RH, Weissman BN, Bancroft L, et al. 2010. ACR appropriateness criteria on metastatic bone disease. *J Am Coll Radiol* 7(6):400–91.

47. Bäuerle T, Semmler W. 2009. Imaging response to systemic therapy for bone metastases. *Eur Radiol* 19(10):2495–507.

18

Ilio-Sacral Pathology

Ian Crosbie, John E. Madewell, and Paul O'Sullivan

CONTENTS

18.1 Introduction

The sacrum is a complex-shaped osseous structure present at the base of the axial spine. This bone plays a vital role in weight-bearing in the ambulant adult. Because of its shape and position, lesions of the sacrum are often slow to present, as there is considerable room from tumor growth in the pelvis. Nonspecific symptoms such as vague lower back pain are frequent early manifestations of lesions in this bone. Fractures and inflammatory diseases often affect the sacrum, in addition to bone-specific tumors and systemic malignancies. Plain radiography is frequently used in initial evaluation, but its efficacy is limited as sacral lesions are often difficult to visualize; because of the shape of the bone itself, its position deep in the pelvis, the presence of overlying soft-tissue structures and the presence of fecal material and bowel gas in the sigmoid colon and rectum.

In this chapter, we have attempted to describe the anatomy, embryology, and the pathological processes frequently encountered in the sacrum. Because of the difficulty in evaluating the sacrum at plain radiographic imaging, computed tomography (CT) is frequently employed. CT provides excellent soft-tissue contrast and bone resolution, in addition to providing three-dimensional (3D) reconstruction of focal lesions if required. CT imaging is the main focus of this chapter with occasional reference to plain radiography and other forms of cross-sectional imaging where appropriate.

18.2 Adult Anatomy

The human sacrum is triangular in appearance with five vertebral segments known as S1 to S5 that are fused together. The sacrum has a curved convex posterior margin articulating with the L5 vertebral body superiorly, coccyx inferiorly, and the iliac bones bilaterally. Caudally the osseous protuberance is known as the sacral promontory flanked on either side by the sacral ala. Anatomical variation exists between the male and female pelvis. The female sacrum is shorter and wider compared to the male pelvis with a more pronounced anterior angulation with the consequence of widening the female pelvic cavity. Both anteriorly and posteriorly the sacrum has four pairs of sacral foramina for the transmission of spinal nerves S1–S4 (Figure 18.1a and b). The spinal canal terminates at the caudal margin of the posterior sacrum in a foramen known as the sacral hiatus; this allows for the passage of the S5 nerve root [1,2].

The sacrum acts as a central base through which large forces are transferred and dissipated to the lower limbs, providing vertical and rotational stability for the pelvis to bear the load of the upper body [3]. The sacroiliac joints (SIJs) are large auricular-shaped joints that are pivotal in providing the lateral stability for the sacrum to perform this function. The SIJs are composed of two elements an inferior cartilaginous joint and an upper fibrous articulation. The cartilaginous component contains a capsule and synovial lining with fibrocartilage located on the ilial articulation and hyaline cartilage on the sacral articulation [4].

The sacrum provides attachments for ligamentous and muscular complexes that acts to reinforce the SIJs. This complex includes: the anterior/posterior SI ligaments, sacrotuberous, sacrospinous and anterior/posterior sacrococcygeal ligaments along with the piriformis and the coccygeus muscles. A nerve plexus known as the sacral plexus is located anterior to the sacral ala and medial to the psoas muscle. The plexus is composed of the anterior rami of the L4 to S4 spinal nerves. The lumbrosacral trunk (L4 and L5) combined with S1, S2, and S3 form the sciatic nerve anterior to the piriformis muscle. The sacral plexus also forms the pudendal nerve from nerve roots S2–S4. We will discuss the pathology of the sacrum and the appearance on CT.

18.3 Spinal Embryology

To aid in the understanding of sacral congenital defects, we present a brief outline of spinal embryology. Fetal development starts during gastrulation with the formation of a trilaminar embryonic disc, which provides a template for the formation of the primitive streak, notochord, ectoderm, mesoderm, and endoderm. The mesoderm and the notochord contribute to the formation of the spinal column [5]. The major role of the notochord is to induce mesodermal differentiation.

The migration of epiblastic cells from the primitive streak results in the formation of the mesoderm and the endoderm. At this time point, there is simultaneous migration of cells from the primitive node resulting in the formation of the notochord [6]. On formation of the notochord the mesoderm lateral to the notochord separates into three separate entities, the paraxial, intermediate, and lateral mesoderm [6]. A total of 44 somites originate from the paraxial mesoderm, with each somite dividing to become a sclerotome and a dermatomyotome. The sclerotomes are responsible for the formation of the osseous spine and at 4 weeks gestation the sclerotome act to encase the notochord and neural tube (derived from ectodermal cells) [6]. Each sclerotome is described as having a cranial half composed of loosely packed cell and a caudal half of tightly packed cells, interposed between the two cellular groups is a cell free space. The cell free space of the sclerotome forms the annulus fibrous of the developing intervertebral disc and the notochord forms the nucleus pulposus [7]. Between each cell free space the compact cellular half from the cranial sclerotome and a loosely packed cellular half from the caudal sclerotome fuse in a process known as segmentation to form the centrum [5]. The centrum is responsible for the formation of the vertebral body. Cells from the sclerotome migrate posteriorly next to the neural tube, resulting in the formation of the posterior vertebral arches.

During the first 8 weeks of gestation following cellular migration, the notochord will disintegrate and primary ossification centers form at the centrum and at each side of the posterior vertebral arch [6]. Postpartum five secondary ossification centers form: one for the extremity of the spinous process, one for the tip of each transverse process, and one for the upper and lower surfaces of the vertebral body. The two elements of the posterior vertebral arch begin to fuse in the first year of life, continuing cephalad to the cervical region; this is completed by year six. Fusion of the posterior arch and the centrum begins in year three, proceeding caudal to the lumbar region; this is completed by year eight [6].

The development of the central nervous system starts during the third week of gestation growing parallel with the osseous spine. The nervous system originates from

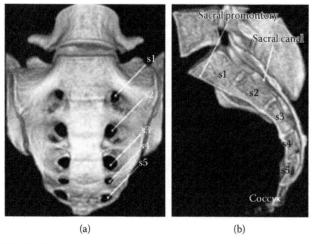

FIGURE 18.1
CT of normal sacrum, volume-rendered images. (a) anteroposterior view and (b) lateral view.

surface ectoderm, with the neural crest becoming the peripheral nervous system and the neural tube becoming the central nervous system [8].

The paraxial mesoderm contributing to the development of the vertebral bodies is also involved in the concurrent development of skeletal muscle and skin. The intermediate and lateral mesoderms are responsible for the development of the urogenital, pulmonary, and cardiac systems. Hence, a mesodermal default that results in spinal developmental anomalies frequently results in congenital defects in an alternative organ system [9].

18.4 Congenital Sacral Defects

18.4.1 Transitional Vertebra

Transitional vertebrae are commonly encountered on imaging of the lumbrosacral spine. The L5 vertebrae can be included in the sacrum, "sacralized," and the S1 vertebrae can be included in the lumbar vertebrae, "lumbarized," Transitional vertebrae rarely result in clinical symptoms, but irritation of adjacent soft tissues with enlarged transverse processes can result in symptoms [10]. The most important aspect of transitional vertebrae is to detect their presence before surgical marking to avoid surgical therapy on the incorrect vertebrae or intervertebral disc space.

18.4.2 Spina Bifida

Neural tube defects are secondary to failure of the neural tube to close during the fourth week of gestation with the resulting failure of overlying structures to form anatomically [5]. The most common neural tube defect is spina bifida. Spina bifida may present at any vertebral level. The most common site is at the lumbrosacral region where the final closure of the neural tube occurs [11]. A number of subgroups exist including spina bifida occulta, spina bifida with meningocele, spina bifida with meningomyelocele, and the most severe type myeloschisis. If not clinically obvious, cutaneous signs of overlying hair growth, lipomas, cysts, or hemangiomas may indicate an underlying neural tube defect [12]. Ultrasound (US), CT, and magnetic resonance imaging (MRI) can be used for imaging. MRI remains the best imaging technique to evaluate neural involvement. For imaging osseous defects, CT is the best. However, this patient population age limits its use, because of the concerns of radiation exposure.

18.4.3 Sacral Agenesis

The incidence of sacral agenesis is rare, ranging from 0.01 to 0.05 per 1000 live births [13,14]. Sacral agenesis is a part of border classification of spinal anomalies referred to as caudal regression syndrome. This refers to a spectrum of aplastic vertebral malformations ranging from agenesis of the coccygeal vertebrae to more pronounced anomalies that include the agenesis of the sacrum or lumbar vertebrae and lower limb malformations. The majority of defects involve only the sacrum so the term "sacral agenesis" has been used synonymously with caudal regression syndrome [15]. The precise etiology of this entity is not known but gestational hyperglycemia is a suggested cause [15,16].

During gestation, a cell mass at the caudal region of the primitive streak, known as the caudal eminence creates the caudal notochord, ectoderm, mesoderm, and endoderm, responsible for generating the somites caudal to somite 30 [15,17]. These somites form the vertebral bodies caudal to and including S2, hence insults to the caudal eminence usually results in subtotal sacral agenesis with the preservation of S1. This finding was observed by Emani-Naeini et al., [18]. Pang et al., [15] and Renshaw [19]. A system for the classification of sacral agenesis was established by Rensahw [18]. The classification includes four groups: Type 1, partial or total unilateral sacral agenesis; Type 2, partial sacral agenesis with bilaterally symmetrical defects and stable articulation between the ilia and a normal or hypoplastic S1 vertebral body; Type 3, total sacral and variable lumbar agenesis with the ilia articulating with the lowest lumbar vertebral body; Type 4, total sacral and variable lumbar agenesis with the inferior endplate of the most caudal vertebrae resting above either a fused ilia or an iliac amphiarthrosis.

Sacral agenesis is associated with multiorgan abnormalities involving the respiratory, genitourinary, and gastrointestinal tracts; a known association exists with VACTERL (vertebral abnormality, anal imperforation, tracheoesophageal fistula, renal and limb anomalies), Mermaid, and Currarino syndromes [20–22].

The external body dysmorphisms include shortening of the intergluteal cleft, buttock dimples, and flattening of the buttocks with a small gluteal mass [15]. The pelvic transverse diameter is reduced in a type 4 deformity because of the ilia articulating or begin fused. Two groups of neurological deficits exist, a static and a dynamic group. The static group is secondary to developmental dysplasia of neural and myotomal elements [23]. The dynamic group neurological deficits are progressive because of intraspinal anomalies, for example, dural stenosis or tethered spinal cord [23]. The motor neurological abnormalities tend to parallel the severity of osseous abnormality, except for when a synchronous meningomyelocele is present. The sensory neurological deficits appear independent to the severity of the osseous abnormality [17].

CT imaging is optimal for detection of underlying boney defect; however, MRI is the main imaging modality for the identification of neural defects.

18.5 Tumors

Based on the anatomical structures of the sacrum, tumors can involve the cauda equnia, meninges, cartilage, and bone; these tumors are varied and are summarized in Table 18.1.

The clinical presentation of sacral tumors is often delayed because of the limited symptoms and signs in the early stages of disease. One of the earliest presentations is nonspecific back pain. Clinical exam can be limited because of the osseous structure of the sacrum and pelvis. Subtle neurology may be the only sign of significant underlying pathology. Plain film radiology has been shown to have low sensitivity in the detection of sacral tumors [23]. Hence, axial imaging is essential for the detection and diagnosis of sacral tumors.

TABLE 18.1

Tumors of the Sacrum

	Benign	Malignant
Meningeal/neuronal	Schwannoma	Ependymoma
	Neurofibroma	Drop metastases
	Meningoma	
Bone	GCT	Metastases
	ABC	MM
	OO	Plasmacytoma
	Osteoblastoma	Lymphoma/leukemia
	Osteochondroma	Chordoma
	Lipoma	CS
	Chondromyxoid fibroma	ES
	Bone island	Fibrosarcoma
	Teratoma	Osteosarcoma
		Malignant fibrous histocytoma
		Carcinoid

Sacral metastases are the most common sacral tumors outnumbering the volume of primary tumors [24,25]. The most common primary benign tumors are giant cell tumors (GCTs) and the commonest primary malignant tumors are chordomas [26].

18.5.1 Meningeal/Neuronal Tumors

18.5.1.1 Benign

18.5.1.1.1 Neurofibroma/Schwannoma

Neurofibromas have no true capsule and contain Schwann cells, fibroblasts, and commonly collagen. Neurofibromas can range in size from a small mass to a large plexiform tumor. About 90% are sporadic and are not associated with neurofibromatosis type1 (NF1). Most neurofibromas are benign, between 3% and 5% of neurofibromas may undergo malignant transformation. The potential risk of malignant transformation exists most frequently in the large plexiform type associated with NF1 [27]. Schwannomas are surrounded by a capsule and arise solely from Schwann cells. Schwannomas are rare in the sacrum; however, if present, they can become large and cause local osseous destruction—giant cell Schwannoma. On CT imaging, neurofibromas and Schwannomas are both isodense with the spinal cord, showing moderate contrast enhancement and can result in adjacent bone remodeling and widening of the neural foramen (Figure 18.2a and b).

18.5.1.1.2 Meningeal Cysts

Benign meningeal cysts are common within the sacrum. Two forms of meningeal cysts exist, a communicating and a noncommunicating form in relation to the subarachnoid space. The most common form known as a Tarlov cyst communicates with the subarachnoid space, the less common form known as a sacral meningeal cyst

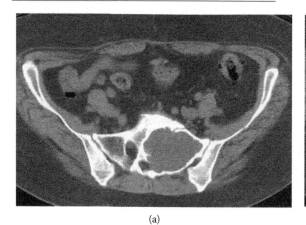

(a)

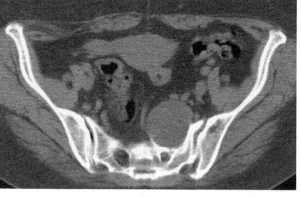

(b)

FIGURE 18.2

A 60-year-old male with benign Schwannoma of sacrum. (a) Axial noncontrast CT shows expansile lytic lesion in left side of sacrum. (b) Slightly more cranial image shows smooth circular nature of benign Schwannoma.

does not communicate with the subarachnoid space [28]. Meningeal cysts are usually asymptomatic and are frequently identified on CT imaging of the pelvis and lumbrosacral spine forming a fluid attenuating cyst within the sacrum. Cases of sacral meningoma are reported within the literature but the occurrence is infrequent, a single case report suggests that sacral meningomas have a more aggressive clinical course [29].

18.5.1.2 Malignant

18.5.1.2.1 Ependyomas

Ependyomas are malignant tumors arising from ependymal cells. Two forms exist, cellular and myxopapillary. The latter arises from ependymal cells involving the conus, filum terminale, and cauda equina and can involve the sacral spinal canal. On CT imaging, an isodense intradural mass is present with infrequent thinning of the pedicles and scalloped vertebral bodies. There is avid homogenous enhancement with the administration of contrast [30]. Dropped metastases from the central nervous systems can involve the dependent sacral spinal canal and meninges, primary sources for metastases include glioblastoma multiforme, choroid plexus tumors, germinoma, and primitive neuroectodermal tumors (PNTs).

18.5.2 Bone Tumors

18.5.2.1 Benign

18.5.2.1.1 Giant Cell Tumor

GCT is a rare neoplasm of bone accounting for 5% of all primary bone tumors in adults [31]. GCTs most frequently present in the third and fourth decade of life with a slight predominance in females. The sacrum is the fourth most common site for GCT [32], representing the second most common primary sacral tumor after chordoma [33]. GCTs are benign tumors composed of osteclast-like multinucleated macrophages; however, transformation to a high-grade malignancy occurs in 1%–3% of patients and lung metastases have been reported in up to 5% [34]. GCTs are often difficult to visualize at plain radiography (as are many sacral tumors) because of the prominent overlying bowel gas of the sigmoid colon and rectum, and the inherent curvature of the sacrum. Sacral GCTs are lytic expansile lesions based centrally that extend to the sacral alae displaying a narrow zone of transition with well-defined peripheral margins, usually nonsclerotic (Figure 18.3a and b). GCTs are highly vascular with avid contrast enhancement. On noncontrast CT, there can be central hypoattenuation because of necrosis.

18.5.2.1.2 Aneurysmal Bone Cyst

Aneurysmal bone cysts (ABCs) were first described in 1942 by Jaffe and Lichenstein, with the description of expansile blood-filled cysts with adjacent bone remodeling [35]. ABCs of the sacrum are infrequent representing 3% of ABCs [36] (Figure 18.4). ABCs are composed of blood-filled cysts separated by septae of varying thickness, often containing fluid–fluid levels caused by blood sedimentation following hemorrhage. Fluid–fluid levels suggest the diagnosis but are not pathognomonic as fluid–fluid levels can also occur in other tumors including GCTs, osteoblastomas, and teleangiectatic osteogenic sarcomas [37]. ABCs are not lined by endothelium and hence do not represent anatomical vascular channels, the majority of ABC are considered primary lesions; however, some are thought to be secondary to trauma or an underlying neoplasm [38]. On CT imaging, ABCs are balloon-like expansile masses containing multiple rounded cysts with fluid–fluid levels extending into the epidural space. There is an "eggshell" cortex and a narrow nonsclerotic zone of transition.

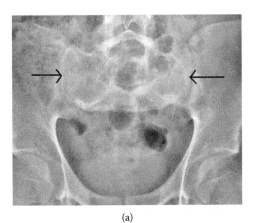
(a)

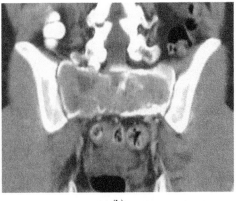
(b)

FIGURE 18.3
A 45-year-old male with GCT of sacrum. (a) Plain radiograph of pelvis poorly shows 8 cm lytic lesion in S1 and bilateral sacral ala (between arrows). (b) Coronal postcontrast CT pelvis readily shows large, expansile, lytic lesion.

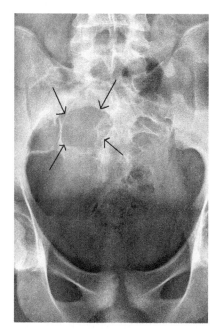

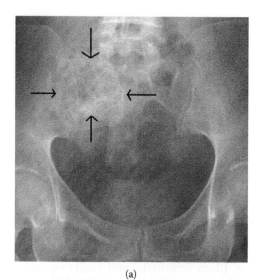

(a)

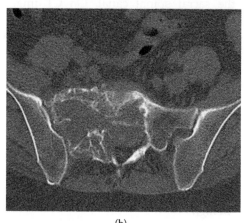

(b)

FIGURE 18.4
A 22-year-old male with an ABC. Plain film poorly shows a 3 cm, circular lytic lesion right side sacrum (arrows).

18.5.2.1.3 Osteoid Osteoma

The majority of osteoid osteomas (OO) present in the second decade of life with a male predominance, only 2% of OO affect the sacrum [26]. OO have a vascular central nidus composed of interconnected trabecular bone and vascularized fibrous connective tissue. The nidus is surrounded by reactive cortical bone measuring 1.5 cm in size. The classic symptoms include night pain that is relieved with salicylates. CT imaging shows a central lytic nidus ± a central sclerotic focus often next to a nutrient vessel surrounded by a sclerotic reaction. Osteoblastomas are similar to an OO, the gross differentiating factor is a size of greater than 1.5 cm [39]. Osteoblastomas predominately involve the posterior elements of the vertebral body. Histological appearances of an osteoblastoma are similar but less organized when compared to OO. CT imaging shows an expansile well-circumscribed lesion in the neural arch with a sclerotic rim and a narrow zone of transition. An aggressive subgroup of osteoblastomas have been described, typically aggressive osteoblastomas have a wide zone of transition and result in osseous cortical defects similar to osteosarcomas (OSA).

18.5.2.1.4 Cavernous Hemangioma

Cavernous hemangiomas (CHs) have a prevalence of 10%. CH most frequently occurs in the thoracic spine with rare sacral involvement [40]. CHs are thin-walled sinusoidal channels that are separated by boney trabeculae. These lesions are usually asymptomatic. CT imaging of a typical hemangioma shows a hypodense lesion in the vertebral body with vertically aligned trabeculae

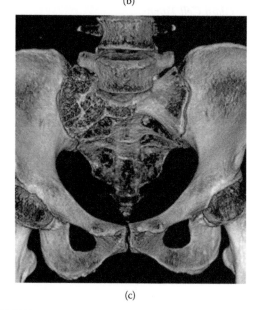

(c)

FIGURE 18.5
A 52-year-old male with large hemangioma. (a) Plain film shows the sclerotic lesion in the right side of the sacrum (arrows). (b) Noncontrast axial CT (bone windows) readily shows 4 cm, irregular, expansile, lytic lesion. (c) Volume-rendered 3D auction shows lesion in right sacral ala.

resulting in a "polka dot" appearance on axial imaging. Occasionally, aggressive lesions are seen, which cause bony expansion (Figure 18.5a through c), or extra osseous extension and result in neurological deficits.

18.5.2.1.5 Osteochondroma

Osteochondroma is an osteocartilaginous out growth that is contigous with the normal boney cortex, which may have an overlying cartilaginous cap. These benign lesions are more frequently seen in the extremities, with growth typically in the opposite direction of the normal epiphysis. Vertebral and sacral involvement is rare; however, in hereditary multiple exostosis (Figure 18.6) vertebral involvement has a prevalence of 9% predominantly located at the posterior arch [41].

18.5.2.1.6 Teratoma

Teratomas are a benign germ cell neoplasms arising from derivatives of ectoderm, endoderm, and mesoderm. The majority of sacrococcygeal teratoma (SCT) are present at birth with an estimated incidence of approximately 1:40,000 live births and a 4:1 female predominance [42]. Most infantile SCT have an external component however some tumors can be completely internal, classification of SCT by Altman is based on the degree of tumor externalization [43]. Presacral masses are present on CT with mixed cystic/solid components and internal calcifications ranging from small foci to formed teeth or small bones. The solid components have heterogenous attenuation and enhance with contrast administration.

18.5.2.2 Malignant

18.5.2.2.1 Metastases

Hematopoietic bone marrow reserves a significant blood supply into adult life and the distribution of hematopoietic marrow plays an important role in the distribution of osseous metastases. The adult sacrum contains hematopoietic marrow and is a frequent site of metastatic disease of visceral and hematological primary malignancies; metastases are the most common malignant lesion to occur within the sacrum. Osteolytic metastases include renal cell and thyroid carcinomas, osteoblastic metastases classically arise from prostate carcinoma; however, breast (Figure 18.7) and lung (Figure 18.8) can produce sclerotic and/or mixed radiological appearances [44]. CT imaging shows regions of either lytic or sclerotic change with variable enhancement patterns with the administration of contrast. Frequently present

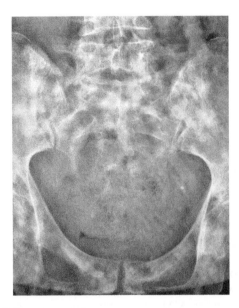

FIGURE 18.7
A 65-year-old female with diffuse breast metastases. Plain radiograph of the sacrum shows the innumerable sclerotic metastases throughout the sacrum and adjacent pelvic bones.

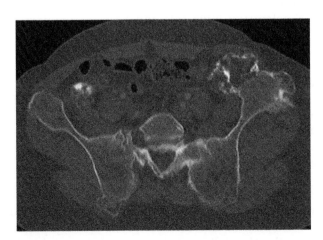

FIGURE 18.6
A 36-year-old-female with hereditary multiple bony exostosis. Axial noncontrast CT (bone windows) shows many large exostosis.

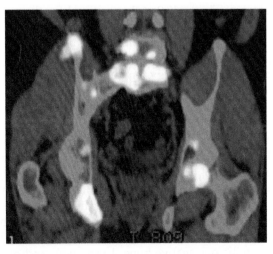

FIGURE 18.8
A 68-year-old female with diffuse bony metastases in non-small cell lung cancer. Coronal fused positron emission tomographic CT image of pelvis shows many flurodeoxyglucose avid metastases.

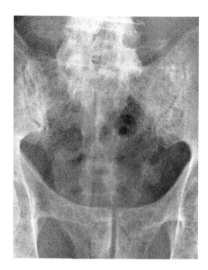

FIGURE 18.9
A 76-year-old male with MM. Plain radiograph shows a diffuse, highly lucent, lytic pattern throughout all the sacral and adjacent bony structures, in marrow packing of extensive MM.

and readily identifiable on CT are soft-tissue masses in the paravertebral or epidural spaces. Careful attention should be made not to overlook a pathological fracture when performing CT of the sacrum.

18.5.2.2.2 Multiple Myeloma

Multiple myeloma (MM) is a neoplastic disorder of plasma B cells with the resultant overproduction of monoclonal immunoglobulins and replacement of normal fatty bone marrow. Plasmacytoma are the monostotic form of MM and often preceding multifocal disease. Plasmacytoma are commonly expansile lytic lesions with extra osseous soft-tissue component and associated cortical disruption. MM produces multiple lytic lesions within the spine that frequently involves the sacrum (Figure 18.9). CT is optimal for the evaluation of vertebral body destruction and fractures associated with MM [45] (Figure 18.10). The differentiation of MM and diffuse metastatic disease based on imaging can be difficult; histology remains the gold standard for this differentiation.

18.5.2.2.3 Primary Lymphoma

Primary lymphoma of bone (PLB) is approximately 5% of all extra nodal lymphomas and 3%–7% of malignant bone lesions [46]. The majority of PLB are diffuse large B cell type as classified by the World Health Organization [47]. Lymphoma of the sacrum is rare; Unni et al. [29] reported 34 sites of sacral disease in a series of 694 bone lymphomas, this included 267 PLB. Imaging shows lytic lesions with permeative bone destruction, and often a soft-tissue mass, which may be extensive (Figure 18.11). Frequently but not always present, is a wide zone of transition without a sclerotic margin.

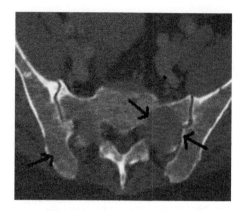

FIGURE 18.10
A 62-year-old female with MM. Axial noncontrast CT (bone windows) shows many "punched-out" lytic lesions (arrows) of sacrum and pelvis.

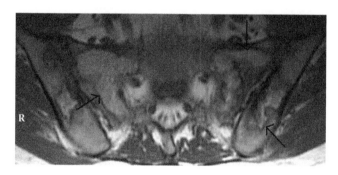

FIGURE 18.11
A 59-year-old male with lymphoma of bone. Axial T2-weighted MRI of sacrum shows several bony infarctions producing a "geographic" pattern (arrows) in the sacrum and pelvis.

18.5.2.2.4 Chordoma

Chordomas arise from notochord remnants, occurring in a midline or a paramedian location about the axial spine. Chordomas involve the sacrococcygeal region in 50%–60% of cases and accounts for 2%–4% of sacral tumors making it the most common primary sacral malignancy [28]. Chordomas are slow growing to a potentially large size and become symptomatic by spreading into adjacent soft tissues as a destructive lytic lesion (Figure 18.12a and b). These tumors are capable of crossing the adjacent joint spaces to involve the ileum or lumbar vertebrae. On CT imaging, there is usually a soft-tissue component with internal calcifications (Figure 18.13a and b), there is variable soft-tissue enhancement with the administration of contrast. Regions of internal hypoattenuation are frequent consistent with the myxoid properties of the tissue.

18.5.2.2.5 Ewing's Sarcoma

Ewing's sarcoma (ES) is a malignant small, round, blue cell tumor. These tumors predominantly present before the age of 30 years, with a male to female ratio of 2:1. Primary ES typically present in the flat bones of the pelvis and the proximal diaphyses of long bones,

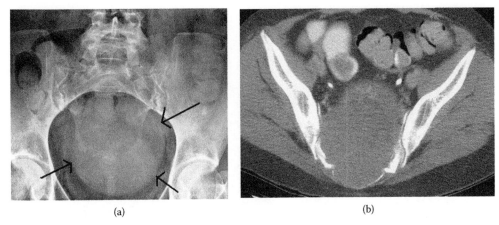

FIGURE 18.12
A 42-year-old male with a large chordoma. (a) Plain radiograph shows a large, circular, dense, tumor projected centrally over the pelvis (arrows), obscuring a lytic area in the sacrum. (b) Axial postcontrast CT of pelvis shows the large destructive near-fluid attenuation chordoma arising from the sacrum.

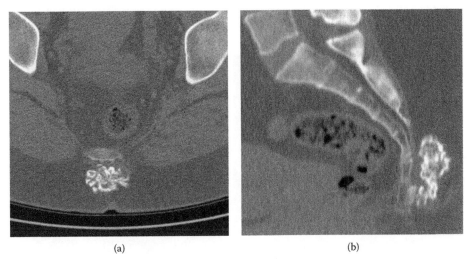

FIGURE 18.13
A 22-year-old male with a grade 2 CS arising from a sacral bony exostosis. (a) Axial noncontrast CT (bone windows) shows the dense, coarse, spiculation of the exostosis. (b) Sagittal noncontrast CT (bone windows) shows the origin in the inferior sacrum dorsally.

involvement of the spine is less typical, but the sacrum is the most common site of spinal disease [28]. PNT, a neural crest tumor, has a radiological appearance that is undifferentiated from that of ES. Appearances show a lytic lesion centered on the sacrum with permeative bone destruction, osseous expansion, wide zone of transition and an ill-defined aggressive appearing margin often with an accompanying soft-tissue mass.

18.5.2.2.6 Chondrosarcoma

Chondrosarcoma (CS) are neoplastic tumors that produce varying degrees of cartilaginous matrix. These tumors range from low, intermediate to high-grade lesions, with varying degrees of well-differentiated cartilage present. Decreasing amounts of well-differentiated cartilage are seen as the tumor spectrum extends from low to high-grade malignancy. Primary CS arise de novo and secondary CS arise from a preexisting benign lesion such as an

enchondroma or osteochondroma (Figure 18.14a and b). CS of the sacrum is unusual; one series reporting 2% of 1041 cases of CS involving the sacrum [29]. At the initial presentation of pelvic CS, the tumors can be large (Figure 18.15a and b) because of a delay in the onset of clinical symptoms [48]. Imaging reveals a lobulated-lytic mass containing chondroid matrix with internal septae and calcifications, these lesions can penetrate the cortex resulting in epidural and paravertebral extension.

18.5.2.2.7 Osteosarcoma

OSA rarely affect the sacrum and are typically seen in the long bones of the extremities. OSA can arise on a background of prior therapeutic radiotherapy or Paget's disease [49]. Like other primary tumors of the sacrum, they initially present with nonspecific symptoms of low-back pain. As this malignant tumor grows, increasing symptomatology occurs due to intra-osseous extension

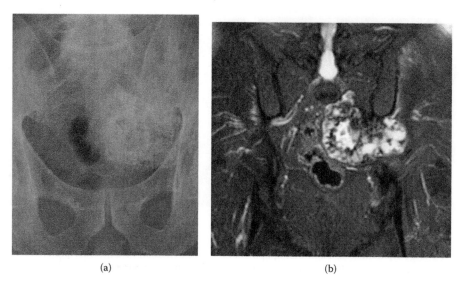

(a)   (b)

FIGURE 18.14
A 70-year-old male with well-differentiated sacral CS. (a) Plain radiograph shows the dense cartilaginous calcification arising from the 7 cm left side sacral tumor. (b) Coronal T2-fat saturated MRI of the pelvis shows the extensive smooth, homogenous pattern seen in the well-differentiated cartilage of the tumor.

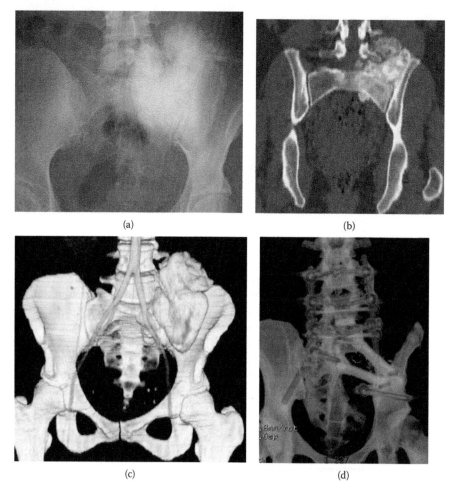

(a)   (b)

(c)   (d)

FIGURE 18.15
A 35-year-old female with osteosarcoma of the sacrum. (a) Plain radiograph shows diffuse "new-bone" formation in the left side of the sacrum from the tumor. (b) Coronal CT image shows the 6 cm partially calcified tumor arising from the sacrum. (c) A 3D volume-rendered image eloquently shows the extent of the tumor and its relationship to adjacent vascular structures. (d) A 3D volume-rendered image shows postoperative appearance, with partial left side sacral and iliac bone resection, lumbar, sacral and iliac bone hardware fixation.

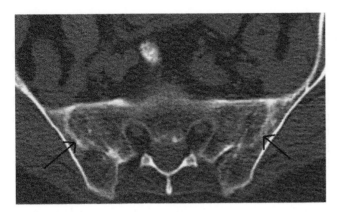

FIGURE 18.16
A 32-year-old male with Crohn's disease. Axial noncontrast CT pelvis shows fused SIJs (arrows).

and compression of adjacent structures, which prompts imaging. These malignant tumors produce marked periostitis, a bony-matrix, and soft-tissue mass. The dense bone produced in OSA may be seen at plain radiography (Figure 18.16a), but is readily identified on CT imaging (Figure 18.16b and c), in addition to the periostitis and soft-tissue mass.

18.5.2.3 Inflammatory Conditions

18.5.2.3.1 Seronegative Spondyloarthropathies

The seronegative spondyloarthropathies (SAs) are the leading cause of inflammatory change of the SI joints. SA produces significant abnormalities at the cartilaginous joints and enthesis, resulting in enthesitis or enthesopathy, with subsequent bony erosions and new-bone proliferation, providing the basis for bony SI joint ankylosis [50]. Clinical entities included in this group are ankylosing spondylitis, enteropathic spondylitis (Figure 18.17), psoriathic arthritis, reactive arthritis, and undifferentiated SA [51].

The characterization of SIJ SA is based on the presence or absence of; joint symmetry, joint space preservation, joint ankylosis, and subchondral sclerosis [52]. Ankylosing spondylitis and enteropathic spondylitis typically result in bilateral symmetrical SIJ disease, initiating with erosive changes progressing to sclerosis and joint ankylosis. Very rarely, these entities result in asymmetric or unilateral SIJ pathology. Psoriathic and reactive arthritis presents as unilateral or bilateral SIJ disease, starting as erosive changes and subsequent sclerosis but rarely joint ankylosis. When presenting as bilateral disease, asymmetry is usually present differentiating these conditions from ankylosing or enteropathic spondylitis.

Osteitis condensans ilii is a benign entity involving the iliac articulation of the SIJ, mainly affecting females before the fourth decade, often occurring postpartum. No proven etiology has been identified; however, the

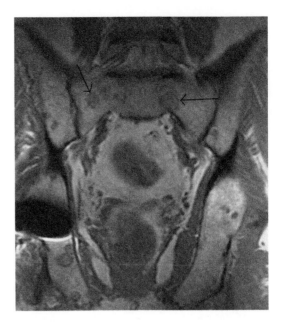

FIGURE 18.17
A 55-year-old male with sarcoid. Coronal T1 MRI sacrum shows several low-signal, focal, irregular lesions (arrows) in the sacrum, which when biopsied showed noncaseating granulomata.

most common theory suggested is that mechanical strain of the SIJ leads to premature joint degeneration and arthritis. Bilateral symmetrical subchondral sclerotic changes are present in the iliac bones, the sclerotic changes have a triangular shape (the apex is oriented cephalad). The ilial articulation is located anterior to the sacrum and the SIJ, giving the false impression of SIJ sclerosis suggesting a diagnosis of sacroiliitis [53].

The SIJ, as like any other synovial joint, can be affected by osteoarthritis (OA). OA can be unilateral, bilateral symmetrical or bilateral asymmetrical. Imaging feature of OA of the SIJs includes subchondral cysts, subchondral sclerosis, and joint space narrowing and osteophyte formation.

18.5.2.3.2 Sarcoidosis

Other inflammatory conditions can also rarely affect the sacrum. Sarcoidosis does have osseous manifestations, typically producing the "lace-like" lytic pattern seen in the phalanges. Unusually, it is seen in other bones such as the sacrum (Figure 18.18). It is often an incidental histological finding in suspicious lesion post biopsy. Appearances at CT can be lytic, sclerotic, or mixed lytic and sclerotic, when present the differential diagnosis includes infection, primary and secondary neoplasms [54].

18.5.2.3.3 Paget's Disease

Paget's disease is an osteometabolic disorder of bone with osteoclastic and osteoblastic hyperactivity resulting bone remodeling. This bone remodeling results in cortical expansion and replacement of cancellous bone by coarsened thickened. Paget's disease affects the

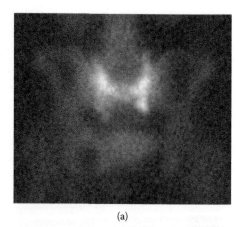

(a)

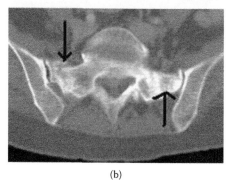

(b)

FIGURE 18.18

A 78-year-old female with bilateral insufficiency fractures of the sacral ala. (a) Radionucleotide bone scan shows increased uptake at the fracture sites producing the "H" of the "Honda" sign. (b) Axial noncontrast CT shows the "step-defect" and sclerosis (arrow) at the fracture site.

pelvis in up to 75% of cases [55]. When involving the sacrum, it is commonly polyostotic; however, isolated sacral involvement can occur [55]. Three distinct phases of the disease exist: a lytic phase, in which osteoclasts predominate; a mixed lytic-sclerotic phase, in which osteoblasts begin to appear superimposed on osteoclastic activity; and a sclerotic phase, in which osteoblastic activity gradually declines. Elevation of serum alkaline phosphatase with a normal serum calcium and phosphate suggest a diagnosis of Paget's disease. Radiologically the diagnosis of Paget's disease is based on the phase of disease. In the lytic phase cortical thinning and lytic lesions are observed. In the later phases, thickening of the trabeculae and cortex is readily identifiable with deformity of anatomical shape. Cortical expansion with the sacrum results in narrowing of the sacral foramina and the sacral canal. Changes in appearance on follow-up imaging may suggest neoplastic transformation, most frequently to an osteosarcoma.

18.5.2.3.4 Fractures

Fractures of the sacrum can be divided into three categories; traumatic, insufficiency, and stress fractures. It is estimated that sacral fractures occur in 45% of patients

with pelvic fractures [56]. Sacral fractures are classified into three zones based on the classification system described by Denis et al. 1988 [57]. Zone 1, fractures lateral to the neural foramina; Zone 2, fractures passing through the neural foramina; and Zone 3, fractures medial to the neural foramina and involve the spinal canal. Transverse fractures of the sacrum traverse all three zones described by Denis et al., separate classifications of transverse fracture have been developed by Roy-Camille et al. [58] and Strange-Vognsen et al [59]. Zone 1 fractures because of location rarely result in neurology, Zone 2 extending through the neural foramina may present with ipsilateral neurology. Zone 3 and transverse fractures are associated with bilateral neurological damage, including bowel and urinary incontinence [60].

Traumatic sacral fractures tend to occur because of high-energy injuries, and often accompany other pelvic bone fractures because of the anatomic osseous ring of the pelvis. Alternatively, insufficiency fractures can occur with minimal or no trauma, this injury pattern is most frequent in the older patient group with underlying bone demineralization, predominantly osteoporotic females [61]. Insufficiency fractures are frequent in the sacral alae and can also occur in patients with osteoporosis or prior sacral radiotherapy [62]. Stress fractures of the sacrum are rare, first described by Volpin et al. [63] in 1989, identifying military recruits with sacral wing stress fractures. Sacral stress fractures now are reported more frequently, mainly in long-distance runners. Postulated causes for sacral stress fractures include leg length discrepancies and asymmetrical movement of the hips, SI structures, and the lower spine [64].

On plain film radiographs, fractures of the sacrum can be difficult to diagnosis because of the angulation of the sacrum, overlying bowel gas and soft tissues, and the frequent association with other bony pelvic injuries. In additional radiographic views, including pelvic inlet/outlet views [65] and lateral views, [60] can improve the visualization of the sacrum and diagnostic yield. Radionuclide bone scan is very useful producing a classic "H-shaped" region (the "Honda" sign) of uptake in insufficiency fractures (Figure 18.19a). High-resolution CT (Figure 18.19b) readily detects subtle cortical breaks in sacral ala fractures, and allows for accurate diagnosis and classification of sacral fractures. However, in elderly patients with severe osteoporosis, bone mineral density may be so reduced that pelvic fractures are still not visualized on CT imaging. MRI is the gold standard in this situation.

18.5.2.3.5 Infection

Pyogenic sacral osteomyelitis, sacral epidural abscesses, and SIJ arthritis can develop from direct open sacral

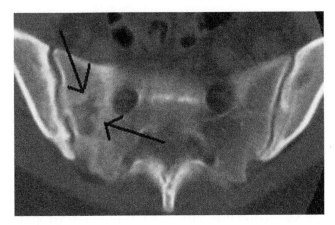

FIGURE 18.19
A 40-year-old female with osteomyelitis of the sacrum. Axial noncontrast image (bone windows) shows a permeative lytic lesion (arrow) with surrounding sclerosis in the right side of the sacrum.

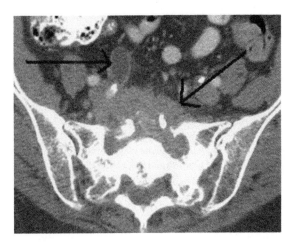

FIGURE 18.20
A 38-year-old male with an inflammatory mass from osteomyelitis of the sacrum. Axial noncontrast CT (soft-tissue windows) shows marked sclerosis throughout the sacrum from infection, in addition to the inflammatory mass arising at its anterior aspect. The mass is producing right side hydroureter (arrows).

trauma, from adjacent soft-tissue infections, from iatrogenic instrumentation, and from hematogenous spread of bacteria [66,67]. Pyogenic infections of the sacrum are rare with the entire axial skeleton accounting for only 2%–7% of all patients with osteomyelitis. Suggestions exist that the incidence of axial spinal infections are increasing, likely related to the increase in iatrogenic instrumentation, intravenous drug abuse and the reemergence of tuberculosis secondary to HIV. Conditions that compromise the immune response are believed to increase the risk of osseous sacral infections; these include long-term steroids, diabetes mellitus, malnutrition, organ transplant, congenital immune compromise, and intravenous drug abuse.

The onset of symptoms is usually insidious, with lower back pain the most common presentation. Because of its rarity and vague initial signs and symptoms, diagnosis is often delayed. Imaging is important in establishing the initial diagnosis. Plain radiographs, radionuclide examinations, and cross-sectional imaging are useful in imaging work-up. On CT imaging, there is often lytic destructive osseous abnormality (Figure 18.20) with periosteal and intramedullary reaction. Presacral soft-tissue masses are frequently associated with chronic infective processes in the sacrum. These soft-tissue masses can be difficult to distinguish from a sacral neoplasm, obliteration of the surrounding fat planes is associated with an infective source and is a useful discriminating sign. Collections with fluid–fluid can be present surrounding the sacrum or in the epidural space suggestive of synchronous soft-tissue abscess formation. Chronic infective changes include sclerotic foci, sequestration, and involucrum. Infective processes in the SIJ are usually unilateral. Image-guided biopsies are useful in the confirmation of the diagnosis and establishing the causative organism.

18.6 Summary

The sacrum is a unique bone at the base of the axial skeleton, which due to its position, size, shape, and function is prone to a range of pathology. Several particular developmental lesions (e.g., spina bifida) are frequently seen in the sacrum. There is a range of benign and malignant tumors particular to the sacrum (e.g., GCT and chordoma). The sacrum is an important site of inflammation (e.g., sacroileitis) and infection in the immunosuppressed (e.g., chronic osteomyelitis). Fractures of the sacrum are also not uncommon (e.g., posttraumatic or insufficiency). Knowledge of the CT radiological appearance of pathology typically affecting the sacrum will improve the radiologist's diagnostic acumen and should lead to more accurate and rapid diagnosis.

References

1. Moore KL, Agur AMR, Dalley AF. *Essential Clinical Anatomy.* 3rd ed. Philadelphia, PA: Lippincott, 2007.
2. Netter F. *Atlas of Human Anatomy.* 5th ed. Philadelphia, PA: W.B. Saunders, 2010.
3. Dreyfuss P, Dreyer SJ, Cole A, Mayo K. Sacroiliac joint pain. *J Am Acad Orthop Surg.* 2004;12:255–665.
4. Bowen V, Cassidy JD. Macroscopic and microscopic anatomy of the sacroiliac joint from embryonic life until the eighth decade. *Spine.* 1981;6:620–628.
5. O'Rahilly R. *Human Embryology and Teratology.* New York: John Wiley & Sons, 1996.

6. Moore KL, Persaud TVN. *The Developing Human: Clinically Oriented Embryology.* 6th ed. Philadelphia, PA: W.B. Saunders Company, 1998.

7. Trout J, Buckwalter JA, Moore KC, Landas SK. Ultrastructure of the human intervertebral disc. *Tissue Cell.* 1982;14:359–369.

8. Weston JA. Regulation of neural crest cell migration and differentiation. In: Gerhart J, ed. *Cell Interactions and Development.* New York: John Wiley & Sons, 1982:150–170.

9. Jaskwhich D, Ali RM, Patel TC, Green DW. Congenital scoliosis. *Curr Opin Pediatr.* 2000;12(1):61–66.

10. Banna M. *Clinical Radiology of the Spine and the Spinal Cord.* Gaithersburg, MD: Aspen, 1985:61–64.

11. Bendo JA, Spivak J, Cally D, Letko L. *Orthopaedics: A Study Guide.* New York: McGraw-Hill, 1999.

12. Drolet BA. Cutaneous signs of neural tube dysraphism. *Pediatr Clin North Am.* 2000;47(4):813–823.

13. Andrish J, Kalamchi A, MacEwen GD. A clinical evaluation of its management, heredity, and associated anomalies. *Clin Orthop Relat Res.* 1979;139:52–57.

14. Caird MS, Hall JM, Bloom DA, Park JM, Farley FA. Outcome study of children, adolescents, and adults with sacral agenesis. *J Pediatr Orthop.* 2007;27(6):682–685.

15. Pang D. Sacral agenesis and caudal spinal cord malformations. *Neurosurgery.* 1993;32(5):755–778.

16. Stroustrup SA, Grable I, Levine D. Case 66: caudal regression syndrome in the fetus of a diabetic mother. *Radiology.* 2004;230(1):229–233.

17. Muller F, O'Rahilly R. The development of the human brain, the closure of the caudal neuropore, and the beginning of secondary neurulation at stage 12. *Anat Embryol (Berl).* 1987;176(4):413–430.

18. Emani-Naeini P, Rahbar Z, Nejat F, Kajbafzadeh A, El Khashab M. Neurological presentation, imaging findings and associated anomalies in 50 patients with sacral agenesis. *Neurosurgery.* 2010;67(4):894–900.

19. Renshaw TS. Sacral agenesis. A classification and review of twenty-three cases. *J Bone Joint Surg.* 1978;60A:373–383.

20. Bauer SB. Neuropathic dysfunction of the lower urinary tract. In: Wein AJ, Kavoussi LR, Novick AC, Partin AW, Peters CA, eds. *Campbell-Walsh Urology.* Vol 4. 9th ed. Philadelphia, PA: W.B. Saunders, 2007:3644–3647.

21. White RI, Klauber GT. Sacral agenesis: analysis of 22 cases. *Urology.* 1976;8(6):521–525.

22. Guidera, KJ, Raney E, Ogden JA, Highhouse M, Habal M. Caudal regression: a review of seven cases including mermaid syndrome. *J Pediatr Orthop.* 1991;11(6):743–747.

23. Murphey MD, Andrews CL, Flemming DJ, Temple HT, Smith WS, Smirniotopoulos JG. Primary tumors of the spine: radiologic-pathologic correlation. *Radiographics.* 1996;16:1131–1158.

24. Disler DG, Miklic D. Imaging findings in tumors of the sacrum. *AJR Am J Roentgenol.* 1999;173:1699–1706.

25. Llauger J, Palmer J, Amores S, Bague S, Camins A. Primary tumors of the sacrum: diagnostic imaging. *AJR Am J Roentgenol.* 2000;174:417–424.

26. Unni KK. *Dahlin's Bone Tumors: General Aspects and Data on 11,087 Cases.* 5th ed. Philadelphia, PA: Lippincott-Raven, 1997.

27. Simou N, Zioga A, Zygouris A, Pahatouridis D, Charalabopoulos K, Batistatou A. Plexiform neurofibroma of the cauda equina: a case report and review of the literature. *Int J Surg Pathol.* 2008;16(1):78–80.

28. Paulsen RD, Call GA, Murtagh FR. Prevalence and percutaneous drainage of cysts of the sacral nerve root sheath (Tarlov cysts). *AJNR Am J Neuroradiol.* 1994;15:293–297.

29. Rutherford SA, Linton KM, Durnian JM, Cowie RA. Epidral meningoma of the sacral canal. Case report. *J Neurosurg Spine.* 2006 Jan;4(1):71–74.

30. Asazuma T, Toyama Y, Suzuki N, Fujimura Y, Hirabayshi K. Ependymomas of the spinal cord and cauda equina: an analysis of 26 cases and a review of the literature. *Spinal Cord.* 1999;37(11):753–759. Review.

31. Mendenhall WM, Zlotecki RA, Scarborough MT, Gibbs CP, Mendenhall NP. Giant cell tumor of bone. *Am J Clin Oncol.* 2006;29:96–99.

32. Martin C, McCarthy EF. Giant cell tumour of the sacrum and the spine: series of 23 cases and a review of the literature. *Iowa Orthop J.* 2010;30:69–75.

33. Diel J, Ortiz O, Losada RA, Price DB, Hayt MW, Katz DS. The sacrum: pathologic spectrum, multimodality imaging, and subspecialty approach. *Radiographics.* 2001;21(1):83–104.

34. Thomas DM, Skubitz T. Giant-cell tumour of bone. *Curr Opin Oncol.* 2009;21:338–344.

35. Jaffe HL, Lichtenstein L. Solitary unicameral bone cyst with emphasis on the roentgen picture, the pathologic appearance, and the pathogenesis. *Arch Surg.* 1942;44:1004–1025.

36. Mirra JM. Aneurysmal bone cyst. In: Mirra JM, Picci P, Gold RH, eds. *Bone Tumors. Clinical, Radiologic, and Pathologic Correlations.* 2nd ed. Philadelphia, PA: Lea and Febiger, 1989:1267–1311.

37. Tsai JC, Dalinka MK, Fallon MD, Zlatkin MB, Kressel HY. Fluid-fluid level: a nonspecific finding in tumors of bone and soft tissue. *Radiology.* 1990;175:779–782.

38. Kransdorf MJ, Sweet DE. Aneurysmal bone cyst: concept, controversy, clinical presentation, and imaging. *AJR Am J Roentgenol.* 1995;164:573–580.

39. Harrop JS, Schmidt MH, Boriani S, Shaffrey CI. Aggressive "benign" primary spine neoplasms: osteoblastoma, aneurysmal bone cyst and giant cell tumour. *Spine (Phila Pa 1976).* 2009;34(suppl 22):S39–S47.

40. Fox MW, Onofrio BM. The natural history and management of symptomatic and asymptomatic vertebral hemangiomas. *J Neurosurg.* 1993;78:36–45.

41. Giudicissi-Filho M, de Holanda CV, Borba LA, Rassi-Neto A, Ribeiro CA, and de Oliveira JG. Cervical spinal cord compression due to an osteochondra in hereditary multiple exostosis: case report and review of the literature. *Surg Neurol.* 2006;66(suppl 3):S7–S11.

42. Azizkhan RG. Teratomas and other germ cell tumors. In: Grosfeld JL, Fonkalsrud EW et al., eds. *Pediatric Surgery.* 6th ed. Philadelphia, PA: Mosby, 2006:554–574.

43. Altman RP, Randolph JG, Lilly JR. Sacrococcygeal teratoma: American Academy of Pediatrics Surgical Section Survey—1973. *J Pediatr Surg.* 1974;9:389–398.

44. Resnick D, Kransdorf MJ. *Bone and Joint Imaging.* Philadelphia, PA: W.B. Saunders, 2005.

45. Hanrahan CJ, Christensen CR, Crim JR. Current concepts in the evaluation of multiple myeloma with MR imaging and FDG PET/CT. *Radiographics.* 2010;30(1):127–142.

46. Dubey P, Chul SH, Besa PC, Fuller L, Cabanillas F, Murray J et al. Localized primary malignant lymphoma of bone. *Int J Radiat Oncol Biol Phys.* 1997;37:1087–1093.

47. Jaffe ES, Harris NL, Stein H, Vardiman JW, editors. World Health Organization Classification of Tumours. *Pathology and Genetics of Tumors of Haematopoietic and Lymphoid Tissues.* Lyon: IARC Press, 2001.

48. Pring ME, Weber KL, Unni KK, Sim FH. Chondrosarcoma of the pelvis: a review of sixty- four cases. *J Bone Joint Surg Am.* 2001; 83-A (11):1630–1642.

49. Haibach H, Farrell C, Ditrich FJ. Neoplasms arising in Paget's disease of bone: a study of 82 cases. *Am J Clin Pathol.* 1985;83:594–600.

50. Shaibani A, Workman R, Rothschild BM. The significance of enthesopathy as a skeletal phenomenon. *Clin Exp Rheumatol.* 1993;11:399–403.

51. Resnick D. Rheumatoid arthritis and the seronegative spondyloarthropathies: radiographic and pathologic concepts. In: Resnick D, ed. *Diagnosis of Bone and Joint Disorders.* 4th ed. Philadelphia, PA: W.B. Saunders, 2002:837–890.

52. Brower AC, Kransdorf MJ. Evaluation of disorders of the sacroiliac joint. *Appl Radiol.* 1992;21:31–42.

53. Mitra R. Osteitis condensans ilii. *Rheumatol Int.* 2010;30(3):293–296. Epub 2009 Aug 27.

54. Binicier O, Sari I, Sen G, Onen F, Akkoc N, Manisali M et al. Axial sarcoidosis mimicking radiographic sacroiliitis. *Rheumatol Int.* 2009;29(3):343–345. Epub 2008 Aug 14.

55. Smith SE, Murphey MD, Motamedi K, Mulligan ME, Resnik CS, Gannon FH. Radiologic spectrum of Paget disease of bone and its complications with pathologic correlation. *Radiographics.* 2002;22(5):1191–1216.

56. Mehta S, Auerbach JD, Born CT, Chin KR. Sacral fractures. *J Amer Acad Orthop Surg.* 2006;14(12):656–665.

57. Denis F, Davis S, Comfort T. Sacral fractures: an important problem: Retrospective analysis of 236 cases. *Clin Orthop Relat Res.* 1988;227:67–81.

58. Roy-Camille R, Saillant G, Gagna G, Mazel C. Transverse fracture of the upper sacrum: Suicidal jumper's fracture. *Spine.* 1985;10(9):838–845.

59. Strange-Vognsen HH, Lebech A. An unusual type of fracture in the upper sacrum. *J Orthop Trauma.* 1991;5(2):200–203.

60. Gibbons KJ, Soloniuk DS, Razack N. Neurological injury and patterns of sacral fractures. *J Neurosurg.* 1990;72:889–893.

61. Saraux A, Valls I, Guedes C, Baron D, LeGoff P. Insufficiency fractures of the sacrum in elderly subjects. *Rev Rhum Engl Ed.* 1995;62:582–586.

62. Rafii M, Firooznia H, Golimbu C, Horner N. Radiation induced fractures of the sacrum: CT diagnosis. *J Comput Assist Tomogr.* 1988;12:231–235.

63. Volpin G, Milgrom C, Goldsher D, Stein H. Stress fractures of the sacrum following strenuous activity. *Clin Orthop.* 1989;243:184–188.

64. Holtzhausen LM, Noakes TX. Stress fractures of the sacrum in two distance runners. *Clin J Sports Med.* 1992;2:139–142.

65. Routt ML Jr, Simonian PT, Swiontkowski MF. Stabilization of pelvic ring disruptions. *Orthop Clinic North Am.* 1997;28(3):369–388.

66. Ziai WC, Lewin JJ 3rd. Update in the diagnosis and management of central nervous system infections. *Neurol Clin.* 2008;26(2):427–468.

67. Kourbeti IS, Tsiodras S, Boumpas DT. Spinal infections: evolving concepts. *Curr Opin Rheumatol.* 2008;20(4):471–479.

19

Upper and Lower Extremities

Jonelle M. Petscavage-Thomas

CONTENTS

19.1 Introduction

Advances in computed tomography (CT) technology over the past decade and the increasing availability of the modality, particularly in emergency room (ER) departments, have resulted in increased use of CT for musculoskeletal imaging. Radiographs remain the primary modality for diagnosing fractures, monitoring progress of healing, assessing for hardware complications, and for initial evaluation of the majority of musculoskeletal complaints. However, CT is a valuable tool for further fracture characterization and treatment planning, detection of radiographically occult fractures, visualization of the degree of union about an arthrodesis or fracture, and diagnosis of hardware related complications. Recent advances have shown utility for early detection of crystal load in gout and in guidance for radiofrequency ablation of osteoid osteoma.

Multichannel helical CT in musculoskeletal imaging has several benefits. Rapid imaging can be performed with very thin sections, important in hemodynamically unstable trauma patients. The speed of image acquisition enables imaging without need for sedation or anesthesia in claustrophobic patients or patients prone to movement. The image reformation capability of CT allows scanning in nonanatomical, comfortable positions while still obtaining image quality adequate for diagnostic interpretation [1]. Multiplanar reformations (MPR) with three-dimensional (3D) visualization provide increased detail and spatial relationships around orthopedic hardware, not available on radiographs or magnetic resonance imaging (MRI).

Section 19.2 will detail indications for imaging of the extremities (Table 19.1), review common pathology and classification systems visualized on CT, and discuss optimal CT imaging techniques.

19.2 Fracture Imaging

Indications for CT imaging of fractures include

1. Diagnosis of radiographically occult fractures when their presence alters management
2. Preoperative planning
3. Assessment after external or internal reduction
4. Evaluation of degree of union

19.2.1 Lower Extremity

19.2.1.1 Pelvic Ring and Acetabulum

Pelvic ring fractures usually occur after high-energy blunt trauma, such as motor vehicle collisions and falls. Reviews of large trauma registries have found an incidence of pelvic ring fractures of 8%–9.3% [2]. In hemodynamically stable patients with polytrauma, the current Modified Advanced Trauma Life Support Guidelines recommend omitting an anteroposterior radiograph of the pelvis [1]. Thus, detection of pelvic fractures is performed from the CT images. CT is advantageous in simultaneously evaluating hemorrhage, neurovascular injury, and solid organ damage, which contribute to mortality rates of between 8.6% and 50% [2]. Multiplanar reformation (MPR) and 3D images enable surgical planning, identification of intra-articular fragments, and improved delineation of spatial relationships.

For polytrauma patients receiving a chest, abdomen, and pelvis scan to exclude visceral injury, normal soft tissue protocols should be adapted to also acquire diagnostic bone images. This prevents double irradiation of the patient. Means of adaption include a higher peak voltage of 120–140 kVp to penetrate bone, using a pitch

TABLE 19.1

CT Indications

Indications or CT of Extremities
Fractures
Radiographically occult
Characterization for surgery
Treatment Planning
Assessment of Fixation
Evaluation of union
Arthrodesis Union
Joint Replacement
Periprosthetic fracture
Osteolysis
Femoral-tibial rotation
Preoperative planning
Heterotopic ossification
Overstuffing radial head
Tarsal Coalition
Gout Crystal Detection
Osteoarthritis
Acroiliitis
Neoplasm
Characterization
Pathological fracture
Biopsy guidance
Radiofrequency Ablation
Arthrography
Tendon Tear
Chondrosis
Labral Tear
Meniscus Tear
Soft Tissue Infection
femoral Version
Tibial Torsion

of less than 1, and acquiring both sharp kernel (B70) and smooth kernel (B10) data sets [3]. Pelvis images can be retroreconstructed into a bone algorithm.

No standard protocol is agreed upon across hospitals, but generally, reformatted images can be acquired at 3-mm thickness with an interval of 3 mm in axial, coronal, and sagittal planes. Thin detector collimation should be used for thin-slice reconstruction (2 mm or less) to obtain high-quality MPR images. The straight axial reformat field of view should include the iliac crests through the lesser trochanters and ischial tuberosities. Straight coronal reformats should extend from behind the gluteal muscles anteriorly to the symphysis and sagittal images should cover both hips.

The Young-Burgess classification system is used to describe the mechanism of traumatic pelvic fractures (Figure 19.1) [4]. Four main types include lateral compression, anteroposterior compression, vertical shear, and combined mechanical injury. Hemorrhage is most commonly

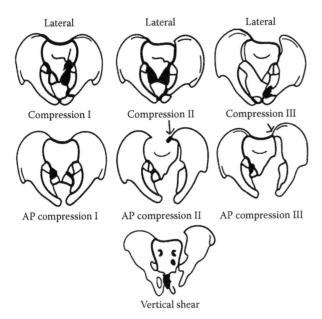

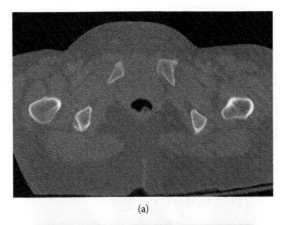

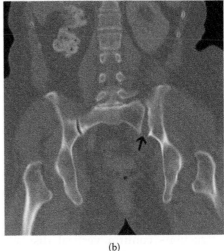

FIGURE 19.1
Illustration of Young–Burgess classification of pelvic ring fractures.

associated with anteroposterior (AP) compression and vertical shear mechanisms. The predominant feature of AP compression injury is pubic diastasis with or without disruption of the sacroiliac (SI) joints. The rotational stability of the pelvis primarily depends on the integrity of the SI ligaments. Normally, the pubic symphysis should be less than 1 cm wide and the SI joint space 2–4 mm wide.

AP compression injuries are divided into three types. Type I injuries are stable and involve less than 2.5 cm of diastasis of the pubis, either at the symphysis or through vertically oriented pubic rami fractures. Type II injuries include anterior diastasis greater than 2.5 cm with diastasis in one or both SI joints. Thus, there is incomplete posterior arch disruption and rotational instability (open-book). However, since the posterior ligaments are intact, there is still vertical stability. Type III injuries involve the posterior SI ligaments, resulting in both a vertically and rotationally unstable pelvis (Figure 19.2).

Lateral compression injuries are suggested by horizontal overlapping fractures of the superior and inferior pubic rami with ipsi- or contralateral vertically oriented sacral buckle fractures (Figure 19.3). Type I results from lateral compression to the sacrum, with ipsilateral sacral strut compression fractures. Type II involves lateral compression to the ilium with ipsilateral posterior iliac fracture. Type III typically occurs in motor vehicle collision rollovers and combines a lateral compression type I or II pattern with a contralateral AP compression injury. These result in an unstable internally rotated hemipelvis.

Vertical shear injuries often result from fall from a height and are also unstable. They can be purely ligamentous or involve vertical fractures of the pubic rami with cranial displacement (Figure 19.4). CT axial images

FIGURE 19.2
(a) Type III anteroposterior compression injury. Axial computed tomography (CT) in bone windows shows greater than 2.5 cm of diastasis at the pubis. (b) Coronal CT in bone windows shows diastasis of posterior aspect of left SI joint (arrow).

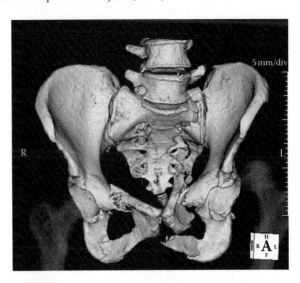

FIGURE 19.3
Lateral compression injury. 3D reformation of the pelvis shows vertically oriented left superior and inferior pubic rami fractures and ipsilateral sacral buckle fracture.

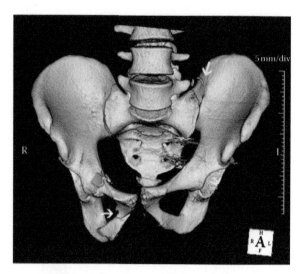

FIGURE 19.4
Vertical shear injury. 3D reformation of the pelvis shows vertically oriented inferior and superior right pubic rami fractures (white arrow) and left sacral fracture (yellow arrow) with diastasis and cranial displacement of the pelvis at these fractures.

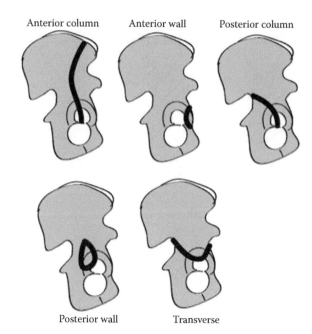

FIGURE 19.5
Illustration of Letournel elementary acetabular fracture classification system.

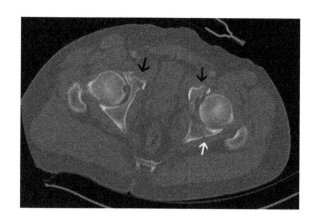

FIGURE 19.6
Elementary and associated acetabulum fractures: axial CT in bone windows shows an elementary anterior column fracture of right acetabulum (black arrow). Associated fracture of anterior (black arrow) and posterior columns (white arrow) of left acetabulum is also present.

are useful in evaluating integrity of the anterior and posterior aspects of the SI joints to differentiate between types of pelvic injuries. Inlet 3D reconstructions assist in assessing the degree of AP displacement of the hemipelvis, pelvic rotation, and pelvic brim integrity. Outlet 3D reconstructions confirm vertical displacement of the hemipelvis and involvement of the sacral neural foramina [3].

About 30%–40% of pelvic ring fractures involve the acetabulum [1]. CT is superior to radiography in diagnostic accuracy and treatment planning of acetabular fractures. The Letournel classification system is the most widely used method for assessing fracture pattern, planning treatment, and evaluating outcomes [5]. Although the system is based on AP and Judet radiographs, higher interobserver agreement has been found with CT imaging with MPR and 3D reconstructions.

The Letournel system divides acetabular fractures into two main groups: elementary and associated fractures. Elementary fractures are fractures in which a part or all of one column of the acetabulum is detached (Figure 19.5). The five types of elementary fractures are posterior wall, posterior column, anterior wall, anterior column (Figure 19.6), and transverse acetabular fractures. Associated fractures are defined as those including at least two of the elementary forms. Potential combinations include (1) T-shaped, (2) posterior wall and column, (3) transverse and posterior (4) anterior column or wall with a hemitransverse posterior component, and (5) both column fractures (Figure 19.6) [5]. Radiologists should note intra-articular bone fragments and associated soft tissue hematoma.

19.2.1.2 Sacrum

Sacral fractures occur in 45% of all pelvic fractures, with less than 5% as isolated injuries [6,7]. Mechanism of injury is primarily high-energy trauma. About 25% of sacral fractures are associated with neurological consequence [8]. CT is superior for detecting sacral fractures often obscured by overlying bowel gas on radiographs. CT with 1- or 2-mm-thin acquisitions and coronal and sagittal reconstructions is the standard of care for evaluating sacral fractures.

The zonal classification system of Denis describes fractures intrinsic to the sacrum [9]. Zone I sacral fractures are the most common and are isolated to the sacral ala. Zone II fractures pass through the neural foramina (Figure 19.7). Zone III extends centrally into the sacral spinal canal. Zone III sacral fractures have a 60% rate of associated symptomatic neurological deficits and 76% of patients have bowel, bladder, or sexual dysfunction.

The Isler system classifies fractures at the lumbosacral junction. These are often difficult to diagnose because of overlapping bowel gas, again making CT invaluable. Type I fractures are lateral to the L5-S1 facet. Type II fractures run through the L5-S1 facet. Type III fractures are medial to the facet, crossing into the neural arch. These can result in significant disability. If bilateral, these may result in lumbosacral dissociation [6].

19.2.1.3 Femoral Neck

Osteoporotic hip fractures are regarded as the most common severe type of fall-related injury among older adults. Over 95% of proximal femur fractures occur in the elderly. They are associated with high morbidity, mortality, and impairment of quality of life. Their incidence continues to rise as life expectancies also increase. Worldwide, the total number of hip fractures is expected to surpass 6 million by the year 2050. These fractures typically result from minor falls, which impart torsional or shearing stress to the bone. Approximately 37% of proximal femoral fractures are intracapsular, 49% intertrochanteric, and 14% subtrochanteric in location [10,11,12].

CT with three-plane imaging may be useful in detecting radiographically occult fractures in osteoporotic patients (Figure 19.8). However, even with CT, the resolution of osteoporotic trabecular bone is limiting and fractures may not be apparent. Although MRI has increased sensitivity, CT is faster to obtain and less expensive, particularly in the ER [13].

Femoral neck fractures are described by the Garden classification system (Figure 19.9) [14]. Type I fractures are incomplete subcapital fractures. Type II fractures are

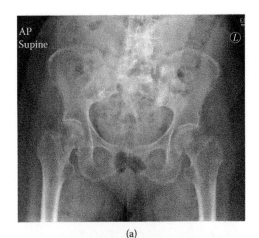

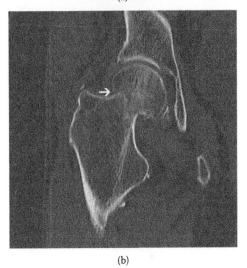

(b)

FIGURE 19.8
(a) Radiographically occult hip fracture. Anteroposterior radiograph of the pelvis in an 81-year-old woman with diffuse pain after fall was interpreted initially as negative. (b) Osteoporotic subcapital fracture. Coronal CT of the right hip in bone window shows a complete, mildly impacted subcapital fracture of her right femur and osteoporosis.

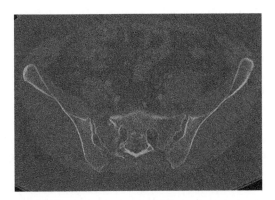

FIGURE 19.7
Isolated sacral fracture. Axial CT in bone window shows Denis Zone II right sacral fracture involving the neural foramin.

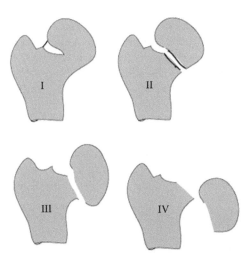

FIGURE 19.9
Illustration of Garden classification of femoral neck fractures.

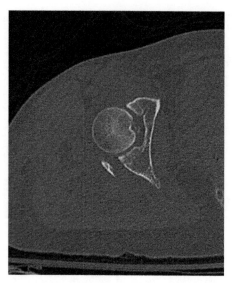

FIGURE 19.10
Hip dislocation. Axial CT in bone window of the right hip after relocation of posterior hip instability shows intra-articular bone fragments and a posterior acetabular wall fracture.

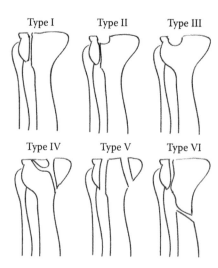

FIGURE 19.11
Illustration of Schatzker classification scheme of tibial plateau fractures.

complete, nondisplaced fractures of the femoral neck. Type III Garden fractures are complete, partially displaced subcapital fractures. The femoral shaft is externally rotated and the femoral neck is in varus alignment. A type IV fracture is fully displaced and the femur is externally rotated and superiorly displaced. Garden type IV fractures are unstable with a poor prognosis. CT is useful in assessing the degree of fracture comminution for surgical planning, postoperatively determining the extent of union, and evaluating for the complication of avascular necrosis. The incidence of osteonecrosis and nonunion in Garden type III and IV fractures is 25%.

Finally, in posterior dislocations at the hip joint, CT has been shown useful in assessing the congruity of reduction, femoral head osteochondral impaction fractures, and intra-articular fragments (Figure 19.10). Presence of loose fragments predisposes to continued instability and secondary arthrosis. Undetected femoral head fractures may result in avascular necrosis, early arthritis, and posttraumatic osteolysis. In addition, CT helps characterize and plan treatment of posterior acetabular wall fractures, the most common fractures associated with posterior dislocation [15]. Hip dislocations that spontaneously reduce are suggested by the Baltimore bubble sign, seen as air in the joint on CT [16]. This is postulated to represent intracapsular nitrogen bubbles resulting from the vacuum created by forcible distraction associated with dislocation.

19.2.1.4 Tibial Plateau

Over 1 million ER visits each year in the United States are due to acute knee trauma. Several studies have shown that radiographs are unreliable in depicting all

injuries and fail to correlate with clinical findings in up to 25% of patients. Fractures of the tibial plateau can be subtle if the fracture is nondepressed or the patient is osteoporotic. CT with 3D reconstructions more accurately depicts tibial plateau fractures in 43% of cases and modifies surgical plan in 59% of patients. CT has 80% sensitivity and 98% specificity for showing osseous avulsions and excluding associated ligamentous injuries in tibial plateau fractures [17–21].

CT protocol includes 120 kV, thin reconstructions, and at thickest 3-mm coronal and sagittal reformations. The axial plane should be prescribed parallel to the axis of the tibial plateau and scanned from the suprapatellar region to below the tibial tubercle [3].

The Schatzker classification system is the most commonly used by surgeons to characterize tibial plateau fractures (Figure 19.11) [22]. The Schatzker system includes six types of fractures based on pattern, location, and presence of a metaphyseal fracture. Type I fractures involve the lateral tibial plateau without depression. Type II fractures are lateral plateau fractures with depression of >4 mm as measured from the normal medial plateau to the point of lateral depression (Figure 19.12). Type II fractures account for 25% of all tibial plateau fractures, are often seen in patients with osteopenia, and have associated medial collateral ligament or medial meniscus injury in 20% of patients. Type III fractures are compression fractures of the lateral (IIIA) or central (IIIB) tibial plateau.

Type IV fractures involve the medial tibial plateau. Around 10% are associated with a fracture dislocation and have increased the likelihood of injury to the peroneal nerve or popliteal vessels. Bicondylar tibial plateau fractures without metadiaphyseal discontinuity comprise type V, whereas plateau fractures with diaphyseal continuity are termed type VI. Differentiation of type V and VI is aided by spatial relationships provided by MPR (Figure 19.13). About 20%–30% of type VI Schatzker fractures are associated with ligamentous injury. In general, increasing grade reflects higher energy imparted to the bone, greater severity, and worse prognosis [23].

19.2.1.5 Distal Tibia

Radiographs underestimate the size and displacement of posterior malleolus fractures. Although CT is not required for evaluation of all ankle fractures, it has been proven useful for assessing the extent of posterior malleolus

plafond involvement, which requires surgery if greater than 25%. CT is also useful for assessment of pilon fractures, which are comminuted intra-articular fractures of the distal tibial articular surface (Figure 19.14). CT has been shown to influence management in 60% of patients with pilon fractures and increase interobserver and intraobserver agreement on treatment plans [24].

A triplane fracture is one seen in three different planes [25]. These include an axial injury through the distal tibial physis, a sagittal component through the distal tibia epiphysis, and a coronal component posteriorly through the distal tibia metaphysis (Figure 19.15). Triplane fractures

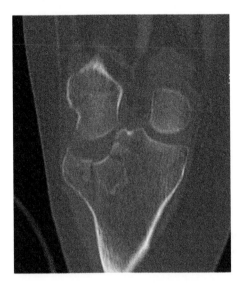

FIGURE 19.12
Schatzker type II fracture. Coronal CT in bone window shows depressed fracture of the lateral tibial plateau.

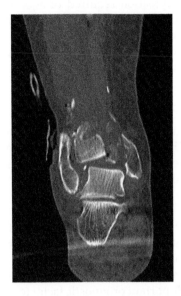

FIGURE 19.14
Pilon fracture. Coronal CT in bone window shows a highly comminuted intra-articular fracture of the distal tibia with areas of angulation, displaced intra-articular fragments, gapping, and articular step-off. An oblique distal fibula fracture is also present.

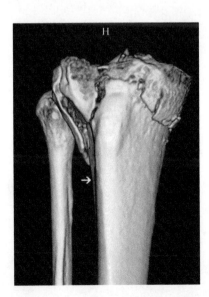

FIGURE 19.13
Schatzker type VI fracture. 3D reconstructed CT image shows the fracture line extending into the diaphysis (arrow) differentiating between type V and VI fractures.

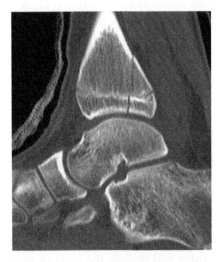

FIGURE 19.15
Triplane fracture. Sagittal CT in bone window shows a fracture line extending through the distal tibia epiphysis and metaphysis as well as an AP directed fracture through the physis.

account for 5%–10% of pediatric intra-articular injuries and 15% of physeal injuries. CT is an adjunct for improved spatial relation of fragments [26]. Treatment involves reduction to avoid physeal arrest, and minimize angular deformity, early arthrosis, leg-length discrepancy, and joint stiffness.

As with other joints, thin detector collimation should be used to generate thin axial images reconstructed with 50% overlap. Many institutions scan both ankles to provide an intrinsic normal reference. In addition, imaging the ankle with the knee in flexion produces high-quality MPR images of the tibial plafond due to the principle of obliquity. The principle of obliquity means that for the volumetric acquisition required of a joint, the affected joint should be placed at an oblique angle relative to the gantry to allow for the maximum number of slices to traverse the joint surface. If it is parallel, fewer slices traverse the cortical surfaces [27].

19.2.1.6 Calcaneus

The calcaneus is the most commonly fractured tarsal bone. 70%–75% of calcaneal fractures are intra-articular, involving the subtalar joint [28]. These generally result from an axial load producing both shear and compression fracture lines. CT with MPR and 3D imaging has become the standard imaging modality to guide in management of intra-articular calcaneal fractures. For the classification of intra-articular fractures, reformatted images parallel and perpendicular to the posterior facet of the sagittal reformatted images are obtained.

The most important prognostic factor to assess on CT is the integrity of the posterior subtalar joint. The Sanders classification system is the most commonly used by surgeons to describe intra-articular fractures (Figure 19.16). Sanders type I fractures are nondisplaced. Type II fractures involve two articular pieces, with A through C subcategories depending on medial or lateral location of the main fracture line. Type III fractures involve three pieces with a dispersed middle fragment. Sanders type IV fractures are highly comminuted (Figure 19.17). Both type II and III fractures have relatively good or excellent surgical outcomes in 70% of patients [29–31].

It is important to evaluate the trochlear process on reformatted images since the peroneus longus tendon courses under this groove and is at risk of injury or dislocation in 25%–48%. In addition, the flexor hallucis longus tendon integrity should be assessed as it passes under the sustentaculum tali. Volume-rendered (VR) images are more useful and time efficient than MRP to visualize the tendon–bone relationships.

Extra-articular fractures account for 25%–30% of calcaneal fractures and include the anterior process, body, sustentaculum tali, peroneal tubercle, lateral process, and posterior calcaneus not involving the posterior facet [29–31].

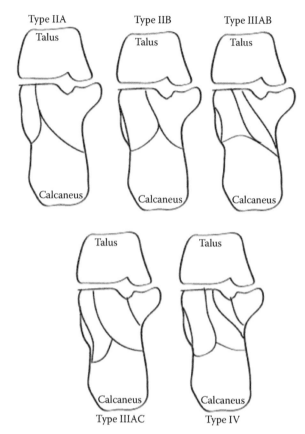

FIGURE 19.16
Illustration of Sanders classification scheme of intra-articular calcaneus fractures.

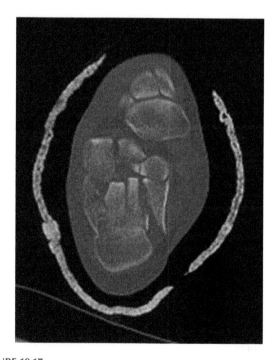

FIGURE 19.17
Sanders type IV fracture: Axial CT image in bone window of the calcaneus shows comminuted intra-articular calcaneus fracture.

19.2.1.7 Talus

The talus consists of a head and body connected by a neck. A forced dorsiflexion of the talus against the anterior tibia often results in a talar neck fracture (Figure 19.18), such as slamming a foot on the brake to prevent a motor vehicle collision. The Hawkins classification describes talar neck fractures. Type I is nondisplaced, type II occurs with distraction and subluxation of the posterior subtalar joint, and type III involves tibiotalar and subtalar dislocation. Surgical reduction with internal fixation is crucial to prevent avascular necrosis, which occurs in 20%–50% of type II and 80%–100% of type III fractures. CT is useful for imaging the degree of comminution, displacement, articular congruity of the subtalar joint, and in identifying unsuspected extension into the talonavicular joint and posterior process [31–33].

CT is also helpful for posterior process fractures of the talar body, since radiographs are insensitive. CT is often needed to diagnose talar head fractures, which are nondisplaced because of the strong intertarsal ligaments. Transchondral fractures involve the subchondral bone and cartilage. The Burnt and Hardy system divides these into four stages. Stage I is a compression fracture. Stage II involves a partial osteochondral fracture. Stage III involves complete injury, and stage IV involves detached loose lesions. Up to 58% of these were missed by radiographs in one study but were identified by CT, thus validating its use. In addition, CT allows detection of loose bodies on the sagittal and coronal images.

19.2.1.8 Lisfranc Joint

The Lisfranc joint is the articulation between the forefoot and the midfoot. It consists of the five tarsometatarsal joints and one ligament, running from the lateral aspect of the medial cuneiform to the medial and plantar aspects of the second metatarsal base. Lisfranc injuries occur in low-energy, sports-related events in athletes or motor vehicle and industrial accidents. Mechanisms involve a direct blow or forced plantar flexion combined with rotation [34].

Approximately 20% of Lisfranc injuries are missed on initial radiographs and are one of the most common reasons for malpractice lawsuits against radiologists and ER physicians [35]. When using CT instead of radiographs, LeClere et al. showed an overall change of diagnosis in 85.6%, treatment plan in 84.2%, and postoperative weight-bearing plan in 87.7%. Detecting these injuries is crucial to prevent posttraumatic arthrosis, dorsalis pedis artery and/or deep peroneal nerve damage, and flatfoot deformity with instability [34].

In a Lisfranc fracture dislocation, there may be dorsolateral dislocation of the lateral four or all five metatarsal bases (homolateral). Alternatively, the 1st metatarsal may dislocate in the opposite direction (divergent). Isolated medial dislocation of the 1st metatarsal may also occur. Other complex patterns with variable plantar and dorsal dislocation are possible. With more severe trauma, associated cuboid and cuneiform fractures may be present (Figure 19.19). Soft tissue windows should be used to assess the integrity of the Lisfranc ligament, which is a soft tissue attenuation band extending from the lateral aspect of the 1st cuneiform to the medial base of the 2nd metatarsal bone.

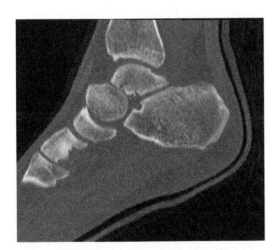

FIGURE 19.18
Talar neck fracture. Sagittal CT image in bone window shows a vertical fracture through the talar neck with rotation of the distal fragment and subluxation at the talonavicular joint.

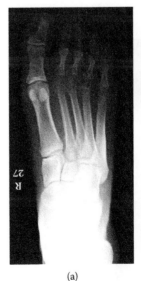
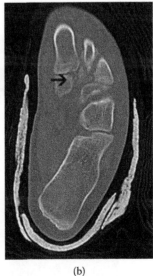

(a)   (b)

FIGURE 19.19
(a) Lisfranc injury. Anteroposterior radiograph of the right foot demonstrates questionable bone fragment at base of second metatarsal bone. (b) Axial CT in the patient in bone window demonstrates the fragment is real as well as a fracture of the medial cuneiform (arrow) with several loose bone fragments and lateral dislocation of the second metatarsal in respect to the cuneiforms.

19.2.2 Upper Extremity

19.2.2.1 Scapula and Humerus

1% of all fractures involve the scapula, and usually result from high-energy trauma. 80%–85% have associated injuries, such as rib fractures, pulmonary injury, humeral fractures, brachial plexus injury, skull fracture, and vascular injury. Nearly half of scapula fractures involve the body and spine while 25% involve the glenoid neck. Radiographs of the scapula only detect acromion, spine, and body fractures. 3D CT images can assess scapula fractures in all six anatomical regions. In addition, there is similar sensitivity and specificity of images reconstructed from the chest CT versus those reconstructed from a dedicated scapula CT. Thus, the chest CT images obtained in a trauma patient can be used to create quality images of the scapula [36,37].

Glenoid cavity fractures are described by the classification scheme of Goss; type I injuries involve the glenoid rim, II–V involve the glenoid fossa, and type VI include comminuted injuries. Instability is suspected if the fracture is displaced >10 mm or if at least one-fourth of the anterior glenoid cavity or one-third of the posterior aspect of the glenoid cavity is involved. This warrants surgical management to prevent persistent subluxation of the humeral head [36].

In fracture dislocations, CT can show radiographically occult bony bankart lesions and Hill–Sachs lesions (Figure 19.20). Preoperative CT has been shown to accurately depict the need for bone grafting repair of a bony bankart in 96% of cases. Other studies have confirmed, showing 93% sensitivity and

79% specificity and high correlation between CT and arthroscopy for the severity of anterior bone loss in bankart lesions [38]. CT arthrography can be simultaneously used to depict soft tissue bankart lesions and associated ligament tears.

Proximal humerus fractures usually occur through the surgical neck. Anatomic neck fractures are rare but have a poor prognosis due to disruption of the blood supply. Radiographs remain the primary approach of diagnosis and characterization. CT is particularly helpful when radiographs underestimate the degree of displacement, such as with tuberosity fractures or head-splitting fractures. CT with 3D reconstructions provides the most complete overlapping-free presentation of fractures. The Neer classification is the most commonly used system to describe proximal humeral fractures. However, several studies have shown that CT did not improve interobserver reliability of Neer fracture classification [39–41].

Distal humeral fractures at the elbow associated with severe comminution, bone loss, and osteopenia benefit from CT evaluation for surgical planning. 3D imaging improves the intraobserver agreement of fracture characterization.

19.2.2.2 Distal Radius

Fracture of the distal radius is the most common forearm fracture, usually occurring after a fall onto an outstretched hand. CT is used to plan operative repair or resolve uncertain findings on conventional radiographs. American College of Radiology (ACR) appropriateness criteria give a rating of 9 (1–9 scale) to CT of the wrist without contrast for surgical planning of comminuted, intra-articular distal radius fractures. On CT, radial height should be measured, radial inclination assessed, intra-articular loose fragments identified, and stability of the distal radial ulnar joint confirmed.

19.2.2.3 Carpus

Carpal fractures account for 18% of hand and wrist fractures and 6% of all fractures. Fractures may be overlooked due to the complexities of carpal anatomy. Studies have shown that 30% of fractures were not prospectively diagnosed on radiographs, suggesting that CT should be considered after negative radiographic findings (Figure 19.21). CT has a sensitivity and specificity of 89% and 97%, respectively, and negative predictive value of 97%–99% for ruling out a fracture. CT of the wrist should be obtained with a small field of view (<25 cm) and thin-slice reconstruction (0.5 mm) to provide isotropic sampling from which MPR images can be obtained in any plane, such as long axis of the scaphoid [3,42–43].

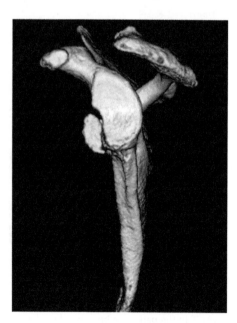

FIGURE 19.20
Bankart fracture. 3D reconstruction of the scapula shows size and orientation of osseous bankart injury after anterior shoulder dislocation.

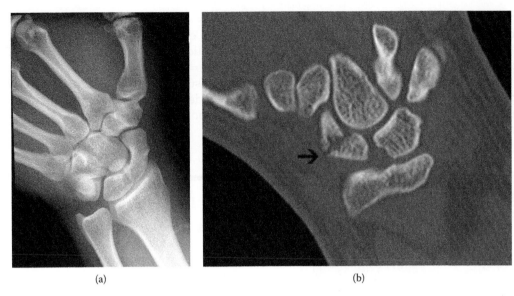

(a)   (b)

FIGURE 19.21

(a) Radiographically occult scaphoid fracture. Anteroposterior wrist radiograph does not show lucent fracture line. (b) Scaphoid waist fracture. Coronal CT in bone window in the same patient clearly shows mildly displaced scaphoid waist fracture (arrow). This is at risk of avascular necrosis (AVN) and nonunion.

Scaphoid fractures account for 70% of all carpal fractures. These are most common in active 20- to 30-year-old men after a hyperextension mechanism. Nearly 80% involve the scaphoid waist. Fractures of the waist and proximal pole are important to diagnosis as they risk avascular necrosis in 15%–30% because of the retrograde blood supply to these regions. In the ER, a clinically suspected scaphoid fracture is often treated with immobilization of the wrist and follow-up even if radiographs are negative. CT is more reliable and accurate than radiographs for assessing displacement of scaphoid fractures [44–45].

Other carpal fractures are less common, but if there is clinical suspicion or pain, CT provides the advantages of MPR and 3D imaging to better visualize complex carpal anatomy.

19.3 Imaging Technique in Patients with Fixation Hardware

Evaluation of hardware can be limited because of metal artifacts that appear as streak or sunburst patterns. Thinner detector collimations, increased peak voltage and tube current settings, and reducing pitch values can help ameliorate partial volume artifacts. For reconstructions, a smooth or soft tissue reconstruction algorithm (kernel) also reduces metal artifacts. Thick reformatted slices reduce severity of metal artifacts. Lowest amount of artifact is present around titanium hardware while cobalt chromium alloys produce the most [3,27,46].

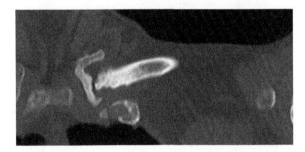

FIGURE 19.22

Nonunion fracture. Coronal CT in bone window of the left clavicle shows nonunion of the medial clavicle fracture 16 months after initial injury. Evaluation of the joint was limited on radiographs due to overlying pulmonary, cardiovascular, and costochondral structures.

19.3.1 Determination of Fusion

Nonunion occurs when healing at a fracture site, osteotomy, or arthrodesis ends before establishment of continuity of bridging bone. It is clinically suspected when pain or tenderness persists at a fracture for greater than 6 months in tibia fractures, 6 months at arthrodesis, and 6–12 months for femoral neck fractures. Contributing factors to delayed and nonunion include vascular impairment, inadequate immobilization and fixation, interposition of soft tissue or bone fragments at the fracture site, and infection.

Radiographs are the routine method of assessing healing but are less accurate than CT. However, radiographs both under- and overestimate the degree of fusion by 19%. CT with multiplanar reformatting is particularly helpful in fractures with surrounding hardware and in the sternoclavicular (Figure 19.22), subtalar, and tibiotalar joints (Figure 19.23), which have complex post-surgical anatomy and overlapping of bone that may be on standard radiographs [47].

For scaphoid fractures, which pose an increased risk of avascular necrosis of the proximal pole, there is poor interobserver reliability of radiographs for signs of union. CT agreement for identifying scaphoid fracture union and avascular necrosis (AVN) has reported sensitivity of 78%, specificity of 96%, and accuracy of 84% (Figure 19.24) [48].

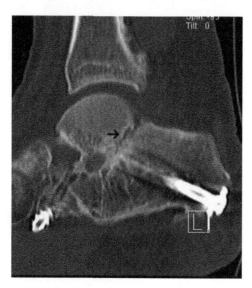

FIGURE 19.23
Nonunion arthrodesis. Sagittal CT of the hindfoot in bone windows 14 months after posterior subtalar arthrodesis with screw shows more than two-thirds of the joint is not fused, consistent with nonunion. CT is very helpful around orthopedic hardware and in the subtalar joint due to its spatial anatomy.

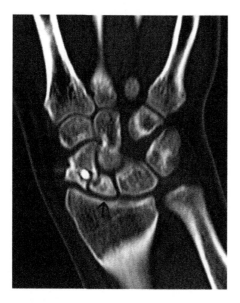

FIGURE 19.24
Scaphoid AVN. Coronal CT in bone window shows nonunion across the scaphoid waist fracture and sclerosis (arrow) of the proximal pole, consistent with AVN.

Roberts et al. showed 100% sensitivity and specificity for characterizing nonunion on CT by using a fusion ratio of >33% as nonunion and >67% as union. The ratio = 100 × (sum of lengths of fused segments on all slices/sum of lengths of joint surface) [49]. Ultimately, sites and degree of osseous bridging should be described in the report whether or not a ratio is measured.

19.4 CT Imaging of Arthroplasty

Total hip, knee, and shoulder arthroplasty are the most common joint replacement surgeries. More than 3 million are placed annually. The number has continued to rise over the past two decades. Thus, radiologists will encounter more short- and long-term complications and CT will become more valuable in assessment of new designs and complications.

For imaging around joint replacements, use of soft tissue (smooth) reconstruction is important because images reconstructed with bone kernel often cause blackout (a dark rim) around the metal. Wide window settings (>6000) help in visualizing periprosthetic bone. Milliamperes per second (mAs) should be increased to 350–450 in adults and up to 600 if there are bilateral arthroplasties. In addition, lower pitch settings to reduce cone beam artifacts with multichannel scanners, narrow detector element collimation, and increased peak killivoltage (140) all aid in optimizing quality. Most data are reconstructed using 1- 1.5-mm-thick slices with 50% overlap. Adequate quality MPR can be created using 1.5- 2-mm-thick slices in sagittal and coronal planes [46].

19.4.1 Periprosthetic Fractures

Most fractures around joint replacements occur after trauma. Other causes include aseptic loosening, fractures through areas of osteolysis, and infection. CT is helpful in assessing the exact extension of periprosthetic fractures around joint implants. In addition, CT assists in detection of residual bone volume and hardware integrity. Depiction of both degree of displacement and integrity of the prosthesis is important in whether a surgical plate is placed across the fracture or revision prosthesis is implanted.

19.4.2 Particle Disease and Osteolysis

The majority of major total joint arthroplasty and some smaller joint replacements include polyethylene in their component design. Wear of polyethylene particles, and less often methyl methacrylate cement, can incite a foreign-body reaction, resulting in osteolysis of the adjacent bone. This is also known as aggressive granulomatosis, particle disease, and histiocytic osteolysis. The process results in continued bone destruction and component loosening. Polyethylene wear with loosening is the most common cause of long-term failure in the three main joint replacements.

CT is the most accurate modality for measuring osteolytic lesion volume. CT features of focal osteolysis include multiple, expansile, oval, or round radiolucencies, which are conglomerated into lobular shapes (Figure 19.25). Cortex adjacent to the osteolysis is thin and discontinuous. Metallosis is another rare condition unique to joint replacements that can result in osteolysis. It involves infiltration of periprosthetic soft tissues and bone by metallic wear debris. The debris instigates a local inflammatory response with synovitis and cytokine-mediated osteolysis. Since radiographic signs may be absent in more than half of the cases, CT may aid in diagnosis. Cases showing imaging findings of metallosis on CT are sparsely documented in literature, but include high-density material outlining the joint capsule or bursa, metallic debris, and high-density joint effusions (Figure 19.26) [52].

A novel complication of the new generation of metal-on-metal total hip and resurfacing prostheses is Adverse Reaction to Metal Debris (ARMD), including aseptic lymphocytic vasculitis-associated lesion (ALVAL). The mechanism is hypothesized to be release of metal ions from the prosthesis that incites a type IV hypersensitivity response in the local soft tissues. Patients often present with pain, soft tissue necrosis, or complex fluid or soft tissue collections. Although MR with metal artifact reduction is the technique of choice, CT can also be obtained. Typical appearances of ARMD include solid collections or fluid collections with capsules >3mm in thickness. These tend to be located along the periprosthetic regions of the anterior hip capsule and posterolateral margin of the femur [53].

Another increasing use of CT for total knee arthroplasty is assessment of femoral–tibial component rotational malalignment. Rotational malalignment can result in patellar maltracking, anterior knee pain, premature polyethylene wear, and flexion instability. A biomechanical study showed increased tibial cortex strain at 10° of rotational malalignment [54].

The femoral rotational alignment is the transepicondylar axis, which is the line running from the lateral epicondylar prominence to the medial epicondylar sulcus. It is typically in 3° of external rotation. On a CT axial image or 3D reformatted image, this line is drawn to assess the femoral component rotation (Figure 19.27a). There is variation as to where the tibial rotational line should be drawn, but one method is to draw a line along the posterior border of the tibial component. Another is the tibial tubercle and the insertion of the posterior

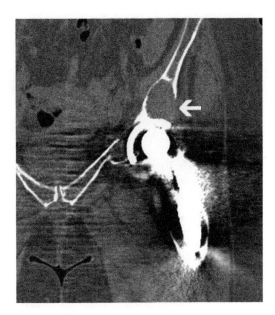

FIGURE 19.25
Particle disease. Coronal CT in bone window of the left hip arthroplasty shows large area of osteolysis of the superior acetabular roof (arrow). The femoral head is also superiorly, asymmetrically positioned, consistent with polyethylene liner wear.

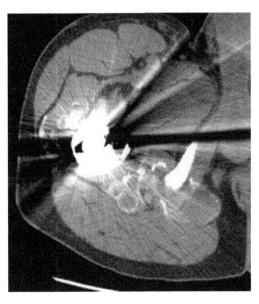

FIGURE 19.26
Metallosis. Axial CT in soft tissue windows of the right hip shows cystic collections with metal lined walls adjacent to the hip arthroplasty. At surgery, the patient had frank metallosis.

cruciate ligament on the posterior border of the tibia as reference points. The two lines are superimposed to determine any mismatch and quantify the angle (Figure 19.27b) [55,56].

Reverse total shoulder arthroplasty (RTSA) is more frequently placed over the past decade for patients with a nonfunctioning rotator cuff with pain, secondary arthropathy, or the inability to lift the arm above

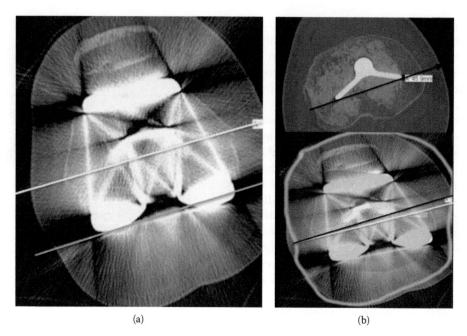

(a)   (b)

FIGURE 19.27
(a) Femoral rotation. Axial CT of a knee arthroplasty at the level of the femur shows the transepicondylar axis (yellow line) is parallel to the posterior aspect of the femoral component (blue line), a normal finding. (b) Tibia rotation. A line is drawn along the posterior aspect of the tibial component (top) and superimposed at the level of the transepicondylar axis. The angle between these two lines should be less than 10°.

the horizontal (pseudoparalysis). Its unique design consists of a semiconstrained ball and socket that moves the center of rotation of the joint more distal and medial to improve the leverage of the deltoid muscle for control over humeral motion. The humeral component consists of a proximal cup-shaped portion and metal stem. A radiolucent polyethylene insert sits in this cup portion and articulates with the glenosphere, which is the rounded metal ball of the prosthesis that attaches to a baseplate (metaglene) secured to the native glenoid.

This unique design poses new types of complication, in addition to the complications seen with the anatomical total and hemiarthroplasties. Unique complications of RTSA include disassembly of humeral or glenosphere-metaglene components (Figure 19.28), migration of the metaglene within the joint due to loosening, malpositioning of fixation screws, scapular and acromial base stress fractures, scapular notching due to impingement, and inferior scapular erosions. The erosions occur due to repetitive contact of the medial aspect of the humeral component with the inferior border of the scapula. Standard radiographs may be of low sensitivity in depicting the unique scapular related complications.

Additional use of CT in shoulder replacements includes measurement of the glenoid version. Typically, the arthritic glenoid is retroverted and

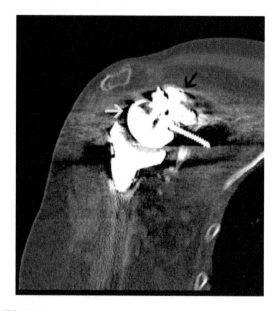

FIGURE 19.28
Complication reverse total shoulder arthroplasty. Coronal CT image in bone windows of a reverse total shoulder arthroplasty shows that the glenosphere (yellow arrow) is disengaged from the metaglene baseplate and screws (black arrow).

restoration to neutral version is recommended for optimal functional outcomes in shoulder arthroplasty. Before CT, glenoid version was measured on axillary radiographs. However, radiographs are ineffective in

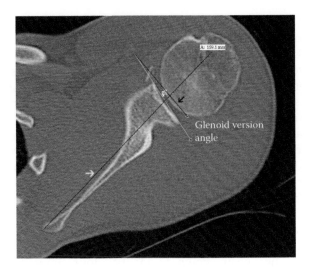

FIGURE 19.29
Glenoid version. Axial CT image in bone windows at the level of the left scapular spine, 1–2 slices below the coracoid. A line is drawn along the scapular spine and a perpendicular created to this. The angle between the perpendicular line and a line along the glenoid surface (blue line) is the glenoid version angle.

measuring version due to overlapping bones, variable radiographic technique, and complexity of scapular anatomy.

Friedman defined glenoid version as the angle between a line drawn from the medial border of the scapula to the center of the glenoid and the line perpendicular to the face of the glenoid on the axial 2D CT slice at or just below the tip of the coracoid (Figure 19.29) [57]. However, axial 2D CT version measurements depend on the relation of the plane of the scapula to the axis of the CT scanner. One study showed greater than 5° difference in measurements of version between 2D CT and 3D CT images in nearly 50% of patients [58,59].

Thus, 3D CT is suggested as the most accurate pre-operative means of assessing glenoid version and morphology. On a 3D CT, a vertical line can be drawn on the 3D surface of the glenoid face, centered in the AP direction (Figure 19.30a). A transverse 2D plane is then generated perpendicular to the midpoint of the vertical line passing through the scapular axis (center of glenoid and tip of scapular spine) to obtain an image for glenoid version angle measurement (Figure 19.30b) [60].

Uses of CT in elbow joint replacement include evaluation of bridging versus nonbridging heterotopic ossification, capitellar osteoarthritis and erosions, and overstuffing of the radial head thickness in the radiocapitellar joint, findings reported after radial head arthroplasty.

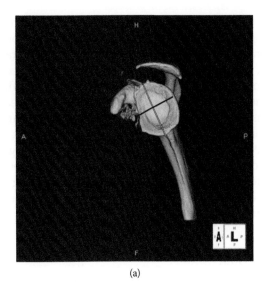

(a)

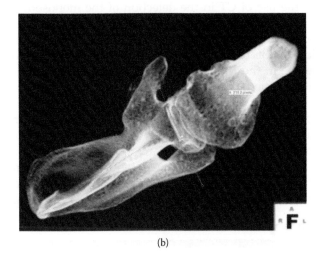

(b)

FIGURE 19.30
(a) 3D volume rendered image of the glenoid face shows method for version calculation. A vertical line (yellow) is drawn on the 3D surface of the glenoid face, centered in the Anteroposterior direction. A transverse 2D plane is generated perpendicular to the midpoint of the vertical line (black) to pass through the scapular axis. (b) Glenoid version angle is then measured at the level of the transverse plane using the Friedman technique for the 2D CT slice. Here, the angle measures 13°, which is abnormal.

19.5 Joint Pain and Assessment

19.5.1 Tarsal Coalition

Tarsal coalitions are abnormal unions of two or more bones of the hindfoot and midfoot. They affect up to 1% of the population and typically present in the second decade of life as a cause of rigid flatfoot with pain. The most common forms are talocalcaneal and calcanealnavicular coalitions. They can be fibrous, cartilaginous, or osseous. Up to 50% of coalitions are bilateral. CT is the study of choice to further detail the extent of a coalition, osseous versus nonosseous composition, and secondary arthritic changes that influence whether arthrodesis is required or resection is feasible. CT has been shown to be more cost effective than MRI for imaging of tarsal coalitions. Osseous coalitions on CT are relatively easy to confirm. A bony bar bridges the two bones (Figure 19.31). In some cases of nonosseous coalition, changes may be subtle, with narrowing of the space between the two bones and mild marginal reactive bone changes [61,62].

19.5.2 Gout

The past few years have produced a flurry of research for the use of CT in the detection of the monosodium urate (MSU) crystal deposits of gout. Gout is the most common crystal arthropathy, resulting from precipitation of MSU crystals in the joint. It affects up to 6 million people in the United States. Peak incidence is in middle age men, with the first metatarsophalangeal joint involved by 50% of cases. Definitive diagnosis requires polarized light microscopy of fluid aspirated from the joint. However, joint aspiration can be difficult and may not occur during the acute flare.

Dual-energy CT has the potential of confirming gout before classic radiographic changes occur as well as monitoring response to treatment. A dual-energy

CT has two x-ray tubes and allows simultaneous acquisition at two different energy levels to create two different datasets simultaneously. An image-based two-material decomposition algorithm of datasets is performed to separate calcium from MSU, using soft tissue as the baseline. Material with high anatomic number has a higher change in attenuation than material with low atomic number, such as gout, and is displayed with different colors. Technique involves 140 kV and 55 mAs for tube A and 80 kV and 243 mAs for tube B. Collimation of 0.6 mm reconstructed to 0.75 mm transverse thick slices obtained at 80 kV and 140 kV is performed with a parameter ratio to 1.28. 3D images can be made and viewed in 360° around any axis [63–65].

CT has been shown to identify four times more locations of involvement by MSU crystals than clinical examination. It also allows high accuracy to detect disease at a preclinical stage, allowing treatment to prevent articular and bony damage, making regression easier to achieve. On CT, the areas of MSU will be shown by the specified color (Figure 19.32) while calcium will appear as a different color due its higher attenuation value.

19.5.3 Sacroiliac Joints

Spondyloarthropathy is a term for the group of five chronic inflammatory diseases primarily affecting the axial skeleton. These are ankylosing spondylitis,

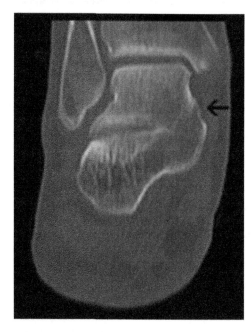

FIGURE 19.31
Coalition. Coronal CT image in bone window of the ankle shows osseous coalition (arrow) of the talus and calcaneus.

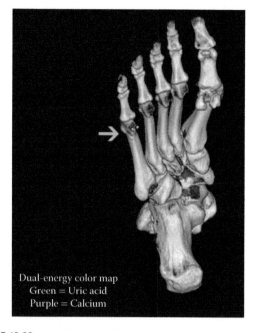

FIGURE 19.32
Gout. Dual-energy CT volume-rendered image shows gout at the fifth metatarsophalangeal (MTP) joint as green and calcium as purple.

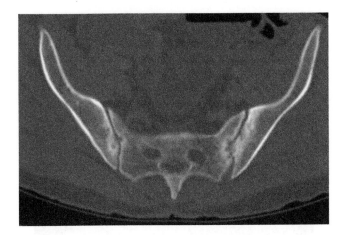

FIGURE 19.33
Sacroiliitis. Axial CT in bone windows shows bilateral sclerosis, erosions, and narrowing of the sacroiliac joints.

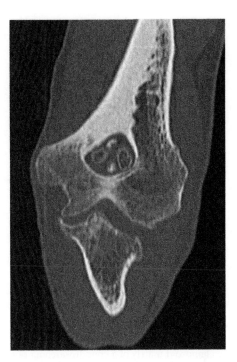

FIGURE 19.34
Osteoarthritis. Coronal CT in bone windows shows several osteochondral bodies in the olecranon fossa of the elbow. Narrowing and subchondral sclerosis is seen of the ulnohumeral joint.

reactive arthritis, psoriatic arthritis, arthritis associated with chronic inflammatory bowel disease, and undifferentiated spondyloarthropathy. MRI is most sensitive for imaging acute inflammatory findings while CT is more sensitive for depicting chronic changes such as erosions, sclerosis, ankylosis, and bone formation. The SI joints are characteristically involved in these arthropathies. CT findings of sacroiliitis initially include joint space widening, followed by narrowing with sclerosis along the iliac side of the joints. Later, erosions, with a postage-stamp appearance will be seen with increasing sclerosis and narrowing (Figure 19.33). In late stages, CT will show fusion across the joints. The process may be unilateral or bilateral. CT is also helpful in guiding therapeutic injections of the SI joints because it enables localization of unfused areas for needle entry.

19.5.4 Osteoarthritis

Osteoarthritis is the most common type of arthritis in the world, with primary degenerative forms and secondary forms. In patients with osteoarthritis, CT can be used for preoperative planning, detection of intra-articular loose bodies, and further evaluation of the severity of the disease. A recent study by Zubler showed that CT is 79% accurate compared to 67% for radiographs in detecting loose bodies in the joint space and detailing the degree of osteoarthritis in the elbow joint (Figure 19.34). CT with 3D reconstructions also assists operative planning for patients who require arthroplasty to treat their osteoarthritis.

Some centers are scanning both feet in simulated weight-bearing to assess the true effects of loading on flatfoot deformity, detect rotational movements among tarsal bones, and guide pre-operative planning for future hindfoot and/or midfoot arthrodesis.

19.6 Skeletal Tumors

Radiographs remain the mainstay of initial evaluation of a suspected primary or secondary bone tumor. CT is helpful to evaluate tumor matrix (Figure 19.35), detect lesions in difficult-to-evaluate areas, such as the sacrum and bony pelvis, determine extension across the epiphysis, and detect periosteal or endosteal reactions. CT can also be combined with a CT angiogram to further define tumor vascularity. CT is also of value in evaluating for an underlying neoplasm in suspected pathological fractures.

Several lesions have characteristic, highly specific CT appearances, such as osteoid osteoma, unicameral bone cysts, aneurysmal bone cysts, osteochondromas, osteosarcoma, Ewing's sarcoma, and chondroblastoma. Osteoid osteoma is a benign bone tumor frequently found in adolescent males. Patients present with pain worst at night but relieved by aspirin. Lesions may be cortically based, medullary, or subperiosteal in location. More than 50% are found in the femur or tibia. AT CT, the nidus of an osteoid osteoma is a well defined, round or oval cortical lucency usually less than 1.5 cm in diameter (Figure 19.36). An area of high attenuation representing mineralized osteoid may be present centrally in 50% of cases. Reactive sclerosis is often present and the

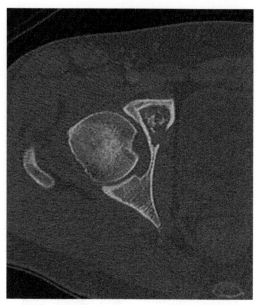

FIGURE 19.35
Tumor matrix. Axial CT image in bone window of the right hip shows ring and arc chondroid matrix of a chondrosarcoma of the anterior column of the acetabulum with cortical break through.

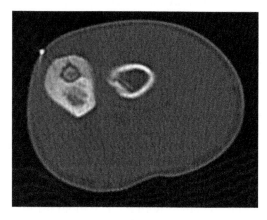

FIGURE 19.36
Osteoid osteoma. Axial CT image in bone windows shows cortical thickening, lucent round area, and central sclerotic nidus of an osteoid osteoma.

hypervascular nidus enhances. CT is better than MRI at depicting the nidus [66].

Over the past decade, CT-guided radiofrequency ablation has become the method of choice for treatment of osteoid osteoma. Benefits of radiofrequency ablation include that the procedure can be performed in 90 minutes and daily activities can be resumed immediately. Contraindications to ablation include lesions in the hand, in the spine <1 cm away from vital structures, pregnancy, infection, and coagulopathy.

The procedure is performed with general, spinal, or propofol-induced anesthesia. Multiple thin-section CT

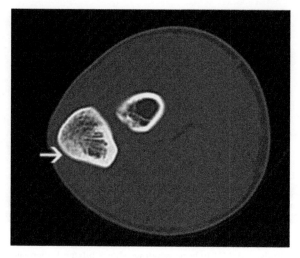

FIGURE 19.37
Ablation outcome. Axial computed tomography image in bone window of the same patient 1 year after radiofrequency ablation shows sclerosis at the site of the osteoid osteoma, consistent with successful outcome.

images are obtained to localize the lesion. For lesions >1 cm, multiple skin entry points are required for success. Preferred approach is an angle perpendicular to the cortical surface, avoiding adjacent neurovascular structures. Grounding pads are put in place to inhibit current transmission through the patient. A bone biopsy system is used to gain access to the lesion, perform biopsy, and guide electrode placement. Thermal heating is applied with RF electrode at target temperature of 90°C. Ablation is performed for 4–6 minutes, though larger lesions may require multiple cycles. Clinical success is between 89% and 98% for primary treatment. Imaging at 2 months to 2 years shows partial or complete replacement of the nidus with sclerotic bone (Figure 19.37). Residual tumor is suggested by persistent radiolucency at the ablated site [67].

CT is also useful for percutaneous biopsy. This is a safe and accurate method to obtain tissue diagnosis with a relatively low complication rate of 1.1% compared to that of 16% for open biopsy. However, care must be taken to avoid seeding malignant cells along the needle track, especially if that tract would require resection of the needle track en bloc with the tumor at limb-sparing reconstructive surgery [68,69].

Most percutaneous needle bone biopsies can be performed under conscious sedation and local anesthesia. Standard CT-guided biopsy planning is obtained with markers on the skin and sterile technique. An 11- or 14-gauge coaxial bone biopsy system with an eccentric drill tip is used for sclerotic lesions and lesions with an intact cortex. A 16-gauge biopsy needle (Quick-Core) is used to sample a soft tissue mass external to bone, but also works well through a 14-gauge bonopty to biopsy a soft tissue mass within bone [68,69].

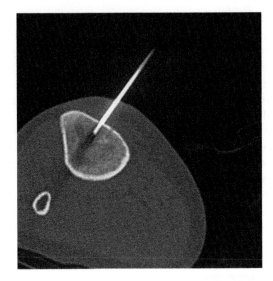

FIGURE 19.38
CT-guided bone biopsy. Axial CT of the proximal tibia shows a bonopty needle system in place for biopsy of permeative lesion. The needle approach is based on compartmental anatomy so not to seed tumor cells or preclude surgical route.

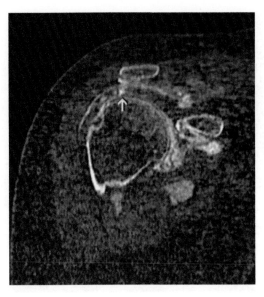

FIGURE 19.39
Rotator cuff tear. CT arthrogram coronal image shows focal area of vertically oriented contrast extending through a full thickness tear of the supraspinatus muscle (arrow).

Core samples should be taken to determine cell type and grade, which are needed for diagnosis of a primary bone tumor. If there are both soft tissue and bone components, both should be sampled. If a lesion is mineralized, sample the least mineralized portion as this usually has highest atypia. It is optimal to use the shortest path between the skin and lesion that avoids neurovascular and joint structures, lung, bowel, and organs. Needle path must be close to the incision and should not traverse an uninvolved compartment, joint, or neurovascular bundle (Figure 19.38).

A recent retrospective review of CT arthrography for suspected intra-articular hip pathology showed 90% sensitivity and 100% specificity for labral tear, 88% sensitivity and 100% specificity for chondrosis of the acetabulum, and 94% sensitivity and 100% specificity in evaluation of femoral chondrosis [71]. In the knee, CT arthrography has been shown to have sensitivity and specificity of 98% and 94%, respectively, for the detection of meniscal abnormalities. The sensitivity and specificity for the detection of unstable meniscal tears has been reported as 97% and 90%, respectively [72].

Ultimately, most centers will continue to use MR arthrography, but radiologists should recognize that CT arthrography is of high accuracy and an option for patients with contraindications to MR.

19.7 CT Arthrography

Although most arthrograms are performed with MRI, there are patients who have contraindications to MRI, such as claustrophobic patients or those with metal implants. MDCT has high accuracy and good interobserver reliability for diagnosis of superior labral anterior-posterior (SLAP) lesions. Sensitivity is 94%–97% and specificity is 72%–77%. Most common false positive or negative results involve differentiation of SLAP type II lesions and a sublabral recess [70]. Excellent correlation has also been shown for use of CT arthrography in diagnosis of rotator cuff tears. Highest sensitivity and specificity are found for supraspinatus and infraspinatus tears. On CT, the presence of the contrast within the normal tendon fibers (Figure 19.39), filling gaps in the articular cartilage, or contour of the labrum suggests a focal tear.

19.8 Infection

About 1.98 million patients have a musculoskeletal infection per year. Rates and severity are higher in inner city hospitals and immunosuppressed patients. Although plain radiographs can detect periosteal reaction, periarticular osteopenia, and erosions, they typically are not positive for at least 7–14 days. Thus, MRI or CT is useful for early detection of infection and prevention of joint destruction. Although MR may provide higher sensitivity and early demonstration of bone marrow edema, it is not often immediately available in the ER, is time consuming, and is more expensive. CT provides analysis of compartmental anatomy, thereby helping to distinguish the various patterns of musculoskeletal infection.

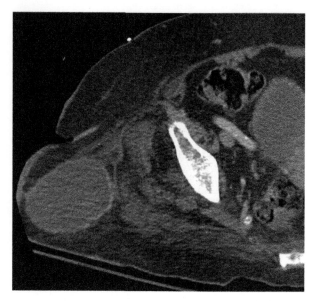

FIGURE 19.40
Abscess. Axial CT in soft tissue window of the right gluteal region shows a rim-enhancing fluid collection in the subcutaneous tissues with mild adjacent stranding of the subcutaneous fat. This was aspirated and cultures were positive for bacterial infection.

Cellulitis is an acute infection of the dermis and subcutaneous tissues usually resulting from disruption of the skin and invasion by microorganisms that may be indigenous flora, such as *Staph aureus*, or exogenous bacteria. CT can be used to distinguish between superficial and deep cellulitis. CT findings include skin thickening, septation of the subcutaneous fat, and thickening of underlying superficial fascia. In deep infections, an abscess may be present. On CT, these appear as well-demarcated fluid collections with rim-enhancing pseudocapsules (Figure 19.40) [73].

Necrotizing fasciitis is a rare, progressive, rapidly spreading infection of the deep fascia with secondary necrosis of the subcutaneous tissues. The condition is a surgical emergency as the mortality rate is 70%–80%, often due to delayed diagnosis. Thus, CT is useful for quick imaging assessment. CT shows gas in the subcutaneous tissues from gas-forming anaerobic organisms, thickening of fascia, fluid collections along deep fascial sheaths, and extension of edema into the intermuscular septa and muscles. Lack of fascial enhancement on CT delineates necrosis from nonemergent forms of fasciitis [73].

Infectious myositis is an infection of skeletal muscle that often only involves a single muscle but can be multifocal in 11%–43% cases. The most common site of involvement is the quadriceps muscle, followed by gluteus and iliopsoas. CT findings include enlargement and decreased attenuation of the affected muscle with effacement of surrounding fat [73].

Osteomyelitis may result from hematogenous spread or direct or contiguous inoculation. Most common sites are the tibia, wrist, femur, ribs, and spine. CT features include periosteal reaction, low-attenuation areas in the medullary canal, trabecular coarsening, and focal cortical erosions. Extramedullary fat–fluid level is a rare but specific sign that indicates cortical breach by the infection. CT is better than MR for chronic osteomyelitis and demonstration of cortical destruction and gas [73].

Finally septic arthritis is an infection that can result in irreversible joint damage within 48 hours of onset of infection. This is due to proteolytic enzymes of the white blood cells that flood the infected synovial space. CT features of septic arthritis include joint effusion, bone erosions, synovitis, and fat–fluid levels.

19.9 Tibial Torsion and Femoral Version

Measurements of femoral version and tibial torsion are important for correcting leg-length discrepancies and performing derotational osteotomy in patients with congenital or posttraumatic abnormalities. Tibial torsion is the anatomic twist of the proximal versus distal articular axis of the tibial bone around the longitudinal axis. Femoral version is the torsion of the proximal femur relative to the distal femur.

CT images should be obtained with the patient supine, feet first, legs flat on the table, as close together as possible. A very long AP plane scout is taken from above the hips to below the ankles. Helical images of 5 mm thickness at 5-mm intervals are obtained. Three small slabs are acquired covering both hips above the femoral heads through the lesser trochanters, the knees just above the femoral physis through the top of the tibias, and just above the syndesmosis of the ankle through the talar dome [74].

Using the method of Jend (Figure 19.41), the section of the proximal tibia is taken immediately distal to the knee joint and proximal to the fibular head. A line of reference is drawn tangent to the dorsal border of the tibia on this slide. In the distal tibia, the section immediately proximal to the talocrural joint is chosen to make a distal line of reference formed by joining the center of a circle fitted to the tibial pilon with the midpoint of a line across the fibular notch of the tibia. An angle between each reference line and the horizontal plane are made. If both angles are pointing in external rotation, then the tibial torsion is equal to the subtraction between them. If the knee is externally rotated and ankle internally rotated, the torsion is the sum of the angles [75–77].

Femoral version is measured by drawing a line in the distal femur as a tangent to the femoral condyles and proximally through the center of the femoral head and

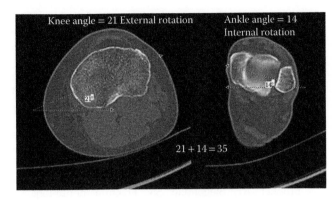

FIGURE 19.41
Tibial torsion. Axial CT images from a CT scanogram show an angle measurement of 21° internal rotation along proximal tibial axis in respect to horizontal. The plafond angle to horizontal is 14° internal rotation. In this case, the angle is additive to result in 35° of external tibial torsion.

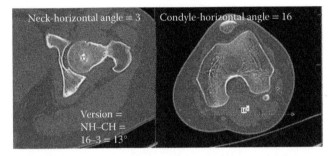

FIGURE 19.42
Femoral anteversion measurements. Axial CT images from a scanogram show the femora neck horizontal angle is 3° anteversion while the condyle to horizontal angle is 16° internal rotation. These are subtracted to give 13° of internal rotation.

neck to the horizontal (Figure 19.42). The angle of the neck relative to the condyles is the anteversion obtained by subtraction. If the femoral condyles are internally rotated, then the angles are added together [75–77].

19.10 Conclusion

CT plays a significant role in imaging of the upper and lower extremities. Most scans are performed for fracture evaluation. Other uses include arthritis, complications of joint replacement, infection, percutaneous biopsy, and leg rotation assessment. The majority of scans do not require administration of intravenous contrast. Additionally, technique can be used to optimize image quality around orthopedic hardware. The future is promising, with use of CT to identify crystals of gout and guide surgical placement of orthopedic hardware.

References

1. Adelaar RS. The treatment of complex fractures of the talus. *Orthop Clin North Am.* 1989 Oct;20(4):691–707.
2. Badillo K, Pacheco JA, Padua SO, Gomez AA, Colon E, Vidal JA. Multidetector CT evaluation of calcaneal fractures. *Radiographics* 2011 Jan–Feb;31(1):81–92.
3. Bahrs C, Rolauffs B, Sudkamp NP et al. Indications for computed tomography (CT-) diagnostics in proximal humeral fractures: a comparative study of plain radiography and computed tomography. *BMC Musculoskeletal Disord.* 2009 Apr 2;10:33.
4. Baumhauer JF, Alvarez RG. Controversies in treating talus fractures. *Orthop Clin North Am.* 1995 Apr;26(2):335–351.
5. Bonin JG. Sacral fractures and injuries to the cauda equina. *J Bone Joint Surg Br.* 1945;27:113–127.
6. Bryce CD, Davison AC, Lewis GS. Two-dimensional glenoid version measurements vary with coronal and sagittal scapular rotation. *J Bone Joint Surg Am.* 2010;92(3):692–699.
7. Buckwalter KA, Rydberg J, Kopecky KK, Crow K, Yan EL. Musculoskeletal imaging with multislice CT. *AJR.* 2001;176(4):979–986.
8. Buckwalter KA, Parr JA, Choplin RH, Capello WN. Multichannel CT imaging of orthopedic hardware and implants. *Semin Musculoskelet Radiol.* 2006;10(1):86–97.
9. Budge MD, Lewis GS, Schaefer E, Coquia S, Flemming DJ, Armstrong AD. Comparison of standard two-dimensional and three-dimensional corrected glenoid version measurements. *J Shoulder Elbow Surg.* 2011;20(4):577–583.
10. Buijze GA, Wijffels MEE, Guitton TG et al. Interobserver reliability of computed tomography to diagnose scaphoid waist fracture union. *J Hand Surg.* 2012;37(2):250–254.
11. Chai JW, Hong SH, Choi JY et al. Radiologic diagnosis of osteoid osteoma: from simple to challenging findings. *Radiographics* 2010;30(3):737–749.
12. Chang KP, Center JR, Nguyen TV, Eisman JA. Incidence of hip and other osteoporotic fractures in elderly men and women: Dubbo osteoporosis epidemiology study. *J Bone Miner Res.* 2004;19(4):532–536.
13. Chesbrough RM. Strategic approach fends off charges of malpractice: program provides tips for avoiding litigation. *Diagn Imaging.* 2002;24:44–51.
14. Cobb JP, Dixon H, Dandachli W, Iranpour F. The anatomical tibial axis reliable rotational orientation in knee replacement. *J Bone Joint Surg Br.* 2008;90(8):1032–1038.
15. Crim JR, Kjeldsberg. Radiographic diagnosis of tarsal coalition. *AJR.* 2004 Feb;182(2):323–328.
16. Daftary A, Haims AH, Baumgaertner MR. Fractures of the calcaneus: a review with emphasis on CT. *Radiographics* 2005;25(5):1215–1226.
17. Denis F, Davis S, Comfort T. Sacral fractures: an important problem. Retrospective analysis of 236 cases. *Clin Orthop Relat Res.* 1988;227:67–81.
18. Desai MA, Peterson JJ, Garner HW, Kransdorf MJ. Clinical utility of dual-energy CT for evaluation of tophaceous gout. *Radiographics* 2011;31(5):1365–1375.

19. Dorsey ML, Liu PT, Roberts CC, Kile TA. Correlation of arthrodesis stability with degree of joint fusion on MDCT. *AJR.* 2009;192(2):496–499.

20. Durkee NJ, Jacobson J, Jamadar D, Karunakar MA, Morag Y, Hayes C. Classification of common acetabular fractures: radiographic and CT appearance. *AJR.* 2006;187(4):915–925.

21. Espinosa LA, Jamadar DA, Jacbson JA et al. CT-Guided biopsy of bone: a radiolgists's perspective. *AJR.* 2008;190(5):W283–W289.

22. Fayad LM, Johnson P, Fishman EK. Multidetector CT of musculoskeletal disease in the pediatric patient: principles, techniques, and clinical applications. *Radiographics* 2005;25(3):603–618.

23. Fayad LM, Carrino JA, Fishman EK. Musculoskeletal infection: role of CT in the emergency department. *Radiographics* 2007;27(6):1723–1736.

24. Gerster JC, Landry M, Dufresne L, Meuwly JY. Imaging of tophaceous gout: computed tomography provides specific images compared with magnetic resonance imaging and ultrasonography. *Ann Rehum Dis.* 2002;61(1):52–54.

25. Goss TP. Scapular fractures and dislocations. Diagnosis and treatment. *J Am Acad Orthop Surg.* 1995;3(1):22–33.

26. Griffith JF, Antonio GE, Yung PSH et al. Prevalence, pattern, and spectrum of glenoid bone loss in anterior shoulder dislocation: CT analysis in 218 patients. *AJR.* 2008;190(5):1247–1254.

27. Haapamaki VV, Kiuru MJ, Koskinen SK. Multidetector CT in shoulder fractures. *Emerg Radiol.* 2004;11(2):89–94.

28. Haapamaki VV, Kiuru MJ, Koskinen SK. Ankle and foot injuries: analysis of MDCT findings. *Am J Roentgenol.* 2004;183(3):615–622.

29. Hernandez RJ, Tachdjian MO, Poznanski AK, Dias LS. CT determination of femoral torsion. *AJR.* 1981;137(1):97–101.

30. Hoenecke JR, Hermida JC, Flores-Hernandez C, D'Lima DD. Accuracy of CT-based measurements of glenoid version for total shoulder arthroplasty. *J Shoulder Elbow Surg.* 2010;19(2):166–171.

31. Insall JN, Scuderi GR, Komistek RD, Math K, Dennis DA, Anderson DT. Correlation between condylar lift-off and femoral component alignment. *Clin Orthop Relat Res.* 2002;(403):143–152.

32. Isler B. Lumbosacral lesions associated with pelvic ring injuries. *J Orthop Trauma.* 1990;4(1):1–6.

33. Johnell O, Kanis J. Epidemiology of osteoporotic fractures. *Osteoporos Int.* 2005;16:S3–S7.

34. Kaewlai R, Avery LL, Asrani AV, Abujudeh HH, Sacknoff R, Novelline RA. Multidetector CT of carpal injuries: anatomy, fractures, and fracture-dislocations. *Radiographics* 2008;28(6):1771–1784.

35. Kalia V, Fishman EK, Carrion J, Fayad LM. Epidemiology, imaging, and treatment of Lisfranc fracture-diloscations revisited. *Skeletal Radiol.* 2012;41(2):129–136.

36. Kessler O, Lacatusu E, Sommers MB, Mayr E, Bottlang M. Malrotation in total knee arthroplasty: effect on tibial cortex strain captured by laser based strain acquisition. *Clin Biomech. (Bristol, Avon)* 2006;21(6):603–609.

37. Kilcoyne RF, Shuman WP, Matsen FA 3rd, Morris M, Rockwood CA. The Neer classification of displaced proximal humeral fractures: spectrum of findings on plain radiographs and CT scans. *AJR.* 1990;154(5):1029–1033.

38. Kim YJ, Choi JA, Oh JH, Hwang SI, Hong SH, Kang HS. Superior labral anteroposterior tears: accuracy and interobserver reliability of multidetector CT arthrography for diagnosis. *Radiology* 2011;260(1):207–215.

39. Krestan CR, Noske H, Vasilevska V et al. MDCT Versus digital radiograph in the evaluation of bone healing in orthopedic patients. *AJR.* 2006;186(6):1754–1780.

40. Kuhlman JE, Fishman EK, Magid D, Scott WW Jr, Brooker AF, Siegelman SS. Fracture nonunion: Ct assessment with multiplanar reconstruction. *Radiology* 1988;167(2):483–488.

41. Letournel E. Acetabulum fractures: classification and management. *ClinOrthop Rel Res.* 1980;151:81–106.

42. Liporace FA, Yoon RS, Kubiak EK et al. Does adding computed tomography change the diagnosis and treatment of tilleaux and triplane pediatric ankle fractures. *Orthopedics* 2012;35:2e208–2e212.

43. Looney RJ, Boyd A, Totterman S et al. Volumetric computerized tomography as a measurement of periprosthetic acetabular osteolysis and its correlation with wear. *Arthritis Res.* 2002;4(1):59–63.

44. Lowery RBW. Fractures of the talus and calcaneus. *Curr Opin Orthop.* 1994;5:24–32.

45. Lozano-Calderon S, Blazar P, Zurakowski D, Lee SG, Ring D. Diagnosis of scaphoid fracture displacement with radiography and computed tomography. *J Bone Joint Surg.* 2006;88(12):2695–2703.

46. Lubovsky O, Liebergall M, Mattan Y, Weil Y, Mosheiff R. Early diagnosis of occult hip fractures MRI versus CT scan. *Injury* 2005;36(6):788–792.

47. Lutzner J, Krummenauer F, Gunther KP, Kirschner S. Rotational alignment of the tibial component in total knee arthroplasty is better at the medial third of tibial tuberosity than at the medial border. *BMC Musculoskelet Disord.* 2010;11:57.

48. Manaster BJ. From the RSNA refresher courses. Total hip arthroplasty: radiographic evaluation. *Radiographics* 1996;16(3):645–660.

49. Markhardt BK, Gross JM, Monu JU. Schatzker classification of tibial plateau fractures: use of CT and MR imaging improves assessment. *Radiographics* 2009;29(2):585–597.

50. Mehta S, Auerbach JD, Born CT, Chin KR. Sacral fractures. *J Am Acad Orthop Surg.* 2006;14(12):656–665.

51. Moon SK, Park JS, Jin W, Ryu KN. CT Findings of traumatic posterior hip dislocation after reduction. *J Korean Radiol Soc.* 2008;58:617–622.

52. Mui LW, Engelsohn E, Umans H. Comparison of CT and MRI in patients with tibial plateau fracture: can CT findings predict ligament tear or meniscal injury? *Skeletal Radiol.* 2007;36(2):145–151.

53. Mustonen AO, Koskinen SK, Kiuru MJ. Acute knee trauma: analysis of multidetector computed tomography findings and comparison with conventional radiography. *Acta Radiol.* 2005;46(8):866–874.

54. Newman JS, Newberg AH. Congenital Tarsal coalition: multimodality evaluation with emphasis on CT and MR imaging. *Radiographics* 2000;20(2):321–332.

55. Nicolaou S, Yong-Hing CJ, Galea-Soler S, Hou DJ, Louis L, Munk P. Dual energy CT as a potential new diagnostic tool in the managemetn of gout in the acute setting. *AJR.* 2010;194(4):1072–1078.

56. Ohashi K, El-Khoury GY. Musculoskeletal CT: recent advances and current clinical applications. *Radiol Clin N Am.* 2009;47(3):387–409.

57. Ohashi K, El-Khoury GY, Bennett DL. MDCT of tendon abnormalities using volume-rendered images. *AJR.* 2004;182(1):161–165.

58. Rosenthal D, Callstrom MR. Critical review and state of the art in interventional oncology: benign and metastatic disease involving bone. *Radiology* 2012;262(3):765–780.

59. Tanner DA, Kloseck M, Crilly RG, Chesworth B, Gilliland J. Hip fracture types in men and women change differently with age. *BMC Geriatr.* 2010;10:12.

60. Schneider B, Laubenberg J, Jemlich S, Groene K, Weber HM, Langer M. Measurement of femoral antetorsion and tibial torsion by magnetic resonance imaging. *Br J Radiol.* 1997;70(834):575–579.

61. Stiell IG, Greenberg GH, Wells GA et al. Prospective validation of a decision rule for the use of radiography in acute knee injuries. *JAMA.* 1996;275(8):611–615.

62. Stiell IG, Greenberg GH, Wells GA et al. Derivation of a decision rule for the use of radiography in acute knee injuries. *Ann Emerg Med.* 1995;26(4):405–413.

63. Stuberg W, Temme J, Kaplan P, Clarke A, Fuchs R. Measurement of tibial torsion and tight-foot angle using goniometry and computed tomography. *Clin Orthop Relat Res.* 1991;272:208–212.

64. Tadros AM, Lunsjo K, Czechowski J, Corr P, Abu-Zidan FM. Usefulness of different imaging modalities in the assessment of scapular fractures caused by blunt trauma. *Acta Radiol.* 2007;48(1):71–75.

65. Temple CL, Ross DC, Bennett JD, Garvin GJ, King GJ, Faber KJ. Comparison of sagittal computed tomography and plain film radiography in a scaphoid fracture model. *J Hand Surg.* 2005;30(3):534–542.

66. Verma A, Su A, Golin AM, O'Marrah B, Amorosa JK. A screening method for knee trauma. *Acad Radiol.* 2001;8(5):392–327.

67. Watura R, Cobby M, Taylor J. Multislice CT in imaging of trauma of the spine, pelvis, and complex foot injuries. *Br J Radiol.* 2004;77:S46–S63.

68. Wechsler RJ, Schweitzer ME, Karasick D, Deely DM, Glaser JB. Helical CT of talar fractures. *Skeletal Radiol.* 1997;26(3):137–142.

69. Welling RD, Jacobson JA, Jamadar DA, Chong S, Caoili EM, Jebson PJ. MDCT and radiography of wrist fractures: radiographic sensitivity and fracture patterns. *AJR.* 2008;190(1):10–16.

70. Wicky S, Blaser PF, Blanc CH, Leyvraz PF, Schnyder P, Meuli RA. Comparison between standard radiography and spiral CT with 3D reconstruction in the evaluation, classification and management of tibial plateau fractures. *Eur Radiol.* 2000;10(8):1227–1232.

71. Young JW, Burgess AR, Brumback RJ, Poka A. Pelvic fractures: value of plain radiography in early assessment and management. *Radiology* 1986;160(2):445–451.

20

Pathology of the Muscles and Soft Tissues

Mohamed Jarraya, Daichi Hayashi, Ali Guermazi, and Frank Roemer

CONTENTS

20.1 Introduction

Compared to magnetic resonance imaging (MRI) and ultrasound, computed tomography (CT) has method-inherent disadvantages in visualizing soft tissue pathology and thus may not necessarily be the first choice for imaging soft tissue pathology. However, its widespread availability, multiplanar reconstruction (MPR) possibilities due to isotropic image acquisition, speed of examination, and excellent patient tolerance make it probably the most important imaging tool in daily clinical practice [1].

After a brief review of technical considerations, we will describe the main commonly encountered soft tissue pathologies in which CT may have an impact in the initial diagnosis and overall management.

CT certainly is the primary diagnostic method in suspected acute hemorrhage as it is rapidly and widely available and is capable of visualizing active bleeding. In addition, it has an important role in characterizing soft tissue lesions. CT may provide a comprehensive assessment of these lesions including detailed visualization of matrix mineralization and the patterns of cortical and marrow involvement [1–3]. The role of CT in the diagnosis and in the differential diagnosis of ossifying tumors and pseudotumors will be discussed. For juxtaosseous lesions, CT provides useful information on the lesions' growth rate by analyzing the detailed structure of cortical bone and bone marrow. For lipomatous lesions, CT provides valuable clues in regard to anatomical locations and tissue involvement and helps differentiate benign from malignant lesions. CT helps distinguish the involvement of different anatomical structures in soft tissue infection, and it is an important guide in treatment planning.

20.2 Technical Considerations

Advanced multi-detector CT (MDCT), with its very fast image-acquisition time of large volumes and submillimetric section thickness, has become the norm in the clinical routine. Isotropic data sets and thin-section scanning allow for different types of postprocessing, such as MPRs, minimum intensity projections (MIPs), and volume rendering technique, which can provide comprehensive information about the internal architecture of a mass, as well as its shape and anatomical relationships. While noncontrast images provide information on tissue densities and mineralization patterns, contrast-enhanced scans give important clues on the vascularization of a specific lesion. Typically, contrast material is administered at a rate of 2–4 mL/s with a typical scan delay of 30–80 seconds to characterize vascularization of a lesion [1]. Serial acquisitions, including nonenhanced, early (arterial), portal venous, and late scans may be necessary especially in the evaluation of acute hemorrhage. Two dimensional MPRs and MIPs are commonly applied in CT angiography. Dual-source CT offers improved temporal resolution and allows for tissue characterization applying image acquisition at dual energies [4]. This feature has recently been shown to be effective for the detection and characterization of

urate deposits, helping to identify subclinical tophus deposits [5]. Additionally, CT is commonly used to guide biopsy of soft tissue tumors.

20.3 Muscular Hematomas

Hematomas of skeletal muscle are observed either after a trauma or spontaneously. Spontaneous hemorrhage is commonly seen in patients with coagulopathy (hemophilia in particular), ruptured aneurysms, or in those receiving anticoagulant treatment or as a postangiographic complication. Iliopsoas and rectus abdominis muscles are major and well-documented sites of spontaneous muscle hemorrhage, especially in patients on anticoagulation therapy [6–8].

In early stages, the diagnosis of acute intramuscular hematoma is usually straightforward on CT. Acute hematoma is easily recognized as a collection of high-attenuation density, enlarging the muscle, and contained within well-defined borders, tracking between but not through fascial planes (Figure 20.1). Occasional fluid–fluid levels may be seen, corresponding to areas of erythrocyte sedimentation. Injection of contrast media may detect focal contrast extravasation, indicating active hemorrhage (Figure 20.2). Moreover, MDCT angiography is often necessary for preembolization planning. With time, the hematoma becomes progressively less dense, and CT findings become less specific. Although historical and physical examination findings remain important, relying on clinical history and ancillary imaging studies only may fail to provide a specific diagnosis. Indeed, chronic hematomas can be easily confused with an abscess or necrotic masses, such as high-grade sarcomas [9]. In such cases, only percutaneous aspiration permits differentiation of hematomas from other

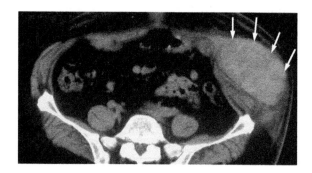

FIGURE 20.1
Spontaneous hemorrhage of the lateral abdominal wall in a 60-year-old man under anticoagulation therapy. Axial unenhanced computed tomography (CT) image displays a large hyperdense hematoma in the left lateral abdominal wall (arrows).

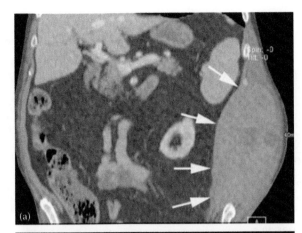
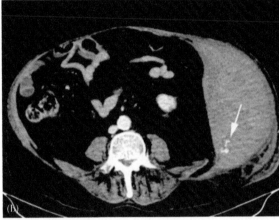

FIGURE 20.2
Spontaneous extraperitoneal hematoma of the lateral abdominal wall under anticoagulation therapy in a 53-year-old man. (a) Coronal reformation of contrast-enhanced CT scan shows extensive hematoma in the left lateral abdominal wall pushing the peritoneum and intra-abdominal organs to the right (large arrows). (b) Axial contrast-enhanced CT image shows focal contrast extravasation indicating active hemorrhage at the time of image acquisition (small arrow).

20.4 Tumors and Tumor-Like Lesions

Soft tissue tumors arise from the mesenchyme, which differentiates during embryonic and fetal development to become fat, skeletal muscle, peripheral nerves, blood vessels, and fibrous tissue [10]. Soft tissue tumors are histologically classified according to the soft tissue component that comprises the lesion [10,11]. On this basis, the World Health Organization (WHO) classification distinguishes nine groups of soft tissue tumors (adipocytic, fibroblastic/myofibroblastic, so-called fibrohistiocytic, smooth muscle, pericytic, skeletal muscle, vascular, chondro-osseous, uncertain differentiation) [12]. Some of these tumors will be highlighted here due to the role CT has in the diagnostic process. We will focus

on adipocytic tumors and hemangiomas for their relatively high prevalence and their typical patterns of CT imaging appearance. Chondro-osseous tumors and myositis ossificans, which are classified as a fibroblastic/myofibroblastic tumor, will also be covered.

20.4.1 Lipomatous Tumors

20.4.1.1 Lipomas

Lipomas are composed of mature fat cells and are often difficult to differentiate from surrounding fatty tissue. They usually present as circumscribed, encapsulated masses. They are most commonly located in the subcutaneous tissue. Superficial lipomas are usually well-circumscribed and small with a greatest diameter <5 cm. They are commonly located in the upper back and neck, shoulder, abdomen, and proximal portion of the extremities. Lipomas are well-vascularized, but this feature may not be readily apparent, owing to vascular compression due to the distended adipocytes [13]. Other mesenchymatous elements, such as fibrous tissue, cartilage, bone, myxoid tissue, and smooth muscle may be present, giving rise to a wide range of histologic variants, such as fibrolipoma, myxolipoma, myolipoma, angiomyolipoma, chondroid lipoma, and osteolipoma [13].

A typical lipoma presents as a homogenous mass of fat density measuring −130 to −70 HU, and does not show any enhancement on CT after intravenous (IV) contrast administration (Figure 20.3). Regular thin septations can appear as strands of soft tissue density. Their width may be unmeasurable. A nonlipomatous component can alter the typical CT appearance, making the differential diagnosis with well-differentiated liposarcoma sometimes complicated.

Heterotopic lipomas develop in association with tissue other than adipose. Examples include intramuscular, intermuscular, tendon sheath, joint, and parosteal lipomas.

20.4.1.1.1 Intramuscular Lipoma

Intramuscular lipoma is commonly seen in patients over 40 years of age and involves the muscles of the extremities (thigh, trunk, shoulder, and upper arm) [13]. The quadriceps is the most commonly affected muscle, followed by the deltoid [14]. Usually, the clinical picture is one of a painless slow-growing mass. In contrast to its subcutaneous counterpart, which is encapsulated and easily removable, intramuscular lipoma tends to infiltrate surrounding tissue. For this reason, it is sometimes referred to as "infiltrating lipoma." Indeed, during surgery, this lesion is more commonly found to be attached or infiltrated into

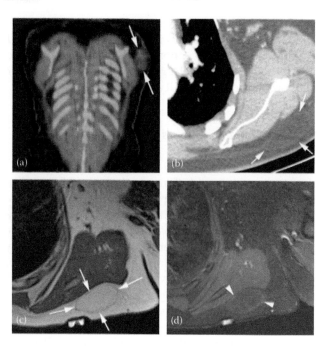

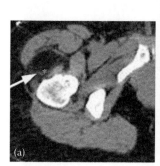

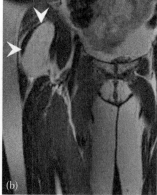

FIGURE 20.4
Intramuscular lipoma of the gluteus minimus in a 45-year-old man. (a) Axial unenhanced CT image shows a fat-isodense (asterisk) mass arising from the gluteus minimus muscle with a streak of soft tissue within the lesion (arrow). (b) Coronal T_1-weighted MRI depicts a fat-isointense uninodular mass (arrowheads).

FIGURE 20.3
Posterior thoracic wall lipoma in a 61-year-old woman with a lipoma of the right thigh. The initial tumor was resected, and the patient presented for restaging 6 months later. (a) 18F-fluorodeoxyglucose (FDG) positron emission tomography (PET) shows mild glucose accumulation in subcutaneous soft tissue in the left scapular region (arrows). (b) Contrast-enhanced axial CT image shows fat-isodense lesion in the posterior subcutaneous tissue adjacent to teres minor muscle (arrows). No apparent enhancing solid or nodular parts of lesion are depicted. (c) Additional T_1-weighted non-enhanced magnetic resonance imaging (MRI) shows fat-isointense lesion (arrows). (d) T_1-weighted contrast-enhanced fat-suppressed image depicts very mild peripheral enhancement (arrowheads). Based on these imaging findings, a definite diagnosis could not be established. Total surgical excision was performed and histologic and immunologic assessment showed no evidence of malignancy.

20.4.1.1.2 Intermuscular Lipomas

Intermuscular lipoma is less frequent than its intramuscular counterpart and may be grossly defined as a deep-seated lipoma arising between muscular layers, without involvement of muscle fibers or tendency to invade the surrounding tissue [14]. Although intermuscular and intramuscular lipomas are similar in regard to age distribution and location, with quadriceps and deltoid most commonly affected, the distinction between these lesions may be helpful for surgical planning since intermuscular lipomas are less infiltrating and thus more easily resected [14]. The typical CT appearance is one of a fat density mass, separating muscular layers, with thin dense streaks, along the central fat, consisting of fibrous tissue of the intermuscular space. These streaky structures are continuous and of relatively uniform thickness, in contrast to those displayed by intramuscular lipoma, which are of varying thickness and discontinuous [14].

20.4.1.1.3 Parosteal Lipoma

Although parosteal lipoma is extremely rare and represents only 0.3% of all lipomas [13,15], its imaging appearance is characteristic. Parosteal lipoma is contiguous with underlying periosteum and shows, typically, a broad-based attachment to the subjacent bone [13]. The lesion is often well-encapsulated except at the site of adherence to bone. The usual age of diagnosis is between 40 and 60 years. The most frequent sites are the arm, forearm, thigh, and calf, adjacent to the diaphysis and metaphyseal junction. Parosteal lipomas are usually slow growing, large masses, generally asymptomatic, measuring up to 20 cm [13]. Occasional osseous changes at the site of attachment, such as bone projections, cortical erosions, and periosteal reaction, may be seen on plain radiographs [13]. The most common osseous manifestation is an irregular osseous excrescence into the soft

the surrounding tissue, making its release difficult, and which increases the risk of recurrence [14]. The size varies greatly from less than 3 cm to more than 20 cm.

On CT, intramuscular lipomas are round or fusiform and rarely dumbbell-shaped. They are most commonly well-defined but may display infiltrative margins [13]. The central fat density is usually accompanied by streaks of soft tissue density, corresponding to either muscle or fibrous tissue (Figure 20.4) [13]. These streaky structures may be interrupted, and their thickness is variable. They are reported to be more distinctive on CT scans than on MRI [14] and demonstrate no enhancement in most cases. Nonetheless, the absence of contrast enhancement is better analyzed on MRI. Uninodularity and absence of contrast enhancement suggest benignity but are not 100% reliable [14]. Table 20.1 shows differential diagnostic criteria that may help to distinguish intramuscular lipoma from intermuscular lipoma and low-grade liposarcoma.

TABLE 20.1

Differential Diagnostic Criteria between Lipoma and Liposarcoma

	Lipoma	Intramuscular Lipoma	Intermuscular Lipoma	Well-Differentiated Liposarcoma
Location	Subcutaneous fat (back, shoulder, neck, arm, thigh, abdomen)	Within muscle (thigh, shoulder, arm)	Between muscle fasciae (thigh, shoulder, arm)	Within muscle or interfascial (thigh, retroperitoneum)
Size	<5 cm (80%) <10 cm (95%)	Frequently >5 cm		Rarely <5 cm
Margins	Well-defined	Infiltrating/well-defined	Well-defined	Usually well-defined
Shape	Uninodular	Uninodular (>85%)	Lobulated	Multinodular
Septa or nodules	Absent or <2 mm	Discontinuous streaks of variable thickness	Thin, regular, and continuous streaks	Thick (>2 mm), linear or nodular streaks
Enhancement	No	No/faint	No/faint	Strong

Source: Data from Nishida J et al., *J Orthop Sci.*, 12(6):533–541, 2007 and Cotten A, *JBRBTR*, 85(1):14–19, 2002.

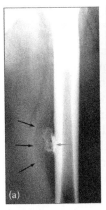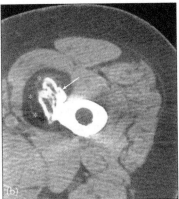

FIGURE 20.5
Parosteal lipoma in a 42-year-old man. (a) Anteroposterior radiograph of the femur demonstrates a bony protuberance (gray arrow) at the surface of the shaft of the femur surrounded by a radiolucent halo (black arrows). (b) Axial CT scan of the femur confirms lipomatous (asterisks) and ossific (white arrow) components of the lesion.

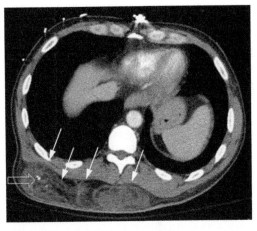

FIGURE 20.7
Subcutaneous liposarcoma in a 28-year-old man presenting with pain after falling from a ladder. Axial contrast-enhanced MDCT image shows an expansive subcutaneous, fat-containing mass (arrows), with soft tissue–equivalent streaks and calcifications (empty arrow).

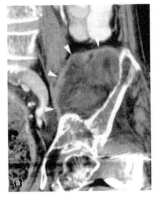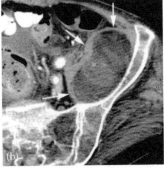

FIGURE 20.6
Intramuscular well-differentiated liposarcoma in a 50-year-old man. (a) Coronal contrast-enhanced multi-detector CT (MDCT) image shows an inhomogeneous, fat-containing, expansive mass adjacent to the left iliac crest (arrowheads). (b) Axial image clearly shows intramuscular location within iliac muscle (arrows) and enhancement of intralesional thick streaks (asterisk). Diagnosis was histologically confirmed and the lesion was resected.

tissue with variable width of base. CT demonstrates, typically, a well-marginated mass of fat attenuation, delineating clearly the bony excrescences and the adjacent bony cortex (Figure 20.5). Ossification and fibrocartilage foci with enchondral ossification may be present, resulting in an osteochondromatous appearance. The lack of medullary continuity into the osseous outgrowth differentiates this entity from osteochondroma [13].

20.4.1.2 Liposarcoma

Liposarcoma is the second most common soft tissue sarcoma, accounting for 10% to 18% of all malignant soft tissue tumors [13,16]. Liposarcoma commonly arises in the fifth and sixth decades and is preponderant in men. The clinical manifestation depends more on location than histological type. Well-differentiated liposarcoma and myxoid liposarcoma are the two most frequent types [13]. Liposarcoma usually presents as a well-circumscribed, lobulated, and painless mass, growing over the years until reaching a very large size. Pain or functional disturbances are very late complaints. Liposarcomas occur more commonly in deep structures than in the subcutaneous fat [13]. The extremities are most commonly affected, especially the thigh, followed by retroperitoneum. The prognosis depends on the histologic type. The imaging features are extremely variable and also depend on the histological type. About 50% of liposarcomas do not have any detectable fat on imaging [17]. For this reason, the appearance of liposarcomas on CT is frequently nonspecific.

20.4.1.2.1 Well-Differentiated Liposarcoma

Well-differentiated liposarcoma grossly resembles lipoma. Although the amount of radiologically identifiable fat is variable, a well-differentiated liposarcoma is frequently composed of more than 75% of fat, while the more dedifferentiated types contain less than 25% [18]. On CT, it presents as a well-marginated mass with attenuation values equal to those of simple fat, with some thickened (more than 2 mm wide), linear or nodular, soft tissue septae, which enhance after IV administration of contrast material (Figures 20.6 and 20.7) [19]. Calcifications may be seen and are more common in this subtype than other variants of liposarcoma [19]. Intramuscular lipoma is the main differential diagnosis (see Table 20.1).

20.4.1.2.2 Dedifferentiated Liposarcoma

Although dedifferentiated liposarcoma has no specific presentation that distinguishes it from well-differentiated liposarcoma, this subtype may be suspected when a nonlipomatous component appears, in a previously known, well-differentiated liposarcoma [13].

FACTS TO REMEMBER

- The diagnosis of a simple lipoma is usually straightforward on CT images.
- Lipomas containing mesenchymal elements other than fatty tissue (such as fibrolipoma, myxolipoma, etc.) are difficult to distinguish from well-differentiated liposarcomas on both CT and magnetic resonance images.
- Benign intramuscular lipomas may show infiltrative margins.
- The most important imaging features that help differentiate a benign lipomatous tumor from a liposarcoma are location (superficial vs. deep), size, internal composition (presence of thick nonlipomatous septa or nodules), contrast-enhancement pattern, and shape of the lesion (uninodular vs. multinodular).

20.4.1.2.3 Other Types of Liposarcomas

Myxoid liposarcoma, as well as round cell and pleomorphic liposarcomas, may contain little or no fat [19] and are difficult to diagnose on imaging. Myxoid liposarcoma may manifest as a mass that is less attenuating than the surrounding muscle, sometimes cystic [13]. Pleomorphic and round cell liposarcomas are very difficult to distinguish from other sarcomas, using both CT and MRI [13].

20.4.2 Peripheral Nerve Sheath Tumors

20.4.2.1 Benign Nerve Sheath Tumors

Benign nerve sheath tumors are subdivided into two different morphological groups with different histopathological features: schwannoma and neurofibroma.

20.4.2.1.1 Schwannoma

Schwannomas represent approximately 5% of benign soft tissue neoplasms [21]. They may occur at all ages and are most prevalent between 20 and 50 years. Sporadic occurrences are common. The most common topographical locations of schwannomas include the spinal root, the cervical plexus, and the vagus, peroneal, and ulnar nerves [21,22]. Small schwannomas may be asymptomatic, but signs of nerve or nerve root compression are possible when the lesion reaches a sufficient size. Nonenhanced CT scans show well-circumscribed homogenous lesions, which are hypo- to isodense relative to muscle. However, inhomogeneous appearance with low-density portions is frequently seen in larger tumors. As a rule, there are usually no hyperdense parts of schwannomas [21,23,24]. On contrast-enhanced scans, most schwannomas become iso- or hyperdense relative to muscle. Nonenhancing cystic or necrotic areas are found in large schwannomas and are a valuable element in the differentiation of neurofibromas, malignant peripheral nerve sheath tumors (MPNSTs), and enlarged lymph nodes [24].

20.4.2.1.2 Neurofibromas

Three types of neurofibromas are usually described: localized, diffuse, and plexiform. The localized type is the most common. It is not associated with neurofibromatosis type 1 (NF1), and occurs between 20 and 30 years of age [25]. The diffuse type is uncommon and affects primarily children. Plexiform neurofibromas are pathognomonic of NF1 and usually develop in early childhood [21]. CT displays hypodense lesions with occasional hyperdense central areas (target sign), which corresponds to dense bands of collagen tissue, produced by fibroblasts [23]. On enhanced CT scans, neurofibromas usually do not show enhancement but may display a cloudy area of enhancement in some cases [21,24]. Retroperitoneal plexiform neurofibromas have characteristic features. They are typically bilateral, symmetric low-attenuation masses in the parapsoas or presacral location [21]. Asymmetry in size suggests the possibility of a malignant tumor of the nerve sheath [26].

20.4.2.2 Malignant Peripheral Nerve Sheath Tumors

MPNSTs represent about 6% of all malignant soft tissue tumors [16]. They may occur sporadically, with no sex predominance. However, in up to 50% of the tumors, NF1 is associated. In this case, MPNST is four times more frequent in men than in women [27]. MPSNT typically affect the large nerves of the neck and proximal extremities (including the sciatic nerve, brachial plexus, and sacral plexus), as well as the retroperitoneum, mediastinum, and viscera [28]. Clinically, MPSNT present as enlarging masses. Sudden enlargement of a preexisting neurofibroma in the setting of NF1 should be viewed with a great suspicion of malignant transformation and lead to immediate diagnostic workup [21]. Metastases ensue within 2 years of the diagnosis and are most common in the lung [29].

CT is of little help in demonstrating the malignant nature of MPSNT. CT displays some common findings with other neurogenic tumors: fusiform shape and the longitudinal orientation along the parent nerve. Criteria that help in establishing the diagnosis of MPSNT are a large mass, inhomogeneity in texture, ill-defined margins, invasion of fat planes, perilesional edema, irregular bone destruction, involvement of lymph nodes, and pleural effusion [21].

FACTS TO REMEMBER

- Tumors of the peripheral nerves comprise schwannomas, neurofibromas, and MPNSTs.
- Imaging findings suggestive of neurogenic tumors are fusiform shape, low attenuation on CT, entering and exiting nerve roots, and target sign.
- Criteria that can be of help in establishing the diagnosis of MPNSTs include a large mass (>5 cm), inhomogeneous tumor architecture (due to areas of necrosis and hemorrhagic foci), ill-defined margins, perilesional edema, heterogeneous enhancement, irregular bone destruction, and involvement of lymph nodes.
- Schwannomas, neurofibromas, and MPNST can all occur in patients with neurofibromatosis.

20.4.3 Extraskeletal Chondro-Osseous Tumors

20.4.3.1 Benign Extraskeletal Chondro-Osseous Tumors

20.4.3.1.1 Soft Tissue Chondroma

Soft tissue chondroma usually presents as a small, well-defined nodule that is composed of focal areas of cartilage without any attachment to bone. It is distinct from other lesions containing cartilage such as lipoma with metaplastic cartilage. Soft tissue chondroma may be seen in patients of any age although it is most common in the third through sixth decade [30]. Distal extremities (i.e., hands and feet) are, by far, most frequently affected [31]. This predilection in topography has raised the hypothesis that repeated microtrauma is probably a provoking factor [31]. Grossly, soft tissue chondromas present as well-demarcated and lobulated lesions, seldom exceeding 2 to 3 cm in the greatest dimension [31,32]. Focal fibrosis, ossification, and myxoid changes are possible, as well as focal hemorrhage and granuloma formation [32]. Older lesions may contain diffuse calcifications, predominantly at the center of the nodule [32,33]. Patients usually present with a slowly growing mass with pain and tenderness [30]. On palpation, the chondroma is usually firm and mobile. Local surgical resection is the treatment of choice, but recurrences may be seen in 15% to 25% of the cases [30,32,34].

Soft tissue chondroma appears on CT as a well-demarcated soft tissue mass. Calcifications are observed in 33% to 77% of cases [30,32,35]. Calcifications are most typically curvilinear, outlining the soft tissue lobules [32]. Punctate or mixed punctuate and curvilinear pattern may also be observed [30,31]. Secondary osseous changes of the adjacent bone, such as reactive cortical sclerosis, have been reported [30,31].

Clinical and radiologic features that help in establishing a diagnosis of extraskeletal chondroma are the small size of the lesion despite its long history, its characteristic location in a distal extremity, and the nature of its calcification, as described above. The diagnosis, however, must be confirmed by histopathologic examination.

20.4.3.1.2 Extraskeletal Osteoma

Extraskeletal osteoma is an extremely rare benign lesion that consists of mature lamellar bone, containing a Haversian system and bone marrow. It nearly always occurs in the head, usually in the posterior portion of the tongue [32]. Symptoms are related to the mass effect of the lesion. Conventional radiography and CT show a densely ossified mass with mature osseous architecture in the soft tissues [36]. Surgical treatment seems to be curative [32].

20.4.3.2 *Extraskeletal Osteosarcoma*

Extraskeletal osteosarcoma is a rare, malignant mesenchymal neoplasm that produces osteoid, bone, or chondroid material and is located in the soft tissue without attachment to the skeleton. It represents approximately 1.2% of all soft tissue sarcomas [37]. The pathogenesis is poorly understood, mainly because of the rarity of the tumor. Mechanical injury has been suggested as a causative agent [38,39]. The occurrence of extraskeletal osteosarcoma in the setting of myositis ossificans is controversial, in spite of the published reports; most of them are poorly documented [40,41]. Nonetheless, radiation-induced extraskeletal osteosarcoma is a well-recognized entity that may appear 4 years or more after radiotherapy [41].

Unlike osteosarcomas of bone, which occur mainly during the first two decades of life, the mean age of diagnosis of extraskeletal osteosarcoma varies between 47 and 54 years [37,42]. Generally, the tumor presents as a progressively enlarging soft tissue mass, fixed to the underlying tissues, and painful in about one-third of the patients [41]. The duration of symptoms varies from a few weeks to several months, with a mean of 6 months [37]. Most common locations are the muscles of the thigh and retroperitoneum, followed by the large muscles of the pelvic and shoulder girdles [41]. The prognosis of this tumor is poor. Indeed, the majority of the patients succumb to metastatic growth within a period of 2 or 3 years after the initial diagnosis [41,43]. The most common sites of metastases are lung, lymph nodes, bone, and soft tissue [41].

Imaging findings consist of a soft tissue mass with spotty to massive calcifications, depending on the amount of mineralization, and no evidence of bone involvement. On conventional radiography and CT, calcifications are present in about half of the cases [44]. CT is superior to radiography for the detection of small amounts of calcification and determination of the degree of mineralization. The spatial distribution of mineralization is an important feature on CT: greatest at the center and least at the periphery, whereas the opposite is true for myositis ossificans. Additionally, CT provides good visualization of necrosis within the tumor and CT angiography may show hypervascularization of the tumor. CT presents valuable information in regard to the distribution of the calcifications, which is particularly helpful for the differential diagnosis with myositis ossificans (Table 20.2).

20.4.4 Myositis Ossificans

According to the last revision of the WHO classification of soft tissue tumors in 2002, myositis ossificans has been classified as a fibroblastic/myofibroblastic lesion instead of a chondro-osseous lesion [11]. Myositis ossificans is a heterotopic bone formation, which occurs in soft tissue in different circumstances (e.g., genetic diseases, post-trauma, postsurgery, etc.). Three entities of myositis ossificans have been identified in the literature and are discussed in this chapter: myositis ossificans progressiva, myositis ossificans circumscripta (MOC), and neurogenic myositis ossificans.

20.4.4.1 *Myositis Ossificans Progressiva*

Myositis ossificans progressiva, also called fibroplasia ossificans progressiva, is a rare disorder of the connective tissue, characterized by a massive progressive deposition of heterotopic bone around multiple joints. Its

TABLE 20.2

Clinical and Radiological Features of Osseous Tumors and Pseudotumors

	Myositis Ossificans Progressiva	Neurogenic Myositis Ossificans	Myositis Ossificans Circumscripta	Extraskeletal Osteosarcoma
Cause	Genetic	Probably microtrauma caused by passive mobilization	Probably trauma	Unknown, radiation
Clinical context	Early in life, beginning at 3 years of age Characteristic skeletal malformations (short great toe and thumb)	Bedridden, comatose patients with central nervous system insults: trauma, inflammation, etc.	Young active adults Inconstant history of trauma	Mean age: fourth to fifth decade
Sites	Neck, then upper spine, and shoulder girdle	Around joints with frequent attachment to the joint capsule	Muscles of thigh, upper arm, and buttock (prone to trauma)	Thigh, retroperitoneum, large muscles of pelvic and shoulder girdles
CT Appearance	*Early:* fascial edema with small scattered foci of ossifications *Later:* ossification encircling the muscle	Single or multiple heterotopic bone fragments frequently attached to the capsule Demineralized bone	Mineralization from periphery to center: "zoning pattern" in mature lesions	Mineralization predominantly at the center of the lesion

occurrence is usually sporadic and probably related to an overexpression of bone morphogenetic protein 4 [45]. First symptoms occur at about age 3 years and manifest either as a palpable soft tissue swelling and stiffness of the neck [46] or as a palpable soft mass adjacent to the upper spine and shoulder girdle [47]. The initial changes are frequently painful and may be accompanied by local inflammatory changes [48]. The tissue swelling corresponds to edema of the fascial planes. The ossification process can occur quickly, within 3 to 4 weeks [46]. Characteristic congenital abnormalities, such as short great toes and short thumbs, are almost invariably present and have important diagnostic value [49]. Over the years, the heterotopic bone deposition progresses from cranial to caudal, and from axial to appendicular skeleton, resulting in major stiffness and disability [47]. Scoliosis is frequent and may result in respiratory complications, which worsen the prognosis.

Although radiographic observations are useful in diagnosing and following patients with myositis ossificans progressiva, conventional radiography is relatively insensitive to the extent of changes, especially early in the disease. CT can demonstrate early swelling of fascial planes. Heterotopic ossification appears initially as small foci scattered randomly throughout the fascia [46] and progressively encircles the muscle. The early imaging appearance, that is, fascial swelling with adjacent foci of ossification, is distinct from that of other forms of myositis ossificans (neurogenic and posttraumatic), allowing early diagnosis and therefore prevention of aggravating factors (trauma and biopsy) [46]. In advanced cases, CT helps in evaluating the extent of the disease (Figure 20.8). Although surgical removal is usually contraindicated, limited surgery may occasionally be performed to restore a specific function [46]. In that case, CT provides a precise definition of changes, helping surgical planning.

20.4.4.2 Myositis Ossificans Circumscripta

Although sometimes called myositis ossificans traumatica, MOC is preceded by a history of mechanical trauma in only half of cases [41]. MOC may be seen at any age, but more frequently in young active adults, predominantly men, especially in their second and third decades [32,50]. MOC occurs predominantly in the muscles of the thigh, buttock, and upper arms, which correspond to muscles most easily traumatized in young adults [50]. The physiopathology is unclear, but when a history of trauma is present, it can be assumed that the process begins with tissue necrosis and/or hemorrhage, followed by exuberant reparative fibroblastic/myofibroblastic activity and vascular proliferation leading to progressive osseous formation [51].

Histologically, MOC is characterized by a distinct zonal pattern, which reflects different degrees of cellular maturation [52]. The innermost portion of the lesion is composed of immature, richly vascular fibroblastic tissue. The intermediate zone contains varying amounts of osteoid rimmed by osteoblasts. Toward the periphery, the osteoid increasingly undergoes calcification and evolves into mature lamellar bone [52]. Characteristically, bone formation is most prominent at the margins of the lesion. Late lesions consist exclusively of mature lamellar bone [51].

Imaging features of MOC correspond to the histological findings. The early stage is characterized by muscle edema, usually confined to a single muscle group, with preservation of the anatomic planes. MRI is usually more contributive than CT at this phase. Calcifications develop between 4 and 6 weeks after the initial trauma and result in a "mature" lesion. In the intermediate stage, these calcifications are irregular and subtle but over time lamellar bone forms at the periphery of the lesion and proceeds toward its center [32,52]. The CT displays well this centrifugal pattern of progressive

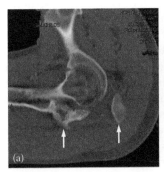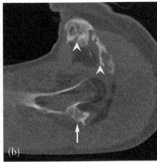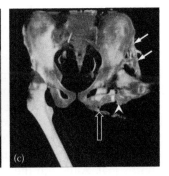

FIGURE 20.8
Myositis ossificans progressiva in a 17-year-old man. (a) Oblique reformation following the long axis of femur. Heterotopic ossification of left middle gluteus is depicted (arrows). Note the demineralization of the femoral head due to immobility. (b) Calcification at the insertion of the gluteus medius muscle (arrow) and the adductors (arrowheads). (c) Volume-rendered image: calcification of the middle gluteus (arrows), adductors (arrowhead), and gracilis (empty arrow) is shown. Note the demineralization of the femoral head due to immobility. (Courtesy of Dr. Robert Yves Carlier, Raymond Poincare Hospital, Garches, France.)

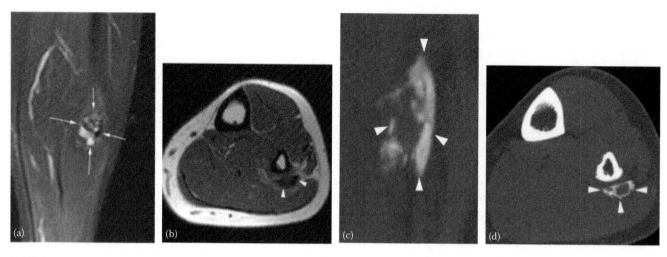

FIGURE 20.9
Myositis ossificans circumscripta (MOC) presenting as a painless left calf mass in a 43-year-old woman. (a) Coronal proton density-weighted MRI shows a well-defined heterogeneous lesion with mixed hyper- and hypointense aspect (arrows) that suggest a chondroid lesion. (b) Axial T_1-weighted image shows homogeneous hypointensity of the lesion (arrowheads). (c and d) Coronal and axial CT images depict a well-defined peripheral ossification suggesting rather a myositis ossificans. The peripheral disposition of the calcification with central low density of the lesion illustrate the "zoning pattern" (arrowheads).

mineralization with peripheral mature ossification recognized as "zoning" pattern (Figures 20.9 through 20.11). This characteristic appearance is essential in differentiating late-stage MOC from other mineralized lesions, especially extraskeletal osteosarcoma. Osteosarcomas show denser calcification in the central area, while MOC has pronounced calcification at the periphery. Because of its self-limiting nature, therapy of MOC is mostly conservative when there is no painful restricted motion. Biopsy is not needed to establish a definite diagnosis.

20.4.4.3 Neurogenic Myositis Ossificans

First described by Dejereine and Ceillier in paraplegic patients [53], neurogenic myositis ossificans usually occurs in bedridden and comatose patients with varied underlying neurological disorders such as spinal cord or head injury and other protracted diseases of the central nervous system [54]. It is a disabling condition affecting large joints and characterized by two complications: limitation of joint mobility and neurovascular compromise. The location and incidence depend on the underlying disease. Shoulders and elbows are more often affected after head injury, whereas hip and knee are more frequently affected in patients with spinal injury [55,56]. After head injury, symptoms usually develop within 2 to 3 months [54]. Although the physiopathology is unclear, many hypotheses have been suggested. One suggests that the induction of enchondral ossification may result from repeated tendinous or muscular microtrauma caused by passive mobilization of the paralyzed limb during rehabilitation [57]. Surgical removal

of mature heterotopic bone is often required to regain functional range of movement and release neurovascular structures. However, surgical treatment is risky because of potential complications including injury to demineralized bones or to compressed or entrapped neurovascular structures within the lesion [58–60].

CT displays heterotopic ossification of variable size, located indifferently in the anterior, posterior, or lateral aspects. Extensive ossification may surround the joint. Neurogenic myositis ossificans may present as a single bony bridge or as several bone fragments. Contact with the joint capsule and bone is frequently seen and may be focal or extensive (Figure 20.12) [54]. Before the advent of multislice CT, various techniques were used, such as scintigraphy, to assess degree of maturation of the heterotopic bone, and phlebography and arteriography were used to identify vascular structures. Now, these techniques have been replaced by contrast-enhanced MDCT [54]. Three-dimensional reconstructions are useful to evaluate the relationship between the vessels and the ossification (Figure 20.13). Precise identification of nerves remains difficult, especially in the presence of a bulky osseous lesion. Nonetheless, CT may sometimes display the entrapped nerve within the osseous lesion. CT has also been proposed as an alternative to densitometry for the assessment of bone demineralization to evaluate the risk of intraoperative fracture (Figure 20.14) [54].

20.4.5 Soft Tissue Metastases

Although soft tissues, and in particular skeletal muscles, represent about 40% of the total body weight, metastases to soft tissue seldom appear: a rate of 1% of

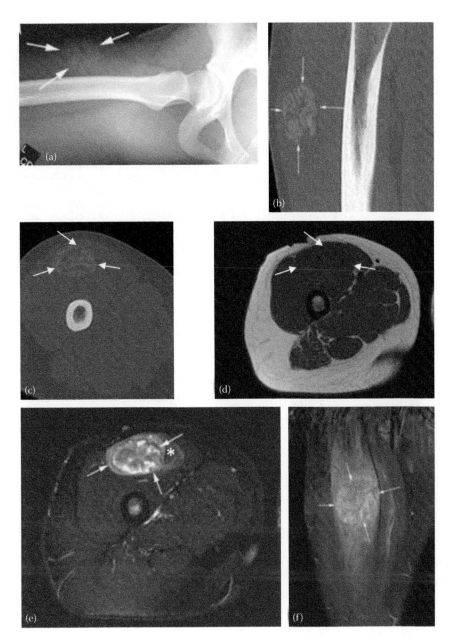

FIGURE 20.10

MOC in a 22-year-old woman who noted, incidentally, a solid mass at the anterior right thigh that was movable beneath the surface. There was no history of trauma. (a) Plain radiograph of the right thigh depicted a lobulated calcified mass of mixed opacity in the anterior soft tissues of the thigh without contact with the anterior femoral cortex (arrows). (b and c) Sagittal and axial unenhanced CT images show a peripherally calcified lesion in the rectus femoris (arrows). (d) Axial T_1-weighted unenhanced MRI. The lesion appears hypointense to muscle. (e) Axial T_2-weighted fat-suppressed image shows lesion with mixed hypo- and hyperintense parts and further depicts a peripheral sclerotic rim (arrows). Note perifocal muscle edema (asterisks). (f) After contrast administration, marked inhomogeneous enhancement is observed (arrows). Note the "zoning pattern" (peripheral disposition of the calcification) is better seen on CT than MRI.

all neoplasms is reported [61]. The reasons for this rarity may be related to blood flow, tissue pressure, and metabolism. Blood turbulence, following physical exercise, may be responsible for the destruction of tumor cells. Additionally, metabolites like lactic acid may create an environment that is hostile to carcinogenesis [62,63]. It has been demonstrated that trauma may favor

development of metastases [64], probably because of increased adherence of tumor cells to vessels resulting from endothelial damage [61]. Nonetheless, the exact incidence and prevalence are probably underestimated because of statistical biases. For instance, autopsic studies that included microscopic metastatic foci showed a prevalence of soft tissue metastases as high as 52% [65,66].

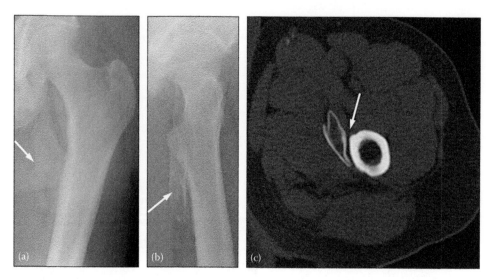

FIGURE 20.11
Myositis ossificans in a 31-year-old man. (a) Anteroposterior and (b) lateral radiographs of the femur demonstrate a mature ossification in the soft tissues in proximity to the shaft of the proximal femur (arrows). The radiographs do not allow for definite localization of the lesion. (c) Axial CT scan of the proximal femur clearly shows that the ossification is separated from the bone with a cleavage plane (arrow). It is also easier to see that the pattern of ossification is denser at the periphery.

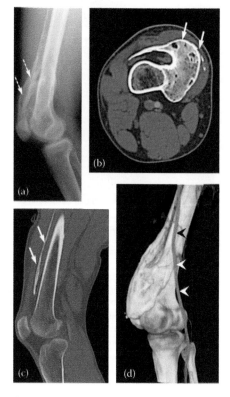

FIGURE 20.12
Neurogenic myositis ossificans of the anterior compartment of the right thigh in a 25-year-old man. (a) Plain radiograph. Extensive soft tissue ossification of the anterior compartment of the thigh (dashed arrows). (b and c). Axial and sagittal contrast-enhanced CT images visualize the heterotopic ossification (arrows) and its attachment to the femoral diaphysis. (d) Volume rendering technique image shows the distal femoral artery (black arrowhead) and popliteal artery coursing distant to the ossification (white arrowheads). (Courtesy of Dr. Fabio Roffi, Raymond Poincare Hospital, Garches, France.)

Soft tissue metastases commonly develop in the muscles neighboring the trunk such as paravertebral, gluteal, abdominal wall, and thigh muscles [61]. Overall, the most common tumors exhibiting soft tissue metastases are lung, renal, and colon primaries [67,68]. The most common histological diagnosis is adenocarcinoma predominantly from lung and gastrointestinal tract [69], while sarcomas are an uncommon cause of metastases to the skeletal muscle [61]. Bone-forming muscle metastases have been linked to gastric adenocarcinoma or to breast, ovary, thyroid, colon, bladder, skin, and prostate cancers or to osteogenic sarcomas (Figure 20.15) [70–73]. Skeletal muscle metastases often present as a firm and tender mass deeply rooted within the muscle and with a diameter of more than 5 cm. Pain is more commonly seen in skeletal muscle metastases than in sarcomas [61,74].

Metastasis to skeletal muscle generally appears on CT as an area of decreased attenuation with a varying degree of delineation [71,73]. Sometimes detection is difficult, and a lesion may be suspected only from a slight asymmetry of soft tissues when compared with the opposite side (Figure 20.16). Enhancement may be either homogeneous or heterogeneous, but rim enhancement with a central hypoattenuating area is the most frequently reported feature (Figures 20.17 and 20.18) [75]. Peritumoral hypoattenuation may be observed and represents peritumoral edema. Muscular abscess presents in a similar fashion and is the primary differential diagnosis. In the presence of the typical focal clinical findings, bacteremia, or a history of IV drug abuse, an abscess is the most likely diagnosis of an intramuscular rim-enhancing hypoattenuating mass [75]. However,

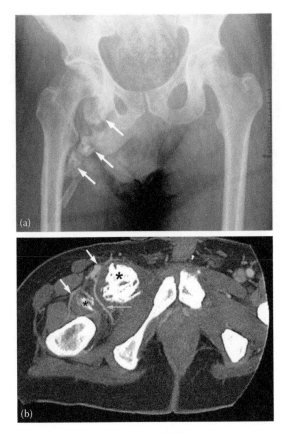

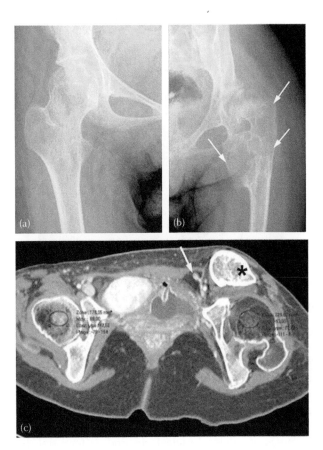

FIGURE 20.13

Neurogenic myositis ossificans of the anterior part of the right hip in a 30-year-old man. (a) Anteroposterior radiograph of the pelvis shows several heterotopic bone fragments medially to the right femoral head (arrows). (b) Axial contrast-enhanced CT for preoperative evaluation shows heterotopic ossifications at the anteromedial aspect of the thigh (asterisks) pushing the femoral vessels laterally (white arrows). A branch of the femoral artery is trapped between the heterotopic bone (gray arrow). (Courtesy of Dr. Fabio Roffi, Raymond Poincare Hospital, Garches, France.)

FIGURE 20.14

Neurogenic myositis ossificans of the anterior aspect of the left hip in a 32-year-old woman after head injury. (a and b) Plain radiographs of the right and left hips. The right hip is normal. On the left side: soft tissue ossification around the hip (arrows) with demineralization of the femoral head compared to the right side. (c) Axial contrast-enhanced CT image shows a heterotopic ossification in the anterior aspect of the hip (asterisk), pushing the femoral vessels medially (arrows). The left femoral head is demineralized (mean density = −53 HU) compared to the right side (mean density = 88 HU). (Courtesy of Dr. Fabio Roffi, Raymond Poincare Hospital, Garches, France.)

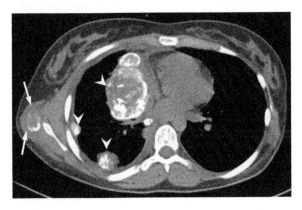

FIGURE 20.15

Axial MDCT image without contrast injection in a 30-year-old man with a history of right femur osteosarcoma, presenting with pain and palpable mass of right thoracic wall. The CT shows a calcified lesion enlarging the latissimus dorsi consistent with an osteosarcoma (arrows). Note multiple pleural metastases with massive areas of mineralization (arrowheads). The pattern of mineralization is central in small parietal lesions and anarchic in the juxtamediastinal mass.

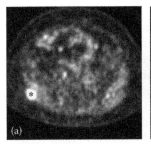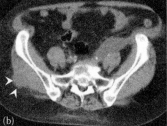

FIGURE 20.16

Right middle gluteal metastasis in a 61-year-old woman with mucoepidermoid carcinoma of the cervix. (a) Axial FDG PET/CT image displays a right gluteal lesion showing avid uptake (asterisk). (b) Axial MDCT image without contrast enhancement shows a slightly hypodense lesion causing an asymmetry of the middle gluteal muscle (arrowheads).

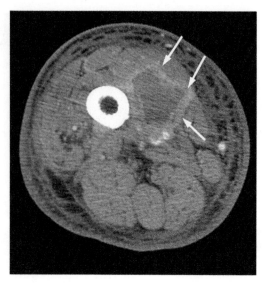

FIGURE 20.17
A 73-year-old man with gastric adenocarcinoma presenting with right thigh swelling and a palpable mass. (a and b) Axial and coronal contrast-enhanced MDCT images show a hypodense lesion with peripheral enhancement (arrows), consistent with metastasis.

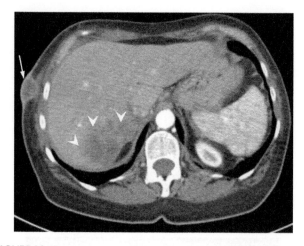

FIGURE 20.18
Cutaneous metastasis in a 57-year-old woman with breast cancer. Axial contrast-enhanced MDCT image shows a right subcutaneous lesion, with central hypodensity and peripheral enhancement (arrow). Note also hepatic metastases (arrowheads).

in the absence of such clinical findings in an oncologic patient, metastases must be considered and biopsy is required to provide the final diagnosis [75]. Moreover, diagnosis of calcified metastases and differential diagnosis with myositis ossificans is easier on CT than on MRI [61]. Positron emission tomography/CT, which is increasingly prescribed for the evaluation and follow-up of cancer patients, is the most sensitive imaging method for the detection of soft tissue metastases [76].

20.4.6 Intramuscular Hemangiomas

Intramuscular hemangiomas are the most common benign neoplasms of the muscle [77] and constitute 10% of all benign vascular tumors. The majority are discovered by 30 years of age, although many are detected by the end of the first decade of life. The most common presenting symptom is pain, ranging from a few weeks to several years in duration. Intramuscular hemangiomas have a predilection for the trunk and extremities. The head and neck are also a common site of involvement. Macroscopically, intramuscular hemangiomas are well-circumscribed unencapsulated lesions with areas of white fibrous connective tissue intermixed with endomysium and perimysium of the muscle, intimately growing with the myofibers. Histologically, they are characterized by ectatic blood-filled spaces that often develop dystrophic calcifications as the neoplasm enlarges. Phleboliths are classic findings on conventional radiographs or CT but are only seen in 20% to 50% of the cases [78,79]. The classification of these lesions is based primarily on the size and morphology of vessels and includes capillary,

venous, cavernous, mixed, and arteriovenous types. When the hemangioma has direct contact with bone, pressure effects may be seen, either as bone resorption or as reactive new bone formation [80]. Osseous changes in contact with hemangioma may be classified into three types: periosteal, cortical, and medullar [80].

Multiple imaging tools are used to characterize hemangiomas. Radiography and MRI are normally used together. Radiographs may show soft tissue thickening, phleboliths, and periosteal reaction. MRI is the most precise imaging tool for determining the extent of the lesion, as well as the nature of its different components (such as adipose tissue and fibrous septae) and may also contribute to determining the flow in ectatic vessels. Nonetheless, CT may serve as a useful adjunct to MRI. CT typically shows a mottled low-density pattern, caused by the fatty, fibrous, and vascular tissue components. Venous malformation, characterized by slow flow and pooling of blood, presents as a soft tissue mass with phleboliths and serpentine vascular components enhancing after IV contrast injection, unless they are thrombosed [81,82]. High flow vascular malformations such as fistulae and arteriovenous malformation show large feeding arteries in addition to draining vessels [83]. When the hemangioma is adjacent to bone, CT may show periosteal changes that are commonly nonaggressive appearing: solid, continuous, and undulating, reflecting a slow-growing mass. Aggressive-appearing periosteal changes, with short periosteal spiculations, are less common. Cortical surface changes include erosion and thickening. Intramedullary sclerosis and osteopenia may also be seen and represent medullary changes [80]. Moreover, MDCT venography has been reported to be of great value in patients with mixed capillary and venous

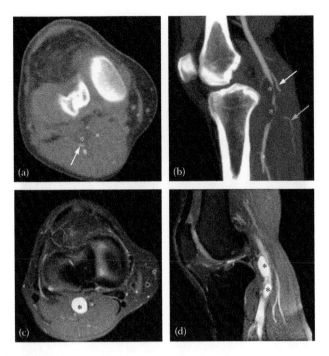

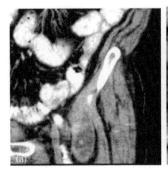

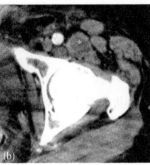

FIGURE 20.20

Iliopsoas (iliopectineal) bursitis in a 52-year-old woman. (a and b) Coronal and axial contrast-enhanced MDCT images. (a) Fluid-equivalent density inside a mass laterally adjacent to the femoral neurovascular bundle (asterisk). (b) The fluid-containing mass shows close relation to the anterior hip joint (asterisk). In 15% of individuals there is iliopsoas bursal communication with the hip joint.

FIGURE 20.19

Adventitial cystic disease of the popliteal artery in a 50-year-old woman presenting with intermittent claudication of the right lower limb. (a) Axial image and sagittal maximum intensity projection (b) image from MDCT angiography. A fluid-equivalent lesion is observed in the popliteal fossa (asterisks) following the popliteal artery, significantly narrowing its lumen. Note collateralization (gray arrow) with dilation of the sural artery (white arrow). (c and d) Axial and sagittal T₂-weighted fat-suppressed MR images confirm the cystic nature of the lesion. (Courtesy of Dr. Nicolas Naggara, Avicenne Hospital, Bobigny, France.)

vascular malformations by revealing the anatomy and extent of aberrant venous drainage patterns [84,85].

20.4.7 Synovial Cystic Lesions

Synovial cystic lesions are divided into four groups based on the combination of the anatomical and histological composition: synovial cyst, ganglion cyst, bursa de novo, and bursitis [86]. Although these lesions are much better studied on ultrasound or MRI, they are very common findings, easily detected on CT. However, it has to be kept in mind that CT is not the primary diagnostic tool for characterizing these lesions.

20.4.7.1 Synovial Cyst and Ganglia

Synovial cyst is a herniation of the synovial membrane through the joint capsule, always communicating with the adjacent joint. Synovial cyst is caused by an accumulation of articular fluid with subsequent elevation of intra-articular pressure, which results in a synovial fluid herniation within the joint capsule. A typical example

is Baker's cyst, in which the synovial breach is located between the gastrocnemius muscle and the semimembranous tendon. Other locations such as spine, shoulders, hands, and feet are less frequent. Synovial cyst and ganglion cyst are believed to be variants of the same disease spectrum, although this theory is subject to controversy [86]. Both types are para-articular and have similar histological composition. However, unlike synovial cysts, ganglion cysts are not always in communication with the joint cavity. Ganglion cysts may be located anywhere around the joint, most frequently in fat, muscles, and bone, but also around arteries and nerves, resulting in adventitial cystic disease (Figure 20.19), or may present as a perineuronal or intraneuronal cyst.

In CT, both synovial and ganglion cysts appear as cystic lesions around the joint. Rim enhancement may be seen after IV contrast injection [87]. CT arthrography can demonstrate the communication of the cyst with the joint cavity, sometimes on delayed images (up to 2 hours after injection) [88]. However, when the communication is very narrow or when intra-cystic fluid is highly viscous, cysts may fail to fill [87].

20.4.7.2 Bursa de Novo (Adventitious Bursa) and Bursitis

While bursitis is an inflammation of a "true" bursa occurring due to chronic mechanical friction, or is observed in infectious or rheumatoid diseases, bursa de novo represents inflammation of connective tissue in areas subject to chronic frictional irritation [86]. On CT, bursitis and bursa de novo appear as well-delineated hypodense structure in a predisposed location. A common example is iliopsoas bursitis, which is secondary to chronic microtrauma of the iliopsoas tendon from overuse and hyperactivity (Figure 20.20). Other examples include chronic frictional infrapatellar bursitis and adventitious bursa of the medial side of the first metatarsophalangeal joint due to chronic friction over a hallux valgus [86].

20.4.8 Soft Tissue Extension of Osseous Tumors

Both primary and secondary bone tumors may invade surrounding soft tissues. However, soft tissue involvement may also be the predominant feature with little involvement of bone. This is observed especially in Ewing sarcoma and bone surface tumors. In this case, CT may help to prove the osseous origin, showing an erosion of the cortex (Figure 20.21). Moreover, CT may be useful for the analysis of tumoral matrix in case of osseous or cartilaginous tumor (parosteal osteosarcoma, parosteal chondrosarcoma) [89].

20.4.9 Endometriosis Mimicking Soft Tissue Tumors

Endometriosis is defined as tissue resembling the endometrium occurring outside the uterus, commonly in the pelvis and the abdomen. Its occurrence in the subcutaneous tissue and skeletal musculature has been reported [90,91]. Although the pathogenesis of endometriosis is multifold, subcutaneous endometriosis of the abdominal wall is known to occur in cesarean section and abdominopelvic incisional scars as a result of direct implantation of endometrial tissue at the time of surgery. The fluctuation of clinical symptoms with the menstrual cycle is a highly important element for the diagnosis of endometriosis. Subcutaneous endometriosis can best be detected by the use of CT or ultrasound, but neither can differentiate endometrioma from a mass of similar density, such as hematoma, lymphoma, sarcoma, or desmoid tumor. CT shows a nonspecific hypodense lesion that enhances after contrast injection. While its ovarian counterpart is typically hyperintense in T_1 and hypointense in T_2-weighted images, abdominal wall endometriosis may be isointense or slightly hyperintense to muscle in T_1- and T_2-weighted images. Enhancement is frequent on both MRI and CT (Figure 20.22). The clinical context of a hemorrhagic lesion in synchronization with a menstrual cycle is paramount in establishing the diagnosis.

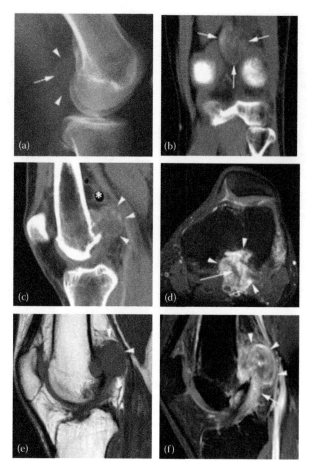

FIGURE 20.21
Periosteal osteosarcoma of the posterior metaphyseal femur in a 37-year-old patient presenting with a painless palpable mass in the popliteal fossa. (a) Lateral radiograph shows soft tissue attenuation in the popliteal fossa adjacent to posterior femoral cortex (arrowheads). No obvious osseous involvement is seen. A small calcification seems to delineate the lesion posteriorly (arrow). (b) Coronal contrast-enhanced MDCT image shows well-defined solid mass with inhomogeneous enhancement suggestive of a tumor (arrows). (c) Sagittal reformation delineates posterior border of mass (arrowheads) and suggests infiltration of posterior femoral cortex anteriorly (no arrow). Note air collection superiorly adjacent to lesion after biopsy (asterisk). (d) Axial contrast-enhanced T_1-weighted fat-suppressed MRI shows avid enhancement of lesion and definite infiltration of tumor into the posterior femur (arrowheads). Note central necrosis reflected as nonenhancing center of lesion (arrow). (e) Sagittal T_1-weighted nonenhanced image depicts mass as homogeneous hypointense mass clearly showing bony involvement (arrowhead). Adjacency to the popliteal vessels suggests extra-articular involvement. (f) Corresponding sagittal T_1-weighted fat-suppressed contrast-enhanced image shows posterior delineation of lesion (arrowheads) and also involvement and infiltration of dorsal parts of proximal anterior cruciate ligament. Tumor was treated with local total resection.

20.5 Nontumoral Soft Tissue† Calcifications

Soft tissue calcifications may be either metastatic or dystrophic. Metastatic calcifications do not refer to tumoral or malignant etiologies; they occur when calcium phosphorus product is greater than 70 mg/dl [92]. Amorphous calcium phosphate and calcium hydroxyapatite crystals are, then, deposited in multiple locations. On CT, large periarticular amorphous fluid–fluid levels may be identified. Other signs may be present

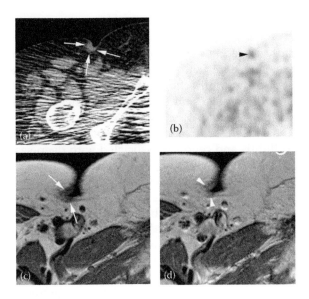

FIGURE 20.22
Extrapelvic subcutaneous endometriosis in a 36-year-old woman. Painless mass in the right groin presenting with intermittent hemorrhagic discharge. (a) Axial nonenhanced CT scan shows cutaneous and subcutaneous well-defined mass in right groin (arrows). (b) Corresponding FDG PET image shows increased glucose uptake in this area (black arrowhead). Corresponding nonenhanced (c) and enhanced (d) T_1-weighted MRI shows the lesion as hypointense horseshoe-like formation (arrows) with avid enhancement (arrowheads) in correlation with intermittent bleeding in synchronization with the menstrual cycle. A diagnosis of endometriosis was established and consequent total resection of lesion was performed.

and are related to the etiology. For instance, secondary hyperparathyroidism shows additional diffuse arterial calcification [93].

Dystrophic calcifications occur in different disorders, in damaged or inflamed soft tissues. These calcifications may present a characteristic radiologic appearance, depending on the etiology. Calcinosis circumscripta and calcinosis universalis are two types of collagen vascular diseases with characteristic radiologic appearances. Calcinosis circumscripta refers to small well-defined localized calcium deposits around phalangeal tufts in systemic sclerosis (scleroderma) that are easily detected on plain radiography. Calcinosis universalis is most commonly noted in dermatomyositis and is characterized, on CT, by diffuse sheet-like deposition of calcium involving the muscles, subcutaneous tissues, and fascial planes.

In crystal deposition disorders, the deposition of monosodium urate, calcium pyrophosphate dehydrate, or hydroxyapatite crystals, which may lead to intra-articular and periarticular calcifications, is characteristic. These crystal disorders may occur as primary abnormalities or secondary to underlying diseases. In patients with tophaceous gout, early detection of urate deposits in subclinical tophus deposits may be

displayed with dual-energy CT [5]. In patients with calcium pyrophosphate deposition disease (CPDD), calcifications may occur in cartilage, synovium, or soft tissues around the knee, wrist, and the symphysis pubis. These calcifications may be detected incidentally or associated with symptoms. In most instances, CPDD is idiopathic; however, it may be seen with metabolic diseases, including primary hyperparathyroidism, gout, and hemochromatosis. In hydroxyapatite deposition disease, the calcification is usually periarticular, occurring especially in tendons. These depositions may be asymptomatic or lead to painful episodes termed calcific tendonitis [94]. Hydroxyapatite deposition may be seen anywhere, but most frequently around the shoulder [94]. Conventional radiography is usually sufficient to make the diagnosis. When performed, CT may show associated cortical erosion. Moreover, CT may be useful if the hydroxyapatite deposit occurs in the longus colli muscle, in which case the clinical presentation may be misleading.

20.5.1 Acute Calcific Prevertebral Tendonitis

Acute calcific tendonitis is also known as calcific retropharyngeal tendonitis and calcific tendonitis of the longus colli muscle. It has been reported in adults between 21 and 81 years old but occurs most frequently in the third through the sixth decade [95]. The longus colli muscle is a paired flexor of the neck and occupies the bulk of prevertebral space together with longus capitis [96]. Anteriorly, the deep cervical fascia delimits the prevertebral space and separates it from the retropharyngeal space [97]. Due to this close proximity, acute calcific tendonitis of the longus colli tendon may mimic a retropharyngeal inflammatory or infectious process. Its clinical presentation is usually associated with acute or subacute onset of pain of the neck, sore throat, odynophagia, and mild fever [98]. Clinical examination may reveal a pharyngeal swelling. Moreover, blood tests may show a mild elevation of erythrocyte sedimentation rate and a mildly elevated white blood cell count. All these findings may be suggestive of a retropharyngeal infectious process and thus CT evaluation becomes necessary.

Typical CT findings consist of a soft tissue swelling of the prevertebral and retropharyngeal space with calcifications within the superior-most fibers of the longus colli tendon at the level of C1, close to the site of tendon insertion (Figure 20.23) [96,97]. However, calcification levels as low as C5–C6 disc have also been reported [99]. These calcifications are homogeneous, amorphous, roughly ovoid, quite variable in size, and without trabeculation, which allow them to be differentiated from heterotopic ossification or accessory ossicles. The greater contrast resolution of CT makes it a more sensitive technique

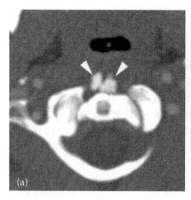
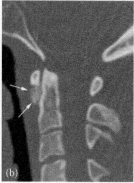

FIGURE 20.23
Acute retropharyngeal calcific tendinitis in a 40-year-old man presenting with acute onset of anterior neck pain and odynophagia. (a) Axial CT image shows prevertebral calcifications adjacent to the dens axis at the insertion site of the superior oblique fibers of the longus colli muscle (arrowheads). Note also prevertebral soft tissue swelling. Air-filled hypopharynx is marked with an asterisk. (b) Sagittal reformation confirms calcium deposit inferior to anterior part of the atlas and anteriorly to the dens axis (arrows). These findings represent self-limiting calcium hydroxyapatite deposition. The diagnosis was established on the basis of imaging findings and characteristic clinical presentation.

than radiography for the detection of such calcifications [96,100]. Additionally, the presence of an effusion along the retropharyngeal space has been described [96]. Since the principal differential diagnosis is a retropharyngeal abscess, important negative signs to look for are the absence of enhancing wall around the fluid and the absence of suppurative retropharyngeal lymph nodes with low-attenuation centers [96]. Therapeutic management is nonsteroidal anti-inflammatory medication, analgesics, and IV steroids for the most painful cases [98].

20.6 Infectious Pathology

Soft tissue infection can take many forms depending on the tissue involved: cellulitis, fasciitis, myositis, and soft tissue abscess are typical manifestations. CT plays an important role in the assessment of soft tissue infections especially in a context of emergency. CT provides an analysis of compartmental anatomy, which helps distinguish various patterns of soft tissue infection and guide treatment planning.

20.6.1 Cellulitis

Cellulitis is an acute infection of dermis and subcutaneous tissues that occurs following disruption of the skin.

It results in pain, edema, and warmth erythema. Patients with peripheral vascular diseases or diabetes are particularly susceptible to this type of infection since minor injuries and damaged skin of the feet may serve as a point of entry for infection. Patients with foreign bodies such as IV catheter and orthopedic hardware are also susceptible to cellulitis.

CT is used to accurately differentiate between superficial cellulitis and cellulitis associated with deep-seated infection. Further, CT is applied to rule out abscess formation that may require drainage or surgery. In uncomplicated cellulitis, CT shows thickened skin, septations, and increased density of subcutaneous fat [101]. Clinical correlation is required since bland subcutaneous edema due to heart failure may have a similar appearance. If the infection spreads to deeper tissues, deep cellulitis, myositis, necrotizing fasciitis, or osteomyelitis can occur. In geriatric patients, cellulitis of the lower extremities is more likely to develop into thrombophlebitis. In this case, contrast-enhanced CT may help identify the extent of the thrombus [101].

20.6.2 Necrotizing Fasciitis

Necrotizing fasciitis is a life-threatening surgical emergency. It is a progressive, rapidly spreading infection of the deep fasciae, with secondary necrosis of the subcutaneous tissues. Because of the increase of the number of immunocompromised patients, necrotizing fasciitis is becoming more frequent [101]. It can occur secondary to a skin breach (trauma, pressure sore, or around foreign bodies in surgical wounds), but may also be idiopathic, as in scrotal necrotizing fasciitis (Fournier's gangrene) (Figure 20.24). Necrotizing soft tissue infections are often accompanied by gas-forming necrotizing bacteria in combination with gram-negative organisms [102].

CT plays a vital role in suggesting the diagnosis early, in visualization of the anatomical extent, and in initiating rapid and successful treatment. The imaging findings are similar but more severe than in cellulitis with involvement of deeper structures. Although it is not observed in all cases, the presence of gas in the subcutaneous tissue is a distinguishing sign of necrotizing fasciitis. Other CT findings are thickening of the affected fasciae and fluid collections along the deep fascial sheaths [101]. The absence of enhancement of the fascia confirms the presence of necrosis and helps in distinguishing nonnecrotizing from necrotizing fasciitis. Nonnecrotizing fasciitis does not require emergency surgery but affected patients need to be followed at short intervals as necrosis can potentially occur at a later stage.

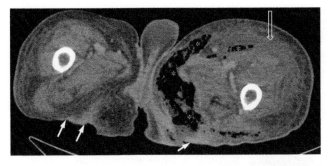

FIGURE 20.24
Necrotizing fasciitis of the left thigh secondary to ischial pressure sore in a 60-year-old man. Axial contrast-enhanced CT shows densification of the subcutaneous tissue with perimuscular fluid collection (empty arrow), presence of gas in the subcutaneous tissue (asterisks), and the loss of substance at both sides: pressure sores (arrows), which served as points of entry to the infection. (Courtesy of Dr. Nicolas Naggara, Avicenne Hospital, Bobigny, France.)

20.6.3 Infectious Myositis

Infectious myositis is an acute, subacute, or chronic infection of the skeletal muscle that is most often seen in young adults. The most common responsible organism is *Staphylococcus aureus* (77% of cases) [103]. It is sometimes reported as the most common musculoskeletal complication of AIDS [104]. Other risk factors are strenuous activity or rhabdomyolysis and muscle trauma, in which case a hematoma may form and act as a nidus infection. Skin infections, infected insect bites, and underlying diabetes mellitus can also lead to pyomyositis. Typically, only a single muscle is involved. The most common site is the quadriceps muscle, followed by the gluteal and iliopsoas muscles [103].

Pyomyositis is characterized by three stages: (1) the invasive stage, in which edema in the affected muscle leads to pain; (2) the suppurative phase, in which the patient develops a fever and, if not treated, leads to an abscess formation; and (3) the late stage, which is potentially life threatening and leads to toxicity and sepsis [103].

CT displays enlargement and decreased attenuation of the affected muscle with effacement of surrounding fat planes. Involvement of a muscle group that is disproportionate to the involvement of subcutaneous tissue helps distinguish myositis from primary cellulitis [101]. Intramuscular fluid collection may be observed, and contrast injection helps differentiate viable musculature and demonstrates a rim-enhancing abscess if present. Moreover, CT can help guide treatment such as aspiration and drainage of muscle abscess. Untreated pyomyositis may lead to a compartment syndrome, osteomyelitis, and septic arthritis [101].

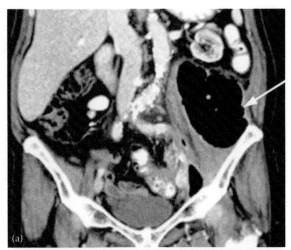
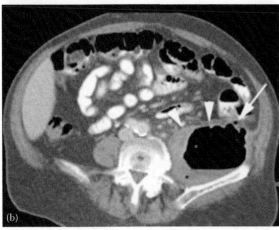

FIGURE 20.25
Large pelvic abscess in a 61-year-old woman. (a) Coronal contrast-enhanced MDCT image shows a large mass (arrow) with a central air collection (asterisk), adjacent to the left iliac crest involving the psoas muscle. (b) Axial CT image displays a fluid level inside the air collection (asterisk), as well as a thickened and enhancing capsule of the abscess (arrowheads). Note the small diverticulum of the descending colon communicating with the mass (arrow); the abscess resulted from perforated diverticulitis.

20.6.4 Soft Tissue Abscess

Secondary to bacterial infection, an abscess may form, particularly in immunocompromised patients. The most commonly isolated pathogen is *S. aureus*. CT shows a well-demarcated fluid collection with a peripheral pseudocapsule displaying rim enhancement. Treatment of soft tissue abscess consists of appropriate antibiotics and percutaneous drainage (Figures 20.25 through 20.28). Additionally, CT may provide important information regarding the origin and the extent of spread of the infectious process. In psoas abscesses, for example, CT may show signs of discitis, urinary infection or stasis, perforated diverticulitis, appendicitis, and Crohn's disease, which may require different treatment approaches.

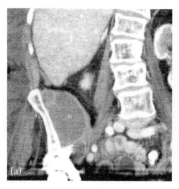
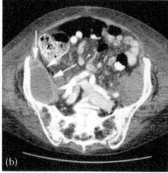
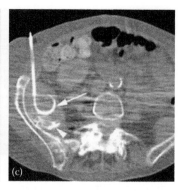

FIGURE 20.26
Iliac muscle abscess in a 55-year-old man who presented with fever and right-side pelvic pain. (a) Coronal contrast-enhanced MDCT image of the abdomen shows a fluid-filled mass involving the right iliac muscle with an enhancing capsule (asterisk), which is characteristic of an abscess. (b) Enhancing and thickened abscess capsule is well depicted in this axial image (arrows). Hypoattenuation is also seen contralaterally, representing early stage of abscess formation (no arrows). (c) CT-guided interventional drainage of the abscess: a pigtail catheter is placed in the center of abscess using Seldinger procedure (arrow). Contrast administration via catheter shows correct position and filling of abscess with contrast (arrowhead).

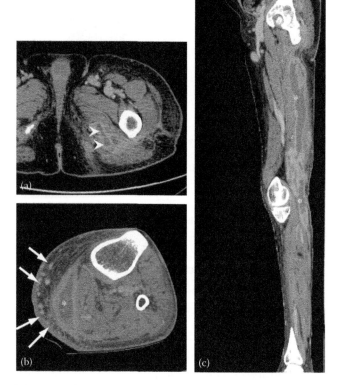

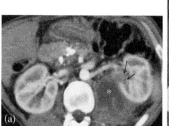
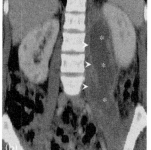

FIGURE 20.28
Extensive left psoas abscess secondary to focal bacterial nephritis in a 65-year-old man. (a) Axial contrast-enhanced CT image shows hypodense collection of the left psoas (asterisk), in direct contact with an area of decreased attenuation of the left kidney, related to a foci of bacterial nephritis (arrows). (b) Coronal-enhanced CT image shows the abscess (asterisks) with peripheral rim enhancement (arrowheads) extending along the whole length of the left psoas.

20.7 Conclusion

Although CT does not provide the best contrast and resolution for soft tissue evaluation, it is a valuable diagnostic tool due to its wide availability and high accuracy in detecting and assessing patterns of calcifications. CT also allows tissue characterization due to x-ray attenuation, for example, fluid, adipose tissue, hemorrhage, as well as the possibility of angiographic studies. It can be useful in the emergency context or as an adjunct to MRI for the evaluation of soft tissue changes in nonemergency situations. CT plays an important role not only in the assessment of

FIGURE 20.27
Abscess of the left lower leg in a 50-year-old man. (a and b) Axial contrast-enhanced images at the level of the buttock and upper leg showing a fluid collection extending from the gluteus minimus muscle (arrowheads). Note the densification of the subcutaneous fat and dilation of superficial veins because of venous compression (arrows) peripheral to the collection (asterisk). (c) Sagittal reformation shows the fluid collection with peripheral enhancement, extending along the posterior compartment of the thigh and the popliteal fossa (asterisks).

soft tissue infections but also in the detection of hemorrhage and for treatment planning. Moreover, radiologists should be aware of the added value of CT, in conjunction with MRI, in the diagnosis and management of soft tissue masses. CT may be diagnostic in characterizing calcified lesions due to high-resolution visualization of the mineralization pattern. In lipomatous tumors, CT may provide important information and helps to distinguish benign from malignant lesions, due to location (superficial vs. deep), size, internal composition (presence of thick nonlipomatous septa or nodules), contrast-enhancement pattern, and shape of the lesion.

References

1. Subhawong TK, Fishman EK, Swart JE, Carrino JA, Attar S, Fayad LM. Soft-tissue masses and masslike conditions: What does CT add to diagnosis and management? *AJR Am J Roentgenol.* 2010; 194(6):1559–1567.

2. West AT, Marshall TJ, Bearcroft PW. CT of the musculoskeletal system: What is left is the days of MRI? *Eur Radiol.* 2009; 19(1):152–164.

3. Mori T, Fujii M, Akisue T, Yamamoto T, Kurosaka M, Sugimura K. Three-dimensional images of contrast-enhanced MDCT for preoperative assessment of musculoskeletal masses: Comparison with MRI and plain radiographs. *Radiat Med.* 2005; 23(6):398–406.

4. Donnino R, Jacobs JE, Doshi JV, Hecht EM, Kim DC, Babb JS et al. Dual-source versus single-source cardiac CT angiography: Comparison of diagnostic image quality. *AJR Am J Roentgenol.* 2009; 192(4):1051–1056.

5. Choi HK, Al-Arfaj AM, Eftekhari A, Munk PL, Shojania K, Reid G et al. Dual energy computed tomography in tophaceous gout. *Ann Rheum Dis.* 2009; 68(10):1609–1612.

6. Cherry WB, Mueller PS. Rectus sheath hematoma: Review of 126 cases at a single institution. *Medicine (Baltimore).* 2006; 85(2):105–110.

7. Balkan C, Kavakli K, Karapinar D. Iliopsoas haemorrhage in patients with haemophilia: Results from one centre. *Haemophilia.* 2005; 11(5):463–467.

8. Sasson Z, Mangat I, Peckham KA. Spontaneous iliopsoas hematoma in patients with unstable coronary syndromes receiving intravenous heparin in therapeutic doses. *Can J Cardiol.* 1996; 12(5):490–494.

9. Gomez P, Morcuende J. High-grade sarcomas mimicking traumatic intramuscular hematomas: A report of three cases. *Iowa Orthop J.* 2004; 24:106–110.

10. Kransdorf MJ and Murphey MD. Origin and classification of soft tissue tumors. In: *Imaging of soft tissue tumors.* Philadelphia, PA: Lippincott Williams & Williams; 2006:1–5.

11. Wu JS, Hochman MG. Soft-tissue tumors and tumorlike lesions: A systematic imaging approach. *Radiology.* 2009; 253(2):297–316.

12. Fletcher CD, Unni KK, Mertens F. *WHO classification of tumour: Pathology and genetics of tumours of soft tissue and bone.* Lyon, France: IARC; 2002.

13. Vanhoenacker FM, Marques MC, Garcia H. Lipomatous tumors. In: Enzinger FM, Weiss SW, eds. *Imaging of soft tissue tumors.* 3rd ed. Berlin, New York: Springer; 2006:227–261.

14. Nishida J, Morita T, Ogose A, Okada K, Kakizaki H, Tajino T et al. Imaging characteristics of deep-seated lipomatous tumors: Intramuscular lipoma, intermuscular lipoma, and lipoma-like liposarcoma. *J Orthop Sci.* 2007; 12(6):533–541.

15. Goldman AB, DiCarlo EF, Marcove RC. Case report 774. Coincidental parosteal lipoma with osseous excresence and intramuscular lipoma. *Skeletal Radiol.* 1993; 22(2):138–145.

16. Kransdorf MJ. Malignant soft-tissue tumors in a large referral population: Distribution of diagnoses by age, sex, and location. *AJR Am J Roentgenol.* 1995; 164(1): 129–134.

17. deSantos LA, Goldstein HM, Murray JA, Wallace S. Computed tomography in the evaluation of musculoskeletal neoplasms. *Radiology.* 1978; 128(1):89–94.

18. Peterson JJ, Kransdorf MJ, Bancroft LW, O'Connor MI. Malignant fatty tumors: Classification, clinical course, imaging appearance and treatment. *Skeletal Radiol.* 2003; 32(9):493–503.

19. Jelinek JS, Kransdorf MJ, Shmookler BM, Aboulafia AJ, Malawer MM. Liposarcoma of the extremities: MR and CT findings in the histologic subtypes. *Radiology.* 1993; 186(2):455–459.

20. Cotten A. [Imaging of lipoma and liposarcoma]. *JBR-BTR.* 2002; 85(1):14–19.

21. Parizel PM, Geniets C. Tumors of peripheral nerves. In: Enzinger FM, Weiss SW, eds. *Imaging of soft tissue tumors.* 3rd ed. Berlin, New York: Springer; 2006:227–261.

22. Enzinger FM, Weiss SW. Benign tumors of peripheral nerves. In: Enzinger FM, Weiss SW, eds. *Soft tissue tumors.* 3rd ed. St. Louis, MO: Mosby; 1995:821–888.

23. Kumar AJ, Kuhajda FP, Martinez CR, Fishman EK, Jezic DV, Siegelman SS. Computed tomography of extracranial nerve sheath tumors with pathological correlation. *J Comput Assist Tomogr.* 1983; 7(5):857–865.

24. Chui MC, Bird BL, Rogers J. Extracranial and extraspinal nerve sheath tumors: Computed tomographic evaluation. *Neuroradiology.* 1988; 30(1):47–53.

25. Donner TR, Voorhies RM, Kline DG. Neural sheath tumors of major nerves. *J Neurosurg.* 1994; 81(3):362–373.

26. Bass JC, Korobkin M, Francis IR, Ellis JH, Cohan RH. Retroperitoneal plexiform neurofibromas: CT findings. *AJR Am J Roentgenol.* 1994; 163(3):617–620.

27. Meis-Kindblom JM, Enzinger FM. *Color atlas of soft tissue tumors.* St. Louis, MO: Mosby-Wolfe; 1996.

28. Osborn AG. Miscellaneous tumors, cysts and metastases. In: *Diagnostic neuroradiology.* St. Louis, MO: Mosby; 1994:626–670.

29. Ghosh BC, Ghosh L, Huvos AG, Fortner JG. Malignant schwannoma. A clinicopathologic study. *Cancer.* 1973; 31(1):184–190.

30. Zlatkin MB, Lander PH, Begin LR, Hadjipavlou A. Soft-tissue chondromas. *AJR Am J Roentgenol.* 1985; 144(6):1263–1267.

31. Kransdorf MJ, Meis JM. From the archives of the AFIP. Extraskeletal osseous and cartilaginous tumors of the extremities. *Radiographics.* 1993; 13(4):853–884.

32. Degryse HR, Aparisi F. Extrasqueletal cartilaginous and osseous tumors. In: De Schepper AM, ed. *Imaging of soft tissue tumors*. 3rd ed. Verlag Berlin Heidelberg: Springer; 2006:355–377.

33. Enzinger FM, Weiss SW. Cartilaginous soft tissue tumors. In: Enzinger FM, Weiss SW, eds. *Soft tissue tumors*. 3rd ed. St. Louis, MO: Mosby; 1995:991–1012.

34. Chung EB, Enzinger FM. Chondroma of soft parts. *Cancer*. 1978; 41(4):1414–1424.

35. Dahlin DC, Salvador AH. Cartilaginous tumors of the soft tissues of the hands and feet. *Mayo Clin Proc*. 1974; 49(10):721–726.

36. Schweitzer ME, Greenway G, Resnick D, Haghighi P, Snoots WE. Osteoma of soft parts. *Skeletal Radiol*. 1992; 21(3):177–180.

37. Allan CJ, Soule EH. Osteogenic sarcoma of the somatic soft tissues. Clinicopathologic study of 26 cases and review of literature. *Cancer*. 1971; 27(5):1121–1133.

38. Lee JH, Griffiths WJ, Bottomley RH. Extraosseous osteogenic sarcoma following an intramuscular injection. *Cancer*. 1977; 40(6):3097–3101.

39. Lorentzon R, Larsson SE, Boquist L. Extra-osseous osteosarcoma: A clinical and histopathological study of four cases. *J Bone Joint Surg Br*. 1979; 61-B(2):205–208.

40. Jarvi OH, Kvist HT, Vainio PV. Extraskeletal retroperitoneal osteosarcoma probably arising from myositis ossificans. *Acta Pathol Microbiol Scand*. 1968; 74(1):11–25.

41. Enzinger FM, Weiss SW. Osseous soft tissue tumors. In: Enzinger FM, Weiss SW, eds. *Soft tissue tumors*. 3rd ed. St. Louis, MO: Mosby; 1995:1013–1037.

42. Chung EB, Enzinger FM. Extraskeletal osteosarcoma. *Cancer*. 1987; 60(5):1132–1142.

43. Bane BL, Evans HL, Ro JY, Carrasco CH, Grignon DJ, Benjamin RS et al. Extraskeletal osteosarcoma. A clinicopathologic review of 26 cases. *Cancer*. 1990; 65(12):2762–2770.

44. Vanhoenacker FM, Van de Perre S, Van Marck E, Somville J, Gielen J, De Schepper AM. Extraskeletal osteosarcoma: Report of a case with unusual features and histopathological correlation. *Eur J Radiol*. 2004; 49(3):97–102.

45. Shafritz AB, Shore EM, Gannon FH, Zasloff MA, Taub R, Muenke M et al. Overexpression of an osteogenic morphogen in fibrodysplasia ossificans progressiva. *N Engl J Med*. 1996; 335(8):555–561.

46. Reinig JW, Hill SC, Fang M, Marini J, Zasloff MA. Fibrodysplasia ossificans progressiva: CT appearance. *Radiology*. 1986; 159(1):153–157.

47. Cohen RB, Hahn GV, Tabas JA, Peeper J, Levitz CL, Sando A et al. The natural history of heterotopic ossification in patients who have fibrodysplasia ossificans progressiva. A study of forty-four patients. *J Bone Joint Surg Am*. 1993; 75(2):215–219.

48. Singleton EB, Holt JF. Myositis ossificans progressiva. *Radiology*. 1954; 62(1):47–54.

49. Smith R, Russell RG, Woods CG. Myositis ossificans progressiva. Clinical features of eight patients and their response to treatment. *J Bone Joint Surg Br*. 1976; 58(1):48–57.

50. McCarthy EF, Sundaram M. Heterotopic ossification: A review. *Skeletal Radiol*. 2005; 34(10):609–619.

51. Kransdorf MJ, Meis JM, Jelinek JS. Myositis ossificans: MR appearance with radiologic–pathologic correlation. *AJR Am J Roentgenol*. 1991; 157(6):1243–1248.

52. Weiss SW, Goldblum JR, Folpe AL. Osseous soft tissue tumors. In: Enzinger FM, Weiss SW, eds. *Soft tissue tumors*. 5th ed. St Louis, MO: Mosby; 2002:1039–1061.

53. Dejerine M, Ceillier A. Three cases of osteoma: juxtamuscular and interfascicular periosteal ossifications in paraplegics by traumatic lesion of spinal cord. *Rev Neurol*. 1918; 25:159–172.

54. Carlier RY, Safa DM, Parva P, Mompoint D, Judet T, Denormandie P et al. Ankylosing neurogenic myositis ossificans of the hip. An enhanced volumetric CT study. *J Bone Joint Surg Br*. 2005; 87(3):301–305.

55. Bravo-Payno P, Esclarin A, Arzoz T, Arroyo O, Labarta C. Incidence and risk factors in the appearance of heterotopic ossification in spinal cord injury. *Paraplegia*. 1992; 30(10):740–745.

56. Mielants H, Vanhove E, de Neels J, Veys E. Clinical survey of and pathogenic approach to para-articular ossifications in long-term coma. *Acta Orthop Scand*. 1975; 46(2):190–198.

57. Izumi K. Study of ectopic bone formation in experimental spinal cord injured rabbits. *Paraplegia*. 1983; 21(6):351–363.

58. Della Santa DR, Reust P. [Heterotopic ossification and ulnar nerve compression syndrome of the elbow. A report of two cases]. *Ann Chir Main Memb Super*. 1990; 9(1):38–41.

59. Brooke MM, Heard DL, de Lateur BJ, Moeller DA, Alquist AD. Heterotopic ossification and peripheral nerve entrapment: Early diagnosis and excision. *Arch Phys Med Rehabil*. 1991; 72(6):425–429.

60. Gallien P, Nicolas B, Le Bot MP, Robineau S, Rivier I, Sarkis S et al. [Heterotopic ossification and vascular compression]. *Rev Rhum Ed Fr*. 1994; 61(11):823–828.

61. De Schepper A, Khan S, Alexiou J, De Beuckeleer L. Soft tissue metastasis. In: Enzinger FM, ed. *Imaging of soft tissue tumors*. Berlin; New York: Springer; 2006:447–458.

62. Magee T, Rosenthal H. Skeletal muscle metastases at sites of documented trauma. *AJR Am J Roentgenol*. 2002; 178(4):985–988.

63. Seely S. Possible reasons for the high resistance of muscle to cancer. *Med Hypotheses*. 1980; 6(2):133–137.

64. Alexander JW, Altemeier WA. Susceptibility of injured tissues to hematogenous metastases: An experimental study. *Ann Surg*. 1964; 159:933–944.

65. Buerger LF, Monteleone PN. Leukemic-lymphomatous infiltration of skeletal muscle. Systematic study of 82 autopsy cases. *Cancer*. 1966; 19(10):1416–1422.

66. Willis RA. *The spread of tumours in the human body*. London: Butterworths; 1952:284–285.

67. Araki K, Kobayashi M, Ogata T, Takuma K. Colorectal carcinoma metastatic to skeletal muscle. *Hepatogastroenterology*. 1994; 41(5):405–408.

68. Avery GR. Metastatic adenocarcinoma masquerading as a psoas abscess. *Clin Radiol*. 1988; 39(3):319–320.

69. Tuoheti Y, Okada K, Osanai T, Nishida J, Ehara S, Hashimoto M et al. Skeletal muscle metastases of carcinoma: A clinicopathological study of 12 cases. *Jpn J Clin Oncol*. 2004; 34(4):210–214.

70. Peh WC, Shek TW, Wang SC, Wong JW, Chien EP. Osteogenic sarcoma with skeletal muscle metastases. *Skeletal Radiol.* 1999; 28(5):298–304.

71. Herring CL, Jr., Harrelson JM, Scully SP. Metastatic carcinoma to skeletal muscle. A report of 15 patients. *Clin Orthop Relat Res.* 1998; 355:272–281.

72. Narvaez JA, Narvaez J, Clavaguera MT, Juanola X, Valls C, Fiter J. Bone and skeletal muscle metastases from gastric adenocarcinoma: Unusual radiographic, CT and scintigraphic features. *Eur Radiol.* 1998; 8(8):1366–1369.

73. Schultz SR, Bree RL, Schwab RE, Raiss G. CT detection of skeletal muscle metastases. *J Comput Assist Tomogr.* 1986; 10(1):81–83.

74. Damron TA, Heiner J. Distant soft tissue metastases: A series of 30 new patients and 91 cases from the literature. *Ann Surg Oncol.* 2000; 7(7):526–534.

75. Pretorius ES, Fishman EK. Helical CT of skeletal muscle metastases from primary carcinomas. *AJR Am J Roentgenol.* 2000; 174(2):401–404.

76. Nguyen NC, Chaar BT, Osman MM. Prevalence and patterns of soft tissue metastasis: Detection with true whole-body F-18 FDG PET/CT. *BMC Med Imaging.* 2007; 7:8.

77. Agamanolis DP, Dasu S, Krill CE, Jr. Tumors of skeletal muscle. *Hum Pathol.* 1986; 17(8):778–795.

78. Cohen EK, Kressel HY, Perosio T, Burk DL, Jr., Dalinka MK, Kanal E et al. MR imaging of soft-tissue hemangiomas: Correlation with pathologic findings. *AJR Am J Roentgenol.* 1988; 150(5):1079–1081.

79. Engelstad BL, Gilula LA, Kyriakos M. Ossified skeletal muscle hemangioma: Radiologic and pathologic features. *Skeletal Radiol.* 1980; 5(1):35–40.

80. Ly JQ, Sanders TG, Mulloy JP, Soares GM, Beall DP, Parsons TW et al. Osseous change adjacent to soft-tissue hemangiomas of the extremities: Correlation with lesion size and proximity to bone. *AJR Am J Roentgenol.* 2003; 180(6):1695–1700.

81. Murphey MD, Fairbairn KJ, Parman LM, Baxter KG, Parsa MB, Smith WS. From the archives of the AFIP. Musculoskeletal angiomatous lesions: Radiologic–pathologic correlation. *Radiographics.* 1995; 15(4):893–917.

82. Ramon F. Tumors and tumor-like lesions of blood vessels. In: Schepper D, ed. *Imaging of soft tissue tumors.* Berlin: Springer; 2006:263–282.

83. Chan FP, Rubin GD. MDCT angiography of pediatric vascular diseases of the abdomen, pelvis, and extremities. *Pediatr Radiol.* 2005; 35(1):40–53.

84. Bastarrika G, Redondo P, Sierra A, Cano D, Martinez-Cuesta A, Lopez-Gutierrez JC et al. New techniques for the evaluation and therapeutic planning of patients with Klippel-Trenaunay syndrome. *J Am Acad Dermatol.* 2007; 56(2):242–249.

85. Mavili E, Ozturk M, Akcali Y, Donmez H, Yikilmaz A, Tokmak TT et al. Direct CT venography for evaluation of the lower extremity venous anomalies of Klippel-Trenaunay syndrome. *AJR Am J Roentgenol.* 2009; 192(6):W311–W316.

86. Vanhoenacker FM, Van Goethem JWM, Vandevenne JE, Shahabpour M. Synovial tumors. In: Schepper AMD, ed. *Imaging of soft tissue tumors.* Berlin; New York: Springer; 2006:311–323.

87. Steiner E, Steinbach LS, Schnarkowski P, Tirman PF, Genant HK. Ganglia and cysts around joints. *Radiol Clin North Am.* 1996; 34(2):395–425, xi–xii.

88. Malghem J, Vande berg BC, Lebon C, Lecouvet FE, Maldague BE. Ganglion cysts of the knee: Articular communication revealed by delayed radiography and CT after arthrography. *AJR Am J Roentgenol.* 1998; 170(6):1579–1583.

89. Chaabane S, Bouaziz MC, Drissi C, Abid L, Ladeb MF. Periosteal chondrosarcoma. *AJR Am J Roentgenol.* 2009; 192(1):W1–W6.

90. Gitelis S, Petasnick JP, Turner DA, Ghiselli RW, Miller AW, 3rd. Endometriosis simulating a soft tissue tumor of the thigh: CT and MR evaluation. *J Comput Assist Tomogr.* 1985; 9(3):573–576.

91. Stein L, Elsayes KM, Wagner-Bartak N. Subcutaneous abdominal wall masses: Radiological reasoning. *AJR Am J Roentgenol.* 2011; 198(2):W146–W151.

92. Stewart VL, Herling P, Dalinka MK. Calcification in soft tissues. *JAMA.* 1983; 250(1):78–81.

93. Contiguglia SR, Alfrey AC, Miller NL, Runnells DE, Le Geros RZ. Nature of soft tissue calcification in uremia. *Kidney Int.* 1973; 4(3):229–235.

94. Hayes CW, Conway WF. Calcium hydroxyapatite deposition disease. *Radiographics.* 1990; 10(6):1031–1048.

95. Kaplan MJ, Eavey RD. Calcific tendinitis of the longus colli muscle. *Ann Otol Rhinol Laryngol.* 1984; 93 (3 Pt 1):215–219.

96. Eastwood JD, Hudgins PA, Malone D. Retropharyngeal effusion in acute calcific prevertebral tendinitis: Diagnosis with CT and MR imaging. *AJNR Am J Neuroradiol.* 1998; 19(9):1789–1792.

97. Omezzine SJ, Hafsa C, Lahmar I, Driss N, Hamza H. Calcific tendinitis of the longus colli: Diagnosis by CT. *Joint Bone Spine.* 2008; 75(1):90–91.

98. Bladt O, Vanhoenacker R, Bevernage C, Van Orshoven M, Van Hoe L, D'Haenens P. Acute calcific prevertebral tendinitis. *JBR-BTR.* 2008; 91(4):158–159.

99. Park SY, Jin W, Lee SH, Park JS, Yang DM, Ryu KN. Acute retropharyngeal calcific tendinitis: A case report with unusual location of calcification. *Skeletal Radiol.* 39(8):817–820.

100. Hall FM, Docken WP, Curtis HW. Calcific tendinitis of the longus coli: Diagnosis by CT. *Am J Roentgenol.* 1986; 147:742–743.

101. Fayad LM, Carrino JA, Fishman EK. Musculoskeletal infection: Role of CT in the emergency department. *Radiographics.* 2007; 27(6):1723–1736.

102. Ozalay M, Ozkoc G, Akpinar S, Hersekli MA, Tandogan RN. Necrotizing soft-tissue infection of a limb: Clinical presentation and factors related to mortality. *Foot Ankle Int.* 2006; 27(8):598–605.

103. Bickels J, Ben-Sira L, Kessler A, Wientroub S. Primary pyomyositis. *J Bone Joint Surg Am.* 2002; 84-A(12): 2277–2286.

104. Bahebeck J, Bedimo R, Eyenga V, Kouamfack C, Kingue T, Nierenet M et al. The management of musculoskeletal infection in HIV carriers. *Acta Orthop Belg.* 2004; 70(4):355–360.

21

Computed Tomography-Based Interventional Radiology in the Musculoskeletal System

Fernando Ruiz Santiago, Luis Guzmán Álvarez, and María del Mar Castellano García

CONTENTS

21.1 Introduction

Although interventional radiology in the musculoskeletal system can be performed based on physical anatomic landmark, it is safer performed under imaging guidance. Fluoroscopy, ultrasound, computed tomography (CT), and magnetic resonance (MR) can be used with different advantages and drawbacks.

CT combines fast imaging acquisition and a superior anatomic resolution of the bone tissue allowing a precise localization of the target. Contrast in soft tissues can be enhanced by iodine dye. Compartmental anatomy can be clearly defined, and the exact course of a needle tract can be accurately planned to avoid entering uninvolved compartments.

The main disadvantage of CT guidance is the risk derived of radiation. Slice acquisitions are performed repetitively on the same anatomic area with absorbed doses up to 1.6 Gray [1]. If fluoro-CT is available, the risk of radiation affects both the patient and the interventionist [2]. Nevertheless, in-room time can be significantly reduced by 32% [3].

21.2 General Patient Preparation

Informed patient consent after detailed explanation of the procedure and potential complications should be obtained before the intervention. Unless emergency, it must be signed by the patient or legal tutor before the procedure.

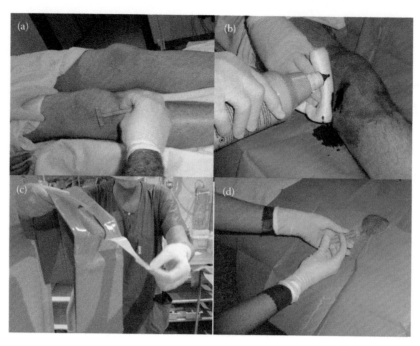

FIGURE 21.1
(a) Shaving of the skin. (b) Antiseptic application. (c) Exposure of the drape adherent surface. (d) Drape delineating the interventional area.

A close coagulation study is mandatory before any interventional procedure. Procedures are contraindicated with platelet levels <100,000/mm³, prothrombin time <70%, and international normalized ratio (INR) >1.4.

High INR is usually due to liver disease or coumarin intake. Coumarin must be replaced by heparin 5–7 days before the procedure. INR can also be reversed by administering vitamin K or fresh plasma. In case of patients taking medication inhibiting platelet aggregation (e.g., acetylic salicylic acid, clopidogrel), medication should be retrieved 7–10 days before the procedure.

Physiologic monitoring including pulse oximetry and pulse rate is routinely used in all procedures performed by administering local anesthesia. Intermittent automatic blood pressure is also monitored if other kind of anesthesia is administered. Detection of changes in cardiac rate, oxygen saturation, or blood pressure allows early application of corrective measures.

21.3 Local Site Preparation

All musculoskeletal procedures require strict adherence to standards of sterility. Microbial contamination of the intervention site may lead to nosocomial infection. Skin entrance point preparation is of paramount importance. Shaving immediately before the intervention compared to shaving within 24 hours preoperatively was associated with a lower local infection risk because microscopic cuts in the skin can serve as foci for bacterial multiplication [4]. The patient's skin is prepared by applying an antiseptic in concentric circles using sterile gauzes, beginning in the area of the proposed entrance point.

Sterile drapes are carefully placed all over the patient respecting aseptic principles and delineating the intervention field (Figure 21.1). The surgical drapes can have an adhesive aperture or margin protected with paper strips, which have to be removed prior to fixing the drape to the patient's skin.

At the end of the interventional procedure, the incision or needle entry point on the skin must be cleaned again with antiseptic and covered with a sterile dressing.

21.4 Pharmacological Agents for Interventions

Local anesthesia is usually enough for most of the procedures performed in CT. Nevertheless, conscious sedation, nerve blockage, or epidural or general anesthesia must be considered in long or painful procedures. Most of the children receive general anesthesia.

Local anesthetic agents are commonly used for infiltrative injection to get local pain control. Added with the injectate, they help to reduce joint pain. Most commonly used for this purpose are amide-linked group of anesthetics (lidocaine, mepivacaine, bupivacaine, and ropivacaine). Their duration of action without epinephrine is medium for lidocaine (30–60 minutes) and mepivacaine (45–90 minutes) and long for bupivacaine (120–140 minutes) and ropivacaine (120–360 minutes).

Sedation can be reached by intravenous administration of benzodiazepines, for example, midazolam (1–5 mg can be administered), and it is specially indicated in anxious patients. Opioids are used when local anesthesia or nerve block do not avoid a very painful procedure. Fentanyl (from 0.02 to 0.15 mg) is used for analgesia and sedation.

Antibiotics should be administered intravenously before some of the procedures to prevent infection. The purpose of antibiotic coverage is to decrease the chance of seeding bacteria into poorly vascularized sites such as the disk or necrotic tissue. We routinely administer 2 g cefazolin before the most complicated procedures, such as vertebroplasty and thermal ablation. Also, in some risky patients, inmunodepressed or with heart diseases, antibiotherapy is advised, even in minor intervention.

Corticosteroids have a long history in the treatment of painful joints. Most commonly used are particulate (triamcinolone acetonide and methylprednisolone acetate) and freely soluble corticoids (betamethasone and dexamethasone sodium phosphate). Potency for milligram of particulate corticoids is fivefold lower than for soluble corticoids. Nevertheless, duration of action is superior for insoluble corticoids because of their chemical nature. As ester preparations, they require hydrolysis by cellular esterases to release the active moiety and consequently last longer in the joint than do nonester soluble preparations, which are quickly taken up with rapid onset of effect and concomitant shorter duration of action [5].

Hyaluronic acid is currently used for the symptomatic treatment of mild to moderate osteoarthritis, mainly at the hip, knee, ankle, and shoulder joints. It is normally found in healthy cartilage and synovial fluid. Injections are intended to supplement the deficiency of natural hyaluronic acid in degenerative joints, cushioning the blow of the joint and helping to reduce pain and restore mobility and flexibility. We administer 3 cc (60 mg) in a single injection. Symptoms usually relieve and improvement is expected to last at least 6 months.

21.5 Needles

Many types of needles are available. Availability, familiarity, and cost are the factors that might influence the choice, but the main reason should be the success rate of the procedure. The gauge and length may influence the success in many procedures. There are two measurement systems. In the gauge (G) system, there is an inverse relationship between the number and the caliber of the needle. This system allows a small range of variability between manufacturers about the dimensions of the inner and outer diameters of the needles and catheters [6]. In the French (F) system, there is a direct relationship between the caliber of the needle and its number. One French is equivalent to 0.33 mm. The appropriate choice of needles and catheters may take years of experience and may change with technological innovations.

For cementoplasty, we use bevelled needles with a notch in the hub indicating the bevelled face. This notch is located in the outer cannula and also serves to fit the stylet by locking inside a metal protrusion on the stylet (Luer-Lock). The stylet must be rotated to unlock before withdrawing. Wings located at the base of the cannula facilitate removal and rotation of the needle. Three gauges are available: 10, 13, and 15 G. We preferentially use 13 G for most of the vertebroplasty procedures, preserving 10 G to cases we need to obtain a coaxial thicker biopsy before cementation (Figure 21.2).

In bone lesions, the selection of the needle is mainly based on the hardness of the bone. We generally use a coaxial system, where an outer shorter guide needle is introduced first until the edge of the lesion and a thinner longer one is used to perform the procedure through the introductory cannula. In most of the bone lesions, we choose a bevelled 10 or 13 G vertebroplasty introductory needle. Then, coaxial biopsy is performed with 13 G Bard Ostycut needle or 15 G OptiMed coaxial bone biopsy cannula. The last sampling can be performed with the introductory needle that is advanced inside the

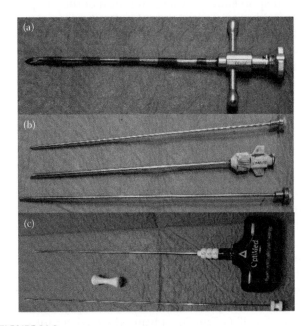

FIGURE 21.2

(a) Vertebroplasty needle. (b) Bard Ostycut needle set. (c) OptiMed needle set.

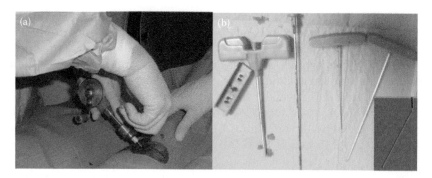

FIGURE 21.3
(a) Manual drill of a bone lesion. (b) BiopsyBell fully remove set. The fully stylet end (insert) is a thin bar of stainless steel that cuts the specimen inside the cannula.

lesion if its consistency is supposed to not be hard, such as in osteolytic or medullary lesions.

The Bard Ostycut set consists of a two-part biopsy cannula, an obturator to push out the sample and a self-locking aspiration syringe to implement sample aspiration. The biopsy cannula consists of an outer cannula with an eccentric bevel at the tip and an inner trocar-type stylet. After removing the stylet, the biopsy sample can be obtained by deepening and rotating clockwise the outer cannula inside the lesion. The threaded tip of the cannula facilitates introduction. Nevertheless, we can also introduce the cannula hitting with a hammer.

The OptiMed coaxial bone biopsy cannula consists of an outer cannula with saw tooth tip and three troughs in the distal end to improve attachment of the biopsy specimen. The cannula is mainly introduced rotating in a clockwise direction, but tapping with a hammer can be of help in some cases. For removal of the sample, an inlet guide is mounted onto the distal end of the cannula and the sample is pushed out in a retrograde way inserting an ejector mandrin through the mounted inlet guide.

In sclerotic bone with thickened cortex or periosteal reaction, care should be taken to minimize the risk of breaking the needles. In these cases, we use two methods. First, we can use a manual or battery-activated drill to open the path to the aforementioned needles. Second, we can use a large bore introductory needle, 8 G BiopsyBell fully remove bone marrow biopsy needle. An inner stylet facilitates penetration of the cortex. After removal of the stylet, the cannula is introduced between 1 and 2 cm. Then the fully needle is introduced and the set cannula-fully is turned twice 360° to cut the sample. The sample is pushed out by inserting an extractor stylet inside the cannula (Figure 21.3).

In soft tissues or lytic bone lesion with soft-tissue component, we prefer to perform the biopsy with automatic 14 to 18 G Tru-Cut, advanced trough an introductory needle of the same length of the armed Tru-Cut.

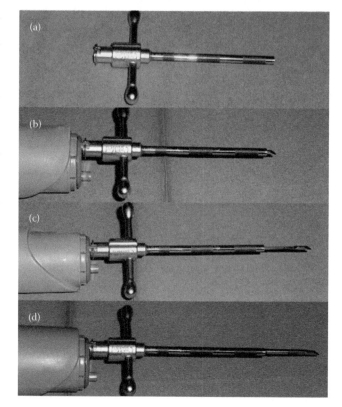

FIGURE 21.4
(a) The cannula of the needle has been cut to the same length of the armed Tru-Cut (b). (c) The inner needle, characterized by a trough in its end, has been fired. (d) The outer needle covers the trough and cuts the sample out.

The introductory needle is approached to the edge of the lesion and the Tru-Cut penetrates a known depth, 11 or 22 mm, inside the lesion. Changes in the obliquity of the introductory needle allow us to obtain different samples with only one entrance point. The cannula of the introductory needle is manually cut by specialized personnel, to match the appropriate length of the armed Tru-Cut, and sterilized before use (Figure 21.4).

The Tru-Cut biopsy needle has an inner component with a trough at the edge of the distal end. When fired by the gun, a core of tissue falls inside the trough. Then, the outer component cuts the core out of the surrounding tissue capturing the sample.

For facet and caudal injections, we prefer 22 G needles with Quincke tip (cutting open bevel). A key/slot arrangement of stylet and cannula hubs facilitates proper needle bevel orientation. For epidural injection or myelography small gauge, 25–27 G and a pencil-point tip can be used. For thinner needles, an introducer may be necessary to direct the needle to the appropriate path.

21.6 CT Guidance

CT guidance provides both precision and safety. It contributes at every stage of the procedure such as the following:

1. Pre-procedure: assessment of the size, configuration, and anatomic localization of the target for selection of the appropriate tools and planning the safest approach to the lesion that avoids sensitive neurovascular structures.
2. Intra-procedure: monitoring of the introductory needles during the procedure and ensuring the correct positioning during all the process.

The anatomic area under study must be centered with the inner laser line of the gantry and marked as zero in the numerical display to reduce table displacement and match the numerical displacement of the anatomic slices with the gantry display number (Figure 21.5). The whole area of interest is imaged to confirm the preselected optimal route of entrance. Because the operating position of the patient can be different to the pre-procedure study, the most appropriate path to the lesion might be changed at this moment. The table is moved to the numerical position of the selected slice and the skin marked with a felt pen matching the laser light beam. The precise entry point may be chosen by using a grid, either commercially or homemade, taped to the skin. Nevertheless, for most of the musculoskeletal procedures, the intramuscular needle used for local anesthesia can be used for selecting the most appropriate way. Injecting a small amount of anesthetic in each step, we reach a more progressive and comfortable anesthesia of the soft tissues. In deep anatomic areas, we use a long spinal needle for infiltration of the tissues not reached by the intramuscular needle.

In the vicinity of sensitive anatomic structures (blood vessels, nerves), damage should be avoided by introducing the needle in short, careful steps.

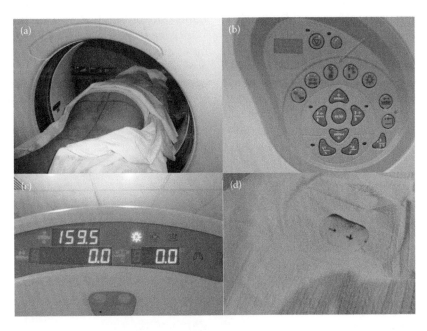

FIGURE 21.5
(a) Patient is centered with the inner laser line. (b) The table displacement is set to zero with the appropriate button (arrow). (c) The numerical display of the gantry marks zero displacement. (d) With a felt pen the entrance point level, matching the target slice displacement with the inner laser line, has been marked.

3. Post-procedure: follow-up of patients is preferentially made by means of MR imaging (MRI) in order to minimize the radiation dose.

21.7 Complications

Any invasive procedure must be managed with the maximum quality criteria to minimize the risk of complications. Complications can be secondary to the puncture or to the medication used. The puncture can lead to vascular injury with hemorrhage, nerve injury, pneumothorax, or infection (Figure 21.6).

Complications secondary to drugs include anaphylactic (idiosyncratic) reaction to iodinated contrast material or anesthetic. The amino ester groups of anesthetics (procaine, tetracaine, and benzocaine) have been used for a long time and are known to have a higher allergic potential than amide-linked groups of anesthetics (lidocaine, mepivacaine, bupivacaine, and ropivacaine).

Anesthetic agents can be toxic, mainly if they are used in inappropriate doses or route. Inadvertent intravascular injection is the most common cause of local anesthetic toxicity. Central nervous system complications include excitation, seizures, depression with a cessation of convulsions and the onset of unconsciousness, and respiratory depression or arrest. Cardiovascular effects are primarily those of direct myocardial depression and bradycardia, which may lead to cardiovascular collapse.

Reported local complications of corticoids at spinal level include arachnoiditis, meningitis, and paraparesis/paraplegia. Arachnoiditis is thought to be secondary to intradural or intrathecal injection that should be avoided. Neurologic deficit have been attributed to particulate corticoids when, inadvertently, injected intra-arterial. At the extremities, they have been related with local tissue atrophy, tendon rupture, and cartilage damage. Systemic effects include flushing and increased blood glucose level.

21.8 Classification of the Procedures

Procedures performed under CT guidance can be classified as diagnostic, therapeutic, or intended to both purposes. CT can also be used to perform regional anesthesia before different procedures because of its ability to identify the epidural space and peripheral nerves.

21.9 Diagnostic Procedures

21.9.1 Biopsy

Biopsy is indicated in diagnosing tumors and infectious conditions. Fine-needle aspiration biopsy, ≥20 G, can be enough to aspirate inside an abscess, although only aseptic pus can be obtained and histologic analysis is not possible. For that reason, in suspected infectious process, we usually approach the lesion with an introductory 13 G needle and target the lesion coaxially, as many times as we need, with a 15 G trephine to obtain fluid and bone or soft-tissue material for microbiological and pathological analysis. In the first case, the sample is put into a sterile tube. For pathological analysis, the sample is fixed in 10% formalin introduced in small plastic perforated containers that avoid dispersion of the tissue (Figure 21.7).

Incisional biopsy is considered the gold standard in bone and soft-tissue tumors with reported diagnostic accuracy between 94% and 98%. However, when tumors are located in the spine, retroperitoneum, or other deep-seated areas of the trunk, or are close to vital organs and neurovascular bundles, open biopsy becomes not only highly invasive but may also cause various complications.

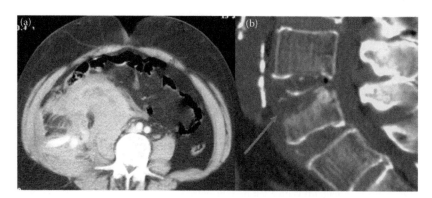

FIGURE 21.6
Retroperitoneal hematoma (a) and spondylodiscitis (arrow in b) secondary to vertebral biopsy.

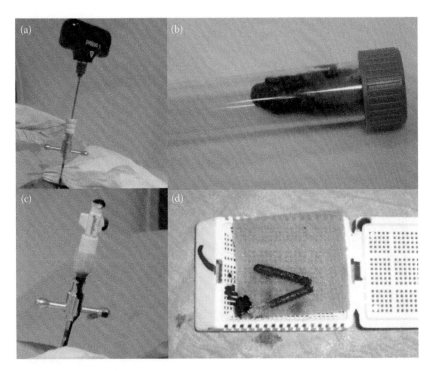

FIGURE 21.7
(a) Coaxial biopsy for an infectious condition. (b) Tube containing the sample. (c) Coaxial biopsy for a tumor. (d) The core biopsy specimens are introduced in a small plastic container.

The introduction of CT guidance in the 1970s, combined with improvements in the ability to handle smaller tissue samples, did much to expand the safety and effectiveness of percutaneous biopsy [7]. It not only helps to avoid neurovascular bundles and vital organs, but also confirms that the needle tip is correctly positioned at the targeted site.

Before indicating a biopsy, all prior imaging studies and patient history must be carefully reviewed, considering the differential diagnoses of the lesion as well as the probable diagnosis. The route of biopsy or type of biopsy to be performed are planned to avoid sensitive neurovascular structures.

Appropriate selection of biopsy needles according to the properties of individual tumors is of paramount importance in strengthening the diagnostic yield. Core biopsy is performed either with spring-activated cutting needles (Tru-Cut) in combination with a biopsy gun or with manually activated cutting needles or trephines.

We recommend at least four core biopsies for soft-tissue tumors and three core biopsies for bone tumors. Nevertheless, quite often, the tissue is very friable, like in some metastases and myeloma, and only hemorrhagic soft-tissue material can be sent to pathologist.

Depending on the localization of the bone lesion, different approaches are available.

Vertebral body biopsies can be approached by a transpedicular or extrapedicular way. For disk biopsy, a posterolateral approach is mostly used. A coaxial system allows obtaining multiple samples with only one entrance point. We use a combination of 13–15 G needles for the disk and small vertebral bodies. For larger vertebral bodies, we can also use a combination of 10–13 G needles.

At cervical level, a right anterolateral approach has been advocated. Even for C1–C2 vertebral bodies, a transoral way has been described. Nevertheless, a contrast-enhanced CT scan may facilitate other choices tailored for each location, including posterior or lateral access (Figure 21.8).

Biopsy of a potential metastasis has different considerations compared with biopsy of a primary bone tumor. For metastases, when surgical treatment is not an option, the route is less important because seeding is not the main concern and the shortest and most direct path to the lesion may be used. If a limb primary bone tumor is suspected, we are forced to choose a well-established approach in the theoretical surgical way because the biopsy path must be resected en bloc with the tumor at the definite time of the limb sparing surgery. The needle should not traverse an uninvolved compartment, joint, or neurovascular bundle, mainly when these adjacent structures are needed for reconstruction [8] (Figure 21.9).

At the shoulder girdle, the deltoid and pectoral muscles are used to reconstruct the shoulder. Therefore, the posterior compartment, with the axillary nerve that innervates the deltoid muscle must be avoided. Ideally, lesions are approached through the anterior third of the deltoid muscle between the cephalic vein and the

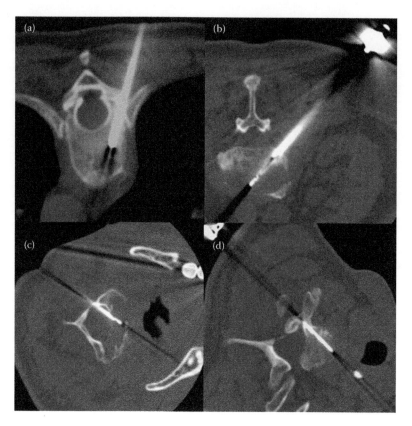

FIGURE 21.8
(a) Transpedicular biopsy at thoracic level. (b) Extrapedicular biopsy at lumbar level. (c) Extrapedicular intra-canal biopsy of C2. (d) Transpedicular biopsy of C7.

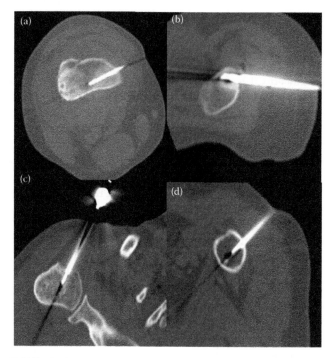

FIGURE 21.9
(a) Medial approach for biopsy of the distal femur in a patient with osteosarcoma. (b) Lateral approach in proximal femur. (c) Anterior approach for an upper humeral chondrosarcoma. (d) Lateral approach in humeral shaft.

biceps tendon. At the humeral shaft, entrance just posterior to the biceps muscle and the cephalic vein, through the brachialis muscle or the distal portion of the deltoid muscle is recommended. At the distal humerus, entrance can be performed directly through the medial or lateral epicondyle [9].

At the forearm, the interosseous membrane forms a natural barrier to the spread of tumor between the extensor and flexor compartments. Transection of the interosseous membrane during biopsy should be avoided [10].

The gluteal musculature and rectus femoris are essential pelvic structures, needed for good functional outcomes. These muscles must be avoided by entering the ileum anteriorly or posteriorly.

The rectus femoris and quadriceps tendon are essential structures for knee function and should be avoided. Care must also be taken to avoid contaminating the knee joint compartment. Ideally, lateral or medial approaches to a femoral lesion are preferred. The lateral approach is preferred when the vastus lateralis muscle is involved without involvement of the medial neurovascular structures. The needle should enter anterior to lateral intermuscular septum for most of the femoral masses, unless there was posterior extension of the mass. If a lesion is close to the femoral vessels, a medial approach facilitates vessel exploration. The needle should enter a line

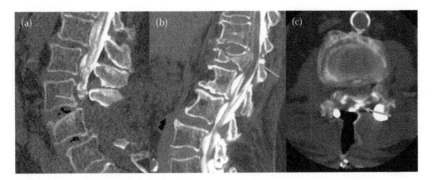

FIGURE 21.10
Myelography. (a) Canal stenosis (arrow). (b) Medullar impingement secondary to a vertebral fracture. (c) Postoperative cerebrospinal fluid fistula (arrow).

overlying the vastus medialis muscle and the adductor tubercle of the femur [9].

At the leg, the medial aspect of the tibia lies immediately beneath the skin and avoid contaminating the extensor or flexor compartments. Both compartments are separated by the interosseous membrane that constitutes a natural barrier to tumor spread. At the fibula, the needle should enter a longitudinal line just anterior to the septum between the peroneus muscles and the soleus muscle [9].

In general, superior results are obtained with lesions in the extremities or pelvis compared with those in the spine [11]. A meta-analysis concluded that the accuracy and complication rates of spinal biopsies increased with the inner diameter of the needles [12]. Reported accuracy of CT-guided biopsy in bone tumors is about 90%, higher in malign than benign tumors, in metastases than in primary tumors, in lytic than sclerotic lesions [13]. Yield in infectious diseases is generally lower, mainly due to antibiotic intake before the procedure [8].

Even though the rate of diagnosis of benignity and malignancy is high, a definitive diagnosis is occasionally difficult to make in cases with tumors such as osteosarcomas containing numerous giant cells and telangiectatic osteosarcomas. Contrast helps to select the appropriate area to biopsy enhancing the vascular and solid parts of the tumors.

21.9.2 Myelography

CT myelography is mainly indicated when MRI is contraindicated, such as in patients with pacemaker, and when conventional CT do not get a conclusive diagnosis. It still plays a role in depicting suspected leakage of cerebrospinal fluid (CSF) or traumatic injury of cervical nerve roots [14].

Appropriate injection of 10–15 cc of contrast can be made through the interspinous space by physical palpation, but CT guidance offers visual evidence of the exact localization of the needle. The patient is in prone position with a pillow under the belly to increase separation of the posterior apophysis of the spine. After introduction of the contrast, a CT scan is performed at the prone position that nicely depicts the anterior aspect of the thecal sac and nerve roots. Another scan in supine position is recommended to elucidate injuries to the posterior part of the thecal sac, mainly when we are looking for postoperative fistula. CT myelography is able to detect any leakage of contrast-enhanced CSF and compression of neural structures (Figure 21.10).

21.10 Diagnostic and Therapeutic Procedures

21.10.1 Arthrography

Arthrography can be performed based on anatomical landmark or under fluoroscopy, ultrasound, or CT guidance. In our hospital, most of these procedures are performed with fluoroscopy guidance, followed by CT and MRI in this order to complete the diagnostic workup. We introduce a mixture of saline with iodine contrast and a small amount of gadolinium (Table 21.1). The mixture can be added with 1–5 cc 2% mepivacaina and 20–40 mg triamcinolone for therapeutic purposes.

TABLE 21.1

Means Values of Mixture Components Used for Arthrography

	Arthrography			
Joint	Saline	Dye	Gadolinium (mg)	Mepivacaine (cc)
Shoulder	10	5	0.2	2
Elbow	4	2	0.1	1
Wrist[a]	4	2	0.1	1
Hip	10	5	0.2	2
Knee	30	10	0.4	5
Ankle	4	2	0.1	1

[a] For wrist, we follow this order: Distal radioulnar joint, 1 cc; midcarpal joint, 1–2 cc; radiocarpal joint, 3–4 cc.

We consider both techniques, CT and MRI, complementary. Nevertheless, CT arthrography (CTA) provides some advantages over MRI, mainly based in the submillimeter resolution capability of current generation multi-detector scanners. CTA provides an excellent contrast between bone, hyaline cartilage, and intra-articular iodinated contrast material. Therefore, morphologic changes of cartilage can be depicted with high resolution. Osteochondral loose bodies are shown as negative defects inside the contrast media. Calcified osteochondral bodies can also be defined, but may be confounded with contrast media if previous X-ray film or noncontrast CT is not available. MRI may detect these osteochondral loose bodies.

We prepare two syringes; one for iodine contrast and another with a mixture of saline, anesthetic, and gadolinium. Both syringes are connected to a fluid extension catheter tube with three-way stopcock. The intra-articular position of the needle is confirmed when the contrast media distribute inside the joint away from the needle tip. Then, filling of the joint is performed alternating the injection of the two syringes until the patient refers bloated feeling of the joint. Only for wrist joint, we connect each syringe to an independent tube. Because of small capacity of the joints, the remaining contrast of the tube could avoid injection of an appropriate amount of saline–gadolinium mixture (Figure 21.11).

Hyaluronic acid is nowadays injected in osteoarthritis to delay progression of cartilage damage. Although it can be done based on anatomical landmark or under ultrasound guidance, quite often we perform this procedure with CT. After inserting the needle inside the joint, it is connected to fluid extension catheter tube with three-way stopcock connected to a syringe filled with a mixture of saline and iodine contrast.

Anesthetic and/or corticoids added to the mixture are optional. The other cock is connected to a syringe with 3 cc (60 mg) of hyaluronic acid. First, we check the intra-articular position of the needle injecting a small amount of dye. The hyaluronic acid in injected after this confirmatory test and filling of the joint is completed with the mixture of saline and iodine contrast. Higher pressure is necessary to inject the hyaluronic acid. Diagnostic arthrography gets a nice picture of the real state of the joint that may be used as anatomical basis for evaluating the progression of the lesions.

21.10.2 Diagnostic and Therapeutic Procedures at the Intervertebral Disk

Discography can be performed under fluoroscopy or CT. As diagnostic test, it should be reserved to confirm unresolved disk-related pain in patients who have failed other diagnostic tests or are being considered for spine fusion. Clinical response is classified after contrast injection as no pain or pressure only, pain dissimilar to clinical symptoms, pain similar to clinical symptoms, or exact reproduction of symptoms [15].

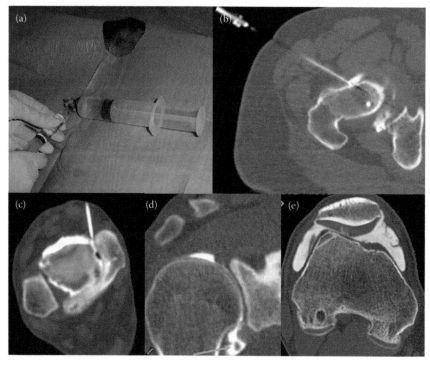

FIGURE 21.11
Arthrography. (a) Syringes and tube during the procedure. (b) Hip arthrography. (c) Ankle arthrography. (d) Osteochondral fragment in the axillary recess of the shoulder (arrow). (e) Chondral fissures in the patellar cartilage (arrow).

If positive, injection of a mixture of anesthetic and corticoids can be used as therapeutic procedure, mainly in degenerate disk with subchondral edema in MRI [16]. Other minimal invasive spine treatments, such as percutaneous disk ablation, chemonucleolysis, percutaneous laser disk decompression, and electrothermal therapy can be performed after successful test because, when correlated to a positive discography, their results seem to be better [17] (Figure 21.12).

Distribution of the contrast inside the disk gives a nice picture of the disk anatomy before surgical or percutaneous treatment. The normal discogram usually shows the appearance of a "cotton ball" or a "hamburger bun" in the center of the disk. Tears of the annulus fibrosus are classified as radial (from the nucleus pulposus to the annulus fibrosus), concentric (between lamellas of annulus fibrous), and transverse (annular tears at the apophyseal rings) (Figure 21.12).

Most of the percutaneous disk treatment procedures aim to reduce pressure of the nucleus pulposus creating a free space that allow the herniated fragment to come back, reducing mechanical irritation of the nerve roots and nerve endings at the annulus fibrosus. This decompression can be mechanical (automated percutaneous lumbar discectomy), chemical (ozone and discogel), and thermal (radiofrequency and laser). Approach to the disk is posterolateral at dorsal and lumbar level and right anterolateral at cervical level [18].

Percutaneous disk decompression is indicated when nucleus pulposus is still contained by the annulus fibrosus, diagnosed by CT or MRI, with associated clinical sign of radicular pain severer than spinal pain and decreased sensitivity, reflex, and motor response. After 6 weeks of medical treatment and, at least, one selective periradicular injection, no significant improvement is reached [19].

21.10.3 Spinal Injections

Pain at the spine can have many sources, including the facet joints, the sacroiliac (SI) joint, the intervertebral disk, the vertebral body, and the pars interarticularis, by themselves or by stimulating the neural structures. Interventional procedures used to treat the underlying disorder can also be considered diagnostic test when they resolve or reduce pain by acting on the suspected painful target as determined by prior imaging techniques.

The most useful technique in planning spinal injection is MRI. Increased intra-articular fluid and subchondral bone marrow edema in facet joints are associated with instability of the involved segment and the presence of symptoms. Modic type I changes usually mean subchondral endplate edema and correlate with pain and instability [20]. When MRI is not available or contraindicated, increased uptake in TC99 bone scan may be helpful in tailoring the percutaneous procedure. Synovial cysts extending into paravertebral tissues can also be painful and, if they extend into the spinal canal, may result in nerve compression.

Targets feasible to percutaneous spinal injections are facets joint, nerve roots, and epidural space. If successful, injections can be performed up to three times a year.

Facet joint syndrome refers to the pain originating in the facet joints. The facet joints contain sensitive nerve fibers that are thought to be a potential transmitter of back

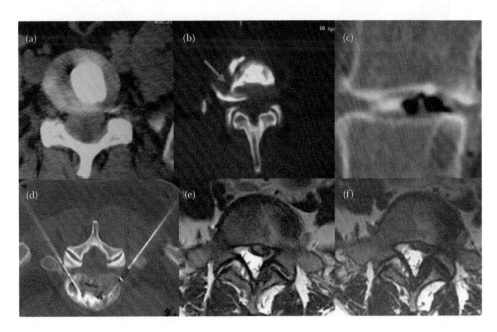

FIGURE 21.12
Discography. (a) Normal disk with dye confined to the nucleus pulposus. (b) Radial tear (arrow). (c) Degenerative disk. (d) Percutaneous disk radiofrequency ablation. Herniate disk before (e) and after ablation (f).

pain. Each facet joint has a dual innervation, one nerve from the dorsal rami above and one from the same level. Injections can be used to diagnose and treat this source of pain. In diagnostic test, local anesthetic is injected and the duration of pain relieve is compared with the theoretical time of action of the anesthetic. In therapeutic injection, a mixture of anesthetic and corticosteroid is administered. We usually use a mixture of 1 cc 2% mepivacaine, 20 mg triamcinolone, and 1 cc iodine contrast in each lumbar facet joint. At cervical and dorsal facets we inject 3-4 mg betamethasone per joint instead triamcinolone.

Facet joint injection is performed on an outpatient basis under local anesthesia and does not require premedication. Nevertheless, monitoring of the patients during the procedure is advised to detect early and treat any complication, such as vasovagal reactions. Although facet injection can be performed under fluoroscopy guidance, CT allows a safe control of the collocation of the needle tip and injected fluid distribution by mixing it with iodine contrast. This is especially relevant when there is synovial or ganglion cyst arising from the joints or located in the interspinous space, for example, in Baastrup disease. In these cases, the ganglion cyst must be drained first and later injected with the mixture of anesthetic and corticoids. A thicker

needle (14 G) is usually used for drainage because of the characteristic gelatinous dense content of the ganglia. Normal communication of the ganglia and facets joint is the rule (Figure 21.13).

For cervical injection, the patient may be positioned supine or in lateral decubitus. For dorsal or lumbar injection, the patient is placed in the prone position over a cushion device. A diagnostic CT scan is performed. Skin marker can be placed over the skin as reference guide to choose the entry point. The spinous apophyses can also be used to accomplish this task. A 22 G spinal needle is directed toward the joint itself. At dorsal level, direct access to the joint may not be possible, because of frontal orientation of the joint space, and a periarticular injection must be performed. At lumbar level, the lower recess of the joint can get an easier intra-articular access. Direct injection in the space between both facets can be hampered by a narrow articular space or by the presence of osteophytes. The inferior recess, when the lower end of the facet contact with the lamina, allows an easy intra-articular filling. Nevertheless, distribution of the drugs, either intra-articular or periarticular, has little influence in the amelioration of pain [21].

SI joint injection is a similar therapeutic procedure to facet joint injection. This procedure is performed with

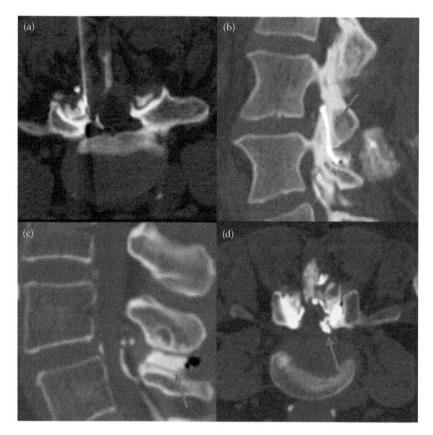

FIGURE 21.13
(a) Facet joint injection. (b) Intra- (arrow) and extraarticular distribution of the dye. (c) Filling of interspinous ganglia in Baastrup disease (arrow). (d) Filling of a juxtafacet cyst (arrow).

either CT or fluoroscopic guidance, with the patient in prone position. The same agents are used as in facet joint injection: a local anesthetic and corticosteroid mixture. SI joint injection has shown to be of benefit in seronegative spondyloarthropathies and degenerative joint disease. The efficacy is superior when there is no articular effusion [22] and when both intra- and periarticular injection are performed [23].

Anesthetic epidural block is routinely used to provide anesthesia before performing other invasive or surgical procedures in the lower spine, pelvis, or lower extremities. Combined with corticoids, it can be used to provide pain control to patients suffering of back pain secondary to degenerative disease.

Epidural space can be targeted through a caudal or lumbar approach. In caudal injection, the needle is introduced through the sacral hiatus, between the two sacral cornua, with slight cranial angulations. Therefore, entrance point must be 1–2 cm caudal to selected target of the spinal canal. Once the needle tip is inside the spinal canal, we advance it a few millimeters inside the sacral canal. Before injection, we must check that the tip bevel is oriented in a cranial direction. We normally inject 12 mg betamethasone 6 cc saline, 2 cc 2% mepivacaine, and 2 cc iodine contrast. Several CT slices are acquired after injecting 2 cc to check that distribution of the fluid is in the appropriate way. Sometimes, we find resistance because of contact of the needle tip with bone. In these cases, the needle must be moved back slightly.

The lumbar approach can be performed through the interlaminar space or through a transforaminal path. Extra pillows under the abdomen can be used to increase the interspinous space. CT images are checked prior to knowing what choice is more suitable. In the first case, we prefer to cross bilaterally the ligamentum flavum and, passing between the thecal sac and nerve roots, to advance the needle tips until the edge of the disk. Then, a mixture of 2 cc 2% mepivacaine, 3-6 mg betamethasone and 1–2 cc iodine contrast is injected in each side. At the epidural level, nonparticulate corticoids, such as betamethasone or dexamethasone sodium phosphate, are preferred to particulate corticoids, such as triamcinolone, because these particles may lead to soft-tissue calcification if they are not perfectly dissolved [5]. Sometimes, if we are not able to reach the anterior epidural space, the posterior epidural space, between the ligamentum flavum and the thecal sac, can be used to inject the mixture.

In the transforaminal approach, we also try to touch the posterior border of the disk or the upper vertebral body, medial to the exiting spinal nerve. We introduce the same mixture as we have described earlier. This approach is also used to perform a selective nerve root block in cases of nerve inflammation secondary to surgery or nerve entrapment secondary to foraminal stenosis, in spondylolisthesis and disk or facet pathology. In these cases, it is not mandatory to touch the disk or the vertebral body and the needle may only approach the back of the root itself. As a general rule, patients who do not respond to spinal nerve root block are unlikely to respond to surgery at that level (Figure 21.14).

Because of the relatively low rate of serious adverse events described after cervical transforaminal nerve

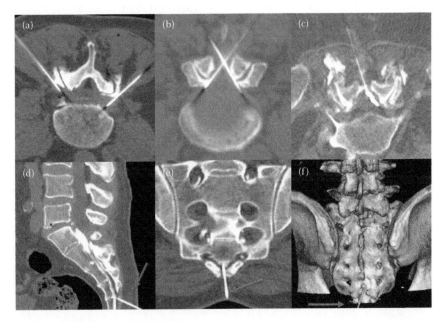

FIGURE 21.14
(a) Epidural transforaminal injection. (b) Bilateral interlaminar anterior epidural injection. (c) Posterior interlaminar epidural injection. (d–f) Caudal Injection. Sagittal (d), coronal (e), and three-dimensional reconstruction (f).

root injections, we have abandoned it. These complications include transient or permanent tetraplegia, brain infarctions leading to death, arterial dissection, or cortical blindness. The postulated mechanism is that ascending and deep cervical arterial branches, which can occasionally supply radicular and segmental medullary arteries to spinal cord, can enter the external opening of the posterior aspect of the foramen and be injected during transforaminal injection. Vascular injury can be the result of direct puncture of the arteries, vasospasm, or embolism from particulate corticoids. Therefore, at cervical, dorsal, and upper lumbar level, we perform only facet injections or a dorsal extraforaminal indirect injection [24].

Tailbone pain and visceral pain that affect the distal structures of the pelvis can be treated by blocking the nerve fibers at the level of the impar ganglion. The impar ganglion is a solitary retroperitoneal structure located anterior to the sacrococcygeal junction. It can be approached through a trans- or para-sacrococcygeal approach. CT can be used as an imaging method to identify the ganglion and guide the needle in impar ganglion blockage. A mixture of anesthetic and corticoids is administered. Contrast helps to delineate fluid distribution [25] (Figure 21.15).

21.10.4 Bone Injections

Other bone lesions can be punctured and injected with corticoids to reduce intralesional pressure and inflammatory changes and promote healing. It is mainly performed in benign tumors and pseudotumors when they are symptomatic, as an alternative to surgical treatment. Lesions, such as intraosseous ganglion cyst, nonossifying fibroma, unicameral bone cyst, giant cell reparative granuloma, and eosinophilic granuloma, can be treated in this way [26].

Intralesional corticosteroid injections may cause cessation of bone resorption by apoptotic action on osteoclast-like cells and reduce osteoclasts production of lysosomal proteases [27] (Figure 21.16).

21.11 Therapeutic Procedures

21.11.1 Neurolysis

After successful relieving of pain with facet joint injections has been demonstrated but the patient becomes again symptomatic and treatment with nonsteroidal analgesic has not proven effective enough, a more definitive treatment can be achieved by rhizolysis. The facet joints are innervated by the dorsal spinal root through its medial branch. The inferior part of the joint receives fibers of the same level and the superior part from the root of the vertebra above it [28]. Therefore, treatment of a painful facet joint includes neurolysis of the medial branch at the same level and the level above.

Permanent neurolysis can be achieved by injection of ethanol or phenol, but control of the distribution of the liquids is not easy. More controlled neurolysis can be accomplished by radiofrequency ablation under CT guidance, guarantying a reliable positioning of the probe. For medial branch neurolysis, the target lies at the junction between the superior articular and transverse processes. The use of sensory and motor pulse stimulation identifies the nerve position and verifies that there is no motor branch involved [17] (Figure 21.17).

After appropriate collocation of the needles, the electrodes are introduced coaxially and connected to the generator. A single dispersive pad electrode is adhered to the thigh skin, close to the buttock.

For radiofrequency (RF) ablation, 90–120 seconds heating of continuous RF, reaching 90°C per position can be sufficient. Nevertheless, pulsed RF get the same effect, without raising the temperature above 40°C–45°C, reducing the risk of producing reactive neuromas or superficial burns. Treatment lasting 120 seconds is usually enough [29].

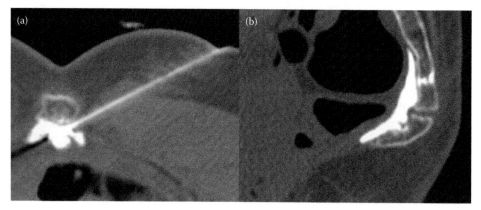

FIGURE 21.15
(a) Impar ganglion injection. (b) Distribution of the dye anterior to sacrococcygeal junction.

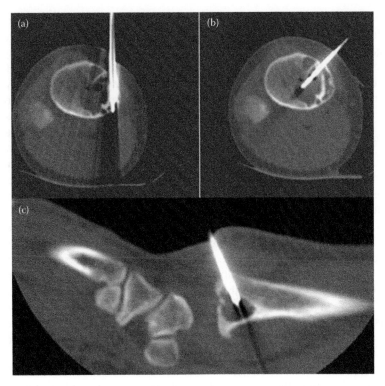

FIGURE 21.16
(a, b) Biopsy and corticoids injection in a symptomatic nonossifying fibroma. (c) Injection of intraosseous ganglia of the distal ulna.

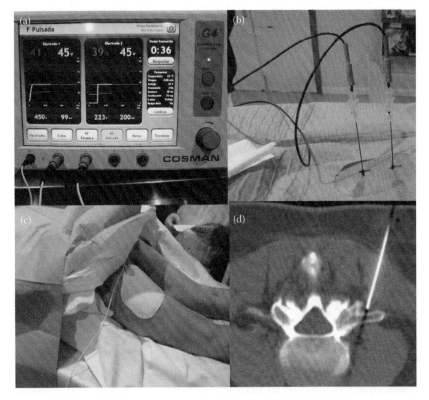

FIGURE 21.17
Radiofrequency ablation in facet joints syndrome. (a) Monitor display of the generator. (b) Electrodes inserted through the needles. (c) Dispersive electrode on the buttocks. (d) CT showing the needle tip in the right place.

RF ablation can also be used to treat root ganglions at the neural foramina for treating chronic unresolved radiculitis. Other root ganglions, such as stellate ganglion at cervical level, the thoracic sympathetic chain, or the lumbar sympathetic chain, can be treated to resolve painful or dystrophic syndromes.

21.11.2 Thermal Ablation

Thermal methods for tumor treatment (RF, cryoablation) have become important palliative and, in some cases, curative modalities [30].

At present, RF treatment for osteoid osteoma is the only one that constitutes the initial procedure of choice. Nevertheless, other benign and malign bone or soft-tissue tumors and pseudotumors are also suitable for RF thermal ablation. In these cases, treatment can be intended to be palliative or curative. Curative treatment implies that the tumor has been completely ablated. Palliative treatment aims to reduce symptoms and debulk tumor mass [31].

The principle of RF ablation is a transformation of electromagnetic energy (RF) into thermal energy. The RF device comprises an electric generator connected to an active electrode (antenna) and two grounding pads. The grounding pads have to be adhered to the skin at an equal distance to the treatment area. As the active electrode is usually positioned using an introductory needle, the guide cannula has to be withdrawn as far as possible to avoid its contact with the active electrode tip before RF activation, because heating of the cannula can burn the pathway and skin. The electrical circuit is formed in the patient by placing the electrode tip at the target tissue and the grounding pads at the skin as dispersive electrodes. The generator produces an alternating current at the tip of the active electrode in the tumor; the current exits through grounding pads placed on the skin and returns to the generator (Figure 21.18).

For bone tumors, we consider a rod monopolar electrode that can be inserted through a cannula inside the bone most appropriate. Different lengths of the active tips are available (0.7 mm–3 cm). In small lesions, for example, osteoid osteoma, we perform a manual dry ablation at 90° in 6 minutes. In bigger lesions with osteolysis and soft-tissue component, we adapt the length of the active tip to the lesion size although many localization may be necessary to complete ablate the lesion. Internal perfusion of the electrode with saline in resistance mode is another effective method of enlarging the area of necrosis during RF ablation. Nevertheless, real temperature in target tissue is only displayed at the end of the ablation, when the generator and the saline infusion pump are stopped. The procedure is considered correct if the temperature reaches over 55°. We also use internal perfusion when treating soft-tissue tumors.

Other options to treat larger lesions do exist. We can apply the RF energy exclusively in the target tissue by using bipolar or multipolar RF devices. In this case, grounding pads are not necessary. Multitined expandable electrodes can be used in soft lesions where an array of multiple thin electrodes can expand from a larger needle cannula in an umbrella or Christmas tree shape.

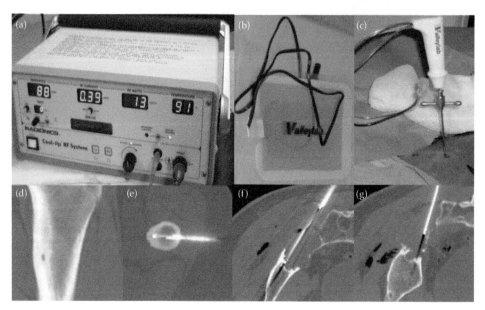

FIGURE 21.18
Radiofrequency thermal ablation. (a) Monitor display of the generator. (b) Electrode grounding pad. (c) Active electrode in place through the introductory cannula. (d) Osteoid osteoma of the proximal femur. (e) Electrode tip in place during ablation. (f, g) Large lytic metastatic thyroid lesion ablated at different places.

21.11.3 Vertebroplasty

In this procedure, polymethyl methacrylate, a cement-like substance, is injected into a pathologic vertebral body, most of the time an osteoporotic vertebral fracture, but also to treat pain related to vertebral tumors, benign or malign, with or without fracture.

Most of the vertebroplasty procedures are performed under fluoroscopy guidance using a C-arm or biplane fluoroscopy. Nevertheless, when there are few vertebral bodies to treat, the procedure may be amenable to be performed in the CT room. In these cases, the intervention begins with CT and is followed by fluoroscopy. The needles are usually placed through the pedicles in the posterior border of the vertebral bodies under CT guidance and the final introduction of the needles and the injection of cement are performed under fluoroscopy guidance with a C-arm introduced in the CT room. When we are going to treat fractures of the cervical–thoracic transitional area, use of CT is warranted because of the poor visualization of these vertebrae on fluoroscopy. In these cases, the needles are left in their final place through an extrapedicular way at the center of the vertebral body under CT guidance. Injection of a small quantity of cement is performed by fluoroscopy guidance around the needle tip. Quite often, a quick CT scan control is needed to check the real distribution of the cement and decide to stop or follow with the injection of cement. At thoracic level, if the pedicles are too narrow, a more lateral approach can be performed, passing through the costovertebral junction (Figure 21.19).

Performing phlebography prior to cement injection is optional, with authors considering it as a useful tool that predicts possible routes of leakage, while other authors consider it a time-consuming technique, with no predictive value, that may cloud the injection of cement. We do not perform phlebography routinely at our institution. We prefer to slowly inject the cement. If venous leakage happens, we try to change the bevel orientation or to retract the needle a little bit. If leakage persists, the needle has to be removed and changed by a new one in case we do not reach an appropriate vertebral body filling by the contralateral needle. At the end of the procedure, the stylet is reintroduced in the cannula and advanced under fluoroscopic monitoring to deliver the remaining cement out of the needle lumen, prior to its withdrawal [32].

We prefer to use bevelled needle because the needle bevel can be used to adjust slightly the direction of the needle. The needle tip tends to penetrate opposed to the bevelled face. Therefore, we begin the approach by the pedicle with the tip directed from its outer to inner margin. If the needle tip touches the inner cortical of the pedicle before reaching the vertebral body, turning the bevel to the inner cortical margin of the pedicle allows as more room to reach the vertebral body without entering the spinal canal. Inside the vertebral body, we use the bevel to project the cement distribution to the

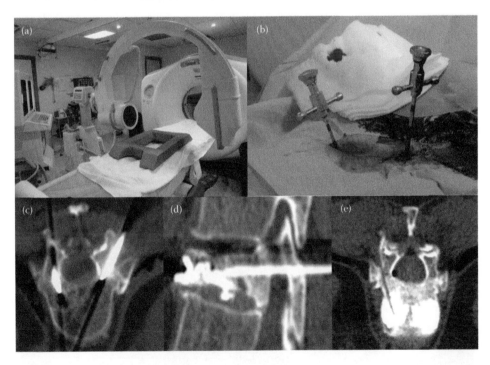

FIGURE 21.19
Vertebroplasty. (a) CT room ready to start. We can see the C-arm in place and the cushion to accommodate the patient. (b) Needles in place. (c) The needle tip is in the posterior border of the vertebral body. (d) Sagittal view of the needle in its final place. (e) Final result.

appropriate direction, although other factors, such as vertebral compaction and clefts, may hamper a homogenous distribution.

In suspected malignancies, a biopsy can be performed prior to vertebroplasty. A trephine is coaxially advanced to the vertebral body through the vertebroplasty needle when its tip is in the posterior border of the vertebral body.

This procedure is associated with a low morbidity rate. Less than 1% of patients with non-neoplastic lesions and only 5%–8% of patients with neoplastic lesions have morbidity, which may include local pain, rib pain, spinal stenosis, nerve root compression, and intravascular extension of acrylic. Isolated cases of symptomatic pulmonary embolism or paraplegia have been described.

21.11.4 Abscess and Fluid Drainage

Primary and postoperative fluid collections in muscles and articular and periarticular locations can now be safely treated percutaneously. Percutaneous drainage consists in the placement of a catheter to provide continuous drainage of a fluid collection. It is indicated when a circumscript fluid collection is detected in contrast-enhanced CT scan.

After applying anesthesia to the soft tissues, sufficient incision of the skin and the subcutaneous tissue with a scalpel is mandatory to avoid sticking the sheath and drainage catheter.

For CT drainage, we recommend the Seldinger technique. First, a needle covered by a long-dwell flexible sheath is inserted into the fluid collection. After removal of the inner needle, a flexible guide wire is coiled within the abscess cavity. The flexible sheath is removed and dilator rigid sheaths are used to create a corridor to the drainage catheter, around the guide wire. Although many authors recommend dilating the path up to 2 F larger than the drainage catheter diameter, most of the time it is enough to dilate with a dilator of the same diameter than the catheter that is most tightly introduced over the guide wire, reducing the reflux of fluid around the catheter. It is important to ensure that all side holes of the drainage catheter lie within the fluid collection (Figure 21.20).

The trocar technique is more difficult to use in CT scans because of the hard nonflexible stylet introduced inside the catheter. This lack of flexibility may hamper the performance of control images because the entrance set can touch the gantry walls.

After successful placement of the drainage catheter, the patient is sent back to the ward where the catheter bag is left to drainage by gravity. The drainage should be irrigated approximately three times per day with sterile saline by the nursing staff to avoid clogging.

Success can be hampered in chronic tuberculous abscess because of the existence of a thickened wall that does not collapse spontaneously. After failure of percutaneous drainage, surgical debridement is warranted [33].

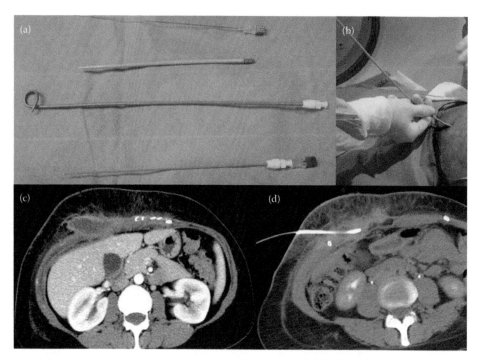

FIGURE 21.20
Abscess drainage. (a) Catheter and needles. (b) Introduction of the catheter. (c) Abscess in the anterior abdominal wall. (d) Catheter in place.

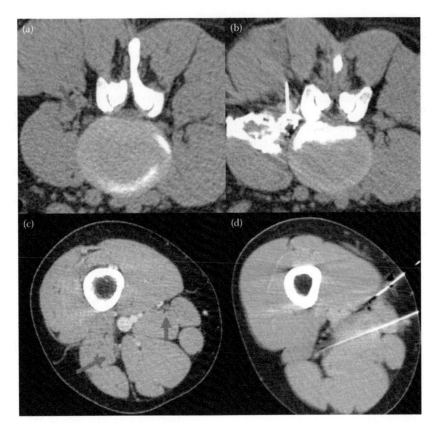

FIGURE 21.21
(a) Lumbar plexus identified at L4–L5 level. (b) Block under CT guidance, before a hip tumor ablation. (c) The sciatic and internal saphenous nerves are identified. (d) Block under CT guidance.

21.12 Regional Anesthesia

Although interest in using imaging guidance to perform regional anesthesia has focused in ultrasound, CT can also accomplish this task, mainly in difficult access, such as lumbosacral plexus.

The aim of image guidance is to approach the needle tip to the selected nerve and check the appropriate distribution of the anesthetic. It is considered a way of reducing the quantity of anesthetic needed to achieve a successful block [34].

Psoas compartment injection led to a safe block of three nerves of the lower limb in only one injection (femoral, lateral femorocutaneous, and obturator nerves) and it is mainly indicated in hip interventions. Anatomical studies have demonstrated that the lumbar plexus is located inside the psoas muscle at L4–L5 level [35]. CT is helpful in identifying nerves and checking anesthetic distribution. We normally use for this block 20 cc 2% mepivacaine, 10 cc saline, and 5 cc iodine dye (Figure 21.21).

Other nerves can be identified on CT and blocked when necessary under CT guidance, mainly if local anesthesia and slight sedation is not enough to follow an initiated procedure that resulted unexpectedly painful. Lower limb nerves feasible to block under CT guidance include sciatic, femoral, internal saphenous, tibial, and peroneous.

References

1. Tsalafoutas IA, Tsapaki V, Triantopoulou C et al. CT-guided interventional procedures without CT fluoroscopy assistance: patient effective dose and absorbed dose considerations. *AJR* 2007; 188: 1479–1484.

2. Yu L, Liu X, Leng S et al. Radiation dose reduction in computed tomography: techniques and future perspective. *Imaging Med* 2009; 1: 65–84.

3. Carlson SK, Bender CE, Classic KL et al. Benefits and safety of CT fluoroscopy in interventional radiologic procedures. *Radiology* 2001; 219: 515–520.

4. Mangran AJ, Horan TC, Pearlson ML et al. Guideline for prevention of surgical site infection. *Infect Control Hosp Epidemiol* 1999; 20: 247–278.

5. MacMahon PJ, Eustace SJ, Kavanagh EC. Injectable corticosteroid and local anesthetic preparations: a review for radiologists. *Radiology* 2009; 252(3): 647–661.

6. Wonsik A, Jae-Hyon B, Young-Jin L. The "gauge" system for the medical use. *Anesth Analg* 2002; 95: 1119–1128.

7. Rosenthal DI. The future of MSK interventions. *Skeletal Radiol* 2011; 40: 1133–1136.

8. Tsukushi S, Nishida Y, Yamada Y et al. CT-guided needle biopsy for musculoskeletal lesions. *Arch Orthop Trauma Surg* 2010; 130: 699–703.

9. Liu PT, Valadez SD, Chivers FS et al. Anatomically based guidelines for core needle biopsy of bone tumors: implications for limb-sparing surgery. *Radiographics* 2007; 27: 189–206.

10. Espinosa LA, Jamadar DA, Jacobson JA et al. CT-guided biopsy of bone: a radiologist's perspective. *AJR* 2008; 190: W283–W289.

11. Hau A, Kim I, Kattapuram S et al. Accuracy of CT-guided biopsies in 359 patients with musculoskeletal lesions. *Skeletal Radiol* 2002; 31: 349–353.

12. Nourbakhsh A, Grady JJ, Garges KJ. Percutaneous spine biopsy: a meta-analysis. *J Bone Joint Surg Am* 2008; 90: 1722–1725.

13. Hryhorczuk AL, Strouse PJ, Biermann JS. Accuracy of CT-guided percutaneous core needle biopsy for assessment of pediatric musculoskeletal lesions. *Pediatr Radiol* 2011; 41: 848–857.

14. Yoshikawa T, Hayashi N, Yamamoto S et al. Brachial plexus injury: clinical manifestations, conventional imaging findings, and the latest imaging techniques. *Radiographics* 2006; 26: 133–143.

15. Sachs BL, Vanharanta H, Spivey MA et al. Dallas discogram description. A new classification of CT/discography in low-back disorders. *Spine* 1987; 12(3): 287–294.

16. Fayad F, Lefevre-Colau MM, Rannou F et al. Relation of inflammatory modic changes to intradiscal steroid injection outcome in chronic low back pain. *Eur Spine J* 2007; 16: 925–931.

17. Kelekis AD, Somonb T, Yilmaz H et al. Interventional spine procedures. *Eur J Radiol* 2005; 55: 362–383.

18. Andreula CF, Simonetti L, De Santis F et al. Minimally invasive oxygen-ozone therapy for lumbar disk herniation. *AJNR Am J Neuroradiol* 2004; 24: 996–1000.

19. Gangi A, Dietemann JL, Mortazavi R et al. CT-guided interventional procedures for pain management in the lumbosacral spine. *Radiographics* 1998; 18: 621–633.

20. Ruiz Santiago F, Castellano García MM, Guzmán Álvarez L. Computed tomography and magnetic resonance imaging for painful spinal column: contributions and controversies. *Radiología* 2011; 53(2): 116–133.

21. Hechelhammer L, Pfirrmann CW, Zanetti M et al. Imaging findings predicting the outcome of cervical facet joint blocks. *Eur Radiol* 2007; 17: 959–964.

22. Liliang PC, Lu K, Weng HC et al. The therapeutic efficacy of sacroiliac joint blocks with triamcinolone acetonide in the treatment of sacroiliac joint dysfunction without spondyloarthropathy. *Spine* 2009; 34: 896–900.

23. Borowsky CD, Fagen G. Sources of sacroiliac region pain: insights gained from a study comparing standard intra-articular injection with a technique combining intra- and peri-articular injection. *Arch Phys Med Rehabil* 2008; 89: 2048–2056.

24. Sutter R, Pfirrman CWA, Zanetti M et al. CT-guided cervical nerve root injections: comparing the immediate post-injection anesthetic-related effects of the transforaminal injection with a new indirect technique. *Skeletal Radiol* 2011; 40: 1603–1608.

25. Datir A, Connell D. CT-guided injection for ganglion impar blockade: a radiological approach to the management of coccydynia. *Clin Radiol* 2010; 65: 21–25.

26. Scaglietti O, Marchetti PG, Bartolozzi P. The effects of methylprednisolona acetate in the treatment of bone cysts: results of three years follow-up. *J Bone Joint Surg* 1979; 61-B: 200–204.

27. Carlos R, Sedano HO. Intralesional corticosteroids as an alternative treatment for central giant cell granuloma. *Oral Surg Oral Med Oral Pathol Oral Radiol Endod* 2002; 93: 161–166.

28. Cohen SP, Raja SN. Pathogenesis, diagnosis, and treatment of lumbar zygapophysial (facet) joint pain. *Anesthesiology* 2007; 106(3): 591–614.

29. Kornick C, Kramarich S, Lamer JT, Sitzman BT. Complications of lumbar facet radiofrequency denervation. *Spine* 2004; 29(12): 1352–1354.

30. Ruiz Santiago F, Castellano García MM, Guzmán Álvarez L et al. Percutaneous treatment of bone tumors by radiofrequency thermal ablation. *Eur J Radiol* 2011; 77: 156–163.

31. Ruiz Santiago F, Castellano García MM, Martínez Montes JL. Treatment of bone tumours by radiofrequency thermal ablation. *Curr Rev Musculoskelet Med* 2009; 2: 43–50.

32. Ruiz Santiago F, Pérez Abela A, Guzmán Álvarez L et al. Pain and functional outcome after vertebroplasty and kyphoplasty. A comparative study. *Eur J Radiol* 2010; 75(2): e108–e113.

33. Dinc H, Ahmetoglu A, Baykal S et al. Image-guided percutaneous drainage of tuberculous iliopsoas and spondylodiskitic abscesses: midterm results. *Radiology* 2002; 225: 353–358.

34. Marhofer P, Greher M, Kapral S. Ultrasound guidance in regional anaesthesia. *Br J Anaesth* 2005; 94(1): 7–17.

35. Farny J, Drolet P, Girard M. Anatomy of the posterior approach to the lumbar plexus block. *Can J Anaesth* 1994; 41: 480–485.

Section IV

Special Applications

22

CT in Pediatrics: A Guide for Optimization

Erich Sorantin and Sabine Weissensteiner

CONTENTS

22.1 Differences between Children and Adults: Relevant for Pediatric CT

Children differ in many aspects from adults—psychology as well as communication, anatomy, proportions, physiology, and radiation sensitivity, just to name a view [1–3]. Most of them can be explained by changes during growth and maturation.

One has to consider that for children, hospitals visits can be stressful—a very unusual building with unfamiliar paintings, people are busy and strangely dressed, everywhere waiting for a call is necessary, and much more. If children use the same waiting area as adults, then the confrontation with handicapped and disabled adults, or intensive care patients can induce anxiety. Computed tomography (CT) machines are huge for children, the CT tunnel may not attract children, positioning on the CT couch is uncomfortable, no movements are allowed, and even several times breath-holding is mandatory.

Therefore, children should be investigated in a calm and quite environment maybe in the morning or at the end of the regular working time, where there is no hurry and there is time for adaption. The surroundings should be friendly for children with paintings and posters. Video screens showing cartoons in the waiting area are useful too.

Mass matters - in adults the body.... weight shows a variation from 40 to 160 kg, thus representing a mass factor of 4. In children, the body weight starts at 300–400 g in premature babies and the obese youngster may have more than 120 kg of body weight—therefore, a mass factor of about 300–400 has to be considered. Additionally, not only the frank mass differences are important but also everything is changing during growth and maturation: for example, skeleton calcifies by age (babies and toddlers have more cartilage components within bones), less muscle mass, white matter of the central nervous system exhibits less fatty contents in babies (lack of myelinization), the last generation of alveoli develop after the third of life, and so on. Therefore, in children, there is an age-dependent decreased overall density as well as reduced relative density differences (e.g., bones with more cartilage, less muscle mass, and less fat). For CT protocols, the overall density of the body must be transformed to exposure settings.

Body proportions are different from adults—the head is bigger and reaches its final size by about 12 years. The relative big head explains the higher incidence of the cranial injuries in small children and most cervical spine fractures occur above the cervical vertebral body of C IV [4,5]. A special type of injury within the cervical spine is represented by SCIWORA—this is an acronym for "Spinal Cervical Injury without Radiographic Abnormality" [6]. The occurrence of SCIWORA is due to the reduced elasticity of the cervical column as compared to the spinal cord. In small children, the chest is short and the abdomen is bigger and therefore the upper abdominal organs are more exposed. Using regular pelvic seat belts for fixation, instead of an appropriate child car seat, results in severe upper abdominal injuries like pancreatic lacerations or small bowel injuries.

Children grow—thus demanding for higher oxygen input as compared to adults (two times more) [1]. Since the tidal volume as well as the cardiac stroke volume per kilogram of body weight is identical to adults, children breathe two times more often and the heart rate is doubled in comparison to adults. The increased circulation time and the reduced distance between cubital veins and the arterial system makes major adoptions of the intravenous (i.v.) contrast injection necessary. Using new CT technologies like volume scanners, the i.v. contrast injection approaches a "hit or miss" event. At the authors' institution, a spreadsheet was developed (Figure 22.1), which does the necessary calculations as well as computes the

pediatric optimized glomerular filtration rate and assists in calculation of the newest CT dose index, namely, the "Size-Specific Dose Estimates (SSDE) in Pediatric and Adult Body CT Examinations" (AAPM Report No. 204) [7].

Radiation sensitivity is increased in children compared to adults—a factor of three to four and even more is discussed [8]. Radiation-induced cancer represents the most serious side effect; Figure 22.2 demonstrates the additional lifetime risk to die from a radiation-induced cancer for both sexes [9].

Moreover, in children, head and extremities are more susceptible to radiation than in adults (Figure 22.3), which can be explained by the maturation of brain as well as more red bone marrow within the appendicular skeleton.

It is clear from the preceding discussion that all components of the "Imaging Chain" (Figure 22.4) have to be optimized for a pediatric CT [2,5].

Pediatric CT - Calculation i.v.CM, GFR, SSDE

Patient	firstname surname	study date	17.05.2012			Size-Specific Dose Estimates (SSDE) (Th. + Abd.)			
age(years)	4	sex	female			AP(mm)	LAT(mm)	32 PMMA corr.factor	16 PMMA corr.factor
flow (ml/s)	2,0	creatinine (mg/dl)	0,9			126,90	199,90		
weight (kg)	30					sum(cm)		32,7	2,08	1,02
height (cm)	118	GFR(ml/min/1,73m$^{2)}$	131,111						
0,9% NaCl(ml/kg)	3				16 cm PMMA	CTDI$_{vol}$		2,20	SSDE(mGy)	2,24

contrast media volume (ml)				corrective factor				
Age: <1a	2,5			neck	1,6	liver	0,8	2,2
Age 1-2a	2			chest	1,2	pelvis	2,2	
Age >2age	1,5			Abdomen	2,8	kidneys	0,8	4,8

Organ	KM Volume 300mg/ml	KM Volume 350mg/ml (>40kg)	Delay	0,9%NaCl	comment
Head	45,0	use 300mg/ml	50,0	50,0	mastoiditis, sinus venous thrombosis, orbital phlegmon
Neck	45,0	use 300mg/ml	54,0	50,0	> 40kg Delay 70s
Chest	30,0	use 300mg/ml	27,0	50,0	> 40kg Delay 30s
Abdomen	45,0	use 300mg/ml	63,0	50,0	> 40kg Delay 70s
Liver arterial	30,0	use 300mg/ml	18,0	50,0	> 40kg Delay 25
Liver (late)	45,0	use 300mg/ml	49,5	50,0	> 40kg Delay 70s
PELVIS	45,0	use 300mg/ml	49,5	50,0	> 40kg Delay 70s
Kidney (arterial)	30,0	use 300mg/ml	18,0	50,0	> 40kg Delay 20s
kidneys (clearance)	45,0	use 300mg/ml	108,0	50,0	
CTA 1 system	30,0	use 300mg/ml	Bolustrackiung	50,0	
CTA 2 systems	45,0	use 300mg/ml	Bolustrackiung	50,0	
CTA carotis	45,0	use 300mg/ml	Bolustrackiung	50,0	
Head(brain death)	58,5	use 300mg/ml	20,0	50,0	diagnosis of brain dead

FIGURE 22.1
Screenshot of the spreadsheet developed at the authors' institution for i.v. contrast calculations as well as computation of the pediatric glomerular filtration rate (green region) and SSDE (pink region).

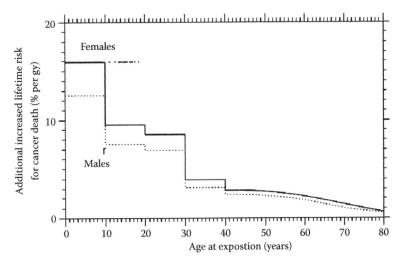

FIGURE 22.2
Plot of age (*x*-axis) versus additional lifetime risk to die from a radiation-induced cancer (% per Gy) for both sexes. One can see that during infancy there is a considerable higher risk. (Modified after (The German Commission on Radiological Protection. Diagnostic imaging in children—Radiation protection, justification and effectiveness—Recommendation of the Commission on Radiological Protection. http://www.ssk.de/de/werke/2006/volltext/ssk0608.pdf.)

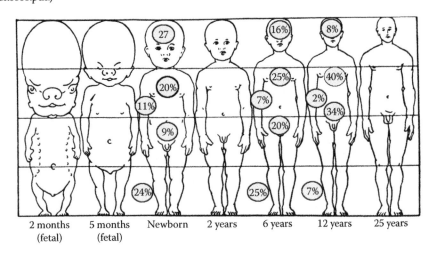

FIGURE 22.3
Image demonstrates the differences of proportions in children. The head predominance can be recognized easily. Numbers in gray circles correspond to the relative radiation sensitivity. You can see that in newborns, in contradiction to adults, head and extremities are more susceptible. (Adapted from Sorantin, E., *Besonderheiten der Computertomographie im Kindesalter*, Georg Thieme Verlag, Stuttgart, New York, 2010.)

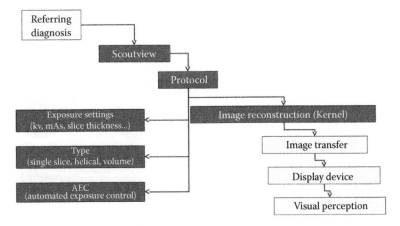

FIGURE 22.4
Components of a CT examination—black boxes with white characters can be manipulated on the CT machine's console.

Take home points: Children are not small adults, differences can be explained by growing and maturation, thus leading to increased radiation sensitivity.

22.2 Differences in CT Technology and Dose Factors

In the past years, there was a steady increase in multidetector CT (MDCT) usage [10]. The technology has developed from single slice to 4 slices to 8, 16, 32, 40, 64, up to 320 slices. The improved speed of the new scanners has also led to new applications (e.g., perfusion CT) as well as improved patient throughput and workflow.

Scanning parameters that affect CT-derived radiation dose include scanner geometry, tube current and voltage, scanning modes, scan length, collimation, table speed and pitch, gantry rotation time, and shielding [11,12].

The distance between the focal spot of the X-ray tube and the isocenter of the scanner depends on scanner geometry, since tube-focus-axis distance is specific for a particular machine. If all scanning parameters on two different CT scanners are the same, a long-geometry scanner will produce less interaction with the patient and increase image noise than a short-geometry scanner. Transferring protocols from one scanner type to another must be done with caution [11].

Tube current relates linearly to dose → double mAs (product of tube currenet (mA) and time (seconds))

means double dose. Furthermore, dose depends on square from voltage, meaning a reduction from 120 kV → 80 kV indicates that 80 kV is just 2/3 from 120 kV. Computation of (2/3)2 leads to 4/9, which is ≈50%. Collimation (slice thickness) is inverted related to dose → half slice thickness needs double dose for same noise. General speaking noise is inversely related to the square root of mA, rotation time, and slice thickness.

All helical MDCTs suffer from overranging and overbeaming, which are less prominent in volume scanners [3]. Use of MDCT scanner results in some amount of unused radiation beyond the beginning and end of the imaging region. For this reason, adaptive collimation techniques have been developed that open the collimation at the beginning of the scan and close it at its end. For children and short-range scans, it is usually not advisable to use the maximum detector width during spiral scanning [11,2].

In single-slice CT, a high pitch is an advantage for providing the best compromise between slice thickness and radiation dose. However, in multislice CT, the effect of pitch depends on the manufacturer. If the mAs are adjusted with varying pitch and the effective mAs are constant, then the radiation should remain constant as well. High pitch has the advantage of a shorter scan time and less motion artifacts but provides more overranging [13].

An increase in the pitch decreases the duration of radiation exposure to the anatomic part being scanned. With MDCT scanners, beam collimation, table speed, and pitch are interlinked parameters that affect the diagnostic quality of an imaging study [14].

Nowadays, replacement of filtered back projection by statistical reconstructions offers new and wide fields of dose reduction (Figures 22.5 and 22.6).

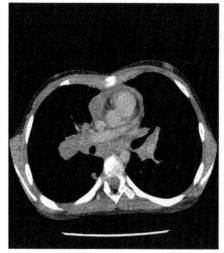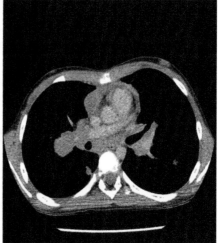

FIGURE 22.5
A 10-year-old boy CT of the chest due to suspicion of lymphoma. Left part of the image was generated by statistical reconstruction; right part by conventional filtered back projection, scan parameters were identical. It can be seen that using the same dose image quality is higher in the left part, and stripe artifacts are less within the spinal area, thus offering challenges for dose reduction.

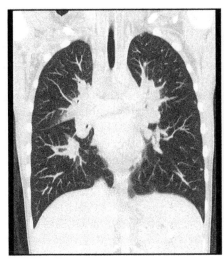
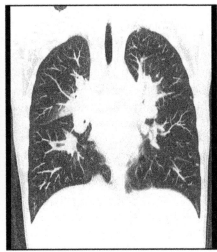

FIGURE 22.6
Same case as in Figure 22.5, coronal "maximum intensity projections"—again for left part statistical reconstruction was used and for the right side conventional back projection scan parameters were identical. As in Figure 22.5, image quality is higher due to lower noise level.

Take home points: Due to differences in CT scanner technology parameter sets cannot be transferred from one machine to another.

22.3 Optimization for Pediatric CT

Enteric opacification in children is a controversial discussed topic [15]. Therefore, it is not possible to give a general recommendation. At the authors' institution, enteric opacification is only used in nonsedated children.

Correct positioning represents an unspecific but very important tool for optimization of image quality. Patients should be placed comfortably in the center of the scanner to minimize radiation. Moreover, in head scans, care should be taken not to include the fixation device for the head basket, since this part is usually made of iron or similar material. Thus, artifacts are created, and if automated exposure control (AEC) is used, dose will be increased due to higher absorption. Arms up in chest CT decreases attenuation, improves image quality, and saves dose.

Bismuth shielding of eyes and chest was suggested, but there is a substantial discussion about usage in pediatric patients—an excellent overview can be found in Kim et al. [16]. It is noted that some basic facts have to be considered: first, to avoid artifacts, bismuth should never be placed directly on the skin, a 2-cm foam rubber padding should be placed between the bismuth and skin (Figure 22.7). Second, if bismuth shielding is used with AEC, dose can be increased due to the higher

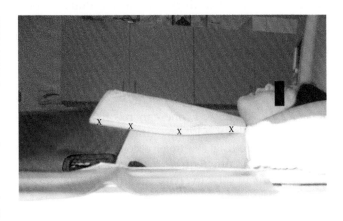

FIGURE 22.7
Girl positioned for chest CT—between the bismuth shield and skin a foam rubber padding (marked by black "x") is placed.

absorption. Third, it is the authors' personal experience that depending on the vendor structural noise can be induced. One solution can be to use only z-axis modulation for AEC and do not place the bismuth shielding during the topogram but during the scan, thus cheating the system. Preferably, there should be phantom measurements to confirm the reduction for a dedicated CT system.

Another issue is getting children to tolerate the CT examination. As a starter, vascular access should not be done within the examination room but before the examination to give the child time to adapt. As already mentioned, patients should be placed comfortably and it is advisable that there is an attracting point in the examination room, which can be fixed by the child's eyes.

In order not to overstress the child's patience, everything should be set as complete as possible at the CT console before calling the child into the examination room. Despite all these maneuvers, sedation will be sometimes necessary. One has to outweigh radiation against impact of the CT examination on patient management. It is the authors' opinion that there is no sense to radiate a child without appropriate diagnostic output. Different types of sedation are suggested and discussed in the literature [15,17,18,19].

Tight topogram and scan length represent another clue to dose savings. If, for example, chest CT examinations are reviewed for scan length, there can be notably "overscanning"—in the authors' experience (unpublished data) up to 40%. To follow the "ALARA" (As Low As Reasonably Achievable) principle, the selection of scan parameters plays a crucial role. One of the most important steps is represented by selecting the appropriate slice thickness for viewing—as already mentioned, half slice thickness means double noise, thus doubled mAs are needed for compensation [2]. The Shannon–Nyquist theorem tells us in short that we always need double resolution [20]. Applying this principle to CT means that for clear visualization of a, for example, 3-mm nodule, a slice thickness of 1.5 mm is sometimes required. Thanks to the introduction of helical and volume CT, one can reconstruct overlapping slices without adding radiation to the patient—so in the preceding example, reconstructing a 3-mm slice every 1.5 mm (equal to increment of 1.5 mm) would result in 50% overlap, thus the nodule should be detectable.

Increased contrast can be achieved by selecting a voltage of 80 kV, which lowers the dose by 50% as compared to 120 kV settings. Theoretically mAs would have to be doubled for compensation of the lowered dose, but due to the inherited better signal-to-noise-ratio, tube current needs only to be increased by about 60%–70%, which represents a good starting point depending on the clinical question and body part examined. Phantom examinations are extremely helpful for calibration of the CT used.. At a voltage of 80 kV, Hounsfield units (HU) change and despite water stays at 0 HU; Due to increased absorption values of all other organs are increased., Thus..... making appropriate adaption of bolus tracking thresholds necessary. It is our own experience that the following thresholds are appropriate for CT angiography (region of interest [ROI] in aorta): 120 kV → 300 HU, 100 kV → 350 HU, and 80 kV → 400 HU. Those values can only be applied if the CT machine starts *immediately* without any delay at the reached threshold and there is an appropriate sized vascular access. If there is a delay between reaching the threshold and scan start, due to tube repositioning, values have to be lowered. A good starting point is the check for the difference in thresholds when performing a CT angiography of the aorta (e.g., for aortic aneurysms) and of the pulmonary arteries (e.g., for pulmonary embolism). Since in babies and small children, delay times are shortened in comparison to adults (e.g., in CT angiography 5–10 seconds), this difference has to be increased in those patients—meaning to start at a lower threshold. But it has to be repeated, the actual delay has to be measured at a particular CT machine. If venous approach is done by a tiny needle, reduction of suggested thresholds by 30% has to be considered.

The advantage of the increased contrast at a voltage of 80 kV can be further exploited for i.v. contrast medium reduction [21]. To avoid beam hardening artifacts, contrast medium with an iodine content of 300 mg/mL is mixed with physiological saline at a ratio of 1:2 and injected at a rate of 1–2 mL/s. As a result, usually 4–8 mL of i.v. contrast medium is usually sufficient for CT angiography in babies and small children (see Figures 22.8 and 22.9)

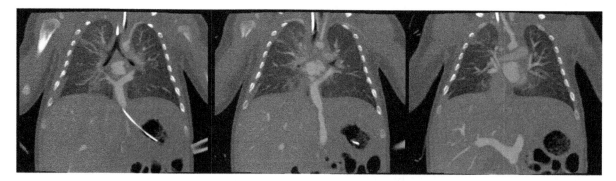

FIGURE 22.8
A 6-week-old boy suffering from total abnormal pulmonary venous return. After cardiac surgery, a retrocardial vein could be still found at echocardiography. CT angiography was performed for presurgical anatomic mapping showing clearly that only the lower pulmonary veins were still forming the retrocardial vein draining infradiaphragmatically into the portal vein. CT scanning was done in volume mode (AquilionOne, Toshiba Medical Systems, Japan) and only 4 mL of i.v. contrast medium was used.

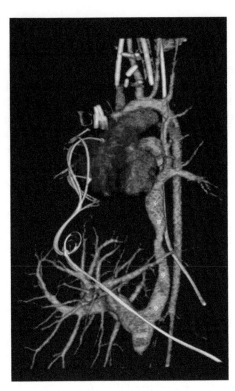

FIGURE 22.9
Same child as in Figure 22.8, 3D reconstruction using volume rendering. White asterisks mark the retrocardial vein draining into the portal vein.

Take home points: Image quality optimization must cover all parts of a CT examination besides correct exposure settings—from children-friendly environment, preparation (enteric opacification, vascular access, sedation, and shielding), positioning, and minimizing the child's retention time within the CT machine and examination room.

22.4 General CT Protocol Suggestions and Special Indications

Generation of pediatric CT protocols is a demanding, creative task. Several factors have to be considered. Children do not grow linearly, therefore equidistant steps in kilogram body weight or in age do not make sense. A practical solution is to adapt the dose according to the following schema examinations of the trunk: 0–3 months, 3–6 months, 6–12 months, 1–3 years, 3–6 years, 6–10 years, 10–14 years, and older. For head examinations, only few groups are necessary: 0–6 months, 6 months to 2 years, 2–10 years, and adults.

All age-dependent schedules assume that particular patients are of normal bodyshape for age. These

schedules fail if the patient is malnourished or obese. As a general rule, a tight dose regimented is prone to fail if the patient does not fit into the basic assumptions. Therefore, organizational difficulties have to be included in considerations like who is doing the exam (always the same team on same machine) or different people on different machines or a combination of both factors.

One of the easiest ways for saving radiation is the reduction of the manufacturer's presets in tube currents by 25%–30% even in adult patients. As a general rule, multiphase examinations should be avoided in children, since, depending on the imaging environment, they are rarely needed.

Tube current: Several suggestions were made. One of the most recent was published by the "Society for Pediatric Radiology" (SPR—http://www.pedrad.org) called "Image Gently Campaign" [22]. Those suggestions start from an ideal examination in adult patients, and for tube current adoption, reduction factors are given. But it has to be kept in mind that always a voltage of 120 kV is used. As a general rule, abdominal CT needs 50% dose more than a chest CT (=150% of chest CT) or vice versa a chest CT needs 66% of an abdominal CT [23].

Tube voltage: For babies, a tube voltage of 80 kV should be used and afterwards up to puberty 100 kV can be chosen. The high-resolution kernel needs special attention, since in some machines, they do not work as expected at a tube voltage of 80 kV or 100 kV, again the most simple thing is to try it on phantoms. Since by lowering tube voltage the dose will be lowered by square (see Section 22.2), this can be first compensated by increasing the tube current in the same amount, for example, lowering tube voltage from 120 kV to 80 kV = 2/3 × 120 means that only $(2/3)2 = 4/9 \approx 50\%$ of dose is applied, thus theoretically tube current must be doubled. As mentioned already in Section 22.3, due to the increased contrast in 80 kV an increase by 60%–70% represents a good starting point with the potential of further lowering.

The scout view can be regarded as forgotten part of a CT examination, but it offers several ways to reduce the radiation burden [2]. Putting the tube below the table will save about two-thirds of dose; this can be achieved by almost all newer CT systems. Moreover, vendors must deliver their systems with fixed exposure settings for the scout view, but there is no reason to use the same dose for all ages. In the authors' experience, not adapted settings for scout view can be deliver the same amount of radiation as the whole scanning in a small child. Therefore, this step must be optimized and patient adapted too. Another possibility of unwanted radiation excess is represented by the bolus tracking—those values need to be adapted too.

In special indications or CT examinations, "low-dose" protocols might be used; some examples are given in the following discussion.

Hydrocephalus—Shunt control: Besides ultrasound in neonates and babies, for sure an indication for magnetic resonance imaging (MRI), but depending on the environment, CT can be sometimes necessary. As a simple rule, tube current can be just half of normal. In any case of diagnostic uncertainty about liquor pedesis, one or two slices with the normal tube current settings should be sufficient to clarify.

Craniostenosis: Tube current should be lowered to 30%–50% of normal values since in craniostenosis the skull is interesting, thus representing a high contrast situation. To overcome noise for 3D rendering, images should be reconstructed using a soft kernel.

Cystic Fibrosis: Again only half of the tube current for standard examinations, slice thickness 1–2 mm. In this situation, AEC needs special attention; if AEC is targeted to 1–2-mm slice thickness, dose will be elevated. So let the AEC be at slice thickness of the standard examination, for example, 3–5 mm.

Funnel Chest: Reduce tube current to at least 50% of standard examination.

Musculoskeletal CT: For hips reduce tube current to 50% of standard pelvic examination, for knees and ankles reduce by 70%. In case of forefoot examinations, X-rays will be attenuated by the whole forefoot because of the upright position of the forefoot. Therefore starting with standard hip tube currents, followed by lowering in 20% steps is advisable.

"Stone CT": For confirmation of stones within the urinary tract, ultrasound should be the first imaging modality. If CT is necessary, reduce tube current by 50%–60%.

Take home points: Cluster different ages and weights in different CT protocols. Abdominal CT needs.... abdominal CT needs 50% more dose than chest CT (= 150% from chest). Think on "low-dose" CT protocols.

22.5 Diagnostic Reference Levels

The radiological protection principle of dose limits used for exposure of workers and the general public does not apply to medical exposures for patients. To assist in the optimization process of medical exposure to patients,

the concept of diagnostic reference level (DRL) has been introduced [12].

Computed tomography dose index (CTDI) and/or dose–length product (DLP) are the quantities proposed as DRLs for CT. The main objectives of DRL are to improve a regional, national, or local dose distribution by identifying and reducing the number of unjustified high or low values and getting an optimum range of values for a specified medical imaging protocol. In this context, CTDI and DLP measurements should be part of the dose optimization program in a CT department. Determination of local DRLs should be done using a sample of 10 standard-sized patients, for example, the common head CT. The mean values of these results have to be compared with the skull DRL from organizations like EMAN, ICRP or the National Institute of Radiation Protection. The upper DRL borders are generated by taking the third quartile value of a survey. Third quartile represents the threshold where 75% of the institutional values are below. If the own levels are higher than nationally or internationally set DRL, appropriate corrective actions should be applied to reducing the dose to the skull [14]. In several nationwide surveys in Germany, the DRLs for adult and pediatric patients have been evaluated by the Federal Office for Radiation Protection—Bundesamt für Strahlenschutz (BfS)—the latest version of which being published in 2010. Table 22.1 is extracted and translated from the original document and presents $CTDI_{vol}$ and DLP. It provides DRLs for pediatric patients in six different age categories [24].

Take home points: For typical and frequent examinations, the delivered dose should be compared with DRLs. Own dose values should be well below; if this is not the case, the whole "Imaging Chain" needs reevaluation including a medical physicist.

22.6 Teamwork

Today's CT machines offer various options; thus, examinations can be tailored to patient needs. As mentioned already in Section 22.1, growing and maturing represents another dimension in pediatric CT. Considering the "Imaging Chain" (see Figure 22.4), it becomes clear that a successful pediatric CT is depending on teamwork—from staff at the departments counter to radiographers, radiologists, and transcriptionists. A chain is strong as its individual parts. If, for example, counter

TABLE 22.1

DRLs for Pediatric CT Examinations/Scan

Examination	Age/Weight	CTDI$_{vol}$-16 (mGy)[a]	CTDI$_{vol}$-32 (mGy)[a]	DLP-16 (mGy × cm)	DLP-32 (mGy × cm)
Brain	Newborn	27		300	
	≤1 year	33		400	
	2–5 years	40		500	
	6–10 years	50		650	
	11–15 years	60		850	
	>15 years	65		950	
Facial bones (tumor diagnosis)	Newborn	9		70	
	≤1 year	11		95	
	2–5 years	13		125	
	6–10 years	17		180	
	11–15 years	20		230	
	>15 years	22		250	
Chest	≤5 kg (newborn)	3	1.5	40	20
	6–10 kg (≤1 year)	4	2	60	30
	11–20 kg (2–5 years)	7	3.5	130	65
	21–30 kg (6–10 years)	10	5	230	115
	31–50 kg (11–15 years)		8		230
	51–80 kg (>15 years)		12		400
Abdomen	≤5 kg (newborn)	5	2,5	90	45
	6–10 kg (≤1 year)	7	3.5	170	85
	11–20 kg (2–5 years)	12	6	330	165
	21–30 kg (6–10 years)	16	8	500	250
	31–50 kg (11–15 years)		13		500
	51–80 kg (>15 years)		20		900

Source: Translated from Federal Office for Radiation Protection. www.BFS.de. Updated Diagnostic Reference Levels for Diagnostic and Interventional Radiology. June 22, 2010. http://www.bfs.de/de/ion/medizin/referenzwerte02.pdf.

Note: The numbers "16" and "32" mean the standard phantom used for CT dosimetry with a diameter of 16 cm (head and child body) or a diameter of 32 cm (body).

[a] For orientation.

staff are busy, people accompanying the patients, such as parents, get more anxious and frightened, thus creating a bad emotional environment for the child with consecutive negative outlook for the planned examination. Skilled radiographers, having already prepared everything in advance, including parameters on the CT console, represent a further clue to a successful examination.

The generation of CT protocols needs special attention, as described in the previous pages. Radiographers and radiologists must act as a team and have to adapt the given general guidelines to the local requirements.

Take home points: A successful CT examination can only be achieved using teamwork, all participating professions must cooperate.

22.7 Summary

In conclusion, pediatric CT represents a higher complexity due to changing body composition and a mass factor of more than 300. Before doing a CT examination in a child, ultrasound and MRI should be used first. Best radiation protection can be achieved by *not doing a CT*.

Proper patient positioning; shielding; a tight scout view with adopted exposure values; and adequate scan settings including scan mode, slice thickness, voltage tube current, as well as reconstruction parameter are essential prerequisites. Dose values for typical examinations should be checked periodically and compared to international reference values. Moreover, after hardware updates or installation of a new machine, all available features for reducing radiation must be evaluated. A set of appropriate phantoms is helpful for these tasks.

References

1. Sorantin E, Coradello H, Wiltgen, M. Computer-assisted mechanical ventilation of newborn infants. *Anaesthesist* 1992; 41, 342–345.
2. Sorantin E, Weissensteiner S, Hasenburger G, Riccabona M. CT in children—dose protection and general considerations when planning a CT in a child. *European Journal of Radiology* 2012;ISSN 1872-7727. doi:10.1016/j.ejrad.2011.11.041. http://www.ncbi.nlm.nih. gov/pubmed/22227258 Last assessed June 28, 2012.
3. Sorantin E, Riccabona M, Stücklschweiger G, Guss H, Fotter R. Experience with volumetric (320 rows) pediatric CT. *European Journal of Radiology* 2012;ISSN 1872-7727. doi:10.1016/j.ejrad.2011.12.001. http://www.ncbi.nlm.nih .gov/pubmed/22227261. Last accessed June 28, 2012.
4. Nitecki S, Moir C R. Predictive factors of the outcome of traumatic cervical spine fracture in children. *Journal of Pediatric Surgery* 1994;29(11):1409–11. http://www.ncbi .nlm.nih.gov/pubmed/7844708?dopt = Abstract. Last accessed May 14, 2012.
5. Sorantin E. Soft-copy display and reading: what the radiologist should know in the digital era. *Pediatric Radiology* 2008;38(12):1276–84. ISSN 0301-0449. doi:10 .1007/s00247-008-0898-6. http://www.ncbi.nlm.nih. gov/pubmed/18548242. Last accessed May 12, 2012.
6. Pang D, Wilberger J E J. Spinal cord injury without radiographic abnormalities in children. *Journal of Neurosurgery* 1982;57(1):114–29. http://www.ncbi.nlm.nih.gov/pubmed /7086488?dopt = Abstract. Last accessed May 14, 2012.
7. AAPM Reports 204: Size-Specific Dose Estimates (SSDE) in pediatric and adult body CT examinations 2011. http://www .aapm.org/pubs/reports/RPT_204.pdf, Last accessed June 22, 2012.
8. Abrams H L. BEIR VII Report 2006. http://www.stanford.edu/dept/news/pr/2005/pr-abrams-102605.html, Last accessed June 23, 2012.
9. The German Commission on Radiological Protection. Diagnostic imaging in children - radiation protection, justification and effectiveness.2006. http://www.ssk .de/SharedDocs/Beratungsergebnisse_PDF/2006/ BildgebendeDiagnostik_Kind.html, Last assessed June 29, 2012.
10. EMAN-European Medical Alara Network. "WG 1: Optimisation of Patient Exposure in CT Procedures". 2012. http://www.eman-network.eu/IMG/pdf/WG1_ Synthesis_doc-2.pdf, Last assessed May 15, 2013.
11. ICRP—International Commission on Radiation Protection. *Managing Patient Dose in Multi-Detector Computed Tomography (MDCT)*, 1st Edition 2007. http://store.elsevier .com/ICRP-Publication-102-Managing-Patient-Dose-in-Multi-Detector-Computed-Tomography-MDCT/isbn-9780702030475/, Last accessed July 4, 2012.
12. ICRP—International Commission on Radiation Protection. Radiological protection in paediatric diagnostic and interventional radiology. 2011. http://www.icrp.org/docs/ Radiological%20Protection%20in%20Paediatric%20 Diagnostic%20and%20Interventional%20Radiology.pdf. Last assessed July 4, 2012.
13. Frush D P, Soden B, Frush K S, Lowry C. Improved pediatric multidetector body CT using a size-based color-coded format. *AJR. American Journal of Roentgenology* 2002;178(3):721–6. ISSN 0361-803X. http://www.ncbi.nlm .nih.gov/pubmed/11856705. Last accessed June 21, 2012.
14. EMAN-European Medical Alara Network. WG 1: Optimisation of patient exposure in CT procedures. 2011 http://www.icrp.org/docs/Radiological%20 Protection%20in%20Paediatric%20Diagnostic%20 and%20Interventional%20Radiology.pdf, Last accessed July 4, 2012.
15. Mahmoud M, McAuliffe J, Donnelly L F. Administration of enteric contrast material before abdominal CT in children: current practices and controversies. *Pediatric Radiology* 2011;41(4):409–12. ISSN 1432-1998. doi:10.1007/s00247-010-1960-8. http://www.ncbi.nlm .nih.gov/pubmed/21221564. Last accessed June 28, 2012.
16. Kim S, Frush D P, Yoshizumi T T. Bismuth shielding in CT: support for use in children. *Pediatric Radiology* 2010;40(11):1739–43. ISSN 1432–1998. doi:10.1007 /s00247-010-1807-3.http://www.ncbi.nlm.nih.gov /pubmed/20734038. Last accessed June 30,, 2012.
17. Macias C G, Chumpitazi C E. Sedation and anesthesia for CT: emerging issues for providing high-quality care. *Pediatric Radiology* 2011;41 Suppl 2:517–22. ISSN 1432-1998. doi:10.1007/s00247-011-2136-x. http://www. ncbi .nlm.nih.gov/pubmed/21847733. Last accessed June 22, 2012.
18. Starkey E, Sammons H M. Sedation for radiological imaging. *Archives of Disease in Childhood. Education and Practice Edition* 2011;96(3):101–6. ISSN 1743-0593. doi:10.1136/adc.2008.153072. http://www.ncbi.nlm.nih .gov/pubmed/20675522. Last accessed June 22, 2012.
19. Becke K, Landsleitner B, Reinhold P, Schmitz B, Strauss J, Philippi-H¨ohne C. [Diagnostic and interventional operations in childhood: anesthesiology management]. *Der Anaesthesist* 2010;59(11):1013–20. ISSN 1432-055X. doi:10.1007/s00101-010-1781-z. http://www.ncbi .nlm .nih.gov/pubmed/20922357. Last accessed June 22, 2012.
20. Nyquist–Shannon sampling theorem.2012. http:// en.wikipedia.org/wiki/Nyquist%E2%80%93Shannon_ sampling_theorem Last accessed June 26rd 2012.
21. Sorantin E, Weissensteiner S, Koestenberger M. "Newborn with minor respiratory distress". Case of the week.2012. Aunt Minnie Europe. http://www.auntminnieeurope .com/index.aspx?sec=edu_n&sub=cases&pag=case&UI D=3J50QTAF. Last accessed June 26, 2012.
22. SPR - Image Gently: How to Develop CT Protocols for Children. 2007. http://www.pedrad.org/associations/5364 /files/Protocols.pdf, Last assessed July 3rd, 2012.
23. Sorantin E. Trainer Kinderradiologie (Training for Pediatric Radiology), chapter 1.5 Special features of computed tomography in children", p 23 – 30. Georg Thieme Verlag, Stuttgart–New York, 1st edition, 2010.
24. Federal Office for Radiation Protection. www.BFS.de. Updated Diagnostic Reference Levels for Diagnostic and Interventional Radiology. June 22, 2010. http://www.bfs .de/de/ion/medizin/referenzwerte02.pdf . Last assessed July 1, 2012.

23

Forensic Medicine

Garyfalia Ampanozi, Lars C. Ebert, Michael J. Thali, and Patricia M. Flach

CONTENTS

23.1 Introduction

Autopsy (from "autos" and "opsis" (from the greek verb: orao/oro) meaning "self" and "to see") is the gold standard procedure in forensic investigations of the deceased. It consists of dissecting the body and organs, and sampling tissues to reveal lethal pathological alterations, macro- and microscopically, respectively. External examination of both deceased and living persons is performed to describe and document surface alterations, especially traumatic ones, indicative of the type of instruments used or direction and strength of the force applied.

Forensic pathologists are historically great anatomists and the art of dissection and macroscopic recognition of the abnormal are individual characteristics. Forensic pathology is the field of medicine with the least technical and technological progress [1]. Handmade schemes and drawings were enhanced by digital photography, and new histological stainings were introduced, but this cannot be compared to the progress that other medical specialties have experienced.

Forensic pathology was revolutionized with the introduction of radiological techniques. However, the evolution of radiology and forensic pathology did not happen simultaneously. Postmortem imaging was introduced into forensics, since the discovery of the x-rays by Wilhelm Conrad Röntgen in 1895. The first case of forensic radiology known is the gunshot injury to the leg of Mr. Tolson Cunning. The projectile could be detected radiological and was removed consecutively. The x-ray film was even admitted to the court as evidence [2]. In 1977, the first postmortem computed tomography (PMCT) was reported in a case of gunshot injury to the head [3].

In 2000, the idea of the Virtopsy® project (www.virtopsy.com), with the objective, noninvasive documentation of the deceased by means of PMCT, was launched in Bern, Switzerland, by Prof. Dirnhofer and Prof. Thali, both former directors of the Institute of Forensic Medicine in collaboration with Prof. Vock, former director of the Department of Interventional, Pediatric and Diagnostic Radiology of the Inselspital, University Hospital of Bern. This recent approach provided totally new perspectives for the traditional field of forensic pathology. PMCT, PMCT angiography (PMCTA), postmortem magnetic resonance (PMMR), computed tomography (CT)-guided minimally invasive needle biopsy, and high-resolution surface scanning of both corpses and objects were implemented and inaugurated a new era in forensics [4,5].

Using teleradiological methods, the acquired images can be sent at the time of the investigation to experts around the world for consultation, or recalled even after many years and reevaluated. Three-dimensional (3D) reconstructions of pathologies gained from scan data are easily understood by medical laypersons, which is of relevance in the courtroom [6]. It also provides information from body regions that are not easy or very time consuming to dissect, like the craniocervical junction, vertebral column, small pelvis, and the extremities. Forensic imaging is nondestructive and non- or at least minimally invasive and adds valuable information to the forensic examination.

23.2 Workflow

The workflow of postmortem imaging depends on the facilities of the forensic institute. If no CT scanner is available, collaboration with the radiology department of a hospital or a private praxis could be the solution [7,8]. Ideally, all cases delivered to the forensic institute are being scanned before autopsy. If cases have to be selected, standardized selection protocols have to be set (e.g., homicides, gunshot injuries, children). If there is a possibility of PMMR imaging (PMMRI), selected cases with specific indications undergo a PMMR examination. If superficial patterned injuries are present surface scanning can be performed for documentation. For histological examinations of tissue changes, CT-guided needle biopsy can deliver tissue samples (both see Section 23. 6).

If vessel pathologies or lesions are suspected, a PMCTA should be performed after the unenhanced PMCT [9–13]. Usually the femoral artery and vein are being cannulated and the cannulas are connected to a modified heart–lung machine, roller or embalming pump. Lacking any blood circulation and vessel distension, contrast medium has to be delivered mixed with a carrier substance, which can be either oil based or polyethylenglycol. Both contrast medium mixtures have advantages and disadvantages [10]. Contrast medium mixture is injected into the vessels under controlled pressure (if a modified heart–lung machine is available) and scans are performed each after arterial and vein injection. A third, dynamic scan has also been proposed during an additional contrast medium administration [12]. Targeted organ or regional angiographies have been also proposed and described in the literature [14–16].

However, prior to any PMCTA procedure it is essential to preserve blood, urine, or any other samples for toxicological examinations.

Finally, all postmortem imaging information has to be reported to the pathologist performing the autopsy.

23.3 Identification

One of the most important tasks for a forensic pathologist and the very first step in the postmortem examination procedure is the identification of the deceased. DNA profiling, fingerprints comparison, and dental data comparison are considered the most secure methods [17]; however, in the routine setting, methods such as confrontation with family members, tattoos, and comparison with ID-cards photographs are often used.

The biological profile of unknown remains found is based on anthropological criteria. Postmortem imaging can provide information regarding human origin of the remains, age, height, and sex [18–21].

PMCT provides documentation of the dentition of the deceased, which can be adjusted regarding angle and perspective to antemortem dental x-rays for comparison. The procedure is fast and even if no antemortem data are available at the time of the scan, the post-processing modalities of a CT dataset allow for future comparison and counter-expertise because of feasible data storage and its noninvasive character compared to destructive autopsy [22–25].

The basic principle of radiologic identification is to compare ante- and postmortem data. Based on that, not only dental information, but almost all anatomical marks and characteristics can be reconstructed from PMCT datasets and used for identification purposes. Paranasal sinuses architecture and their characteristic appearance in CT examinations is a very good example, as their form does not change during adult life, if not affected from pathology [26]. Frequent use of CT in clinical settings provides increasingly antemortem imaging data to compare with postmortem acquired scans [27]. Skeletal abnormalities, postsurgery characteristics, medical implants, and other individual features can be used for identification purposes [28,29]. Furthermore, the role of PMCT in Disaster Victim Identification protocols has been commented extensively in the literature [17,21,26,30,31]. The availability of mobile CT units, which were already exploited in the postmortem setting [32], makes it even more feasible in these cases.

23.4 Differences of Forensic Radiology Compared to Clinical Radiology

23.4.1 General Issues on Postmortem Imaging

Contrary to clinical scans, radiation hygiene is no issue in forensic radiology and the examiner does not have to bother with motion artifacts. Still, during image-guided biopsy, radiation exposure to the personnel should still be kept as low as possible by using appropriate techniques similar to clinical radiology. In addition, decompositional gas, foreign material, and maggot/insect infestation are typical postmortem problems that may even impair image quality. In a forensic setting typically full body scans are performed, which leads to larger scan volumes that are to be investigated.

Forensic radiology poses different problems than clinical radiology, for example, identification of the corpse; detection of medical malpractice; and location and identification of foreign materials such as projectiles, incidental internal metal parts such as a broken tip of a knife, implants or large objects stuck in the body in cases of impalement [4,33].

In the past decade, typical, nonpathologic postmortem signs on postmortem imaging have been identified as there are typical postmortem changes that occur in cadavers. A radiologist who is only used to read clinical images may easily misinterpret these changes. Basically, with death immediate breakdown of cellular barriers begins and decomposition alters the soft tissue. Consequently, these findings on postmortem imaging may mimic antemortem pathologies [34].

23.4.2 Decomposition and Gas Embolism

Initial sign of putrefaction is gas accumulation within the portal venous and hepatobiliary system, which needs to be differentiated from gas embolism [35–38]. Decomposition occurs in the organs and the soft tissue as well as in the vasculature and involves usually the whole body. In the brain, tissue decomposition creates a typical "swiss-cheese" sign (Figure 23.1). However, decompositional gas may also appear to be position-dependent and will then dominate the ventral parts of the body because of gravity. In addition, putrefaction may lead in a later stage to liquefaction and relapse of parenchymal organs and fluid accumulation within body cavities (Figure 23.2) [34]. Therefore, in decomposed bodies, fluid within the thoracic or abdominal cavity should not be mistaken for pleural effusion or ascites and has to be noted as physiological postmortem change. In contrast, gas or air embolism is only located within the vascular structures and the heart chambers (Figure 23.3). Both internal imaging findings, decomposition and gas embolism, are best seen on PMCT and

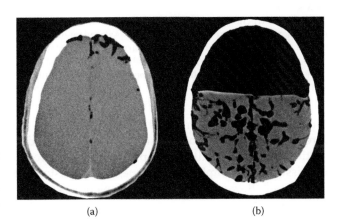

(a)   (b)

FIGURE 23.1

(a) Early position-dependent decompositional gas in the anterior part of the brain. (b) Further putrefaction will lead in later stages to the typical "swiss-cheese" sign with gas accumulation within the brain tissue and vasculature. Note the liquefaction and relapse of the brain within the skull.

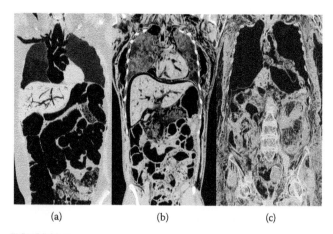

FIGURE 23.2
(a) Air embolism with little signs of initial decomposition in the liver. The remaining soft tissue shows no signs of putrefaction. Note the typical air-filled heart chambers and supraaortal vessels. (b) Progressed decomposition with symmetric gas distribution within the soft tissue, the vasculature, and complete air-filled, autolytic tissue of the pancreas. In addition, there is gas in the abdominal cavity due to putrefaction and not caused by perforation of air-containing structures. (c) Late stage of decomposition with liquefaction of the lung tissue and vast lyses of most of the organs in a case of exhumation after 4 months being buried in the ground.

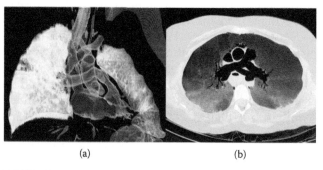

FIGURE 23.3
(a) 3D-reconstruction (angulated slab) of air-containing structures of the thorax in a case of gas embolism. (b) Axial view of the same case at the level of the air-filled pulmonary trunc and arteries, the aorta and caval vein with extensive air embolism only located within the vascular system and the heart chambers. There are no significant signs of decomposition.

especially gas embolism needs to be suspected by the forensic pathologist to be investigated by a special dissection method. In badly decomposed bodies, the residual tissue, for example, brain tissue, will be dislocated and literally flow out and an in situ depiction is not feasible anymore.

23.4.3 Postmortem Position Changes

The radiological investigator always has to take into account that organs may be displaced when interpreting images. Hemo- and pneumothorax may compress and dislocate lung tissue and a shot or sharp-injury

wound canal may be disguised and not be in the trajectory of the entrance and exit wound. In addition, the position of the body during the inflicted trauma is usually not static and this must be kept in mind when virtually reconstructing a wound channel [34].

23.4.4 Imaging of the Head

Immediately after death, a loss of the corticomedullary differentiation on PMCT similar to a generalized stroke occurs, which should not be mistaken with antemortem brain edema [39]. However, brain edema despite the physiological postmortem changes is difficult to differentiate on PMCT but may be facilitated by additional PMMR [40,41].

A normal postmortem finding is the hyperdense sinus and cortical veins and should not be confused with the antemortem "hyperdense sinus" sign as seen in venous thrombosis. This finding is related to position-dependent sedimentation effects [42]. However, the hyperdense cortical veins may simulate slight subarachnoidal hemorrhage and may be ruled out by adding a PMCTA procedure or PMMR (Figure 23.4) [9,10,13]. In frozen bodies, the brain tissue will appear very hypodense in the center and the gyri will be emphasized (Figure 23.5).

23.4.5 Imaging of the Thorax

In external inspection, livor mortis of the skin is a well-known finding in forensic pathology. On imaging, internal livor mortis occurs position-dependent within the lungs with ground-glass opacification (Figure 23.6) [43]. However, discriminating between pathologies such as concomitant pulmonary edema, aspiration, and pneumonia may be difficult and only detectable after postmortem ventilation techniques [44–46].

Bilateral symmetric ventral rib fractures or a sternal cross fracture are typical in cases of resuscitation and are often not because of prior trauma. In addition, so-called incomplete or buckle rib fractures are frequently detected by PMCT in consequence of anterior compressive force to the chest, for example, after external cardiac massage, and show a cortical disruption to the inner side of the rib while maintaining the outer side, usually located in the anterior third of the rib [47,48]. Sedimentation effects within the large vessels such as the aorta lead to the "hyperdense aortic wall" sign and collapse of the aorta to "vanishing aorta" in, for example, cases of major blood loss [34,49,50].

Hyperdense formation in the pulmonary trunc and both pulmonary arteries is a nonspecific finding on PMCT and should not be interpreted as antemortem pulmonary embolism as cause of death. Unenhanced PMCT solely does not allow for diagnoses of pulmonary embolism, as postmortem clotting (cruor) appears

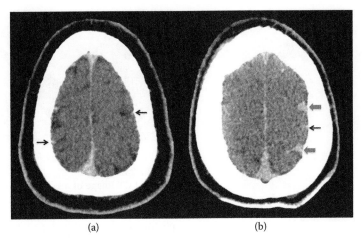

FIGURE 23.4
(a) Typical postmortem finding of a hyperdense sinus and cortical veins (black arrows) in a natural cause of death due to intravascular sedimentation effects. (b) A case with trauma to the head presenting with slight subarachnoid hemorrhage (gray arrows), which may be misinterpreted as postmortem normal hyperdense cortical veins (black arrow).

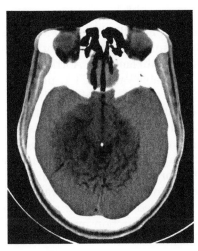

FIGURE 23.5
Typical appearance of frozen brain tissue with a hypodense center according to the frozen part and normal postmortem brain tissue adjacent to it.

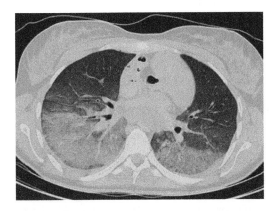

FIGURE 23.6
Note the normal postmortem finding of internal livor mortis in posterior position-dependent areas of the lung due to supine position of the corpse.

similar to antemortem clots. Dilatation of the right atrium and ventricle is unspecific and may occur in, for example, general agonal blood congestion and in drowning [51].

23.4.6 Imaging of the Abdomen

Air distension of the stomach is typical after resuscitation and fluid distension of the stomach and duodenum typical in cases of drowning [52]. Initial decomposition with gas in the liver, hepatobiliary, and portal venous system should not be mistaken with pneumatosis intestinalis as seen in clinical patients but is a frequent normal postmortem finding [35–38]. The same applies to intramural gas in the intestines (Figure 23.7). Unenhanced PMCT is limited in detection of lesions of the parenchymal organs and heterogeneous tissue is indicative for organ laceration [53–55]. Adjacent fluid accumulation with hyperdense sedimentation effects will substantiate potential parenchymal injury [56]. Heat related thermal tissue changes lead to protrusion of the intestines and is related to thermal impact and not to trauma [57].

23.4.7 Malpractice

Frequently, there are misplaced endotracheal tubes detected on imaging either incidental in only one main bronchus during resuscitation attempts or in the mediastinum because of ruptured airways [34]. However, this finding is only documented on imaging as typically all the medical devices are removed before autopsy and external inspection will not reveal such a potential malpractice. The same principle applies for other medical tubes or devices such as thoracic drainage that may not have reached the target organ or cavity (Figure 23.8).

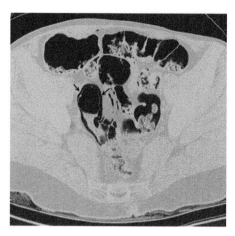

FIGURE 23.7
Intramural gas in the intestines (here sigmoid colon, black arrows) frequently noted in the course of decay and not a sign of ante mortem pathology such as ischemia/pneumatosis intestinalis.

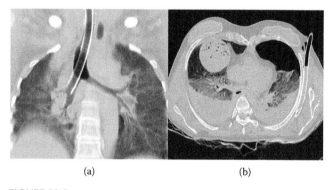

FIGURE 23.8
(a) Misplacement of an endotracheal tube during resuscitation with the tip located deep in the right main bronchus. (b) Misplacement of a thoracic tube in the soft tissue of the chest and not correctly located within the "chest" instead of "lung" cavities. Besides note the bilateral pleural effusion, pneumothorax, and additional inner livores of the lung.

23.5 Answering Forensic Questions

23.5.1 Natural Causes of Death

A person who died because of natural causes will undergo a forensic examination, if the circumstances of death are sudden and unknown and/or suspicious. The goal of postmortem imaging in such cases is the exclusion of trauma and involvement of other persons/third-party influence.

Cardiovascular diseases form the vast majority of natural causes of death. Cardiac deaths were the most common causes of natural deaths in a forensic institute, in all age groups, as of a large study published in 2007 [58]. In PMCT, coronary artery calcification can be detected easily. However, calcification is not an evidence of cardiac ischemia. Noncalcified atheromatic plaques, coronary stenosis, and coronary occlusion because of

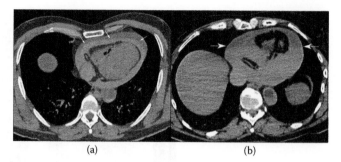

FIGURE 23.9
(a) Axial CT image of a heart tamponade after myocardial rupture. Note the two-layered blood around the heart ("double ring" or "armored heart" sign, arrows in a). The deceased had been complaining of chest and back pain two days before he died. (b) Axial CT image of a heart tamponade as a result of an aortic dissection and rupture in the pericardial sac. Note the sedimentation of the corpuscular blood particles (arrows in b). No "double ring sign" is seen in this case.

thrombosis can be seen only after injection of contrast medium or with PMMRI [59–61]. PMCTA enables the depiction of suspicious locations for significant coronary stenosis and thrombosis. Aortic or coronary aneurysms are detectable on PMCTA, unenhanced PMCT usually offers too little detail of the vasculature to detect vessel pathologies reliably. Aortic dissections as another natural cause of death are precisely detected on PMCTA and even the intimal tear can be located. Fresh myocardial infarction cannot be visualized with PMCT solely, except for chronic, already calcified, infarction scars or focal thinning of the myocardium. Therefore, PMMR is considered the current method of choice to detect myocardial infarction by means of postmortem imaging [62,63].

Cardiac tamponade can occur after rupture of the ascending aorta, ruptured myocardial infarction, coronary artery rupture, etc. PMCT offers an easy possibility to detect hemopericardium in cases of cardiac tamponade. Often, a "double ring" sign is seen, whereas in other cases only sedimentation of corpuscular blood particles is noticed [64] (Figure 23.9).

It is believed that the "double ring" or "hyperdense armored heart" sign is present in cases where death did not occur instantly. The volume of blood in the pericardial sack can be assessed reliably with segmentation techniques [65].

Pulmonary embolism is not unusual in forensic pathology cases. PMCT is not reliable in diagnosing this cause of death. Hyperdense formations within the pulmonary truncation are frequently seen on PMCT, but cannot be differentiated from physiological postmortem clotting (cruor; see also Section 23.4.5). At this point in time, either image-guided biopsy, eventually PMMR, or dissection is the only valid manner to confirm or rule out pulmonary embolism.

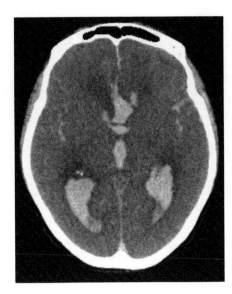

FIGURE 23.10
Axial PMCT image of the head. Subarachnoidal hemorrhage after rupture of an aneurysma of the circle of Willis.

Sudden natural deaths with causes located in the central nervous system are common: they can occur because of epilepsy, fatal intracranial hemorrhages, infections (e.g., meningitis), malignomas, etc. Spontaneous nontraumatic subarachnoid hemorrhage is commonly related to a ruptured arterial aneurysm (Figure 23.10) and intra-axial hemorrhage in the basal ganglia region usually is caused by hypertensive bleeding. On postmortem imaging, it is sometimes challenging to differentiate whether an intracranial hemorrhage was nontraumatic or secondary to fall after a prior pathological incidence.

Abdominal aortic aneurysm rupture and dissection, nontraumatic splenic rupture, metastasis, and gastrointestinal hemorrhages are natural causes of death, just to mention some, that can be encountered by the forensic pathologist. The presence of fluid in the abdominal cavity, inhomogeneous organ parenchyma, and gastrointestinal tract, that is isodense to blood, can be some indicators of abdominal pathology. Although it is extremely difficult to depict the cause of death, PMCT contributes in these cases primarily to the work of the forensic pathologist by including or excluding traumatic injuries.

There is a variety of causes of sudden natural death because of respiratory system disease. Tension-pneumothorax (after rupture of emphysematic bullae) is an excellent example of how PMCT can support the autopsy planning and execution for correct documentation of the fatal finding (special preparation of the thoracic soft tissues is needed, so that the pleural cavity will be opened below the surface of water and gas bubbles ascending to the surface can be seen [66]).

Bronchiectasia and chronic emphysema (as a manifestation of chronic obstructive pulmonary disease) can also be found.

23.5.2 Blunt Force Injury

The impact of blunt force on the human body causes a variety of external and internal injuries. Externally, the following alterations are described [67]:

- Abrasions: are superficial injuries of the epidermis. In some cases it is extremely difficult to define when the abrasion occurred, especially in the perimortem time period (minutes before and after death). Presence of epidermal flakes allows determination of the direction of the impact.
- Contusions: require exsanguination of blood from injured vessels in deeper skin layers.
- Lacerations: are characterized by tears of the skin. They must be differentiated from injuries with sharp instruments (see Section 23.5.4).

Besides the timing of the occurrence of injuries, an important forensic aspect regarding external injuries because of blunt force is the ability to draw conclusions toward the instrument used. Progress in postmortem imaging techniques in recent years allows for 3D documentation of patterned skin lesions and matching of them to blunt force instruments [68–70] (The surface scanning technique is explained in Section 23.6.1).

23.5.2.1 Head and Spinal Injuries

Usually at the side of the impact, cephalic hematomas are indicative of blunt force application.

Skull fractures are well-depicted on PMCT. It is superior in comparison to the classical autopsy in complex fractures, where small osseous fragments can be unintentionally or even scattered during scalp removal and especially in facial fractures (Figure 23.11). The preparation of the facial soft tissues is a very time-consuming procedure and is not performed in a routine base. Forensic principles such as Puppe's rule, according to which new fracture lines end when they meet preexisting fracture lines, allow for sequential ordering of the injuries [71]. Fractures above the maximal diameter of the head (the imaginary line where a hat rests, the hat-brim line) are results of blunt force directed from above (e.g., blow with an object), whereas falls on the ground (however, not from height) result to impact with the most prominent marks of the cranium [72].

Fractures of the anterior vertebrae with dislocation of the fragmented parts can be seen after traffic fatalities,

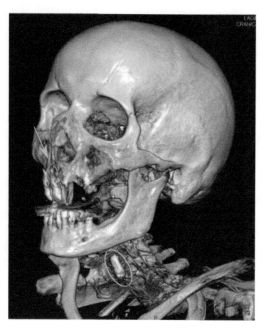

FIGURE 23.11
Three-dimensional volume rendering of the head. Maxilla fracture (arrow) and dislocated swallowed tooth above the epiglottis (encircled).

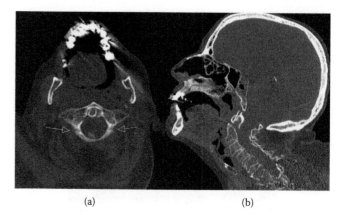

(a)   (b)

FIGURE 23.12
(a) Axial PMCT image at the height of atlas vertebra. Fractures of the posterior arches of C1 indicated by the arrows. (b) Sagittal PMCT image. Fracture of the odontoid process of the C2 vertebra. Odontoid fractures are difficult to see during autopsy.

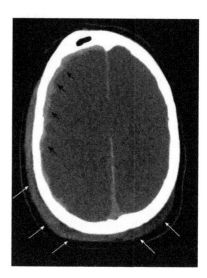

FIGURE 23.13
Craniocerebral trauma after fall from stairs. Axial PMCT image of the head. Extended hemorrhage of the right scalp (white arrows) and right subdural hematoma (black arrows).

falls from height, or other blunt forces applied, and are not problematic in autopsy documentation. However, fractures of the middle and posterior column such as vertebral process are extremely difficult to detect during autopsy. Instead, indications as hemorrhages of the surrounding soft tissues can be found. PMCT allows for documentation of difficult to dissect regions and depiction of injury in routinely nondissected body parts (Figure 23.12).

Cerebral injury and hemorrhages can occur either with or without fractures of the skull. Epidural hemorrhages are typically biconvex, usually combined with a skull fracture and often located temporoparietally, and are in many cases combined with a midline shift toward the other side according to their expansive character. The blood is in the majority of the cases of arterial origin (meningeal artery) but may also be venous. An artificial epidural hematoma, the so-called heat epidural, can also occur after exposure to fire (Section 23.5.6).

Subdural hemorrhages occur more often and are less related to skull fractures [73]. They are caused by rupture of the bridging veins and collection of blood in the subdural space (Figure 23.13). In the clinical setting a "lucent" time interval is described before onset of symptoms for both epi- and subdural hemorrhages. Subdural hemorrhages are also seen in cases of "shaken baby syndrome," and depiction of the ruptured veins can succeed after application of contrast medium on PMCTA [74].

Exsanguination of blood in the subarachnoid space can have natural (see Section 5.1) or traumatic causes.

Unfortunately, this cannot be clearly differentiated in all cases, even if PMCTA is applied. Rupture of an intracranial aneurysm and subsequent subarachnoid hemorrhage may cause an incident (fall, traffic fatality, etc.) but may also be the result of it.

Cerebral contusions, lacerations, and intracerebral hemorrhages are often seen after head injury. It is of great importance to the forensic pathologist to be able to characterize a brain traumatic lesion as a "coup" or "contre-coup" injury. Briefly, a coup injury appears beneath the impact side, whereas a contre-coup lesion is seen at the diametrically opposite part of the brain. Contre-coup lesions are usually present when a moving head hits a fixed surface (e.g., falling to the ground) (Figure 23.14).

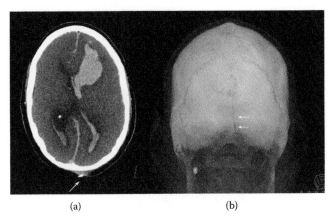

(a)   (b)

FIGURE 23.14
Craniocerebral injury after fall to the ground. Occipital galeal hematoma (white arrow on a) and contre-coup injury of the left frontal brain parenchyma. Hemorrhage into the side ventricles and midline shift towards the right side. At the side of the impact, a linear fracture line (arrows on b).

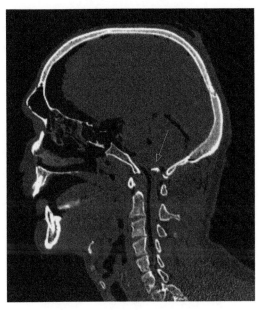

FIGURE 23.15
Sagittal PMCT image of a pedestrian fatality. Small bone fragments penetrating the brainstem (arrow). Note the skull base fractures as well as fractures of the frontal sinus walls with concomitant pneumencephalon.

In all cases, the cause of death can be either direct trauma of regions with importance for living functions, such as the brainstem (Figure 23.15), or a subsequent result of the trauma, such as edema, tonsilar herniation, secondary brainstem hemorrhage, anoxia, and so on.

23.5.2.2 Strangulation

Strangulation is a special form of blunt force applied to the neck. It can be distinguished into strangulation with bare hands or with a ligature and hanging. In the

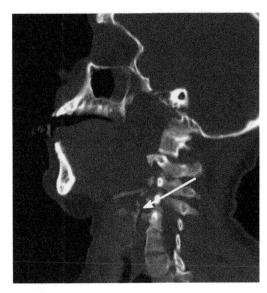

FIGURE 23.16
Blunt force applied to the neck. Sagittal PMCT image at the level of the thyroid cartilage. The right superior horn is fractured and slightly dislocated (arrow).

first case, the manner of death is always homicidal, as one cannot manually strangle himself: once the consciousness is lost, the hands will loose and blood flow will take place again. The strangulation with ligature can be homicidal or self-inflicted (the ligature has to be set tight and fix). Hangings are in the majority of the cases suicidal. Accidental hanging is in some cases also possible, and hanging as a judicial execution is nowadays rare if not nonexisting. The body can be hanging free (complete suspension) or some parts of it can touch the ground (incomplete suspension) and the rope can be seen posteriorly, anteriorly, or at one side of the neck. Typical autopsy signs of strangulation are petechial bleeding in the mucosa above the plane of the strangulation, congestion of the head (in cases where some arterial blood flow remains, whereas the venous outflow is blocked), and bleeding in the soft tissues of the neck. On the skin, the mark of the ligature or rope or evidence of manual strangulation, such as ecchymosis or small abrasions, can be found. Osseous alterations like fractures of the hyoid bone and/or the thyroid cartilage are of great importance (Figure 23.16) [71,75].

23.5.2.3 Thoracic and Abdominal Injuries

Thoracic blunt force trauma results commonly in traffic incidents, falls from height, or after active sustain by a blunt object from another person. Rib fractures, thoracic vertebral fractures, lung lacerations and/or contusions, heart lacerations, aortic ruptures, and presence of blood or gas in the thoracic cage can be seen (Figure 23.17). The cause of death can be in such cases direct trauma of the heart, lethal extravasation of blood, restriction of

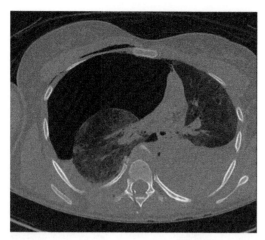

FIGURE 23.17
Axial PMCT image. Blunt force injury to the chest after a pedestrian-vehicle collision. Extended hemothorax predominantly on the left side and a large right-sided pneumothorax causing mediastinal shift to the left.

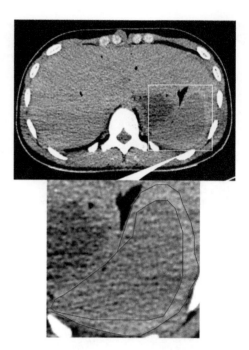

FIGURE 23.18
Axial PMCT image of a motor vehicle fatality at the height of the liver and spleen. Note the hematoma around the spleen (marked red in the magnified figure), which is indicative of a traumatic spleen rupture. No further free abdominal fluid was found.

the cardiac function (e.g., in a tension pneumothorax), restriction of the respiration, etc.

The presence of parenchymatous organs in the abdomen (e.g., liver, spleen, kidneys) leads to blood exsanguinations, when severe abdominal injury is present. Although even small volumes of free blood in the abdominal cavity can be found with PMCT, it is usually very difficult to locate the injured organ in noncontrast images. Sometimes perifocal hemorrhage to the organs into the soft-tissue, hematomas in close proximity of the organ's surface [76], or alterations of the density of the parenchyma can be indicative of injury (Figure 23.18) [77]. PMCTA and PMMR can provide valuable information in such cases.

The volume of the extravasated blood is significant, as ex- or ensanguination can be the cause of death. Segmentation techniques allow for reliable estimations of free blood volumes in the abdominal cavity [78].

In a study published recently [79], the utility of the vertebral process fractures in determining whether a pedestrian was overrun or not is being discussed. The authors conclude that bilateral fractures of transverse process are a possible sign for an overrun, whereas unilateral fractures are not specific. It must be noted that these fractures are much better seen and documented with PMCT examination than autopsy.

23.5.2.4 Extremities

Although usually nonlethal, trauma located to the extremities is forensically very important. In traffic injuries, the so-called Messerer wedge or butterfly fractures (Figure 23.19) of the lower extremities indicate the side of the impact and the direction of the applied force [71].

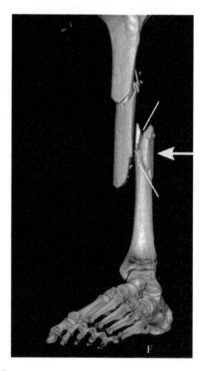

FIGURE 23.19
Three-dimensional volume rendering of a left tibia. The fibula was digitally removed. This pedestrian was hit by a car from behind and slightly left. The Messerer-wedge fragment is an indication for the direction of the applied force (arrow shows the direction of the force). The base of the butterfly wedge represents the direct side of the impact.

23.5.3 Gunshot Injury

From a forensic point of view, in cases of gunshot injuries, aspects like the differentiation of entrance and exit wound, the number of shots, the presence of fragments of the projectile, the pathway of the projectile inside the body, the firing distance and direction, and the type of weapon and/or projectile used are of great importance. The use of plain x-rays in such cases is being recommended by many forensic books, mostly for metal fragments localization [80,81].

CT is an excellent tool for depicting the characteristic features of gunshot injuries. It is superior compared to plain x-rays mostly for allowing 3D reconstructions and exact localization in space [82].

When the projectile passes through bones, the description of the wound channel can be easier, as bony fragments and/or metallic fragments of the projectile itself follow the course of the projectile and disperse along the forming path. Gas bubbles embedded in the soft tissues of either the skin and/or musculature, or the parenchyma of the organs, are also indicative of the gunshot tract, under the condition that decomposition processes allow for it. In some cases, hemorrhage along the wound track may be detected (Figure 23.20).

Gunshot injuries to the head represent a distinct category of cases. In fact, the entrance and exit wounds in such cases can be well-differentiated based on PMCT findings, which have been widely described in the literature [83]. The entrance wound is usually cone shaped with the osseous defect of the tabula interna being larger

than the defect of the tabula externa (Figure 23.21), whereas the opposite is seen at the site of the exit wound (Figure 23.22). Next to the entrance wound, bony flakes can usually be found along the path of the projectile through the brain (Figure 23.23). Resulting fracture patterns with either linear or radial fracture lines follow Puppe's rule [84]. Compared to the gold standard, the autopsy, PMCT has the advantage of showing the spatial position of even the smallest fragments, which is usually lost when removing the scalp [83,85–87].

The estimation of the firing distance can be challenging. The presence of gunshot residues not only is

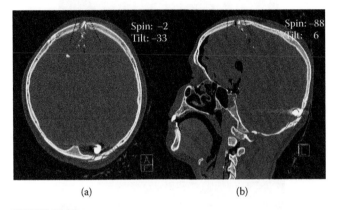

(a) (b)

FIGURE 23.21
(a) Oblique axial and (b) sagittal PMCT image of a penetrating gunshot injury to the head. The projectile is lodged occipitally. Note the characteristics of the entrance wound: the defect of the tabula interna is larger than that of the tabula externa (dotted lines) and multiple bony flakes/fragments are scattered along the brain parenchyma.

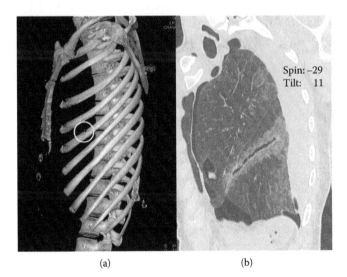

(a) (b)

FIGURE 23.20
Penetrating gunshot injury to the thorax. (a) Three-dimensional volume rendering of the left thoracic cage. Osseous defect of the fifth left rib (yellow circle) and final position of the projectile (marked blue) dorsally at the level of the left shoulder, after perforating the left scapula. (b) Oblique sagittal PMCT image of the left lung. The gunshot path through the left lower lung lobe is well depicted.

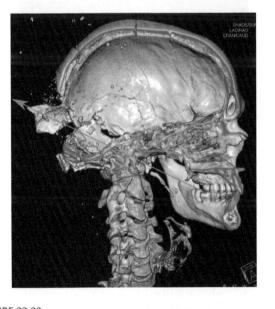

FIGURE 23.22
Three-dimensional volume rendering of a gunshot injury through the oral cavity. The entrance wound was located at the soft palate, the projectile passed through the skullbase and exited occipitally (green arrow).

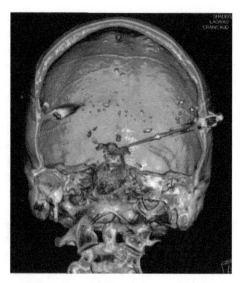

FIGURE 23.23
Three-dimensional volume rendered image of a skull after a suicidal gunshot injury. The projectile entered the cranial cavity at the right temporal area and exited it at the left side. End position of the projectile underneath the scalp at the left temporal area. Multiple osseous and metal fragments along the path.

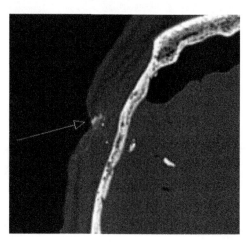

FIGURE 23.24
Axial PMCT image, suicidal gunshot to the head. Hyperintense gunshot residues (arrow) reveal a firing distance from close proximity. Note the traumatic pneumencephalon.

a supplementary indication of an entrance wound, but also allows for determining the contact, or very close range of the gunshot. Radiopaque particles (Figure 23.24) can be found in these cases at the soft tissues of the entrance wound [88]. A wider firing range is more difficult to be estimated based solely on PMCT findings. Evidence gained from external examination of the body and the scene of death should be always taken into consideration.

People lacking training in forensics could be mistaken by considering as the pathway of the projectile a direct, straight line between entrance and exit wound

or entrance wound and end position of the projectile inside the body. In fact, the wound channel is not always easy to describe on PMCT images. The movement of the living body, the relational position of the internal organs, and the phase of vital functions such as breathing or heart beating affect the course a projectile will follow. Internal ricocheting on osseous structures and projectile embolization should also be considered. In the latter case, the projectile or fragments of it enters the systemic blood circulation and can be found at any location [89].

23.5.4 Sharp Force Injury

Sharp instruments can produce either cut or stab wounds or both. In general, a cut injury is wider on the skin surface than deeper in the soft tissues, whereas a stab injury the opposite. They can be differentiated from blunt force lacerations based on the absence of bruising of their edges (exception: bruising produced by the handle of a knife), the absence of tissue bridges or strands connecting the edges of the wound (the wound margins are "clean"), and sometimes the presence of sharp injury on the underlying osseous structures [67]. There are a variety of instruments that can produce such injuries: blades with double or single cutting edges, scissors, screwdrivers, or even glass fragments, sharp edged metals, and so on.

There are many limitations when examining a sharp force injury. First of all, the depth of the wound does not necessarily correspond to the length of the instrument used. It is possible (and in most cases a fact) that the stabbing organ is being pushed deeper than its length, because of the elasticity of the skin and the underlying soft tissues. On the other hand, the length of the dermal trauma does not always correspond to the width of the instrument used. Here, the skin cleavage lines (Langer's lines) play an important role [90].

PMCT is helpful in locating a possibly retained broken part (usually the tip) of the instrument used, which can lead to its identification. It can also depict osseous lesions and trauma of the cartilages. Usually, at the site of the injury, gas collections in the soft tissues and disturbance of their continuity are the only signs of a sharp force wound. Estimating the depth of the wound on PMCT and drawing conclusions regarding the weapon used should be done thoughtfully [91].

Blood loss and gas embolism are common causes of death in cases of sharp trauma. As mentioned before, gas is very easily documented in PMCT. Fatal hemorrhage on the other hand is a cause of death based principally on the experience of the forensic pathologist (minimal livor mortis, pale color of the organs). A sign described in PMCT in fatal blood loss cases is the collapse of the great vessels [53].

The distinction between homicidal or suicidal sharp force fatalities is necessary. In suicidal cases, the wounds are located to the frontal body part for obvious reasons. There are in some cases initial, nonlethal wounds and there is no evidence of defense injuries. PMCTA allows for documentation of the injured blood vessels (Figure 23.25) [92–94].

23.5.5 Drowning

According to the widely used definition proposed by Roll: "death by drowning is the result of a hampering of the respiration by obstruction of mouth and nose by a fluid medium (usually water)" [95].

Drowning is a difficult diagnosis in forensic pathology. A body found in water is a true drowning case only after all other possible causes of death have been excluded. These other causes of death include natural causes (either while being in water or before getting into it), traumatic causes (again, either while being in water or before getting into it), and reflex-death in water [96]. There are controversial theories regarding the pathophysiology of drowning, but analyzing these is beyond the scope of this chapter. In general, the presence of fresh water in the alveoli leads to the absorption of it (because of its lower osmolarity in comparison to the blood) and inevitably to hypervolemia and hemodilution. In contrast, drowning in seawater leads to hemoconcentration (as water moves from blood to the alveoli).

Intraalveolar edema is usually also seen in both cases ("edema aquosum").

A distinct type of emphysema, the "emphysema aquosum," is the result of the presence of water in the bronchi, which induces acute overinflation; valvular mechanisms of bronchospasm have been described [96]. The lung volume is increased and after opening the thoracic cavity during autopsy, the lungs are often seen "kissing" each other over the mediastinum (Figure 23.26). In some cases, imprints of the ribs can be seen on the lung surface [97].

Hyperperfused areas are synchronously mixed leads to the typical mosaic-pattern appearance of the lungs in drowning cases on imaging (Figure 23.27). Areas in PMCT of ground glass opacity correspond to the hyperperfused lung regions, whereas more lucent areas correspond to emphysematous lung regions [52].

The presence of froth is often the first sign described in the drowning—chapters of forensic books. It consists of the drowning medium, air, and proteinaceous exudate [96,98]. It can be found in very fresh bodies exceeding from mouth and nostrils, and filling the airways.

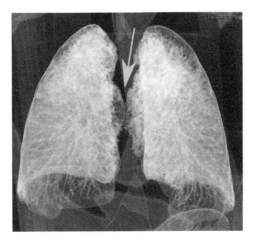

FIGURE 23.26
Volume rendering of the lungs in a drowning case. Note the "kissing" effect of the frontal parts of the lungs (arrow).

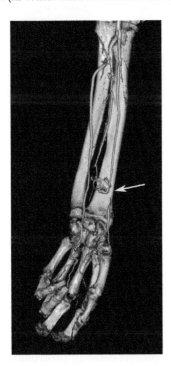

FIGURE 23.25
PMCTA with 3D reconstruction of the left upper extremity. Sharp force injury of the soft tissue and the left arteria radialis. Extravasation of contrast medium at the site of the injury (arrow).

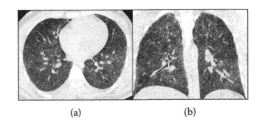

(a)   (b)

FIGURE 23.27
Axial (a) and coronal (b) PMCT image showing diffuse hyper- and hypoventilated areas of the lung parenchyma (mosaic pattern). Drowning in fresh water.

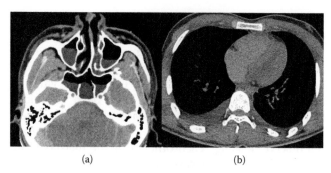

FIGURE 23.28
(a) Axial PMCT image showing fluid levels in the maxillary and sphenoid sinuses. (b) Pleura effusions (predominance in the right thoracic cavity) after accidental drowning in fresh water.

Presence of drowning fluid in the paranasal sinuses is a very often finding in drowning cases (Figure 23.28a). In some cases, high-density material, corresponding to sand, can be found in the airways and paranasal sinuses [52,97].

During the drowning process, some amount of the drowning medium can be swallowed and may lead to fluid distension in the stomach and duodenum. Wydler's sign (the presence of three-layered fluid in stomach) is another characteristic but nonspecific sign of drowning.

Pleural effusions may also play a supportive role in diagnosing death by drowning, but are usually not seen in the early postmortem period [99,100] (Figure 23.28b). Right atrial dilatation has also been described as a possible drowning sign (due to elevated resistance in the pulmonary artery); however, nonspecific.

Further drowning findings like the presence of Paltauf-spots (hemolytic spots, larger than the Tardieu-spots described in asphyxia) and the detection of diatoms in the lungs or other organs cannot be assessed with imaging modalities like PMCT. However, image-guided needle biopsy may deliver histology for detection of diatoms.

23.5.6 Fire-Related Deaths

Finding a body in a fire scene retrieves a variety of forensically relevant questions: Who was the victim? Are there any signs of vitality during the fire? Are there any traumatic findings? If so, were they induced ante- or postmortem? What was the cause of death? PMCT can assist significantly to the identification of the deceased [101], as described previously, and also to revealing foreign bodies, in some cases directly related to the cause of death [102].

The calculation of the extent of burns on the human body is based on the "rule of nines," which is also known in clinical praxis. The degree of the thermal injury is

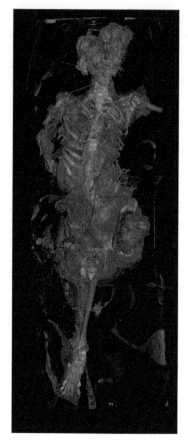

FIGURE 23.29
Charred body, with multiple fire-induced fractures of both the upper and lower extremities and the head. Organ protrusion through abdominal wall.

defined as first, second, third, and fourth depending on whether the fire-related damage affects superficially the skin, its partial thickness, the full thickness of the skin, and further deeper the musculature and bones, respectively [103].

The impact of thermal energy on human body causes many of the characteristics of the external appearance of a burned body (Figure 23.29). It is important to underline that these are postmortem phenomena:

- The skin contracts and ruptures, which results in heat-induced postmortem wounds that must be differentiated from antemortem ones (there is no evidence of vital reactions, but it is still a challenging task for the forensic pathologist).

- The torso is initially distended because of the effect of heat on the internal organs and body fluids, and later the abdominal and/or thoracic wall is ruptured causing protrusion and exposure of the organs.

- The muscles of the upper and lower extremities are contracted, leading to a characteristic "pugilistic" fencing position. Furthermore, amputations can occur and heat fractures of the bones are not uncommon. The cancellous bone rarefies leading finally to postmortem heat fractures. They are usually with smooth edges, in contrast to antemortem fractures. Subcutaneous hematomas add information of traumatic impacts, but are better detected on PMMR. On the skull, parts of the tabula externa can be absent or dislocated.

- The internal organs are shrunken (they are being described as "puppet organs") [103].

- Postmortem hematomas can be found with the mostly described being the "heat epidural hematoma" (Figure 23.30). It is a result of the shift of fluid from the diploe and the venous sinuses when the skullcap is in direct contact with the thermal impact. The differentiation between a real antemortem epidural hematoma of traumatic etiology and the postmortem one relies on the exclusion of presence of traumatic injury such as skull fracture. Furthermore, it does not usually exceed the cranial sutures if it is antemortem in origin [104]. Knight also describes the level of carboxyhemoglobin (COHb) as an indicator: a postmortem epidural hematoma should have similar concentration of COHb to the blood.

There is evidence that preexisting trauma of the skull can be recognized even after cremation [105]. Collecting human remains from a scene of fire can be challenging, as the fragmentation of bones and the context of the remains may cause problems [106]. To answer the very important, from a forensic point of view, question of whether the person died before or during the fire, signs of vitality have to be looked for [107]. The most significant ones are

- The level of COHb in the blood. The concentration of COHb should be elevated if the person was alive and inhaled carbon monoxide, which is a product of incomplete combustion. The absence of COHb does not mean that the person was necessarily dead before the fire (e.g., a fire in outer space or old people), but the strong positive COHb in blood is a sign of vitality during the fire. The blood and internal organs have in those cases a cherry-pink coloration.

- Soot in the airways, preferably down to the small bronchi. Soot is unlikely to be found in the trachea and bronchi without respiratory function.

- Soot in the stomach (because swallowing is a vital function). In PMCT the inhalation or swallowing of radiopaque debris can be depicted.

- Thermal injury of the pharynx, larynx, and airways (swelling, inflammatory reaction). This finding actually confirms the presence of the deceased in close proximity to the heat source, whereas the previous findings only suggest presence of fire fumes.

- External findings such as burn blisters, crow's feet around the eyes, or petechial hemorrhages have been disputed as strong evidences.

23.5.7 Intoxication

Fatalities because of toxic substances overdose are not a rare issue in institutes of forensic medicine. Either accidentally or intentionally (suicides), these fatalities include a large number of chemical substances like alcohol, drugs, and medicines. Describing all forensic aspects of intoxication is far beyond the scope of this chapter. In PMCT, an indication of fatal intoxication is the presence of radiopaque stomach content, which may correspond to ingestion of medication (Figure 23.31). Suspicious hyperdense material can be seen sometimes also in the duodenum, or even further in the intestine [108–110].

Recently, a study published by Rohner et al. suggests the urinary bladder volume as an indicator of intoxication. The authors found that PMCT is a reliable method for calculating the urine volume and also that there was a statistically significant correlation between urinary bladder distension and cases of intoxication. Axial urinary bladder diameter, as measured in PMCT, of more than 10 cm indicates positive toxicology results with a specificity of 95%, according to this study [111].

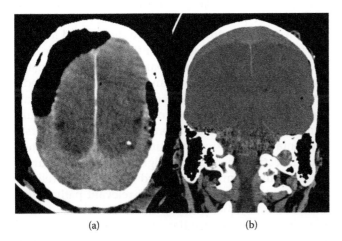

(a) (b)

FIGURE 23.30
Postmortem phenomena in charred bodies: Heat epidural hematoma. (a) Axial PMCT (b) Coronal PMCT.

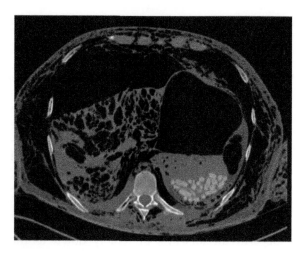

FIGURE 23.31
Axial PMCT image at the level of the stomach. In the stomach, a large quantity of radiopaque structures (pills) can be seen. Note the vast postmortem alteration of soft tissues and liver parenchyma because of decomposition.

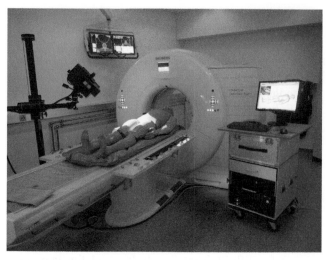

FIGURE 23.32
Surface scanner (left) scanning the body on the CT table (middle). The scanner (Atos Triple Scan, Gesellschaft für Optische Messtechnik, GOM, Germany) delivers a high-resolution surface model of the body, displayed on the scanners control system (right).

23.6 Other Modalities

23.6.1 Surface Scanning

Although CT and MR are imaging modalities well-suited for finding and displaying injuries, they are quite limited in visualizing body surfaces and superficial injury patterns. This is the case for two reasons. First, the resolution is not sufficient to incorporate detailed surface information such as small abrasions or bite marks. Second, these modalities do not provide color information. It is standard practice to use digital photography to document these findings; this however, comes with a loss of information since a 3D object is documented with a 2D imaging technique. Furthermore, it does not allow the integration of different modalities (such as laser scans of the crime scene).

Several surface documentation techniques exist to overcome these problems (e.g., laser scanning, photogrammetry, fringe pattern), all of them generating a 3D surface model with color information (Figure 23.32). In contrast to CT and MR that consists of voxels (volume pixels), surface models are built up by polygons (points in space that are connected), which makes it possible to import these models into 3D animation software such as Maya or 3D Studio Max. Here, they can be combined with digital 3D scans of crime scenes, suspected injury inflicting instruments, or structures and polygonal reconstructions of underlying anatomical structures from CT or MR datasets [69,112]. For being able to relate superficial injuries to damages visible on imaging, the fusion of datasets has to be as precise as possible. Surface scans of deceased are therefore performed on the CT couch, to have the same position of the body in both modalities. In addition, the deceased is prepared with radiopaque markers that are visible in all modalities that are to be fused (i.e., surface scan and CT scan). Based on this information, both datasets can be related to each other (registration). Crime scene reconstruction and surface scanning requires a multidisciplinary cooperation of police experts, forensic pathologist, radiologists, and engineers.

23.6.2 Minimally Invasive Postmortem Needle Biopsy

Some pathologies require examination on a cellular level with specific stainings, for which the resolution of CT is clearly not sufficient. If tissue changes are visible or suspected on imaging, a minimally invasive needle biopsy can be performed. For multiple specimen acquisition, a coaxial needle is placed to the desired location and is used as a needle guide for the biopsy needle after removal of the inner trocar. Apart from being minimally invasive (and therefore minimally destructive), needle biopsies allow for precise placement based on CT data and therefore the correlation of CT findings with results from histological examinations. Needle biopsy is usually contamination free and minimizes contact to potentially infectious body fluids significantly. An accuracy of less than 5 mm is considered sufficient for reliably retrieving tissue samples of most relevant pathologies. Different techniques exist to make use of CT data to accurately place the needles. After identifying the target, the introducer needle can be placed manually under CT guidance [113], by using surgical navigation systems [114] (as used in neurosurgery or orthopedic surgery) or

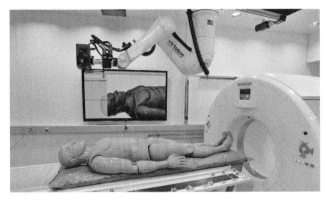

FIGURE 23.33
Virtobot with mounted Surface scanner, scanning the body on the CT table. The scanner (Atos Compact Scan, Gesellschaft für optische Messtechnik (GOM), Germany) delivers a high-resolution surface model of the body, displayed on the screen in the background.

with the help of robotic systems [115,116] (Figure 23.33). After retrieval, tissue samples are stained and analyzed to identify the cellular pathology.

The accuracy of manual needle placement is strongly user-dependent and can, depending on the technique, require x-ray exposure to the radiologist. Since the needle is placed within the current scanning plane of the CT, the insertion angle is limited to the possible gantry tilt if high accuracy is desired. Surgical navigation systems on the other hand use optical tracking systems to gather positional information about tools and body and give visual feedback on a computer screen on how to insert the needle. Surgical navigation is less user-dependent than manual insertion, and comes without radiation exposure and allows for any needle insertion angle. Robotic systems can be used to support manual insertion or to fully automate the process.

23.7 Forensic Radiology in Living Persons

23.7.1 Drug Mules

Smuggling and trafficking of illicit drugs by means of internal concealment is a risky but practiced way across the world by so-called drug-mules. Commonly, the term "body packer" is used to describe any kind of internal drug container concealment. However, there are more precise definitions that should be used [117–119]. A body packer is a courier who swallows a large amount of drug packets (weight usually approximately 5–10 g) for smuggling and hides them in the alimentary tract (meaning the stomach, small and large intestines). Although, a body pusher usually conceals

even larger drug containers within the body cavities (rectum, vagina), a body stuffer "mini packer" is typically a trafficker or user who ingests small amounts of cocaine pellets (1–2 g) when required by the risk of imminent capture by the police. Nevertheless, there are sometimes combinations of body packing and pushing or body stuffing and pushing. In Asia, the authorities have to deal with more Methamphetamine smuggling whereas Europe and the United States are more confronted with cocaine and heroin in cases of drug carriers [120].

Momentarily the gold standard for securing evidence in drug carriers is collecting the drug containers in the feces of the detained suspect. Nevertheless, the authorities also rely on imaging in order to accelerate the management of the suspect and to address also medical issues as the pack may rupture or leak [121–126].

Plain radiography (DR) is a radiological tool, which is widely accepted and used to detect the internal payload of drug carriers (Figure 23.34) [127,128]. However, studies showed that there is a high insecurity with a wide variety of sensitivity and specificity [118]. The reading radiologists frequently tend to underreport the amount of drug containers or to misjudge other structures for drug containers as they are usually not familiar with appearance of drug containers on imaging. In addition, there are often a multitude of sequential radiographs performed to document the rate of clearance and to finally get a negative result to transfer the perpetrator to prison. Sonography may be useful but is examiner-dependent and only conclusive when detecting drug containers [129]. A negative exam in sonography does not rule out internal drugs. Magnetic resonance imaging (MRI) is expensive and rarely available and the patient has to be compliant during the exam, which makes this method negligible. CT on the other hand comes with initial higher radiation dose but offers the most accurate method to detect even tiny internal drug containers in body stuffers (Figure 23.35) [118,130–133]. However, sequel exams may be obviated and even low-dose unenhanced CT protocols may be used, which finally may result in lower radiation that several DRs and may even cut health system costs due to immediate reliable results.

On DR and CT are there some well-described signs such as the "double-condom" and "halo" sign that occur because of inevitable air inclusion during manufacturing [119,127,134,135]. The double condom sign is created if the pack is projected longitudinally or the halo sign if imaged transverse. The "rosette" sign (due to trapped air at the twisted end of a pack) is not easy assessable on plain radiograph [119,127,134,135]. Other known signs such as "tic-tac" sign and "parallelism" sign are created by parallel arrangement of longitudinal packs within

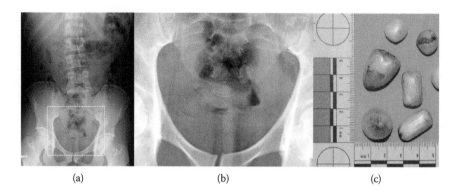

(a)   (b)   (c)

FIGURE 23.34

Clinical images. (a) DR of a body pusher with 2 drug containers located in the rectum. (b) Magnified view of the small pelvis. Note the typical double-condom and halo sign due to inevitable air in the pack during manufacture. One container is smaller and cone-shaped and the other one is a typical longitudinal body pack weighting about 10–12 g. The longitudinal packs show in addition the typical air-filled reservoir of the tip of a condom used as wrapping. (c) Excreted drug packs showing a similar cone-shaped container as in image a and b. The small pellets are similar to those shown in Figure 23.35.

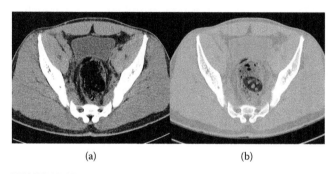

(a)   (b)

FIGURE 23.35

Clinical images. (a) Abdominal window. Hardly detectable small pellets wrapped in one large container surrounded by feces in the rectum. The small pellets have only a dense center and adjacent wrapping and layers appear to be hypodense. (b) Pulmonary window. Alteration of the window reveals the 4 pellets in a case of body pushing.

the large bowel. Geometrical-shaped suspicious gas formation projecting over the rectum may be an indicator for internal drug containers but is rather an unreliable sign. Table 23.1 summarizes the diagnostic clues on DR and CT. Nevertheless, knowledge about the shape, manufacture, and wrapping of the several drug containers is crucial for the radiologist to know what to look for [118,119].

23.7.2 Strangulation Victims

Recent literature reported a sensitivity and specificity of 70% in assessing life-threatening strangulation on MR in surviving victims [137]. The MR images are even admissible at court and may display injury to the deep layers of the neck, the larynx, and the subcutaneous tissue even more precise than external inspection and photodocumentation alone. Frequently, there are

TABLE 23.1

Diagnostic Clues on DR and CT in "Drug Mules" Cases

Pearls on DR

Magnify images to detect even small drug containers

Investigate the complete alimentary tract (from stomach to rectum)

Use white bone to black bone inversion

Supine imaging in body packers and pushers to decrease summation over the small pelvis

Upright imaging to detect small floating pellets on the fluid–air level in the stomach in body stuffers

Pearls on CT

Window alteration from abdominal to pulmonary window to detect iso- to hypodense packs [136]

no or little signs of the physical assault to the neck and therefore additional MRI is a handy tool to display life-threatening events and to even discriminate those from nonlife—threatening attacks [34,137–140]. However, MR scan should be performed at latest within the first 72 hours after the assault to preserve actual findings before reconvalescence.

Based on the study by Christe et al. (2009) the radiological imaging of the neck in cases of strangulation can be divided into three layers: superficial, middle, and deep zone [137]. The so-called danger zone is the middle layer containing the deep nerve-vessel sheath, muscles, lymph nodes, and salivary gland, which is followed by the deep zone containing the larynx and perilaryngeal tissue. In addition, bilateral impact on the middle to deep zone aggravates the clinical symptoms and may easily end up in a life-threatening event. MR provides an objective documentation of life-threatening strangulation events [138].

Read-out of the neck should detect hemorrhage or respectively edema intra-, subcutaneous, intramuscular, perilaryngeal, and parapharyngeal signal alterations on T2 and TIRM sequences. Special focus should be on the platysma as it appears frequently thickened and signal altered as a specific sign for strangulation according to Yen et al. [139] (Figure 23.36). In addition, signal changes within the sterno-cleidomastoid, strap and dorsal neck muscles have to be assessed. Glottic edema is not so frequently seen. Bold hyperintense signal on TIRM and T2 sequences in the salivary glands, lymph nodes, and the thyroid gland have to be interpreted as hemorrhageous [137,138]. However, additional focus should be on the supraaortal vasculature to detect rupture and dissection.

CT and CTA in living persons allow for easier depiction in an emergency of vascular lesions, especially in cases of suspected vessel dissection. Subtle changes to the soft tissue and the platysma may be missed more easily. On the other hand, detection of osseous or cartilaginous injuries of the larynx is facilitated by CT compared to MRI [34,140,141]. Therefore, the two modalities supplement each other.

23.7.3 Nonaccidental Injury-Child Abuse

Child abuse accounts for the number one traumatic cause of death in children [142]. Death after nonaccidental injury (NAI) usually occurs due to brain edema in sequel to shaken impact syndrome with intracranial hemorrhage (mainly subdural bleeding), diffuse axonal injury with/without retinal hemorrhage, or ischemic lesion due to strain trauma to the myelon (Figures 23.37 and 23.38) [143]. Multiple hematomas and/or fractures of different age have to raise suspicion for nonaccidental trauma [144] both in living and deceased victims. However, etiologies such as accidental trauma, benign enlargement of the subarachnoid spaces, coagulopathy (hemophilia, leukemia), metabolic (Glutaric aciduria type 1, Menkes syndrome, kinky hair syndrome) and skeletal abnormalities have to be ruled out.

Radiological images such as DR, CT, and MR play an important role in diagnostics and will even eventually be admitted to court as evidence in living as well as in deceased victims.

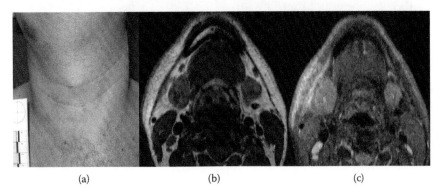

(a)   (b)   (c)

FIGURE 23.36
Clinical images (a) External inspection in a surviving victim after bimanual strangulation. There is a soft-tissue hematoma on the right mandible angle. However, there are no other external findings except for superficial abrasions and scratches. (b) Axial T1w image at the level of the submandibular glands below the mandible angle. Note the hypointense thickening of the right platysma with adjacent slight hemorrhage in the subcutaneous tissue. (c) Axial TIRM sequence with corresponding hyperintense signal alterations. The deep nerve-vessel sheath is not affected.

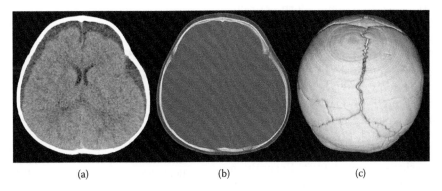

(a)   (b)   (c)

FIGURE 23.37
Clinical images. (a) CT of a 3-year-old girl with bilateral chronic subdural hemorrhage in a surviving case of NAI. (b) CT in a bone window with according osseous reconstruction kernel showing suspicious potential fracture lines in the occipital region. (c) Three-dimensional reconstruction of the skull showing a multitude of fairly symmetric, accessory sutures with typical zigzag patterns and sclerotic borders and no fractures in this case. There was no adjacent soft tissue swelling detectable.

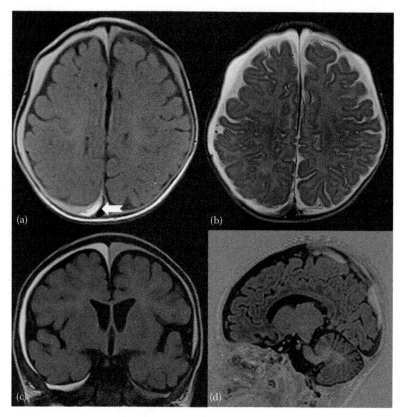

FIGURE 23.38
Clinical images. (a) Axial, T1w slice with bilateral subdural hemorrhage in a 1-year and 9-month-old boy. Note the focal acute to subacute bleeding on the right adjacent to the superior sagittal sinus (white arrow). (b) Axial T2w image at the same level as image a. According to fresh hemorrhage there is a hypointense signal change next to the superior sagittal sinus. (c) Coronal fluid attenuated inversion recovery sequence. Note the more hyperintense signal in the subdural bleeding of the right hemisphere compared to the left hemispheric subdural hemorrhage due to different ages of the bleeding. (d) Sagittal inversion recovery sequence displaying a hyperintense signal neighboring the superior sagittal sinus on the right according to the acute to subacute components of the bleeding.

23.8 Conclusions

Nowadays numerous Forensic Institutes own CT scanners and/or have implemented PMCT examinations in their routine work. To name some, Bern, Zurich, and Lausanne in Switzerland, Baltimore (MD) and Albuquerque (NM) in the United States, Melbourne in Australia, Tsukuba in Japan, London and Leicester in the United Kingdom, Toulouse and Marseille in France, Institutes in Germany, Italy, Poland, Malaysia and many more. Large studies and systematic reviews comparing postmortem imaging and autopsy can be found in the literature [145,146]. Postmortem imaging is present in the most significant international forensic meetings with sessions devoted to it. Recently, a new society was formed, the International Society of Forensic Radiology and Imaging (www.isfri.org), which also underlines the great interest of the forensic scientific community.

Acknowledgments

The authors thank Nicole Schwendener and Robert Breitbeck for their contribution to this work.

References

1. Dirnhofer R, Jackowski C, Vock P et al. (2006) VIRTOPSY: Minimally invasive, imaging-guided virtual autopsy. *Radiographics*. 26:1305–1333.
2. Brogdon BG, Lichtenstein JE (2011) Forensic radiology in historical perspective. In: Thali MJ, Viner MD, Brogdon BG (eds) *Brogdon's Forensic Radiology*, 2nd ed. CRC Press, Boca Raton, FL.
3. Wullenweber R, Schneider V, Grumme T (1977) A computer-tomographical examination of cranial bullet wounds [in German]. *Z Rechtsmed*. 80:227–246.

4. Thali MJ, Yen K, Schweitzer W et al. (2003) Virtopsy, a new imaging horizon in forensic pathology: Virtual autopsy by postmortem multislice computed tomography (MSCT) and magnetic resonance imaging (MRI)—a feasibility study. *J Forensic Sci.* 48:386–403.

5. Thali MJ, Dirnhofer R, Vock P (2009) The Virtopsy Approach. 3D Optical and Radiological Scanning and Reconstruction in Forensic Medicine. CRC Press, Boca Raton, FL.

6. Ampanozi G, Zimmermann D, Hatch GM et al. (2012) Format preferences of district attorneys for post-mortem medical imaging reports: Understandability, cost effectiveness, and suitability for the courtroom: A questionnaire based study. *Leg Med (Tokyo).* 14:116–120.

7. Persson A, Lindblom M, Jackowski C (2011) A state-of-the-art pipeline for postmortem CT and MRI visualization: From data acquisition to interactive image interpretation at autopsy. *Acta Radiol.* 52:522–536.

8. Levy AD, Harcke HT (2011) Integrating imaging and autopsy. In: Levy AD, Harcke HT (eds) *Essentials of Forensic Imaging. A Text Atlas.* CRC Press, Boca Raton, FL.

9. Grabherr S, Gygax E, Sollberger B et al. (2008) Two-step postmortem angiography with a modified heart-lung machine: Preliminary results. *AJR Am J Roentgenol.* 190:345–351.

10. Ross S, Spendlove D, Bolliger S et al. (2008) Postmortem whole-body CT angiography: Evaluation of two contrast media solutions. *AJR Am J Roentgenol.* 190:1380–1389.

11. O'Donnell C, Hislop-Jambrich J, Woodford N et al. (2012) Demonstration of liver metastases on postmortem whole body CT angiography following inadvertent systemic venous infusion of the contrast medium. *Int J Legal Med.* 126:311–314.

12. Grabherr S, Doenz F, Steger B et al. (2011) Multi-phase post-mortem CT angiography: Development of a standardized protocol. *Int J Legal Med.* 125:791–802.

13. Jackowski C, Persson A, Thali MJ (2008) Whole body postmortem angiography with a high viscosity contrast agent solution using poly ethylene glycol as contrast agent dissolver. *J Forensic Sci.* 53(2):465–468.

14. Saunders SL, Morgan B, Raj V et al. (2011) Targeted postmortem computed tomography cardiac angiography: Proof of concept. *Int J Legal Med.* 125:609–616.

15. Roberts IS, Benamore RE, Peebles C et al. (2011) Technical report: Diagnosis of coronary artery disease using minimally invasive autopsy: Evaluation of a novel method of post-mortem coronary CT angiography. *Clin Radiol.* 66:645–650.

16. Rutty G, Saunders S, Morgan B et al. (2012) Targeted cardiac post-mortem computed tomography angiography: A pictorial review. *Forensic Sci Med Pathol.* 8:40–47.

17. Jackowski C, Thali M (2009) Radiologic identification. In: Thali MJ, Dirnhofer R, Vock P (eds) *The Virtopsy Approach. 3D Optical and Radiological Scanning and Reconstruction in Forensic Medicine.* CRC Press, Boca Raton, FL.

18. Bassed RB, Hill AJ (2011) The use of computed tomography (CT) to estimate age in the 2009 Victorian Bushfire Victims: A case report. *Forensic Sci Int.* 205:48–51.

19. Ciaffi R, Gibelli D, Cattaneo C (2011) Forensic radiology and personal identification of unidentified bodies: A review. *Radiol Med.* 116:960–968.

20. Barrier P, Dedouit F, Braga J et al. (2009) Age at death estimation using multislice computed tomography reconstructions of the posterior pelvis. *J Forensic Sci.* 54:773–778.

21. O'Donnell C, Iino M, Mansharan K et al. (2011) Contribution of postmortem multidetector CT scanning to identification of the deceased in a mass disaster: Experience gained from the 2009 Victorian bushfires. *Forensic Sci Int.* 205:15–28.

22. Birngruber CG, Obert M, Ramsthaler F et al. (2011) Comparative dental radiographic identification using flat panel CT. *Forensic Sci Int.* 209:e31–e34.

23. Jackowski C, Aghayev E, Sonnenschein M et al. (2006) Maximum intensity projection of cranial computed tomography data for dental identification. *Int J Legal Med.* 120:165–167.

24. Jackowski C, Wyss M, Persson A et al. (2008) Ultra-high-resolution dual-source CT for forensic dental visualization-discrimination of ceramic and composite fillings. *Int J Legal Med.* 122:301–307.

25. Thali MJ, Markwalder T, Jackowski C et al. (2006) Dental CT imaging as a screening tool for dental profiling: Advantages and limitations. *J Forensic Sci.* 51:113–119.

26. Ruder TD, Kraehenbuehl M, Gotsmy WF et al. (2012) Radiologic identification of disaster victims: A simple and reliable method using CT of the paranasal sinuses. *Eur J Radiol.* 81:e132–e138.

27. Haglund WD, Fligner CL (1993) Confirmation of human identification using computerized tomography (CT). *J Forensic Sci.* 38:708–712.

28. Dedouit F, Telmon N, Costagliola R et al. (2007) New identification possibilities with postmortem multislice computed tomography. *Int J Legal Med.* 121:507–510.

29. Silva RF, Botelho TL, Prado FB et al. (2011) Human identification based on cranial computed tomography scan: A case report. *Dentomaxillofac Radiol.* 40:257–261.

30. Sidler M, Jackowski C, Dirnhofer R et al. (2007) Use of multislice computed tomography in disaster victim identification— advantages and limitations. *Forensic Sci Int.* 169:118–128.

31. Blau S, Robertson S, Johnstone M (2008) Disaster victim identification: New applications for postmortem computed tomography. *J Forensic Sci.* 53:956–961.

32. Hayakawa M, Yamamoto S, Motani H et al. (2006) Does imaging technology overcome problems of conventional postmortem examination? A trial of computed tomography imaging for postmortem examination. *Int J Legal Med.* 120:24–26.

33. Vock P (2009) Intravital versus postmortem imaging. In: Thali MJ, Dirnhofer R, Vock P (eds) *The Virtopsy Approach.* CRC Press, Taylor & Francis Group, Boca Raton, FL.

34. Flach PM, Ross SG, Christe A et al. (2010) Clinical and forensic radiology are not the same. In: Thali MJ, Viner MD, Brogdon BG (eds) *Brogdon's Forensic Radiology,* 2nd ed. CRC Press, Taylor & Francis, Boca Raton, FL.

35. Keil W, Bretschneider K, Patzelt D et al. (1980) Air embolism or putrefaction gas? The diagnosis of cardiac air embolism in the cadaver. *Beitr Gerichtl Med.* 38:395–408.

36. Jackowski C, Sonnenschein M, Thali MJ et al. (2007) Intrahepatic gas at postmortem computed tomography: Forensic experience as a potential guide for in vivo trauma imaging. *J Trauma.* 62:979–988.

37. Patzelt D, Lignitz E, Keil W et al. (1979) Diagnostic problem of air embolism in a corpse. *Beitr Gerichtl Med.* 37:401–405.

38. Pedal I, Moosmayer A, Mallach HJ et al. (1987) Air embolism or putrefaction? Gas analysis findings and their interpretation. *Z Rechtsmed.* 99:151–167.

39. Takahashi N, Satou C, Higuchi T et al. (2010) Quantitative analysis of brain edema and swelling on early postmortem computed tomography: Comparison with antemortem computed tomography. *Jpn J Radiol.* 28:349–354.

40. Añon J, Remonda L, Spreng A et al. (2008) Traumatic extra-axial hemorrhage: Correlation of postmortem MSCT, MRI, and forensic-pathological findings. *J Magn Reson Imaging.* 28(4):823–836.

41. Yen K, Lövblad KO, Scheurer E et al. (2007) Postmortem forensic neuroimaging: Correlation of MSCT and MRI findings with autopsy results. *Forensic Sci Int.* 15;173(1):21–35.

42. Takahashi N, Satou C, Higuchi T et al. (2010) Quantitative analysis of intracranial hypostasis: Comparison of early postmortem and antemortem CT findings. *AJR Am J Roentgenol.* 195:W388–W393.

43. Shiotani S, Kohno M, Ohashi N et al. (2004) Non-traumatic postmortem computed tomographic (PMCT) findings of the lung. *Forensic Sci Int.* 139:39–48.

44. Shiotani S, Kobayashi T, Hayakawa H et al. (2011) Postmortem pulmonary edema: A comparison between immediate and delayed postmortem computed tomography. *Leg Med (Tokyo).* 13:151–155.

45. Germerott T, Preiss US, Ebert LC et al. (2010) A new approach in virtopsy: Postmortem ventilation in multislice computed tomography. *Leg Med (Tokyo).* 12:276–279.

46. Aghayev E, Christe A, Sonnenschein M et al. (2008) Postmortem imaging of blunt chest trauma using CT and MRI: Comparison with autopsy. *J Thorac Imaging.* 23:20–27.

47. Yang KM, Lynch M, O'Donnell C (2011) "Buckle" rib fracture: An artifact following cardio-pulmonary resuscitation detected on postmortem CT. *Leg Med (Tokyo).* 13:233–239.

48. Love JC, Symes SA (2004) Understanding rib fracture patterns: Incomplete and buckle fractures. *J Forensic Sci.* 49:1153–1158.

49. Shiotani S, Kohno M, Ohashi N et al. (2002) Hyperattenuating aortic wall on postmortem computed tomography (PMCT). *Radiat Med.* 20:201–206.

50. Christe A, Flach P, Ross S et al. (2010) Clinical radiology and postmortem imaging (Virtopsy) are not the same: Specific and unspecific postmortem signs. *Leg Med (Tokyo).* 12:215–222.

51. Shiotani S, Kohno M, Ohashi N et al. (2003) Dilatation of the heart on postmortem computed tomography (PMCT): Comparison with live CT. *Radiat Med.* 21(1):29–35 and 21(2).

52. Christe A, Aghayev E, Jackowski C et al. (2008) Drowning—post-mortem imaging findings by computed tomography. *Eur Radiol.* 18:283–290.

53. Aghayev E, Sonnenschein M, Jackowski C et al. (2006) Postmortem radiology of fatal hemorrhage: Measurements of cross-sectional areas of major blood vessels and volumes of aorta and spleen on MDCT and volumes of heart chambers on MRI. *Am J Roentgenol.* 187:209–215.

54. Kelly J, Raptopoulos V, Davidoff A et al. (1989) The value of non-contrast-enhanced CT in blunt abdominal trauma. *Am J Roentgenol.* 152:41–48.

55. Christe A, Ross S, Oesterhelweg L et al. (2009) Abdominal trauma—sensitivity and specificity of postmortem non-contrast imaging findings compared with autopsy findings. *J Trauma.* 66:1302–1307.

56. Jackowski C, Thali M, Aghayev E et al. (2005) Postmortem imaging of blood and its characteristics using MSCT and MRI. *Int J Legal Med.* 19:1–8.

57. Levy AD, Harcke HT, Getz JM et al. (2009) Multidetector computed tomography findings in deaths with severe burns. *Am J Forensic Med Pathol.* 30:137–141.

58. Christiansen LR, Collins KA (2007) Natural death in the forensic setting. a study and approach to the autopsy. *Am J Forensic Med Pathol.* 28:20–23.

59. Michaud K, Grabherr S, Doenz F et al. (2012) Evaluation of postmortem MDCT and MDCT-angiography for the investigation of sudden cardiac death related to atherosclerotic coronary artery disease. *Int J Cardiovasc Imaging.* 28(7):1807–1822. doi:10.1007/s10554-012-0012-x.

60. Ruder TD, Bauer-Kreutz R, Ampanozi G et al. (2012) Assessment of coronary artery disease by post-mortem cardiac MR. *Eur J Radiol.* 81(9):2208–2214 doi:10.1016/j.ejrad.2011.06.042.

61. Jackowski C, Hofmann K, Schwendener N et al. (2012) Coronary thrombus and peracute myocardial infarction visualized by unenhanced postmortem MRI prior to autopsy. *Forensic Sci Int.* 214:e16–e19.

62. Jackowski C, Christe A, Sonnenschein M et al. (2006) Postmortem unenhanced magnetic resonance imaging of myocardial infarction in correlation to histological infarction age characterization. *Eur Heart J.* 27:2459–2467.

63. Jackowski C, Warntjes MJ, Berge J et al. (2011) Magnetic resonance imaging goes postmortem: Noninvasive detection and assessment of myocardial infarction by postmortem MRI. *Eur Radiol.* 21:70–78.

64. Shiotani S, Watanabe K, Kohno M et al. (2004) Postmortem computed tomographic (PMCT) findings of pericardial effusion due to acute aortic dissection. *Radiat Med.* 22:405–407.

65. Ebert LC, Ampanozi G, Ruder TD et al. (2012) CT based volume measurement and estimation in cases of pericardial effusion. *J Forensic Leg Med.* 19:126–131.

66. Saukko P, Knight B (2004) The forensic autopsy. In: Saukko P, Knight B (eds) *Knight's Forensic Pathology*, 3rd ed. Edward Arnold Ltd, London.

67. Saukko P, Knight B (2004) The pathology of wounds. In: Saukko P, Knight B (eds) *Knight's Forensic Pathology*, 3rd ed. Edward Arnold Ltd, London.

68. Naether S, Buck U, Campana L et al. (2012) The examination and identification of bite marks in foods using 3D scanning and 3D comparison methods. *Int J Legal Med*. 126:89–95.

69. Buck U, Naether S, Braun M et al. (2007) Application of 3D documentation and geometric reconstruction methods in traffic accident analysis: With high resolution surface scanning, radiological MSCT/MRI scanning and real data based animation. *Forensic Sci Int*. 170:20–28.

70. Buck U, Albertini N, Naether S et al. (2007) 3D documentation of footwear impressions and tyre tracks in snow with high resolution optical surface scanning. *Forensic Sci Int*. 171:157–164.

71. Bolliger SA, Ross S, Thali MJ (2009) Postmortem imaging of blunt trauma. In: Thali MJ, Dirnhofer R, Vock P (eds) *The Virtopsy approach. 3D Optical and Radiological Scanning and Reconstruction in Forensic Medicine*. CRC Press, Boca Raton, FL.

72. Bratzke H (2007) Stumpfe gewalt. In: Madea B (ed) *Praxis Rechtsmedizin*, 2nd ed. Springer, Heidelberg.

73. Saukko P, Knight B (2004) Head and spinal injuries. In: Saukko P, Knight B (eds) *Knight's Forensic Pathology*, 3rd ed. Edward Arnold Ltd, London.

74. Stein KM, Ruf K, Ganten MK et al. (2006) Representation of cerebral bridging veins in infants by postmortem computed tomography. *Forensic Sci Int*. 163:93–101.

75. Saukko P, Knight B (2004) Fatal pressure on the neck. In: Saukko P, Knight B (eds) *Knight's Forensic Pathology*, 3rd ed. Edward Arnold Ltd, London.

76. O'Donnell C, Bedford P, Burke M (2011) Massive hemoperitoneum due to ruptured ectopic gestation: Postmortem CT findings in a deeply frozen deceased person. *Leg Med (Tokyo)*. 13:245–249.

77. Yamazaki K, Shiotani S, Ohashi N et al. (2006) Comparison between computed tomography (CT) and autopsy findings in cases of abdominal injury and disease. *Forensic Sci Int*. 162:163–166.

78. Ampanozi G, Hatch GM, Ruder TD et al. (2012) Postmortem virtual estimation of free abdominal blood volume. *Eur J Radiol*. 81(9):2133–2136 doi:10.1016/j.ejrad.2011.09.014

79. Martos V, Jackowski C (2012) Bilateral fractures of transverse processus: A diagnostic sign of overrun? *Forensic Sci Int*. 219(1-3):244–247 doi:10.1016/j.forsciint.2012.01.013

80. Saukko P, Knight B (2004) Gunshot and explosion deaths. In: Saukko P, Knight B (eds) *Knight's Forensic Pathology*, 3rd ed. Edward Arnold Ltd, London.

81. Di Maio VJM (1999) *Gunshot Wounds. Practical Aspects of Firearms, Ballistics, and Forensic Techniques*, 2nd ed. CRC Press, Boca Raton, FL.

82. Harcke HT, Levy AD, Abbott RM et al. (2007) Autopsy radiography: Digital Radiographs (DR) vs Multidetector Computed Tomography (MDCT) in high-velocity gunshot-wound victims. *Am J Forensic Med Pathol*. 28:13–19.

83. Thali MJ, Yen K, Vock P et al. (2003) Image-guided virtual autopsy findings of gunshot victims performed with multi-slice computed tomography (MSCT) and magnetic resonance imaging (MRI) and subsequent correlation between radiology and autopsy findings. *Forensic Sci Int*. 138:8–16.

84. Viel G, Gehl A, Sperhake JP (2009) Intersecting fractures of the skull and gunshot wounds. Case report and literature review. *Forensic Sci Med Pathol*. 5:22–27.

85. Tartaglione T, Filograna L, Roiati S et al. (2011) Importance of 3D-CT imaging in single bullet craniocephalic gunshot wounds. *Radiol Med*. 117(3):461–470. doi: 10.1007/s11547-011-0784-4.

86. Levy AD, Abbott RM, Mallak CT et al. (2006) Virtual autopsy: Preliminary experience in high-velocity gunshot wound victims. *Radiology*. 240:522–528.

87. Levy AD, Harcke HT (2011) Gunshot wounds. In: Levy AD, Harcke HT (eds) *Essentials of Forensic Imaging, A Text-Atlas*. CRC Press, Boca Raton, FL.

88. Stein KM, Bahner ML, Merkel J et al. (2000) Detection of gunshot residues in routine CTs. *Int J Legal Med*. 114:15–18.

89. Bolliger SA, Kneubuehl BP, Thali MJ (2011) New developments in gunshot analysis. In: Thali MJ, Viner MD, Brogdon BG (eds) *Brogdon's Forensic Radiology*, 2nd ed. CRC Press, Boca Raton, FL.

90. Byard RW, Gehl A, Tsokos M (2005) Skin tension and cleavage lines (Langer's lines) causing distortion of ante- and postmortem wound morphology. *Int J Legal Med*. 119:226–230.

91. Bolliger SA, Thali MJ (2009) Sharp trauma. In: Thali MJ, Dirnhofer R, Vock P (eds) *The Virtopsy Approach. 3D Optical and Radiological Scanning and Reconstruction in Forensic Medicine*. CRC Press, Boca Raton, FL.

92. Ruder TD, Ketterer T, Preiss U et al. (2011) Suicidal knife wound to the heart: Challenges in reconstructing wound channels with post mortem CT and CT-angiography. *Leg Med (Tokyo)*. 13:91–94.

93. Bolliger SA, Preiss U, Glaeser N et al. (2010) Radiological stab wound channel depiction with instillation of contrast medium. *Leg Med (Tokyo)*. 12:39–41.

94. Brunel C, Fermanian C, Durigon M et al. (2010) Homicidal and suicidal sharp force fatalities: Autopsy parameters in relation to the manner of death. *Forensic Sci Int*. 198:150–154.

95. Roll HF (1918) Leerboek der Gerechtelijke Geneeskunde voor de scholen tot opleiding van Ind. artsen, 's-Gravenhage, Martinus Nijhoff.

96. Saukko P, Knight B (2004) Immersion deaths. In: Saukko P, Knight B (eds) *Knight's Forensic Pathology*, 3rd ed. Edward Arnold Ltd, London.

97. Levy AD, Harcke HT (2011) Death by drowning and bodies found in water. In: Levy AD, Harcke HT (eds) *Essentials of Forensic Imaging, A Text-Atlas*. CRC Press, Boca Raton, FL.

98. Levy AD, Harcke HT, Getz JM et al. (2007) Virtual autopsy: Two- and three-dimensional multidetector CT findings in drowning with autopsy comparison. *Radiology*. 243:862–868.

99. Piette MHA, De Letter EA (2006) Drowning: Still a difficult autopsy diagnosis. *Forensic Sci Int*. 163:1–9.

100. Yorulmaz C, Arican N, Afacan I et al. (2003) Pleural effusion in bodies recovered from water. *Forensic Sci Int*. 136:16–21.

101. Woisetschläger M, Lussi A, Persson A et al. (2011) Fire victim identification by post-mortem dental CT: Radiologic evaluation of restorative materials after exposure to high temperatures. *Eur J Radiol.* 80:432–440.

102. Sano R, Hirawasa S, Kobayashi S et al. (2011) Use of postmortem computed tomography to reveal an intraoral gunshot injuries in a charred body. *Leg Med (Tokyo).* 13:286–288.

103. Spendlove D, Thali MJ (2009) Heat and burns. In: Thali MJ, Dirnhofer R, Vock P (eds) *The Virtopsy Approach. 3D Optical and Radiological Scanning and Reconstruction in Forensic Medicine.* CRC Press, Boca Raton, FL.

104. Thali MJ, Yen K, Plattner T et al. (2002) Charred body: Virtual autopsy with multi-slice computed tomography and magnetic resonance imaging. *J Forensic Sci.* 47:1326–1331.

105. Pope EJ, Smith OC (2004) Identification of traumatic injury in burned cranial bone: An experimental approach. *J Forensic Sci.* 49:431–440.

106. Ubelaker DH (2009) The forensic evaluation of burned skeletal remains: A synthesis. *Forensic Sci Int.* 183:1–5.

107. Bohnert M, Werner CR, Pollak S (2003) Problems associated with the diagnosis of vitality in burned bodies. *Forensic Sci Int.* 135:197–205.

108. Aghayev E, Jackowski C, Christe A et al. (2010) Radiopaque stomach contents in postmortem CT in suicidal oral medication intoxication: Report of three cases. *J Forensic Leg Med.* 17:164–168.

109. Burke MP, O'Donnell C, Bassed R (2012) The use of postmortem computed tomography in the diagnosis of intentional medication overdose. *Forensic Sci Med Pathol.* 8(3):218–236 doi:10.1007/s12024-011-9292-z.

110. Leth PM, Worm-Leonhard M (2008) Tablet residues in stomach content found by routine postmortem CT. *Forensic Sci Int.* 179:e16–e17.

111. Rohner C, Franckenberg S, Schwendener N et al. (2013) New evidence for old lore - urinary bladder distension on post-mortem computed tomography is related to intoxication. *Forensic Sci Int.* 10;225(1-3):48–52.

112. Bolliger MJ, Buck U, Thali MJ (2011) Reconstruction and 3D visualisation based on objective real 3D based documentation. *Forensic Sci Med Pathol.* 8(3):208–217 doi: 10.1007/s12024-011-9288-8

113. Aghayev E, Thali MJ, Sonnenschein M et al. (2007) Postmortem tissue sampling using computed tomography guidance. *Forensic Sci. Int.* 166:199–203.

114. Aghayev E, Ebert LC, Christe A et al. (2008) CT database-based navigation for post-mortem biopsy—a feasibility study. *J Forensic Leg Med.* 15:382–387.

115. Cleary K, Melzer A, Watson V et al. (2006) Interventional robotic systems: Applications and technology state-of-the-art. *Minim Invasive Ther Allied Technol.* 15:101–113.

116. Ebert LC, Ptacek W, Naether S et al. (2010) Virtobot—a multi-functional robotic system for 3D surface scanning and automatic post mortem biopsy. *Int J Med Robot.* 6:18–27.

117. Booker RJ, Smith JE, Rodger MP (2009) Packers, pushers and stuffers-managing patients with concealed drugs in UK emergency departments: A clinical and medicolegal review. *Emerg Med J.* 26:316–320.

118. Flach PM, Ross SG, Ampanozi G et al. (2011) "Drug mules" as a radiological challenge: Sensitivity and specificity in identifying internal cocaine in body packers, body pushers and body stuffers by computed tomography, plain radiography and Lodox. *Eur J Radiol.* 81(10):2518–2526 doi:10.1016/j.ejrad.2011.11.025.

119. Flach PM, Ross SG, Thali MJ (2010) Forensic and clinical usage of X-rays in body packing. In: Thali MJ, Viner MD, Brogdon BG (eds) *Brogdon's Forensic Radiology*, 2nd ed. CRC Press, Taylor & Francis Group, Boca Raton, FL.

120. United Nations Office on Drugs and Crime (UNODC) (2010). http://www.unodc.org/unodc/en/data-and-analysis/ WDR-2010.html, accessed March 2012.

121. Goertemoeller S, Behrman A (2006) The risky business of body packers and body stuffers. *J Emerg Nurs.* 32:541–544.

122. June R, Aks SE, Keys N et al. (2000) Medical outcome of cocaine bodystuffers. *J Emer Med.* 18:221–224.

123. Schaper A, Hofmann R, Bargain P et al. (2007) Surgical treatment in cocaine body packers and body pushers. *Int J Colorectal Dis.* 22:1531–1535.

124. Gsell M, Perrig M, Eichelberger M et al. (2010) Body-packer & body-stuffer-a medical challenge. *Praxis.* 99:533–544.

125. Heinemann A, Miyaishi S, Iwersen S et al. (1998) Body-packing as cause of unexpected sudden death. *Forensic Sci Int.* 92:1–10.

126. Bulstrode N, Banks F, Shrotria S (2002) The outcome of drug smuggling by "body packers"—the British experience. *Ann R Coll Surg Engl.* 84:35–38.

127. Algra PR, Brogdon BG, Marugg RC (2007) Role of radiology in a national initiative to interdict drug smuggling: The Dutch experience. *AJR.* 189:331–336.

128. Traub SJ, Hoffman RS, Nelson LS (2003) Body packing—the internal concealment of illicit drugs. *N Engl J Med.* 349:2519–2526.

129. Hierholzer J, Cordes M, Tantow H et al. (1995) Drug smuggling by ingested cocaine-filled packages: Conventional x-ray and ultrasound. *Abdom Imaging.* 20:333–338.

130. Meyers MA (1995) The inside dope: Cocaine, condoms, and computed tomography. *Abdom Imaging.* 20:339–340.

131. Schmidt S, Hugli O, Rizzo E et al. (2007) Detection of cocaine filled packets-diagnostic value of unenhanced CT. *Eur J Radiol.* 67:133–138.

132. Maurer MH, Niehues SM, Schnapauff D et al. (2011) Low-dose computed tomography to detect body-packing in an animal model. *Eur J Radiol.* 78:302–306.

133. Pache G, Einhaus D, Bulla S et al. (2012) Low-dose computed tomography for the detection of cocaine body packs: Clinical evaluation and legal issues. *Rofo.* 184:122–129.

134. Hergan K, Kofler K, Oser W (2004) Drug smuggling by body packing: What radiologists should know about it. *Eur Radiol.* 14:736–742.

135. Niewiarowski S, Gogbashian A, Afaq A et al. (2010) Abdominal X-ray signs of intra-intestinal drug smuggling. *J Forensic Leg Med.* 17:198–202.

136. Sengupta A, Page P (2008) Window manipulation in diagnosis of body packing using computed tomography. *Emerg Radiol.* 15:203–205.

137. Christe A, Thoeny H, Ross S et al. (2009) Life-threatening versus non-life-threatening manual strangulation: Are there appropriate criteria for MR imaging of the neck? *Eur Radiol.* 19:1882–1889.

138. Christe A, Oesterhelweg L, Ross S et al. (2010) Can MRI of the neck compete with clinical findings in assessing danger to life for survivors of manual strangulation? A statistical analysis. *Leg Med (Tokyo).* 12:228–232.

139. Yen K, Vock P, Christe A et al. (2007) Clinical forensic radiology in strangulation victims: Forensic expertise based on magnetic resonance imaging (MRI) findings. *Int J Legal Med.* 121:115–123.

140. Yen K, Thali MJ, Aghayev E et al. (2005) Strangulation signs: Initial correlation of MRI, MSCT, and forensic neck findings. *J Magn Reson Imaging.* 22:501–510.

141. Kempter M, Ross S, Spendlove D et al. (2009) Postmortem imaging of laryngohyoid fractures in strangulation incidents-first results. *Leg Med (Tokyo).* 11:267–271.

142. Cullen PM (2012) Paediatric trauma. *Contin Educ Anaesth Crit Care Pain.* 12(2):1–5 doi: 10.1093/bjaceaccp/mks010.

143. Jaspan T (2008) Current controversies in the interpretation of non-accidental head injury. *Pediatr Radiol.* 38:S378–S387.

144. Sanchez T, Stewart D, Walvick M et al. (2010) Skull fracture vs. accessory sutures: How can we tell the difference? *Emerg Radiol.* 17:413–418.

145. Roberts IS, Benamore RE, Benbow EW et al. (2012) Postmortem imaging as an alternative to autopsy in the diagnosis of adult deaths: A validation study. *Lancet.* 379:136–142.

146. Scholing M, Saltzherr TP, Fung Kon Jin PH et al. (2009) The value of postmortem computed tomography as an alternative for autopsy in trauma victims: A systematic review. *Eur Radiol.* 19:2333–2341.

24

Dental Scan and Odontoiatric Applications

Ashu Seith Bhalla, Kalyanasundaram Srinivasan, and Pankaj Gupta

CONTENTS

24.1 Dental CT Technique

Dental computed tomography (CT) protocol involves the acquisition of axial data with the highest possible resolution coupled with curved and orthoradial multiplanar reconstructions (MPRs). This high resolution imaging is essential as the dental pathologies can be very subtle.

Patient should be instructed not to swallow or move the jaw during the scan. If, despite counseling, such movements are likely, patient may be instructed to bite a cotton roll to achieve immobilization. Scanning is done in supine position with slight extension of the neck. The head should be positioned symmetrically and strapped.

Dental CT may be performed on a conventional CT, spiral CT, or a multislice CT scanner. Multi-detector array CT (MDCT) with its faster imaging capabilities and ability to obtain volumetric data has become the standard now. After acquisition of thin axial slices (up to 1 mm), dental CT reformatting protocols allow the extensive evaluation of the dental and periodontal disease. The axial data are acquired parallel to the alveolar ridge and para-axial and panoramic images are reconstructed. The former are especially useful for planning and measurement of implants and the latter simulate a panoramic radiograph allowing accurate assessment of relationship of tumor and cysts to the roots of teeth, mandibular canal, and maxillary antra.

A low-dose CT technology that is specifically applied to the dental and maxillofacial region is a cone beam x-ray CT (CBCT). In CBCT systems, the x-ray beam has a conical geometry that is in contrast to conventional fan-beam geometry of MDCT. The conical geometry allows an entire volumetric dataset to be acquired with a single rotation of the gantry, against multiple axial slices in MDCT. Another difference between CBCT and MDCT is the isotropic nature of acquisition and reconstruction in cone beam systems. Compared with MDCT, CBCT reduces the effect of partial volume averaging and can improve the spatial resolution of high-contrast structures in any viewing plane. Imaging time is short, typically 20–40 seconds. The compact structure of CBCT is suitable for use in an office-based setting. The limiting factor, however, is the contrast resolution that suffers from an increase in x-ray scatter. This limits the evaluation of soft tissue. Moreover, the streak artifacts from dental fillings can degrade image quality. At present, CBCT is applied to solve complex diagnostic and therapeutic planning issues, including craniofacial fractures, implant planning, orthodontics, and others.

24.2 Cysts, Tumors, and Tumor-Like Lesions

24.2.1 Introduction

A diverse variety of benign and malignant lesions arise in jaw bones. They may arise from dental elements, bone, or mesenchymal components [1]. Many classifications have been proposed, which are mostly based on the cell of origin and aggressiveness of the lesion. The classification published by World Health Organization (WHO) in 1992 divided tumors into benign and malignant types and further subdivided based on the odontogenic tissue types [2]. Table 24.1 shows a simplified classification of jaw lesions.

TABLE 24.1

Benign and Malignant Lesions of the Mandible

Cystic lesions
  Odontogenic
    Periapical cyst
    Dentigerous cyst
    KCOT
  Nonodontogenic
    Simple bone cyst
    ABC
    Stafne's cyst
Solid lesions
  Benign Odontogenic
    Odontoma
    Ameloblastoma
    Odontogenic myxoma
    Calcifying epithelial odontogenic tumor
    Cementoblastoma
    Adenomatoid odontogenic tumor
  Benign Nonodontogenic
    Osseous lesions
      Ossifying fibroma
      Periapical cemental dysplasia
      Florid COD
      Torus
      Osteoma
      FD
    Nonosseous lesions
      Central giant cell granuloma
      Central hemangioma
      Arteriovenous malformations
  Malignant
    Odontogenic—Ameloblastic carcinoma
    Nonodontogenic—osteosarcoma, metastasis, myeloma,
      squamous cell carcinoma, lymphoma, leukemia,
      chondrosarcoma, etc.

Source: Modified from Dunfee BL, Sakai O, Pistey R, Gohel A, *Radiographics*, 26(6), 2006.

Odontogenic lesions develop during or after the formation of teeth. These lesions could be solid or cystic and benign or malignant. Odontogenic cysts may be developmental, inflammatory, or neoplastic in origin. Odontogenic tumors are mostly benign and include a broad spectrum of lesions such as ameloblastoma, odontoma, and odontogenic myxoma. Malignant odontogenic lesions are very rare. Benign nonodontogenic lesions may be osseous or fibro-osseous in nature. Malignant nonodontogenic lesions include primary malignant bone tumors, metastasis, multiple myeloma, secondary involvement from tumors of oral cavity. In addition, tumor-like lesions such as fibrous dysplasia (FD), vascular lesions such as arteriovenous malformations, and metabolic conditions such as brown tumor can occur in jaw bones.

Clinically, many of these lesions are asymptomatic and are discovered incidentally at routine radiography. The most common symptoms are jaw swelling and pain. Other symptoms include tooth mobility, deformity, and facial asymmetry. Malignant lesions often present with paresthesia over chin due to mandibular canal involvement. Few patients present with bleeding or with signs and symptoms of secondary infection.

Even after the advent of modern imaging modalities, panoramic radiographs still remain the screening modality for jaw lesions. Panoramic radiographs provide a curved-plane tomogram of maxilla and mandible including teeth [[3]]. They are highly sensitive in detecting the lesion and depicting the tooth resorption and relation of the lesion to inferior alveolar canal. Other extraoral radiographs such as lateral oblique and posteroanterior (PA) are also used for evaluation. The radiographic features of cysts and tumors are often nonspecific and are overlapping. Cross-sectional imaging modalities such as CT and magnetic resonance imaging (MRI) are commonly used for further workup. Multi-detector MDCT is presently a robust technique for diagnosis and surgical planning of jaw lesions. Three-dimensional (3D) postprocessing techniques such as MPRs and volume-rendered technique (VRT) are used for evaluating the extent of lesions, cortical integrity, and relation to surrounding structures. MRI is used for the evaluation of bone marrow and extraosseous soft-tissue component. However, MRI is not optimal for detecting calcified foci or cortical destruction.

24.3 Approach to the Diagnosis of Jaw Lesions

The imaging appearances of many jaw lesions are nonspecific and overlap with each other. The patient's age, clinical presentation, and a systematic analysis of radiographs and CT can aid in narrowing the differential diagnosis. Systematic analysis of the lesions includes evaluation of location, relation to dentition and alveolar canal, density/attenuation of the lesion, cortical integrity, and soft-tissue involvement [4,5].

Location: Majority of the lesions arise in posterior mandible owing to more vascular nature of this region. However, few lesions have a propensity to involve anterior mandible, which include giant cell reparative granuloma, cemento-osseous dysplasia (COD), simple bone cyst, and brown tumor.

Relation to dentition: Few odontogenic lesions are typically seen in relation to the apices of teeth, that is, periapical in location, which include radicular cyst, cementoblastoma, and periapical cemental dysplasia. Dentigerous cysts are typically pericoronal, that is, related to crown of tooth. Odontogenic lesions such as ameloblastoma, pindborg tumor, odontoma, and keratocystic odontogenic tumor (KCOT) are associated with an impacted tooth.

Relation to inferior alveolar canal: The lesions with epicenter above the canal are likely odontogenic and the lesions below the canal are nonodontogenic in origin [6].

Margins: Benign lesions are usually well circumscribed, and inflammatory or malignant lesions are ill-defined.

Cortical integrity and soft tissue: Benign lesions are generally expansile with cortical thinning, whereas malignant or locally aggressive lesions cause cortical destruction with soft-tissue component. Presence of periosteal reaction is suggestive of osteomyelitis (OM) or malignant etiology.

Density/attenuation of the lesion: On CT, the lesions may be lytic, sclerotic, or mixed in density. Majority of the lesions are lytic, which may be well circumscribed or poorly defined. The remaining lesions may be sclerotic or mixed and the differentials include a variety of neoplastic and inflammatory conditions. A simplified approach to jaw lesions based on the density is shown in Table 24.2. We have used this approach to organize this chapter which also helps in better understanding of the entities along with their differential diagnosis.

24.3.1 Well-Defined Lytic Lesions: Odontogenic Cysts

24.3.1.1 Periapical (Radicular) Cyst

Periapical cyst is the most common odontogenic cystic lesion of the jaw. It is associated with dental caries that cause inflammation of pulp cavity leading to pulp necrosis. The infection then reaches apex of tooth resulting in apical periodontitis and granuloma formation with subsequent development of periapical cyst. The lesion appears as a well-defined unilocular lytic lesion in the periapical region associated with carious tooth [7,8]. The term residual cyst is used for a periapical cyst that remains after surgical intervention.

24.3.1.2 Dentigerous Cyst (Follicular Cyst)

Dentigerous cyst is the most common noninflammatory odontogenic cystic lesion occurring in jaw. The lesion appears as a well-defined unilocular lytic lesion associated with an unerupted tooth (Figure 24.1). The crown of unerupted tooth is usually seen projecting into cyst and the roots are located outside the lesion [9]. The cyst wall is attached to cementoenamel junction of the tooth. The lesion is commonly located in the maxillary or mandibular third molar region. The wall of dentigerous cyst

TABLE 24.2

Radiological Approach of Jaw Lesions

Well-defined lytic lesions	
Odontogenic	*Nonodontogenic*
Radicular cyst	Incisive canal cyst
Dentigerous cyst	Simple bone cyst
KCOT	ABC
Ameloblastoma	Stafne's cyst
Odontogenic myxoma	Giant cell reparative granuloma
	Central hemangioma
	Eosinophilic granuloma
Poorly defined lytic lesions	
Odontogenic	*Nonodontogenic*
Ameloblastic carcinoma	Osteosarcoma
	Metastases
	Myeloma
	Direct tumor extension
	OM
Mixed density lesions	
Odontogenic	*Nonodontogenic*
Calcifying epithelial odontogenic tumor	COF
AFO	FD
Adenomatoid odontogenic tumor	COD
	Chronic OM, Osteosarcoma
Sclerotic lesions	
Odontogenic	*Nonodontogenic*
Odontoma	Osteoma
Cementoblastoma	Osteochondroma, Torus

Source: Modified from Neyaz Z, Gadodia A, Gamanagatti S, Mukhopadhyay S, *Singapore Med J.*, 49(2), 2008.

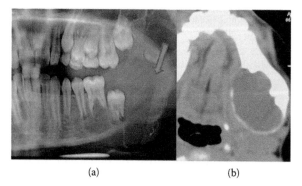

(a)   (b)

FIGURE 24.1
Dentigerous cyst. Orthopantomogram (OPG) (a) and axial computed tomography (CT) (b) images reveal a well-defined lytic lesion (arrow) in the left mandible in the region of molars causing buccolingual expansion with intact cortex. The lesion is noted to be in relation to crown of unerupted molar. In fact, the patient had a history of resection a few years back suggesting a recurrent dentigerous cyst.

may occasionally show ameloblastic transformation that is termed as mural ameloblastoma [10]. The treatment options include enucleation for small lesions and surgical drainage with marsupialization for large lesions.

The differential diagnosis for dentigerous cyst includes KCOT and unicystic ameloblastoma. Both KCOT and unicystic ameloblastoma often have an associated impacted tooth and may mimic dentigerous cyst.

24.3.1.3 Keratocystic Odontogenic Tumor

KCOT was previously known as odontogenic keratocyst. The WHO's 2005 edition of histological classification [11] of odontogenic tumors has defined KCOT as "a benign uni- or multicystic intra-osseous tumor of odontogenic origin, with a characteristic lining of parakeratinized stratified squamous epithelium and potentially aggressive, infiltrative behavior." It can occur at any age but more commonly in second and third decades. On CT, the lesion is seen as a well-defined uni- or multilocular cystic lesion with corticated margins and commonly seen in posterior body and ramus of mandible (Figure 24.2). The lesion characteristically shows mediolateral expansion along the axis of the mandible [6]. The lesion is often locally aggressive and may show areas of cortical perforation or destruction. The inferior alveolar canal may be inferiorly displaced or destroyed. Root resorption may be noted in adjacent teeth. The thick cheesy contents may appear as hyperdense areas within the lesion. There may be few daughter cysts adjacent to the main lesion. Most KCOTs possess destructive potential, with a high recurrence rate after resection [12].

The differential diagnosis includes simple bone cyst (SBC), unicystic ameloblastoma, and dentigerous cyst. The presence of scalloped superior border and absence of resorption or displacement of adjacent roots help in differentiation of SBC from KCOT. Unicystic ameloblastoma is radiologically indistinguishable from KCOT and should be included in the differential diagnosis of

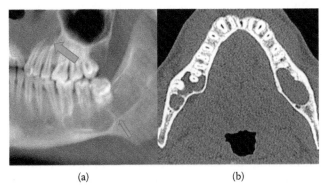

(a)   (b)

FIGURE 24.2
Keratocystic odontogenic tumor (KCOT). OPG (a) shows multiple unilocular well-defined lytic lesions involving the left half of the mandible (thin arrow) and maxilla (thick arrow). Axial CT image (b) shows the cystic nature of these lesions as well as the lesions on the right side. Multiple keratocystic odontogenic tumors are seen in the setting of basal cell nevus syndrome.

KCOT. In 30% of cases, KCOT may be associated with an unerupted tooth and mimics dentigerous cyst.

Multiple KCOTs (Figure 24.2) are seen in basal cell nevus syndrome (Gorlin–Goltz syndrome), which is an autosomal dominant disorder. Other findings associated with this syndrome include midfacial hypoplasia, prognathism, mental retardation, and calcification of falx cerebri [13].

24.3.2 Well-Defined Lytic Lesions: Nonodontogenic Cysts

24.3.2.1 Incisive Canal Cyst

Incisive canal cyst or nasopalatine duct cyst is a nonodontogenic developmental cystic lesion. It is derived from the embryological remnants of the nasopalatine duct that is enclosed within the incisive canal and normally disappears before birth. The lesion is asymptomatic and often diagnosed incidentally on panoramic radiographs. The lesion presents as a well-defined unilocular lytic lesion located anteriorly in the midline between the roots of maxillary central incisors [14]. Unlike in periapical cyst, the incisors are vital and the lamina dura and periodontal ligament space are intact.

24.3.2.2 Aneurysmal Bone Cyst

Aneurysmal bone cyst (ABC) is a rare nonodontogenic neoplasm involving mandible more commonly than maxilla. WHO classification [11] has defined ABC as "an expanding osteolytic lesion consisting of blood filled spaces separated by connective tissue septae containing trabeculae of osteoid tissue and giant cells." Most cases occur in children and adults in their second and third decades [15]. The incidence is more common in females, and clinically they present with a rapidly increasing painless swelling. On imaging, the lesion appears as a well-defined multilocular, expansile lytic lesion with ballooning of cortex. CT shows multiple fluid–fluid levels that are pathogonomic for the diagnosis of ABC. The fluid levels represent sedimentation of red blood cells within blood-filled cavities [16].

Secondary ABCs are associated with various primary disorders of the jaw such as giant cell reparative granuloma, FD, chondroblastoma, telangiectatic osteosarcoma, etc.

24.3.2.3 Simple Bone Cyst

Simple bone cyst or traumatic bone cyst is an intraosseous pseudocyst that lacks an epithelial lining. It is believed to arise secondary to trauma and tooth extraction resulting in intramedullay hemorrhage and

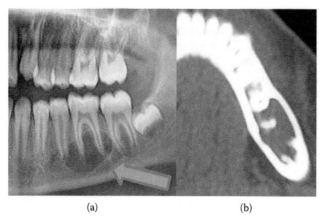

FIGURE 24.3
Simple bone cyst. OPG (a) of the left half of the mandible reveals a well-defined round lytic lesion involving the body of the mandible that appears fluid attenuation on axial CT (b) and shows no significant expansion. The lesion is related to the roots of multiple teeth and there are no carious teeth changes differentiating the lesion from radicular cyst.

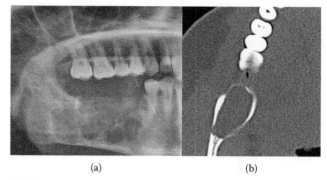

FIGURE 24.4
Multilocular ameloblastoma. OPG (a) reveals a well-defined multiloculated lesion involving the right half of the body of mandible with multiple missing teeth. Axial CT (b) shows the buccolingual expansion in one of the components of the lesion.

subsequent resorption [17]. It commonly occurs in posterior mandible in the premolar and molar regions. On imaging, it presents as a unilocular lytic lesion and has a characteristic scalloped superior border that extends between the roots of adjacent teeth [18]. The teeth show minimal displacement and do not show resorption of roots (Figure 24.3). The differential diagnosis includes KCOT and dentigerous cyst. The superior scalloped border of the lesion favors the diagnosis of simple bone cyst, whereas mediolateral expansion of the lesion along the curve of mandible and resorption of adjacent teeth favor KCOT. Dentigerous cyst is typically associated with crown of an unerupted tooth, whereas SBC is not associated with an unerupted tooth.

24.3.2.4 Lingual Salivary Gland Inclusion Defect (Stafne's Cyst)

Stafne's cyst is a pseudocyst and is seen as a focal concavity in the lingual cortex of mandible near the mandibular angle. The defect often contains fat and occasionally an aberrant lobe of submandibular salivary gland [19].

24.3.3 Well-Defined Lytic Lesions: Odontogenic Tumors

24.3.3.1 Ameloblastoma

Ameloblastoma is a benign odontogenic tumor that arises from enamel-forming cells of odontogenic epithelium [9]. These lesions constitute about 10% of odontogenic tumors and typically present in third and fourth decades of life [10]. Ameloblastomas commonly occur in ramus and posterior body of mandible; however, they can occur in maxilla. Ameloblastomas

are classified into two types based on the radiological appearance—multicystic and unicystic.

Multicystic variety is the most common type and radiologically presents as a multilocular lytic lesion with internal septations producing honeycomb appearance [20]. The lesions show both buccolingual and mediolateral expansion (Figure 24.4). It often shows areas of cortical perforation or frank destruction [21]. On contrast-enhanced CT images, these lesions show mixed solid and cystic areas of varying proportions. The differential diagnosis of this variety includes odontogenic myxoma and KCOT. The predilection to involve the maxilla more than mandible and the presence of well-developed internal osseous trabeculae differentiate myxoma from other odontogenic lesions. KCOT can occasionally be multilocular and radiologically mimics ameloblastoma. The presence of solid-enhancing areas favors the diagnosis of ameloblastoma, as KCOT does not have solid components.

Unicystic ameloblastoma is a rare variant that accounts for about 6%–19% of all ameloblastomas. This variety is usually less aggressive than the multicystic type and occurs in younger age group [22]. They present as a unilocular lytic lesion usually in the posterior mandible (Figure 24.5). Unicystic ameloblastoma is radiologically indistinguishable from KCOT and both occur in the same age group.

Desmoplastic ameloblastoma is a rare variant of ameloblastoma that presents in fourth and fifth decades of life. It is most commonly seen in anterior mandible. On imaging, the lesion is seen as an ill-defined mixed lytic–sclerotic lesion [23]. It shows areas of coarse calcifications with cortical destruction. Fibro-osseous lesions and osteosarcoma should be included in the differential diagnosis of this variant.

Malignant ameloblastoma is referred to as histologically benign ameloblastoma with evidence of distant metastasis [24].

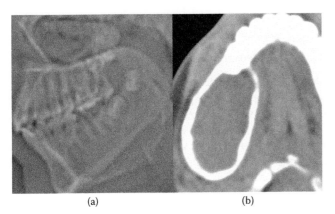

(a)   (b)

FIGURE 24.5
Unilocular ameloblastoma. Lateral oblique scanogram (a) image shows an expansile unilocular lesion arising from the mandibular body. Axial CT (b) confirms the unilocular nature of the lesion. Note that the lesion contains solid tissue having the same density as tongue muscles.

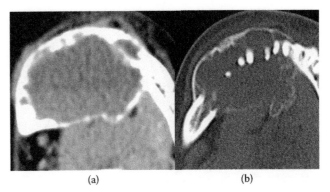

(a)   (b)

FIGURE 24.6
Central giant cell reparative granuloma. Axial CT in soft-tissue window (a) shows an expansile lytic lesion of the right anterior mandible extending to the left side. The lesion is solid with heterogeneous appearance. Bone window (b) shows marked buccolingual expansion with thinned out cortex.

24.3.3.2 Odontogenic Myxoma

Odontogenic myxomas are benign odontogenic tumor that manifests in second and third decades of life. They are more commonly seen in females and show a predilection to involve maxilla more than mandible. On CT, they are indistinguishable from ameloblastoma and present as a multilocular expansile lytic lesion. They show internal osseous trabeculae and thin septations producing honeycomb appearance [25]. They are often locally aggressive and show areas of cortical perforation or destruction. The adjacent teeth may show displacement or resorption. The differential diagnosis includes ameloblastoma, KCOT, and central giant cell reparative granuloma. Ameloblastomas generally present at a later age than myxomas and are more common in mandible. The presence of solid-enhancing areas favors the diagnosis of ameloblastoma. Dynamic contrast-enhanced MRI may be used for differentiating these two lesions, as myxomas show delayed enhancement due to myxoid stroma present in them [26]. KCOT occurs in the same age group as that of myxoma and occasionally present as a multicystic lesion. However, KCOTs do not have well-developed trabeculae and are purely cystic. CGRG commonly occur in anterior mandible and show homogeneous or heterogeneous enhancement of the matrix with areas of hemorrhage or secondary ABC formation.

24.3.4 Well-Defined Lytic Lesions: Nonodontogenic Tumor

24.3.4.1 Central Giant Cell Reparative Granuloma

Central giant cell reparative granuloma is an uncommon nonodontogenic lesion that is considered to be a reactive process to a previous trauma to the jaw bones. They typically manifest in adolescents and young adults less than 30 years of age. They occur more commonly in females [27]. The most common location is the bone from anterior mandible to first molars with a tendency to cross midline. The imaging appearance of CGRG is typically unilocular or multilocular expansile lytic lesion with fine trabeculations in the anterior mandible, which may cross midline [28]. The matrix may show heterogeneous enhancement (Figure 24.6). Areas of hemorrhages may be seen on noncontrast images. Secondary ABC formation in not an uncommon finding in CGRG. Aggressive lesions may show cortical perforation or destruction. There may be resorption or displacement of adjacent teeth.

The differential diagnosis includes KCOT, hemangioma, ameloblastoma, and myxoma. KCOT usually occurs in posterior mandible and is typically cystic, whereas CGRG occurs in anterior mandible and the matrix is usually solid, which may show cystic degeneration. Hemangiomas typically occur in children and show moderate to intense enhancement of the matrix. Brown tumor of hyperthyroidism is radiologically and pathologically indistinguishable from CGRG [9]. Brown tumor generally presents in middle-aged adults and has radiological changes in other bones with abnormal laboratory values.

24.3.4.2 Central Hemangioma

Central hemangioma is a rare nonodontogenic lesion that occurs in children. It is considered to be a vascular neoplasm that is composed of disorganized masses of endothelium-lined vessels and sinusoidal spaces filled with blood [29]. Most of the cases occur in mandible, and only a few cases have been reported in maxilla. The lesion commonly presents as a multilocular lytic

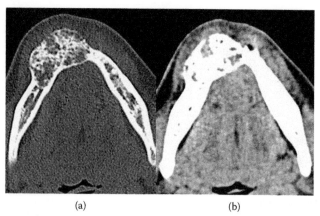

(a)   (b)

FIGURE 24.7
Hemangioma. Axial CT images in bone window (a) and soft-tissue window (b) shows an expansile lytic lesion involving the right side of the mandible near the midline with multiple "honeycomb"-like spaces.

lesion expanding posterior body or ramus of mandible producing a soap-bubble or honeycomb appearance (Figure 24.7). They show moderate to intense enhancement on postcontrast images [30]. Hemorrhagic foci may be noted within the lesion.

24.3.4.3 Eosinophilic Granuloma

Eosinophilic granuloma is a benign form of Langerhans cell histiocytosis and usually occurs in children or young adults. Multiple or solitary lesions may be seen. On imaging, the lesions are smooth, regular or irregular lytic, and are commonly seen in ramus of mandible. Associated floating teeth may be seen due to loss of periodontal bone support [31].

24.3.5 Poorly Defined Lytic Lesions: Odontogenic

24.3.5.1 Ameloblastic Carcinoma

Ameloblastic carcinoma is a rare malignant odontogenic epithelial neoplasm and may arise de novo or from a pre-existing odontogenic lesion. It commonly involves the posterior mandible and less often the maxilla [32]. It exhibits malignant features on histology, with or without metastasis [33]. The tumor presents as a multilocular lytic lesion with extensive cortical destruction and soft-tissue extension. The lesion may be mixed solid-cystic or purely solid showing enhancement on contrast enhanced images. The term ameloblastic carcinoma should be differentiated from malignant ameloblastoma. Ameloblastic carcinoma is a histologically malignant tumor, whereas malignant ameloblastoma is a histologically benign ameloblastoma with evidence of distant metastasis [24].

24.3.6 Poorly Defined Lytic Lesions–Nonodontogenic

24.3.6.1 Osteosarcoma

Osteosarcoma, the primary malignant tumor can radiologically present as a poorly defined lytic permeative destruction with or without soft-tissue involvement. CT underestimates the extent of involvement of marrow space by the tumor when compared with MRI. The imaging features of osteosarcoma have been discussed in Section 24.3.8.5.

24.3.6.2 Acute Osteomyelitis

Acute OM appears as an ill-defined lytic permeative type of destruction with or without periosteal reaction [6]. The adjacent soft tissue often shows inflammatory changes. The radiologic differentiation from primary malignant tumors is difficult as the imaging findings overlap. Acute OM has been dealt in detail in Section 24.4

24.3.6.3 Direct Tumor Extension

Malignant lesions originating from the oral cavity and maxillary antrum can secondarily involve mandible and maxilla, respectively. They usually appear as a saucer-shaped erosive defect in lingual or buccal cortex associated with a soft-tissue mass [34]. They may also manifest as multiple lytic foci, which may eventually coalesce into a larger irregular lesion. There is usually no evidence of a bony sclerotic reaction or periosteal reaction in such lesions.

24.3.6.4 Metastases

Malignant tumors of breast, kidney, lung, and prostate can metastasize to jaw bones. The posterior body and angle of mandible are commonly affected due to the presence of high marrow volume and vascularity [34]. On CT imaging, an ill-defined lytic destruction with or without soft-tissue component is seen. The area of destruction within the mandible may be localized, bilateral, or diffuse. Metastases from breast and prostate can produce mixed lytic–sclerotic or purely sclerotic areas.

24.3.6.5 Myeloma

Multiple myeloma is a malignant neoplasm of plasma cells, which occurs most frequently in patients of 40–70 years of age [34]. Mandible is affected more than the maxilla, with posterior body and angle being commonest sites. Myeloma of jaw bones occurs in two forms: diffuse and solitary plasmocytoma. Diffuse form is characterized by multiple punched-out, lytic lesions without any

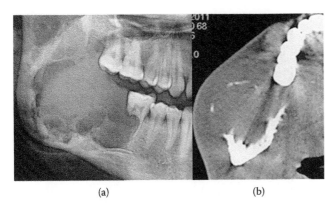

(a)   (b)

FIGURE 24.8
Plasmacytoma. OPG image of the right half of the mandible (a) shows a markedly expansile lytic lesion of the angle of mandible with loss of the superior cortex and multiple teeth. Axial CT (b) confirms the expansile nature of the lesion with breech of the overlying cortex.

surrounding bone reaction. Bone expansion is typically absent in this variety. Solitary plasmocytoma is a localized form of myeloma, which may progress to multiple myeloma [35]. Solitary plasmocytoma may present as a unilocular or multilocular lytic lesion mimicking many odontogenic and nonodontogenic tumors (Figure 24.8). It can also present as an ill-defined lytic lesion involving the mandible with enhancing soft-tissue component. In such cases, differentiation from metastasis, malignant odontogenic, and nonodontogenic lesions is difficult.

24.3.7 Mixed Density Lesions: Odontogenic

24.3.7.1 Calcifying Epithelial Odontogenic Tumor (Pindborg Tumor)

Calcifying epithelial odontogenic tumor (CEOT) is a rare benign odontogenic tumor that is composed of epithelial cells in a fibrous stroma. The deposition of extracellular amyloid-like substance and concentric calcified deposits (Liesegang rings) are pathognomic histopathological findings [36]. Patients usually present at 30–50 years of age. Many of these lesions are located in posterior mandible and are often associated with an unerupted tooth. The imaging appearance of CEOT is typically a uni- or multilocular expansile lytic lesion with an associated unerupted tooth [37]. Multiple calcific densities are seen either scattered within the lesion or clustered near the crown of impacted tooth. The differential diagnosis includes ameloblastic fibro-odontoma (AFO), adenomatoid odontogenic tumor, ossifying fibroma, and ameloblastoma.

24.3.7.2 Ameloblastic Fibro-Odontoma

AFO is an uncommon odontogenic tumor that is composed of a mixture of ameloblastic tissue and complex odontoma. It usually manifests in second and third

decades of life. Clinically, the patient presents with a painless swelling. Radiologically, the lesion appears as a well-defined unilocular lytic lesion with densely calcified tissues seen within [38].

The differential diagnosis includes complex odontoma, CEOT, cement-ossifying fibroma, and adenomatoid odontogenic tumor. Complex odontoma is often radiologically indistinguishable from AFO and sometimes considered to be a continuum of differentiation. The odontomas are surrounded by a thin radiolucent space, whereas in AFO, the amount of radiolucent space exceeds the calcified tissues [6].

24.3.7.3 Adenomatoid Odontogenic Tumor

Adenomatoid odontogenic tumor is a rare odontogenic tumor that is seen more common in females. Most cases are diagnosed in the second decade of life [39]. This tumor has a predilection to involve the maxilla more than mandible. The lesion appears as a well-defined lytic lesion with areas of punctuate calcifications. The tumor is associated with an unerupted tooth mimicking a dentigerous cyst. In dentigerous cyst, the wall is attached to the cementoenamel junction and crown projects into the cyst, whereas AOT extends beyond cementoenamel junction and may include the roots. The differential diagnosis includes CEOT, cemento-ossifying fibroma (COF) and AFO.

24.3.8 Mixed Density Lesions: Nonodontogenic

24.3.8.1 Fibrous Dysplasia

FD is an idiopathic, slowly progressing benign disorder in which the medullary bone is replaced by abnormal fibro-osseous tissue. FD usually presents in adolescents and young adults. Three basic forms of FD are recognized: monostotic (affecting one bone), polyostotic form (affecting multiple bones), and McCune–Albright syndrome [40]. McCune–Albright syndrome is characterized by polyostotic FD with associated skin pigmentation and precocious puberty and is seen exclusively in females.

Craniofacial FD is usually monostotic, with maxilla being the most commonly affected site. However, multiple sites can be affected, extending contiguously in a flowing manner across the sutures. The imaging appearance on CT depends on the amount of matrix mineralization. The lesions are usually ill-defined and may be homogeneously hyperdense producing ground-glass appearance or heterogeneous showing mixed hyper- and hypodense areas (Figure 24.9). CT shows expansion of the involved bone with cortical thinning [41]. The bone expansion is usually fusiform in the mandible, and more complex in the maxilla, reflecting the more complex

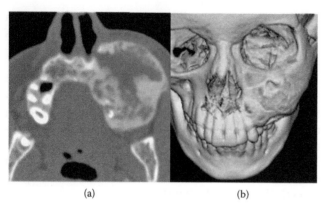

(a)   (b)

FIGURE 24.9
Fibrous dysplasia (FD). Axial CT (a) shows an ill-defined mixed lytic–sclerotic lesion involving the left maxilla with extension across the midline and involvement of part of the right maxilla. Note the expansion of the left maxilla with ground glass matrix. Image obtained by volume-rendered technique (b) shows the extent of the lesion to better advantage.

anatomy of the latter. Another characteristic feature of expansion in FD is that the underlying morphology of the bone is maintained. Maxillary lesions often expand into maxillary sinus causing complete obliteration of the sinus [42]. Lesions involving infra-orbital ridge of maxilla produce upward displacement of the orbital floor. The inferior alveolar canal is usually displaced superiorly and there may be loss of lamina dura. The disease is usually self-limiting, often not progressing after third decade of life. Malignant transformation is a rare complication and is seen in less than 1% of cases and the patients should be kept in regular follow-up.

24.3.8.2 Cemento-Ossifying Fibroma

COF is an encapsulated benign neoplasm consisting of fibrous tissue with varying amounts of bony trabeculae. It typically manifests during third and fourth decades of life [43]. COF occurs more commonly in the mandible, in the molar, and in the premolar regions. CT shows a well-circumscribed, expansile lesion often surrounded by a hyper- or hypodense rim. The matrix attenuation depends on the amount of mineralized tissue, the early lesions appear lytic (Figure 24.10) and the attenuation increases as the lesions mature (Figure 24.11). Mandibular COF often exhibits bowing of inferior border of mandible. The main differential diagnosis of COF is FD. The imaging features favoring COF include well-circumscribed margins and convex shape of outer wall of the involved bone [40]. FD generally blends with surrounding bone, and morphology and shape of the involved bone is preserved. Other differentials include calcified epithelial odontogenic tumor, AFO, and adenomatoid odontogenic tumor.

Juvenile aggressive ossifying fibroma or psammomatoid ossifying fibroma is a variant of COF, which

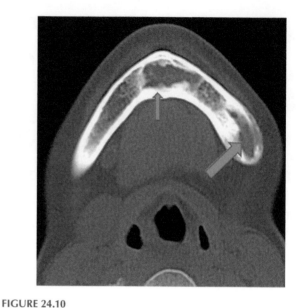

FIGURE 24.10
Cement-ossifying fibroma. Axial CT image of the mandible in bone window shows two lytic lesions in the midline and the left half of the mandible. The matrix of the midline lesion shows few high density areas (small arrow) whereas the one on the left side shows diffuse homogeneous ground glass matrix (large arrow). The lesions were found to be cement-ossifying fibromas on histopathology and these lesions show matrix attenuation depends on the amount of mineralized matrix.

typically occurs in adolescents and younger adults [44]. It typically occurs in sinonasal tract and behaves in a locally aggressive manner with extensive cortical destruction. On imaging, the tumor shows soft tissue admixed with fibro-osseous component. Multiple round or oval calcified foci representing psammomatoid bodies are also seen within the lesion.

24.3.8.3 Cemento-Osseous Dysplasia

COD arises because of proliferation of connective tissue within periodontal membrane [45]. It is usually diagnosed in third and fourth decades of life. It is of two types: periapical and florid dysplasia.

- Periapical COD: It arises around the apices of vital tooth with a predilection for mandibular incisors. The lesion appears as a well-defined lucent lesion in the early stages and becomes progressively radiodense as the lesion matures [46]. The differential diagnosis of this entity includes periapical cyst for early stages and cementoblastoma for later stages of COD. Periapical cyst is formed around the apices of caries tooth whereas COD is formed around a vital tooth. In cementoblastoma, the periodontal space is obliterated by the attachment of the mass to the roots, whereas in periapical COD, the periodontal ligament space is intact.

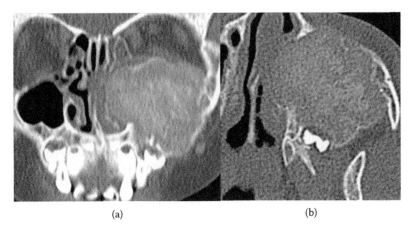

FIGURE 24.11
Ossifying fibroma. Coronal (a) and axial images (b) show a well-defined expansile lesion involving the left half of the mandible with mass effect on the left maxillary sinus and the nasal cavity. The lesion shows diffusely mineralized matrix, giving the lesion a sclerosed appearance.

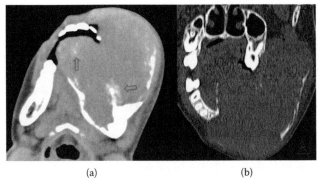

(a)   (b)

FIGURE 24.12
Juvenile ossifying fibroma. Axial (a) and coronal CT (b) of a 10-year-old girl reveals a markedly expansile lytic lesion involving the body and left half of the mandible. The lesion is solid and show few round areas of calcified matrix (arrows).

- Florid COD: It is characterized by multiple periapical lesions that involve the entire mandible (Figure 24.12).

24.3.8.4 Chronic Osteomyelitis

Chronic OM is radiologically seen as a mixed lytic–sclerotic lesion with periosteal reaction and sequestrum formation. The differential diagnosis includes osteosarcoma, FD, and COD. Chronic OM has been discussed in detail in Section 24.4.

24.3.8.5 Osteosarcoma

Osteosarcoma is an osteoid-producing primary malignant bone tumor rarely affecting the jaw bones. It constitutes about 6%–9% of all osteosarcomas affecting the skeleton. The peak age of incidence is third decade of life, unlike osteosarcoma of long bones, which peaks in second decade. Several predisposing factors such as radiation, trauma, FD, and Paget's disease have been implicated in the pathogenesis of this tumor [34]. The

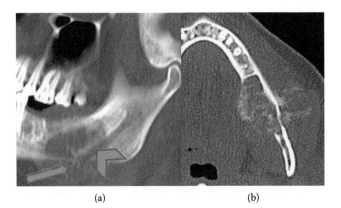

(a)   (b)

FIGURE 24.13
Osteosarcoma. OPG image (a) of the left half of the mandible shows a permeative lytic lesion involving the angle and ramus of the mandible. The erosion of inferior part of the mandibular canal (arrow head) and the inferior cortex (arrow) are well shown. Axial CT image in bone window (b) shows aggressive periosteal reaction on both the buccal and lingual cortical aspects of the left mandible. Also note the soft-tissue mass. There are areas of amorphous calcification within the matrix of the lesions suggestive of osteosarcoma.

most common location is posterior mandible; however, they can arise in maxilla. Radiologically, three patterns of bone destruction have been described: (1) osteolytic pattern, producing ill-defined lytic permeative areas (Figure 24.13), (2) osteoblastic pattern, which is the most common type encountered in jaw and is seen as sclerotic areas, and (3) mixed pattern, which has mixed lytic and sclerotic areas. A sunburst type of periosteal reaction caused by radiating mineralized spicules can be seen.

CT shows the pattern of destruction and extent of soft-tissue involvement. However, the extent of tumor spread within the marrow space is better shown by MRI [34]. Radical surgery with adjuvant chemotherapy or radiotherapy is the treatment of choice.

24.3.9 Hyperattenuating/Sclerotic Lesions: Odontogenic

24.3.9.1 Odontoma

Odontomas are characterized by abnormal proliferation of various odontogenic tissues and hence considered to be a hamartoma, rather a neoplasm [6]. They are typically diagnosed in second decade of life. There are two types of odontomas: compound and complex.

- Compound odontomas are composed of multiple well-formed teeth-like structures or "denticles." They commonly occur in anterior jaw and are often associated with an unerupted tooth.
- Complex odontoma is composed of conglomerate mass of irregular calcified tissues with a thin radiolucent space surrounding the calcified mass. They are also associated with unerupted tooth and are commonly located in posterior jaw. Differential diagnosis include AFO, COF, periapical cemental dysplasia and cementoblastoma. In odontoma, the calcified mass is surrounded by a thin lucent space (Figure 24.14); whereas in AFO, large amount of lucent space is seen, which exceeds the odontoma component. Periapical cemental dysplasia and cementoblastoma are densely calcified masses and are attached to roots of teeth, whereas odontomas are found occlusal or overlapping the involved teeth. COF is differentiated from complex odontoma because of the propensity to occur in older age, and they are less sclerotic than odontomas.

24.3.9.2 Cementoblastoma

Cementoblastoma is a benign neoplasm characterized by the formation of cementum-like mass in the molar or premolar region [9]. The lesion is usually solitary and is attached to the root of the tooth. The lesion appears as a well-defined densely calcified mass and surrounded by a radiolucent rim of uniform width. Cementoblastoma has to be differentiated from periapical COD. Both lesions are seen as a densely calcified mass seen at the root apices. In cementoblastoma, the periodontal space is obliterated by the attachment of the mass to the roots, whereas in periapical COD, the periodontal ligament space is intact.

24.3.10 Hyperattenuating/Sclerotic Lesions: Nonodontogenic

24.3.10.1 Osteoma

Osteomas are benign, slow growing osseous tumors composed of mature compact and/or cancellous bone. They are usually found in craniofacial skeleton more commonly in frontal and ethmoidal sinuses. Among jaw bones, mandible is affected more often than maxilla. Two types of osteomas are described depending on the location: central osteoma that arises from endosteum and peripheral osteoma that arises from periosteum. CT shows a well-circumscribed sclerotic mass in the mandible (Figure 24.15). In peripheral osteoma, the lesion is attached to the surface of mandible by broad base or pedicle [46].

Multiple osteomas are seen in Gardner's syndrome, an autosomal dominant disorder characterized by the presence of multiple colonic polyps, epidermoid, sebaceous cysts, desmoid tumors, and supernumerary teeth [47].

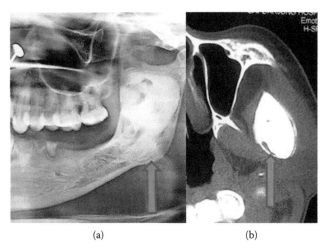

(a) (b)

FIGURE 24.14
Complex odontoma. OPG and axial CT show an ill-defined conglomerate calcified mass (arrows) in the posterior aspect of the left mandible with a radiolucent halo around the lesion.

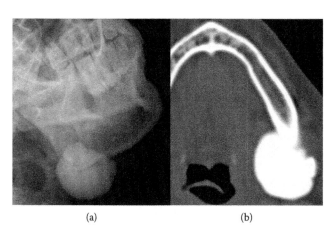

(a) (b)

FIGURE 24.15
Osteoma. Left lateral oblique radiograph (a) and axial bone window CT (b) show a uniformly densely calcified round mass in the left mandible close to its angle.

24.3.10.2 Torus

Tori are localized outgrowths from the surface of maxilla or mandible and are named accordingly. Torus mandibularis arises from the lingual aspect of mandible and are usually bilateral. Torus palatinus is a flat or nodular outgrowth from the midline of hard palate and projects into oral cavity [48].

24.3.10.3 Osteochondroma

Osteochondroma is a bony exostosis projecting from the surface of a bone. It commonly occurs in coronoid and condylar process of mandible [9]. Condylar lesions present with malocclusion, mandibular deviation to the contralateral side and facial asymmetry. CT shows a broad-based or pedunculated bony projection from the condyle. Surgical excision of the mass is the treatment of choice.

The presence of both compact and cancellous bone in osteochondroma differentiates it from torus, which is composed of only compact bone [48].

24.4 Osteomyelitis of Jaw

OM is defined as an inflammatory process involving both cortex and marrow. Mandible is involved more commonly than maxilla. The clinical presentation and imaging appearances depend on the stage of the disease [49].

Acute osteomyelitis: It is usually secondary to periodontal infection or following tooth extraction and may last up to 1 month. Hematogenous OM most commonly affects the maxilla in children. The patients usually present with fever, pain, swelling, and tenderness abutting the mandible. When the inflammatory exudates extend into muscles of mastication, the patients may complain of trismus. In the early stages, ill-defined lytic areas are seen in cancellous bone [50]. There may be erosion and loss of definition of cortical wall of the inferior alveolar canal. As the infection progresses, CT shows cortical plate erosion and the extension of inflammation into surrounding soft tissues. Periosteal new bone formation is seen when the infection spreads into subperiosteal space. Later in the disease course, there may be sclerosis and sequestrum formation. The differential diagnosis of acute OM include osteosarcoma, direct tumor extension from oral cavity, metastases and myeloma. All these lesions can present as an ill-defined lytic lesion. Osteosarcoma and OM are often radiologically indistinguishable and both can also show periosteal reaction.

Direct tumor extension, metastases, and myeloma do not show periosteal reaction.

Chronic osteomyelitis: It can be divided into primary and secondary forms depending on the clinical presentation. Secondary chronic OM results from an inadequately treated acute episode where infection persists in lacunae of necrotic bone. Primary chronic OM results from a chronic low-grade infection and is not preceded by an acute phase. Fever and constitutional symptoms are usually absent in primary form. The characteristic imaging findings in chronic OM include medullary sclerosis, periosteal reaction, and sequestrum formation [50]. The cancellous bone shows increased density, which may either show mixed lytic and sclerotic areas or diffuse sclerosis. Sequestra are pieces of devitalized bone that are not resorbed and they appear dense due to surrounding osteolysis. Sequestra formation is characteristic of chronic OM; however, they may be seen in late acute stages as well. They are more common on buccal aspect and are better shown on CT than on MRI. Periosteal new bone formation causes thickening and mandibular enlargement. The differential diagnosis of chronic OM include osteosarcoma, FD, and COD.

Osteomyelitis with periostitis: It was previously known as Garre OM and is a variant of OM in which a periosteal reaction predominates, resulting in significant cortical thickening. It is usually seen in children and young adults [50].

24.5 Osteoradionecrosis of Mandible

Osteoradionecrosis (ORN) of mandible is an uncommon but serious complication of radiotherapy used for treating head and neck tumors. ORN can also involve hyoid bone, sphenoid bone, and clivus. Maxilla is less commonly involved due to its rich blood supply. The pathogenesis of ORN is complex and is less understood. It is usually seen 1–2 years following radiation therapy. Radiation therapy probably induces endothelial cell death and thrombosis of vessels resulting in impaired vascular and lymphatic flow [51]. The hypoxic state reduces the capacity of irradiated bone to meet its metabolic demands resulting in necrosis of bone and sequestra formation. Secondary infection also plays an important role in the pathogenesis of ORN. The various risk factors associated with development of ORN include total radiation dosage, field size, poor oral hygiene, and presence of dental disease. ORN is likely to occur if the dose is higher than 65–75Gy. Clinically, the patients present with mucositis, ulceration, and exposure of necrotic bone. There may be associated soft-tissue

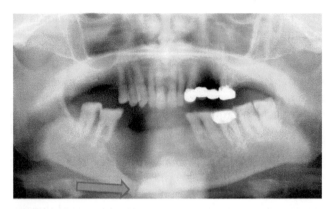

FIGURE 24.16
Osteoradionecrosis. OPG shows lytic destruction with fragmentation of the mandible in the midline. This patient had history of radiation therapy for the advanced carcinoma of the buccal mucosa.

swelling. Other manifestations include pus discharge, pathologic fracture, and orocutaneous fistula.

Mandibular ORN is radiologically characterized by loss of trabeculations and interruptions in the cortical margins of mandible [51]. Panoramic radiographs and CT show mixed lytic and sclerotic areas and pathologic fracture (Figure 24.16). Bone fragments or sequestra are also noted. Intra-osseous air is often seen, which may be due to trapping of air secondary to ulcers, fistulas in soft tissue, or secondary infection. In few patients, soft-tissue swelling and enhancement may be seen surrounding the abnormal bone. Such enhancement is common around the fracture site; however, it may occur in patients even without pathologic fracture. In some patients, ORN can be seen in other sites than the primary tumor, which are exposed to radiation.

In the absence of soft tissue, the osseous changes such as loss of trabeculations, cortical interruption, and bone fragmentation are suggestive of ORN. When there is associated soft-tissue mass, ORN is often confused with recurrence of primary tumor. Most tumor recurrences appear within the first 2 years following treatment, whereas ORN is a late complication and is seen 1–2 years after radiation therapy. When the bone destruction and associated soft-tissue mass is situated at a different site than the primary tumor, a tumor recurrence is less likely.

24.6 Dental Implant Imaging

Dental implant candidates are preoperatively evaluated to determine bone quantity (whether sufficient to accept an implant), precise location of the mandibular canal, maxillary sinuses, and incisive foramen (damage to these vital structures lead to complications).

Conventionally, this assessment relied on several intraoral and extraoral radiographs, panoramic images, and motion tomography [52]. Obvious limitations of these techniques were 2D information and severe distortion, making accurate measurements difficult [53].

The most accurate technique for preoperative evaluation of dental implantation is dental CT [54]. This is because of the ability of this technique to quantify bone in three dimensions, precisely locate adjacent anatomic structures (mandibular canal, dental inferior nerve, incisive foramen, mental foramen, maxillary sinus), and provide information about the quality of available bone.

Basic technique for CT is the same as discussed in Section 24.1. After acquisition of axial data, dental reconstructions used for preoperative evaluation include (1) curved planar reformation (curved MPRs)—sagittal oblique images are most important and (2) panoramic images.

Curved MPRs: The plane and location for reformation is identified on one of the axial images of the maxilla or mandible (Figure 24.17). The axial image for this purpose is obtained approximately at the level of the tooth roots; in patients with edentulism, axial image should be obtained at a level where gum is shown completely. By the application of special software, several contiguous points are placed throughout the center of the mandible or maxilla. These points are connected by the program to generate the curve. The perpendicular lines marked along the superimposed curve indicate the position of the sagittal oblique reformatted images. The numbering of these lines typically starts from the right posterior zone and ends in the left posterior zone; however, the parameters can vary slightly from program to program.

Sagittal oblique images: These are the most important component of dental CT, as they provide detailed information about the shape, angulation, height, and thickness of the alveolar bone. This information is important for implant planning. More than 100 images may be generated that are numbered from right to left.

Panoramic images: The panoramic images are created from superimposed curves (Figure 24.18). From this reformation, several images are generated from back to front on either side of the midline (three in our scanner). Thus, a total of seven images are generated each having a section thickness of 1 mm with a 1-mm interval between consecutive images.

Factors that can lead to implant failure include substandard fixtures, inadequate bone quality, nerve impingement, or infection [54]. Postimplantation imaging, thus, play a role as vital as in preoperative evaluation as it can identify a specific cause of implant failure. For this indication too, CT is the method of choice, and radiographic evaluation remains inadequate.

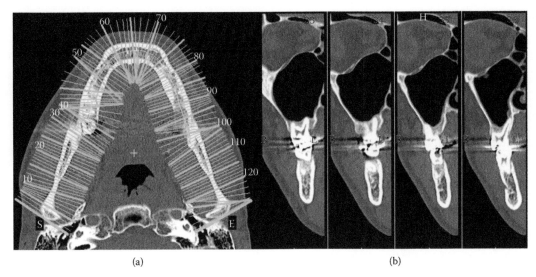

(a) (b)

FIGURE 24.17
Dental implant imaging: sagittal reformatted images. (a) Planning of sagittal oblique reformatted images on an axial image obtained at the level of roots of teeth. A curved central line (yellow) is obtained by joining several dots marked along the mandible. Perpendicular lines (green) are then generated starting from the right side (S). These lines represent the level of the sagittal reformatted images as shown in (b). The numbers marked (33–36) on the stack of four images in (b) represent the position of the perpendicular lines (green) in (a).

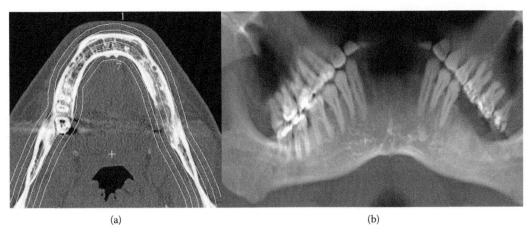

(a) (b)

FIGURE 24.18
Panoramic reconstruction (a) shows the planning of panoramic images. A curved line is placed on an axial image at the same level as for the sagittal reformatted images. Several curved lines (yellow) are generated by the software. A total of seven panoramic images are generated. One of the representative images is shown in (b). This image corresponds to line 3 in (a).

24.7 Temporomandibular Joint Imaging

Temporomandibular joint (TMJ) is a complex articulation that is essential for speech and mastication. A wide variety of disorders (congenital, traumatic, inflammatory, and rarely neoplastic) can affect this joint. The symptoms of TMJ disorders include pain, facial asymmetry, impaired mouth opening, and/or malocclusion. Internal derangement is the most common abnormality of TMJ [55]. It refers to an abnormal relationship, positional as well as functional between the disk and articulating surfaces. Other two conditions that account for the rest of TMJ pathology include trauma and inflammatory arthritis. An important

sequel of TMJ disorders is ankylosis. Various imaging modalities available for evaluation of TMJ include plain radiography, ultrasonography (USG), CT, and MRI.

Conventional radiography is widely available and inexpensive and hence widely used. However, it is far inferior to CT in the evaluation of TMJ. USG has a role in the assessment of the jaw in suspected cases of internal derangement or inflammation; however, use of this modality is indicated by interobserver variability and advent of MDCT and MRI. MDCT has revolutionized imaging in trauma around the skull. Short scan times and volumetric acquisition with MPRs allow CT to play a key role in the assessment of jaw trauma and concomitant osseous injuries. CT also plays an important role in the evaluation

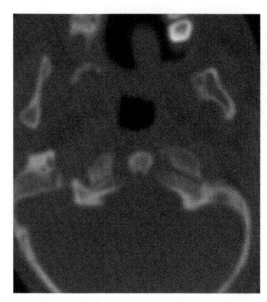

FIGURE 24.19
Mandibular hypoplasia. Axial CT shows hypoplastic left mandible. This 3-year-old girl had other multiple craniofacial anomalies including left external auditory canal and middle hypoplasia, nonpneumatized left mastoid and parotid hypoplasia.

of TMJ arthritides and ankylosis. However, there is little role of CT in the evaluation of internal derangement; MRI is the modality of choice for this indication.

24.7.1 Congenital Disorders

24.7.1.1 Hemifacial Microsomia (Goldenhar Syndrome or Oculo–Auriculo–Vertebral Syndrome)

It is the second most common developmental craniofacial anomaly after cleft lip and palate [7]. Craniofacial involvement is characterized by incomplete development of the ear, nose, soft palate, lip, and mandible. Asymmetric development of the mandible is a diagnostic hallmark of this syndrome.

24.7.1.2 Nonsyndromic Congenital Mandibular Hypoplasia

Mandibular hypoplasia can be congenital or acquired. Congenital hypoplasia results from maldevelopment of the first and second branchial arches (Figure 24.19). Acquired causes include radiation damage, trauma, and hemifacial atrophy. MDCT is valuable in making the diagnosis and surgical planning.

24.7.2 Condylar Hyperplasia

Condylar hyperplasia is a characterized by persistent or accelerated growth of the condyle. It affects young patients. Unilateral condylar enlargement can cause malocclusion and facial asymmetry (Figure 24.20). CT

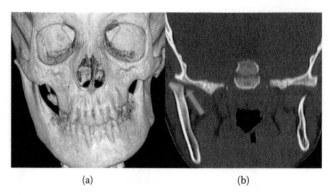

(a)   (b)

FIGURE 24.20
Mandibular hyperplasia. Volume-rendered technique (a) shows asymmetry of the mandible with subtle deviation towards left side. Coronal CT (b) shows hyperplasia of the right mandibular condyle (arrow).

plays an important role in differentiating condylar hyperplasia from chondroma, and osteochondroma may cause similar symptoms and signs.

24.7.3 Trauma

Road traffic accidents, assaults, falls, and sporting injuries account for the majority of cases of mandibular fractures. Condylar process fractures account for 25% of all mandibular fractures. These are classified into fractures of condylar neck and condylar head (extracapsular or intracapsular). Assessment of the type and grade of displacement of bony structures is important in treatment planning. MDCT is the modality of choice. [56]. It allows evaluation of the entire mandible, TMJ, and the maxilla including maxillary sinuses. There are three main types of condylar fractures: diacapitular fracture (i.e., through the head of the condyle), fracture of the condylar neck, and fracture of the condylar base [57]. Fractures of the condylar head are classified as intracapsular or extracapsular; and displaced or undisplaced. CT evaluation enables the radiologist to assess the type and grade of displacement of bony structures, angulation of the fractured fragments, presence of vertical compression, and damage to the soft-tissue structures of the joint. Sequel of trauma include functional disturbances, pain, ankylosis, and degenerative arthritis. Identification of these complications also requires imaging.

24.7.4 Inflammation

Rheumatoid arthritis is the most common inflammatory disease involving the TMJ. Gout, psoriatic arthritis, ankylosing spondylitis, and systemic lupus erythematosus can rarely involve the TMJ. CT plays an important role in the demonstartion of joint space narrowing, cartilage destruction, erosions, and long-term complication of bony ankylosis.

24.7.5 TMJ Ankylosis

Ankylosis refers to fixation or fusion of the joint causing chronic, painless restriction of joint movements. Causes of TMJ ankylosis include trauma, infection, inflammatory arthritis (rheumatoid arthritis, ankylosing spondylitis), and surgery. TMJ ankylosis can be classified into two categories: type I showing medial angulatation of condyle with deformity of articular fossa and a mild-to-moderate amount of new bone formation; and type II with no recognizable condyle or fossa (Figure 24.21) but instead a large mass of new bone [58]. TMJ ankylosis is treated surgically by excision of the ankylosis, with or without graft replacement. Preoperative measurement of the dimensions of the condylar mass is essential for surgical planning. MDCT plays an indispensable role in this evaluation.

24.7.6 Maxillofacial Trauma

Imaging plays an essential role in the pre- and postoperative evaluation of maxillofacial trauma. Plain radiographs play a limited role in the evaluation of injuries in this region, considering the complex 3D anatomy. This is easily overcome with the use of CT. The benefits of CT are already well established in many dental specialties, and several studies have supported the use of CT to the management of trauma to the maxillofacial skeleton. Current MDCT techniques are optimal for fast scanning in the emergency setting. More importantly, the current CT applications provide high-resolution 3D reconstructions that are very important for management planning. The high radiation dose, cost, and limited availability are some limitations to the widespread application of

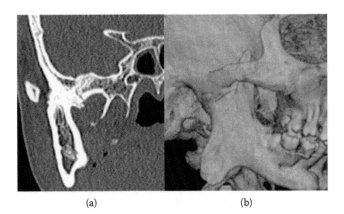

(a)   (b)

FIGURE 24.21
Temporomandibular joint (TMJ) ankylosis. Coronal CT (a) and volume-rendered technique (b) reveal complete loss of right TMJ space with deformity and sclerosis, both of the condyle and the glenoid fossa.

this tool. Recently, CBCT has appeared as an alternative to CT in the trauma setting. CBCT could substantially alter the manner that patients who have potentially complex traumatic fractures are managed [59].

References

1. Dunfee BL, Sakai O, Pistey R, Gohel A. Radiologic and pathologic characteristics of benign and malignant lesions of the mandible. *Radiographics*. 2006;26(6):1751–1768.
2. Kramer IRH, Pindborg JJ, Shear M, eds. Histological typing of odontogenic tumours. In: *World Health Organization—International Histological Classification of Tumours*. 2nd ed. Berlin, Germany: Springer-Verlag, 1992;1–42.
3. Ferreira Júnior O, Damante JH, Lauris JR. Simple bone cyst versus odontogenic keratocyst: differential diagnosis by digitized panoramic radiography. *Dento Maxilla Fac Radiol*. 2004;33(6):373–378.
4. DelBalso AM. An approach to the diagnostic imaging of jaw lesions, dental implants, and the temporomandibular joint. *Radiol Clin North Am*. 1998;36(5):855–890.
5. Bernaerts A, Vanhoenacker FM, Hintjens J, Chapelle K, DeSchepper AM. Imaging approach for differential diagnosis of jaw lesions: a quick reference guide. *JBR-BTR*. 2006;89(1):43–46.
6. Neyaz Z, Gadodia A, Gamanagatti S, Mukhopadhyay S. Radiographical approach to jaw lesions. *Singapore Med J*. 2008;49(2):165–176.
7. Yoshiura K, Weber AL, Scrivani SJ. Cystic lesions of the mandible and maxilla. *Neuroimaging Clin N Am*. 2003;13(3):485–494.
8. Boeddinghaus R, Whyte A. Current concepts in maxillofacial imaging. *Eur J Radiol*. 2008;66(3):396–418.
9. Weber AL, Kaneda T, Scrivani SJ et al. Cysts, tumors, and nontumorous lesions of the jaw. In: Som PM, Curtin HD, eds. *Head and Neck Imaging*. 4th ed. St Louis, MO: Mosby, 2003;930–994.
10. Scholl RJ, Kellett HM, Neumann DP, Lurie AG. Cysts and cystic lesions of the mandible: clinical and radiologic-histopathologic review. *Radiographics*. 1999;19(5):1107–1124.
11. Barnes L, Reichart P, Eveson JW, Sidransky D. *WHO Classification of Tumours: Pathology and Genetics of Head and Neck Tumours*. Lyon, France: IARC Press, 2005.
12. Miles DA, Kaugars GE, Van Dis M, Lovas JG. *Oral and Maxillo Facial Radiology*. Philadelphia, PA: Saunders, 1991.
13. MacDonald-Jankowski DS. Keratocystic odontogenic tumour: systematic review. *Dentomaxillofac Radiol*. 2011;40(1):1–23.
14. Mraiwa N, Jacobs R, Van Cleynenbreugel J et al. The nasopalatine canal revisited using 2D and 3D CT imaging. *Dentomaxillofac Radiol*. 2004;33(6):396–402.
15. Theodorou SJ, Theodorou DJ, Sartoris DJ. Imaging characteristics of neoplasms and other lesions of the jawbones. Part 2. Odontogenic tumor-mimickers and tumor-like lesions. *Clin Imaging*. 2007;31:120–126.

16. Capote-Moreno A, Acero J, García-Recuero I, Ruiz J, Serrano R, de Paz V. Giant aneurysmal bone cyst of the mandible with unusual presentation. *Med Oral Patol Oral Cir Bucal.* 2009;14:E137–E140.

17. Cortell-Ballester I, Figueiredo R, Berini-Aytés L, Gay-Escoda C. Traumatic bone cyst: a retrospective study of 21 cases. *Med Oral Patol Oral Cir Bucal.* 2009;14:E239–E243.

18. Suomalainen A, Apajalahti S, Kuhlefelt M, Hagstrom J. Simple bone cyst: a radiological dilemma. *Dentomaxillofac Radiol.* 2009;38:174–177.

19. Shimizu M, Osa N, Okamura K, Yoshiura K. CT analysis of the Stafne's bone defects of the mandible. *Dentomaxillofac Radiol.* 2006;35:95–102.

20. Kaneda T, Minami M, Kurabayashi T. Benign odontogenic tumors of the mandible and maxilla. *Neuroimaging Clin N Am.* 2003;13(3):495–507.

21. Minami M, Kaneda T, Yamamoto H et al. Ameloblastoma in the maxillomandibular region: MR imaging. *Radiology.* 1992;184(2):389–393.

22. Gupta N, Saxena S, Rathod VC, Aggarwal P. Unicystic ameloblastoma of the mandible. *J Oral Maxillofac Pathol.* 2011;15(2):228–231.

23. Thompson IO, van Rensburg LJ, Phillips VM. Desmoplastic ameloblastoma: correlative histopathology, radiology and CT-MR imaging. *J Oral Pathol Med.* 1996;25:405–410.

24. Berger AJ, Son J, Desai NK. Malignant ameloblastoma: concurrent presentation of primary and distant disease and review of the literature. *J Oral Maxillofac Surg.* 2012;24:212–213.

25. MacDonald-Jankowski DS, Yeung RW, Li T, Lee KM. Computed tomography of odontogenic myxoma. *Clin Radiol.* 2004;59(3):281–287.

26. Asaumi J, Matsuzaki H, Hisatomi M, Konouchi H, Shigehara H, Kishi K. Application of dynamic MRI to differentiating odontogenic myxomas from ameloblastomas. *Eur J Radiol.* 2002;43(1):37–41.

27. Murphey MD, Nomikos GC, Flemming DJ, Gannon FH, Temple HT, Kransdorf MJ. From the archives of AFIP. Imaging of giant cell tumor and giant cell reparative granuloma of bone: radiologic-pathologic correlation. *Radiographics.* 2001;21(5):1283–1309.

28. Jadu FM, Pharoah MJ, Lee L, Baker GI, Allidina A. Central giant cell granuloma of the mandibular condyle: a case report and review of the literature. *Dentomaxillofac Radiol.* 2011;40(1):60–64.

29. Zlotogorski A, Buchner A, Kaffe I, Schwartz-Arad D. Radiological features of central haemangioma of the jaws. *Dentomaxillofac Radiol.* 2005;34(5):292–296.

30. Nagpal A, Suhas S, Ahsan A, Pai K, Rao N. Central haemangioma: variance in radiographic appearance. *Dentomaxillofac Radiol.* 2005;34(2):120–125.

31. Gadodia A, Seith A, Sharma R, Choudhury AR, Bhutia O, Gupta A. Multidetector computed tomography of jaw lesions in children and adolescents. *J Med Imaging Radiat Oncol.* 2010;54(2):111–119.

32. Suomalainen A, Hietanen J, Robinson S, Peltola JS. Ameloblastic carcinoma of the mandible resembling odontogenic cyst in a panoramic radiograph. *Oral Surg Oral Med Oral Pathol Oral Radiol Endod* 2006;101:638–642.

33. Ram H, Mohammad S, Husain N, Gupta PN. Ameloblastic carcinoma. *J Maxillofac Oral Surg.* 2010;9(4):415–419. Epub 2011 Mar 17.

34. Weber AL, Bui C, Kaneda T. Malignant tumors of the mandible and maxilla. *Neuroimaging Clin N Am.* 2003;13(3):509–524.

35. Pisano JJ, Coupland R, Chen SY, Miller AS. Plasmacytoma of the oral cavity and jaws: a clinicopathologic study of 13 cases. *Oral Surg Oral Med Oral Pathol Oral Radiol Endod* 1997;83:265–271.

36. Singh N, Sahai S, Singh S, Singh S. Calcifying epithelial odontogenic tumor (Pindborg tumor). *Natl J Maxillofac Surg.* 2011;2(2):225–227.

37. Venkateswarlu M, Geetha P, Lakshmi Kavitha N. CT imaging findings of a calcifying epithelial odontogenic tumour. *Br J Radiol.* 2012;85(1009):e14–e16.

38. Sumi M, Yonetsu K, Nakamura T. CT of ameloblastic fibroodontoma. *AJR Am J Roentgenol.* 1997;169(2):599–600.

39. Batra P, Prasad S, Parkash H. Adenomatoid odontogenic tumour: review and case report. *J Can Dent Assoc.* 2005;71(4):250–253.

40. Mafee MF, Yang G, Tseng A, Keiler L, Andrus K. Fibro-osseous and giant cell lesions, including brown tumor of the mandible, maxilla, and other craniofacial bones. *Neuroimaging Clin N Am.* 2003;13(3):525–540.

41. MacDonald-Jankowski D. Fibrous dysplasia: a systematic review. *Dentomaxillofac Radiol.* 2009;38(4):196–215.

42. Macdonald-Jankowski DS, Li TK. Fibrous dysplasia in a Hong Kong community: the clinical and radiological features and outcomes of treatment. *Dentomaxillofac Radiol.* 2009;38(2):63–72.

43. More C, Thakkar K, Asrani M. Cemento-ossifying fibroma. *Indian J Dent Res.* 2011;2(2):352–355.

44. Rinaggio J, Land M, Cleveland DB. Juvenile ossifying fibroma of the mandible. *J Pediatr Surg.* 2003;38(4):648–650.

45. Alsufyani NA, Lam EW. Cemento-osseous dysplasia of the jaw bones: key radiographic features. *Dentomaxillofac Radiol.* 2011;40(3):141–146.

46. Yonetsu K, Nakamura T. CT of calcifying jaw bone diseases. *AJR Am J Roentgenol.* 2001;177(4):937–943.

47. Johann AC, deFreitas JB, deAguiar MC, deAraújo NS, Mesquita RA. Peripheral osteoma of the mandible: case report and review of the literature. *J Cranio Maxillofac Surg.* 2005;33(4):276–281.

48. Fonseca LC, Kodama NK, Nunes FC, Maciel PH, Fonseca FA, Roitberg M. Radiographic assessment of Gardner's syndrome. *Dentomaxillofac Radiol.* 2007;36(2):121–124.

49. Yoshiura K, Hijiya T, Ariji E. Radiographic patterns of osteomyelitis in the mandible: plain film/CT correlation. *Oral Surg Oral Med Oral Pathol* 1994;78:116–124.

50. Schuknecht B, Valavanis A. Osteomyelitis of the mandible. *Neuroimaging Clin N Am.* 2003;13(3):605–618.

51. Hermans R. Imaging of mandibular osteoradionecrosis. *Neuroimaging Clin N Am.* 2003;13(3):597–604.

52. Lam EW, Ruprecht A, Yang J. Comparison of two-dimensional orthoradially reformatted computed tomography and panoramic radiography for dental implant treatment planning. *J Prosthet Dent.* 1995;74(1):42–46.

53. Matteson SR, Deahl ST, Alder ME, Nummikoski PV. Advanced imaging methods. *Crit Rev Oral Biol Med.* 1996;7(4):346–395.

54. Saavedra-Abril JA, Balhen-Martin C, Zaragoza-Velasco K, Kimura-Hayama T, Saavedra S, Stoopen ME. Dental multisection CT for the placement of oral implants: technique and applications. *Radiographics* 2010; 30:1975–1991.

55. Sommer JO, Aigner F, Rudisch A, Gruber H, Fritsch H, Millesi W, Stiskal M. Cross-sectional and functional imaging of the temporomandibular joint: radiology, pathology, and basic biomechanics of the jaw. *Radiographics* 2003;23:e14.

56. Som PM, Curtin HD. *Head and Neck Imaging*. St Louis, MO: Mosby, 2003.

57. Cenzi R, Burlini D, Arduin L, Zollino I, Guidi R, Carinci F. Mandibular condyle fractures: evaluation of the strasbourg osteosynthesis research group classification. *J Cranio Fac Surg.* 2009;20:24–28.

58. Aggarwal S, Mukhopadhyay S, Berry M, Bhargava S. Bony ankylosis of the temporomandibular joint: a computed tomography study. *Oral Surg Oral Med Oral Pathol Oral Radiol.* 1990;69(1):128–132.

59. Shintaku WH, Venturin JS, Azevedo B, Noujeim M. Applications of cone-beam computed tomography in fractures of the maxillofacial complex. *Dent Traumatol.* 2009;25:358–366.

25

Dual Energy Computed Tomography: Tissue Characterization

Thomas Flohr and Bernhard Schmidt

CONTENTS

25.1 Principle

Imaging with computed tomography (CT) shows the patient's anatomy in great detail, with excellent spatial resolution and good low-contrast detectability, however, it cannot provide information about the chemical composition of the examined structures. CT is only sensitive to the x-ray attenuation coefficients μ of the examined objects—these are shown as gray-scale differences, scaled in Hounsfield units (HU), in a CT image. Tissues of different chemical composition, but with the same μ, will appear with the same Hounsfield number in the image. As an example, calcified plaques in a vessel can often not be differentiated from the surrounding lumen in the presence of iodinated contrast agent.

This ambiguity is caused by the dependence of the x-ray attenuation coefficient μ in a voxel on both, the mass attenuation coefficient $(\mu/\rho)(E,Z)$ of the material, which is a function of energy E and its atomic number Z, and its mass density ρ.

$$\mu = \frac{\mu}{\rho}(E,Z) \cdot \rho \qquad (25.1)$$

Different materials with different mass attenuation coefficients $(\mu/\rho)(E,Z)$ can show the same attenuation coefficient μ in a CT measurement depending on the value of the mass density ρ.

Additional information obtained by measurements at different x-ray energies E can help to overcome this limitation. Alvarez and Macovski observed that in the typical energy range of the CT x-ray spectra, ranging from 30 to 140 keV, only two absorption processes are relevant, the Compton effect and the photoelectric effect [1]. Both processes have a characteristic energy dependence that is almost independent of the atomic number Z. The mass attenuation coefficient $(\mu/\rho)(E,Z)$ of each material as a function of the photon energy E can be expressed as a linear combination of the pure Compton and pure photo effect cross sections. This model only holds for elements with a K-edge of photo absorption outside the energy range of the CT x-ray spectra. This is fulfilled for the tissues of a human body. The K-edge for iodine in contrast agents at 33 keV is still below the used x-ray photon energies.

As a consequence of the model, all materials and also compounds or mixtures can be decomposed into Compton and photo absorption components. Moreover, $(\mu/\rho)(E)$ of any material can be decomposed into a linear combination of $(\mu/\rho)_1(E)$ and $(\mu/\rho)_2(E)$ of two base materials, 1 and 2, which differ in their photoelectric and Compton characteristics.

The relative contributions of these two base materials to each voxel of interest can be determined, if the x-ray absorption by the object of interest is measured with two different spectra.

25.2 Techniques to Acquire Dual Energy Data

There are several methods to acquire CT data with spectral information. Today's medical CT systems are equipped with solid-state detectors. A scintillation crystal or a ceramic scintillator absorb the x-rays and convert them into visible light, which is then detected by a Si photo diode attached to the backside of the scintillator. These detectors integrate the x-ray flux over the measurement time of a projection (also referred to as reading), with a weighting factor proportional to the energy of the absorbed x-ray quanta. As a consequence, they do not provide energy resolution, and the use of different x-ray spectra is mandatory to acquire spectral CT data. In CT, different x-ray spectra can be realized by using different kV-setting of the x-ray tube. In a standard CT system, the kV-setting of the x-ray tube can be changed either between different CT scans (slow kV-switching), or more rapidly, ideally between the different projections of a CT scan (fast kV-switching). An alternative is the use of dual source CT (DSCT) systems with two x-ray tubes and two corresponding detectors offset by about 90°, which have the potential to acquire dual energy data by operating both x-ray tubes simultaneously at different kV-settings.

Energy-resolving detectors enable the acquisition of spectral CT data with a single polychromatic x-ray spectrum. Pertinent examples are dual layer detectors consisting of two conventional scintillation detectors on top of each other, and direct converting photon counting detectors. So far, only prototype CT systems relying on both detector technologies have been realized. In particular, photon counting detectors are a promising technology for future CT systems.

The most straightforward approach to acquire dual energy CT data is by means of two consecutive axial scans of the same anatomy, one with low tube potential (e.g., 80 kV), the other with high tube potential (e.g., 140 kV). To reduce the time shift between both scans, they can be performed as partial scans (see Figure 25.1).

Another simple method is the use of two consecutive spiral/helical scans of the same anatomy, at different kV-settings and preferably at high pitch for short overall acquisition times. Most commonly 80 and 140 kV are used, because these are typically the lowest and highest kV-settings of a CT x-ray tube, which provide best spectral separation.

The spectral separation achieved with this approach is good. Spectrally resolved CT data can be acquired with standard CT systems, in the full scan field of view

(SFOV) of the respective CT detectors, which is typically 50 cm in diameter. As a downside, the long time interval of at least half a second between the two scans hampers the evaluation of moving organs. Furthermore, dual energy applications requiring iodinated-contrast agent, such as the calculation of iodine maps are very limited because of the varying density of the contrast agent between the two scans.

In clinical practice, slow kV-switching can be used for dual energy imaging in "static" situations, for example, for the characterization of different types of kidney stones, for the differential diagnosis of gout, or for the calculation of monoenergetic images to reduce metal artifacts at a metal-specific high energy (see Figure 25.2).

In a more refined approach, the kV-setting of the x-ray tube is rapidly switched between consecutive projections of the same axial or spiral scan (see Figure 25.3).

Rapid kV-switching was already implemented in a medical CT scanner in 1986 [2] to obtain pseudo-monoenergetic or material specific images. Technical limitations and the lack of clinically relevant applications at those times, however, prevented the routine use of this technology. Meanwhile, with the ongoing process of scanner technology, rapid kV-switching has seen a revival [3].

Rapid kV-switching allows the use of raw data-based dual energy algorithms. Dual energy scans can be performed in the full SFOV of the respective CT scanner. The nearly simultaneous acquisition of low-energy and high-energy projections prevents registration problems because

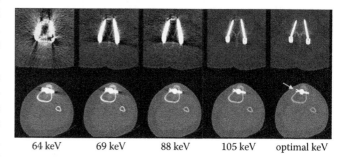

| 64 keV | 69 keV | 88 keV | 105 keV | optimal keV |

FIGURE 25.2
Example of a clinically relevant application of slow kV-switching. Two consecutive spiral scans at 80 kV and at 140 kV are used to compute pseudo-monoenergetic images, with the goal of metal artifact reduction at a metal-specific high energy.

140 kV   Switch kV and mA for equal dose   80 kV

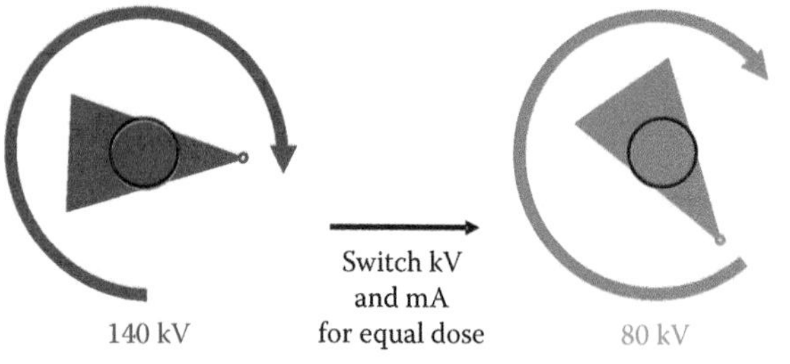

FIGURE 25.1
Principle of slow kV-switching to acquire dual energy CT data.

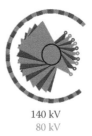

140 kV
80 kV

FIGURE 25.3
Principle of rapid kV-switching to acquire dual energy CT data.

of organ motion or contrast agent dynamics. However, as a downside, the switching time between low and high kV is in the order of a quarter to half a millisecond. Therefore, to acquire a sufficient number of projections at both kV-settings (>800), the method is limited to slower rotation times (0.6 seconds). Furthermore, current tube technology allows switching the voltage between consecutive readings, but not the tube current. Equal dose at 80 and 140 kV can only be achieved if each 80 kV reading is a factor 3–4 longer than the corresponding 140 kV reading. This additionally reduces the number of projections per rotation. Another drawback is the fixed and relatively high tube current that is required to obtain stable switching between both tube potentials (in terms of undershoots and overshoots of both voltage and current, stable shape and size of the focal spot). In one realization, a fixed tube current of 600 mA has to be applied [3,4]. Radiation dose can only be adapted to the clinical application by variation of the spiral pitch and the rotation time.

Dual energy scanning based on rapid kV-switching was commercially introduced by one vendor under the trade name "Gemstone spectral imaging." Its clinical applicability has meanwhile been shown in several studies [3–8] (see Figure 25.4).

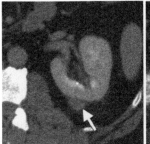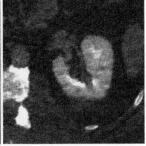

FIGURE 25.4
Example of a contrast-enhanced dual energy kidney scan acquired with fast kV-switching technology. Left: Axial monochromatic 75 keV image shows a 1.8 cm lesion with attenuation of 57 HU along the posterior aspect of the left kidney (arrow). Right: Iodine-density image from iodine–water material-density image pair generated from the same dual energy CT data indicates a lack of iodine enhancement, which is characteristic for a cyst. (From Kaza RK, Platt JF, Cohan RH, Caoili EM, Al-Hawary MM, Wasnik A, *RadioGraphics*, 2:353–369, 2012. With permission.)

Finally, dual energy data can be acquired with DSCT systems. A DSCT is a CT system with two x-ray tubes and the corresponding detectors. Both measurement systems operate simultaneously and acquire scan data at the same anatomical level of the patient (same z-position).

In 2006, the first DSCT was commercially introduced by one vendor (see Figure 25.5).

The two acquisition systems are mounted onto the rotating gantry with an angular offset of 90° for the first-generation DSCT [9] resp. and 95° for the second generation DSCT. Detector A covers the full SFOV of 50 cm diameter, whereas detector B only covers a smaller FOV as a consequence of space limitations on the gantry (26 resp. 33 cm). The shortest gantry rotation time is 0.33 resp. 0.28 seconds. Each of the two rotating envelope x-ray tubes can be operated with independent kV- and mA-settings.

DSCT systems provide significantly improved temporal resolution for cardiothoracic imaging. The shortest data acquisition time for an image corresponds to a quarter of the gantry rotation time [9]. For $t_{rot} = 0.33$ seconds, the temporal resolution of a DSCT system is $t_{rot}/4 = 83$ milliseconds. For the second generation DSCT with $t_{rot} = 0.28$ seconds it is 75 milliseconds, slightly more than a quarter of the gantry rotation time because of the increased angle between both measurement systems (95°). Meanwhile, several clinical studies have shown the potential of DSCT to reliably perform coronary CT angiographic studies also in patients with high and irregular heart rates [10–14].

With a DSCT system, dual energy data can be acquired by simultaneously operating both x-ray tubes at different kV-settings, for example, 80 and 140 kV. The scan parameters can be individually adjusted for both measurement systems, resulting in a flexible choice of scan protocols. The maximum temporal resolution in dual energy mode is half the gantry rotation time, 165 resp. 140 ms, because each of the measurement systems needs to acquire a half-scan data interval. Optimization of the spectral separation is possible by introducing additional prefiltration into the 140 kV beam, for example, by means

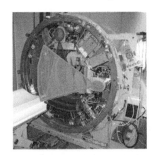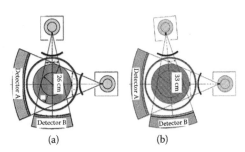

(a)   (b)

FIGURE 25.5
DSCT system with two independent measurement systems. (a) First generation. The system angle between both measurement systems is 90°. (b) Second generation. To increase the SFOV of detector B, a larger system angle of 95° was chosen.

of a filter that can be moved into the beam when needed and moved out for standard applications. An additional tin filter with a thickness of 0.4 mm shifts the mean energy of the 140 kV spectrum behind the bow-tie filter from 69 to 89 keV (see Figure 25.6). The mean energy of the 80 kV spectrum is 52 keV. The tin filter has several benefits. It increases the spectral separation between the low- and the high-energy spectrum, it narrows the 140 kV spectrum (which results in better dose efficiency and less beam hardening artifacts), and it reduces cross-scattering. Primak et al. [15] found that adding tin filtration to the high-kV tube improved the dual energy contrast between iodine and calcium as much as 290%.

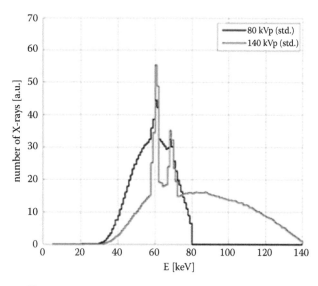

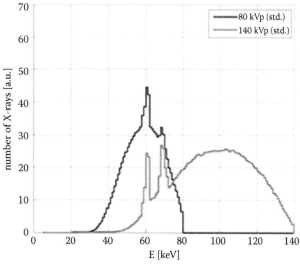

FIGURE 25.6
Standard 80 kV and 140 kV spectra (top). The mean energy of the 140 kV spectrum is 69 keV. 80 kV spectrum and 140 kV spectrum with additional 0.4 mm tin prefiltration (bottom). Note the shift to higher energies. The mean energy is now 89 keV. (Courtesy of S. Kappler, Siemens Healthcare, Forchheim, Germany.)

As a downside, dual energy evaluation with a DSCT is limited to a smaller central SFOV (26 resp. 33 cm diameter). Raw data-based dual energy algorithms are difficult to realize, because high-energy and low-energy projections are not simultaneously acquired at the same z-position. Dual energy algorithms are therefore image-based. Cross-scattered radiation has to be carefully corrected for in order not to degrade the stability of the Hounsfield numbers and—as a consequence—the quality of the image based dual energy evaluation. Furthermore, images of moving objects show slightly different motion artifacts because of the 90° offset between both measurement systems, which may result in registration problems.

Meanwhile, several studies have shown the potential of dual energy scanning with DSCT. Clinical applications include tissue characterization, classification of kidney stones, differential diagnosis of gout, calcium quantification, calculation of pseudo-monochromatic images, and virtual noncontrast images, and quantification of the local blood volume in contrast enhanced scans, in the abdomen as well as in the lungs or in the myocardium [16–28].

25.3 Raw Data-Based versus Image-Based Dual Energy Algorithms

In CT, the line integrals $p = -\ln(I/I_0)$ of the object's x-ray attenuation are measured. I_0 is the primary intensity of the x-ray beam, I is the attenuated density after passing the object. For each ray from the x-ray source to the corresponding detector element, p can be expressed as the sum of two base materials 1 and 2, with

$$p(E) = \left(\frac{\mu}{\rho}\right)_1 (E) \cdot \rho_1 \cdot d_1 + \left(\frac{\mu}{\rho}\right)_2 (E) \cdot \rho_2 \cdot d_2 \quad (25.2)$$

where $\rho_i \cdot d_i$ represents the area density (in g/cm²) of material i. Measuring p at two different x-ray tube voltages allows for the characterization of the two materials. For monochromatic spectra this is achieved by solving the resulting two linear equations for the area densities, whereas for polychromatic spectra a complex but monotonous two-dimensional function has to be inverted [29].

The raw data- or projection data-based approach can then be used to synthesize quasi-monochromatic raw data of the scanned object. Depending on the values selected for the attenuation coefficients μ_1 and

μ_2 of the base materials (most commonly water and Ca, or water and iodine), either material selective or pseudo-monochromatic images free of beam-hardening artifacts can be generated [30]. Many researchers have aimed at expanding and refining raw data-based material decomposition, and it is often claimed that image-based methods are strongly limited by the problem of beam hardening.

However, under conditions that are typically fulfilled in modern CT systems image-based methods are practically equivalent for clinical tasks.

One prerequisite for image-based material decomposition is the validity of the so-called thin absorber model. If we use, for example, water and iodine as the basis materials for image-based dual energy evaluation, the maximum x-ray attenuation coefficient $\mu_I(E)$ and the maximum thickness d_I of the iodine along any measured ray path is expected to be so small that it is valid to assume a linear contribution of the additional nonwater-like attenuation $\mu_I(E)\,d_I$ to the total attenuation. It can be shown that the thin absorber model holds for iodine samples up to 5000 HU·cm in water, which corresponds to the clinical situation of an object with 200 HU iodine enhancement and 25 cm thickness.

In addition, the thin absorber model is based on the concept of an "effective spectrum": the measured absorption is independent of the spatial distribution of the traversed materials along the beam. This means in practice that neither the CT-value of water nor the CT-value of a small iodine sample depends on its position within the scanned object. This is achieved if the scanner is equipped with a bowtie filter of sufficient beam hardening and if the approximately cylindrical patient cross section is centered within the SFOV. In practice, electronics noise, scanner calibration, stability of emitted spectra, cone beam effects, and scattered radiation can have a larger impact on the obtained results than the analysis method.

25.4 Applications

We will focus on image-based techniques for dual energy processing. As shown above, raw data-based algorithms and image-based algorithms are practically equivalent under typical clinical operating conditions. It should be pointed out, however, that image-based dual energy algorithms—unlike raw data-based algorithms—do not automatically remove beam hardening effects, but rely on accurate beam hardening corrections being applied before image reconstruction.

25.4.1 Viewing of Dual Energy Images

A very simple way of processing dual energy data is a linear combination, that is, a weighted subtraction or weighted addition, of the images that are separately reconstructed at the two different beam energies.

By weighted subtraction, material selective images can be obtained equivalent to a base material decomposition in raw data space. Weighted addition has the potential to maximize the contrast-to-noise ratio in case of a contrast-enhanced scan, or to minimize image noise, depending on the relative contribution of the low kV image [31]. Linear combination of low kV and high kV images is also used to restore a more familiar image appearance similar to a standard 120 kV scan. More advanced techniques apply nonlinear blending to contrast-enhanced dual energy images [32]. The higher the CT number of a pixel, the larger is the contribution of the low kV image to that pixel. In areas without contrast agent, both images contribute equally, or the 140 kV image dominates. This method combines the high-iodine contrast of the low kV images with a low image noise level in areas with little or no contrast agent (see Figure 25.7).

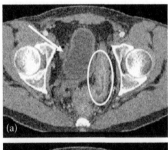

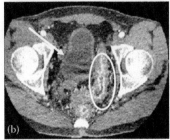

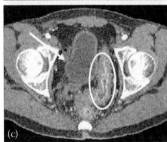

FIGURE 25.7
Example of contrast-enhanced viewing by nonlinear image blending. (a) 140 kV image. (b) 80 kV image. (c) Blended image combining the enhanced contrast of the 80 kV image with the low noise level of the 140 kV image.

25.4.2 Monoenergetic Images

Pseudo-monoenergetic images at arbitrary energies can be obtained from the polychromatic low kV and high kV images, if we assume that the object consists of only two materials in variable concentrations, for example, water and iodine. The concentrations of both materials in each image pixel are calculated by means of an image-based material decomposition. They are multiplied with predicted CT numbers per concentration at the desired energy, and summed up to the final monoenergetic image. Other materials will contribute to both base material images, their CT numbers may therefore not reflect the actual enhancement of the respective material at the desired energy.

In clinical practice, calculation of monoenergetic images can be used to reduce beam hardening artifacts caused by metal objects (Figure 25.8), as long as the metal attenuation is not too high and photon starvation dose not occur.

25.4.3 Differentiation of Two Materials

Dual energy information can be used for a binary distinction between two materials, that is, to classify image pixels as belonging to one of the two materials. A clinically relevant example is the differentiation between bone and iodine-filled vessels in a CT angiographic scan for an automated removal of bone and calcifications from the images.

Dual energy based binary distinction between two materials can be performed by means of a diagram in which the CT number of each image pixel at low kV is plotted as a function of its CT number at high kV. Image pixels containing a mixture of blood and iodine in different

concentrations line up along a straight line in that diagram, with slope >1 because the CT number of iodine is significantly higher at low kV as a consequence of the prevailing photo effect. Image pixels with a mixture of bone marrow and bone (with calcium as the main component) will line up along another straight line with different, smaller slope. By introducing a separation line between both lines, "bone" pixels can be separated from "iodine" pixels (Figure 25.9) and removed from the image data set [33]. A representative clinical example is shown in Figure 25.10.

Another clinical relevant example for dual energy based material differentiation is the distinction between

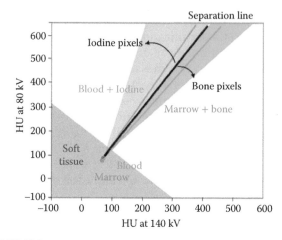

FIGURE 25.9
Principle of image-based distinction between two materials in a dual energy scan, in this case bone and iodine-filled vessels. Image pixels containing a mixture of blood and iodine in various concentrations line up along a straight line (orange), image pixels containing a mixture of marrow and bone line up along another straight line with smaller slope (green). A separation line can be introduced to differentiate between pixels containing mostly iodine and pixels containing mostly bone.

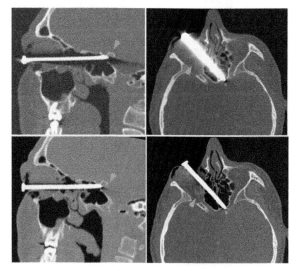

FIGURE 25.8
(Top row) Standard linear blending of the high kV and low kV image of a dual energy scan, showing severe metal artifacts. (Bottom row) Metal artifacts are significantly reduced in pseudo-monoenergetic images at a metal-specific high energy, in this case 106 keV. (Courtesy of Dr. Rajiv Gupta, Massachusetts General Hospital, Boston, MA.)

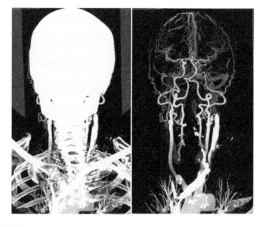

FIGURE 25.10
Automatic dual energy based bone removal in a DSCT angiographic scan of the carotid arteries. (Left) Maximum intensity projection (MIP) of "standard" images, obtained by a linear combination of the low kV and high kV images. (Right) Ca pixels identified by using dual energy information, as shown in Figure 25.9, are removed, and only the iodine-filled vessels remain visible. (Courtesy of M. Pasowicz, The John Paul II Hospital, Krakow, Poland.)

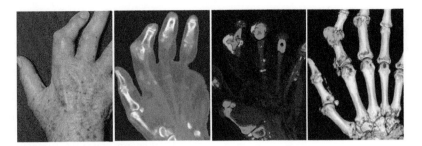

FIGURE 25.11
Dual energy-based differentiation between uric acid and other materials for a differential diagnosis of gout. Uric acid is highlighted in green, Ca is highlighted in blue. (Courtesy of M. Desai, Mayo Clinic Jacksonville, FL.)

uric acid and other materials, for example, for the characterization of kidney stones [17–19,34–36], or the differential diagnosis of gout [37] (see Figure 25.11).

25.4.4 Three-Material Decomposition

Three-material decomposition was first proposed in 1990 [38,39]. For three-material decomposition using only two different spectral measurements, one additional condition must be provided to solve for three unknowns. One solution is to assume volume conservation. The volume fractions of three materials in each image pixel can be expressed as

$$f_1 + f_2 + f_3 = 1 \qquad (25.3)$$

where f_1, f_2, and f_3 are the volume fractions of materials 1, 2, and 3. The mass attenuation of the mixture is then

$$\mu = \left(\frac{\mu}{\rho}\right)_1 (E) \cdot \rho_1 \cdot f_1 + \left(\frac{\mu}{\rho}\right)_2 (E) \cdot \rho_2 \cdot f_2$$
$$+ \left(\frac{\mu}{\rho}\right)_3 (E) \cdot \rho_3 \cdot (1 - f_1 - f_2) \qquad (25.4)$$

This equation can be solved by two measurements, if the densities of the respective materials are known.

A variant of the above method assumes two materials with known density and one material with very high, but unknown density, and negligible volume fraction. A clinically relevant example is a mixture of fat and soft tissue in the body plus an unknown amount of iodinated contrast agent. Instead of decomposing into three fixed points in the CT number diagram, the two data points of the base materials with known density (fat and soft tissue) and the slope of the iodine enhancement vector can be used. This is possible because the addition of small amounts of iodine leads to a similar enhancement for both tissues. Figure 25.12 shows the basic idea of a modified three-material decomposition for the subtraction of iodine from a contrast-enhanced liver scan. Mixtures of the base materials (in this case

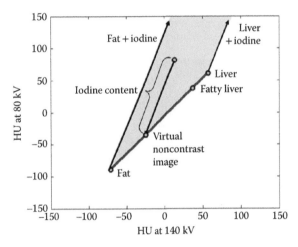

FIGURE 25.12
Basic principle of a modified three-material decomposition: subtraction of iodine from contrast-enhanced CT images of the abdomen.

fatty liver) are located along the line between pure fat and pure liver tissue. If iodine is added, the respective data points in the CT number diagram move in the direction of the iodine enhancement vector. To extract the iodine, each pixel in the CT number diagram is projected onto the line between fat and liver tissue along the direction of the iodine enhancement vector. The length of the displacement vector represents the enhancement attributed to iodine in that pixel. The iodine enhancement values for all pixels are displayed in a so-called iodine map, they can be subtracted from the original contrast-enhanced image to provide a "virtual noncontrast image."

Virtual noncontrast images calculated from dual energy scans may in some cases replace true noncontrast CT images, in this way avoiding an additional CT scan and reducing the radiation dose to the patient. The use of virtual noncontrast images has been described for the detection of urinary calculi, for the differentiation of liver and kidney tumors and adrenal masses, or for the assessment of aortic aneurysms [16–20,26,27,40,41]. A clinical example is shown in Figure 25.13.

In lung applications the iodine map is of particular interest, as it is a surrogate parameter for the blood volume in

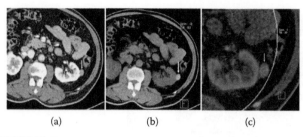

FIGURE 25.13
Characterization of kidney lesions by means of dual energy CT. (a) Linear blending of the high kV and low kV image of a dual energy scan corresponding to a standard 120 kV image reveals a kidney lesion. (b) Virtual noncontrast image shows the lesion to be hyperattenuating. (c) Iodine map shows no sign of iodine-uptake in the lesion, which is most probably benign. (Courtesy of T. Johnson, Klinikum Großhadern, Munich, Germany.)

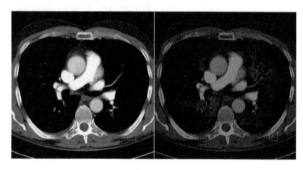

FIGURE 25.14
Visualization of perfusion defects in the lung parenchyma caused by pulmonary embolism. Left: dual energy mixed 80 kV/140 kV image is similar to a standard 120 kV image and shows small embolus occluding subsegmental vessel in right lower lobe. Right: iodine distribution map in the lung parenchyma as a colored overlay (red) on the mixed 80 kV/140 kV image shows wedge-shaped perfusion defect (dark zone) distal to tiny occlusive embolus in right lower lobe. (Courtesy of S. Thieme, Klinikum Großhadern, Munich, Germany.)

the lung parenchyma. It can be used to visualize the extent of perfusion defects caused by pulmonary embolism [23–25,42] (see Figure 25.14). Using inhaled Xenon or Krypton as a contrast agent, lung ventilation can be assessed [43–45].

Dual energy based iodine maps of the myocardium have been used as a surrogate parameter for the myocardial blood volume to evaluate myocardial perfusion defects [21,22,28].

References

1. Alvarez RE, Macovski A. Energy-selective reconstructions in X-ray computerized tomography. *Phys Med Biol.* 1976; 21(5):733–44.
2. Kalender WA, Perman WH, Vetter JR, Klotz E. Evaluation of a prototype dual-energy computed tomographic apparatus. I. Phantom studies. *Med Phys.* 1986; 13(3):334–9.
3. Zhang D, Li X, Liu B. Objective characterization of GE discovery CT750 HD scanner: gemstone spectral imaging mode. *Med Phys.* 2011; 38(3):1178–88.
4. Lv P, Lin XZ, Li J, Li W, Chen K. Differentiation of small hepatic hemangioma from small hepatocellular carcinoma: recently introduced spectral CT method. *Radiology.* 2011; 259(3):720–9.
5. Lee YH, Park KK, Song HT, Kim S, Suh JS. Metal artefact reduction in gemstone spectral imaging dual-energy CT with and without metal artefact reduction software. *Eur Radiol.* 2012 Feb 4 [Epub ahead of print].
6. Lin XZ, Wu ZJ, Tao R, Guo Y, Li JY, Zhang J, Chen KM. Dual energy spectral CT imaging of insulinoma—value in preoperative diagnosis compared with conventional multi-detector CT. *Eur J Radiol.* 2011 Dec 5 [Epub ahead of print].
7. Wu HW, Cheng JJ, Li JY, Yin Y, Hua J, Xu JR. Pulmonary embolism detection and characterization through quantitative iodine-based material decomposition images with spectral computed tomography imaging. *Invest Radiol.* 2012; 47(1):85–91.
8. Kaza RK, Platt JF, Cohan RH, Caoili EM, Al-Hawary MM, Wasnik A. Dual-energy CT with single- and dual-source scanners: current applications in evaluating the genitourinary tract. *RadioGraphics.* 2012; 32:353–69.
9. Flohr TG, McCollough CH, Bruder H, Petersilka M, Gruber K, Süß C, Grasruck M et al. First performance evaluation of a dual-source CT (DSCT) system. *Eur Radiol.* 2006; 16(2): 256–68.
10. Achenbach S, Ropers D, Kuettner A, Flohr T, Ohnesorge B, Bruder H, Theessen H et al. Contrast-enhanced coronary artery visualization by dual-source computed tomography—initial experience. *Eur J Radiol.* 2006; 57(3):331–5.
11. Johnson TRC, Nikolaou K, Wintersperger BJ, Leber AW, von Ziegler F, Rist C, Buhmann S, Knez A, Reiser MF, Becker CR. Dual source cardiac CT imaging: initial experience. *Eur Radiol.* 2006; 16:1409–15.
12. Matt D, Scheffel H, Leschka S, Flohr TG, Marincek B, Kaufmann PA, Alkadhi H. Dual-source CT coronary angiography: image quality, mean heart rate, and heart rate variability. *AJR Am J Roentgenol.* 2007; 189(3):567–73.
13. Leber AW, Johnson T, Becker A, von Ziegler F, Tittus J, Nikolaou K, Reiser M, Steinbeck G, Becker CR, Knez A. Diagnostic accuracy of dual-source multi-slice CT-coronary angiography in patients with an intermediate pretest likelihood for coronary artery disease. *Eur Heart J.* 2007; 28(19):2354–60.
14. Ropers U, Ropers D, Pflederer T, Anders K, Kuettner A, Stilianakis NI, Komatsu S et al. Influence of heart rate on the diagnostic accuracy of dual-source computed tomography coronary angiography. *J Am Coll Cardiol.* 2007; 50(25):2393–8.
15. Primak AN, Giraldo JC, Eusemann CD, Schmidt B, Kantor B, Fletcher JG, McCollough CH. Dual-source dual-energy CT with additional tin filtration: dose and image quality evaluation in phantoms and in vivo. *AJR Am J Roentgenol.* 2010; 195(5):1164–74.
16. Johnson TRC, Krauß B, Sedlmair M, Grasruck M, Bruder H, Morhard D, Fink C et al. Material differentiation by dual energy CT: initial experience. *Eur Radiol.* 2007; 17(6):1510–7.
17. Primak AN, Fletcher JG, Vrtiska TJ, Dzyubak OP, Lieske JC, Jackson ME, Williams JC Jr, McCollough CH. Noninvasive differentiation of uric acid versus non-uric acid kidney stones using dual-energy CT. *Acad Radiol.* 2007; 14(12):1441–7.

18. Scheffel H, Stolzmann P, Frauenfelder T, Schertler T, Desbiolles L, Leschka S, Marincek B, Alkadhi H. Dual-energy contrast-enhanced computed tomography for the detection of urinary stone disease. *Invest Radiol.* 2007; 42(12):823–9.

19. Graser A, Johnson TR, Bader M, Staehler M, Haseke N, Nikolaou K, Reiser MF, Stief CG, Becker CR. Dual energy CT characterization of urinary calculi: initial in vitro and clinical experience. *Invest Radiol.* 2008; 43(2):112–9.

20. Graser A, Becker CR, Staehler M, Clevert DA, Macari M, Arndt N, Nikolaou K et al. Single-phase dual-energy CT allows for characterization of renal masses as benign or malignant. *Invest Radiol.* 2010; 45(7):399–405.

21. Ruzsics B, Lee H, Powers ER, Flohr TG, Costello P, Schoepf UJ. Myocardial ischemia diagnosed by dual-energy computed tomography: correlation with single-photon emission computed tomography. *Circulation.* 2008; 117:1244–5.

22. Ruzsics B. Integrative computed tomography imaging of ischemic heart disease. *J Thorac Imaging.* 2010; 25(3):231–8.

23. Thieme SF, Johnson TRC, Lee C, McWilliams J, Becker CR, Reiser MF, Nikolaou K. Dual-energy CT for the assessment of contrast material distribution in the pulmonary parenchyma. *AJR.* 2009; 193:144–9.

24. Remy-Jardin M, Faivre JB, Pontana F, Hachulla AL, Tacelli N, Santangelo T, Remy J. Thoracic applications of dual energy. *Radiol Clin North Am.* 2010; 48(1):193–205.

25. Bauer RW, Kerl JM, Weber E, Weisser P, Huedayi K, Lehnert T, Jacobi V, Vogl TJ. Lung perfusion analysis with dual energy CT in patients with suspected pulmonary embolism—influence of window settings on the diagnosis of underlying pathologies of perfusion defects. *Eur J Radiol.* 2010; 80(3):e476–82.

26. Coursey CA, Nelson RC, Boll DT, Paulson EK, Ho LM, Neville AM, Marin D, Gupta RT, Schindera ST. Dual-energy multidetector CT: how does it work, what can it tell us, and when can we use it in abdominopelvic imaging? *RadioGraphics.* 2010; 30(4):1037–55.

27. Sommer CM, Schwarzwaelder CB, Stiller W, Schindera ST, Stampfl U, Bellemann N, Holzschuh M et al. Iodine removal in intravenous dual-energy CT-cholangiography: is virtual non-enhanced imaging effective to replace true non-enhanced imaging? *Eur J Radiol.* 2012; 81(4):692–9.

28. Weininger M, Schoepf UJ, Ramachandra A, Fink C, Rowe GW, Costello P, Henzler T. Adenosine-stress dynamic real-time myocardial perfusion CT and adenosine-stress first-pass dual-energy myocardial perfusion CT for the assessment of acute chest pain: initial results. *Eur J Radiol.* 2010 Dec 29 [Epub ahead of print].

29. Cardinal HN, Fenster A. An accurate method for direct dual-energy calibration and decomposition. *Med Phys.* 1990; 17(3):327–41.

30. Stonestrom JP, Alvarez RE, Macovski A. A framework for spectral artifact corrections in x-ray CT. *IEEE Trans Biomed Eng.* 1981; 28(2):128–41.

31. Yu L, Primak AN, Liu X, McCollough CH. Image quality optimization and evaluation of linearly mixed images in dual-source, dual-energy CT. *Med Phys.* 2009; 36(3):1019–24.

32. Holmes DR 3rd, Fletcher JG, Apel A, Huprich JE, Siddiki H, Hough DM, Schmidt B et al. Evaluation of non-linear blending in dual-energy computed tomography. *Eur J Radiol.* 2008; 68(3):409–13.

33. Lell MM, Hinkmann F, Nkenke E, Schmidt B, Seidensticker P, Kalender WA, Uder M, Achenbach S. Dual energy CTA of the supraaortic arteries: technical improvements with a novel dual source CT system. *Eur J Radiol.* 2010; 76(2):e6–12.

34. Qu M, Ramirez-Giraldo JC, Leng S, Williams JC, Vrtiska TJ, Lieske JC, McCollough CH. Dual-energy dual-source CT with additional spectral filtration can improve the differentiation of non-uric acid renal stones: an ex vivo phantom study. *AJR.* 2011; 196:1279–87.

35. Zilberman DE, Ferrandino MN, Preminger GM, Paulson EK, Lipkin ME, Boll DT. In vivo determination of urinary stone composition using dual energy computerized tomography with advanced post-acquisition processing. *J Urol.* 2010; 184(6):2354–9.

36. Stolzmann P, Kozomara M, Chuck N, Müntener M, Leschka S, Scheffel H, Alkadhi H. In vivo identification of uric acid stones with dual-energy CT: diagnostic performance evaluation in patients. *Abdom Imaging.* 2010; 35(5):629–35.

37. Manger B, Lell M, Wacker J, Schett G, Rech J. Detection of periarticular urate deposits with dual energy CT in patients with acute gouty arthritis. *Ann Rheum Dis.* 2012; 71(3):470–2.

38. van Kuijk C, Grashuis JL, Steenbeek JC, Schütte HE, Trouerbach WT. Evaluation of postprocessing dual-energy methods in quantitative computed tomography. Part 1. Theoretical considerations. *Invest Radiol.* 1990; 25(8):876–81.

39. van Kuijk C, Grashuis JL, Steenbeek JC, Schütte HE, Trouerbach WT. Evaluation of postprocessing dual-energy methods in quantitative computed tomography. Part 2. Practical aspects. *Invest Radiol.* 1990; 25(8):882–9.

40. Stolzmann P, Frauenfelder T, Pfammatter T, Peter N, Scheffel H, Lachat M, Schmidt B, Marincek B, Alkadhi H, Schertler T. Endoleaks after endovascular abdominal aortic aneurysm repair: detection with dual-energy dual-source CT. *Radiology.* 2008; 249(2):682–91.

41. Sommer CM, Schwarzwaelder CB, Stiller W, Schindera ST, Heye T, Stampfl U, Bellemann N et al. Dual-energy CT-cholangiography in potential donors for living-related liver transplantation: improved biliary visualization by intravenous morphine co-medication. *Eur J Radiol.* 2011 Jun 20 [Epub ahead of print].

42. Pontana F, Faivre JB, Remy-Jardin M, Flohr T, Schmidt B, Tacelli N, Pansini V, Remy J. Lung perfusion with dual-energy multidetector-row CT (MDCT): feasibility for the evaluation of acute pulmonary embolism in 117 consecutive patients. *Acad Radiol.* 2008; 15(12):1494–504.

43. Park EA, Goo JM, Park SJ, Lee HJ, Lee CH, Park CM, Yoo CG, Kim JH. Chronic obstructive pulmonary disease: quantitative and visual ventilation pattern analysis at xenon ventilation CT performed by using a dual-energy technique. *Radiology.* 2010; 256(3):985–97.

44. Thieme SF, Hoegl S, Nikolaou K, Fisahn J, Irlbeck M, Maxien D, Reiser MF, Becker CR, Johnson TR. Pulmonary ventilation and perfusion imaging with dual-energy CT. *Eur Radiol.* 2010; 20(12):2882–9.

45. Hachulla AL, Pontana F, Wemeau-Stervinou L, Khung S, Faivre JB, Wallaert B, Cazaubon JF et al. Krypton ventilation imaging using dual-energy CT in chronic obstructive pulmonary disease patients: initial experience. *Radiology.* 2012; 263(1):253–9.

26

Computed Tomography Multispectral Imaging

Masahiro Jinzaki, Yoshitake Yamada, Minoru Yamada, and Sachio Kuribayashi

CONTENTS

26.1 Introduction

In a conventional computed tomography (CT) system, an object is usually scanned with 120 kVp x-rays possessing a polychromatic spectrum. The CT number of materials in each voxel is directly related to the ratio of the linear x-ray attenuation coefficient of the material in a voxel to the linear attenuation coefficient of water at the effective x-ray energy and at the voxel location [1]. However, the polychromatic spectrum is more strongly absorbed by the object in the lower-energy x-rays, and thus, the effective x-ray energy changes as it passes through the object: the detected x-ray beam contains the higher-energy portion. This phenomenon is called beam-hardening effective energy shift.

The beam-hardening effective energy shift brought in several problems in single-energy CT images. First, CT numbers may not accurately represent material composition because the effective energy varies with location, and thus, the same material at two different locations in the scan field of view (FOV) could have very different CT numbers. Second, although beam-hardening effective energy shift is corrected by using calibration data measured in specific phantoms and calculated by the specific function during the image reconstruction process in single-energy CT systems, nonlinear artifacts such as shading and dark artifacts occur if beam-hardening correction is insufficient. These artifacts mimic pathologies and lead to misdiagnosis [2–4].

With dual-energy CT (DECT), by obtaining two image data sets in the same anatomic location with two different x-ray spectra, it is possible to analyze energy-dependent changes in attenuation of material and hence obtain material-specific information that would help distinguish between materials having similar linear Hounsfield Unit but different chemical composition [5,6]. In the 1970s and 1980s, dual-energy technology was first implemented; however, its use was limited because of noise in the low kilovolt power images and the length of time required for data acquisition, which led to misregistration. Recent CT technologies that allow for more rapid data acquisition have sparked renewed interest in dual-energy applications.

The original type of DECT was rotate-rotate system, in which the CT gantry fully rotates once to acquire data at the first kilovolt power setting, and then rotates again almost immediately to acquire data at the second kilovolt power setting. The nonsimultaneous nature of data acquisition and low speed are disadvantages of this method. There are three newly developed dual-energy systems. The first one is dual-source CT system (Definition or Definition flush; Siemens Medical Solutions), in which the two orthogonally mounted detectors and tube arrays can operate at a considerably improved rate, nearly simultaneously, and can be set to different tube potentials [7]. The second one is the fast-kVp switching technique (Discovery CT 750 HD, GE Healthcare), which enables rapid and essentially simultaneous acquisition of datasets at two different

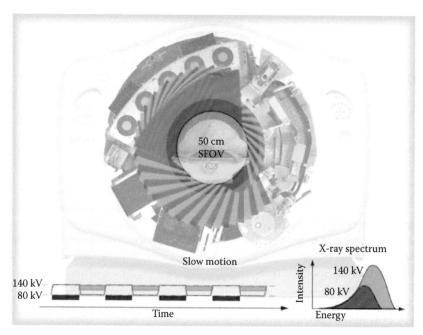

FIGURE 26.1
The scheme of fast-kVp switching dual-energy computed tomography (CT) system. In the fast-kVp switching technology, dynamic switching between 80 and 140 kVp of x-rays are pulsed in less than 0.5 milliseconds. Blue color corresponds to 80 kVp and green color corresponds to 140 kVp.

energies for the same projection angle with one tube and a detector (Figure 26.1) [8–10]. The third one is the dual-layer detector DECT scanner (Brilliance CT, Phillips Healthcare), equipped with a modified detector with two scintillation layers to acquire dual-energy data from a single x-ray source [11]. Among these three, the dual-source CT system and fast-kVp switching technique is available for regular clinical use, but the dual-layer DECT is currently not yet available.

26.2 Principle of Fast-kVp Switching Dual-Energy CT System

The fast-kVp switching technology obtains images with dynamic switching between 80 and 140 kVp of x-rays in less than 0.5 milliseconds with full 50 cm FOV, whereas dual-source technology obtains images with 75–83 milliseconds time delay between 80 and 140 kVp of x-rays. This technology was enabled on the latest 64 slice CT by a high-voltage generator with ultrafast tube voltage switching mechanism, a new garnet crystal scintillator detector with ultrafast speed optical response and data acquisition system with fast sampling capabilities. As a result, the data acquisition system allows more than 2.5 times of data sampling in one gantry rotation compared with a conventional 64 slice CT.

A constant tube current is employed for both kilovolt power as it is not feasible to alternate the tube current (mA) as rapidly as the tube voltage. The exposure time ratio between the 80 and 140 kVp scans is adjusted with 65% of exposure time used for 80 kVp acquisition and 35% for the 140 kVp acquisition to account for the higher x-ray tube output for a given mA at 140 kVp and to maximize contrast-to-noise ratio (CNR) [8]. The tube current choices that are presently available include 260, 275, 360, 375, 550, 600, 630, and 640 mA. In addition to varying gantry rotation times and types of bowtie filters, 66 preset dual-energy protocols are available to select from depending on the patient size and body part to be covered. The advantages of fast-kVp switching DECT are the availability of full 50 cm FOV for dual-energy data analysis and good temporal registration between high- and low-energy data [9].

The acquisition data set of 80 and 140 kVp in the fast-kVp switching technology are treated as coincident projection data both temporally and spatially, because of an extremely small time difference (less than 0.5 milliseconds) between the two data sets. Thus, the fast-kVp switching data acquisition enables mathematically to transform the attenuation measurements into the density of two basis materials in projection data space (using raw data before reconstruction of high- and low-energy images), whereas dual-source data acquisition transform the attenuation measurements in image data base (i.e., after reconstruction of high- and

TABLE 26.1

The Difference between Dual-Source CT and Fast-kVp Switching DECT

	Dual-Source CT	Fast-kVp Switching DECT
Tube	Dual	Single
Detector	Gd oxysulfide	Gemstone
Gantry rotation	300 or 330 ms	350 ms
Time between images	83 or 75 ms	0.3–0.5 ms
FOV	26 cm, 33 cm	50 cm
Reconstruction	Image data base	Projection data base

low-energy images). This projection-based process corrects for multimaterial, beam-hardening effects, which provides accurate material decomposition with material density unit.

The difference between dual-source CT and fast-kVp switching DECT is described in Table 26.1.

26.3 Image Reconstruction: Material Density Image and Virtual Monochromatic Spectral Image

The fast-kVp switching dual-energy scanners generate material density images and virtual monochromatic spectral (VMS) images. Material density images give us new informations, which were not obtained in conventional CT. VMS images are similar to conventional CT images but enable more accurate attenuation measurement and less beam-hardening artifact.

26.3.1 Material Density Image

Each type of material has its own characteristic changing pattern in attenuation between the high- and low-energy spectra, enabling material classification [5]. Materials with higher atomic number such as iodine have a greater change in attenuation with a change in energy as compared to materials with lower atomic number such as calcium or water because of dominant photoelectric effect (Figure 26.2). Thus, materials can be differentiated further by applying different x-ray spectra and analyzing the differences in attenuation, a process that is referred to as material decomposition or material separation. This works especially well in materials with large atomic numbers such as iodine because of the photoelectric effect and makes it beneficial to use the spectral information to differentiate iodine from other materials that do not show this behavior.

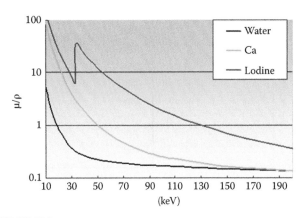

FIGURE 26.2

CT number (mass attenuation coefficient) in different kiloelectron volt. The change in measurement of CT attenuation between low- and high-energy spectra differs depending on material, which enables differentiating iodine and calcium.

Material density image is generated using the hypothesis that the attenuation coefficients of any material can be computed as a weighted sum of the attenuation coefficients of two basis materials that are sufficiently different in atomic number and thus would have different attenuation properties [5,9] Materials other than the chosen basis materials are considered combinations of both material densities. The iodine/water basis material pair is commonly used that would generate an iodine density image and water density image [9,12]. The water density image does not have any image voxels with attenuation similar to iodine, and thus serves as a virtual unenhanced image [9].

Quantitative information in the form of physical density of a selected material can also be derived from dual-energy data. Following decomposition of dual-energy data of a contrast-enhanced scan, quantitative estimation of iodine concentration within each pixel within a selected region of interest (ROI) can be displayed as $mg \cdot mL^{-1}$. The measured iodine density can be used to judge the presence or absence of enhancement within a lesion and also quantify the amount of added iodine into a pixel [13,14].

26.3.2 Virtual Monochromatic Spectral Image

VMS image is also an important component of DECT as well as material density image. VMS image depicts how the imaged object would look if the x-ray source produced only x-ray photons at a single energy (Figure 26.3). If projection-based, beam-hardening correction through two different materials can be done using two different kilovolt power data for the same projection angle, the rigorous beam-hardening correction will enable accurate material density images and mass attenuation coefficients to be obtained in the material decomposition calculation

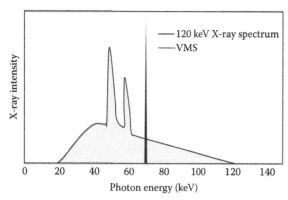

FIGURE 26.3
Polychromatic x-ray versus virtual monochromatic x-ray. Conventional 120 kVp image is polychromatic where 120 keV is a peak. X-ray image at a specific photon energy (kiloelectron volt) is called monochromatic image. The calculation of energy selective monochromatic projection from the dual-energy data produces virtual monochromatic spectral image.

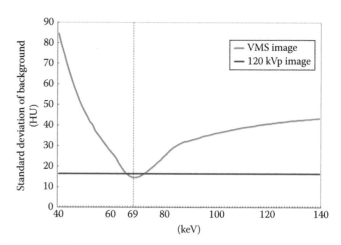

FIGURE 26.5
The mean standard deviation of background noise on VMS images and 120 kVp CT images. Background noise on VMS image was lowest at approximately 70 keV (69 keV), and background noise levels on VMS images in the range of 67–72 keV were significantly lower than those on 120 kVp CT images.

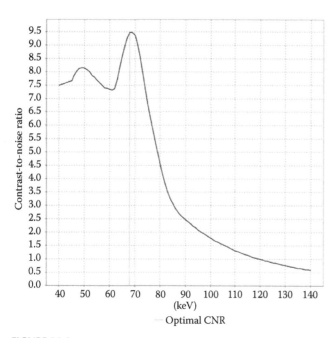

— Optimal CNR

FIGURE 26.4
The optimal kiloelectron volt level of virtual monochromatic spectral (VMS) images. The optimal kiloelectron volt level of VMS images can be automatically shown by placing the region of interests on the evaluated structures.

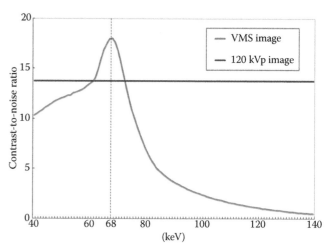

FIGURE 26.6
The mean contrast-to-noise ratio (CNR) on VMS image and 120 kVp CT image. The CNR for each contrast medium concentration was highest at approximately 70 keV (68 keV). The CNR on the VMS images was significantly higher in the range 63–72 keV compared with that on 120 kVp CT images.

process. VMS image can be reconstructed at any kiloelectron volt levels between 40 and 140 keV from a pair of accurate material density images and mass attenuation coefficients. The optimal kiloelectron volt level of VMS images can be determined to optimize the CNR of the evaluated structures on dedicated workstation with Gemstone Spectral Imaging software (Figure 26.4).

VMS image is expected to provide improved image quality by reducing beam-hardening artifacts. According to one study comparing the image quality obtained with

VMS imaging in phantoms with that obtained with 120 kVp CT for a given radiation dose, image noise on VMS images in the range of 67–72 keV was significantly lower than that on the 120 kVp CT images (Figure 26.5), whereas CNR on the VMS images was approximately 30% higher compared to with that on the 120 kVp CT images (Figure 26.6) [15]. VMS image has the potential to replace 120 kVp CT as the standard CT imaging modality, since optimal VMS image at approximately 70 keV may be expected to provide improved image quality (lower image noise and higher CNR).

26.4 Potential Clinical Usefulness

26.4.1 Material Density Image

An iodine density image and water density image are most commonly used in the clinical field. There are several clinical reports regarding iodine images, introduced later. Virtual noncontrast (water density) images provide information equivalent to a true unenhanced image obtained before contrast administration and have a potential to eliminate the true unenhanced scan. The data using fast-kVp switching technology, however, is not yet reported.

Iodine image using fast-kVp switching technology is reported in the field of lung, cardiac, portal vein, kidney, and thyroid. Wu et al. assessed the diagnostic value of pulmonary embolism detection and characterization through quantitative iodine density images in 53 patients [16]. There was a significant difference for the iodine density among normal lung parenchyma (1.89 mg·mL^{-1} [0.85–3.29 mg·mL^{-1}]), nonocclusive perfusion defects (0.83 mg·mL^{-1} [0.44–1.26 mg·mL^{-1}]), and occlusive perfusion defects (0.27 mg·mL^{-1} [0.00–0.62 mg·mL^{-1}]) ($p < .001$). The authors concluded that iodine density images are useful for quantitative depiction of pulmonary blood flow and perfusion defects (Figure 26.7) and that quantification of iodine density may be used as a predictor in distinguishing the presence or absence of pulmonary embolism and the severity of pulmonary embolism [16]. Geyer et al. also evaluated the feasibility of iodine density maps in 14 patients with suspicion of acute pulmonary embolism [17]. On a per patient basis, the sensitivity and specificity of iodine maps compared to CT pulmonary angiography (CTPA) were 80.0% and 88.9%, respectively, whereas on a per segment basis, it was 40.0% and 97.6%, respectively. They concluded that DECT might be a helpful adjunct to assess the clinical severity of pulmonary embolism (PE), especially for assessing the functional relevance of an occlusion of the pulmonary arteries. Hur et al. assessed the diagnostic performance of dual-energy cardiac CT in the detection of left atrial appendage thrombi and differentiation between thrombus and circulatory stasis (false-positive CT findings when an attenuation-based method is used) in patients with stroke, by using transesophageal echocardiography as the reference standard [18]. The mean iodine concentration was 1.23 mg·mL^{-1} ± 0.34 (standard deviation) for thrombus and 3.61 mg·mL^{-1} ± 1.01 for circulatory stasis ($p = .001$). They concluded that iodine imaging is a highly sensitive modality for detecting left atrial appendage thrombus and for differentiating thrombus from circulatory stasis in patients with stroke. With respect to portal vein, Qian et al. reported that iodine imaging, with quantification of thrombus iodine density in the portal venous phase, appears to be

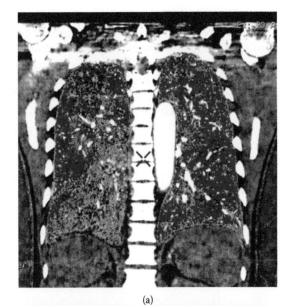

(a)

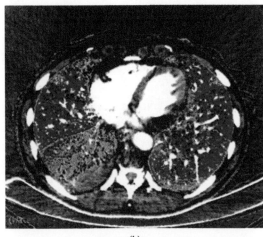

(b)

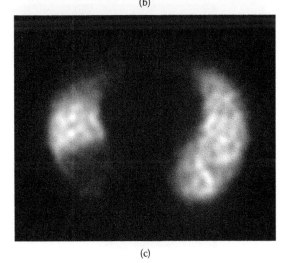

(c)

FIGURE 26.7
Pulmonary perfusion image. Pulmonary perfusion defects in right lower lobe on iodine density image, (a) coronal image and (b) axial image, is well corresponded to the image of lung perfusion scintigraphy (c).

a promising new method for distinguishing neoplastic from bland macroscopic portal vein thrombi [19]. With regard to renal lesions, Kaza et al. reported that iodine density image is highly specific in excluding enhancement and moderately to highly sensitive in detecting enhancement of renal lesions [13] (Figure 26.8). The authors suggest that the iodine density measurement using a threshold of 2 mg·cm^{-3} is most accurate in distinguishing enhancing from nonenhancing renal lesions. Li et al. attempted to quantitatively assess the imaging characteristics of thyroid nodules in iodine density image for differentiation of benign and malignant lesions, and the statistical analysis showed a significant difference between benign (nodular goiters and follicular adenomas) and malignant (papillary carcinomas) groups in iodine concentration [20].

The iodine/calcium basis material pair is also available. This application has potential in evaluating severely calcified coronary arteries, in which the degree of stenosis was difficult to evaluate using the single kilovolt power CT image. According to our study that applied this technology to ex vivo human heart specimen, the significant stenosis in severely calcified legions were clearly shown in the iodine density image, which corresponded well to the CAG findings (Figure 26.9). This technology has just recently been applied to clinical coronary CT scan; thus as of yet, there are no clinical reports on its effectiveness.

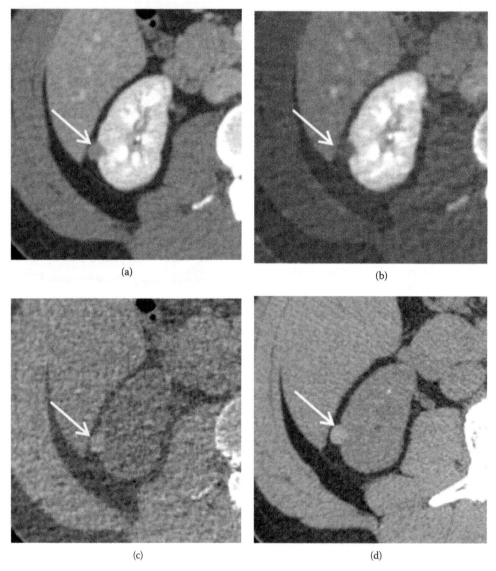

(a)

(b)

(c)

(d)

FIGURE 26.8
Hemorrhagic cyst of kidney. Enhanced CT image (a) shows a hyperdense lesion in the right kidney. Iodine density image (b) shows no iodine content in the lesion, meaning that the lesion is avascular. Water density (virtual unenhanced) image (c) shows persistent hyperdensity in the lesion after the exclusion of iodine content, indicating the finding is consistent with hemorrhagic cyst. This finding is similar to the true unenhanced CT image (d), suggesting that virtual unenehnced CT image has a potential to eliminate the true unenhanced scan.

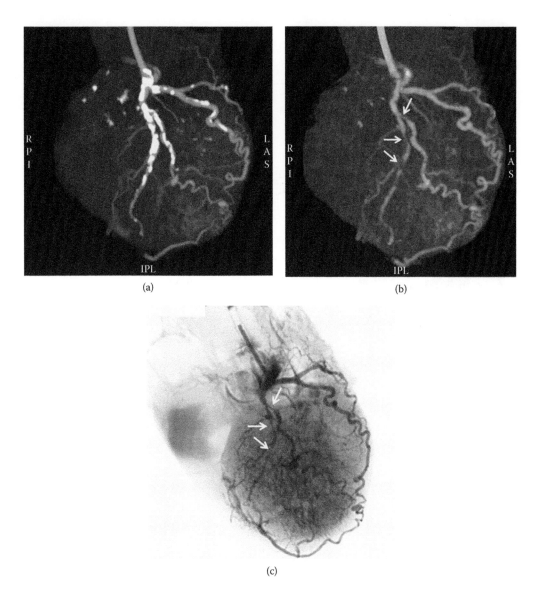

FIGURE 26.9
Severely calcified lesions of coronary arteries in ex vivo human heart. The degree of stenosis could not be evaluated on the maximum intensity projection (MIP) images generated by 120 kVp CT (a) because of severe calcification. The significant stenotic regions in the left anterior descending artery and diagonal branch are clearly shown in the MIP iodine density image (b, arrows) generated by fast-switching, which corresponded well to the CAG findings (c, arrows).

26.4.2 Virtual Monochromatic Spectral Image

There are more reports regarding VMS image than material density image. The fields evaluated in these reports are head, liver, cardiac, portal vein, pulmonary artery, lower limb vein, and stent in aorta. In CT of the brain, Lin et al. reported that the optimal monochromatic level was determined at 70 keV to provide both image noise reduction and beam-hardening artifacts reduction compared with the 140 kVp images [21]. In abdominal CT, we reported that VMS imaging at approximately 70 keV (69–70 keV) yielded the lowest image noise of the liver parenchyma and a high CNR for hypovascular hepatic metastases in the portal-dominant phase (Figure 26.10) [22]. Lv et al. reported that

monochromatic energy level of 40, 50, 60, and 70 keV can increase detectability in small hepatocellular carcinoma by improving CNR values during the late arterial phase and that 70 keV VMS image provides the higher overall image quality [23] In cardiac CT, we investigated the effectiveness of beam-hardening correction using electrocardiography-gated VMS imaging for myocardial imaging (Figure 26.11) [24]. A human ex vivo heart specimen and artificial descending aorta were scanned using both dualkilovolt power and single 120 kVp modes. The myocardial CT values at the posterobasal walls were low dense (49.9 ± 13.5 HU) for the 120 kVp images because of beam-hardening artifact, but 87.1 ± 6.9 HU (P = 0.59) for the 69 keV images that is similar to

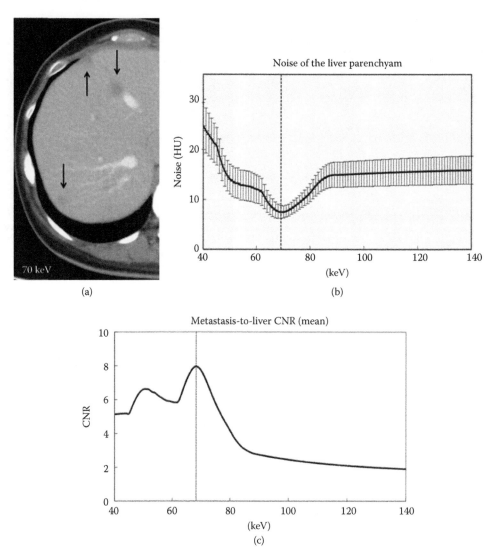

FIGURE 26.10
Hepatic metastases from colon cancer in the portal-dominant phase. VMS imaging at approximately 70 keV (a) yields the lowest image noise of the liver parenchyma (b) and the highest contrast-to-noise ratio (c) for hypovascular hepatic metastases (arrows).

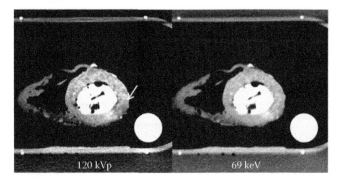

FIGURE 26.11
Myocardial perfusion image in ex vivo human heart. In the 120 kVp CT images (left), the myocardial CT value was lower in the posterobasal wall (arrow) than in the anterior wall. In the CT image with virtual monochromatic imaging at 69 keV (right), the myocardial CT value of the posterobasal wall was almost consistent with that of the other perfused wall.

the CT value in other normal perfused wall. Thus, VMS imaging is appeared to be useful for the correction of CT value deficits induced by beam-hardening that mimics perfusion defects. So et al. also evaluated the minimization of beam-hardening artifact with DECT-generated VMS images to improve perfusion estimates by using phantom models and porcine [25]. They also concluded that, by effectively reducing beam-hardening artifact, 70 keV VMS imaging may permit improved quantitative myocardial CT perfusion compared with the conventional single-energy CT technique. Zhao et al. investigated the effect of VMS image quality of CT portal venography in cirrhosis patients [26]. The authors described that the VMS images at 51 keV were found to provide the best CNR for both the intrahepatic and extrahepatic portal veins. At this energy level, VMS images had about 100% higher CNR than the 140 kVp polychromatic images with 30% noise increase. Yuan et al. compared quantitative and subjective image quality between standard CTPA and 50 keV VMS image with 50% reduced iodine load, by randomizing to one of two protocols: standard CTPA (100–120 kVp) and dual-energy CTPA (VMS imaging at 50 keV) [27]. The authors concluded that VMS imaging at 50 keV enables significant reduction in iodine load CTPA while maintaining compatible single-to-noise ratio, CNR, and effective radiation dose. However, they noted a slight reduction in image quality and increased image noise. Kulkarni et al. studied the performance of VMS imaging in venography in the assessment of lower extremity deep venous thrombosis [28]. Two radiologists evaluated 50 and 70 keV VMS images and found that compared with 70 keV data, 50 keV data yielded 90% increase in intravascular CT attenuation and higher CNR of the deep veins; however, objective noise at 50 keV was higher. They concluded that the 50 keV VMS images increase the confidence in the image interpretation of deep vein thrombosis (DVT) and decrease the number of indeterminate studies compared with 70 keV VMS images. Maturen et al. assessed endoleak detection and conspicuity using low kiloelectron volt VMS imaging [29]. and compared 55 keV VMS imaging with 75 keV VMS imaging. They concluded that sensitivity for endoleak detection and overall endoleak conspicuity ratings were both higher at 55 keV than at 75 keV.

When summarizing these reports so far, the soft-tissue evaluation would be optimal in approximately 70 keV because of higher CNR and lower image noise. On the other hand, the vascular system evaluation would be optimal in approximately 50 keV because of higher CNR, although the image noise is lowest in 70 keV. CNR, defined by the equation $|ROI_{lesion} + ROI_{background}|/SD_{background} \cdot SD_{background}$ is consistently lowest in approximately 70 keV. However, CT attenuation of iodine is very high in lower kiloelectron volt than higher kiloelectron volt, whereas CT attenuation of soft tissue is slightly high in lower kiloelectron volt than higher kiloelectron volt. Thus, CNR of soft tissue is highest in 70 keV, but CNR of vascular system (iodine) may occur to be highest in lower kiloelectron volt (50 keV) than 70 keV.

26.5 Conclusion

The fast-kVp switching technology is a new DECT system, which enables rapid and essentially simultaneous acquisition of datasets at two different energies for the same projection angle with one tube and one detector. The same projection angle acquisition enables the reconstruction images in projection data space, which

results in the rigorous beam-hardening correction and high-quality VMS image.

The clinical usefulness of material density image and VMS image is increasingly reported in many fields. VMS image has the potential to replace 120 kVp CT as the standard CT imaging modality, since optimal VMS image provides improved image quality. Material decomposition image will open the door for CT to enter the field of molecular imaging, which will consequently spark the development of photon-counting CT.

References

1. Hounsfield GN. Computerized transverse axial scanning (tomography). 1. Description of system. *Br J Radiol.* 1973;46:1016–22.
2. Rodriguez-Granillo GA, Rosales MA, Degrossi E et al. Signal density of left ventricular myocardial segments and impact of beam hardening artifact: implications for myocardial perfusion assessment by multidetector CT coronary angiography. *Int J Cardiovasc Imaging.* 2010;26:345–54.
3. Menvielle N, Goussard Y, Orban D et al. Reduction of beam-hardening artifacts in X-ray CT. *Conf Proc IEEE Eng Med Biol Soc.* 2005;2:1865–8.
4. Sun H, Qiu S, Lou S et al. A correction method for nonlinear artifacts in CT imaging. *Conf Proc IEEE Eng Med Biol Soc.* 2004;2:1290–3.
5. Kalender WA, Perman WH, Vetter JR et al. Evaluation of a prototype dual-energy computed tomographic apparatus. I. Phantom studies. *Med Phys.* 1986;13:334–9.
6. Johnson TR, Krauss B, Sedlmair M et al. Material differentiation by dual energy CT: initial experience. *Eur Radiol.* 2007;17:1510–7.
7. Fletcher JG, Takahashi N, Hartman R et al. Dual-energy and dual-source CT: is there a role in the abdomen and pelvis? *Radiol Clin North Am.* 2009;47:41–57.
8. Li B, Yadava G, Hsieh J. Quantification of head and body CTDI(VOL) of dual-energy x-ray CT with fast-kVp switching. *Med Phys.* 2011;38:2595–601.
9. Silva AC, Morse BG, Hara AK et al. Dual-energy (spectral) CT: applications in abdominal imaging. *Radiographics.* 2011;31:1031–46; discussion 47–50.
10. Zhang D, Li X, Liu B. Objective characterization of GE discovery CT750 HD scanner: gemstone spectral imaging mode. *Med Phys.* 2011;38:1178–88.
11. Hidas G, Eliahou R, Duvdevani M et al. Determination of renal stone composition with dual-energy CT: in vivo analysis and comparison with x-ray diffraction. *Radiology.* 2010;257:394–401.
12. Alvarez RE, Macovski A. Energy-selective reconstructions in X-ray computerized tomography. *Phys Med Biol.* 1976;21:733–44.
13. Kaza RK, Caoili EM, Cohan RH et al. Distinguishing enhancing from nonenhancing renal lesions with fast kilovoltage-switching dual-energy CT. *AJR Am J Roentgenol.* 2011;197:1375–81.

14. Chandarana H, Megibow AJ, Cohen BA et al. Iodine quantification with dual-energy CT: phantom study and preliminary experience with renal masses. *AJR Am J Roentgenol.* 2011;196:W693–700.

15. Matsumoto K, Jinzaki M, Tanami Y et al. Virtual monochromatic spectral imaging with fast kilovoltage switching: improved image quality as compared with that obtained with conventional 120-kVp CT. *Radiology.* 2011;259:257–62.

16. Wu HW, Cheng JJ, Li JY et al. Pulmonary embolism detection and characterization through quantitative iodine-based material decomposition images with spectral computed tomography imaging. *Invest Radiol.* 2012;47:85–91.

17. Geyer LL, Scherr M, Korner M et al. Imaging of acute pulmonary embolism using a dual energy CT system with rapid kVp switching: initial results. *Eur J Radiol.* 2012;81:3711–8.

18. Hur J, Kim YJ, Lee HJ et al. Cardioembolic stroke: dual-energy cardiac CT for differentiation of left atrial appendage thrombus and circulatory stasis. *Radiology.* 2012;263:688–95.

19. Qian LJ, Zhu J, Zhuang ZG et al. Differentiation of neoplastic from bland macroscopic portal vein thrombi using dual-energy spectral CT imaging: a pilot study. *Eur Radiol.* 2012;22:2178–85.

20. Li M, Zheng X, Li J et al. Dual-energy computed tomography imaging of thyroid nodule specimens: comparison with pathologic findings. *Invest Radiol.* 2012;47:58–64.

21. Lin XZ, Miao F, Li JY et al. High-definition CT Gemstone spectral imaging of the brain: initial results of selecting optimal monochromatic image for beam-hardening artifacts and image noise reduction. *J Comput Assist Tomogr.* 2011;35:294–7.

22. Yamada Y, Jinzaki M, Tanami Y et al. Virtual monochromatic spectral imaging for the evaluation of hypovascular hepatic metastases: the optimal monochromatic level with fast kilovoltage switching dual-energy computed tomography. *Invest Radiol.* 2012;47:292–8.

23. Lv P, Lin XZ, Chen K et al. Spectral CT in patients with small HCC: investigation of image quality and diagnostic accuracy. *Eur Radiol.* 2012;22:2117–24.

24. Yamada M, Jinzaki M, Kuribayashi S et al. Beam-hardening correction for virtual monochromatic imaging of myocardial perfusion via fast-switching dual-kVp 64-slice computed tomography. *Circ J.* 2012;76:1799–801.

25. So A, Lee TY, Imai Y et al. Quantitative myocardial perfusion imaging using rapid kVp switch dual-energy CT: preliminary experience. *J Cardiovasc Comput Tomogr.* 2011;5:430–42.

26. Zhao LQ, He W, Li JY et al. Improving image quality in portal venography with spectral CT imaging. *Eur J Radiol.* 2012;81:1677–81.

27. Yuan R, Shuman WP, Earls JP et al. Reduced iodine load at CT pulmonary angiography with dual-energy monochromatic imaging: comparison with standard CT pulmonary angiography—a prospective randomized trial. *Radiology.* 2012;262:290–7.

28. Kulkarni NM, Sahani DV, Desai GS et al. Indirect computed tomography venography of the lower extremities using single-source dual-energy computed tomography: advantage of low-kiloelectron volt monochromatic images. *J Vasc Interv Radiol.* 2012;23:879–86.

29. Maturen KE, Kaza RK, Liu PS et al. "Sweet spot" for endoleak detection: optimizing contrast to noise using low keV reconstructions from fast-switch kVp dual-energy CT. *J Comput Assist Tomogr.* 2012;36:83–7.

27

Positron Emission Tomography–Computed Tomography: Concept and General Application

Lale Kostakoglu and Karin Knesaurek

CONTENTS

27.1 Introduction

Positron emission tomography with 2-deoxy-2-[fluorine-18]fluoro-D-glucose integrated with computed tomography (FDG-PET/CT) has been recognized as an effective imaging modality for the staging and restaging of the majority of malignancies. FDG, as a glucose analog, provides functional information based on the increased glucose utilization of cancer cells, thus acts as a proxy for malignant transformation and maintenance of post-therapy tumor viability. Integrated FDG-PET/CT allows for accurate anatomical localization of metabolically active lesions yielding a high sensitivity and specificity in high-grade cancers. At initial staging, FDG-PET/CT synergizes with other morphologic imaging modalities, particularly, contrast-enhanced CT (ceCT) and magnetic resonance imaging (MRI) resulting in a higher test accuracy compared to each individual test alone. In the post-therapy setting, however, FDG-PET/CT alone may be more accurate than other existing imaging techniques. Especially, in patients with high suspicion of recurrent high-grade solid tumors with rising tumor markers, it should be the preferred imaging modality in cases with negative or equivocal conventional imaging findings. During or after therapy, in a number of malignancies, primarily in lymphoma, rapid decrease in FDG uptake within weeks of therapy initiation significantly correlates with favorable survival. However, therapy intensification or de-escalation should not be pursued outside clinical research merely based on FDG-PET findings until more data with long-term follow-up emerge from ongoing clinical trials.

In the last decade, following a considerable technologic evolution, PET has become an integral part of the imaging armamentarium for staging and restaging of almost all cancers. However, the uniform interpretation criteria and standardized PET protocols are yet to be more adequately disseminated to all circles to overcome the limitations of this functional imaging modality. The clinical content of this chapter will include only PET applications in those tumors with extensive literature support. The technical content will cover both established and novel PET technologies, including time-of-flight (TOF) and PET/MRI applications.

27.2 Positron Emission Tomography Systems

27.2.1 The History of PET Imaging

The first application of positron annihilation radiation for medical imaging was reported in 1951 by Sweet [1] at Massachusetts General Hospital (MGH). Gordon L. Brownell along with William H. Sweet and the physics group at MGH developed and built the first brain probe using two opposing sodium iodide (NaI(Tl)) detectors. In the mid-1950s, Ter-Pogossian and Powers [2] of Washington University's Mallinckrodt Institute of Radiology reinstated in biomedical research the use of radiopharmaceuticals labeled with short-lived, cyclotron-produced radioisotopes. In 1960s, invention of CT by Alan Cormack and Godfrey Hounsfield [3,4]

and popularization by investigator, David Kuhl, and colleagues [5] at the University of Pennsylvania in 1959 also strongly contributed to the emergence of PET. The first human PET tomograph was developed by Mike Phelps and Ed Hoffman in 1974. The first images of blood flow (BF), oxygen and glucose metabolism, and F-18 bone scans from this tomograph represented the first published human PET images using the filtered back projection algorithm [6,7]. In 1976, using an application evolved from the work of Louis Sokoloff and colleagues [8], Al Wolf and Joanna Fowler [9], chemists at Brookhaven National Laboratory, developed the radiopharmaceutical, FDG—a development that laid the groundwork for more in-depth research and did much to expand the scope of PET imaging. The 1980s were characterized with the further development in PET instrumentation, as well as in a number of radiopharmaceutical developments, such as development and validation of determining cardiac viability with N-13, ammonia to monitor BF, and FDG to monitor glucose metabolism [10]. Also, the use of PET in the diagnosis, management, and treatment of cancer was extensively investigated. In late 1980s, major imaging companies, such as Siemens and General Electric (GE), entered the PET market. However, during 1980s, the most PET applications had been in research. The turning point in moving PET imaging into clinical domain was the passage of the Food and Drug Administration (FDA) Reform Bill by the U.S. Congress in the fall of 1997 and the first U.S. government reimbursement for PET was announced in January 1998 for lung cancer and cardiovascular disease. Soon after, that coverage was extended to include other cancers such as colorectal cancer, melanoma, and lymphoma. Senator Ted Stevens from Alaska, who was strongly influenced by his friend Michael E. Phelps from UCLA, was a major sponsor of the FDA Reform Bill. In 2000, in United States, the Medicare coverage expanded to include the use of PET in the treatment of six cancers: lung, colorectal, lymph, skin, head and neck, and esophageal. For noncancer indications, coverage includes identifying and treating those cardiac patients who would benefit from coronary revascularization and those epilepsy patients who would benefit from surgery. The other main event in the history of PET imaging, which occurred at the end of 1990s, was development of the PET/CT scanner. The PET/CT scanner was developed by David Townsend, a physicist at the University of Geneva in Switzerland, and Ronald Nutt, electrical engineer and cofounder of CTI company, which is now part of Siemens [11,12]. Even in 1990s, PET scans had been read alongside high-resolution CT or MRI scans [13]. Such combination of PET images with MRI or CT images, or co-registered images, provided both anatomic and metabolic information. The advantages of PET/CT scanners are not only

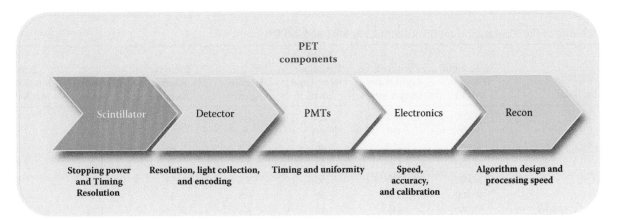

FIGURE 27.1
Basic components of a positron emission tomography (PET) system.

that they provide online, almost perfect co-registration of the PET functional with CT anatomical images, but also that CT provides very fast and accurate attenuation correction (AC) for PET. At present, practically all PET systems come as PET/CT systems. In the last 10 years, the availability and affordability of F-18 FDG also significantly increased and commercial companies are providing F-18 FDG unit doses even to community hospitals and outpatient clinics, which now offer PET services.

27.2.2 Basic Components of PET Systems

The basic components of a PET system are shown in Figure 27.1. These include the scintillator, detector, photomultiplier tube (PMT), electronics, and reconstruction software.

Each of the PET system components shown in Figure 27.1 makes an important contribution to the overall performance of the PET system. Each component has desired characteristics that need to work in harmony with the other components. We can look at the scintillator crystal for example, which is there to stop gamma photons emitted from the patient and relay the signal in a form of light that the detector can distinguish. Scintillators can be made from different crystals that have slightly different properties in terms of stopping power, decay time, light output, emission of light, and so on. The properties of interest for crystals that can be used in PET are given in Table 27.1.

The NaI(Tl) crystal has mostly been used in the past and bismuth germanate ($Bi_4Ge_3O_{12}$, BGO) and gadolinium orthosilicate (Gd_2SiO_5, GSO) have been more common up to very recently. However, at present, practically all manufacturers have chosen lutetium oxyorthosilicate (Lu_2SiO_5, LSO) or lutetium yttrium orthosilicate ($(Lu_{1-y}Y_y)_{2(1-x)}SiO_5$, LYSO) as the scintillator for state-of-the-art PET systems. The reasons are that LSO and LYSO have relatively high linear attenuation coefficients and the shortest decay time (40 ns) among the crystals listed earlier. This short decay time allows the application of TOF methodology in the reconstruction process of images, which significantly reduces the noise in the images and improves contrast. Short decay time also allows scanning with higher count rates, which is important in three-dimensional (3D) mode PET, and leads to shorter acquisition times.

TOF concept was introduced in early 1980s by late Ter-Pogossian [14]. However, at that time, neither electronics nor crystals used in PET detection were suitable for TOF imaging. The key advance that enabled modern TOF PET was the development LSO scintillator, which was discovered in 1991 [15]. Second development was improvement in electronics and PMTs, which also became much faster and enabled production of the first clinically available TOF system Gemini TF by Philips in 2006. The other PET/CT vendors, Siemens and GE, quickly followed and at present, all top of the line PET/CT systems include TOF PET machines.

Design of the detector, which includes the size and shape of the crystals, and the packing and positioning of PMTs, is also very important. Different PMTs have different properties in regard to timing and uniformity. The electronics behind the PMTs determines the speed and accuracy of processing. Finally, the reconstruction algorithms sort the acquired data into readable images, and are frequently being improved by vendors.

27.2.2.1 Current PET/CT Systems

Currently, state-of-the-art PET/CT system consists of the high-performance TOF PET and 128 or higher number of slices CT machine (Figure 27.2).

The characteristics of the PET/CT systems and their comparison can be found on http://www.itnonline.com /comparison-charts?t=PET%20/%20CT%20Systems and Table 27.2 shows the results.

TABLE 27.1

Characteristics of the Most Important Scintillator Crystals Used in PET

Crystal Material	Light Yield (Photons/ MeV)	Emitted Light Wave Length (nm)	Light Emission Decay Time (ns)	Density (g/cm^3)	Effective Atomic Number	Refractive Index	Energy Resolution at 511 keV(%)
NaI(Tl)	38,000	415	230	3.7	51	1.85	10
BGO (Bi$_4$Ge$_3$O$_{12}$)	9,000	480	300	7.1	75	2.15	20
LSO (Lu$_2$SiO$_5$)	26,000	420	40	7.4	66	1.82	15
LYSO (Lu$_{1-y}$Y$_y$)$_{2(1-x)}$SiO$_5$	32,000	430	40	7.1	66	1.82	12
GSO (Gd$_2$SiO$_5$)	13,000	440	50	6.7	59	1.85	15
LaBr$_3$ (5% Ce)	60,000	370	25	5.3	47	1.9	10
LuAP (0.4% Ce) (LuAlO$_3$)	12,000	365	18	8.3	65	1.94	7

Source: Acceptance Testing, Quality Assurance and Quality Control for Positron Emission Tomography Systems, IAEA-TECDOC: 09 May 2008.

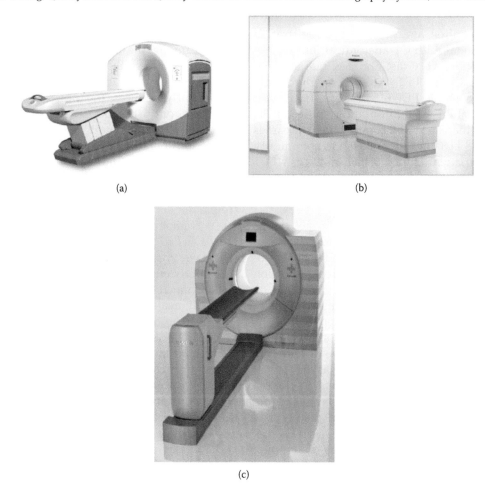

(a)

(b)

(c)

FIGURE 27.2
Current commercial PET/CT scanners. (a) Discovery 690 (GE Healthcare); (b) Gemini TF (Philips Medical Systems); (c) mCT (Siemens Medical Solutions). (All images courtesy of vendors.)

27.2.3 Recent Developments

27.2.3.1 PET/CT Systems

TOF can significantly reduce the signal-to-noise ratio and improve the contrast in clinical images, which leads to better detection of lesions, especially small ones and those in large patients [16]. TOF is based on measuring the difference in arrival time of the two coincidence photons at the detectors to better locate the annihilation position of the emitted positron (Figure 27.3). TOF PET/CT systems require all the components of a PET system (as shown in Figure 27.1) to be state of the art.

It must include fast crystals (e.g., LSO or LYSO), appropriate detectors, very fast PMTs, electronics, and processing computers. TOF reconstruction algorithms require significantly more computing power and time, because for each line of response, it is necessary to perform TOF calculations.

Other recent advances in PET technology are depth of interaction correction, using new detectors, either fast ceramic or other inorganic scintillators, or detectors with higher quantum efficiency, that is, avalanche photodiodes (APDs) and SiPMTs. Also, new reconstruction algorithms, mostly 3D algorithms, have been developed with the inclusion of the TOF information.

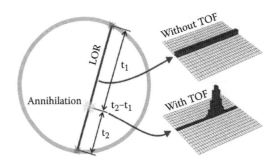

FIGURE 27.3
Illustration of the time-of-flight (TOF) concept. Image elements contributing to a line-of-response (LOR), for conventional PET without TOF and with TOF.

TABLE 27.2

Characteristics of Current Leading PET/CT Systems

Company	GE Healthcare	Philips Healthcare	Siemens Medical Solutions USA, Inc.
Model/product name	Discovery PET/CT 690 Elite	Ingenuity TF (PET/CT)	Biograph TruePoint PET/CT
FDA-cleared, year	Yes	Yes	Yes, 2006, 2007, 2009
Scanner Characteristics			
PET/CT system			
Gantry dimensions, H × W × D (cm)	192 × 226.1 × 140	219 × 239 × 223.7	197 × 234 × 156
Weight, kg (lb)	4,916 (10,834)	4,201 (9,262)	3,212 (7,079)
Power requirements, PET/CT	150 kVA max, 30 kVA average	480 VAC, 50/60 Hz,100 kVA max	4.8 kW PET, 3.2 kW CT
Heat load	6.3 MHU	27,950 BTU/hr	2 kW
Gantry cooling	Air cooled	Air cooled	Yes
Patient port	70 cm	OpenView gantry (70 cm for PET and CT)	70 cm
Transmission source	CT AC	CT	CT
Install time	10 business days approximately	8–10 days	1 week
Patient Handling System			
Vertical travel (cm)	2.5–20.5 below isocenter	35.5	53–96
Patient scan range (cm)	Standard 170; option 200	190	185—with TrueV
Horizontal speed (mm·s⁻¹)	100	150	0–200
Maximum patient weight, kg (lb)	226 (500)	196 (430)	204 (450)
Pallet deflection	N/S	<2 mm	No differential deflection
Gantry controls on front and back of gantry	Yes	4 sets of gantry controls, 2 each side	No
Software Processing			
WB acquisition time, with AC and processing	Physician preference	Approx. <10 min	<15 min
Acquisition modes	3D, 4D	3D, 4D TOF (respiratory gating)	3D
Reconstruction time, 2D mode, 128 × 128, OSEM-IR	N/A	N/A	N/A
Reconstruction time, 3D mode, 128 × 128, Fore-IT- weighted least square (WLS)	3D VUE Point HD: 60 sec; 4D VUE Point HD: 3 min	< 1 min/bed with list mode TOF, concurrent	< 1 min per bed
Event transfer rate	N/S	158 MB/sec	187.5 M events/sec
Correction for contrast in patient	Yes	Yes	Yes
Measured and automated randoms correction	Yes	Yes	Yes
Measured and automated scatter correction	Yes	Yes	Yes

(Continued)

TABLE 27.2   *(Continued)*

Characteristics of Current Leading PET/CT Systems

Company	GE Healthcare	Philips Healthcare	Siemens Medical Solutions USA, Inc.
Simultaneous acquisition/processing	Yes	Yes	Yes
Automated standard uptake value creation	Yes	Yes	Yes
WLS reconstruction	N/S	Yes	Yes
Attenuation weighted iterative reconstruction	Yes	Yes	Yes
One-click whole-body PET protocol	Yes	Yes	Yes
PET Physical Assembly			
Number of detectors	24 rings	28 pixelar modules	192 with TrueV
Number of image planes	47	45 or 90	109 with TrueV
Plane spacing (mm)	3.27 mm	2 or 4	2
Number of crystals	13,824	28,336	32,448 with TrueV
Ring diameter	88.6 cm	90 cm	842 mm
Number of PMTs	1,024 (256 quad-anode)	420	4 per block
Physical axial field of view (FOV) (cm)	15.7	18	21.6 with TrueV
Effective axial FOV in whole body (cm)—3D	N/S	N/S	15 with TrueV
Detector material	LBS	LYSO	LSO
Stopping power for 511 keV photons	High	High	High
Hygroscopic	No	No	No
Crystal size (mm)	$4.2 \times 6.3 \times 25$	$4 \times 4 \times 22$	$4 \times 4 \times 20$
PET Performance			
System sensitivity—3D, kcps/uCi/cc//LLD (NEMA 2001)	7 cps/KBq	7,200 cps/MBq at 10 cm; >19,370 with TOF	7.6//435 keV with TrueV
System sensitivity—2D, kcps/uCi/cc//LLD (NEMA 2001)	N/A	N/A	N/A
Transverse resolution at 1 cm (mm) (NEMA 2001)	NEMA performance standards: 4.9 VUE Point HD: 4	4.5	4.2
Transverse resolution at 10 cm (mm) (NEMA 2001)	NEMA performance standards: 6.3 VUE Point HD: 4.5	5	4.8
Axial resolution at 1 cm (mm) (NEMA 2001)	NEMA performance standards: 5.6 VUE Point HD: 5	4.7	4.5
Axial resolution at 10 cm (mm) (NEMA 2001)	NEMA performance standards: 6.3 VUE Point HD: 5	5.2	5.5
Peak noise equivalent count rate, kcps (NEMA 2001)	130 at 29.5 KBq/ml	N/S	N/S
2D	N/A	N/A	N/A
3D	Yes	118 kcps at 18 KBq/ml (>315 kcps with TOF)	165
Scatter fraction—2D (NEMA 2001)	N/A	N/A	N/A
Scatter fraction—3D (NEMA 2001)	37%	30%	<36%
CT Physical Assembly			
Type of detector	Volara DAS	Solid State—GOS	UltraFast Ceramic
Number elements/channels/fan beam	21,888 elements	128: 43,008 (86,016 effective)	26,880/17,664/11,776/54.4
Generator output	53.2 kW	80 kW (105 kW effective)	50–80 kW
kV-range/mA-range	Max mA at 120 kV is 440 mA	80–140 kVp/20–665 mA	80–140 kV/28–665 mA
Anode heat storage/cooling/min.	6.3 MHU and 284 kHU/min	8 MHU/1,608 kHU/min	5 MHU or 0 MHU/5,000 kHU/min
Tube focal spot	0.9 mm × 0.7 mm; 1.2 mm × 1.1 mm	1×1 mm/0.5×1 mm	0.8×0.5; 0.8×0.7 or 0.6×0.7; 0.8×1.1
Gantry dimensions (cm)	$192 \times 226.1 \times 140$	Integrated, see above	$197 \times 234 \times 156$

TABLE 27.2 (Continued)

Characteristics of Current Leading PET/CT Systems

Company	GE Healthcare	Philips Healthcare	Siemens Medical Solutions USA, Inc.
Gantry weight, kg (lb)	Integrated, see above	Integrated, see above	3,212 (7,079)
CT Image Quality			
LC resolution (20 cm catph./surface)	5 mm at 0.3% at 13.3 mGy	4 mm at 0.3%	5 mm at 3 HU at 16 mGy
CT dose index (dose/100 mAs) B/16 cm phant	Axial head: 18.4 mGy; axial body: 9.3 mGy	11 mGy/100 mAs	6/16 slice 15.7/40/64 slice 4.5
Max HC resolution (2% MTF)	15.4 lp/cm at 0% MTF	24 lp/cm (at cutoff)	24 lp/cm
Standard HC resolution (2% MTF)	8.5 lp/cm at 0% MTF	13 lp/cm (at cutoff)	15.6 lp/cm or 24 lp/cm
CT Scan Parameters			
Scan times (partial)/subsec (partial)	Physician preference	Partial 240 deg: 0.28, 0.33; Full: 0.4,0.5, 0.75, 1, 1.5, 2	Partial: 0.25–0.67; Full: 0.33–1.5
Scan field (cm)	50	Up to 70	70
Number of slices	16	128	6, 16, 40, or 64
Slice thickness (mm)	0.625	0.5–12.5	0.5–14.4
Rotation speed	Full 360 rotational scans in 0.5*, 0.6*,0.7, 0.8*, 0.9*, 1	0.4–2 seconds	0.33–1.5 seconds
Topogram length	N/S	190 cm	128–2,048 mm
Reconstruction time: std/high res/topo	6 FPS/16 FPS	Up to 20 images per sec	6–20 images per second
Scan matrix/display matrix	1,024 × 1,024	512 × 512; 768 × 768; 1,024 × 1,024	512 × 512; 1,024 × 1,024
Max. spiral volume/max. spiral scan time	N/S	190 cm/100 sec	190/100 sec
Console/Computer/Storage			
Host computer	Quad Core Xeon CPU	Dell PC workstation	Windows
User interface	Discovery Elite console	Ingenuity console	syngo
Archival storage	PACS	CD/DVD-R, DVD—RAM	MOD/CD-R/DVD
DICOM 3.0 PET	Yes	Yes	Yes
DICOM 3.0 CT	Yes	Yes	Yes
Special features	N/S	Exclusive state-of-the-art Astonish TF technology for improved lesion detection integrated with iDose4 and results-driven scanning. TOF for short scan times and industry-leading image quality.	High-definition PET with uniform resolution across the FOV. Largest axial FOV available for fast 10-minute PET scans?. Syngo.via ready

27.2.3.2 PET/MRI Systems

Great success of the combined PET and CT systems recently encourage development of PET/MRI systems. The main motivations to combine PET and MR together were an excellent soft-tissue contrast for MRI imaging, the elimination of the added radiation from the CT, and the multifunctional imaging ability of MRI. The first clinically installed whole-body PET/MRI system (Ingenuity TF, Philips Healthcare, Cleveland) was installed in January 2010 at The Mount Sinai Hospital, New York (Figure 27.4a). The system is sequential and consists of TOF PET system (GEMINI TF) and the MRI Achieva 3T X-series system with an innovative rotating bed that accurately positions the patient inside each scanner [17]. Mutual interferences between the two systems have been minimized by separating the gantries: the PET gantry is placed at a distance of 3.0 m from the MR magnet. Additional electromagnetic isolation is provided for the PET detectors and the PMTs, and most of the PET electronics are housed outside the scanner room for further electromagnetic interference isolation. Although the scanner does not provide simultaneous MR and PET imaging, it provides built-in accurate positioning and co-registration of MR and PET images obtained sequentially. At the end of 2010, at the Radiological Society of North America meeting, Siemens introduced Biograph mMRI (Figure 27.4b), which is a first whole-body clinical simultaneous PET/MRI scanner [18]. To create simultaneous system, Siemens used APDs instead of magnetically susceptible PMTs, but also made a sophisticated integration of the PET insert into the MRI system to minimize mutual interference.

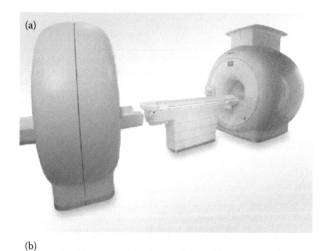

(a)

(b)

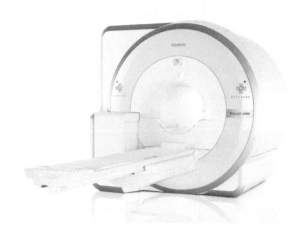

FIGURE 27.4
A whole-body positron emission tomography/magnetic resonance imaging (PET/MRI) system developed by (a) Philips and (b) Siemens.

One of the main challenges in PET/MRI imaging is how to perform MRI-derived AC on PET data. The Philips PET/MRI system uses a specific MR sequence, called atMR, to provide PET AC [19]. The atMR sequence, a T1 weighted sequence that matches the PET dimensions, allows both anatomical detail and AC, similar to a low-dose CT image in a standard PET-CT camera. The attenuation values are obtained by segmenting the atMR images into three segments, lungs, air, and soft tissue. Siemens system in clinical protocols uses a two-point Dixon MR sequence [20], which is used as the basis for AC. The attenuation values are obtained by segmenting the Dixon images into four compartments: air, lung, fat, and soft tissue.

In comparison between PET/CT and PET/MRI, PET/MRI system has advantages in better MRI soft-tissue contrast than CT and significantly less radiation. Also, MRI advanced techniques such as perfusion imaging, diffusion imaging, and MRI spectroscopy can be used. However, the disadvantages of PET/MRI versus PET/

CT are relatively long scanning time and problems related to AC for PET derived from MRI images.

The developments in electronics, detectors, and other technology make both PET/CT and, now also, PET/MRI a very dynamic field, with new developments practically almost every year.

27.3 PET/CT Clinical Oncologic Applications

The clinical indications of FDG-PET/CT imaging have been broadened over the past decade echoing the technologic improvements (Table 27.1). This chapter will review the FDG-PET applications in head and neck, non-small cell lung, breast, esophageal, colorectal, pancreatic, and urogenital cancers, mainly, testicular cancer, gynecologic malignancies, lymphoma, and myeloma (Table 27.2).

27.3.1 Head and Neck Cancer

More than 95% of head and neck malignancies are of squamous cell histology (HNSCC). At initial staging, a high proportion of patients present with locally advanced stage disease with regional nodal metastasis. Following first line therapy, disease recurs in 40% of the patients and 3 year survival is 30%–50% [21].

Intravenous ceCT is often the first-line choice of imaging, but FDG-PET has higher diagnostic accuracy in the staging and detection of local and regional metastases in patients with HNSCC. The reported sensitivity and specificity of FDG-PET/CT for the detection of lymph node metastases are 87%–96% and 80%–99%, respectively, versus 61%–97% and 25%–100% for ceCT [22–24]. In a meta-analysis involving 1236 patients, FDG-PET had a sensitivity of 79% and a specificity of 86% in the overall pretreatment evaluation of patients with HNSCC [25]. However, in the same series, in clinically lymph node-negative patients(N0), FDG-PET detected only half of the lymph node metastases emphasizing the fact that in N0 patients, the size of the metastases are usually below the resolution limit of PET imaging (~7.0 mm) [26–28].

Although distant metastasis usually occurs late during the course of disease, identification of metastatic disease is essential part of the staging process to determine an optimal management strategy. The main advantage of FDG-PET/CT is its ability to accurately identify distant metastases that occur in 10%–15% and synchronous or metachronous primaries in 5%–10% of cases regardless of disease stage with a sensitivity of above 95% [29,30]. Addition of PET/CT to conventional staging leads to changes in tumor–node–metastasis (TNM) classification in approximately 30% and management alterations in 15%–30% of patients [31,32]. A recent prospective study comparing whole-body MRI and FDG-PET/CT demonstrated a 74% concordance for tumor staging, with an 80% concordance for lymph node staging, and a 100% concordance for distant metastasis staging [33]. These results are promising for the combined use of whole-body MRI and PET imaging although further investigation is required for the establishment of this emerging modality.

FDG-PET has significant advantage over CT on the basis of its ability to provide quantitative data, mainly using standardized uptake values (SUVs). A significant disparity is notable between the SUV cutoffs across various studies; however, the results of a recent meta-analysis revealed a better disease-free survival and overall survival in patients with low pre- and posttreatment SUVs than those with high SUVs [34]. The low specificity is one of the cited shortcomings of FDG-PET imaging, as a result of high false-positive results encountered in reactive cervical lymph nodes and inflammatory changes [35].

FDG-PET/CT can also detect the site of a carcinoma of unknown primary tumors (CUP) in 60%–75% of the patients with HNSCC but with a suboptimal sensitivity [32,36–39]. A recent study reported that integrated PET/CT was superior to PET alone in the detection of the primary site of CUP (55% vs. 31%; $p = .04$). However, in view of such a low sensitivity, a negative result should still be further investigated by means of panendoscopy followed by tonsillectomy and blind biopsies [40].

Five-year risk of developing a locoregional recurrence and distant metastasis is high at 30%–50% and 20%–30%, respectively, despite aggressive multimodality therapy [41,42]. After surgical resection, distortion of anatomic landmarks, acute and chronic tissue inflammation, and edema induced by irradiation contribute significantly to the challenges associated with the identification of recurrences. A meta-analysis showed, sensitivity and specificity for recurrent disease: 86% and 73% for PET versus 56% and 59% for CT/MRI [43]. The sensitivity, specificity, and accuracy of FDG-PET/CT in restaging patients with head and neck cancer are 88%, 78%, and 86%, respectively [44] (Table 27.3). It is recommended that delaying FDG-PET/CT until 12 weeks after treatment would allow for acute inflammation to subside as well as any viable tumor to repopulate to a size that could be visualized by current PET technology [45,46]. Although there is no consensus on the role of FDG-PET/CT as surveillance tool, results of a recent study suggested that a second FDG-PET/CT examination appears beneficial 4 to 6 months after the first 3-month posttreatment PET scan for the detection of late recurrences [47].

There have been conflicting results on the role of FDG-PET/CT in the avoidance of planned neck dissection in patients with a negative FDG-PET/CT scan after definitive therapy [48–52]. A negative predictive value of 100%

TABLE 27.3

Clinical Indications of 18F-FDG-PET/CT in Oncology (Except Low-Grade Malignancies)

- Characterization of pulmonary nodules
- Nodal staging for solid tumors
- Evaluating the extent of disease at distant sites (M staging)
- Detection of tumor recurrence after therapy in patients with suspected relapse as a first line tool
- Further evaluation for disease in suspected recurrence when there is no morphological evidence of disease as a second line tool
- Searching for an unknown primary when metastatic disease is the first clinical presentation
- Evaluation of response during ongoing chemotherapy
- Evaluation of response after completion of therapy (both chemotherapy and radiotherapy)
- Direction of biopsy when there is more than one disease site
- Providing a roadmap for high-yield biopsies in large masses to avoid necrotic components
- Presurgical planning to avoid futile interventions as well as providing guidance for effective resection of multiple masses
- Radiotherapy planning with therapeutic

was reported for a complete neck response for post-chemoradiotherapy FDG-PET/CT [53]. Nonetheless, the positive predictive value was less than desirable at around 40%. Consequently, it was suggested that neck dissections be avoided in patients with a complete clinical, radiologic, and PET response while other PET/CT negative patients with an incomplete response by radiologic finding be closely monitored [53].

Although it is outside the scope of this chapter, in dedifferentiated thyroid cancers, the sensitivity of FDG-PET is 85% in cases with rising thyroglobulin and negative I-131 whole-body scans [54]. Hence, FDG-PET/CT alters clinical management in up to 50% of the patients [55–57].

In conclusion, FDG-PET/CT is effective in nodal staging of HNSCC and determination of distant metastases and secondary malignancies. FDG-PET is highly effective in detecting recurrent disease, provided that it is performed with a 12-week delay after completion of chemoradiotherapy. It has a high negative predictive value (NPV) for identification of residual disease and early recurrent disease. Currently, more data are warranted to determine its exact role in deferring planned neck dissection. The sensitivity of FDG-PET/CT is low in the detection of CUP and metastases in N0 necks. Given the paucity of prospective multicenter trials on the role of FDG-PET/CT in the post-chemoradiotherapy setting, the role of FDG-PET/CT as a surveillance tool is yet to be addressed.

27.3.2 Pulmonary Nodules and Non-Small Cell Lung Cancer

FDG-PET emerged as a promising modality for the characterization of pulmonary nodules; however, its specificity significantly varies across studies because of varying prevalence of malignancy versus granulomatous disease in the included patient sample. The pooled sensitivity and specificity of PET for differentiating malignant from a benign pulmonary nodule of any size were 97% and 78%, respectively, with an associated positive likelihood ratio of 4.4 and a negative likelihood ratio of 0.04 [58]. These data suggest that FDG-PET is a useful modality only for excluding the possibility of malignancy but not diagnosing a malignancy because of its high false-positive rate. More recently, in a systematic review of prospective studies, the sensitivity ranged from 79% to 100% and specificity from 40% to 90%, conceivably the wide range can be on the account of different prevalence rates of granulomatous disease and ground-glass opacities, and the lesions size the patient population differences [59].

Accurate staging of non-small cell lung cancer (NSCLC) is imperative in differentiating operable patients from those inoperable who can benefit from neoadjuvant treatment. For detecting mediastinal lymph node metastasis, PET is more sensitive than CT scanning in patients with NSCLC. A meta-analysis and a systematic review reported the sensitivity and specificity of PET for the mediastinal staging of NSCLC to be 74%–84% and 82%–85%, respectively, compared to a similar specificity but a rather inferior sensitivity at 51%–57% for CT [60,61]. Not surprisingly, PET was found to be less sensitive for identifying metastasis in nonenlarged lymph nodes and less specific in enlarged lymph nodes [62–64]. The high NPV of FDG-PET/CT at above 95% for mediastinal lymph node characterization [65–67] suggested an algorithm using FDG-PET and omission of mediastinoscopy in patients with negative FDG-PET/CT results except in patients with central tumors that have a high incidence of occult nodal metastases [68–70], as well as in those with suspected N2 tumors. Biopsy of the enlarged lymph nodes through mediastinoscopy regardless of PET/CT results would also be a rational approach to nodal staging. FDG-PET/CT imaging lands itself as a more relevant modality in the identification of distant metastasis in stage III patients with a reported sensitivity and specificity of 82% and 93%, respectively, in identifying extrathoracic metastasis although tissue confirmation is still warranted in many cases because of suboptimal specificity [65]. The NPVs of the clinical evaluations for brain, abdominal, and bone metastases were above 90%, suggesting that routinely imaging asymptomatic lung cancer patients may not be necessary [61].

FDG-PET results can alter management decisions in 35%–70% of patients by mostly upstaging, thus, allowing for palliative care as well as reducing the number of futile thoracotomies [71–76].

There are conflicting reports about the association of SUVs of the primary tumor with prognosis. Although, in several studies, greater FDG uptake was independently associated with worse prognosis, it was difficult to stratify confounding factors such as host-related risk factors, tumor size, histology, and surgical plan [77–79]. There are also preliminary data that prognosis is relatively favorable in patients with false-negative PET results in malignant lung nodules despite a delay in surgical resection [80,81]. However, these results should be confirmed in prospective series.

Prediction of early response to treatment may affect management significantly. Although the sample sizes were insufficient for defining its role in the prediction of response, the results of several studies have suggested a correlation between early metabolic response after several cycles and best overall response [82–85]. In contrast, some other studies found no association between FDG uptake and survival in patients undergoing neoadjuvant therapy [86,87]. After completion of concurrent chemoradiotherapy or radical radiotherapy, PET-based metabolic response was associated with survival before and after adjustment for other prognostic factors [85,86]. Since the timing of post-therapy PET is crucial, a delay of 3–4 weeks after completion of radiation therapy leads to a more accurate PET result [88].

At restaging, FDG-PET is currently considered complementary to CT for the identification of residual or recurrent disease. However, it has a considerable value in patients with significant distortion of anatomic structures after surgery or radiotherapy [89,90] with a sensitivity of 93%–100% and a specificity of 89%–92% for detecting recurrent NSCLC [91–93]. Notably, the sensitivity and specificity of PET for restaging the mediastinum can vary depending on the location of the involved lymph nodes, with the accuracy being high in anterior mediastinum and suboptimal in the posterior mediastinum [94,95]. Percent reduction in the baseline SUVmax was predictive of a complete pathologic response with an accuracy of 96% [85]. The sensitivity and specificity of FDG-PET using an SUV cutoff of 2.5 were 80% and 75%, respectively, for identifying residual nodal disease highlighting the inadequacy of a binary approach for effectively stratifying response categories [96]. It is yet to be proven, however, whether PET can identify a high-risk group that is more likely to benefit from adjuvant chemotherapy following surgery, or whether early detection of recurrence is associated with a better survival after salvage treatment.

In summary, staging with PET is more accurate than with CT and thus, may reduce the risk of futile thoracotomies. However, it is important to emphasize that positive PET findings should be histopathologically confirmed before ruling out potentially curative surgical resection. A negative FDG-PET study, although associated with a high negative predictive value for nodal staging, may still require confirmatory mediastinoscopy in a patient with central tumors and N2 involvement.

27.3.3 Breast Cancer

FDG-PET has a low sensitivity and high specificity in the detection of locoregional lymph node metastases with considerable heterogeneity across various studies [97,98]. In a recent meta-analysis including 2591 patients, mean sensitivity and specificity of FDG-PET for axillary staging were 63% and 94%, respectively [99]. Nonetheless, in patients with tumors larger than 2.0 cm or who are at a high risk of axillary lymph node metastasis, the data suggest that a negative PET/CT can identify a patient subgroup that can undergo sentinel lymph node biopsy (SLNB) instead of axillary lymph node dissection [100]. However, definitive clinical endpoints are yet to be developed. Consequently, PET/CT cannot replace SLNB whose sensitivity exceeds 95% [101].

The most important role for FDG-PET/CT imaging is the detection of distant metastatic disease in patients with locally advanced breast cancer (LABC) who have a higher chance for distant metastasis compared to those with early stage disease. In fact, the addition of FDG-PET to the standard workup of LABC patients contributed to a better stage stratification in 20%–25% of patients by differentiating true stage III and stage IV disease and detecting unsuspected metastasis [102]. Furthermore, FDG-PET can assess bone dominant metastases, although its performance is lower in osteoblastic compared to osteolytic metastases [103]. FDG-PET/CT has a high overall sensitivity, specificity, and accuracy for the detection of locoregional recurrence and is also more sensitive than the serum tumor marker CA15-3 in detecting disease relapse [104]. A meta-analysis of 808 patients showed an FDG-PET sensitivity and specificity of 93% and 82%, respectively, in recurrent breast cancer patients [105]. PET/CT can alter therapeutic options in 30% of cases with suspected recurrence and distant metastasis, primarily by demonstrating local or distant occult disease missed at other imaging studies [106].

There is evidence in support of a role for the use of FDG-PET as a predictor of pathologic complete response (pCR) for therapy response in LABC patients undergoing neoadjuvant therapy with at least a 90% sensitivity and 75%–85% specificity [107–109]. A decrease in SUVmax of more than 55% compared to the baseline levels predicted histopathological response to chemotherapy for LABC with a sensitivity of 100% and a specificity of 85% in identifying responders after the first cycle [108]. Persistent or elevated metabolic rate measurements (MR-FDG) and tumor BF at midtherapy at a mean of 9 weeks after first chemotherapy cycle predicted pCR [109]. The reported overall survival in non-metabolic responders was 8.8 months, compared with 19.2 months for responders [110]. In patients with bone metastases, a favorable response is usually associated with increase in the osteoblastic component and

decrease in FDG uptake. In a recent publication, both morphologic and metabolic changes in osseous metastases were associated with a favorable therapy response. Multivariate analysis revealed that an increase in the change in SUV was a significant predictor of response duration ($p = .003$) [111].

Recently, dedicated positron emission mammography (PEM) devices have been introduced to fulfill the need for a more sensitive and specific imaging modality for the evaluation of primary breast cancer [112–114]. The FDA has approved a PEM scanner that uses pixelated LYSO crystals (spatial resolution 2.4 mm), also equipped with a stereotactic biopsy system. A prior single center study demonstrated a sensitivity equivalent to that of MRI at 93% in the detection of the primary tumor in breast cancer patients [112]. For unsuspected or multifocal lesions, there was no statistically significant difference between the sensitivities of MRI and PEM (85%), but MRI (98%) tended to detect more lesions [113]. In a recent multicenter comparative effectiveness study of newly diagnosed breast cancer, MRI was more sensitive in depicting contralateral synchronous breast cancer than PEM (93% vs. 73%) [114]. Further studies are necessary to assess the role of these devices in suspicious, multifocal breast lesions to demonstrate their capability in the differentiation between benign and malignant etiologies.

In conclusion, currently, FDG-PET/CT is a useful test in breast cancer patients, but has limitations. PET may miss breast cancer in women with small tumors, and cannot replace sentinel node biopsy or axillary dissection. On the other hand, PET is more sensitive than conventional imaging for detecting metastatic disease and should be considered when staging or restaging women with suspected or known distant metastases. PET may also be useful in evaluating response to therapy, when symptoms are unclear and a change in therapy is considered. However, FDG-PET based evaluation of response is challenging because of the absence of a reproducible, validated, and widely accepted set of standards.

27.3.4 Gastrointestinal Malignancies

27.3.4.1 Esophageal Cancer

In esophageal cancer (EC) patients, endoscopic ultrasound (EUS) is the modality of choice for the evaluation of tumor depth of invasion (T) and locoregional lymph node (N) staging, preferred over FDG-PET/CT and dedicated CT [115–118]. Nonetheless, a significant correlation exists between the SUVs and both the size of the primary and with the depth of tumor penetration [119].

It is now widely recognized that FDG-PET imaging is not highly sensitive in locoregional staging. A meta-analysis [120] reported a pooled sensitivity for the detection of locoregional lymph node metastases of

51% with a pooled specificity of 84% [121]. A prospective comparison of CT, EUS, and FDG-PET [122] demonstrated a higher sensitivity for EUS in the detection of locoregional nodal disease compared to PET and CT (85% vs. 35% vs. 42%). Consequently, FDG-PET remains as an adjunct to conventional imaging modalities for the evaluation of lymph node metastases. Similar to other gastrointestinal (GI) cancers, FDG-PET/CT is the most accurate modality to determine distant metastatic disease with a better sensitivity and specificity. In a systematic analysis, the pooled sensitivity and specificity for the detection of metastatic disease by PET was 67% and 97%, respectively [121]. However, a positive PET finding usually triggers a confirmatory tissue biopsy to avoid false-positive results [123,124]. In a meta-analysis, the hazard ratios for disease recurrence and death were 2.5 and 1.9, respectively, for those with a higher than median tumor SUVmax [115] even for those with apparently early stage squamous cell carcinoma [116]. The 5-year overall survival for those with an SUVmax >4.5 was 47% compared to 76% in those with lower SUVs [118]. However, these results could not be replicated in patients with adenocarcinoma of the distal esophagus or gastroesophageal junction (GEJ) [125]. Thus, further validation of SUVmax as an independent predictor of patient outcome is warranted.

The percent change in SUV of the primary tumor after chemotherapy or chemoradiotherapy was investigated to predict therapy response [126–129]. A reduction of 35% from baseline was demonstrated to have a sensitivity and specificity of 93% and 95%, respectively, for the detection of a pathological response [126]. Using this cutoff in patients with locally advanced GEJ tumors undergoing preoperative chemotherapy, 44% with a metabolic response had a pathological response, compared to 5% of metabolic nonresponders [127]. More recently, in same category of patients in the metabolic response evaluation for individualization of neoadjuvant chemotherapy in oesophageal and oesophagogastric adeNocarcinoma (MUNICON) trial, of the metabolic responders (>35% decrease in SUV 2 weeks after treatment initiation) versus nonresponders 58% versus 0% achieved a major histological response [128]. Metabolic nonresponders had a median event-free survival (EFS) of 14 months compared to 30 months in metabolic responders. However, metabolic responders without a pathological response had comparable survival profiles to those of metabolic nonresponders, implying that a metabolic response does not herald an improved survival. In a cross-trial comparison between the original study by Ott et al. and the later trial by Lordick et al. patient survival was unaffected by continuing or discontinuing ineffective chemotherapy and proceeding early to surgery. Further data are required to define the exact role for FGD PET/CT in evaluation of response in EC patients before a tailored approach can be established [127,128].

Not surprisingly, FDG-PET is a sensitive tool for the detection of EC recurrences, with a sensitivity and specificity of 94% and 82%, respectively, versus 81% and 82% for conventional modalities [130]. Although the sensitivity for local, regional, and distant sites of metastases were high at 97%, 86%, and 90.5%, respectively, the specificity was lower for locoregional recurrence at 50% versus ≥90%, respectively [131]. PET was also superior to CT in the detection of local metastasis [132].

27.3.4.2 Colorectal Cancer

Further staging of colorectal cancer patients who are candidates for definitive surgical treatment for metastatic disease is essential for proper management [133]. FDG-PET/CT is highly sensitive and specific for intrahepatic colorectal metastasis and the most sensitive imaging modality for the identification of extrahepatic tumors. In multiple systematic reviews and meta-analyses [134–137], FDG-PET was found to be significantly more sensitive at 88%–95% than anatomic modalities followed by MRI yielding a sensitivity at approximately 75% [134–138]. However, more recent data suggest that contrast-enhanced MRI is more sensitive for detection of small hepatic metastases [139–141] but with a caveat of inferior specificity compared to FDG-PET/CT [140]. These data are also outdated by the application of novel methodologies such as superparamagnetic iron oxide-enhanced MRI that is deemed to be superior to gadolinium-enhanced MRI especially in small lesions [134,135,140]. In a meta-analysis, although specificities were similar (95%–96% vs. 87%–97%) for hepatic lesions, PET/CT had higher sensitivity (91%–100% vs. 78%–94%) and specificity (75%–100% vs. 25%–98%) than CT [137]. In a systematic review, in patients with apparently resectable hepatic metastases, occult extrahepatic disease was detected by FDG-PET in about 20% of patients [142]. It should be emphasized that the likelihood of PET-based detection of extrahepatic metastasis increases with disease severity (e.g., high tumor burden as evidenced by multiple hepatic metastases, lymph node metastases) [143–145]. FDG-PET alters management in 25% of patients, essentially reducing the rate of futile hepatic resections as a result of the discovery of extrahepatic disease [143–148]. In some cases, liver resection is performed along with resection of lung metastasis or isolated metastasis at other sites [143,144,148]. Nonetheless, staging with FDG-PET does not increase the number of survivors after liver resection but the proportion of survivors by eliminating patients who would not benefit from surgery [149].

After primary curative treatment, for the patients with rising carcinoembryonic antigen but normal cross-sectional imaging, FDG-PET is the standard care imaging tool for identification of occult recurrent disease

[150–154], both in hepatic and extrahepatic sites. The overall reported average sensitivity and specificity for detecting recurrent disease are 89%, and 92%, respectively [12]. For local recurrence, PET/CT has better accuracy than CT (sensitivity, 93%–100% vs. 0%–100% and specificity 98% vs. 98%) [138]. The course of management can change in up to 60% of patients on the basis of PET findings [152,155,156].

In summary, staging with FDG-PET is recommended as standard practice for detection of intrahepatic and extrahepatic colorectal metastases in patients scheduled for hepatic resection. FDG-PET should be used in combination with MRI, when possible, to increase the sensitivity for small hepatic metastases. FDG-PET reduces futile laparotomies and to a lesser extent futile hepatectomies. FDG-PET should be used to stage patients with synchronous or metachronous colorectal hepatic metastases with the expectation that management will be altered. False negative findings can occur in small tumors (<1.0 cm) [143,144,147,157,158], after recent chemotherapy [148], and in mucinous tumors [158].

27.3.4.3 Pancreatic Adenocarcinoma

Cystic pancreatic lesions are increasingly being recognized as a significant challenge to cross-sectional imaging. In the differentiation of benign versus malignant cystic disease of the pancreas, FDG-PET was found superior to CT with respect to sensitivity, specificity, and positive and negative predictive values, at 94%, 94%, 89%, and 97%, respectively; corresponding values for CT were 65%, 88%, 73%, and 83% [159]. FDG-PET has a lower sensitivity than EUS, but a higher specificity than all other modalities, and highest positive predictive value and overall accuracy [160]. In a larger study, comparing PET with CT and MRI, the sensitivity of PET was lower than that of CT but higher than that of MRI (91% CT vs. 82% PET vs. 78% MRI), and PET had the highest specificity and positive predictive value among the three modalities.

At staging, FDG-PET is inferior to thin-slice CT and EUS in delineating the anatomical boundaries of the primary tumor to determine resectability. Similarly, PET is poorly sensitive for the detection of locoregional lymph node metastases, with a sensitivity ranging from 50% to 75% [161,162]. Similar to other malignancies, FDG-PET is highly sensitive for the detection of hepatic and bone metastases, but not for the peritoneal spread [162,163].

Semiquantitative analysis using SUV of 4 as a cutoff at baseline showed promising results for risk stratifying patients into two distinct groups [159,164]. Furthermore, in patients with locally advanced disease who undergo neoadjuvant chemoradiotherapy, a metabolic response was associated with a significantly

longer survival than otherwise (23.2 months vs. 11.3 months) [165,166]. The significance of these preliminary results within the context of management changes, however, is not assessable in the absence of effective treatment regimens. Of note, the SUVs were significantly higher in carcinomas compared to those of chronic pancreatitis (mean SUVmax, 6.4 vs. 3.6) ($p < .001$) [167].

The sensitivity of FDG-PET for detection of local recurrence, abdominal lymph node metastasis, and peritoneal carcinomatosis is approximately 85% [168]. FDG-PET/CT appears superior to anatomic modalities in the detection of recurrent disease within the tumor bed, but ceCT or MRI have better discriminatory power within the hepatic parenchyma [169]. Thus, addition of ceCT to PET in the same session may lead to further gains in the detection sensitivity [168,170,171]. False positives may occur, after instrumentation of the biliary tree, or in cases with bile duct dilations. Delayed PET may aid in the differentiation of benign from malignant lesions [172]. Glycemic control also increases the sensitivity of PET by as much as 50% [173].

In summary, for the esophageal, gastric, and colonic malignancies, depth of invasion and lymph node metastases cannot be optimally evaluated by FDG-PET scans. However, FDG-PET imaging is a standard practice in lymph node staging of the cancers of the esophagus. However, the niche for FDG-PET imaging in GI malignancies is the identification occult metastatic disease in locally advanced malignancies or detection of extrahepatic disease in those undergoing hepatic resections, which may then change the treatment plan. Preliminary studies suggested promising results in the prediction of therapy but more data are warranted to justify its use and determine an incremental benefit.

27.3.5 Gynecologic Malignancies

27.3.5.1 Cervical Cancer

There has been a growing interest in applications of FDG-PET imaging in gynecologic malignancies to provide better care and improve patient outcome. Cervical cancers are mainly of squamous cell histology and spread by direct invasion into the parametrium and adjacent organs and through lymphatic invasion involves the pelvic, para-aortic (PALN), and supraclavicular lymph nodes. Hematogenic spread to distant solid organs or bone is rare. Surgical staging with lymphadenectomy is more accurate than the clinical staging, using the International Federation for Gynecology and Obstetrics (FIGO) system, but is controversial as there is no proof for a survival benefit [174].

FDG-PET/CT is not a highly sensitive imaging modality to differentiate between various depths of tumor invasion within the cervical stroma to allow for omission of radiotherapy following radical hysterectomy [175]. Pelvic lymph node metastasis is the most important prognostic factor rendering radical hysterectomy futile if the suspected lymph nodes are proven positive by histopathology. Similar to other malignancies, FDG-PET is superior to other modalities in identifying distant metastasis in patients with locally advanced stage disease [176–181]. In this population, detection of otherwise unknown extrapelvic disease may lead to abandoning plans of definitive chemoradiotherapy. The sensitivity of FDG-PET in the identification of PALN metastases is 95% [179], which may have a high clinical relevance in precise definition of radiotherapy fields [182,183]. Moreover, salvage therapy plans may be obviated by the discovery of disseminated disease. Currently, there is no established role for quantitative measurements using SUVmax in the grading of the tumor aggressiveness and in predicting stromal invasion or pelvic lymph node metastasis [175].

Determination of disease prognosis through PET/CT-based risk stratification may alter treatment strategies with an ultimate goal of improving outcome. Despite the absence of a proven survival benefit, PET/CT can detect recurrent disease in asymptomatic patients [184–187]. However, more data are warranted to determine whether PET as a routine diagnostic imaging modality is beneficial.

27.3.5.2 Ovarian Cancer

More than 50% of ovarian cancer patients are diagnosed at an advanced stage with rather unfavorable prognosis [188,189]. Commonly, the tumor spreads into the peritoneal cavity rather than involving lymph nodes [190,191] and metastases to distant and extra-abdominal organs are relatively uncommon except in the late course of the disease. The mainstay of ovarian cancer treatment involves optimal neoadjuvant chemotherapy and cytoreductive surgery [192–196]. Although the overall response rate is about 80%, majority of the patients will ultimately succumb to progressive disease.

In characterization of asymptomatic adnexal masses, FDG-PET has no proven superiority over morphologic modalities with a reported sensitivity of only 60% and a specificity of 75% [197,198]. Although its sensitivity increases in cases presenting with elevated CA125 serum levels [199], the role of FDG-PET in the characterization of adnexal masses is yet to be validated. For the staging of ovarian carcinoma, FDG-PET provides additional information improving the accuracy of CT [200–202] essentially proving useful in evaluating for distant metastases as well as equivocal lesions [202,203]. Moreover, the improved staging specificity provided

with the use of PET/CT compared to CT (91% vs. 64%) was striking in distinguishing between stages IIIC–IV and I–IIIB cancer [202,204]. In this context, the combined use of FDG-PET with ceCT was reported to increase the overall sensitivity from 40% to 70% at no cost to specificity [203]. Thus, integrated PET/ceCT may be helpful in the identification of patients for whom optimal debulking surgery is planned.

In the post-therapy setting, the sensitivity (80%–100%) of FDG-PET/CT for detecting recurrent ovarian cancer is higher than its specificity (42%–100%) [205–208]. Combination of FDG-PET and CA-125 titers in monitoring epithelial ovarian cancer apparently increased the sensitivity to above 95% when conventional imaging studies were equivocal [209–211]. PET/CT was able to detect active disease at relatively low levels of CA-125 [212,213] resulting in significant management changes in 40%–60% of patients with suspected ovarian cancer recurrence [213–216]. However, small-volume disease, omental carcinomatosis of multiple coalescing subcentimeter lesions, mucinous, and cystic tumors may give rise to false negative findings [206,207,217,218]. A higher test accuracy was reported when PET was performed with ceCT compared with each test alone (79% vs 74% vs 61%) [214].

27.3.5.3 Endometrial Cancer

The overall survival rate for endometrial cancer is favorable at 75%–90% for stage I patients on the account of early detection [219]. To date, no significant benefit was obtained with the use of CT, MRI, and FDG-PET imaging in the preoperative evaluation of endometrial cancer. At initial stage, endometrial cancer most commonly metastasizes to the regional lymph nodes. The morphologic techniques have a relatively low sensitivity at 18%–66% for detecting nodal metastases [220–223]. For FDG-PET imaging, a trend toward a higher sensitivity was reported for detecting lymph node metastases [224]. The sensitivity for detecting metastatic lesions is 67% for lesions measuring 5–9 mm and 93% for lesions measuring ≥10 mm. PET is also more sensitive than either CT or MRI for identifying other extranodal metastatic disease (~85% vs. 70%).

In view of data showing no survival benefit with systematic pelvic lymphadenectomy, preoperative staging with CT or PET scan does not seem to offer additional benefit. Despite a recommendation for complete surgical staging by FIGO, no survival benefit has, thus far, been suggested; therefore, many surgeons perform only selective lymph node dissection. In the absence of comparative data between PET/CT staging and surgical staging, further definition of the role of PET in cervical cancer staging is not possible at present.

Recurrence in the vagina and isolated pelvic lymph nodes can be successfully treated, but recurrence at distant sites are rarely salvageable [225,226]. FDG-PET provides improved sensitivity and specificity compared to CT in recurrent endometrial cancer, leading to a change of management in about 40% of patients [180]. Hence, FDG-PET imaging can be used as the preferred modality in the case of suspicious recurrence to identify disease sites.

In summary, FDG-PET/CT in the staging of cervical and ovarian cancer may increase the staging accuracy when combined with ceCT; however, further studies with larger patient populations are warranted to definitively prove its clinical value. However, the niche for FDG-PET/CT lies in its ability to identify extrapelvic spread and distant metastases to guide the decision for abandoning surgical intervention for chemoradiotherapy or administration of neoadjuvant chemotherapy as the first-choice treatment prior to surgery. FDG-PET/CT is an effective imaging modality in the early detection of recurrent gynecologic cancers.

27.3.6 Lymphoma

The common lymphoma histologies, including Hodgkin lymphoma (HL), diffuse large B-cell lymphoma (DLBCL), and follicular lymphoma (FL), are uniformly FDG avid yielding a high diagnostic sensitivity of 90%–100% for PET/CT imaging [227–230]. However, the sensitivity of PET can be as low as 50% for the other subtypes of indolent lymphoma including extranodal marginal zone lymphoma and chronic lymphocytic leukemia/small lymphocytic lymphoma [231–236]. FDG-PET is particularly helpful in identifying the site of transformation to a higher grade histology with more than 80% certainty, especially when SUVmax exceeds 10 in an individual lesion [237,238].

Ann Arbor staging, the most widely used staging system [239,240], but does not include FDG-PET imaging as a recommended staging test for lymphoma. However, recommendations may change in the near future considering the superiority of FDG-PET over CT as a staging tool as evidenced by results of a meta-analysis revealing a pooled sensitivity and a false-positive rate of 91% and 10%, respectively, on a patient-based analysis [241]. On a lesion basis, the maximum joint sensitivity and specificity (96%) far exceeded corresponding values for ceCT [228,233,241–245]. FDG-PET typically leads to upstaging in about 30% of patients, but stage migration from early to advanced stage disease occurs in less than 15% of patients [228,242–252]. This is clinically relevant with the recent trend of de-escalating treatment and limiting radiotherapy to only involved lymph nodes that require a highly accurate test to determine the extent of disease. A diagnostic strategy of combining FDG-PET

with ceCT may be reasonable in patients with advanced stage disease and abdominal lymphomas for delineating lymph nodes from adjacent bowel loops and vasculature [244–246]. Evaluation for bone marrow involvement (BMI) is one of the dilemmas in lymphoma management as BMI upstages disease and may change treatment approach. The sensitivity of PET in detecting BMI is high in HL (~90%) but moderate in aggressive non-Hodgkin lymphoma (NHL) (~75%) and low in low-grade lymphomas (~50%) [247–253]. The lower sensitivity in NHL is probably on the basis of presence of discordant diffuse small-cell lymphoid infiltrates in DLBCL, low-grade histology in the latter, and diffuse uptake pattern in both [230,254–256]. Given the rare occurrence of BMI and early-stage HL [257–259], bone marrow biopsy should be restricted to patients with suspected sites detected on a staging FDG-PET, those with NHL, as well as those with advanced stage or unfavorable HL.

27.3.6.1 Evaluation of Therapy Response

Post-therapy FDG-PET imaging proved to be a good predictor for disease recurrence [96–103] with significantly disparate relapse-free survivals between PET-negative (85%–95%) and PET-positive patients (0%–5%) in HL and aggressive NHL populations [260–267]. Consequently, in the revised Integrated International Workshop Criteria, the terminology of "complete remission/unconfirmed" has been eliminated by better tissue characterization provided by FDG-PET imaging. Currently, those patients without metabolic evidence of residual disease are classified as CR regardless of CT findings. Similar results are also emerging for untreated FL patients after 4 or 6 cycles of induction chemoimmunotherapy indicating that posttreatment PET positive patients are likely to relapse earlier than PET-negative patients [212,268].

FDG-PET showed a prognostic value in patients with relapsed/refractory HL or DLBCL undergoing salvage chemotherapy prior to autologous stem cell transplantation (ASCT) [268–272]. A recent meta-analysis of HL and DLBCL patients reported a 3-year progression-free survival (PFS) for positive versus negative functional imaging was 23% versus 69%, respectively ($p < .0001$) [273]. More recently data were confirmed with PET-positive disease yielding significantly inferior 3-year PFS or EFS (31%–41%) compared with patients who had PET-negative results following salvage chemotherapy prior to ASCT (75%–82%) [268–272].

27.3.6.2 Early Response Evaluation during Therapy

Persistent FDG uptake after a few cycles of chemotherapy is associated with a high relapse rate (50%–100%) while the relapse rate is usually low (~10%) in those with a negative interim PET [274–279]. A meta-analysis reported a sensitivity of 81% and a specificity of 97%, for an interim FDG-PET study in advanced-stage HL, and a sensitivity of 78% and a specificity of 87% in DLBCL [279]. Recent studies provided further support for the role of PET in advanced stage HL, in the prediction of ultimate outcome although in early stage HL enthusiasm for interim PET imaging has been tempered with no clear difference noted between PET-2 positive and negative patients with respect to PFSs low [280–288]. In limited stage nonbulky HL patients treated with ABVD, no significant difference PFS between interim PET-positive and negative groups could be demonstrated (87% vs. 91%; $p = .57$) [267] when end-chemotherapy PET was highly predictive of PFS (94% vs. 54%; $p < .0001$). It should be emphasized that the effectiveness of therapy affects the predictive value of diagnostic tests, namely less efficacious therapy regimens yield higher false negative results [265,266]. In addition, treatment intensification schemes executed after a positive interim PET result negate the positive predictive value of PET [268–270]. In such a randomizing setting in HL, based on interim PET, the negative and PPV for predicting 2-year PFS were 96% and 16%, respectively ($p < .0001$). Another adaptive therapy trial in advanced-stage HL, using not only interim-PET results but also the international prognostic score (IPS), reported a 10-year PFS was 83% in patients with positive interim PET compared with 93% for those with a negative interim study (ns) suggesting that unfavorable outcomes can be overcome by therapy intensification [269].

In DLBCL, although there was early evidence that an interim would predict PFS, the results of later studies varied significantly among patient groups, particularly in the PET-positive cohorts. The 2-year PFS for the PET-negative group was 82%–93% versus 0%–43% for PET-positive group [289–291]. These differences in PET results can be attributed to differences in follow-up periods, patient populations, and types of treatments employed, that is, chemotherapy alone or with immunotherapy. More recently, interim PET after four cycles of chemoimmunotherapy was found to yield a considerably high false-positive rate (87%) proven by and 51% of these patients remained progression free after consolidation therapy during the follow-up period [292]. In contrast, in a phase II trial of interim PET-adapted therapy of B cell lymphoma patients, the favorable outcome achieved here in historically poor-risk patients warrants further, more definitive investigation of treatment modification based on early PET scanning [293]. There are multiple ongoing PET-adapted randomized trials whose results will be shedding more light onto the clinical use of interim PET in both HL and DLBCL.

Interim PET should be performed at least 10–15 days after the start of chemotherapy to avoid false-positive results induced by inflammatory response that maximizes at day 10 of chemotherapy [294,295]. After completion of therapy, a 3–4 week window should be allowed to minimize confounding by inflammation. The time interval between radiation therapy and FDG-PET should not be less than 4 weeks and ideally should be 6–8 weeks. The widely recognized challenge to the interim PET is the so-called "minimal residual uptake" phenomenon [275–277]. The threshold for a positive interim PET scan has increased over the years to increase the specificity of PET readings. Definition of a positive interim PET scan has evolved from any uptake above background to uptake intensity that is equal to that seen in the mediastinal blood pool (MBP) structures [294], and more recently to an intensity exceeding the background in the liver [296–298]. The criteria defined by the imaging subcommittee of the International Harmonization Project in lymphoma for post-therapy PET scans use the MBP as an internal reference for lesions 2.0 cm or larger [294]. More recently, a graded system "Deauville five-point scale" was proposed to accommodate different positivity thresholds for better tuning of the test specificity [296–298]. These criteria have recently been validated in a multicenter study of a retrospective cohort of 260 advanced-stage HL patients treated with ABVD [299]. After a mean follow-up of 27 months, the 3-year PFS of PET-2 positive and negative patients were 28% and 95%, respectively ($p < .001$). The binary concordance between paired reviewers for positive versus negative results was "very good" (Cohen's k: 0.84).

27.3.6.3 Recurrent Lymphoma

In a meta-analysis, the sensitivity and specificity of FDG-PET in predicting disease relapse for HL were 50%–100% and 67%–100%, respectively, and for NHL 33%–77% and 82%–100%, respectively [300]. The majority of relapses are diagnosed clinically in aggressive NHL; however, HL relapses may be more commonly detected by FDG-PET imaging [301–303]. However, survival does not appear to be affected by mode of detection. Frequent FDG-PET follow-up is not necessary in patients with early-stage nonbulky, low-risk HL, given recurrence rates of less than 15% [304,305].

In summary, FDG-PET reliably detects disease resistance early in the course of therapy, its effectiveness as a surrogate for chemoresistance or chemosensitivity has been proven at interim evaluation only in advanced stage HL. Furthermore, there is no evidence to suggest that an early change of therapy in poorly responding patients will translate into a survival benefit. Prospective, randomized, multicenter trials are underway to further define the benefit of individualized therapies using FDG-PET as a surrogate for tumor therapy response.

27.3.7 Myeloma

Multiple myeloma is a malignant plasma cell disorder characterized by serum calcium elevation, renal insufficiency, anemia, and osteolytic lesions. However, FDG-PET proved more sensitive than whole-body x-ray (WBXR) surveys at staging or restaging [306–313] by revealing at least 50% more lesions. Importantly, MRI has a proven superiority in detecting myeloma in the spine and pelvis, especially when there is diffuse bone infiltration [306,309,311,314–317].

There is paucity of data investigating the value of FDG-PET imaging in response evaluation after initial therapy [306,316,318–320]. In prospective studies, a correlation was demonstrated between baseline SUVs (SUV > 4.2) and survival [320]. In addition, the presence of more than three FDG-avid focal lesions at baseline was an independent parameter associated with inferior survival (30-month EFS, 66% vs. 87%). For defining complete remission, normalization of FDG uptake was a better prognostic marker than M-protein (30-month EFS 89% vs. 63%), even in patients with poor cytogenetics [319]. There is only limited information on the value of FDG-PET scan in evaluating nonsecretory multiple myeloma [309,321], an entity in which PET can identify disease presence in the absence of positive laboratory tests. The inconsistent interpretation criteria, however, require standardization to clearly define focal and diffuse skeletal and extramedullary uptake. Although visual assessment of FDG-PET images remain the mainstay for diagnosis and response assessment, quantitative analysis with SUVs would allow for an objective assessment, thereby minimizing inter-observer variations.

In summary, FDG-PET with its clearly higher sensitivity should replace the currently recommended WBXR as the gold standard imaging modality. FDG-PET is less sensitive than MRI for detecting bone disease in the spine and pelvis; however, the potential impact of whole-body MRI on clinical management remains to be explored. Using FDG-PET/CT with or without MRI will probably upstage patients with smoldering myeloma but the clinical consequences of upstaging are unclear in light of current international myeloma working group (IMWG) guidelines [322]. For response assessment, complete normalization of FDG uptake before ASCT correlates with better survival; hence, PET may be preferable over MRI to confirm rapid metabolic normalization when the latter continues to be positive for prolonged periods after therapy. However, it is essential that these prior results be prospectively validated in large patient samples using uniform protocol guidelines and interpretation criteria to justify possible management changes, particularly, in view of the emerging novel treatment options.

27.3.8 Urogenital Cancers

27.3.8.1 Testicular Cancer

Contrast-enhanced CT imaging is currently the imaging procedure of choice for staging of testicular cancer patients although ultrasound, MRI, and FDG-PET/CT have specific roles in the clinical management of these patients [323,324]. Approximately 30% of patients have small metastatic deposits in nonenlarged lymph nodes seen on CT [323,324]. The identification of retroperitoneal lymph node involvement is important because stage I disease is treated with surgical treatment while patients with stage II disease receive chemotherapy [325]. The sensitivity of FDG-PET in the detection of retroperitoneal nodal metastases in seminomatous and nonseminomatous testicular cancer varies between 67% and 91% but is slightly better than that of CT [324,326–330]. However, both CT and FDG-PET are limited by their ability to detect small lesions in nonseminomatous germ cell tumors [326–328]. Although FDG-PET/CT at initial staging of early stage disease is promising, an incremental benefit is yet to be proven for its adoption in clinical practice. A rational use of FDG-PET would be in patients with suspected distant metastases to accurately determine the site of metastases [331].

Approximately one-third of patients with early stage nonseminomatous germ cell tumors will relapse within the first year after orchidectomy [325]. It was suggested that FDG-PET may have a role in the detection of recurrent disease in patients with rising tumor markers and no evidence of active disease on CT [331–333]. Despite a high positive predictive value at ~90%, the negative predictive value of FDG-PET was suboptimal at only 50%, particularly in patients with mature teratoma [327,333].

Similar to lymphoma, post-therapy masses are common and it has been estimated that almost half of the patients with a residual post-therapy mass seen on CT undergo unwarranted surgical resection [15]. FDG-PET can help characterize residual masses in seminomas with a superior specificity and sensitivity of 100% and 80%, respectively, compared to ~75% and ~70%, respectively, for CT [334–336]. FDG-PET performed within 8 weeks of orchidectomy yielded false-negative results in 30% of patients who relapsed with a median follow-up of 12 months [337]. Therefore, FDG-PET alone cannot be used as a substitute for retroperitoneal lymph node dissection to distinguish between stage I and stage II disease.

Several studies have addressed the favorable role of serial FDG-PET for prediction of treatment response in germ cell tumor patients undergoing salvage high-dose chemotherapy [335,336,338]. The sensitivities and specificities for prediction of therapy response were 100% and 67% for FDG-PET, 62% and 80% for CT and/or MRI, and 83% and 100% for normalization of tumor markers [335]. In a recent study of a large group of patients, PET sensitivity, specificity, negative predictive value, and positive predictive value were 82%, 90%, 95%, and 69%, respectively, when PET was performed at least 6 weeks after the end of chemotherapy [336]. The PET accuracy significantly improved from 73% to 88% when PET performance was compared within 6 weeks and beyond 6 weeks after therapy ($p = .032$). Although these results suggest a role for FDG-PET as a tool for clinical decision-making prospective, multicenter data are warranted to confirm these results.

27.3.8.2 Renal Cell Carcinoma

FDG-PET does not provide more useful information than CT for the characterization of renal masses because of its limited sensitivity at 60% compared with >90% for CT [339]. However, it may have a role in identification of retroperitoneal lymph node, lung, or bone metastases and renal bed recurrence, because of a higher specificity compared to CT [340]. FDG-PET may be also useful to assess tumor response to therapy, at metastatic sites [341–343]. Recent reports have indicated that high FDG uptake may herald a worse outcome compared with less FDG-avid RCC lesions [344]. However, FDG may not be the ideal radiotracer for imaging renal cell cancer. Other molecules including a [124]I-labeled chimeric antibody cG250, which targets the tumor-associated protein carbonic anhydrase IX, are in investigation for the detection of clear cell renal cancer [345].

27.3.8.3 Prostate Cancer

Currently, there is no established role for FDG-PET/CT in the assessment of osseous and soft-tissue metastases of prostate cancer, as well as in the detection of recurrent disease probably owing to the relatively low metabolic rate of the tumor [346–350]. However, there is some evidence to suggest that FDG-PET can identify active osseous disease versus quiescent lesions as well as those with osteoclastic activity [351]. Currently, there are no data proving a therapy efficacy based on FDG uptake changes after treatment [352] in castrate-resistant metastatic disease. Given the limitations of FDG-PET imaging in the management of prostate cancer, other PET tracers are under investigation. These include phospholipids in the cell membrane of tumor cells representing the rate of tumor cell replication such as F-18 labeled choline, radiolabeled amino acid tracers such as anti-1-amino-3-^{18}F-fluorocyclobutyl-1-carboxylic acid (^{18}F-FACBC), and PSMA targeting molecules such as 18F-DCFBC [353,354].

27.3.8.4 Bladder Cancer

Currently, there is no established role for FDG-PET/CT imaging in the staging of bladder cancer, mainly because of the physiological urinary excretion of the tracer [355]. Although the sensitivity of FDG-PET is better than CT in the detection of pelvic nodal metastases, it still remains at 46% with a specificity of 97% [356,357]. FDG-PET/CT might be more helpful in patients with suspected distant metastasis [358]. Reports also suggest a role for FDG-PET in identification of the site of recurrent disease [357,359]. However, FDG may not be the ideal radiotracer as other radiotracers such as ^{11}C-acetate for the assessment of bladder cancer or its metastasis [360].

27.3.9 NaF Bone Imaging

Although F-18 labeled NaF was developed in the 1960s as a bone imaging radiotracer, introduction of more practical and less costly radiotracers, that is, Tc-99m-labeled bone agents, stunned its growth until at present. The recent availability of PET scanners and the favorable imaging performance of NaF have ignited a renewed interest in NaF as a routine bone-imaging agent. The uptake mechanism of NaF is similar to that of diphosphonates with chemisorption into bone crystals with the formation of fluoroapatite [361,362]; however, its higher first pass extraction by the bones and unbound status to proteins provide grounds for obtaining high-quality scans as early as 1 hour after injection with similar dosimetry profile to MDP bone scan [362–365]. Integrated PET/CT improves the specificity and overall accuracy of skeletal NaF PET [366,367]. It was also noted that sclerotic lesions with higher CT Hounsfield units (HUs) yielded negative results and there was a negative correlation between SUV and HU measurements [368]. In prospective series, NaF-PET was more accurate in detecting skeletal metastases than bone scintigraphy (99% versus 64%–74%) on a lesion basis, but on a patient basis, the differences were smaller [369,370]. The sensitivity of NaF-PET was the same for osteoblastic prostate cancer metastases as it was for osteolytic metastases from lung and thyroid carcinomas [364]. When NaF was compared with planar bone scintigraphy with single photon emission computed tomography (SPECT) of the spine [371], there was not a significant difference in the accuracy between SPECT and PET (94% vs. 99%). However, a larger study in lung cancer patients showed a statistical difference between PET and SPECT (99% vs. 87.5%). In a more recent study, NaF-PET was compared with FDG-PET/CT and planar bone scintigraphy in NSCLC [372]. In this group of patients, more skeletal metastatic lesions were detected with FDG-PET/CT than with NaF-PET overall. Although FDG-PET/CT was more accurate than bone scintigraphy, it remains uncertain whether it can also replace NaF-PET in staging the skeleton in lung cancer. It was also postulated to combine the two tracers to optimize diagnostic information [373,374]. A multicenter study is underway in the United States comparing NaF-PET with Tc-99m MDP in routine skeletal staging in patients with breast cancer, prostate cancer, and NSCLC [375]. This large collaborative project will be of great interest in addressing unanswered questions regarding skeletal staging with NaF. Moreover, therapeutic interventions targeting neoplastic bone diseases should be assessed for their effectiveness in future clinical trials.

27.3.10 General Pitfalls

It is important to consider some pitfalls of FDG-PET/CT imaging for more accurate scan interpretation. False-negative results may be obtained in lesions smaller than 7 mm, in tumors with a low metabolic rate (e.g., well-differentiated prostate, thyroid, and hepatocellular carcinoma; low-grade lymphoma; and mucinous carcinomas), and suboptimal preparation of patients with diabetes, non-fasting, steroid administration, immediately after cytotoxic or cytostatic treatments that may interfere with glucose transport into the cell. Waiting at least 4 weeks after the last cycle of chemotherapy is recommended to avoid false-negative results from metabolic stunning. In addition, activated macrophages, neutrophils, and fibroblasts in infectious/inflammatory processes and granulation tissues demonstrate significant FDG accumulation. Hence, interpretation of FDG-PET studies in the post-therapy requires special attention to minimize a false-positive result.

27.3.11 Radiotherapy Planning

The difference between the dose that is required for tumor control and normal tissue tolerance, so-called "therapeutic window," is an important concept for radiotherapy. To effectively increase the tumor control with no increase in toxicity, accurate definition of tumor borders is of pivotal importance. Improved accuracy in the determination of gross tumor volume (GTV) may allow for dose escalation to tumor and reduced dose to critical structures to improve local control [376–380], but, given its low discriminatory value, CT may lead to undertreatment of metabolically active disease. In this regard, FDG-PET/CT has been used for selection of candidates for definitive radiotherapy and delineation of radiation therapy volume [378]. It has been reported that the GTV is statistically significantly larger with FDG-PET/CT–based assessment than with CT-based assessment [381]. PET/CT is generally more accurate in detection of lymph node and distant metastases, radiation therapy can be designed to target positive nodes

selectively [378,379]. The CT component of PET may also be used for radiation therapy planning if acquired using the proper dedicated CT protocol. Overall, the addition of FDG-PET to CT in radiation therapy planning may lead to changes in the target volumes in 20%–60% of patients [11,103,376,377,382–385].

One important issue to consider is the false-positive PET findings in up to 39% of patients, which should be confirmed by histology, probably with the help of EUS-FNA, when possible [386,387]. Whether PET-based radiotherapy planning will result in improved outcomes such as survival or locoregional tumor control is yet to be proven with ongoing trials.

27.3.12 Positron Emission Tomography/ MRI and the Future

Integrated PET/MRI in oncologic applications is an emerging modality that is increasingly gaining recognition in oncologic and imaging circles, however, the available data are rather limited to justify a role for it particularly in the presence of extensive data on PET/CT. Based on its high soft-tissue contrast, MRI has the ability to define soft-tissue pathology and differentiate between various depths of tumor penetration for assessing local tumor infiltration at staging or relapse [388–392]. In preoperative planning of tumor resection, the combination of MRI and FDG-PET can determine a well-delineated tumor-free surgical margin for surgically resectable tumors [392]. FDG-PET with its superior metabolic tissue characterization may provide significant staging and prognostic information with clear management consequences. In this context, FDG-PET/CT apparently has a higher sensitivity for the detection of lymph node metastases, compared to whole-body MRI [393–395]. MRI, especially when incorporating diffusion-weighted sequences, can identify bone marrow infiltration [396] with a higher sensitivity than FDG-PET [397–400] and also before the development of anatomic changes noted on CT. This is highly relevant for myeloma, lymphoma, and bone metastasis in solid tumors [388,389]. In lymphoma, the addition of diffusion-weighted MRI may significantly increase the accuracy of whole-body MRI for primary staging [401]; this may not be impressive, however, in view of the success or FDG-PET/CT in lymphoma. Nonetheless, in low-grade lymphomas and in lymphomas with variable FDG accumulation such as mantle cell lymphoma, PET/MRI may be preferable. Particularly, on the basis of the lack of radiation exposure of MRI compared with CT, this integrated modality may also be preferred for patients with curable lymphomas such as HL and DLBCL.

Functional PET/MRI coupled with diffusion-weighted and chemical shift imaging is a promising tool for response assessment in lymphoma patients [401]. In addition, diffusion-weighted MRI was shown to provide a measure of tumor cellularity, thus, may be used in the assessment of chemotherapy response in solid tumors [402]. This is a worthwhile area to perform prospective research to prove an incremental role for PET/MRI. MRI, with diffusion-weighted imaging, might also be a valuable tool in disease restaging, which has been shown to detect all residual nodal disease that were positive on FDG-PET/CT [403]. Theoretically, the combination of size criteria with ADC analysis and PET findings may decrease the false-positive rate associated with FDG-PET/CT alone.

In summary, FDG-PET integrated with MRI can be a preferable TNM staging tool for various cancers including head and neck cancer, soft-tissue and bone sarcomas, and pelvic cancers including gynecologic cancers. It also offers significant promise in characterizing hepatic lesions and brain tumors. The PET/MRI may be able to guide surgical planning and provide prognostic information with a positive impact to patient management and outcome. The benefits that could be derived from this novel modality with respect to staging and restaging of cancers compared to PET/CT applications are yet to be discovered in a sufficiently large scale.

With the emerging effective treatment options, the future directions for PET/CT will probably expand in the area of response assessment. It is likely that well-designed, multicenter clinical trials will facilitate the approval of approved clinical indications in the ongoing or post-therapy setting. More importantly, although integrated PET-CT has been widely adopted in clinical practice, standardization of image acquisition protocols and image interpretation have not kept up pace with expansion in PET application [404,405]. Although PET offers uniquely superior quantitative data for tracer biology and kinetics, PET quantitative applications have not been fully exploited in many oncology fields whose applications may be invaluable in the therapy response assessment. However, considering the nonspecific uptake mechanism of FDG, the most unmet need is in the area of novel PET radiotracers. Development of novel tracers for evaluation of tumor angiogenesis, tumor hypoxia, tumor cell proliferation, and tumor receptors will undoubtedly increase the applications of PET/CT as well as PET/MRI, if they are proven more specific with a minimal cost at sensitivity.

References

1. Sweet WH. The use of nuclear disintegration in diagnosis and treatment of brain tumors. *N Engl J Med.* 1951;245:875–878.

2. Ter-Pogossian MM, Powers WE. The use of radioactive oxygen-15 in determination of oxygen content in malignant neoplasmas. In: Valk PE ed. *Radioisotopes in Scientific Research*, Pergamon Press: London 1958.

3. Cormack AM. Representation of a function by its line integrals, with some radiological applications. *J Appl Phys.* 1963;34:2722–2727; Reconstruction densities from their projections, with applications in radiological physics. *Phys Med Biol.* 1973;18:195–207.

4. Hounsfield GN. Computerized transverse axial scanning (tomography). Part I: description of system. Part II: clinical applications. *Brit J Radiol.* 1973;46:1016–1022.

5. Kuhl D, Edwards R. Image separation radioisotope scanning. *Radiology.* 1963;80:653–661.

6. Phelps ME, Hoffman E, Mullani N, Higgins C, Ter-Pogossian M. Design considerations for a positron emission transaxial tomograph (PET III). *IEEE Trans Biomed Eng.* 1976;NS-23:516–522.

7. Hoffman E, Phelps M, Mullani N, Higgins C, Ter-Pogossian M. Design and performance characteristics of a whole body transaxial tomograph. *J Nucl Med.* 1976;17:493–503.

8. Sokoloff L, Reivich M, Kennedy C et al. The [14C] deoxyglucose method for the measurement of cerebral glucose utilization: theory, procedure and normal values in the conscious and anesthetized albino rat. *J Neurochem.* 1977;28:897–976.

9. Ido T, Wan CN, Casella JS et al. Labeled 2-deoxy- D-glucose analogs: 18F labeled 2-deoxy-2-fluoro-D-glucose, 2-deoxy-2-fluoro-D-mannose and 14C-2deoxy-2-fluoro-D-glucose. *J Labeled Compds Radiopharmacol.* 1978;14:175–183.

10. Schwaiger M, Brunken R, Grover-McKay M et al. Regional myocardial metabolism in patients with acute myocardial infarction assessed by positron emission tomography. *Am Coll Cardiol.* 1986;8:800–808.

11. Nutt R. 1999 ICP Distinguished Scientist Award. The history of positron emission tomography. *Mol Imaging Biol.* 2002;4:11–26.

12. Townsend DW. Dual-modality imaging: combining anatomy and function. *J Nucl Med.* 2008;49:938–955.

13. Knešaurek K, Ivanovic M, Machac J, Weber DA. Medical image registration. *Europhysics News.* 2000;31(4):5–8.

14. Ter-Pogossian MM, Ficke DC, Yamamoto M, Hood JT. Design characteristics and preliminary testing of Super-PETT I, a positron emission tomograph utilizing photon time-of-flight information (TOF PET). Proceedings of the Workshop on Time of Flight Tomography. St. Louis, MO. 1982. pp. 37–41.

15. Melcher CL, Schweitzer JS. Cerium-doped lutetium orthosilicate: a fast, efficient new scintillator. *IEEE Trans Nucl Sci.* 1992;NS-39:502–505.

16. Karp JS, Suleman S, Daube-Witherspoon ME, Muehllehner G. The benefit of time-of-flight in PET imaging: experimental and clinical results. *J Nucl Med.* 2008;49:462–470.

17. Zaidi H, Ojha N, Morich M et al. Design and performance evaluation of a whole-body Ingenuity TF PET-MRI system. *Phys Med Biol.* 2011;56:3091–3106.

18. Dels G, Furst S, Jakoby B et al. Performance measurements of the siemens mMR integrated whole-body PET/MR scanner. *J Nucl Med*. 2011;52:1–9.
19. Schulz V, Torres-Espallardo I, Renisch S et al. Automatic, three-segment, MR-based attenuation correction for whole-body PET/MR data. *Eur J Nucl Med Mol Imaging*. 2011;38:138–152.
20. Dixon WT. Simple proton spectroscopic imaging. *Radiology*. 1984;153:189–194.
21. Jemal A, Siegel R, Ward E et al. Cancer statistics, 2008. *CA Cancer J Clin*. 2008;58:71–96.
22. Schöder H, Yeung HWD. Positron emission imaging of head and neck cancer, including thyroid carcinoma. *Semin Nucl Med*. 2004;34:180–197.
23. Jeong HS, Baek CH, Son YI et al. Use of integrated 18F-FDG PET/CT to improve the accuracy of initial cervical nodal evaluation in patients with head and neck squamous cell carcinoma. *Head Neck*. 2007;29:203–210.
24. Kubicek GJ, Champ C, Fogh S et al. FDG-PET staging and importance of lymph node SUV in head and neck cancer. *Head Neck Oncol*. 2010;2:19.
25. Kyzas PA, Evangelou E, Denaxa-Kyza D, Ioannidis JPA. 18F-flurodeoxyglucose positron emission tomography to evaluate cervical node metastases in patients with head and neck squamous cell carcinoma: a meta-analysis. *J Natl Cancer Inst*. 2008;100:712–720.
26. Stoeckli SJ, Steinert H, Pfaltz M, Schmid S. Is there a role for positron emission tomography with 18F-fluorodeoxyglucose in the initial staging of nodal negative oral and oropharyngeal squamous cell carcinoma. *Head Neck*. 2002;24:345–349.
27. Myers LL, Wax MK, Nabi H, Simpson GT, Lamonica D. Positron emission tomography in the evaluation of the N0 neck. *Laryngoscope*. 1998;108:232–236.
28. Agarwal V, Branstetter BF IV, Johnson JT. Indications for PET/CT in the head and neck. *Otolaryngol Clin North Am*. 2008;41:23–49.
29. Kim SY, Roh JL, Yeo NK et al. Combined 18F-fluorodeoxyglucose- positron emission tomography and computed tomography as a primary screening method for detecting second primary cancers and distant metastases in patients with head and neck cancer. *Ann Oncol*. 2007;18:1698–1703.
30. Stokkel MP, Moons KG, ten Broek FW, van Rijk PP, Hordijk GJ. 18F-flurodeoxyglucose dual-head positron emission tomography as a procedure for detecting simultaneous primary tumors in cases of head and neck cancer. *Cancer*. 1999;86:2370–2377.
31. Connell CA, Corry J, Milner AD et al. Clinical impact of, and prognostic stratification by, F-18 FDG PET/CT in head and neck mucosal squamous cell carcinoma. *Head Neck*. 2007;29:986–995.
32. Lonneux M, Hamoir M, Reychler H et al. Positron emission tomography with [18F]fluorodeoxyglucose improves staging and patient management in patients with head and neck squamous cell carcinoma: a multicenter prospective study. *J Clin Oncol*. 2010;28:1190–1195.
33. O'Neill JP, Moynagh M, Kavanagh E, O'Dwyer T. Prospective, blinded trial of whole-body magnetic resonance imaging versus computed tomography positron emission tomography in staging primary and recurrent cancer of the head and neck. *J Laryngol Otol*. 2010;124:1274–1277.
34. Xie P, Li M, Zhao H, Sun X, Fu Z, Yu J. (18)F-FDG PET or PET-CT to evaluate prognosis for head and neck cancer: a meta-analysis. *J Cancer Res Clin Oncol*. 2011;137:1085–1931.
35. Fogarty GB, Peters LJ, Stewart J, Scott C, Rischin D, Hicks RJ. The usefulness of fluorine 18-labelled deoxyglucose positron emission tomography in the investigation of patients with cervical lymphadenopathy from an unknown primary tumor. *Head Neck*. 2003;25:138–145.
36. Wong WL, Chevretton EB, McGurk M et al. A prospective study of PET-FDG imaging for the assessment of head and neck squamous cell carcinoma. *Clin Otolaryngol Allied Sci*. 1997;22:209–214.
37. Lowe VJ, Dunphy FR, Varvares M et al. Evaluation of chemotherapy response in patients with advanced head and neck cancer using [F-18]flurodeoxyglucose positron emission tomography. *Head Neck*. 1997;19:666–674.
38. Lapela M, Grénman R, Kurki T et al. Head and neck cancer: detection of recurrence with PET and 2-[F-18]fluoro-2-deoxy-D-glucose. *Radiology*. 1995;197:205–211.
39. Schwartz DL, Ford E, Rajendran J et al. FDG-PET/CT imaging for preradiotherapy staging of head-and-neck squamous cell carcinoma. *Int J Radiat Oncol Biol Phys*. 2005;61:129–136.
40. Keller F, Psychogios G, Linke R et al. Carcinoma of unknown primary in the head and neck: comparison between positron emission tomography (PET) and PET/CT. *Head Neck*. 2011;33:1569–1575.
41. Bernier J, Domenge C, Ozsahin M et al. Postoperative irradiation with or without concomitant chemotherapy for locally advanced head and neck cancer. *N Engl J Med*. 2004;350:1945–1952.
42. Cooper JS, Pajak TF, Forastiere AA et al. Postoperative concurrent radiotherapy and chemotherapy for high-risk squamous-cell carcinoma. Radiation Therapy Oncology Group 9501/Intergroup. *N Engl J Med*. 2004;350:1937–1944.
43. Klabbers BM, Lammertsma AA, Slotman BJ. The value of positron emission tomography for monitoring response to radiotherapy in head and neck cancer. *Mol Imaging Biol*. 2003;5:257–270.
44. Halpern BS, Yeom K, Fueger BJ, Lufkin RB, Czernin J, Allen-Auerbach M. Evaluation of suspected local recurrence in head and neck cancer: a comparison between PET and PET/CT for biopsy proven lesions. *Eur J Radiol*. 2007;62:199–204.
45. Horiuchi C, Taguchi T, Yoshida T et al. Early assessment of clinical response to concurrent chemoradiotherapy in head and neck carcinoma using fluoro-2-deoxy-d-glucose positron emission tomography. *Auris Nasus Larynx*. 2008;35:103–108.
46. Ryan WR, Fee WE Jr, Le QT, Pinto HA. Positron-emission tomography for surveillance of head and neck cancer. *Laryngoscope*. 2005;115:645–650.
47. Ito K, Yokoyama J, Kubota K, Morooka M, Shiibashi M, Matsuda H. 18F-FDG versus 11C-choline PET/CT for the imaging of advanced head and neck cancer after combined

intraarterial chemotherapy and radiotherapy: the time period during which PET/CT can reliably detect non-recurrence. *Eur J Nucl Med Mol Imaging.* 2010;37:1318–1327.

48. Nayak JV, Walvekar RR, Andrade RS et al. Deferring planned neck dissection following chemoradiation for stage IV head and neck cancer: the utility of PET-CT. *Laryngoscope.* 2007;117:2129–2134.

49. Yao M, Smith RB, Graham MM et al. The role of FDG PET in management of neck metastasis from head-and-neck cancer after definitive radiation treatment. *Int J Radiat Oncol Biol Phys.* 2005;63:991–999.

50. Ong SC, Schöder H, Lee NY et al. Clinical utility of 18FFDG PET/CT in assessing the neck after concurrent chemoradiotherapy for locoregional advanced head and neck cancer. *J Nucl Med.* 2008;49:532–540.

51. Gourin CG, Williams HT, Seabolt WN, Herdman AV, Howington JW, Terris DJ. Utility of positron emission tomography- computed tomography in identification of residual nodal disease after chemoradiation for advanced head and neck cancer. *Laryngoscope.* 2006;116:705–710.

52. Tan A, Adelstein DJ, Rybicki LA et al. Ability of positron emission tomography to detect residual neck node disease in patients with head and neck squamous carcinoma after definitive chemoradiotherapy. *Arch Otolaryngol Head Neck Surg.* 2007;133:435–440.

53. Rabalais AG, Walvekar R, Nuss D et al. Positron emission tomography-computed tomography surveillance for the node-positive neck after chemoradiotherapy. *Laryngoscope.* 2009;119:1120–1124.

54. Horn J, Lock-Andersen J, Sjostrand H, Loft A. Routine use of FDG-PET scans in melanoma patients with positive sentinel node biopsy. *Eur J Nucl Med Mol Imaging.* 2006;33:887–892.

55. Nahas Z, Goldenberg D, Fakhry C et al. The role of positron emission tomography/computed tomography in the management of recurrent papillary thyroid carcinoma. *Laryngoscope.* 2005;115:237–243.

56. Palmedo H, Bucerius J, Joe A et al. Integrated PET/CT in differentiated thyroid cancer: diagnostic accuracy and impact on patient management. *J Nucl Med.* 2006;47:616–624.

57. Shammas A, Degirmenci B, Mountz JM et al. 18F-FDG PET/CT in patients with suspected recurrent or metastatic well-differentiated thyroid cancer. *J Nucl Med.* 2007;48:221–226.

58. Gould MK, Jett JR, Sloan JA et al. Accuracy of positron emission tomography for diagnosis of pulmonary nodules and mass lesions: a meta-analysis. *JAMA.* 2001;285(7):914–924.

59. Ung YC, Maziak DE, Vanderveen JA et al. 18Fluorodeoxyglucose positron emission tomography in the diagnosis and staging of lung cancer: a systematic review. *J Natl Cancer Inst.* 2007;99(23):1753–1767.

60. Silvestri GA, Gould MK, Margolis ML et al. Noninvasive staging of non-small cell lung cancer: ACCP evidenced-based clinical practice guidelines (2nd edition). *Chest.* 2007;132(Suppl 3):178S–201S.

61. Toloza EM. Noninvasive staging of non-small cell lung cancer: a review of the current evidence. *Chest.* 2003;123(90010):137S–146S.

62. Nomori H, Watanabe K, Ohtsuka T, Naruke T, Suemasu K, Uno K. The size of metastatic foci and lymph nodes yielding false-negative and false-positive lymph node staging with positron emission tomography in patients with lung cancer. *J Thorac Cardiovasc Surg.* 2004;127(4):1087–1092.

63. Bille A, Pelosi E, Skanjeti A et al. Preoperative intrathoracic lymph node staging in patients with non-small-cell lung cancer: accuracy of integrated positron emission tomography and computed tomography. *Eur J Cardiothorac Surg.* 2009;36(3):440–445.

64. Gould MK, Kuschner WG, Rydzak CE et al. Test performance of positron emission tomography and computed tomography for mediastinal staging in patients with non-small-cell lung cancer: a meta-analysis. *Ann Intern Med.* 2003;139(11):879–892.

65. Pieterman RM, van Putten JW, Meuzelaar JJ et al. Preoperative staging of non-small-cell lung cancer with positron-emission tomography. *N Engl J Med.* 2000;343:254–261.

66. Verhagen AF, Bootsma GP, Tjan-Heijnen VC et al. FDG-PET in staging lung cancer: how does it change the algorithm? *Lung Cancer.* 2004;44(2):175–181.

67. Vansteenkiste JF, Stroobants SG, De Leyn PR et al. Lymph node staging in non-small-cell lung cancer with FDG-PET scan: a prospective study on 690 lymph node stations from 68 patients. *J Clin Oncol.* 1998;16:2142–2149.

68. Jett JR. How to optimize staging in early non-small cell lung cancer. *Lung Cancer.* 2002;38:S13–S16.

69. Kramer H, Groen HJ. Current concepts in the mediastinal lymph node staging of nonsmall cell lung cancer. *Ann Surg.* 2003;238:180–188.

70. Sarraf N, Aziz R, Gately K et al. Pattern and predictors of occult mediastinal lymph node involvement in non-small cell lung cancer patients with negative mediastinal uptake on positron emission tomography. *Eur J Cardiothorac Surg.* 2008;33:104–109.

71. van Tinteren H, Hoekstra OS, Smit EF et al. Effectiveness of positron emission tomography in the preoperative assessment of patients with suspected non-small-cell lung cancer: the PLUS multicentre randomised trial. *Lancet.* 2002;359(9315):1388–1392.

72. Fischer B, Lassen U, Mortensen J et al. Preoperative staging of lung cancer with PET-CT. *N Eng J Med.* 2009;361:32–39.

73. Maziak DE, Darling GE, Inculet RI et al. Positron emission tomography in staging early lung cancer: a randomized trial. *Ann Intern Med.* 2009;151(4):221–228. W-48.

74. Viney RC, Boyer MJ, King MT et al. Randomized controlled trial of the role of positron emission tomography in the management of stage I and II non-small-cell lung cancer. *J Clin Oncol.* 2004;22(12):2357–2362.

75. Herder GJ, Kramer H, Hoekstra OS et al. Traditional versus up-front [18F] fluorodeoxyglucose-positron emission tomography staging of non-small-cell lung cancer: a Dutch cooperative randomized study. *J Clin Oncol.* 2006;24(12):1800–1806.

76. Gupta NC, Graeber GM, Bishop HA. Comparative efficacy of positron emission tomography with fluorodeoxyglucose in evaluation of small (<1 cm), intermediate (1 to 3 cm), and large (>3 cm) lymph node lesions. *Chest.* 2000;117:773–778.

77. Paesmans M, Berghmans T, Dusart M et al. Primary tumor standardized uptake value measured on fluorodeoxyglucose positron emission tomography is of prognostic value for survival in non-small cell lung cancer: update of a systematic review and meta-analysis by the European Lung Cancer Working Party for the International Association for the Study of Lung Cancer Staging Project. *J Thorac Oncol.* 2010;5(5):612–619.

78. Nair VS, Krupitskaya Y, Gould MK. Positron emission tomography 18F-fluorodeoxyglucose uptake and prognosis in patients with surgically treated, stage I non-small cell lung cancer: a systematic review. *J Thorac Oncol.* 2009;4(12):1473–1479.

79. Nair VS, Barnett PG, Ananth L, Gould MK, Veterans Affairs Solitary Nodule Accuracy Project Cooperative Studies Group. PET scan 18F-fluorodeoxyglucose uptake and prognosis in patients with resected clinical stage IA non-small cell lung cancer. *Chest.* 2010;137(5):1150–1156.

80. Marom EM, Sarvis S, Herndon JE 2nd, Patz EF Jr. T1 lung cancers: sensitivity of diagnosis with fluorodeoxyglucose PET. *Radiology.* 2002;223(2):453–459.

81. Barnett PG, Ananth L, Gould MK. Cost and outcomes of patients with solitary pulmonary nodules managed with PET scans. *Chest.* 2010;137:53–59.

82. Lee DH, Kim SK, Lee HY et al. Early prediction of response to first-line therapy using integrated 18F-FDG PET/CT for patients with advanced/metastatic non-small cell lung cancer. *J Thorac Oncol.* 2009;4(7):816–821.

83. Weber WA, Petersen V, Schmidt B et al. Positron emission tomography in non-small-cell lung cancer: prediction of response to chemotherapy by quantitative assessment of glucose use. *Clin Oncol.* 2003;21(14):2651–2657.

84. Hoekstra CJ, Stroobants SG, Smit EF et al. Prognostic relevance of response evaluation using [18F]-2-fluoro-2-deoxy-D-glucose positron emission tomography in patients with locally advanced non-small-cell lung cancer. *J Clin Oncol.* 2005;23(33):8362–8370.

85. Cerfolio RJ, Bryant AS, Winokur TS, Ohja B, Bartolucci AA. Repeat FDG-PET after neoadjuvant therapy is a predictor of pathologic response in patients with non-small cell lung cancer. *Ann Thorac Surg.* 2004;78(6):1903–1909.

86. Tanvetyanon T, Eikman EA, Sommers E, Robinson L, Boulware D, Bepler G. Computed tomography response, but not positron emission tomography scan response, predicts survival after neoadjuvant chemotherapy for resectable non-small-cell lung cancer. *J Clin Oncol.* 2008;26:4610–4616.

87. Pottgen C, Levegrün S, Theegarten D et al. Value of 18F-fluoro-2-deoxy-D-glucose-positron emission tomography/computed tomography in non-small-cell lung cancer for prediction of pathologic response and times to relapse after neoadjuvant chemoradiotherapy. *Clin Cancer Res.* 2006;12(1):97–106.

88. Cerfolio RJ, Bryant AS. When is it best to repeat a 2-fluoro-2-deoxy-D-glucose positron emission tomography/computed tomography scan on patients with non-small cell lung cancer who have received neoadjuvant chemoradiotherapy? *Ann Thorac Surg.* 2007;84(4):1092–1097.

89. Port J. Positron emission tomography scanning poorly predicts response to preoperative chemotherapy in non-small cell lung cancer. *Ann Thorac Surg.* 2004;77(1):254–259.

90. Xu X, Yu J, Sun X et al. The prognostic value of 18F-fluorodeoxyglucose uptake by using serial positron emission tomography and computed tomography in patients with stage III nonsmall cell lung cancer. *Am J Clin Oncol.* 2008;31(5):470–475.

91. Bury T, Corhay JL, Duysinx B et al. Value of FDG-PET in detecting residual or recurrent nonsmall cell lung cancer. *Eur Respir J.* 1999;14:1376–1380.

92. Hellwig D, Gröschel A, Graeter TP et al. Diagnostic performance and prognostic impact of FDG-PET in suspected recurrence of surgically treated non-small cell lung cancer. *Eur J Nucl Med Mol Imaging.* 2006;33:13–21.

93. Hicks RJ, Kalff V, MacManus MP et al. The utility of (18)F-FDG PET for suspected recurrent non-small cell lung cancer after potentially curative therapy: impact on management and prognostic stratification. *J Nucl Med.* 2001;42:1605–1613.

94. Cerfolio RJ, Ojha B, Mukherjee S, Pask AH, Bass CS, Katholi CR. Positron emission tomography scanning with 2-fluoro-2-deoxy-d-glucose as a predictor of response of neoadjuvant treatment for non-small cell carcinoma. *J Thorac Cardiovasc Surg.* 2003;125(4):938–944.

95. Rebollo-Aguirre AC, Ramos-Font C, Villegas Portero R, Cook GJ, Llamas Elvira JM, Romero Tabares A. Is FDG-PET suitable for evaluating neoadjuvant therapy in non-small cell lung cancer? Evidence with systematic review of the literature. *J Surg Oncol.* 2010;101(6):486–494.

96. Cerfolio RJ, Bryant AS, Ojha B. Restaging patients with N2 (stage IIIa) non-small cell lung cancer after neoadjuvant chemoradiotherapy: a prospective study. *J Thorac Cardiovasc Surg.* 2006;131(6):1229–1235.

97. Schirrmeister H, Kühn T, Guhlmann A et al. Fluorine-18 2-deoxy-2-fluoro-D-glucose PET in the preoperative staging of breast cancer: comparison with the standard staging procedures. *Eur J Nucl Med.* 2001;28:351–358.

98. Greco M, Crippa F, Agresti R et al. Axillary lymph node staging in breast cancer by 2-fluoro-2-deoxy-D-glucose-positron emission tomography: clinical evaluation and alternative management. *J Natl Cancer Inst.* 2001;93:630–635.

99. Cooper KL, Harnan S, Meng Y et al. Positron emission tomography (PET) for assessment of axillary lymph node status in early breast cancer: a systematic review and meta-analysis. *Eur J Surg Oncol.* 2011;37:187–198.

100. Heusner TA, Kuemmel S, Hahn S et al. Diagnostic value of full-dose FDG PET/CT for axillary lymph node staging in breast cancer patients. *Eur J Nucl Med.* 2009;36:1543–1545.

101. Veronesi U, DeCicco C, Galimberti VE et al. A comparative study on the value of FDG-PET and sentinel node biopsy to identify occult axillary metastases. *Ann Oncol.* 2007;18:473–478.

102. van der Hoeven JJ, Krak NC, Hoekstra OS et al. 18F-2-fluoro-2-deoxy-d-glucose positron emission tomography in staging of locally advanced breast cancer. *J Clin Oncol.* 2004;22:1253–1259.

103. Uematsu T, Yuen S, Yukisawa S et al. Comparison of FDG PET and SPECT for detection of bone metastases in breast cancer. *AJR.* 2005;184:1266–1273.

104. Dirisamer A, Halpern BS, Flöry D et al. Integrated contrast-enhanced diagnostic whole-body PET/CT as a first-line restaging modality in patients with suspected metastatic recurrence of breast cancer. *Eur J Radiol.* 2010;73:294–299.

105. Isasi CR, Moadel RM, Blaufox MD. A meta-analysis of FDG-PET for the evaluation of breast cancer recurrence and metastases. *Breast Cancer Res Treat.* 2005;90:10512.

106. Eubank WB, Mankoff D, Bhattacharya M et al. Impact of FDG PET on defining the extent of disease and on the treatment of patients with recurrent or metastatic breast cancer. *AJR Am J Roentgenol.* 2004;183:479–486.

107. Smith IC, Welch AE, Hutcheon AW et al. Positron emission tomography using [(18)F]-fluorodeoxy-D-glucose to predict the pathologic response of breast cancer to primary chemotherapy. *J Clin Oncol.* 2000;18:1676.

108. Schelling M, Avril N, Nährig J. Positron emission tomography using (18)F]Fluorodeoxyglucose for monitoring primary chemotherapy in breast cancer. *J Clin Oncol.* 2000;18:1689–1695.

109. Dunnwald LK, Gralow JR, Ellis GK et al. Tumor metabolism and blood flow changes by positron emission tomography: relation to survival in patients treated with neoadjuvant chemotherapy for locally advanced breast cancer. *J Clin Oncol.* 2008;26:4449–4457.

110. Dose Schwarz J, Bader M, Jenicke L. Early prediction of response to chemotherapy in metastatic breast cancer using sequential 18F-FDG PET. *J Nucl Med.* 2005;46:1144–1150.

111. Tateishi U, Gamez C, Dawood S, Yeung HW, Cristofanilli M, Macapinlac HA. Bone metastases in patients with metastatic breast cancer: morphologic and metabolic monitoring of response to systemic therapy with integrated PET/CT. *Radiology.* 2008;247:189–196.

112. MacDonald L, Edwards J, Lewellen T, Haseley D, Rogers J, Kinahan P. Clinical imaging characteristics of the positron emission mammography camera: PEM Flex Solo II. *J Nucl Med.* 2009;50;1666–1675.

113. Schilling K, Narayanan D, Kalinyak JE et al. Positron emission mammography in breast cancer presurgical planning: comparisons with magnetic resonance imaging. *Eur J Nucl Med Mol Imaging.* 2010;38:23–36.

114. Berg WA, Madsen KS, Schilling K et al. Comparative effectiveness of positron emission mammography and MRI in the contralateral breast of women with newly diagnosed breast cancer. *AJR Am J Roentgenol.* 2012;198:219–232.

115. Pan L, Gu P, Huang G, Xue H, Wu S. Prognostic significance of SUV on PET/CT in patients with esophageal cancer: a systematic review and meta-analysis. *Eur J Gastroenterol Hepatol.* 2009;21:1008–1015.

116. Rizk N, Downey RJ, Akhurst T et al. Preoperative 18[F]-fluorodeoxyglucose positron emission tomography standardized uptake values predict survival after esophageal adenocarcinoma resection. *Ann Thorac Surg.* 2006;81:1076–1081.

117. van Westreenen HL, Plukker JT, Cobben DC, Verhoogt CJ, Groen H, Jager PL. Prognostic value of the standardized uptake value in esophageal cancer. *AJR Am J Roentgenol.* 2005;185:436–440.

118. Omloo JM, Sloof GW, Boellaard R et al. Importance of fluorodeoxyglucose-positron emission tomography (FDG-PET) and endoscopic ultrasonography parameters in predicting survival following surgery for esophageal cancer. *Endoscopy.* 2008;40:464–471.

119. Kato H, Kuwano H, Nakajima M et al. Comparison between positron emission tomography and computed tomography in the use of the assessment of esophageal carcinoma. *Cancer.* 2002;94:921–928.

120. van Westreenen HL, Cobben DC, Jager PL et al. Comparison of 18F-FLT PET and 18F-FDG PET in esophageal cancer. *J Nucl Med.* 2005;46:400–404.

121. van Westreenen HL, Westerterp M, Bossuyt PM, et al. Systematic review of the staging performance of 18F-fluorodeoxyglucose positron emission omography in esophageal cancer. *J Clin Oncol.* 2004;22:3805–3812.

122. Luostarinen ME, Viljanen T, Färkkilä MA, Salo JA. Adenocarcinoma of the esophagus and the esophagogastric junction: positron emission tomography improves staging and prediction of survival in distant but not in locoregional disease. *J Gastrointest Surg.* 2004;8:988–996.

123. Muijs CT, Schreurs LM, Busz DM et al. Consequences of additional use of PET information for target volume delineation and radiotherapy dose distribution for esophageal cancer. *Radiother Oncol.* 2009;93:447–453.

124. Leong T, Everitt C, Yuen K et al. A prospective study to evaluate the impact of FDG-PET on CT-based radiotherapy treatment planning for oesophageal cancer. *Radiother Oncol.* 2006;78:254–261.

125. Rizk NP, Tang L, Adusumilli PS et al. Predictive value of initial PET-SUVmax in patients with locally advanced esophageal and gastroesophageal junction adenocarcinoma. *J Thorac Oncol.* 2009;4:875–879.

126. Weber WA, Ott K, Becker K et al. Prediction of response to preoperative chemotherapy in adenocarcinomas of the esophagogastric junction by metabolic imaging. *J Clin Oncol.* 2001;19:3058–3065.

127. Ott K, Weber WA, Lordick F et al. Metabolic imaging predicts response, survival, and recurrence in adenocarcinomas of the esophagogastric junction. *J Clin Oncol.* 2006;24:4692–4698.

128. Lordick F, Ott K, Krause BJ et al. PET to assess early metabolic response and to guide treatment of adenocarcinoma of the oesophagogastric junction: the MUNICON phase II trial. *Lancet Oncol.* 2007;8:797–805.

129. Gillham CM, Lucey JA, Keogan M et al. (18)FDG uptake during induction chemoradiation for oesophageal cancer fails to predict histomorphological tumour response. *Br J Cancer.* 2006;95:1174–1179.

130. van Vliet EP, Steyerberg EW, Eijkemans MJ, Kuipers EJ, Siersema PD. Detection of distant metastases in patients with oesophageal or gastric cardia cancer: a diagnostic decision analysis. *Br J Cancer.* 2007;97:868–876.

131. Guo H, Zhu H, Xi Y et al. Diagnostic and prognostic value of 18F-FDG PET/CT for patients with suspected recurrence from squamous cell carcinoma of the esophagus. *J Nucl Med.* 2007;48:1251–1258.

132. Teyton P, Metges JP, Atmani A et al. Use of positron emission tomography in surgery follow-up of esophageal cancer. *J Gastrointest Surg.* 2009;13:451–458.

133. Mayo SC, Pawlik TM. Current management of colorectal hepatic metastasis. *Expert Rev Gastroenterol Hepatol.* 2009;3:131–144.

134. Bipat S, van Leeuwen MS, Comans EF et al. Colorectal liver metastases: CT, MR imaging, and PET for diagnosis–metaanalysis. *Radiology.* 2005;237:123–131.

135. Kinkel K, Lu Y, Both M, Warren RS, Thoeni RF. Detection of hepatic metastases from cancers of the gastrointestinal tract by using noninvasive imaging methods (US, CT, MR imaging, PET): a meta-analysis. *Radiology.* 2002;224:748–756.

136. Huebner RH, Park KC, Shepherd JE et al. A meta-analysis of the literature for whole-body FDG PET detection of recurrent colorectal cancer. *J Nucl Med.* 2000;41:1177–1189.

137. Wiering B, Krabbe PF, Jager GJ, Oyen WJ, Ruers TJ. The impact of fluor-18-deoxyglucose-positron emission tomography in the management of colorectal liver metastases. *Cancer.* 2005;104:2658–2670.

138. Patel S, McCall M, Ohinmaa A, Bigam D, Dryden DM. Positron emission tomography/computed tomographic scans compared to computed tomographic scans for detecting colorectal liver metastases: a systematic review. *Ann Surg.* 2011;253:666–671.

139. Kong G, Jackson C, Koh DM et al. The use of 18F-FDG PET/CT in colorectal liver metastases–comparison with CT and liver MRI. *Eur J Nucl Med Mol Imaging.* 2008;35:1323–1329.

140. Rappeport ED, Loft A, Berthelsen AK et al. Contrast-enhanced FDG-PET/CT vs. SPIO-enhanced MRI vs. FDG-PET vs. CT in patients with liver metastases from colorectal cancer: a prospective study with intraoperative confirmation. *Acta Radiol.* 2007;48:369–378.

141. Cantwell CP, Setty BN, Holalkere N, Sahani DV, Fischman AJ, Blake MA. Liver lesion detection and characterization in patients with colorectal cancer: a comparison of low radiation dose non-enhanced PET/CT. *J Comput Assist Tomogr.* 2008;32:738–744.

142. Yang YY, Fleshman JW, Strasberg SM. Detection and management of extrahepatic colorectal cancer in patients with resectable liver metastases. *J Gastrointest Surg.* 2007;11:929–944.

143. Fong Y, Saldinger PF, Akhurst T et al. Utility of 18F-FDG positron emission tomography scanning on selection of patients for resection of hepatic colorectal metastases. *Am J Surg.* 1999;178:282–287.

144. Strasberg SM, Dehdashti F, Siegel BA, Drebin JA, Linehan D. Survival of patients evaluated by FDG-PET before hepatic resection for etastatic colorectal carcinoma: a prospective database study. *Ann Surg.* 2001;233:293–299.

145. Schussler-Fiorenza CM, Mahvi DM, Niederhuber J, Rikkers LF, Weber SM. Clinical risk score correlates with yield of PET scan in patients with colorectal hepatic metastases. *J Gastrointest Surg.* 2004;8:150–157.

146. Pawlik TM, Assumpcao L, Vossen JA et al. Trends in nontherapeutic laparotomy rates in patients undergoing surgical therapy for hepatic colorectal metastases timothy. *Ann Surg Oncol.* 2009;16:371–378.

147. Ruers TJM, Wiering B, van der Sijp JRM et al. Improved selection of patients for hepatic surgery of colorectal liver metastases with 18F-FDG PET: a randomized study. *J Nucl Med.* 2009;50:1036–1041.

148. Arulampalam TH, Francis DL, Visvikis D, Taylor I, Ell PJ. FDG-PET for the pre-operative evaluation of colorectal liver metastases. *Eur J Surg Oncol.* 2004;30:286–291.

149. Fernandez FG, Drebin JA, Linehan DC, Dehdashti F, Siegel BA, Strasberg SM. Five-year survival after resection of hepatic metastases from colorectal cancer in patients screened by positron emission tomography with F-18 fluorodeoxyglucose (FDG-PET). *Ann Surg.* 2004;240:438–447.

150. Libutti SK, Alexander HR Jr, Choyke P et al. A prospective study of 2-[18F] fluoro-2-deoxy-D-glucose/positron emission tomography scan, 99mTc-labeled arcitumomab (CEA-scan), and blind second-look laparotomy for detecting colon cancer recurrence in patients with increasing carcinoembryonic antigen levels. *Ann Surg Oncol.* 2001;8:779–786.

151. Zervos EE, Badgwell BD, Burak WE Jr, Arnold MW, Martin EW. Fluorodeoxyglucose positron emission tomography as an adjunct to carcinoembryonic antigen in the management of patients with presumed recurrent colorectal cancer and nondiagnostic radiologic workup. *Surgery.* 2001;130:636–643; discussion 43–44.

152. Flamen P, Hoekstra OS, Homans F et al. Unexplained rising carcinoembryonic antigen (CEA) in the postoperative surveillance of colorectal cancer: the utility of positron emission tomography (PET). *Eur J Cancer.* 2001;37:862–869.

153. Flanagan FL, Dehdashti F, Ogunbiyi OA, Kodner IJ, Siegel BA. Utility of FDG-PET for investigating unexplained plasma CEA elevation in patients with colorectal cancer. *Ann Surg.* 1998;227:319–323.

154. Liu FY, Chen JS, Changchien CR et al. Utility of 2-fluoro-2-deoxy-D-glucose positron emission tomography in managing patients of colorectal cancer with unexplained carcinoembryonic antigen elevation at different levels. *Dis Col Rect.* 2005;48:1900–1912.

155. De Geus-Oei LF, Ruers TJ, Punt CJ, Leer JW, Corstens FH, Oyen WJ. FDG-PET in colorectal cancer. *Cancer Imaging.* 2006;6:S71–S81.

156. Blokhuis TJ, van der Schaaf MC, van den Tol MP, Comans EF, Manoliu RA, van der Sijp JR. Results of radio frequency ablation of primary and secondary liver tumors: long-term follow-up with computed tomography and positron emission tomography-18F-deoxyfluoroglucose scanning. *Scand J Gastroenterol Suppl.* 2004;241:93–97.

157. Simó M, Lomeña F, Setoain J et al. FDG-PET improves the management of patients with suspected recurrence of colorectal cancer. *Nucl Med Commun.* 2002;23:975–982.

158. Truant S, Huglo D, Hebbar M, Ernst O, Steinling M, Pruvot FR. Prospective evaluation of the impact of [18F]fluoro-2-deoxy-D-glucose positron emission tomography of resectable colorectal liver metastases. *Br J Surg.* 2005;92:362–369.

159. Sperti C, Pasquali C, Chierichetti F, Ferronato A, Decet G, Pedrazzoli S. 18-Fluorodeoxyglucose positron emission tomography in predicting survival of patients with pancreatic carcinoma. *J Gastrointest Surg.* 2003;7:953–959; discussion 959–960.

160. Inokuma T, Tamaki N, Torizuka T et al. Evaluation of pancreatic tumors with positron emission tomography and F-18 fluorodeoxyglucose: comparison with CT and US. *Radiology.* 1995;195:345–352.

161. Bares R, Klever P, Hauptmann S et al. F-18 fluorodeoxyglucose PET in vivo evaluation of pancreatic glucose metabolism for detection of pancreatic cancer. *Radiology.* 1994;192:79–86.

162. Diederichs CG, Staib L, Vogel J et al. Values and limitations of 18F-fluorodeoxyglucose-positron-emission tomography with preoperative evaluation of patients with pancreatic masses. *Pancreas.* 2000;20:109–116.

163. Fröhlich A, Diederichs CG, Staib L, Vogel J, Beger HG, Reske SN. Detection of liver metastases from pancreatic cancer using FDG PET. *J Nucl Med.* 1999;40:250–255.

164. Nakata B, Nishimura S, Ishikawa T et al. Prognostic predictive value of 18F-fluorodeoxyglucose positron emission tomography for patients with pancreatic cancer. *Int J Oncol.* 2001;19:53–58.

165. Choi M, Heilbrun LK, Venkatramanamoorthy R, Lawhorn-Crews JM, Zalupski MM, Shields AF. Using 18F-fluorodeoxyglucose positron emission tomography to monitor clinical outcomes in patients treated with neoadjuvant chemo radiotherapy for locally advanced pancreatic cancer. *Am J Clin Oncol.* 2010;33:257–261.

166. Kuwatani M, Kawakami H, Eto K et al. Modalities for evaluating chemotherapeutic efficacy and survival time in patients with advanced pancreatic cancer: comparison between FDG-PET, CT, and serum tumor markers. *Intern Med.* 2009;48:867–875.

167. Koyama K, Okamura T, Kawabe J et al. Diagnostic usefulness of FDG PET for pancreatic mass lesions. *Ann Nucl Med.* 2001;15:217–224.

168. Kitajima K, Murakami K, Yamasaki E et al. Performance of integrated FDG-PET/contrast-enhanced CT in the diagnosis of recurrent pancreatic cancer: comparison with integrated FDG-PET/non-contrast-enhanced CT and enhanced CT. *Mol Imaging Biol.* 2010;12:452–459.

169. Ruf J, Lopez Hänninen E, Oettle H et al. Detection of recurrent pancreatic cancer: comparison of FDG-PET with CT/MRI. *Pancreatology.* 2005;5:266–272.

170. Farma JM, Santillan AA, Melis M et al. PET/CT fusion scan enhances CT staging in patients with pancreatic neoplasms. *Ann Surg Oncol.* 2008;15:2465–2471.

171. Strobel K, Heinrich S, Bhure U et al. Contrast-enhanced 18F-FDG PET/CT: 1-stop-shop imaging for assessing the resectability of pancreatic cancer. *J Nucl Med.* 2008;49:1408–1413.

172. Nakamoto Y, Higashi T, Sakahara H et al. Delayed (18)F fluoro-2-deoxy-D-glucose positron emission tomography scan for differentiation between malignant and benign lesions in the pancreas. *Cancer.* 2000;89:2547–2554.

173. Zimny M, Bares R, Fass J et al. Fluorine-18 fluorodeoxyglucose positron emission tomography in the differential diagnosis of pancreatic carcinoma: a report of 106 cases. *Eur J Nucl Med.* 1997;24:678–682.

174. Lagasse LD, Creasman WT, Shingleton HM, Ford JH, Blessing JA. Results and complications of operative staging in cervical cancer: experience of the Gynecologic Oncology Group. *Gynecol Oncol.* 1980;9(1):90–98.

175. Magne N, Chargari C, Vicenzi L et al. New trends in the evaluation and treatment of cervix cancer: the role of FDG-PET. *Cancer Treat Rev.* 2008;34(8):671–681.

176. Narayan K, Hicks RJ, Jobling T, Bernshaw D, McKenzie AF. A comparison of MRI and PET scanning in surgically staged loco-regionally advanced cervical cancer: potential impact on treatment. *Int J Gynecol Cancer.* 2001;11(4):263–271.

177. Singh AK, Grigsby PW, Dehdashti F, Herzog TJ, Siegel BA. FDG-PET lymph node staging and survival of patients with FIGO stage IIIb cervical carcinoma. *Int J Radiat Oncol Biol Phys.* 2003;56(2):489–493.

178. Yeh LS, Hung YC, Shen YY, Kao CH, Lin CC, Lee CC. Detecting para-aortic lymph nodal metastasis by positron emission tomography of 18F-fluorodeoxyglucose in advanced cervical cancer with negative magnetic resonance imaging findings. *Oncol Rep.* 2002;9(6):1289–1292.

179. Yen TC, Ng KK, Ma SY et al. Value of dual-phase 2-fluoro-2-deoxy-d-glucose positron emission tomography in cervical cancer. *J Clin Oncol.* 2003;21(19):3651–3658.

180. Amit A, Beck D, Lowenstein L et al. The role of hybrid PET/CT in the evaluation of patients with cervical cancer. *Gynecol Oncol.* 2006;100(1):65–69.

181. Grigsby PW. PET/CT imaging to guide cervical cancer therapy. *Future Oncol.* 2009;5(7):953–958.

182. Rose PG, Adler LP, Rodriguez M, Faulhaber PF, Abdul-Karim FW, Miraldi F. Positron emission tomography for evaluating para-aortic nodal metastasis in locally advanced cervical cancer before surgical staging: a surgicopathologic study. *J Clin Oncol.* 1999;17(1):41–45.

183. Wright JD, Dehdashti F, Herzog TJ et al. Preoperative lymph node staging of early-stage cervical carcinoma by [18F]-fluoro-2-deoxy-d-glucose-positron emission tomography. *Cancer.* 2005;104(11):2484–2491.

184. Belhocine T, De Barsy C, Hustinx R, Willems-Foidart J. Usefulness of (18)F-FDG PET in the post-therapy surveillance of endometrial carcinoma. *Eur J Nucl Med Mol Imaging.* 2002;29(9):1132–1139.

185. Brooks RA, Rader JS, Dehdashti F et al. Surveillance FDG-PET detection of asymptomatic recurrences in patients with cervical cancer. *Gynecol Oncol.* 2009;112(1):104–109.

186. Grigsby PW, Siegel BA, Dehdashti F, Rader J, Zoberi I. Posttherapy [18F] fluorodeoxyglucose positron emission tomography in carcinoma of the cervix: response and outcome. *J Clin Oncol.* 2004;22(11):2167–2171.

187. Tran BN, Grigsby PW, Dehdashti F, Herzog TJ, Siegel BA. Occult supraclavicular lymph node metastasis identified by FDG-PET in patients with carcinoma of the uterine cervix. *Gynecol Oncol.* 2003;90(3):572–576.

188. Schutter EM, Kenemans P, Sohn C et al. Diagnostic value of pelvic examination, ultrasound, and serum CA 125 in postmenopausal women with a pelvic mass. An international multicenter study. *Cancer.* 1994;74(4):1398–1406.

189. Schutter EM, Sohn C, Kristen P et al. Estimation of probability of malignancy using a logistic model combining physical examination, ultrasound, serum CA 125, and serum CA 72-4 in postmenopausal women with a pelvic mass: an international multicenter study. *Gynecol Oncol.* 1998;69(1):56–63.

190. Burghardt E, Lahousen M, Stettner H. The significance of pelvic and para-aortic lymphadenectomy in the operative treatment of ovarian cancer. *Baillieres Clin Obstet Gynaecol.* 1989;3(1):157–165.

191. Burghardt E, Pickel H, Lahousen M, Stettner H. Pelvic lymphadenectomy in operative treatment of ovarian cancer. *Am J Obstet Gynecol.* 1986;155(2):315–319.

192. Goff BA, Matthews BJ, Larson EH et al. Predictors of comprehensive surgical treatment in patients with ovarian cancer. *Cancer.* 2007;109(10):2031–2042.

193. Le T, Adolph A, Krepart GV, Lotocki R, Heywood MS. The benefits of comprehensive surgical staging in the management of early-stage epithelial ovarian carcinoma. *Gynecol Oncol.* 2002;85(2):351–355.

194. Eisenkop SM. Commenting on centralizing surgery for gynecologic oncology: a strategy assuring better quality treatment? (89:4–8) by Karsten Munstedt et al. *Gynecol Oncol.* 2004;94(2):605–606 [author reply: 606–607].

195. Munstedt K, von Georgi R, Misselwitz B, Zygmunt M, Stillger R, Künzel W. Centralizing surgery for gynecologic oncology—a strategy assuring better quality treatment? *Gynecol Oncol.* 2003;89(1):4–8.

196. Boente MP, Chi DS, Hoskins WJ. The role of surgery in the management of ovarian cancer: primary and interval cytoreductive surgery. *Semin Oncol.* 1998;25(3):326–334.

197. Grab D, Flock F, Stohr I et al. Classification of asymptomatic adnexal masses by ultrasound, magnetic resonance imaging, and positron emission tomography. *Gynecol Oncol.* 2000;77:454–459.

198. Fenchel S, Grab D, Nuessle K. Asymptomatic adnexal masses: correlation of FDG PET and histopathologic findings. *Radiology.* 2002;223:780–788.

199. Risum S, Hogdall C, Loft A et al. The diagnostic value of PET/CT for primary ovarian cancer—a prospective study. *Gynecol Oncol.* 2007;105(1):145–149.

200. Kitajima K, Murakami K, Yamasaki E et al. Performance of integrated FDG-PET/contrast-enhanced CT in the diagnosis of recurrent uterine cancer: comparison with PET and enhanced CT. *Eur J Nucl Med Mol Imaging.* 2009;36(3):362–372.

201. Yoshida Y, Kurokawa T, Sawamura Y et al. The positron emission tomography with F18 17beta-estradiol has the potential to benefit diagnosis and treatment of endometrial cancer. *Gynecol Oncol.* 2007;104(3):764–766.

202. Castellucci P, Perrone AM, Picchio M. Diagnostic accuracy of 18F-FDG PET/CT in characterizing ovarian lesions and staging ovarian cancer: correlation with transvaginal ultrasonography, computed tomography, and histology. *Nucl Med Commun.* 2007;28:589–595.

203. Kitajima K, Murakami K, Yamasaki E et al. Accuracy of 18F-FDG PET/CT in detecting pelvic and paraaortic lymph node metastasis in patients with endometrial cancer. *Am J Roentgenol.* 2008;190(6):1652–1658.

204. Nam EJ, Yun MJ, Oh YT et al. Diagnosis and staging of primary ovarian cancer: correlation between PET/CT, Doppler US, and CT or MRI. *Gynecol Oncol.* 2010;116:389–394.

205. Pannu HK, Bristow RE, Cohade C, Fishman EK, Wahl RL. PET-CT in recurrent ovarian cancer: initial observations. *Radiographics.* 2004;24:209–223.

206. Torizuka T, Nobezawa S, Kanno T et al. Ovarian cancer recurrence: role of whole-body PET using 18-FDG. *Eur J Nuc Med Mol Imaging.* 2002;29:797–803.

207. Cho SM, Ha HK, Byun JY et al. Usefulness of FDG PET for assessment of early recurrent epithelial ovarian cancer. *AJR Am J Roentgenol.* 2002;179:391–395.

208. Yen RF, Sun SS, Shen YY, Changlai SP, Kao A. Whole body positron emission tomography with 18F-fluoro-2-deoxyglucose for the detection of recurrent ovarian cancer. *Anticancer Res.* 2001;21:3691–3694.

209. Thrall MM, DeLoia JA, Gallion H, Avril N. Clinical use of combined positron emission tomography and computed tomography (FDG-PET/CT) in recurrent ovarian cancer. *Gynecol Oncol.* 2007;105:17–22.

210. Sheng XG, Zhang XL, Fu Z et al. Value of positron emission tomography-CT imaging combined with continual detection of CA125 in serum for diagnosis of early asymptomatic recurrence of epithelial ovarian carcinoma. *Zhonghua Fu Chan Ke Za Zhi.* 2007;42:460–463.

211. Gu P, Pan LL, Wu SQ, Sun L, Huang G. CA125, PET alone, PET-CT, CT and MRI in diagnosing recurrent ovarian carcinoma: a systematic review and meta-analysis. *Eur J Radiol.* 2009;71:164–174.

212. Palomar A, Nanni C, Castellucci P et al. Value of FDG PET/CT in patients with treated ovarian cancer and raised CA125 serum levels. *Mol Imaging Biol.* 2012;14:123–129.

213. Peng NJ, Liou WS, Liu RS, Hu C, Tsay DG, Liu CB. Early detection of recurrent ovarian cancer in patients with low-level increases in serum CA-125 levels by 2-[F-18]fluoro-2-deoxy-D-glucose-positron emission tomography/computed tomography. *Cancer Biother Radiopharm.* 2011;26:175–181.

214. Kitajima K, Murakami K, Yamasaki E. Diagnostic accuracy of integrated FDG-PET/contrast-enhanced CT in staging ovarian cancer: comparison with enhanced CT. *Eur J Nucl Med Mol Imaging,* 2008;35:1912–1920.

215. Mangili G, Picchio M, Sironi S et al. Integrated PET/CT as a first-line re-staging modality in patients with suspected recurrence of ovarian cancer. *Eur J Nucl Med Mol Imaging.* 2007;34:658–666.

216. Fulham MJ, Carter J, Baldey A, Hicks RJ, Ramshaw JE, Gibson M. The impact of PET-CT in suspected recurrent ovarian cancer: a prospective multi-centre study as part of the Australian PET Data Collection Project. *Gynecol Oncol.* 2009;112:462–468.

217. Sebastian S, Lee SI, Horowitz NS et al. PET-CT vs. CT alone in ovarian cancer recurrence. *Abdom Imaging.* 2008;33:112–118.

218. Qayyum A, Coakley FV, Westphalen AC, Hricak H, Okuno WT, Powell B. Role of CT and MR imaging in predicting optimal cytoreduction of newly diagnosed primary epithelial ovarian cancer. *Gynecol Oncol.* 2005;96:301–306.

219. Parkin DM, Bray F, Ferlay J, Pisani P. Global cancer statistics, 2002. *CA Cancer J Clin.* 2005;55(2):74–108.

220. Hricak H, Rubinstein LV, Gherman GM, Karstaedt N. MR imaging evaluation of endometrial carcinoma results of an NCI cooperative study. *Radiology.* 1991;179(3):829–832.

221. Connor JP, Andrews JI, Anderson B, Buller RE. Computed tomography in endometrial carcinoma. *Obstet Gynecol.* 2000;95(5):692–696.

222. Manfredi R, Mirk P, Maresca G et al. Local-regional staging of endometrial carcinoma: role of MR imaging in surgical planning. *Radiology*. 2004;231(2):372–378.

223. Rockall AG, Sohaib SA, Harisinghani MG et al. Diagnostic performance of nanoparticle-enhanced magnetic resonance imaging in the diagnosis of lymph node metastases in patients with endometrial and cervical cancer. *J Clin Oncol*. 2005;23(12):2813–2821.

224. Suzuki R, Miyagi E, Takahashi N et al. Validity of positron emission tomography using fluoro-2-deoxyglucose for the preoperative evaluation of endometrial cancer. *Int J Gynecol Cancer*. 2007;17(4):890–896.

225. Saga T, Higashi T, Ishimori T et al. Clinical value of FDG-PET in the follow up of post-operative patients with endometrial cancer. *Ann Nucl Med*. 2003;17(3):197–203.

226. Park JY, Kim EN, Kim DY et al. Clinical impact of positron emission tomography or positron emission tomography/computed tomography in the posttherapy surveillance of endometrial carcinoma: evaluation of 88 patients. *Int J Gynecol Cancer*. 2008;18(6):1332–1338.

227. Thill R, Neuerburg J, Fabry U et al. Comparison of findings with 18-FDG PET and CT in pretherapeutic staging of malignant lymphoma. *Nuklearmedizin*. 1997;36:234–239.

228. Buchmann I, Reinhardt M, Elsner K et al. 2-(fluorine-18) fluoro-2-deoxy-D-glucose positron emission tomography in the detection and staging of malignant lymphoma. A bicenter trial. *Cancer*. 2001;91:889–999.

229. Elstrom R, Guan L, Baker G et al. Utility of FDG-PET scanning in lymphoma by WHO classification. *Blood*. 2003;101:3875–3876.

230. Ott G, Katzenberger T, Lohr A et al. Cytomorphologic, immunohistochemical, and cytogenetic profiles of follicular lymphoma: 2 types of follicular lymphoma grade 3. *Blood*. 2002;99:3806–3812.

231. Le Dortz L, De Guibert S, Bayat S et al. Diagnostic and prognostic impact of (18)F-FDG PET/CT in follicular lymphoma. *Eur J Nucl Med Mol Imaging*. 2010;37:2307.

232. Wöhrer S, Jaeger U, Kletter K et al. 18F-fluorodeoxyglucose positron emission tomography (18F-FDG-PET) visualizes follicular lymphoma irrespective of grading. *Ann Oncol*. 2006;17:780–784.

233. Jerusalem G, Beguin Y, Najjar F et al. Positron emission tomography (PET) with 18F-fluorodeoxyglucose (18F-FDG) for the staging of low-grade non-Hodgkin's lymphoma (NHL). *Ann Oncol*. 2001;12:825–830.

234. Perry C, Herishanu Y, Metzer U et al. Diagnostic accuracy of PET/CT in patients with extranodal marginal zone MALT lymphoma. *Eur J Haematol*. 2007;79:205–209.

235. Tsukamoto N, Kojima M, Hasegawa M et al. The usefulness of 18Ffluorodeoxyglucose positron emission tomography (18F-FDG-PET) and a comparison of 18F-FDG-PET with 67gallium scintigraphy in the evaluation of lymphoma: relation to histologic subtypes based on the World Health Organization classification. *Cancer*. 2007;110:652–659.

236. Weiler-Sagie M. 18F-FDG avidity in lymphoma readdressed: a study of 766 patients. *J Nucl Med*. 2010;51:25–30.

237. Noy A, Schöder H, Gönen M et al. The majority of transformed lymphomas have high standardized uptake values (SUVs) on positron emission tomography (PET) scanning similar to diffuse large B-cell lymphoma (DLBCL). *Ann Oncol*. 2009;20:508–512.

238. Schoder H, Noy A, Gonen M et al. Intensity of 18fluorodeoxyglucose uptake in positron emission tomography distinguishes between indolent and aggressive non-Hodgkin's lymphoma. *J Clin Oncol*. 2005;23(21):4643–4651.

239. Lister TA, Crowther D, Sutcliffe SB et al. Report of a committee convened to discuss the evaluation and staging of patients with Hodgkin's disease: Cotswald meeting. *J Clin Oncol*. 1989;7:1630–1636.

240. Rosenberg S. Validity of the Ann Arbor staging system classification for the non-Hodgkin's lymphomas. *Cancer Treat Rep*. 1977;61:1023–1027.

241. Isasi CR, Lu P, Blaufox MD. A metaanalysis of 18F-2-deoxy-2-fluoro-D-glucose positron emission tomography in the staging and restaging of patients with lymphoma. *Cancer*. 2005;104:1066–1074.

242. Hutchings M, Loft A, Hansen M et al. Position emission tomography with or without computed tomography in the primary staging of Hodgkin's lymphoma. *Haematologica*. 2006;91:482–489.

243. Schaefer NG, Hany TF, Taverna C et al. Non-Hodgkin lymphoma and Hodgkin disease: coregistered FDG PET and CT at staging and restaging—do we need contrast-enhanced CT? *Radiology*. 2004;232:823–829.

244. Tatsumi M, Cohade C, Nakamoto Y, Fishman EK, Wahl RL. Direct comparison of FDG PET and CT findings in patients with lymphoma: initial experience. *Radiology*. 2005;237:1038–1045.

245. Elstrom RL, Leonard JP, Coleman M, Brown RK. Combined PET and low-dose, noncontrast CT scanning obviates the need for additional diagnostic contrast-enhanced CT scans in patients undergoing staging or restaging for lymphoma. *Ann Oncol*. 2008;19:1770–1773.

246. Rodríguez-Vigil B, Gomez-Leon N, Pinilla I et al. PET/CT in lymphoma: prospective study of enhanced full-dose PET/CT versus unenhanced low dose PET/CT. *J Nucl Med*. 2006;47:1643–1648.

247. Pakos EE, Fotopoulos AD, Ioannidis JP. 18FFDG PET for evaluation of bone marrow infiltration in staging of lymphoma: a meta-analysis. *J Nucl Med*. 2005;46:958–963.

248. Carr R, Barrington SF, Madan B et al. Detection of lymphoma in bone marrow by whole-body positron emission tomography. *Blood*. 1998;91:3340–3346.

249. Moog F, Bangerter M, Kotzerke J, Guhlmann A, Frickhofen N, Reske SN. 18-F-fluorodeoxyglucose-positron emission tomography as a new approach to detect lymphomatous bone marrow. *J Clin Oncol*. 1998; 16:603–609.

250. Moulin-Romsee G, Hindie´ E, Cuenca X et al. 18F-FDG PET/CT bone/bone marrow findings in Hodgkin's lymphoma may circumvent the use of bone marrow trephine biopsy at diagnosis staging. *Eur J Nucl Med Mol Imaging*. 2010;37:1095–1105.

251. Cerci JJ, Pracchia LF, Linardi CC et al. 18F-FDG PET after 2 cycles of ABVD predicts event-free survival in early and advanced Hodgkin lymphoma. *J Nucl Med*. 2010 Sep;51(9):1337–1343.

252. Wu LM, Chen FY, Jiang XX, Gu HY, Yin Y, Xu JR. (18) F-FDG PET, combined FDG-PET/CT and MRI for evaluation of bone marrow infiltration in staging of lymphoma: a systematic review and meta-analysis. *Eur J Radiol.* 2012;8:303–311.

253. Chen YK, Yeh CL, Tsui CC. F-18 FDG PET for evaluation of bone marrow involvement in non-Hodgkin lymphoma: a meta-analysis. *Clin Nucl Med.* 2011;36:553.

254. Schaefer NG, Strobel K, Taverna C, Hany TF. Bone involvement in patients with lymphoma: the role of FDG-PET/CT. *Eur J Nucl Med Mol Imaging.* 2007;34:60–67.

255. Núñez R, Rini JN, Tronco GG, Tomas MB, Nichols K, Palestro CJ. Correlation of hematologic parameters with bone marrow and spleen uptake in FDG PET. *Rev Esp Med Nucl.* 2005;24:107–112.

256. Salaun PY, Gastinne T, Bodet-Milin C et al. Analysis of 18F-FDG PET diffuse bone marrow uptake and splenic uptake in staging of Hodgkin's lymphoma: a reflection of disease infiltration or just inflammation? *Eur J Nucl Med Mol Imaging.* 2009;36:1813–1821.

257. Hutchings M. The role of bone marrow biopsy in Hodgkin lymphoma staging: "to be, or not to be, that is the question"? *Leuk Lymphoma.* 2012;53:523–524.

258. Richardson SE, Sudak J, Warbey V, Ramsay A, McNamara CJ. Routine bone marrow biopsy is not necessary in the staging of patients with classical Hodgkin lymphoma in the 18F-fluoro-2-deoxyglucose positron emission tomography era. *Leuk Lymphoma.* 2012;53:381–385.

259. Hines-Thomas MR, Howard SC, Hudson MM et al. Utility of bone marrow biopsy at diagnosis in pediatric Hodgkin's lymphoma. *Haematologica.* 2010;95:1691–1696.

260. Zinzani PL, Magagnoli M, Chierichetti F et al. The role of positron emission tomography (PET) in the management of lymphoma patients. *Ann Oncol.* 1999;10:1181–1184.

261. Cremerius U, Fabry U, Neuerburg J, Zimny M, Osieka R, Buell U. Positron emission tomography with 18F-FDG to detect residual disease after therapy for malignant lymphoma. *Nucl Med Commun.* 1998;19:1055–1063.

262. Mikhaeel NG, Timothy AR, O'Doherty MJ, Hain S, Maisey MN. 18-FDG-PET as a prognostic indicator in the treatment of aggressive Non-Hodgkin's Lymphoma-comparison with CT. *Leuk Lymphoma.* 2000;39:543–553.

263. Dittmann H, Sokler M, Kollmannsberger C et al. Comparison of 18FDG-PET with CT scans in the evaluation of patients with residual and recurrent Hodgkin's lymphoma. *Oncol Rep.* 2001;8:1393–1399.

264. Spaepen K, Stroobants S, Dupont P et al. Prognostic value of positron emission tomography (PET) with fluorine-18 fluorodeoxyglucose ([18F]FDG) after first line chemotherapy in non-Hodgkins lymphoma: is [18F]FDG PET a valid alternative to conventional diagnostic methods? *J Clin Oncol.* 2001;19:414–419.

265. Mikhaeel NG, Mainwaring P, Nunan T, Timothy AR. Prognostic value of interim and post treatment FDG-PET scanning in Hodgkin lymphoma [abstract]. *Ann Oncol.* 2002;13(Suppl 2):21.

266. Wiedmann E, Baican B, Hertel A et al. Positron emission tomography (PET) for staging and evaluation of response to treatment in patients with Hodgkin's disease. *Leuk Lymphoma.* 1999;34:545–551.

267. Hueltenschmidt B, Sautter-Bihl ML, Lang O et al. Whole body positron emission tomography in the treatment of Hodgkin disease. *Cancer.* 2001;91:302–310.

268. Moskowitz AJ, Yahalom J, Kewalramani T et al. Pretransplantation functional imaging predicts outcome following autologous stem cell transplantation for relapsed and refractory Hodgkin lymphoma. *Blood.* 2010;116:4934–4937.

269. Schot BW, Zijlstra JM, Sluiter WJ et al. Early FDG-PET assessment in combination with clinical risk scores determines prognosis in recurring lymphoma. *Blood.* 2007;109(2):486–491.

270. Moskowitz CH, Yahalom J, Zelenetz AD et al. High-dose chemo-radiotherapy for relapsed or refractory lymphoma and the significance of pre-transplant functional imaging. *Br J Haematol.* 2010;148(6):890–897.

271. Smeltzer JP, Cashen AF, Zhang Q et al. Prognostic significance of FDG-PET in relapsed or refractory classical Hodgkin lymphoma treated with standard salvage chemotherapy and autologous stem cell transplantation. *Biol Blood Marrow Transplant.* 2011;17:1646–1652. Prepublished on 2011/05/24.

272. Svoboda J, Andreadis C, Elstrom R et al. Prognostic value of FDG-PET scan imaging in lymphoma patients undergoing autologous stem cell transplantation. *Bone Marrow Transplant.* 2006;38(3):211–216.

273. Poulou LS, Thanos L, Ziakas PD. Unifying the predictive value of pretransplant FDG PET in patients with lymphoma: a review and meta-analysis of published trials. *Eur J Nucl Med Mol Imaging.* 2010;37:156–162.

274. Hutchings M, Mikhaeel NG, Fields PA, Nunan T, Timothy AR. Prognostic value of interim FDG-PET after two or three cycles of chemotherapy in Hodgkin lymphoma. *Ann Oncol.* 2005;16:1160–1168.

275. Hutchings M, Loft A, Hansen M et al. FDG-PET after two cycles of chemotherapy predicts treatment failure and progression-free survival in Hodgkin lymphoma. *Blood.* 2006;107:52–59.

276. Gallamini A, Rigacci L, Merli F et al. The predictive value of positron emission tomography scanning performed after two courses of standard therapy on treatment outcome in advanced stage Hodgkin's disease. *Haematologica.* 2006;91:475–481.

277. Gallamini A, Hutchings M, Rigacci L et al. Early interim 2-[18F]fluoro-2-deoxy-D-glucose positron emission tomography is prognostically superior to international prognostic score in advanced-stage Hodgkin's lymphoma: a report from a joint Italian-Danish study. *J Clin Oncol.* 2007;25:3746–3752.

278. Zinzani PL, Tani M, Fanti S et al. Early positron emission tomography (PET) restaging: a predictive final response in Hodgkin's disease patients. *Ann Oncol.* 2006;17:1296–1300.

279. Kostakoglu L, Goldsmith SJ, Leonard JP et al. FDG-PET after 1 cycle of therapy predicts outcome in diffuse large cell lymphoma and classic Hodgkin disease. *Cancer.* 2006;107:2678–2687.

280. Zinzani PL, Rigacci L, Stefoni V et al. Early interim 18F-FDG PET in Hodgkin's lymphoma: evaluation on 304 patients. *Eur J Nucl Med Mol Imaging.* 2012 Jan;39(1):4–12. Epub 2011 Sep 6.

281. Straus DJ, Johnson JL, LaCasce AS et al. Doxorubicin, vinblastine, and gemcitabine (CALGB 50203) for stage I/II nonbulky Hodgkin lymphoma: pretreatment prognostic factors and interim PET. *Blood*. 2011; 117:5314–5320.

282. Kostakoglu L, Schoder H, Hall N et al. Interim FDG PET imaging in CALGB 50203 trial of stage I/II non-bulky Hodgkin lymphoma: would using combined PET and CT criteria better predict response than each test alone? *Leuk Lymphoma*. 2012 Mar 12 [Epub ahead of print]

283. LaCasce AS, Zukotynski K, Israel D et al. End-of-treatment but not interim PET scan predicts outcome in nonbulky limited-stage Hodgkin's lymphoma. *Ann Oncol*. 2011 Apr;22(4):910–915. Epub 2010 Oct 15.

284. Le Roux PY, Gastinne T, Le Gouill S et al. Prognostic value of interim FDG PET/CT in Hodgkin's lymphoma patients treated with interim response-adapted strategy: comparison of International Harmonization Project (IHP), Gallamini and London criteria. *Eur J Nucl Med Mol Imaging*. 2011;38:1064–1071.

285. Dann EJ, Blumenfeld Z, Bar-Shalom R et al. A 10-year experience with treatment of high and standard risk Hodgkin disease: six cycles of tailored BEACOPP, with interim scintigraphy, are effective and female fertility is preserved. *Am J Hematol*. 2012;87:32–36.

286. Avigdor A, Bulvik S, Levi I et al. Two cycles of escalated BEACOPP followed by four cycles of ABVD utilizing early-interim PET/CT scan is an effective regimen for advanced high-risk Hodgkin's lymphoma. *Ann Oncol*. 2010;21:126–132.

287. Markova J, Kahraman D, Kobe C et al. Role of [18F]-fluoro-2-deoxy-D-glucose positron emission tomography in early and late therapy assessment of patients with advanced Hodgkin lymphoma treated with bleomycin, etoposide, adriamycin, cyclophosphamide, vincristine, procarbazine and prednisone. *Leuk Lymphoma*. 2012;53:64–70.

288. Gallamini A, Patti C, Viviani S et al. Early chemotherapy intensification with BEACOPP in advanced-stage Hodgkin lymphoma patients with a interim-PET positive after two ABVD courses. *Br J Haematol*. 2011;152:551–560.

289. Haioun C, Itti E, Rahmouni A et al. [18F]Fluoro-2-deoxy-D-glucose positron emission tomography (FDG-PET) in aggressive lymphoma: an early prognostic tool for predicting patient outcome. *Blood*. 2005;106:1376–1381.

290. Mikhaeel NG, Hutchings M, Fields PA, O'Doherty MJ, Timothy AR. FDG-PET after two to three cycles of chemotherapy predicts progression-free and overall survival in high-grade non-Hodgkin lymphoma. *Ann Oncol*. 2005;16:1514–1523.

291. Spaepen K, Stroobants S, Dupont P et al. Early restaging positron emission tomography with (18) F-fluorodeoxyglucose predicts outcome in patients with aggressive non-Hodgkin's lymphoma. *Ann Oncol*. 2002;13:1356–1363.

292. Moskowitz CH, Schöder H, Teruya-Feldstein J et al. Risk-adapted dose-dense immunochemotherapy determined by interim FDG-PET in Advanced-stage diffuse large B-Cell lymphoma. *J Clin Oncol*. 2010;28:1896–1903.

293. Kasamon YL, Wahl RL, Ziessman HA et al. Phase II study of risk-adapted therapy of newly diagnosed, aggressive non-Hodgkin lymphoma based on midtreatment FDG-PETscanning. *Biol Blood Marrow Transplant*. 2009 Feb;15(2):242–248.

294. Juweid ME, Stroobants S, Hoekstra OS et al. Use of positron emission tomography for response assessment of lymphoma: consensus of the Imaging Subcommittee of International Harmonization Project in Lymphoma. *J Clin Oncol*. 2007;25:571–578.

295. Spaepen K, Stroobants S, Dupont P et al. [(18)F]FDG PET monitoring of tumour response to chemotherapy: does [(18)F]FDG uptake correlate with the viable tumour cell fraction? *Eur J Nucl Med Mol Imaging*. 2003;30:682–688.

296. Barrington SF, Qian W, Somer EJ et al. Concordance between four European centres of PET reporting criteria designed for use in multicentre trials in Hodgkin lymphoma. *Eur J Nucl Med Mol Imaging*. 2010;37:1824–1833.

297. Gallamini A, O'Doherty M. Report of satellite workshop on interim-PET in Hodgkin lymphoma: 8th International Symposium on Hodgkin Lymphoma, Cologne, 23 October 2010. *Leuk Lymphoma*. 2011;52:583–586.

298. Meignan M, Gallamini A, Haioun C. Report on the First International Workshop on interim-PET scan in Lymphoma. *Leuk Lymphoma*. 2009;50:1257–1260.

299. Gallamini A, Barrington S, Biggi A et al. International Validation Study of interpretation rules and prognostic role of interim-PET scan in advanced-stage Hodgkin Lymphoma. *Ann Oncol*. 2011;22(Suppl 4) Abstr O47.

300. Terasawa T, Nihashi T, Hotta T, Nagai H. 18F-FDG PET for posttherapy assessment of Hodgkin's disease and aggressive Non-Hodgkin's lymphoma: a systematic review. *J Nucl Med*. 2008;49:13–21.

301. Goldschmidt N, Or O, Klein M, Savitsky B, Paltiel O. The role of routine imaging procedures in the detection of relapse of patients with Hodgkin lymphoma and aggressive non-Hodgkin lymphoma. *Ann Hematol*. 2010 Aug 13. [Epub ahead of print]

302. Zinzani PL, Stefoni V, Tani M et al. Role of [18F]fluorodeoxyglucose positron emission tomography scan in the follow-up of lymphoma. *J Clin Oncol*. 2009;27:1781–1787.

303. Lee AI, Zuckerman DS, Van den Abbeele AD et al. Surveillance imaging of Hodgkin lymphoma patients in first remission: a clinical and economic analysis. *Cancer*. 2010;116:3835.

304. Cheson B. The case against heavy PETing. *J Clin Oncol*. 2009;11:1742–1743.

305. Meyer RM, Gospodarowicz MK, Connors JM et al. Randomized comparison of ABVD chemotherapy with a strategy that includes radiation therapy in patients with limited stage Hodgkin's lymphoma: National Cancer Institute of Canada Clinical Trials Group and the Eastern Cooperative Oncology Group. *J Clin Oncol*. 2005;23:4634–4642.

306. Zamagni E, Nanni C, Patriarca F et al. A prospective comparison of 18F-fluorodeoxyglucose positron emission tomography-computed tomography, magnetic resonance imaging and whole-body planar radiographs in the assessment of bone disease in newly diagnosed multiple myeloma. *Haematologica*. 2007;92:50–55.

307. Adam Z, Bolcak K, Stanicek J et al. Fluorodeoxyglucose positron emission tomography in multiple myeloma, solitary plasmocytoma and monoclonal gammapathy of unknown significance. *Neoplasma.* 2007;54:536–540.

308. Bredella MA, Steinbach L, Caputo G, Segall G, Hawkins R. Value of FDG PET in the assessment of patients with multiple myeloma. *Am J Roentgenol.* 2005;184:1199–1204.

309. Breyer RJ III, Mulligan ME, Smith SE, Line BR, Badros AZ. Comparison of imaging with FDG PET/CT with other imaging modalities in myeloma. *Skelet Radiol.* 2006;35:632–640.

310. Mileshkin L, Blum R, Seymour JF, Patrikeos A, Hicks RJ, Prince HM. A comparison of fluorine-18 fluorodeoxyglucose PET and technetium-99m sestamibi in assessing patients with multiple myeloma. *Eur J Haematol.* 2004;72:32–37.

311. Nanni C, Zamagni E, Farsad M et al. Role of 18F-FDG PET/CT in the assessment of bone involvement in newly diagnosed multiple myeloma: preliminary results. *Eur J Nucl Med Mol Imaging.* 2006;33:525–531.

312. Schirrmeister H, Bommer M, Buck AK et al. Initial results in the assessment of multiple myeloma using 18F-FDG PET. *Eur J Nucl Med.* 2002;29:361–366.

313. Schirrmeister H, Buck AK, Bergmann L, Reske SN, Bommer M. Positron emission tomography (PET) for staging of solitary plasmacytoma. *Cancer Biother Radiopharm.* 2003;18: 841–845.

314. Fonti R, Salvatore B, Quarantelli M et al. 18F-FDG PET/CT, 99mTc-MIBI, and MRI in evaluation of patients with multiple myeloma. *J Nucl Med.* 2008;49:195–200.

315. Hur J, Yoon CS, Ryu YH, Yun MJ, Suh JS. Comparative study of fluorodeoxyglucose positron emission tomography and magnetic resonance imaging for the detection of spinal bone marrow infiltration in untreated patients with multiple myeloma. *Acta Radiol.* 2008;49:427–435.

316. Jadvar H, Conti PS. Diagnostic utility of FDG PET in multiple myeloma. *Skelet Radiol.* 2002;31:690–694.

317. Shortt CP, Gleeson TG, Breen KA et al. Whole-body MRI versus PET in assessment of multiple myeloma disease activity. *Am J Roentgenol.* 2009;192:980–986.

318. Dimitrakopoulou-Strauss A, Hoffmann M, Bergner R, Uppenkamp M, Haberkorn U, Strauss LG. Prediction of progression-free survival in patients with multiple myeloma following anthracycline-based chemotherapy based on dynamic FDG-PET. *Clin Nucl Med.* 2009;34:576–584.

319. Bartel TB, Haessler J, Brown TLY et al. F18-fluorodeoxyglucose positron emission tomography in the context of other imaging techniques and prognostic factors in multiple myeloma. *Blood.* 2009;114:2068–2076.

320. Zamagni E, Patriarca F, Nanni C et al. Prognostic relevance of 18-F FDG PET/CT in newly diagnosed multiple myeloma patients treated with up-front autologous transplantation. *Blood.* 2011 Dec 1;118(23):5989–5995.

321. Durie BGM, Waxman AD, D'Agnolo A, Williams CM. Whole-body 18F-FDG PET identifies high-risk myeloma. *J Nucl Med.* 2002;43:1457–1463.

322. Kyle RA, Durie BG, Rajkumar SV et al. Monoclonal gammopathy of undetermined significance (MGUS) and smoldering (asymptomatic) multiple myeloma: IMWG consensus perspectives risk factors for progression and guidelines for monitoring and management. *Leukemia.* 2010;24:1121–1127.

323. Sohaib SA, Cook G, Koh DM. Imaging studies for germ cell tumors. *Hematol Oncol Clin North Am.* 2011;25:487–502.

324. Chernyak V. Novel imaging modalities for lymph node imaging in urologic oncology. *Urol Clin North Am.* 2011;38:471–481.

325. Stephenson AJ, Aprikian AG, Gilligan TD et al. Management of low-stage nonseminomatous germ cell tumors of testis: SIU/ICUD Consensus Meeting on Germ Cell Tumors (GCT), Shanghai 2009. *Urology.* 2011;78(Suppl 4):S444–S455.

326. Albers P, Bender H, Yilmaz H, Schoeneich G, Biersack HJ, Mueller SC. Positron emission tomography in the clinical staging of patients with stage I and II testicular germ cell tumors. *Urology.* 1999;53:808–811.

327. Spermon JR, De Geus-Oei LF, Kiemeney LA, Witjes JA, Oyen WJ. The role of 18fluoro-2-deoxyglucose positron emission tomography in initial staging and re-staging after chemotherapy for testicular germ cell tumours. *BJU Int.* 2002;89:549–556.

328. Cremerius U, Wildberger JE, Borchers H et al. Does positron emission tomography using 18-fluoro-2-deoxyglucose improve clinical staging of testicular cancer? Results of a study in 50 patients. *Urology.* 1999;54:900–904.

329. Hain SF, O'Doherty MJ, Timothy AR, Leslie MD, Partridge SE, Huddart RA. Fluorodeoxyglucose PET in the initial staging of germ cell tumours. *Eur J Nucl Med.* 2000;27:590–4.

330. De Wit M, Brenner W, Hartmann M et al. [18F]-FDG-PET in clinical stage I/II non-seminomatous germ cell tumours: results of the German multicentre trial. *Ann Oncol.* 2008;19:1619–1623.

331. Lassen U, Daugaard G, Eigtved A, Hojgaard L, Damgaard K, Rorth M. Whole-body FDG-PET in patients with stage I non-seminomatous germ cell tumours. *Eur J Nucl Med Mol Imaging.* 2003;30:396–402.

332. Hain SF, O'Doherty MJ, Timothy AR, Leslie MD, Harper PG, Huddart RA. Fluorodeoxyglucose positron emission tomography in the evaluation of germ cell tumours at relapse. *Br J Cancer.* 2000;83:863–869.

333. Sanchez D, Zudaire JJ, Fernandez JM et al. 18F-fluoro-2-deoxyglucose-positron emission tomography in the evaluation of nonseminomatous germ cell tumours at relapse. *BJU Int.* 2002;89:912–916.

334. Becherer A, De Santis M, Karanikas G et al. FDG PET is superior to CT in the prediction of viable tumour in post-chemotherapy seminoma residuals. *Eur J Radiol.* 2005;54:284–288.

335. De Santis M, Becherer A, Bokemeyer C et al. 2-18fluoro-deoxy-D-glucose positron emission tomography is a reliable predictor for viable tumor in postchemotherapy seminoma: an update of the prospective multicentric SEMPET trial. *J Clin Oncol.* 2004;22:1034–1039.

336. Bachner M, Loriot Y, Gross-Goupil M et al. 2-18fluoro-deoxy-D-glucose positron emission tomography (FDG-PET) for postchemotherapy seminoma residual lesions: a retrospective validation of the SEMPET trial. *Ann Oncol.* 2012;2:59–64.

337. Huddart RA, O'Doherty MJ, Padhani A et al. 18fluorodeoxyglucose positron emission tomography in the prediction of relapse in patients with high-risk, clinical stage I nonseminomatous germ cell tumors: preliminary report of MRC Trial TE22 – the NCRI Testis Tumour Clinical Study Group. *J Clin Oncol.* 2007;25:3090–3095.

338. Pfannenberg AC, Oechsle K, Kollmannsberger C et al. [Early prediction of treatment response to high-dose chemotherapy in patients with relapsed germ cell tumors using [18F]FDG-PET, CT or MRI, and tumor marker]. *Rofo.* 2004;176:76–84.

339. Kang DE, White RL Jr, Zuger JH, Sasser HC, Teigland CM. Clinical use of fluorodeoxyglucose F 18 positron emission tomography for detection of renal cell carcinoma. *J Urol.* 2004;171:1806–1809.

340. Majhail NS, Urbain J, Albani JM et al. F-18 fluorodeoxyglucose positron emission tomography in the evaluation of distant metastases from renal cell carcinoma. *J Clin Oncol.* 2003;21:3995–4000.

341. Lawrentschuk N, Davis I.D, Bolton DM, Scott AM. Functional imaging of renal cell carcinoma. *Nat Rev Urol.* 2010;7:258–266.

342. Revheim ME, Winge-Main AK, Hagen G, Fjeld JG, Fosså SD, Lilleby W. Combined positron emission tomography/computed tomography in sunitinib therapy assessment of patients with metastatic renal cell carcinoma. *Clin Oncol (R Coll Radiol).* 2011;23(5):339–343.

343. Kayani I, Avril N, Bomanji J et al. Sequential FDG-PET/CT as a biomarker of response to Sunitinib in metastatic clear cell renal cancer. *Clin Cancer Res.* 2011; 17:6021–6028.

344. Namura K, Minamimoto R, Yao M et al. Impact of maximum standardized uptake value (SUVmax) evaluated by 18-Fluoro-2-deoxy-D-glucose positron emission tomography/computed tomography (18F-FDG-PET/CT) on survival for patients with advanced renal cell carcinoma: a preliminary report. *BMC Cancer.* 2010;10:667–673.

345. Pryma DA, O'Donoghue JA, Humm JL et al. Correlation of in vivo and in vitro measures of carbonic anhydrase IX antigen expression in renal masses using antibody 124I-cG250. *J Nucl Med.* 2011;52:535–540.

346. Fogelman I, Cook G, Israel O, Van der Wall H. Positron emission tomography and bone metastases. *Semin Nucl Med.* 2005;35:135–142.

347. Schoder H, Herrmann K, Gonen M et al. 2-[18F]fluoro-2-deoxyglucose positron emission tomography for the detection of disease in patients with prostate-specific antigen relapse after radical prostatectomy. *Clin Cancer Res.* 2005;11:4761–4769.

348. Seltzer MA, Barbaric Z, Belldegrun A et al. Comparison of helical computerized tomography, positron emission tomography and monoclonal antibody scans for evaluation of lymph node metastases in patients with prostate specific antigen relapse after treatment for localized prostate cancer. *J Urol.* 1999;162:1322–1328.

349. Nunez R, Macapinlac HA, Yeung HW et al. Combined 18F-FDG and 11C-methionine PET scans in patients with newly progressive metastatic prostate cancer. *J Nucl Med.* 2002;43:46–55.

350. Heicappell R, Muller-Mattheis V, Reinhardt M et al. Staging of pelvic lymph nodes in neoplasms of the bladder and prostate by positron emission tomography with 2-[18F]-2-deoxy-D-glucose. *Eur Urol.* 1999; 36:582–587.

351. Morris MJ, Akhurst T, Osman I et al. Fluorinated deoxyglucose positron emission tomography imaging in progressive metastatic prostate cancer. *Urology.* 2002;59:913–918.

352. Morris MJ, Akhurst T, Larson SM et al. Fluorodeoxyglucose positron emission tomography as an outcome measure for castrate metastatic prostate cancer treated with antimicrotubule chemotherapy. *Clin Cancer Res.* 2005;11:3210–3216.

353. Bauman G, Belhocine T, Kovacs M, Ward A, Beheshti M, Rachinsky I. 18F-fluorocholine for prostate cancer imaging: a systematic review of the literature. *Prostate Cancer Prostatic Dis.* 2012;15:45–55.

354. Zaheer A, Cho SY, Pomper MG. New agents and techniques for imaging prostate cancer. *J Nucl Med.* 2009;50:1387–1390.

355. Kibel AS, Dehdashti F, Katz MD et al. Prospective study of [18F]fluorodeoxyglucose positron emission tomography/computed tomography for staging of muscle-invasive bladder carcinoma. *J Clin Oncol.* 2009;27:4314–4320.

356. Swinnen G, Maes A, Pottel H et al. FDG-PET/CT for the preoperative lymph node staging of invasive bladder cancer. *Eur Urol.* 2010;4:641–647.

357. Liu IJ, Lai YH, Espiritu JI et al. Evaluation of fluorodeoxyglucose positron emission tomography imaging in metastatic transitional cell carcinoma with and without prior chemotherapy. *Urol Int.* 2006;77:69–75.

358. Jadvar H, Quan V, Henderson RW, Conti PS. [F-18]-Fluorodeoxyglucose PET and PET-CT in diagnostic imaging evaluation of locally recurrent and metastatic bladder transitional cell carcinoma. *Int J Clin Oncol.* 2008;13:42–47.

359. Kosuda S, Kison PV, Greenough R, Grossman HB, Wahl RL. Preliminary assessment of fluorine-18 fluorodeoxyglucose positron emission tomography in patients with bladder cancer. *Eur J Nucl Med.* 1997;24:615–620.

360. Moses KA, Zhang J, Hricak H, Bochner BH. Bladder cancer imaging: an update. *Curr Opin Urol.* 2011;21:393–397.

361. Bang S, Baud CA. Topographical distribution of fluoride in iliac bone of a fluoride-treated osteoporotic patient. *J Bone Mineral Res.* 1990;5(Suppl 1):S87–S89.

362. Kurdziel KA, Shih JH, Apolo AB et al. The kinetics and reproducibility of 18F-sodium fluoride for oncology using current PET camera technology. *J Nucl Med.* 2012 Jun 22. [Epub ahead of print]

363. Grant FD, Fahey FH, Packard AB, Davis RT, Alavi A, Treves ST. Skeletal PET with 18F-fluoride: applying new technology to an old tracer. *J Nucl Med.* 2008;49:68–78.

364. Cook GJ. PET and PET/CT imaging of skeletal metastases. *Cancer Imaging.* 2010 Jul 19;10:1–8.

365. Czernin J, Satyamurthy N, Schiepers C. Molecular mechanisms of bone 18F-NaF deposition. *J Nucl Med.* 2010;51:1826–1829.

366. Even-Sapir E, Metser U, Flusser G et al. Assessment of malignant skeletal disease: initial experience with 18F-fluoride PET/CT and comparison between 18F-fluoride PET and 18F-fluoride PET/CT. *J Nucl Med.* 2004;45:272–278.

367. Even-Sapir E, Metser U, Mishani E, Lievshitz G, Lerman H, Leibovitch I. The detection of bone metastases in patients with high risk prostate cancer: 99mTc MDP planar bone scintigraphy, single and multi field of view SPECT, 18F-fluoride PET and 18F-fluoride PET/CT. *J Nucl Med.* 2006;47:287–297.

368. Beheshti M, Vali R, Waldenberger P et al. Detection of bone metastases in patients with prostate cancer by 18F fluorocholine and 18F fluoride PET/CT: a comparative study. *Eur J Nucl Med Mol Imaging.* 2008; 35:1766–1774.

369. Schirrmeister H, Guhlmann A, Elsner K et al. Sensitivity in detecting osseous lesions depends on anatomic localization: planar bone scintigraphy versus 18F PET. *J Nucl Med.* 1999;40:1623–1629.

370. Schirrmeister H, Guhlmann A, Kotzerke J et al. Early detection and accurate description of extent of metastatic bone disease in breast cancer with fluoride ion and PET. *J Clin Oncol.* 1999;17:2381–2389.

371. Schirrmeister H, Glatting G, Hetzel J et al. Evaluation of the clinical value of planar bone scans, SPECT and 18F-labeled NaF PET in newly diagnosed lung cancer. *J Nucl Med.* 2001;42:1800–1804.

372. Kruger S, Buck AK, Mottaghy FM et al. Detection of bone metastases in patients with lung cancer: 99mTc MDP planar bone scintigraphy, 18F-fluoride PET or 18F-FDG PET-CT. *Eur J Nucl Med Mol Imaging.* 2009;36:1807–1812.

373. Hoegerle S, Juengling F, Otte A, Altehoefer C, Moser EA, Nitzsche EU. Combined FDG and F-18 fluoride whole body PET: a feasible two in one approach to cancer imaging. *Radiology.* 1998;209:253–258.

374. Iagaru A, Mittra E, Yaghoubi SS et al. Novel strategy for a cocktail 18F-fluoride and 18F-FDG PET/CT scan for evaluation of malignancy: results of the pilot phase study. *J Nucl Med.* 2009;50:501–505.

375. F-18 PET/CT Versus TC-MDP Scanning to Detect Bone Mets. http://clinicaltrials.gov/ct2/show/NCT00882609?term=NaF+bone&rank=6.

376. Moureau-Zabotto L, Touboul E, Lerouge D et al. Impact of CT and 18F-deoxyglucose positron emission tomography image fusion for conformal radiotherapy in esophageal carcinoma. *Int J Radiat Oncol Biol Phys.* 2005;63:340–345.

377. Konski AA, Cheng JD, Goldberg M et al. Correlation of molecular response as measured by 18-FDG positron emission tomography with outcome after chemoradiotherapy in patients with esophageal carcinoma. *Int J Radiat Oncol Biol Phys.* 2007;69:358–363.

378. De Ruysscher D, Kirsch CM. PET scans in radiotherapy planning of lung cancer. *Radiother Oncol.* 2010;96:335–338.

379. Price PM, Green MM. Positron emission tomography imaging approaches for external beam radiation therapies: current status and future developments. *Br J Radiol.* 2011 Dec;84(Spec No 1):S19–S34.

380. Troost EG, Schinagl DA, Bussink J, Oyen WJ, Kaanders JH. Clinical evidence on PET-CT for radiation therapy planning in head and neck tumours. *Radiother Oncol.* 2010 Sep;96(3):328–334.

381. Deantonio L, Beldì D, Gambaro G. FDG-PET/CT imaging for staging and radiotherapy treatment planning of head and neck carcinoma. *Radiat Oncol.* 2008;3:29.

382. Gillham C, Zips D, Ponisch F et al. Additional PET/CT in week 5–6 of radiotherapy for patients with stage III non-small cell lung cancer as a means of dose escalation planning? *Radiother Oncol.* 2008;88:335–341.

383. Wang D, Schultz CJ, Jursinic PA et al. Initial experience of FDG-PET/CT guided IMRT of head-and-neck carcinoma. *Int J Radiat Oncol Biol Phys.* 2006;65:143–151.

384. Ashamalla H, Rafla S, Parikh K et al. The contribution of integrated PET/CT to the evolving definition of treatment volumes in radiation treatment planning in lung cancer. *Int J Radiat Oncol Biol Phys.* 2005;63:1016–1023.

385. Bradley J, Thorstad WL, Mutic S et al. Impact of FDG-PET on radiation therapy volume delineation in non-small-cell lung cancer. *Int J Radiat Oncol Biol Phys.* 2004;59:78–86.

386. Graeter TP, Hellwig D, Hoffmann K, Ukena D, Kirsch CM, Schäfers HJ. Mediastinal lymph node staging in suspected lung cancer: comparison of positron emission tomography with F-18-fluorodeoxyglucose and mediastinoscopy. *Ann Thorac Surg.* 2003;75:231–235; discussion 235–236.

387. Wallace MB, Pascual JM, Raimondo M et al. Minimally invasive endoscopic staging of suspected lung cancer. *JAMA.* 2008;299:540–546.

388. Buchbender C, Heusner TA, Lauenstein TC, Bockisch A, Antoch G. Oncologic PET/MRI, part 2: bone tumors, soft-tissue tumors, melanoma, and lymphoma. *J Nucl Med.* 2012 Jul 10. [Epub ahead of print].

389. Buchbender C, Heusner TA, Lauenstein TC, Bockisch A, Antoch G. Oncologic PET/MRI, part 1: tumors of the brain, head and neck, chest, abdomen, and pelvis. *J Nucl Med.* 2012;53:928–938.

390. Sinha S, Peach AH. Diagnosis and management of soft tissue sarcoma. *BMJ.* 2010;341:c7170.22.

391. Buchbender C, Heusner TA, Lauenstein TC, Bockisch A, Antoch G. Oncologic PET/MRI, part 1: Tumors of the brain, head and neck, chest, abdomen, and pelvis. *J Nucl Med.* 2012;53:928–938.

392. Yokouchi M, Terahara M, Nagano S et al. Clinical implications of determination of safe surgical margins by using a combination of CT and 18FDG-positron emission tomography in soft tissue sarcoma. *BMC Musculoskelet Disord.* 2011;12:166.

393. Muller-Horvat C, Radny P, Eigentler TK et al. Prospective comparison of the impact on treatment decisions of whole-body magnetic resonance imaging and computed tomography in patients with metastatic malignant melanoma. *Eur J Cancer.* 2006;42:342–350.

394. Pfannenberg C, Aschoff P, Schanz S et al. Prospective comparison of 18F-fluorodeoxyglucose positron emission tomography/computed tomography and whole-body magnetic resonance imaging in staging of advanced malignant melanoma. *Eur J Cancer.* 2007;43:557–564.

395. Laurent V, Trausch G, Bruot O, Olivier P, Felblinger J, Re´gent D. Comparative study of two whole-body imaging techniques in the case of melanoma metastases: advantages of multi-contrast MRI examination including a diffusion weighted sequence in comparison with PET-CT. *Eur J Radiol.* 2010;75:376–383.

396. Yang HL, Liu T, Wang XM, Xu Y, Deng SM. Diagnosis of bone metastases: a meta-analysis comparing 18FDG PET, CT, MRI and bone scintigraphy. *Eur Radiol.* 2011;21:2604–2617.

397. Schmidt GP, Schoenberg SO, Schmid R et al. Screening for bone metastases: whole-body MRI using a 32-channel system versus dual-modality PET-CT. *Eur Radiol.* 2007;17:939–949.13.

398. Liu T, Cheng T, Xu W, Yan WL, Liu J, Yang HL. A meta-analysis of 18FDGPET, MRI and bone scintigraphy for diagnosis of bone metastases in patients with breast cancer. *Skeletal Radiol.* 2011;40:523–531.

399. Imamura F, Kuriyama K, Seto T et al. Detection of bone marrow metastases of small cell lung cancer with magnetic resonance imaging: early diagnosis before destruction of osseous structure and implications for staging. *Lung Cancer.* 2000;27:189–197.

400. Reischauer C, Froehlich JM, Koh DM et al. Bone metastases from prostate cancer: assessing treatment response by using diffusion-weighted imaging and functional diffusion maps—initial observations. *Radiology.* 2010;257:523–531.

401. Lin C, Luciani A, Itti E et al. Whole-body diffusion-weighted magnetic resonance imaging with apparent diffusion coefficient mapping for staging patients with diffuse large B-cell lymphoma. *Eur Radiol.* 2010;20:2027–2038.

402. Schnapauff D, Zeile M, Niederhagen MB et al. Diffusion-weighted echo-planar magnetic resonance imaging for the assessment of tumor cellularity in patients with soft-tissue sarcomas. *J Magn Reson Imaging.* 2009;29:1355–1359.

403. Lin C, Itti E, Luciani A et al. Whole-body diffusion-weighted imaging with apparent diffusion coefficient mapping for treatment response assessment in patients with diffuse large B-cell lymphoma: pilot study. *Invest Radiol.* 2011;46:341–349.

404. Boellaard R, O'Doherty MJ, Weber WA et al. FDG PET and PET/CT: EANM procedure guidelines for tumour PET imaging: version 1.0. *Eur J Nucl Med Mol Imaging.* 2010;37:181–200.

405. Podoloff DA, Ball DW, Ben-Josef E et al. NCCN task force: clinical utility of PET in a variety of tumor types. *J Natl Compr Canc Netw.* 2009;7(Suppl 2):S1–S26.

Section V

CAD Applications

28

Modified Akaike Information Criterion for Selecting the Numbers of Mixture Components: An Application to Initial Lung Segmentation

Ahmed Elnakib, Mohamed Abou El-Ghar, Georgy Gimel'farb, Robert Falk, Jasjit S. Suri, and Ayman El-Baz

CONTENTS

28.1 Introduction

Low-order probabilistic models of visual appearance of each object of interest in a three-dimensional (3D) image, which allow for fast unsupervised online learning of the model and account for nonuniform variations of voxel signals (intensities) because of different scanners and scanning parameters, can considerably enhance the accuracy of medical image segmentation and registration. Frequently, the appearance is described by a 1D empirical marginal probability distribution of intensities, being modeled by a mixture of unimodal components associated each with an individual object of interest. Mixture components with either Gaussian [1] or rarely other analytically learnable parametric unimodal distributions [2] are still the most popular. More precise approximations of an empirical distribution with a linear combination of sign-alternate Gaussians (LCG) [3] or discrete Gaussians (LCDG) [4] also rely on the Gaussian mixture to model prominent dominant modes of the empirical distribution, which relate to the objects of interest.

Nonetheless, a proper number of components for a mixture are typically selected manually, in spite of multiple existing criteria for automatic selection [5–16]. Each deterministic criterion, such as the Akaike's information (AIC) [5–7], Schwarz's Bayesian inference [8], minimum message length (MML) [9,10], classification likelihood

[11], mutual information between the components [12], or greedy mixture learning [13,14], can be applied to decrease sequentially a large initial set of the candidate components or increase their initial small set. However, these methods are too computationally expensive: for instance, the AIC requires the recalculation of the model's log-likelihood for all the exclusions or inclusions of the individual candidates. A few known stochastic techniques, for example, based on resampling [15] or cross-validation [16], are also computationally expensive.

This chapter proposes a more feasible approach combining the automatic selection of the number of components with the expectation-maximization (EM) process of learning a mixture. To compute the log-likelihood of the mixture components for the conventional AIC, one requires the prior knowledge of which component each individual signal belongs to; for example, which voxel signals relate to each mixture component. In many applications, including medical image analysis, such knowledge is usually too imprecise because of ambiguous image boundaries between the objects of interest. An easily computable approximate version of the AIC, called the modified AIC (mAIC), which circumvents this problem, is introduced below and embedded into the iterative EM learning process. In contrast to the modification of the AIC criterion by Ali and Farag [17] that works only with continuous probability mixtures and assumes independent probabilities of the mixture components (which is not the case in medical images), our proposed mAIC can deal with any continuous or discrete probability mixture and does not require the probabilities of the mixture components to be independent.

The selected proper number of the dominant LCG/LCDG components and the EM-based precise modeling of their probability distributions facilitate fast, accurate, and fully automated initial segmentation of lungs from the 3D computed tomography (CT) images. The proposed automated segmentation allows for different CT scanning protocols and can be easily combined with any subsequent spatial image analysis focused on improving the final segmentation. Section 28.2 details the mAIC and describes how it can be embedded into the main EM-loop to both select the proper number and estimate parameters of the mixture components. Experiments confirming that this approach is highly accurate on various synthetic 2D phantoms and in vivo 3D lung CT images, captured with different scanning protocols, are presented in Section 28.3. Section 28.4 concludes the chapter.

28.2 mAIC-Based Estimation of the Number of Components

28.2.1 Basic Notation

Let $Q = \{0,1,\ldots,Q-1\}$ be a finite set of Q scalar signals, for example, voxel-wise gray levels, or intensities in a 3D image. Let $\psi_k(q)$; $\sum_{q \in Q} \psi_k(q) = 1$ denote a k-th component; $k = 1,\ldots, K$, of a K-component Gaussian mixture model of a given empirical probability distribution:

$$\mathbf{P} = \begin{pmatrix} p(q): q \in \mathbf{Q};\ p(q) = \sum_{k=1}^{K} w_k \psi_k(q); \\ \sum_{q \in \mathbf{Q}} p(q) = 1;\ \sum_{k=1}^{K} w_k = 1 \end{pmatrix} \quad (28.1)$$

Where w_k are positive weights or prior probabilities of the components.

For modeling a continuous probability density, each component $\psi_k(q)$ is a Gaussian density function:

$$\psi_k(q) = \phi(q|\theta_k) = \frac{1}{\sqrt{2\pi}\sigma_k} \exp\left(-\frac{1}{2\sigma_k^2}(q-\mu_k)^2\right);\ \int_{-\infty}^{\infty} \phi(u|\theta_k)$$

$du = 1$, with the mean μ_k and the variance σ_k^2. For brevity, these parameters will be denoted $\theta_k = (\mu_k, \sigma_k^2)$. For modeling a discrete distribution, each component is a discrete Gaussian [4]:

$$\psi_k(q) = \begin{cases} \Phi_k(0.5) & q = 0 \\ \Phi_k(q+0.5) - \Phi_k(q-0.5) & q = 1,\ldots,Q-2 \\ 1 - \Phi_k(Q-1.5) & q = Q-1 \end{cases} \quad (28.2)$$

Where $\Phi_k(q) = \int_{-\infty}^{q} \phi(u|\theta_k)du$ is the cumulative Gaussian probability function.

Let $s_n : n = 1,\ldots, N$; $s_n \in \mathbf{Q}$, be N observed signals. Let a binary indicator $\delta_{n:k} \in \{0,1\}$, such that $\sum_{k=1}^{K} \delta_{n:k} = 1$, selects a mixture component in Equation (28.1), which an individual signal s_n actually belongs to. Given a set of all the indicators $\Delta_K = \{\delta_{n:k}: k = 1,\ldots, K; n = 1,\ldots, N\}$ for the components and observations, the complete log-likelihood of the mixture with parameters $\Theta_K = \{\theta_k: k = 1,\ldots, K\}$ of the components is

$$L_c(\Theta_K, \Delta_K) = \frac{1}{N}$$

$$\sum_{k=1}^{K} \sum_{n=1}^{N} \delta_{k:n} \log \psi_k(s_n) = \sum_{k=1}^{K} \sum_{q \in Q} f_{k:q} \log \psi_k(q) \quad (28.3)$$

Where $f_{k:q} = \frac{1}{N} \sum_{n:s_n=q} \delta_{k:n}$ is the empirical probability of signals q produced by the component k.

Then the proper number K^* of components in Equation (28.1) is found [6] by maximizing the conventional $AIC(K) = L_c(\Theta_K, \Delta_K) - M_K$, where M_K is the number of unknown model parameters. In our case with the three parameters (μ_k, σ_k, w_k) per Gaussian component, $M_K = 3K$ and $K^* = \arg \max_K \{L_c(\Theta_K, \Delta_K) - 3K\}$.

The indicator set Δ_K is actually unknown. For the known parameters of the components, there exist straightforward estimates of these indicators:

$$\delta_{n:k} = \begin{cases} 1 & \text{if } k = \arg \max_{k=1,\ldots,K} w_k \psi_k(s_n) \\ 0 & \text{Otherwise} \end{cases} \quad (28.4)$$

However, these binary estimates are too imprecise when both the number and parameters of the components have to be learned. Therefore, we replace each unknown binary indicator $\delta_{n:k}$ with the continuous posterior belief $\beta_{k:q}$ that the observed signal $s_n = q$ belongs to the mixture component k:

$$0 \leq \beta_{k:q} \leq 1;\ \beta_{k:q} = \frac{w_k \psi_k(q)}{\sum_{k=1}^{K} w_k \psi_k(q)} \quad (28.5)$$

and use the "modified" (plausible) log-likelihood:

$L_p(\Theta_K) = \sum_{k=1}^{K} \sum_{q \in \mathbf{Q}} \beta_{k:q} \log \psi_k(q)$ of the model to specify the mAIC:

$$\text{mAIC} = L_p(\Theta_K) - 3\varsigma K \qquad (28.6)$$

where a fixed penalty factor ς accounts for the above approximation of the complete log-likelihood.

28.2.2 Sufficient Monotonicity Condition for the mAIC

Let the mixture components be sorted in the ascending order of their relative weights: $\hat{w}_1 \le \hat{w}_2 \le \dots \le \hat{w}_K$:

$$\hat{w}_k = \frac{\sum\limits_{q \in \mathbf{Q}} \beta_{k:q}}{\sum\limits_{k=1}^{K} \sum\limits_{q \in \mathbf{Q}} \beta_{k:q}} = \frac{1}{Q} \sum\limits_{q \in \mathbf{Q}} \beta_{k:q},$$

so that

$$\sum\limits_{q \in \mathbf{Q}} \sum\limits_{k=2}^{K} \beta_{k:q} = Q(1 - \hat{w}_1)$$

For brevity, let $A = \min\limits_{k \ge 2; q \in \mathbf{Q}} \log \psi_k(q)$ and $B = \max\limits_{q \in \mathbf{Q}} \log \psi_1(q)$. Our idea is to successively remove from the mixture the component of the smallest weight while the mAIC increases, that is, while the difference $\Delta_K = \text{mAIC}(K-1) - \text{mAIC}(K) > 0$.

Provided that the mixture components are only reweighed, but preserve their order after removing the component of the smallest relative weight, the corresponding mAIC values of Equation (28.6) will be as follows:

$$\text{mAIC}(K) = \sum\limits_{q \in \mathbf{Q}} \sum\limits_{k=2}^{K} \beta_{k:q} \log \psi_k(q) + \\ \sum\limits_{q \in \mathbf{Q}} \beta_{1:q} \log \psi_1(q) - 3\varsigma K$$

and

$$\text{mAIC}(K-1) = \frac{1}{1 - \hat{w}_1} \sum\limits_{q \in \mathbf{Q}} \sum\limits_{k=2}^{K} \beta_{k:q} \log \psi_k(q) - 3\varsigma(K-1)$$

so that the difference $\Delta_K = \text{mAIC}(K-1) - \text{mAIC}(K)$ is bounded:

$$\Delta_K = \frac{\hat{w}_1}{1 - \hat{w}_1} \sum\limits_{q \in \mathbf{Q}} \sum\limits_{k=2}^{K} \beta_{k:q} \log \psi_k(q) - \sum\limits_{q \in \mathbf{Q}} \beta_{1:q} \log \psi_1(q) + 3\varsigma$$

$$\ge \frac{\hat{w}_1}{1 - \hat{w}_1}[Q(1 - \hat{w}_1)]A - Q\hat{w}_1 B + 3\varsigma = Q\hat{w}_1(A - B) + 3\varsigma$$

Thus, if the condition

$$Q\hat{w}_1(A - B) + 3\varsigma \ge 0 \qquad (28.7)$$

is satisfied, then $\Delta_K \ge 0$, and the mAIC increases after the adjustment. This simple consideration leads to the proposed Algorithm 28.1 for learning a mixture by embedding the mAIC search for the number of components into the conventional EM-based estimation of the mixture parameters. On the basis of the accurate number and parameters of the mixture components found by Algorithm 28.1, we used the LCDG-based approach [4] for lung segmentation.

ALGORITHM 28.1 UNSUPERVISED EM–mAIC-BASED MIXTURE LEARNING

1. Set an overfitting number K of the mixture components and estimate its initial weights $\hat{w}$ and parameters $\hat{\Theta}$.
2. Apply the expectation step of the EM algorithm and find the component of the smallest weight $\hat{w}$.
   - If there is more than one component with the same weight, perform a principle component analysis and pick the one with the smallest eigenvalue.
3. Check the condition of Equation (28.7) for the selected component:
   - If it is satisfied, remove this component, adjust the remaining weights $\hat{w}$, and apply the maximization step of the EM algorithm.
   - Otherwise, set the components number to current K and terminate the process.
4. Repeat Steps 2 and 3 until the condition of Equation (28.7) is met.

28.3 Experimental Results

To assess the accuracy and robustness of the proposed approach, Algorithm 28.1 has been tested first on synthetic phantoms and then on real 3D axial chest images. To explore variations in signal distributions because of different scanning protocols, the CT slices were collected using two protocols: 1-mm-thick low-dose CT and 2.5-mm-thick high-dose CT. These spiral scans were reconstructed every 4 mm with the scanning pitch of 1 mm. In these experiments, all the mixture parameters, including the number of its components, were estimated automatically. Initially, the number of components, K, is set to twice the number of the automatically detected image histogram peaks, the initial mean values, μ, are set to the locations of the highest peaks and the middle points between each two locations, the initial variance values, σ^2, are set to the number of gray levels divided by 50, and initial weights, w_k, are assumed equiprobable. For comparison, the automatic AIC–EM learning, similar to Algorithm 28.1, except the least informative components are removed using the approximate AIC with the binary indicators of Equation 28.4, was applied to the same test data.

28.3.1 Experiments on Synthetic Phantoms

To mimic real images, our synthetic 2D ones were obtained by using overlapping distributions of signals of complex shape for each class (see Figure 28.1a through d). The numbers of dominant modes (from two to four) corresponding to the ideal regions in Figure 28.1a were known and the random gray values in the range [0, 2048] were generated in line with the probability distributions in Figure 28.1c. As shown in Figure 28.1e, unlike the AIC curves in Figure 28.1f, all the mAIC curves have successfully reached their maximum at the proper number of components. These results highlight the efficiency and advantages of the proposed approach.

28.3.2 Experiments on Real Images

Figure 28.2 shows results for the real 3D low- and high-dose CT lung images. According to the practical experience, the marginal empirical signal distributions in Figure 28.2b have two dominant modes: one for the chest and another for the lungs. The mAIC curve has the prominent maximum at the right number of components on both of the datasets (see Figure 28.2c). Contrastingly, the AIC fails for both the sets, as shown in Figure 28.2d. The poor performance of the AIC criterion is due to the ambiguous region boundaries of the region of interest in the images that leads to an inaccurate estimation of labels (i.e., inaccurate estimation of the indicator function).

The right selection of the number of dominant components and the accurate learning of their distributions make our LCDG-based (see Figure 28.3, which illustrates two examples of LCDG-based modeling of empirical marginal intensity distributions for 3D CT images) lung segmentation more accurate than other known approaches, for example, iterative thresholding (IT) by Hu and Hoffman [18] (Figure 28.4b and c) for the low-dose CT data. High accuracy of our final segmentation after spatial analysis and smoothing of the initial one is confirmed by the Dice similarity coefficient, approaching the ideal value of 1 in Figure 28.4e. It is significantly better than for the IT after the same spatial analysis and smoothing (Figure 28.4d).

The proposed approach provides fast and accurate initial segmentation of medical structures, in particular, 3D lungs. Its present MATLAB® implementation on a quad-core Intel processor (3.2GHz each) with 16 GB of memory and 1 TB hard drive with redundant array of inexpensive disks technology takes 1.30 ± 0.02 seconds for a complete lung CT dataset, whereas the IT takes 5.8 ± 0.1 seconds for the same job. The C/C++ programming environment may considerably reduce this time.

28.4 Conclusion

We proposed and validated a new approach to model a marginal empirical probability distribution of signals with a mixture of unimodal, for example, Gaussian probability distributions. The mixture models are used frequently for describing visual appearance of objects of interest in images, including 3D medical images, either directly or as dominant parts of more accurate LCG and LCDG. The proper number of components in the mixture is selected automatically and concurrently with the conventional iterative EM process of learning other model parameters. Our selection is based on maximization of an approximate version of the well-known AIC, called in the chapter the mAIC, in application to the mixture components. The mAIC is computed in the main EM loop to exclude successively, one by one, the least informative components, starting from their overfitting set. In our experiments, the mAIC showed the marked monotone increase to the prominent maximum at the correct number of the components for the simulated phantoms and at the practically justified number for the in vivo 3D medical images, such as the 3D lung images. Combined with our previous algorithms for precise LCG- or LCDG-based modeling of marginal distributions, this proposal leads to a fully automated modeling framework that can provide fast and accurate initial segmentation of various medical images.

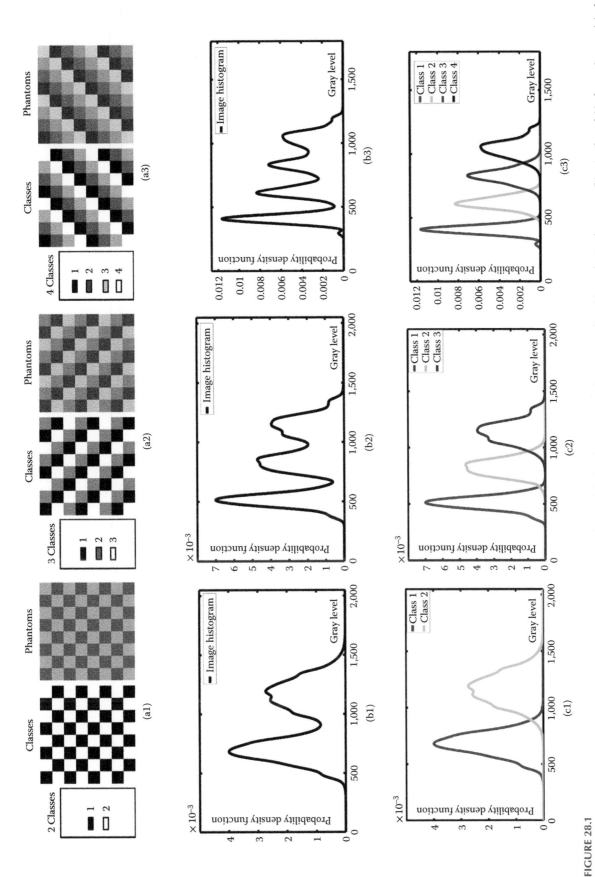

FIGURE 28.1
Experiments on synthetic images with 2 to 4 classes of signals (from left to right): the classes map and corresponding (a) synthetic phantoms, (b) mixed, and (c) class-wise empirical probability distributions of intensities for the phantoms with relative overlaps of 2.2% (column 1); 1.1% and 4.2% (column 2); and 0.7%, 3.0%, and 5.7% (column 3). Each distribution (c) is a linear combination of the dominant DG and sign-alternate subordinate DGs (d). The mAIC values (e), obtained with $\varsigma = 0.05$, reach the maximum at the true number of components, unlike the AIC values (f).

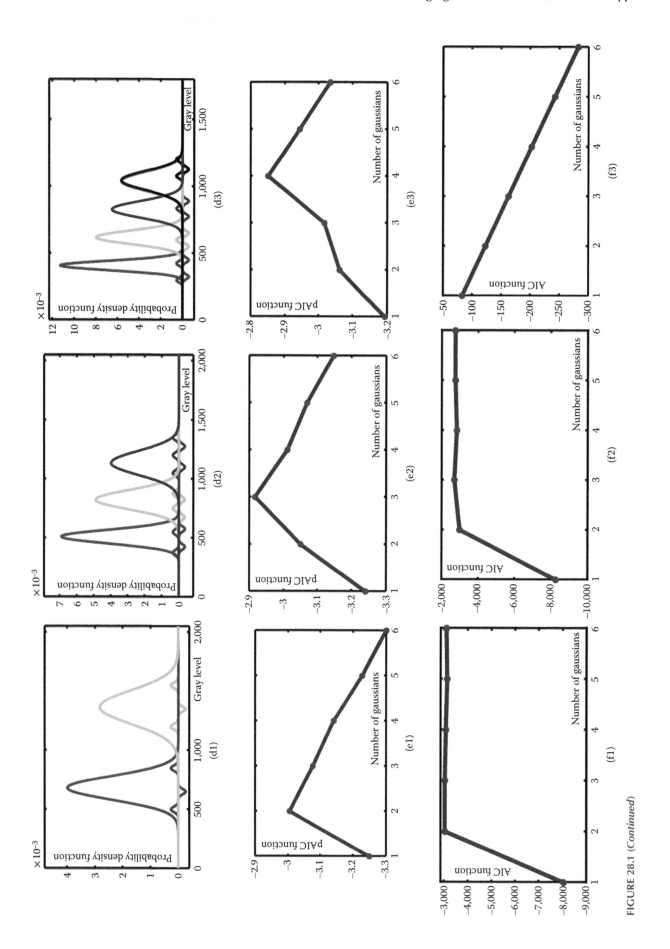

FIGURE 28.1 (*Continued*)

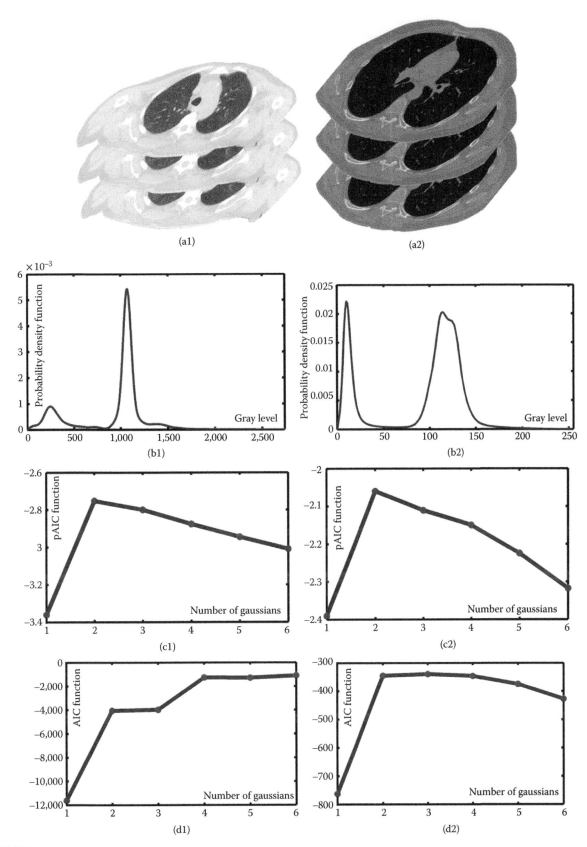

FIGURE 28.2
Modeling of the high-dose (left) and low-dose (right) 3D CT images with different scanning protocols: (a) 3D data, (b) empirical marginal intensity distributions, (c) the corresponding mAIC curves, obtained with $\varsigma = 0.05$, that reach their maximum at the proper number of the dominant DGs, and (d) the corresponding AIC curves.

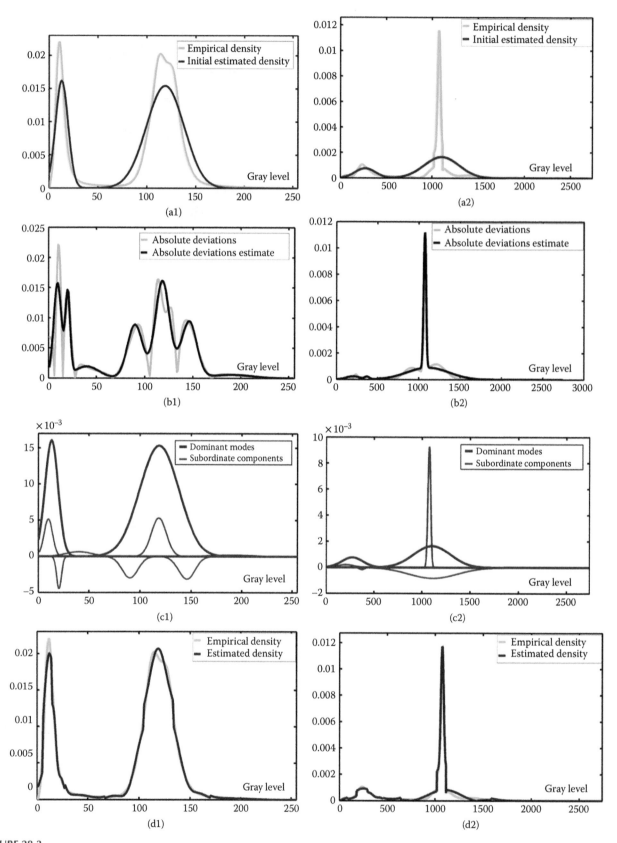

FIGURE 28.3
LCDG modeling of empirical marginal intensity distributions for the low-dose (left) and high-dose (right) 3D CT images with different scanning protocols: (a) the estimated mixture of the dominant DGs, (b) absolute deviations between the dominant mixture and the empirical distribution, (c) the sign-alternate subordinate DGs, and (d) the final estimated LCDG.

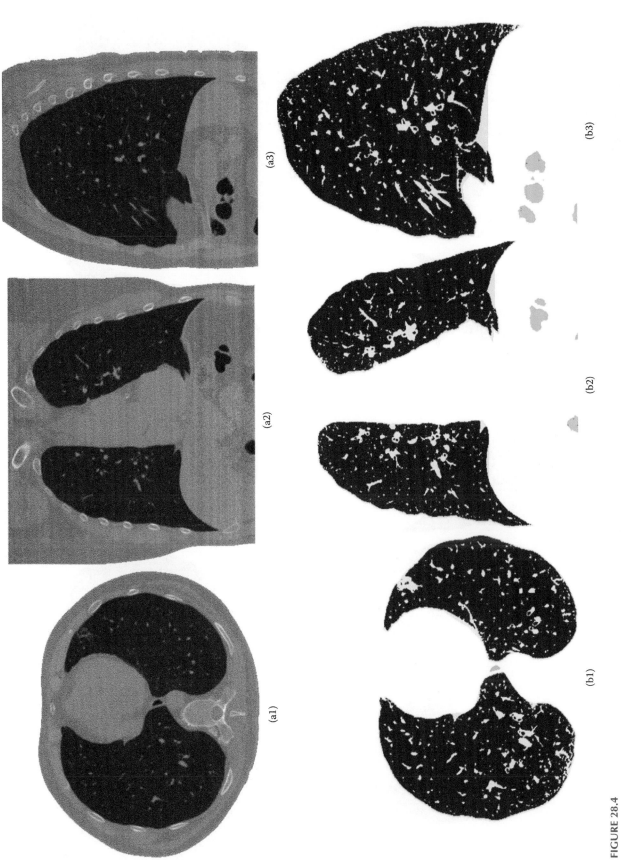

FIGURE 28.4

The 3D lung segmentation results projected onto the axial (A), coronal (C), and sagittal (S) planes: (a) original images; (b) IT, and (c) our initial segmentation, and (d) IT, and (e) our final segmentation after spatial analysis of the initial one. Errors with respect to the expert manual segmentation, are in green (false positive points) and yellow (false negative points).

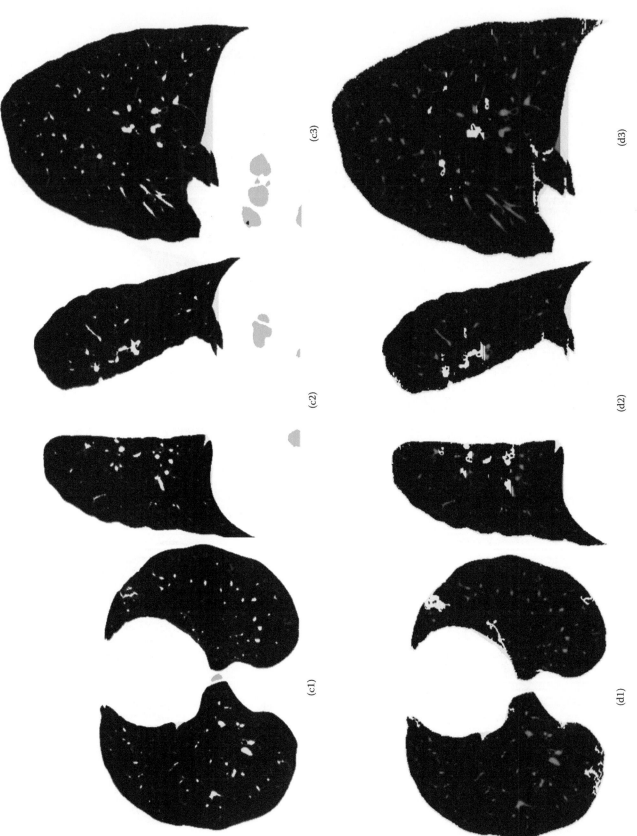

FIGURE 28.4 *(Continued)*

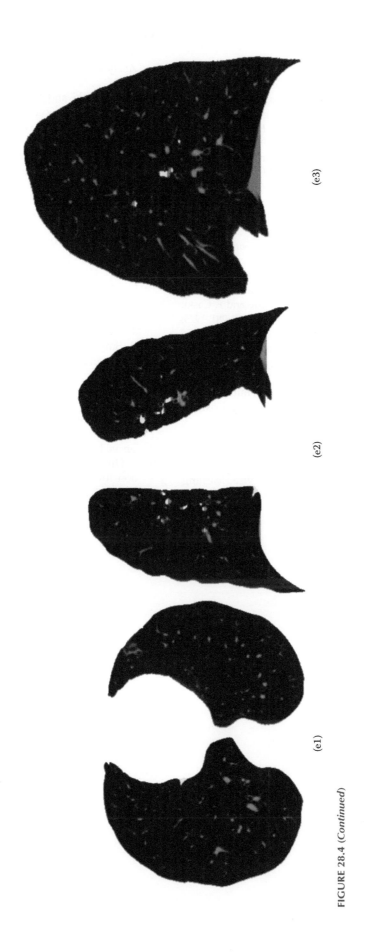

FIGURE 28.4 *(Continued)*

References

1. A. Webb, *Statistical Pattern Recognition, Second Edition.* Chichester, England:John Wiley & Sons, 2002.

2. D. Wilson and J. Noble, "An adaptive segmentation algorithm for time-of-flight MRA data," *IEEE Transactions on Medical Imaging,* vol. 18, no. 10, pp. 938–945, 1999.

3. A. A. Farag, A. El-Baz, and G. Gimel'farb, "Precise segmentation of multi-modal images," *IEEE Transactions on Image Processing,* vol. 15, no. 4, pp. 952–968, 2006.

4. A. El-Baz and G. Gimel'farb, "EM based approximation of empirical distributions with linear combinations of discrete Gaussians," In: *Proceedings of International Conference on Image Processing (ICIP'07),* San Antonio, Texas, pp. 373–376, September 16–19, 2007.

5. H. Akaike, "Information theory and an extension of the maximum likelihood principle," In: *Second International Symposium on Information Theory,* B. N. Petrov and F. Caski, eds., Akademiai Kiado, Budapest, Hungry, pp. 267–281, 1973.

6. F. H. Evans, "Detecting fish in underwater video using the EM algorithm," In: *Proceedings of International Conference on Image Processing (ICIP'03),* Barcelona, Catalonia, Spain, pp. 1029–1032, 2003.

7. M. Volk, M. Nagode, and M. Fajdiga, "Finite mixture estimation algorithm for arbitrary function approximation," *Journal of Mechanical Engineering,* vol. 58, no. 2, pp. 115–124, 2012.

8. G. Schwarz, "Estimating the dimension of a model," *Annals of Statistics,* vol. 6, pp. 461–464, 1978.

9. J. Oliver, R. Baxter, and C. Wallace, "Unsupervised learning using MML," In: *Proceedings of 13th International Conference on Machine Learning,* Bari, Italy, pp. 364–372, 1996.

10. M. A. Figueiredo and A. K. Jain, "Unsupervised learning of finite mixture models," *IEEE Transactions on Pattern Analysis and Machine Intelligence,* vol. 24, pp. 381–396, 2002.

11. C. Biernacki and G. Govaert, "Using the classification likelihood to choose the number of clusters," *Computing Science and Statistics,* vol. 29, no. 2, pp. 451–457, 1997.

12. Z. R. Yang and M. Zwolinski, "Mutual information theory for adaptive mixture models," *IEEE Transactions on Pattern Analysis and Machine Intelligence,* vol. 23, no. 4, pp. 396–403, 2001.

13. A. Likas, N. Vlassis, and J. Verbeek, "The global k-means clustering algorithm," *Pattern Recognition,* vol. 36, pp. 451–461, 2003.

14. J. Verbeek, N. Vlassis, and B. Kröse, "Efficient greedy learning of Gaussian mixture," *Neural Computation,* vol. 15, pp. 469–485, 2003.

15. G. McLachlan, "On bootstrapping the likelihood ratio test statistic for the number of components in a normal mixture," *Journal of Royal Statistical Society Series (C),* vol. 36, pp. 318–324, 1987.

16. P. Smyth, "Model selection for probabilistic clustering using cross-validated likelihood," *Statistics and Computing,* vol. 10, no. 1, pp. 63–72, 2000.

17. A. M. Ali and A. A. Farag, "Density estimation using a new AIC-type criterion and the EM algorithm for a linear combination of Gaussians," In: *Proceedings of International Conference on Image Processing (ICIP'07),* San Antonio, Texas, USA, pp. 3024–3027.

18. S. Hu and E. A. Hoffman, "Automatic lung segmentation for accurate quantization of volumetric X-ray CT images," *IEEE Transactions on Medical Imaging,* vol. 20, no. 6, pp. 490–498, 2001.

29

CAD Computed Tomography Lung Application

Lubomir Hadjiiski and Heang-Ping Chan

CONTENTS

29.1 Introduction

Multi-detector row computed tomography (CT) is an increasingly common modality for imaging of lung diseases. The recent National Lung Screening Trial (NLST) [1] found that low-dose CT offered better diagnostic capabilities and reduced mortality from lung cancer compared to chest x-rays (CXRs). However, a thoracic CT examination using thin-section reconstruction contains hundreds of images, which makes it a demanding task for the radiologists to carefully review them and detect subtle lesions. It is expected that effective computer-aided detection (CADe) and computer-aided diagnosis (CADx) systems can be useful tools to assist radiologists in the process of interpreting lung CT exams. Studies have shown that CADe systems have the promise to serve as a second reader for lung cancer detection. The characterization of lung lesions by radiologists is also a challenging task because of the equivocal features of many malignant and benign lesions. CADx systems for the classification of lesions are under development by a number of research groups. The results reported to date have shown the feasibility for CADx to be used as an aid

to the radiologists for characterization of malignant and benign lung lesions. An important part of CAD development is to evaluate the impact of CAD on the radiologists' performance. A number of observer studies were conducted to assess the effects of CAD. The main focus of this chapter is to review the current status and discuss issues on the evaluation of the effect of CAD (CADe and CADx) on the radiologists for detection and characterization of lung lesions in CT.

29.2 Challenges in Lung Cancer Detection on CT Examinations

In the United States, it is estimated that 226,160 new cases will be diagnosed and 160,340 deaths will result from lung cancer in 2012 [2]. Lung cancer remains the leading cause of cancer deaths for men since the 1950s and for women since 1987. The overall prognosis of lung cancer is very poor. The 5 year survival rate is only about 16% for all stages combined [2]. However, if detected and resected at its earliest stage (stage I), the 5 year survival rate can reach 70% [3–5].

The Early Lung Cancer Action Project (ELCAP) investigated the usefulness of annual low-dose CT screening for lung cancer in a high-risk population and found that low-dose CT can detect four times more malignant lung nodules than CXR and six times more stage I malignant nodules, which are potentially more curable [6]. The subsequent International ELCAP (I-ELCAP) study showed that the 10 year survival of patients who were detected with stage I lung cancer on CT screening and underwent surgical resection within 1 month reached 92%, and concluded that CT screening can detect lung cancer that is curable [7]. However, another multicenter study found that, in comparison with the predictions from a model, there were a 3-fold increase in cancer detection and 10-fold increase in lung resection but no decline in diagnoses of advanced lung cancer or mortality rate [8].

A 33-site randomized controlled study sponsored by the National Cancer Institute (NCI) NLST enrolled 53,454 participants to compare the effect of screening using low-dose helical CT or CXR on the mortality rate of lung cancer patients [1]. In the NLST, a 20% reduction in mortality, relative to CXR, from lung cancer was observed among current or former heavy smokers who were screened with CT. The rate of positive results was higher with low-dose CT screening than with CXR screening by a factor of more than 3.

There is consensus that CT allows the detection of more and smaller lung nodules than CXR. In a study of 446 emphysema patients in the National Emphysema Treatment Trial, 25.6% patients were found to have noncalcified nodules [9]. In ELCAP, 23.3% of the patients were found to have noncalcified nodules by CT, which represented a threefold increase in sensitivity than CXRs [6,9]. This increase in sensitivity comes at the price of an increased workload for radiologists. A major potential difficulty in using helical CT for screening is the dramatic increase in the number of images that need to be interpreted for each case. Another potential difficulty is the additional resources that will be needed for clinical management of the expected screening detected nodules. Different criteria are being used by physicians to manage lung nodules in current clinical practice [6,10]. Many nodules are recommended to be followed up. However, the rate of benign nodules being resected is still high at about 20%–40% [11]. A study of 426 patients who underwent video-assisted thoracoscopic surgery [12] indicated that 42.5% of these cases were benign. Keagy et al. [13] found that 40% of their patients with benign nodules were subjected to thoracotomy for presumed malignant disease. It is therefore important to establish more reliable criteria to estimate the likelihood of malignancy of the lung nodules based on image information without resorting to invasive procedures, thereby reducing the potential patient morbidity and additional health care costs associated with lung

cancer screening. ^{18}F-fluoro-2-deoxy-D-glucoseenhanced positron-emission tomography scans [14] have been found to provide high sensitivity and good specificity for differentiating nodules as malignant and benign although the procedure will involve radioactivity, relatively high costs, and may not be available in many medical facilities. The I-ELCAP study [7] showed that, with workup protocols that mainly used repeated CT scans to estimate nodule growth, the negative biopsy rate could be as low as 8% in their patient cohort. However, short-term follow-up with repeated CT will further increase radiologists' workload.

Although CT has a much higher sensitivity than CXR, missed cancers are not uncommon in CT interpretation [15–18]. The main causes for missed cancers include detection errors and characterization errors. Detection errors can be attributed to factors such as oversight or failure to detect the lesion among other structures, which can be caused by distraction, inexperience, satisfaction of search effect, and large workload. Characterization errors may be attributed to the difficulty in differentiating malignant lesions from benign nodules. On the one hand, it can cause the radiologist to underestimate the likelihood of malignancy and diagnose a detected malignant nodule as normal or benign. On the other hand, it can cause the radiologist to overestimate the likelihood of malignancy and recommend biopsy for benign lesions.

Double reading may reduce missed diagnosis but it doubles the demand on radiologists' time. Some criteria have been suggested to estimate the likelihood of malignancy of solitary pulmonary nodules [10,19–24]. Computer-assisted classification of malignant and benign lung nodules has been attempted and promising results were reported [25–29]. Gurney et al. [22,30] used Bayesian analysis and an artificial neural network (ANN) [30] to classify radiologist-provided image feature descriptors and clinical features. The classifiers achieved a higher accuracy than subjective classification by radiologists but manual extraction of feature descriptors is both time consuming and subject to inter- and intra-observer variations. In addition, subtle change in nodule volume, especially when the nodule is small, is difficult to detect visually on CT images.

CADe or CADx, in which a computer is trained to automatically detect and characterize the lesions of interest on the images, can be a viable approach to improving the accuracy of lung nodule detection and characterization on CT studies. A CADe system may provide a second opinion by alerting the radiologist to areas of concern, reducing the chance of oversight. CADx techniques have the potential to improve the specificity of cancer detection by estimating the likelihood of malignancy of a detected lesion and predicting which cases are most suitable for a particular management option. In addition, CADe or CADx may reduce inter- and intra-observer variability in image interpretation. A number of studies have shown the usefulness of applying CADe and CADx to the interpretation of thoracic CT scans. Some of these studies are summarized in this chapter.

29.3 Computerized Detection of Lung Nodules

Development of CADe methods for the detection of lung nodules has been an area of interest as the potential of CT for lung cancer screening is recognized. Although the specific computer vision techniques used in the different CADe systems differ, the overall scheme can generally be described in several major steps. First, the lung regions are isolated from other anatomical structures by segmentation of the CT images. Potential juxtapleural nodules attached to the pleura are usually excluded during lung region segmentation and need to be recovered with specific boundary refinement techniques. Nodule detection will be performed only within the lung regions and along their boundaries in the subsequent steps. Nodule enhancement preprocessing may be applied to the lung regions to enhance nodules and suppress other background structures. The lung regions are then pre-screened for nodule candidates. Feature descriptors that can characterize the detected objects are extracted from each nodule candidate. Rule-based and/or other classifiers are trained to classify nodules and false positives (FPs) based on the extracted features. Alternatively, neural network may be trained to differentiate nodules from other lung structures by pattern recognition without extracting individual features. The suspected nodules are then marked on the CT scan and displayed as output of the CAD system (Figures 29.1 and 29.2).

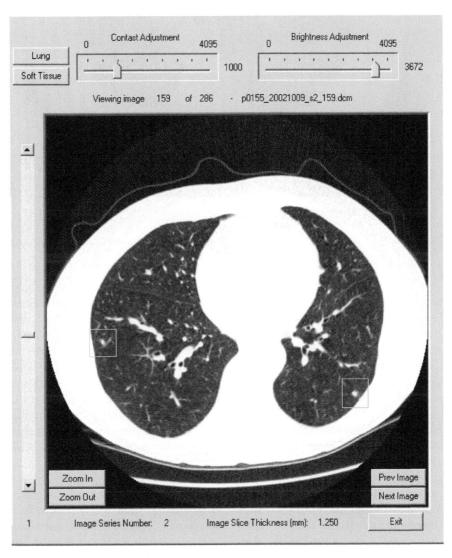

FIGURE 29.1
Computer-aided detection (CADe) system markings of true nodules on a computed tomography (CT) scan.

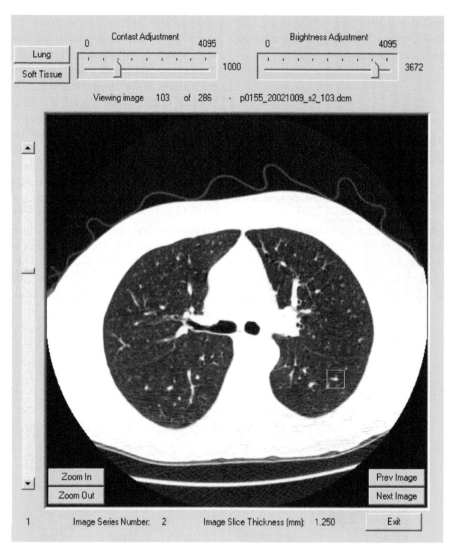

FIGURE 29.2
CADe system marking of a false positive (vessel crossing) on a CT scan.

The performances of various CADe systems for nodule detection on CT scans are summarized in Table 29.1, which includes representative studies from different groups, but it is by no means exhaustive. For additional information and greater details of the CAD technical development, the readers can refer to the number of informative review articles that were published in recent years [31–36].

The performance of a CADe system depends on a number of factors including, but not limited to, (1) the image acquisition and reconstruction parameters of the CT scans; (2) the size of the nodule; (3) the composition and location of the nodule; (4) the reference standard; (5) the data set size; and (6) whether the reported results are obtained from resubstitution (same data set used for training and testing), validation (optimizing system design using the validation results as a guide), or independent testing (test set not used until the system design

is completed and fixed). Radiologists' detection of lung nodules on CT scans is affected also by factors (1) to (5) and some of the information is discussed in Section 29.4; however, the readers should refer to the original literature and the review articles [31–36] for more details.

Because of the many factors that may affect the CADe performance and because the information about the data set and the training and evaluation methods may not have been described thoroughly in the articles, the performances of the different CADe systems generally cannot be directly compared.

One of the challenging processes in the development of CADe or CADx systems is the collection of a sufficiently large data set with ground truth or reference standard that encompasses case samples representative of the patient population. The NCI recognized the need of CAD for lung CT interpretation and supported the Lung Imaging Database Consortium (LIDC) to collect a

TABLE 29.1

Observer Performance Studies for Evaluation of the Effects of CADe on Radiologists' Detection of Lung Nodules in Thoracic CT Examinations

References	No. of CT Exams	Section Thickness/ Interval	Nodule Sizes	Total No. of Nodules	No. of Observers	Reading without CAD	Reading with CAD	p Value
Awai et al. 2004 [46]	50 (36 pos, 14 neg)	7.5 mm	3–29 mm, mean = 8.1 45: 3–10 mm 11: 11–29 mm	56	5 Rad, 5 Resid	AFROC A1: All 0.64 Rad: 0.63 Resid: 0.66	AFROC A1: All 0.67 Rad: 0.66 Resid: 0.68	<0.01 <0.01 0.02
Marten et al. 2004 [47] ICAD(Siemens)	18	0.75/0.6 mm	49: <4 mm 43: 4–9.9 mm 4: >9.9 mm	96 (89 solid, 2 mixed, 5 calcified)	4 Rad, 2 read with CAD	ROC Az: Rad1: 0.71 Rad3: 0.49	ROC Az Rad1: 0.93 Rad3: 0.79	<0.05 <0.05
Marten et al. 2005 [48] ICAD(Siemens)	20	0.75/0.6 mm 2.0/1.2 mm 4.0/2.7 mm	61: <4 mm 58: 4–9.9 mm 15: >9.9 mm	135[a]	2	Az, Sens, FPs/case CAD: 0.80, 74%, 0.79 Rad1: 0.70, 53%, 0.26 Rad2: 0.70, 53%, 0.21	Az, Sens, FPs/case Rad1: 0.93, 93%, 0.11 Rad2: 0.95,91%, 0.05	<0.05 <0.05
Li et al. 2005 [49]	27 (17 pos,10 neg) (LD)	10 mm	6–17 mm mean = 10 mm	18 (6 GGO, 10 mixed, 1 solid)	All 14 Rad: 6 (multiformat), 8 (cine)	Az, Sens 0.763, 52% 0.757, 49% 0.768, 54%	Az, Sens 0.854, 68% 0.862, 71% 0.848, 67%	0.002,0.001 0.04, 0.02 0.01, 0.006
Brown et al. 2005 [50]	8 (6 pos, 2 neg) (LD) (5 cm thorax)	1.25 mm	2.5–12.8 mm mean = 5.2 mm	22	39 chest Rad, 95 nonthoracic Rad, 68 non-Rad	13 readers: Sens, FPs/case 64%, 0.144 JAFROC FOM 0.78	13 readers: Sens, FPs/case 81.9%, 0.173 JAFROC FOM 0.84	<0.01, <0.01 >0.05
Rubin et al. 2005 [51] (Simulation)	20 (19 pos, 1 neg)	1.25/0.6 mm	≥3 mm mean = 5.1 mm	195	3	Sens, FPs/case CAD: 65%, 3 CAD: 76%, 10 Sens: 63% (2 Rads) 50% (indiv Rads)	(Simulation at 65% CAD thresh) Sens: 76%	<0.05
Das et al. 2006 [52]	25 (23 pos, 2 neg)	12 scans: 2/1.5 mm 13 scans: 1.0/0.5 mm	Mean 3.4 mm 89 <5 mm 27 ≥5 mm	116	3	Sens: Rad1: 68% Rad2: 78% Rad3: 82% Sens, FPs/case R2: 73%, 6 NEV: 75%, 8	Sens: R2, NEV Rad1: 79%, 79% Rad2: 90%, 90% Rad3: 84%, 86% (FP rate not reported)	0.005, 0.116 0.081, 0.032 0.123, 0.161
Yuan et al. 2006 [53] (Simulation)	150 (134 pos, 16 neg)	1.25 mm (CAD) 2.5 mm (Rad)	291: <4 mm 310: 4–10 mm 27: >10 mm	628	1	Sens: Rad: 83% R2: 73% @ 3.19 FPs/ case	Predicted sens increase 21.2%	—

Continued

TABLE 29.1 *(Continued)*

Observer Performance Studies for Evaluation of the Effects of CADe on Radiologists' Detection of Lung Nodules in Thoracic CT Examinations

References	No. of CT Exams	Section Thickness/ Interval	Nodule Sizes	Total No. of Nodules	No. of Observers	Reading without CAD	Reading with CAD	p Value
Sahiner et al. 2007 [54]	48 (30 pos, 18 neg)	1.5–3 mm	3–36.3 mm Median = 5.5 mm	70	4	Sens, FPs/case CAD: 79%, 4.9 Rad: 78%, 0.42 JAFROC FOM: 0.83	Sens, FPs/case Rad: 86%, 0.46 JAFROC FOM: 0.88	0.03
Jankowski et al. 2007 [55] LungCare (Siemens)	28 (28 pos)	1 mm	1–30 mm Mean = 3.05 mm	285	1 Rad, 2 Resid	Sens, FPs/case CAD: 38%, 6.8 Thoracic Rad1: 22%, 0.89 Resid1: 30%, 1.07 Resid2: 47%, 2.36	Sens, FPs/case Thoracic Rad1: 35%, 1.89 Resid1: 36%, 1.68 Resid2: 36%, 2.39	0.001 0.136 0.009
Beyer et al. 2007 [42] LungCAD (Siemens)	50 (25 pos, 25 neg)	1.25 mm	1.1–30.9 mm Mean = 3.7 mm	340	4	Sens, FPs/case CAD: 48%, 1.3 Rads: 68%, 1.2	Sens, Second reader: Rads: 75% Concurrent reader: Rads: 68% (FP rate not reported)	0.001 0.45
Hirose et al. 2008 [56] ZIOCAD LE (Ziosoft, Inc)	21 (15 pos, 6 neg)	1 mm	1.5–15 mm Median = 4.5 mm	49	6	Sens, FPs/case CAD: 71%, 0.95 Rads: 40%, 0.14 JAFROC FOM: Rads: 0.390	Sens, FPs/case Rads: 81%, 0.89 JAFROC FOM: Rads: 0.845	0.003 <0.0001
Das et al. 2008 [57] LungCAD (Siemens)	77 (70 pos, 7 neg)	1.5 mm	1.5–25 mm Mean = 5.8 mm 317 ≤4 mm 350 >4 mm	667	2	Sens, FPs/case Full dose: CAD: 72.5%, 4 Rad1: 85.2% Rad2: 61.4% Low dose: CAD: 64.3%, 4 Rad1: 84% Rad2: 63.5%	Sens, FPs/case Rad1: 94.7% Rad2: 89.4% Rad1: 92.6% Rad2: 87.4%	0.0001 0.0001 0.0001 0.0001
Goo et al. 2008 [58]	150 (23 pos)	1–3.2 mm	5.0–18 mm Mean = 12.6 mm	352	5 Rad, 5 Resid	Sens, FPs/case CAD: 80%, 2.96 JAFROC FOM: Rads: 0.71 Resid: 0.68	JAFROC FOM: Rads: 0.79 Resid: 0.77	0.001 <0.001
White et al. 2008 [59] Extended Brilliance Workspace (Philips)	109 (53 pos, 56 neg)	0.9–3 mm	4–30 mm	91	10	Sens CAD: 33%–81% ROC (Az) Rads: 0.867	ROC (Az) Rads: 0.887	<0.05 (for 4 Rads)

Continued

Park et al. 2009 [60]	49 (41 pos, 8 neg [benign])	1 mm	1.0–29 mm Mean = 4.4 mm	514	4	Sens, FPs/case CAD: 48%, 3.4 Rad1: 50.7%, 1.3 Rad2: 50.4%, 0.6 Rad3: 47.2%, 0.6 Rad4: 44.4%, 0.8	Sens, FPs/case Rad1: 62.4%, 1.4 Rad2: 62.4%, 0.7 Rad3: 62.8%, 0.8 Rad4: 60.4%, 1.5	<0.001 <0.001 <0.001 <0.001
Sahiner et al. 2009 [61]	85 (85 pos)	1.25–3 mm	3.0–18.6 mm Median = 4.4 mm	241	6	Sens, FPs/case CAD: 64%, 5.6 Rads: 67%, 0.67 JAFROC FOM: Rads: 0.729	Sens, FPs/case Rads: 75.8%, 0.78 JAFROC FOM: Rads: 0.763	0.003 0.02
Yanagawa et al. 2009 [62] Lung VCAR (GE Healthcare)	48 (48 pos)	0.625 mm	4–30 mm Mean = 6.8 mm	229 (102 GGO, 27 mixed, 100 solid)	3	Sens, FPs/case CAD: 40%, 5.7 Rad1: 59%, 1.4 Rad2: 58%, 0.5 Rad3: 79%, 1.4 JAFROC FOM: Rad1: 0.535 Rad2: 0.634 Rad3: 0.808	Sens, FPs/case Rad1: 76%, 1.9 Rad2: 69%, 0.6 Rad3: 87%, 1.8 JAFROC FOM: Rad1: 0.606 Rad2: 0.662 Rad3: 0.842	0.02 0.04 0.02
Roos et al. 2010 [63]	20 (20 pos)	1.25/0.6 mm	≥3 mm Mean = 5.2 mm	190	3	Sens, FPs/case CAD: 74%, 38.05 Rads: 53%, 1.15 Rad1: 59%, 0.6 Rad2: 57%, 2.1 Rad3: 44%, 0.75	Sens, FPs/case Rads: 69%, 1.45 Rad1: 67%, 0.85 Rad2: 82%, 2.7 Rad3: 60%, 0.8	>0.18 <0.004 <0.03
Kusano et al. 2010 [64]	60 (30 pos, 30 neg)	10.0 mm	5–30 mm	30	3 Thoracic Rads, 5 General Rads, 3 Resid	Sens, FPs/case CAD: 80%, 15 ROC (Az) Thoracic Rads: 0.872 General Rads: 0.864 Resid: 0.875	ROC (Az) Thoracic Rads: 0.910 General Rads: 0.924 Resid: 0.837	<0.05 <0.05 >0.05

LD = low-dose CT, pos = positive, neg = negative, Rad = radiologists, Resid = residents, R2 = CADe system by R2 Technologies, NEV = CADe system by Siemens Medical Solutions.

[a] Subgroup numbers add up to 134 while a total of 135 was given in the article.

large database of lung CT examinations for this purpose [37,38]. The availability of this common database may alleviate some of the problems in comparing different CADe systems although it still depends on how the researchers use the LIDC public data set, namely, whether they use the data set for both training and testing, design the methods and parameters based on the test results on the data set, or reserve the data set for true independent testing.

29.4 Observer Performance Studies for the Effects of CAD on Radiologists

The usefulness of a CADe system depends on its effect on the radiologist's detection performance and, specifically, whether it can improve the radiologist's detection of significant lung nodules in clinical practice. For example, a CADe system that has high standalone performance may not be useful as a second reader if it misses the same type of lesions that radiologists may miss. One way to assess the impact of CAD on radiologists is to conduct prospective and retrospective observer performance studies. Prospective studies are conducted in clinical settings with cases for which the clinical diagnosis is determined by radiologist using CAD compared to decisions made by radiologist without CAD. Prospective studies may be conducted with the cross-sectional design or the longitudinal design, of which the former is considered to be superior [39]. However, despite the fact that two commercial CADe systems for lung nodule detection in CT examinations have been approved by the Food and Drug Administration (FDA) since 2004, no large-scale prospective clinical trial for evaluation of the utility of CADe systems in routine clinical practice has been reported to date. One possible factor is that CADe has not been approved for reimbursement in lung CT so that it has not been widely used, and another factor may be the high cost of conducting prospective studies.

Retrospective observer studies are conducted with prior cases for which the clinical diagnosis has been previously determined and the study results generally do not affect patient care. Retrospective studies are easier to conduct and are usually used for the evaluation of the effect of CAD on radiologists' performance before a prospective clinical trial can be performed. Radiologists' detection of lung nodules on CT scans may be affected by a number of factors including the prevalence of abnormal cases in the study data set and the psychological effects of whether a decision will influence patient care, in addition to other physical factors such as the image acquisition and reconstruction parameters of the CT scans, the nodule size, and the composition

and location of the nodules. Therefore, the absolute performances of the radiologists without and with CADe in these retrospective studies may not be generalized to their performance in clinical settings. However, observer studies were designed to evaluate the relative changes in the radiologists' performance when reading with CAD. The impact of these factors on the relative performances will likely be smaller, although the extent of improvement will certainly depend on the characteristics of the lesions in the data set and whether the CADe system detects lesions that are complementary to those detected by the radiologist.

Observer studies can be designed in different ways. Two commonly used designs are the independent reading design and the sequential reading design [40,41]. In the independent reading design, the radiologist first evaluates the cohort of cases without CAD. At a later time, the radiologist evaluates the same cohort of cases with CAD. The evaluation results without and with CAD are recorded and analyzed. In the sequential reading design, the radiologist initially evaluates a case without CAD and then immediately evaluates the same case with CAD. The evaluation results without and with CAD are also recorded and analyzed. The sequential reading design has been shown to provide a greater statistical power for the observer study [41]. In a detection observer study, the typical radiologist evaluation results are the detected locations of the potential nodules and the likelihood rating for each potential nodule to be a true nodule. The CADe system outputs are displayed on a workstation as annotated marks at the location of the computer-detected nodule candidates. An example of the output of a noncommercial system is shown in Figures 29.1 and 29.2. In a characterization observer study, the typical radiologist evaluation results are the likelihood of malignancy ratings and the clinical action that the radiologist will consider for the lung nodule(s) of interest. The CADx system outputs may be displayed in different ways, such as a number representing the computer-estimated malignancy scores, an estimated likelihood of malignancy, or a relative rating. The commercial CADe systems that have been approved by FDA to be used as a second reader closely resemble the sequential reading design. Most of the reported observer studies are retrospective and the CADe system is used as a second reader (sequential reading design). Beyer et al. [42] compared CADe as a concurrent reader (display of CAD marks immediately in the reading session) with CADe as a second reader (display of CAD marks after the radiologist completed first reading without CAD). They found that a CADe system designed as a second reader was not effective in improving sensitivity if it was used as a concurrent reader. This study indicated that it is important to design CAD system and observer studies based on the specific intended use of the CAD system.

Radiologists' detection of lung nodules on CT scans is affected by many of the factors that influence computerized detection. Some of these factors are summarized in Section 29.4.1.

29.4.1 Data Collection

As can be seen from Table 29.1, the image acquisition and reconstruction parameters of the data sets used in the different studies vary over a wide range. Many studies, especially the early ones, used thick-slice reconstruction that would limit the sensitivity for detection of small nodules. More recent studies tended to use thin-section reconstruction obtained from multi-detector row CT scans with some having submillimeter slice intervals.

Several studies collected the cases from lung cancer screening using low-dose CT, whereas the others are higher dose diagnostic CT scans that may offer higher signal-to-noise ratios and thus better detectability of small nodules.

29.4.1.1 Nodule Characteristics

Nodule characteristics such as size and type have a strong influence on the detection accuracy.

29.4.1.2 Size

Most of the studies included lesions with diameters ranging from 3 to 30 mm, following the size range that radiologists consider to be clinically significant lung nodules. However, some studies only considered nodules greater than 4, 5, or even 10 mm, and others included nodules smaller than 3 mm.

29.4.1.3 Type

Many studies included only noncalcified solid nodules and some might include small fractions of groundglass, mixed, or calcified nodules. Ground-glass nodules are more difficult to detect than solid nodules for both radiologists and CADe systems because of their low CT values.

29.4.1.4 Location

Juxtapleural nodules are usually more difficult for the computer to detect than internal nodules, the proportion of the two types varied in the different data sets used in the studies.

29.4.2 Definition of Reference Standard

Because the presence of most lung nodules is not biopsy-proven, the reference standards for the majority of the cases have to be established by consensus from an expert panel of one or several radiologists. The "truth" relative to which the CADe performance is assessed thus depends on the number and the experiences of the radiologists who provide the reference standards, as well as the consensus process and the criteria to determine truth.

29.4.3 Statistical Analysis of Results

For analysis of the results of the observer studies, the receiver operating characteristic (ROC) analysis, Dorfman–Berbaum–Metz method for analysis of multireader multicase data [43], free-response ROC (FROC) analysis, and jackknife FROC (JAFROC) [44] analysis are frequently used. The sensitivity and specificity at a certain decision threshold (or operating point) may also be reported.

An important step in the design of the observer studies is the collection of a sufficiently large data set with ground truth or reference standard that encompasses case samples representative of the patient population. A larger data set will provide greater statistical power of the study. A representative data set will lead to a more general evaluation of the performance of the radiologists without and with CADe and thus the results of the study will be a closer estimate of their performance to that in the clinical settings. Alternatively, a smaller data set that includes a relatively large proportion of difficult cases, typically of those that can be missed by radiologists, may be used in an observer study to more efficiently show the usefulness of CAD systems in reducing false negative detection by radiologists. Some practical issues of ROC observer study design can be found in the seminal article by Metz [45].

29.5 Observer Studies

A number of retrospective observer performance studies have been conducted as summarized in Table 29.1.

Awai et al. [46] conducted an observer study in which 50 CT examinations were read by 5 board-certified radiologists and 5 residents. They found that the detection performance in terms of the area under the alternative FROC (AFROC) curve was significantly improved with CAD for either group of readers. Marten et al. [47] conducted an observer study to evaluate the performance of a CADe system (Siemens Corporate Research) using 18 thin-section CT cases. Two of the four participating radiologists read without and then with CADe. Both readers showed statistically significant improvement in the area under the ROC curve (A_z). However, it is not clear how the ROC analysis was performed with multiple nodules in a case and how much uncertainty would be introduced by an ROC analysis with a three-point confidence rating scale. The same group [48] also compared the detection performances of the CADe system and two radiologists without and with CADe for 20 cases reconstructed at three different slice thicknesses. They found that the slice thickness of the CT data had much stronger effect on the performance of their CADe system than on that of the radiologists. As a result, CADe improved the radiologists' performance significantly for the 0.75 and 2 mm slice thickness but had only marginal influence at 4 mm slice thickness. Li et al. [49] evaluated the effects of CADe on radiologists' detection of peripheral lung cancers missed in clinical practice. Using two different display formats (multiformat and cine), they found that CADe could improve radiologists' detection sensitivity and A_z regardless of display format.

Brown et al. [50] collected observer data from 202 participants at a Radiological Society of North America annual meeting. The readers read a data set of eight cases without and then with their CADe system and provided confidence ratings for nodule detection. They found that there were statistically significant increases in nodule detection and FP rates for all types of observers. For the 13 readers who finished all 8 cases, the sensitivity and the FP rates increased significantly; their average figure-of-merit (FOM) from JAFROC analysis also increased but did not achieve statistical significance.

Rubin et al. [51] reported a simulated observer study with 20 CT scans and 3 radiologists. The radiologists and the CADe system performed the detection independently. They simulated a radiologist's reading with CADe by assuming an ideal situation in which the radiologist would accept all true positive marks by the CADe but reject all FP marks. The average sensitivity of the radiologists would then increase significantly from 50% to 76% at a CADe system performance of 65% sensitivity and 3 FPs/case. In a follow-up study, Roos et al. [63] reported the results of 3 radiologists evaluating a dataset of 20 cases without and then with their CADe system. They found that there were statistically significant increases in nodule detection for two of the observers. The FP rates were slightly increased for all observers.

In a study by Das et al. [52], the nodule detection sensitivity of 3 radiologists on 25 CT scans without and with CADe was compared. Two commercial CADe systems, one with a sensitivity of 73% at 6 FPs/case and the other with a sensitivity of 75% at 8 FPs/case for this data set, were used. The results showed that the sensitivities of all three radiologists increased although the increase was significant for only one of the three radiologists using either CADe system. The effects of CADe on the readers' FP rates were not discussed. In a follow-up study,

Das et al. [57] compared 2 radiologists on 77 full-dose and simulated low-dose CT scans without and with CADe. A commercial system with a sensitivity of 73% for full dose and a sensitivity of 64% for low dose at 4 FPs/case was used. Both radiologists improved their sensitivity with CADe for the full-dose and the low-dose scans. The improvement was statistically significant. The effects of CADe on the readers' FP rates were not discussed.

Yuan et al. [53] compared the detection accuracy of a commercial CADe system with one radiologist in 150 CT examinations. The radiologist detected 83% of the nodules while the CADe system had a sensitivity of 73% at 3.19 FPs/case. The radiologist had higher sensitivity in detecting peripheral and juxtapleural nodules, but the CADe system was more sensitive to hilar and central nodules. They predicted an increase in the radiologist's sensitivity by 21.2% because of the complementary detection of nodules in different regions of the lungs but no prediction on the FP rate was made.

Jankowski et al. [55] compared the detection accuracy of 1 thoracic radiologist and 2 radiology residents and 28 CT examinations without CAD, with CAD, and with maximum intensity projection (MIP) technique. The radiologist's detection performance was significantly improved when reading with CAD. The performance of one of the residents was also improved with CAD. However, the performance of the other resident with CAD was significantly decreased. All observers improved their performance when using MIP. The radiologist's detection rate with CAD was higher than the detection rate with MIP, but the difference was not statistically significant. The residents' detection performance with MIP was higher than their detection performance with CAD.

Beyer et al. [42] designed an observer study to compare the use of CAD as a concurrent reader and that as a second reader. Four radiologists participated in the study. When CAD was used as a second reader, the detection performance of the radiologists with CAD was significantly improved. However, when CAD was used as a concurrent reader, there was no improvement in radiologists' detection accuracy.

Hirose et al. [56] conducted an observer study with 6 thoracic radiologists and 21 CT examinations (15 abnormal and 6 normal). The detection performance was analyzed with JAFROC methodology. Statistically significant improvement in radiologists' performance was observed with CAD.

Goo et al. [58] performed an observer study with 5 thoracic radiologists and 5 radiology residents using 150 CT examinations (23 confirmed lung cancers by biopsy). The detection performance was analyzed with JAFROC methodology. They observed statistically significant improvement in the detection performance of both thoracic radiologists and residents when they used CAD.

However, the detection performance of both thoracic radiologists and residents for lung cancer without and with CAD remained the same.

White et al. [59] conducted a multicenter observer study with 10 thoracic radiologists from 5 different sites. A data set of 109 CT examinations (53 abnormal) was used and the detection performance of the radiologists was analyzed with ROC methodology. All radiologists improved their performance with CAD. For four of the radiologists, the improvement was statistically significant.

Park et al. [60] compared the detection accuracy of 4 radiologists without CAD, with CAD, and with MIP technique in 49 CT examinations. CAD significantly improved the radiologists' detection performance. Their performance also improved with MIP. The radiologists' detection rate with CAD was higher than their detection rate with MIP although the difference was not statistically significant.

Sahiner et al. [61] conducted an observer study to compare the detection performance of 6 radiologists with and without CAD in 85 CT examinations. The detection performance was analyzed with JAFROC methodology. They found that the average FOM of the radiologists improved with CAD for nodules greater than 3, 4, 5, or 6 mm in diameter, although the increase was significant only for the size thresholds of 3 and 4 mm. The average sensitivity and FP rate at the size threshold of 3 mm for the radiologists also increased significantly by 18.9% and 16.8%, respectively.

Yanagawa et al. [62] conducted an observer study with 3 thoracic radiologists reading 48 CT examinations. The detection performance was also analyzed with JAFROC methodology. Statistically significant improvement in all radiologists' performance was observed with CAD.

Kusano et al. [64] conducted an observer study with 3 thoracic radiologists, 5 general radiologists, and 3 radiology residents using 60 CT examinations (30 abnormal and 30 normal). The detection performance was analyzed with ROC methodology. They observed statistically significant improvement in the performance of the thoracic and general radiologists when they used CAD. However, the performance of the residents with CAD was slightly decreased, but the change was not statistically significant.

The retrospective observer studies showed that even experienced radiologists will overlook some lung nodules in CT scans and CADe can significantly reduce the false negatives. However, the data sets used in these studies to date are relatively small. In two of the studies, the less-experienced observers (residents) had poorer performance with CADe. This can likely be attributed to improper use of CADe, such as using CADe as a first reader or dismissing their own detected nodule if the nodule was not marked by CADe. If the CADe was used as a second reader, it is not possible to have a reduced sensitivity with CADe.

How CAD will affect radiologists' interpretation in clinical practice is still unknown. The management, long-term survival, and mortality rates of patients when their lung cancer is detected at an earlier stage will also play a role in the consideration of implementing CADe for clinical use. The NLST study shows that the detection of small lung cancer at an early stage can significantly reduce the mortality of lung cancer patients. It can be expected that CAD may further enhance the efficacy of CT screening by reducing the false negative rate.

29.6 Computerized Characterization of Lung Nodules

A number of studies have been reported on the development of CADx systems for characterization of malignant and benign lung nodules on CT scans. A few observer studies have been performed to evaluate the effect of CADx on radiologists' characterization of lung nodules, as summarized in Table 29.2. We summarize briefly some of the studies.

Henschke et al. [65] differentiated malignant and benign nodules by a CADx system based on a neural network and feature patterns extracted from the images. The CADx system correctly classified all 14 malignant nodules and 11 of the benign nodules. Kawata et al. [66] showed good separation between 47 malignant and 15 benign nodules from 62 cases. The same group [67] also investigated the feasibility of developing an image-guided decision support system that would retrieve from a reference database nodule images having morphological and internal features consistent with the query nodule. McNitt-Gray et al. [68,69] designed a linear discriminant classifier with texture features in two studies using 31 and 32 nodules. They obtained high classification accuracy ranging from 90.3% to 100%, sensitivity ranging from 88.2% to 100%, and specificity ranging from 92.3% to 100%, depending on the number of texture features used. They cautioned that the results might be overly optimistic because of the small data sets available. Matsuki et al. [70] classified 99 malignant and 56 benign nodules with a neural network trained with 7 clinical parameters and 16 radiologic findings and achieved an A_z value of 0.951. Lo et al. [71] trained a neural network with features that described the shape, size, texture, and vascularity of the 24 malignant and 24 benign lung nodules and achieved an A_z of 0.89.

Armato et al. [72] evaluated a serial approach in which automated nodule detection was followed by automated nodule classification using a low-dose CT data set from

TABLE 29.2

Observer Performance Studies for Evaluation of the Effects of CADx for Characterization of Malignant and Benign Lung Nodules in Thoracic CT Examinations

References	No. of Exams	Section Thickness/ Interval (mm)	Nodule Sizes (mm)	Total No. of Nodules	Malignant	Benign	CAD A_z	No. of Observers	A_z without CAD	A_z with CAD	p Value
Matsuki et al. 2002 [70]	50	2	<30	50	25	25	0.951	12: 4 Rad 4 fellows 4 Resid	0.831 0.933 0.821 0.759	0.959 0.984 0.932 0.961	<0.001 <0.001 <0.001 <0.001
Li et al. 2004, 2006 [75,76]	56	1	6–20	56	28	28	0.831	16: 7 thoracic Rad 9 other Rad	0.785	0.853	0.016
Shah et al. 2005 [78]	28	Not reported	6–54 (mean = 24)	28	15	13	Sens 91%, Spec 67%	8: 2 thoracic 2 general 1 thoracic fellow 3 Resid	0.75	0.81	0.02
Awai et al. 2006 [81]	33	1–1.25	<30	33	18	15	0.795	19: 10 Rad 9 Resid	0.843 0.910 0.768	0.924 0.944 0.901	0.021 0.19 0.009
Way et al. 2010 [85]	152	1–7.5	3–36	256	124	132	0.86	6 thoracic Rad	0.83	0.85	<0.01

Sens = sensitivity, Spec = specificity, Rad = radiologists, Resid = residents

a lung cancer screening program in Japan that contained 401 benign and 69 malignant nodules. The nodule candidates at the output of the automated detection program included 335 of the nodules (59 malignant, 276 benign) among other FPs, which were then input to a classifier to differentiate malignant nodules from the benign nodules and FPs. The classifier achieved an A_z of 0.79. This serial approach of detection followed by classification represents one potential implementation of fully automated analysis of CT scans for lung cancer. Aoyama et al. [73] developed a lung nodule classification scheme using a data set containing 76 cancers and 413 benign nodules from the same source as the study of Armato et al. [72]. With a 10 mm slice thickness, the nodules were covered by only 1–3 slices. They obtained the best performance of A_z of 0.846, which was higher than the average A_z of 0.7 from 17 radiologists reading a subset of the nodules. Using the same data set, Suzuki et al. [74] classified the malignant and benign lung nodules with a multimassive training ANN and achieved an A_z of 0.882 and 100% sensitivity for identifying the malignant nodules. The same group [75,76] further developed their computerized classification by incorporating a linear discriminant classifier [73]. They used a data set of 61 malignant and 183 benign nodules that included ground-glass opacity (GGO), mixed, and solid nodules. The classification accuracy for the three types of nodules using a "leave-one-out" testing method was 0.919, 0.852, and 0.957. The overall accuracy for all nodules (61 malignant and 183 benign nodules) was A_z of 0.937.

Shah et al. [77] compared linear discriminant analysis, quadratic discriminant analysis, a logistic regression classifier, and a decision tree classifier on a data set of 48 malignant and 33 benign nodules on thin-section CT images. The four classifiers achieved an A_z of 0.92, 0.87, 0.88, and 0.68. Using a different data set with 33 malignant and 21 benign nodules, they trained another decision tree classifier with image features and obtained a sensitivity of 91% and a specificity of 67% [78]. The same group [79] designed a computerized classification system with features derived as the difference between the precontrast and the postcontrast features extracted from thin-section CT image data acquired before and after the injection of contrast media, respectively. They compared three classifiers and obtained A_z values ranging from 0.69 to 0.92. Mori et al. [80] analyzed thin-section CT scans obtained at three time points: before, 2 minutes after, and 4 minutes after contrast enhancement. They extracted three features describing the shape and attenuation of the 35 malignant and 27 benign nodules and designed a linear discriminant classifier. They achieved A_z values of 0.91, 0.99, and 1.0 at the three time points.

Awai et al. [81] trained an ANN to differentiate malignant and benign nodules using shape and density features from 34 nodules. The ANN achieved an A_z of 0.795 for a test data set of 18 malignant and 15 benign nodules. Way et al. [82] developed a lung nodule classification system using morphological and texture features extracted from nodules segmented by an automated three dimensional active contour model. The system achieved an A_z of 0.83 in a data set of 44 malignant and 52 benign nodules. In a later study [83], the performance of the CADx was increased to 0.86 with an improved feature space and an enlarged data set of 124 malignant and 132 benign nodules. Hadjiiski et al. [84] incorporated interval change information obtained from serial CT examinations into the feature space for classification of lung nodules. In a data set of 103 temporal pairs of 39 malignant and 64 benign nodules, a linear discriminant classifier achieved an A_z of 0.85, which is significantly higher than that of 0.78 using the features extracted from the current CT scan alone.

29.7 Effect of Computer-Aided Diagnosis on Radiologists' Characterization of Lung Nodules

Several studies have been conducted to evaluate the effects of CADx on radiologists' accuracy for characterization of malignant and benign lung nodules as summarized in Table 29.2.

Matsuki et al. [70] evaluated the usefulness of an ANN-based CADx system for assisting radiologists in characterizing malignant and benign nodules. Three groups of observers including four attending radiologists, four radiologist fellows, and four radiology residents participated in the study. The performance of each of the three groups obtained statistically significant improvement, and the average A_z of all 12 readers improved from 0.831 to 0.959. The improvement was statistically significant. Li et al. [75,76] conducted an observer study using 28 malignant and 28 benign nodules and 16 readers (7 thoracic and 9 other radiologists). A linear discriminant classifier was used in the CADx system that achieved a classification accuracy of $A_z = 0.831$ for these nodules. They found that the performance of every reader increased with CADx and the average A_z improved significantly from 0.785 to 0.853. The radiologists' recommendations were changed by use of CADx in 18% of the readings, of which 68% would have a beneficial effect. In addition, 69% of the changed recommendations regarding biopsy would have a beneficial effect.

Shah et al. [78] conducted a study to evaluate the classification accuracy for 15 malignant and 13 benign nodules by 8 radiologists using image data alone, with additional clinical data and then with CAD output. The CADx system was a decision tree classifier using image features. It had a sensitivity of 91% and a specificity of 67%. The A_z value of each of the eight readers (two thoracic radiologists, two general radiologists, one thoracic radiology fellow, and three radiology residents) increased with CADx. The average A_z for all readers increased significantly from 0.75 (image data and clinical data) to 0.81 with the use of CADx output. Awai et al. [81] evaluated the impact of an ANN-based CADx on radiologists' performance in an observer study for characterization of lung nodules using a data set of 18 malignant and 15 benign nodules. Nineteen readers participated in the observer study, including 10 body imaging radiologists and 9 residents. The average A_z of 19 readers and that of the group of 9 residents increased significantly, whereas the increase in the A_z for the group of 10 radiologists did not achieve significance. Way et al. [83] developed a CADx system for automated segmentation and classification of lung nodules. The CADx system was used in an observer study to compare radiologists' performance without and with CADx [85]. Six thoracic radiologists read a data set of 124 malignant and 132 benign nodules from 152 patients. The average A_z of the six radiologists was found to improve significantly with the use of CADx.

These studies showed the potential of CADx for assisting radiologists in making diagnostic decision for lung nodules in CT examinations. However, the data sets used in these studies were small. The characteristics of the nodules in these data sets would likely be different from case samples randomly drawn from patient population. Many considerations that may affect radiologists' diagnostic decisions in clinical practice will not exist in retrospective studies. How radiologists will respond to the CADx system output in clinical settings cannot be easily predicted from the results of retrospective studies. CADx will have to be evaluated in prospective clinical trials to assess the impact of the computerized classification on biopsy recommendations.

systems and the majority of the other CADe systems have focused on solid lung nodules, whereas nonsolid nodules are more likely to be missed by radiologists and CADe may be more helpful. Only three studies included a substantial fraction of nonsolid nodules [49,62,86], but the sample sizes in these studies were very small. For lung nodule diagnosis, one of the most important pieces of information that radiologists use for assessment of the likelihood of malignancy of a nodule is its growth rate measured in repeated CT examinations. Only one study [84] to date incorporated interval change information into the design of the CADx system. As discussed earlier, the most challenging step in the development of a CADe or CADx system is often the collection of a sufficiently large database for training and testing the computer algorithms and obtaining the reference standard. For lung nodules, the publicly available LIDC database is an invaluable resource that may accelerate new developments for computer-aided nodule detection and diagnosis. However, the database is still not very large and does not include serial CT examinations.

The observer studies performed to date for evaluation of the effect of CAD (CADe and CADx) on the radiologists for detection and characterization of lung lesions on the CT scans are retrospective, using limited data sets and small numbers of observers. Whether a CAD system can improve radiologists' performance in clinical practice will depend on many factors, such as radiologists' experience with and confidence in the CAD system and whether they use the system properly as a second opinion and maintain vigilance in their first reading, in addition to the accuracy of the CAD system. These factors cannot be simulated in retrospective observer performance studies. It is important to study the impact of CAD with properly designed prospective clinical trials. Understanding these issues may help radiologists take best advantage of CAD and improve patient care.

29.8 Summary

From this brief review of the effects of CADe systems for lung nodule detection and the effects of CADx systems for lung nodule characterization on radiologists' interpretation of CT scans, it is apparent that the investigations in these areas are still at an early stage. The technical development of the CADe and CADx systems needs further advancements. Although commercial CADe systems seem to be more mature, the reported studies so far used very limited data sets and their performances in the general patient population have yet to be evaluated. For lung nodule detection, the commercial

References

1. D.R. Aberle, A.M. Adams, C.D. Berg, W.C. Black, J.D. Clapp, R.M. Fagerstrom, I.F. Gareen et al., "Reduced lung-cancer mortality with low-dose computed tomographic screening," *New England Journal of Medicine*, 365, 395–409 (2011).
2. American Cancer Society, "Cancer Facts & Figures 2012," www.cancer.org, (2012).
3. B.J. Flehinger, M. Kimmel, and M.R. Melamed, "Survival from early lung cancer: implications for screening," *Chest*, 101, 1013–1018 (1992).
4. J.C. Nesbitt, J.B. Putnam, G.L. Walsh, J.A. Roth, and C.F. Mountain, "Survival in early-stage lung cancer," *Annals of Thoracic Surgery*, 60, 466–472 (1995).

5. R. Shah, S. Sabanathan, J. Richardson, A.J. Means, and C. Goulden, "Results of surgical treatment of stage I and II lung cancer," *Journal of Cardiovascular Surgery*, 37, 169–172 (1996).

6. C.I. Henschke, D.I. McCauley, D.F. Yankelevitz, D.P. Naidich, G. McGuinness, O.S. Miettinen, D.M. Libby et al., "Early lung cancer action project: overall design and findings from baseline screening," The Lancet, 354, 99–105 (1999).

7. The International Early Lung Cancer Action Program Investigators, "Survival of patients with stage I lung cancer detected on CT screening," *New England Journal of Medicine*, 355, 1763–1771 (2006).

8. P.B. Bach, J.R. Jett, U. Pastorino, M.S. Tockman, S.J. Swensen, and C.B. Begg, "Computed tomography screening and lung cancer outcomes," *JAMA-Journal of the American Medical Association*, 297, 953–961 (2007).

9. S. Adusumilli, E.A. Kazerooni, and T.C. Ojo, "Screening CT for lung cancer: a study of emphysema patients being evaluated for lung volume reduction surgery," *Radiology*, 209(P), 222–223 (1998).

10. S.J. Swensen, J.R. Jett, W.S. Payne, R.W. Viggiano, P.C. Pairolero, and V.F. Trastek, "An integrated approach to evaluation of the solitary pulmonary nodule," *Mayo Clinic Proceedings*, 65, 173–186 (1990).

11. D.E. Midthun, S.J. Swensen, and J.R. Jett, "Clinical strategies for solitary pulmonary nodule," *Annual Review of Medicine*, 43, 195–208 (1992).

12. M.S. Ginsberg, S.K. Griff, B.D. Go, H.H. Yoo, L.H. Schwartz, and D.M. Panicek, "Pulmonary nodules resected at video-assisted thoracoscopic surgery: etiology in 426 patients," *Radiology*, 213, 277–282 (1999).

13. B.A. Keagy, P.J.K. Starek, G.F. Murray, J.W. Battaglini, M.E. Lores, and B.R. Wilcox, "Major pulmonary resection for suspected but unconfirmed malignancy," *Annals of Thoracic Surgery*, 38, 314–316 (1984).

14. N.A. Dewan, C.J. Shehan, S.D. Reeb, L.S. Gobar, W.J. Scott, and K. Ryschon, "Likelihood of malignancy in a solitary pulmonary nodule: comparison of Bayesian analysis and results of FDG-PET scan," *Chest*, 112, 416–422 (1997).

15. J.W. Gurney, "Missed lung cancer at CT: imaging findings in nine patients," *Radiology*, 199, 117–122 (1996).

16. S.D. Davis, "Through the "retrospectoscope": a glimpse of missed lung cancer at CT," *Radiology*, 199, 23–24 (1996).

17. R. Kakinuma, H. Ohmatsu, M. Kaneko, K. Eguchi, T. Naruke, K. Nagai, Y. Nishiwaki, A. Suzuki, and N. Moriyama, "Detection failures in spiral CT screening for lung cancer: analysis of CT findings," *Radiology*, 212, 61–66 (1999).

18. C.S. White, A.I. Salis, and C.A. Meyer, "Missed lung cancer on chest radiography and computed tomography: imaging and medicolegal issues," *Journal of Thoracic Imaging*, 14, 63–68 (1999).

19. A.V. Proto and S.R. Thomas, "Pulmonary nodules studied by computed tomography," *Radiology*, 156, 149–153 (1985).

20. S.S. Siegelman, N.F. Khouri, F.P. Leo, E.K. Fishman, R.M. Braverman, and E.A. Zerhouni, "Solitary pulmonary nodules: CT assessment," *Radiology*, 160, 307–312 (1986).

21. S.J. Swensen and M.D. Silverstein, "The probability of malignancy in the solitary pulmonary nodule," *Archives of Internal Medicine*, 157, 849–855 (1997).

22. J.W. Gurney, "Determining the likelihood of malignancy in solitary pulmonary nodules with Bayesian analysis—Part I. Theory," *Radiology*, 186, 405–413 (1993).

23. J.J. Erasmus, J.E. Connolly, H.P. McAdams, and V.L. Roggli, "Solitary pulmonary nodules: part I. Morphological evaluation for differentiation of benign and malignant lesions," *Radiographics*, 20, 43–58 (2000).

24. J.J. Erasmus, J.E. Connolly, H.P. McAdams, and V.L. Roggli, "Solitary pulmonary nodules: part II. Evaluation of the indeterminate nodule," *Radiographics*, 20, 59–66 (2000).

25. A.W. Templeton, C. Jansen, J.L. Lehr, and R. Hufft, "Solitary pulmonary lesions: computer aided differential diagnosis and evaluation of mathematical methods," *Radiology*, 89, 605–613 (1967).

26. J. Wojtowicz, L. Pietraszkiewicz, and B. Grala, "A trial of differential diagnosis of solitary pulmonary foci on the basis of Bayes's equation with the use of electronic digital computers," *Polish Review of Radiology and Nuclear Medicine*, 34, 694–691 (1970).

27. K.H. Rotte and W. Meiske, "Results of computer-aided diagnosis of peripheral bronchial carcinoma," *Radiology*, 125, 583–586 (1977).

28. F. Edwards, P.S. Schaefer, S. Callahan, G.M. Geoffrey, and R.A. Albus, "Bayesian statistical theory in the preoperative diagnosis of pulmonary lesions," *Chest*, 92, 888–891 (1987).

29. F.H. Edwards, P.S. Schaefer, A.J. Cohen, R.F. Bellamy, L. Thompson, G.M. Graeber, and M.J. Barry, "Use of artificial intelligence for the preoperative diagnosis of pulmonary lesions," *Annals of Thoracic Surgery*, 48, 556–559 (1989).

30. J.W. Gurney, D.M. Lyddon, and J.A. McKay, "Determining the likelihood of malignancy in solitary pulmonary nodules with Bayesian analysis—Part II. Application," *Radiology*, 186, 415–422 (1993).

31. H.P. Chan, L.M. Hadjiiski, C. Zhou, and B. Sahiner, "Computer-aided diagnosis of lung cancer and pulmonary embolism in computed tomography—a review," *Academic Radiology*, 15, 535–555 (2008).

32. L. Saba, G. Caddeo, and G. Mallarini, "Computer-aided detection of pulmonary nodules in computed tomography: analysis and review of the literature," *Journal of Computer Assisted Tomography*, 31, 611–619 (2007).

33. Q. Li, "Recent progress in computer-aided diagnosis of lung nodules on thin-section CT," *Computerized Medical Imaging and Graphics*, 31, 248–257 (2007).

34. B. van Ginneken, C.M. Schaefer-Prokop, and M. Prokop, "Computer-aided diagnosis: how to move from the laboratory to the clinic," *Radiology*, 261, 719–732 (2011).

35. I. Sluimer, A. Schilham, M. Prokop, and B. van Ginneken, "Computer analysis of computed tomography scans of the lung: a survey," *IEEE Transactions on Medical Imaging*, 25, 385–405 (2006).

36. J.G. Goldin, M.S. Brown, and I. Petkovska, "Computer-coded diagnosis in lung nodule assessment," *Journal of Thoracic Imaging*, 23, 97–104 (2008).

37. S.G. Armato, G. McLennan, M.F. McNitt-Gray, C.R. Meyer, D. Yankelevitz, D.R. Aberle, C.I. Henschke, et al., "Lung image database consortium: developing a resource for the medical imaging research community," *Radiology*, 232, 739–748 (2004).

38. S.G. Armato, III, R.Y. Roberts, M.F. McNitt-Gray, C.R. Meyer, A.P. Reeves, G. McLennan, R.M. Engelmann et al., "The lung image database consortium (LIDC): ensuring the integrity of expert-defined "truth"," *Academic Radiology*, 14, 1455–1463 (2007).

39. R.M. Nishikawa and L.L. Pesce, "Computer-aided detection evaluation methods are not created equal," *Radiology*, 251, 634–636 (2009).

40. L.M. Hadjiiski, H.P. Chan, B. Sahiner, M.A. Helvie, M. Roubidoux, C. Blane, C. Paramagul et al., "Improvement of radiologists' characterization of malignant and benign breast masses in serial mammograms by computer-aided diagnosis: an ROC study," *Radiology*, 233, 255–265 (2004).

41. S.V. Beiden, R.F. Wagner, K. Doi, R.M. Nishikawa, M. Freedman, S.-C. Lo, and X.-W. Xu, "Independent versus sequential reading in ROC studies of computer-assist modalities: analysis of component of variance," *Academic Radiology*, 9, 1036–1043 (2002).

42. F. Beyer, L. Zierott, E.M. Fallenberg, K.U. Juergens, J. Stoeckel, W. Heindel, and D. Wormanns, "Comparison of sensitivity and reading time for the use of computer-aided detection (CAD) of pulmonary nodules at MDCT as concurrent or second reader," *European Radiology*, 17, 2941–2947 (2007).

43. D.D. Dorfman, K.S. Berbaum, and C.E. Metz, "ROC rating analysis: generalization to the population of readers and cases with the jackknife method," *Investigative Radiology*, 27, 723–731 (1992).

44. D.P. Chakraborty, "Analysis of location specific observer performance data: validated extensions of the jackknife free-response (JAFROC) method," *Academic Radiology*, 13, 1187–1193 (2006).

45. C.E. Metz, "Some practical issues of experimental design and data analysis in radiological ROC studies," *Investigative Radiology*, 24, 234–245 (1989).

46. K. Awai, K. Murao, A. Ozawa, M. Komi, H. Hayakawa, S. Hori, and Y. Nishimura, "Pulmonary nodules at chest CT: effect of computer-aided diagnosis on radiologists' detection performance," *Radiology*, 230, 347–352 (2004).

47. K. Marten, T. Seyfarth, F. Auer, E. Wiener, A. Grillhösl, S. Obenauer, E.J. Rummeny, and C. Engelke, "Computer-assisted detection of pulmonary nodules: performance evaluation of an expert knowledge-based detection system in consensus reading with experienced and inexperienced chest radiologists," *European Radiology*, 14, 1930–1938 (2004).

48. K. Marten, A. Grillhösl, T. Seyfarth, S. Obenauer, E.J. Rummeny, and C. Engelke, "Computer-assisted detection of pulmonary nodules: evaluation of diagnostic performance using an expert knowledge-based detection system with variable reconstruction slice thickness settings," *European Radiology*, 15, 203–212 (2005).

49. F. Li, H. Arimura, K. Suzuki, J. Shiraishi, Q. Li, H. Abe, R. Engelmann, S. Sone, H. MacMahon, and K. Doi, "Computer-aided detection of peripheral lung cancers missed at CT: ROC analyses without and with localization," *Radiology*, 237, 684–690 (2005).

50. M.S. Brown, J.G. Goldin, S. Rogers, H.J. Kim, R.D. Suh, M.F. McNitt-Gray, S.K. Shah, D. Truong, K. Brown, and J.W. Sayre, "Computer-aided lung nodule detection in CT results of large-scale observer test," *Academic Radiology*, 12, 681–686 (2005).

51. G.D. Rubin, J.K. Lyo, D.S. Paik, A.J. Sherbondy, L.C. Chow, A.N. Leung, R. Mindelzun et al., "Pulmonary nodules on multi-detector row CT scans: performance comparison of radiologists and computer-aided detection," *Radiology*, 234, 274–283 (2005).

52. M. Das, G. Muhlenbruch, A.H. Mahnken, T.G. Flohr, L. Gundel, S. Stanzel, T. Kraus, R.W. Gunther, and J.E. Wildberger, "Small pulmonary nodules: effect of two computer-aided detection systems on radiologist performance," *Radiology*, 241, 564–571 (2006).

53. R. Yuan, P.M. Vos, and P.L. Cooperberg, "Computer-aided detection in screening CT for pulmonary nodules," *American Journal of Roentgenology*, 186, 1280–1287 (2006).

54. B. Sahiner, L.M. Hadjiiski, H.P. Chan, J. Shi, P.N. Cascade, E.A. Kazerooni, C. Zhou et al., "Effect of CAD on radiologists' detection of lung nodules on thoracic CT scans: observer performance study," *Proceedings of SPIE*, 6515, 65151D–1,7 (2007).

55. A. Jankowski, T. Martinelli, J.F. Timsit, C. Brambilla, F. Thony, M. Coulomb, and G. Ferretti, "Pulmonary nodule detection on MDCT images: evaluation of diagnostic performance using thin axial images, maximum intensity projections, and computer-assisted detection," *European Radiology*, 17, 3148–3156 (2007).

56. T. Hirose, N. Nitta, J. Shiraishi, Y. Nagatani, M. Takahashi, and K. Murata, "Evaluation of computer-aided diagnosis (CAD) software for the detection of lung nodules on multidetector row computed tomography (MDCT): JAFROC study for the improvement in radiologists' diagnostic accuracy," *Academic Radiology*, 15, 1505–1512 (2008).

57. M. Das, G. Muehlenbruch, S. Heinen, A.H. Mahnken, M. Salganicoff, S. Stanzel, R.W. Guenther, and J.E. Wildberger, "Performance evaluation of a computer-aided detection algorithm for solid pulmonary nodules in low-dose and standard-dose MDCT chest examinations and its influence on radiologists," *British Journal of Radiology*, 81, 841–847 (2008).

58. J.M. Goo, H.Y. Kim, J.W. Lee, H.J. Lee, C.H. Lee, K.W. Lee, T.J. Kim, K.Y. Lim, S.H. Park, and K.T. Bae, "Is the computer-aided detection scheme for lung nodule also useful in detecting lung cancer?," *Journal of Computer Assisted Tomography*, 32, 570–575 (2008).

59. C.S. White, R. Pugatch, T. Koonce, S.W. Rust, and E. Dharaiya, "Lung nodule CAD software as a second reader: a multicenter study," *Academic Radiology*, 15, 326–333 (2008).

60. E.A. Park, J.M. Goo, J.W. Lee, C.H. Kang, H.J. Lee, C.H. Lee, C.M. Park, H.Y. Lee, and J.G. Im, "Efficacy of computer-aided detection system and thin-slab maximum intensity projection technique in the detection of pulmonary nodules in patients with resected metastases," *Investigative Radiology*, 44, 105–113 (2009).

61. B. Sahiner, H.-P. Chan, L.M. Hadjiiski, P.N. Cascade, E.A. Kazerooni, A.R. Chughtai, C. Poopat et al., "Effect of CAD on radiologists' detection of lung nodules on thoracic CT scans: analysis of an observer performance study by nodule size," *Academic Radiology*, 16, 1518–1530 (2009).

62. M. Yanagawa, O. Honda, S. Yoshida, Y. Ono, A. Inoue, T. Daimon, H. Sumikawa et al., "Commercially available computer-aided detection system for pulmonary nodules on thin-section images using 64 detectors-row CT: preliminary study of 48 cases," *Academic Radiology*, 16, 924–933 (2009).

63. J.E. Roos, D. Paik, D. Olsen, E.G. Liu, L.C. Chow, A.N. Leung, R. Mindelzun et al., "Computer-aided detection (CAD) of lung nodules in CT scans: radiologist performance and reading time with incremental CAD assistance," *European Radiology*, 20, 549–557 (2010).

64. S. Kusano, T. Nakagawa, T. Aoki, T. Nawa, K. Nakashima, Y. Goto, and Y. Korogi, "Efficacy of computer-aided diagnosis in lung cancer screening with low-dose spiral computed tomography: receiver operating characteristic analysis of radiologists' performance," *Japanese Journal of Radiology*, 28, 649–655 (2010).

65. C.I. Henschke, D.F. Yankelevitz, I. Mateescu, D.W. Brettle, T.G. Rainey, and F.S. Weingard, "Neural networks for the analysis of small pulmonary nodules," *Clinical Imaging*, 21, 390–399 (1997).

66. Y. Kawata, N. Niki, H. Ohmatsu, R. Kakinuma, K. Eguchi, M. Kaneko, and N. Moriyama, "Quantitative surface characterization of pulmonary nodules based on thin-section CT images," *IEEE Transactions on Nuclear Science*, 45, 2132–2138 (1998).

67. Y. Kawata, N. Niki, H. Ohmatsu, M. Kusumoto, R. Kakinuma, K. Yamada, K. Mori et al., "Pulmonary nodule classification based on nodule retrieval from 3-D thoracic CT image database," In Medical Image Computing and Computer-Assisted Intervention, C. Barillot, D.R. Haynor, and P. Hellier (Eds.): MICCAI 2004, LNCS 3217, 838–846, 2004. © Springer-Verlag Berlin Heidelberg 2004.

68. M.F. McNitt-Gray, E.M. Hart, N. Wyckoff, J.W. Sayre, J.G. Goldin, and D.R. Aberle, "A pattern classification approach to characterizing solitary pulmonary nodules imaged on high resolution CT: preliminary results," *Medical Physics*, 26, 880–888 (1999).

69. M.F. McNitt-Gray, N. Wyckoff, J.W. Sayre, J.G. Goldin, and D.R. Aberle, "The effects of co-occurrence matrix based texture parameters on the classification of solitary pulmonary nodules images on computed tomography," *Computerized Medical Imaging and Graphics*, 23, 339–348 (1999).

70. Y. Matsuki, K. Nakamura, H. Watanabe, T. Aoki, H. Nakata, S. Katsuragawa, and K. Doi, "Usefulness of an artificial neural network for differentiating benign from malignant pulmonary nodules on high-resolution CT: evaluation with receiver operating characteristic analysis," *American Journal of Roentgenology*, 178, 657–663 (2002).

71. S.C.B. Lo, L.Y. Hsu, M.T. Freedman, F. Lure, and H. Zhao, "Classification of lung nodules in diagnostic CT: an approach based on 3-D vascular features, nodule density distributions, and shape features," *Proceedings of SPIE*, 5032, 183–189 (2003).

72. S.G. Armato, M.B. Altman, J. Wilkie, S. Sone, F. Li, K. Doi, and A.S. Roy, "Automated lung nodule classification following automated nodule detection on CT: a serial approach," *Medical Physics*, 30, 1188–1197 (2003).

73. M. Aoyama, Q. Li, S. Katsuragawa, F. Li, S. Sone, and K. Doi, "Computerized scheme for determination of the likelihood measure of malignancy for pulmonary nodules on low-dose CT images," *Medical Physics*, 30, 387–394 (2003).

74. K. Suzuki, F. Li, S. Sone, and K. Doi, "Computer-aided diagnostic scheme for distinction between benign and malignant nodules in thoracic low-dose CT by use of massive training artificial neural network," *IEEE Transactions on Medical Imaging*, 24, 1138–1150 (2005).

75. F. Li, M. Aoyama, J. Shiraishi, H. Abe, Q. Li, K. Suzuki, R. Engelmann, S. Sone, H. MacMahon, and A.K. Doi, "Radiologists' performance for differentiating benign from malignant lung nodules on high-resolution CT using computer-estimated likelihood of malignancy," *American Journal of Roentgenology*, 183, 1209–15 (2004).

76. F. Li, Q. Li, R. Engelmann, M. Aoyama, S. Sone, H. MacMahon, and K. Doi, "Improving radiologists' recommendations with computer-aided diagnosis for management of small nodules detected by CT," *Academic Radiology*, 13, 943–950 (2006).

77. S.K. Shah, M.F. McNitt-Gray, S.R. Rogers, J.G. Goldin, R.D. Suh, J.W. Sayre, I. Petkovska, H.J. Kim, and D.R. Aberle, "Computer-aided diagnosis of the solitary pulmonary nodule," *Academic Radiology*, 12, 570–575 (2005).

78. S.K. Shah, M.F. McNitt-Gray, K.R. De Zoysa, J.W. Sayre, H.J. Kim, P. Batra, A. Behrashi, K. Brown, L.E. Greaser, and J.M. Park, "Solitary pulmonary nodule diagnosis on CT results of an observer study," *Academic Radiology*, 12, 496–501 (2005).

79. S.K. Shah, M.F. McNitt-Gray, S.R. Rogers, J.G. Goldin, R.D. Suh, J.W. Sayre, I. Petkovska, H.J. Kim, and D.R. Aberle, "Computer aided characterization of the solitary pulmonary nodule using volumetric and contrast enhancement features," *Academic Radiology*, 12, 1310–1319 (2005).

80. K. Mori, N. Niki, T. Kondo, Y. Kamiyama, T. Kodama, Y. Kawada, and N. Moriyama, "Development of a novel computer-aided diagnosis system for automatic discrimination of malignant from benign solitary pulmonary nodules on thin-section dynamic computed tomography," *Journal of Computer Assisted Tomography*, 29, 215–222 (2005).

81. K. Awai, K. Murao, A. Ozawa, Y. Nakayama, T. Nakaura, D. Liu, K. Kawanaka, Y. Funama, S. Morishita, and Y. Yamashita, "Pulmonary nodules: estimation of malignancy at thin-section helical CT—effect of computer-aided diagnosis on performance of radiologists," *Radiology*, 239, 276–284 (2006).

82. T.W. Way, L.M. Hadjiiski, B. Sahiner, H.P. Chan, P.N. Cascade, E.A. Kazerooni, N. Bogot, and C. Zhou, "Computer-aided diagnosis of pulmonary nodules

on CT scans: segmentation and classification using 3D active contours," *Medical Physics*, 33, 2323–2337 (2006).

83. T.W. Way, H.-P. Chan, J. Stojanovska-Nojkova, L. Frank, T.K. Song, E.A. Kazerooni, P.N. Cascade et al., "Effect of computer-aided diagnosis (CAD) on radiologists' characterization of lung nodules on CT: an ROC study," *RSNA Program Book*, 2007, 267 (2007).

84. L.M. Hadjiiski, T.W. Way, B. Sahiner, H.P. Chan, P.N. Cascade, N. Bogot, E.A. Kazerooni, and C. Zhou, "Computer-aided diagnosis for interval change analysis of lung nodule features in serial CT examinations," *Proceedings of SPIE*, 6514, 111–117 (2007).

85. T. Way, H.P. Chan, L. Hadjiiski, B. Sahiner, A. Chughtai, T.K. Song, C. Poopat et al., "Computer-aided diagnosis of lung nodules on CT scans: ROC study of its effect on radiologists' performance," *Academic Radiology*, 17, 323–332 (2010).

86. K.G. Kim, J.M. Goo, J.H. Kim, H.J. Lee, B.G. Min, K.T. Bae, and J.-G. Im, "Computer-aided diagnosis of localized ground-glass opacity in the lung at CT: initial experience," *Radiology*, 237, 657–661 (2005).

30

PET/CT Nodule Segmentation and Diagnosis: A Survey

Behnoush Abdollahi, Ali Cahid Civelek, Xiao-Feng Li, Jasjit S. Suri, and Ayman El-Baz

CONTENTS

30.1 Introduction

Bronchogenic carcinoma normally known as lung cancer is the most frequently diagnosed "major" cancer in the world, and the leading cause of cancer death in the United States. The most recent statistics showed that in 2011, 156,940 Americans died from lung cancer, which accounts for 27% of all cancer deaths in the United States [1]. With the evolution of medical imaging, the accuracy of lung cancer detection, diagnosis, and treatment is largely improved. The role of imaging ranges from screening for lung cancer to staging of the lung cancer.

Tomography is an imaging tool that provides information on what is actually happening inside the body by sections and through the use of any kind of penetrating wave. Positron emission tomography (PET) and computed tomography (CT) are widely used types of tomography that provide information about possible tumors and metastases of the cancer.

PET with the glucose analog, 18F-2-fluoro-2-deoxy-D-glucose (FDG), is becoming more popular in oncology applications such as lung nodule detection and segmentation. It has been shown to be a helpful tool to improve the accuracy of target volume delineation, treatment optimization, and surveillance of tumor recurrence in non-small cell lung cancer (NSCLC). Using CT alone, target volume delineation of lung cancer is prone to interobserver variability, with variations in the gross tumor volume (GTV) definition being as high as 700% in lung tissue [2]. Generally, we can consider that all the lung tumors are spherical, then by decreasing the radius by half, the volume of the tumor decreases by eight; this results in planning a more precise treatment of the tumor cells. Thus, accurate delineation of lung tumors

can improve the effectiveness of treatment and increase the patient's chance of survival.

Recently, co-registration of FDG-PET and CT images are widely taken into consideration, which has made it possible to integrate both functional and anatomical data with only one single scanning procedure. Fusing PET and CT gives the best of both image modalities that are the anatomical information of the CT and the ability to detect cells with abnormal metabolic activity in the PET. PET images give information about the functional activity inside the body while CT images provide the anatomical detail. Hence, usually CT images are needed to retrieve the anatomical information of the tumor lesion, while the existence of the cancer cells can be recognized in PET image.

Integrating PET and CT has made new possibilities for target volume delineation in NSCLC. In addition, incorporating PET improves diagnostic evaluation of pulmonary nodules and staging the mediastinum. Greco et al. [3] have shown that the overall diagnostic accuracy of PET/CT has been shown to be 93%, and having higher diagnostic accuracy than either CT or PET alone.

Figure 30.1 is an axial CT (left) and a fused PET/CT (right) scan of a patient with lung cancer. Left image shows a normal CT component. On the other hand, the right image reveals a region with abnormal FDG uptake. Exact delineation of the tumor and separating it from distal collapsed lung is hardly possible on CT. On the other hand, it has been well perceived that PET/CT provides the ability to differentiate the tumor from atelectasis, and reveals and localizes unsuspected metastases. Fused PET/CT (right image) clearly shows the distinction between the tumor and the distal atelectasis. This clear demonstration of the tumor region optimizes the treatment in the process of radiotherapy.

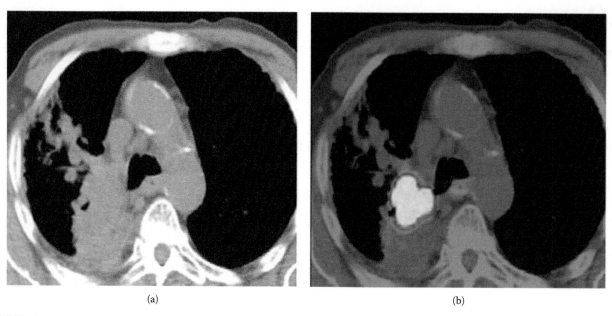

(a)   (b)

FIGURE 30.1
(a) CT scan of a patient with atelectasis lung tumor showing normal lung tissue, whereas the fused PET/CT scan (b) reveals abnormal activity and can identify the location of lesion for metastatic carcinoma. (From Eakin et al., *Imaging* 1, no. 6, 2007. With permission.)

Studies show that in up to 75% of cases, CT underestimated the extent of tumor length and 31% of GTV would be missed to be included in the radiotherapy [4]. Thus, incorporating PET images for lung nodule delineation and tumor diagnosis can be an alternation to the contouring of tumor volumes in CT alone.

This chapter provides an overview of the state-of-the-art methods for computer-automated segmentation and diagnosis of tumor volumes in PET images and fused PET/CT. Before describing the current lung nodule segmentation methods and their various issues that must be confronted, benefits of PET modality in clinical oncology are provided.

30.2 PET/CT Nodule Segmentation

Precise contouring and delineation of functional volumes in PET images are currently considered crucial for nodule segmentation and tumor diagnosis in image-guided oncology applications. In addition, the accurate definition of uptake values within the tumor itself may facilitate assigning dose intensification during intensity-modulated radiotherapy technique.

To extract and characterize volume of interest (VOI) with respect to some input features or expert knowledge, image segmentation methodologies are used that can be classified as manual or automatic. This is known to be a challenging task due to the various characteristics of the images. Manual segmentation methods

require considerable effort and time, and they are highly subjective [5]. On the other hand, automatic segmentation techniques in PET only are not trivial because of low resolution and resulting partial volume effect (PVE) and low contrast ratios.

The widely used quantifier in PET imaging is the standardized uptake value (SUV) that estimates the intensity of the lesion in PET. Large value of the SUV determines that the region is highly metabolically active, which is the indication of cancer cells. SUV of five means that the intensity of the region is five times greater than the average cell. The SUV is calculated either pixel-wise or over a region of interest for each image at time t, as the ratio of tissue radioactivity concentration, $c(t)$, and injected dose at the time of injection divided by body weight:

$$\mathrm{SUV_{BW}} = \frac{c(t)}{\dfrac{\text{injected dose}(t_0)}{\text{body weight}}} \tag{30.1}$$

Alternatively, injected dose may also be corrected by the lean body mass or body surface area [6]:

$$\mathrm{SUV_{BSA}} = \frac{c(t)}{\dfrac{\text{injected dose}(t_0)}{\text{body surface area}}} \tag{30.2}$$

To define tumor volume using SUV, the most straightforward technique is to apply a thresholding-based method, either adaptive, using a priori CT [7], or fixed threshold [5] using values derived from phantom studies. Automatic thresholding-based methods used the

SUV parameter to estimate the optimal threshold that defines the tumor region. Both the maximum SUV and the mean SUV can be easily calculated within the tumor region in addition to the mean SUV to be used as a measurement, but maximum SUV probably gives a less accurate result since it is a single value. Johnstone and Paulino [8] used an SUV of 2.5 to auto-contour the derived GTV. In most thresholding-based methods, first the maximum or the mean SUV is calculated using Equation 30.1 or 30.2, and then based on an arbitrary threshold value relative to the calculated number such as 40%, 42%, or 50% of the maximum SUV, the GTV is delineated [9–14].

Erdi et al. [11] studied the accuracy of lesion definition in FDG-PET in conjunction with CT. Eleven patients were included in this study. PET and CT were registered in the treatment planning system using either manual or automated methods. The planning target volume (PTV) outline obtained from the PET/CT fused images differed from the CT images. In seven out of 11 cases, the PTV volume increased. The increase in PTV is due to inclusion of distant lesions as nodal disease, detected by PET. PET scan showed increased activity in some regions, which was not detected by CT imaging. In four other cases, the PTV decreased. The decrease in the PTV prevents the exposure to unnecessary toxicity without compromising dose coverage in the PTV.

Some other approaches incorporate tumor volume, background activity, and source-to-background (S/B) ratios [15–20].

In an effort to determine the best method for GTV delineation, Nestle et al. [18] compared differences between the delineation philosophies for PET when finding the best threshold to obtain the most appropriate target volume delineation. They compared different GTVs obtained from different methods to look for the optimal thresholding value. Four different GTVs are obtained using four different methods: (1) visual interpretation (GTV_{vis}), (2) applying a threshold of 40% of the SUV_{max} (SUV_{40}), (3) applying a threshold equal to SUV = 2.5 ($GTV_{2.5}$), and (4) using phantom studies and the best fit obtained based on the tumor and background intensities (GTV_{bg}). GTV_{vis}, $GTV_{2.5}$, and GTV_{bg} showed a strong correlation with the CT-derived GTV, whereas the GTV_{vis} was shown to be the unsuitable one. The variability of the differences was found to be due to the tumor inhomogeneity and size. In addition, the time point of the acquisition of the PET scan influences the delineation of the positive tumor region and the tumor size.

Black et al. [16] and Biehl et al. [19] performed a series of phantom studies to determine an accurate and uniformly applicable method for defining a GTV with FDG-PET. They tried to find a regressive function based on phantom experiments, which represent the relationship between the threshold SUV and the mean target SUV. Threshold SUV is the threshold value that yields to the value that matches the one employed in the experiment.

Biehl et al. [19] studied the possibility of presenting a single SUV threshold value for GTV segmentation for NSCLC. Studies are conducted to obtain a 1:1 volumetric correlation between the GTV delineation in CT and PET. The optimal threshold was associated with the tumor size. It is shown that the best match between the two modalities of the CT and the PET was 24 ± 13%. This study shows that due to conditions such as necrosis and hypoxia in NSCLC, a single threshold model cannot be obtained since these conditions create nonuniform uptake to be perceived.

The main limitations of thresholding-based techniques are that they are user and system dependent. They involve user-dependent initializations, pre- and postprocessing, or a priori information like CT. Without having an a priori knowledge, Daisne et al. [15] proposed a method to find the best threshold value based on the relationship between S/B ratio and the isoactivity level to be used from the phantom studies. They showed that a fixed threshold value between 36% and 44% of the maximal activity has been shown to predict well the true volume, but for lesions larger than 4 ml. For lesions smaller than 4 ml or for poorly estimated lesions (S/B below 5.5), such thresholding methods could lead to substantial overestimation of the true volume, even with the knowledge of a priori volume.

Furthermore, thresholding methods do not consider some important factors in the tumor delineation such as target motion due to respiration and cardiac activity. Image noise, poor resolution, and VOI definition affect the calculated SUV. The accuracy of these methodologies in determining the VOI is greatly sensitive to variations in S/B contrast and also the level of the noise. In addition, a single threshold model lacks the incorporation of other factors such as tumor size and nonuniform distribution of FDG activity, thus leads to variable VOI determination. In many cases, due to conditions such as necrosis and hypoxia in NSCLC, a single threshold model cannot be obtained since these conditions create nonuniform uptake value. Experimental measurements of radioactive spheres in a phantom using thresholding-based methods show that the thresholding-based methods are unreliable in the clinical applications ([17–19,21].

To provide more reliable tumor delineation, statistical segmentation techniques cast the tumor segmentation within a statistical framework as an unsupervised classification problem. For a given data set composed of a set of items, a statistical classification framework attempts to give a label to each item with some level of certainty, like in the study by Pham et al. [22]. These algorithms are shown to give better tumor delineation results with respect to thresholding methods. Fuzzy locally adaptive Bayesian (FLAB) [23] and 3-FLAB [24] are segmentation approaches that are combined with a fuzzy measure. Each voxel will be assigned to its appropriate class based on its and its neighbors values. The parameters of noise model are also taken into consideration in the model.

Hatt et al. [23] proposed a FLAB segmentation method for automatic lesion volume delineation in PET. This method is assessed on spherical volumes acquired of the phantom and also realistic nonuniform and nonspherical volumes. The reported volume error is between 5% and 15%. Comparing this method with thresholding methods and fuzzy C-Means (FCM) [25] algorithms, FLAB performed better results for lesions less than 2 cm and for lesions with inhomogeneous activity distributions. FLAB is a Bayesian-based image segmentation approach that allows for automatic noise modeling since it is an unsupervised statistical methodology. In statistical segmentation methods, the parameters of the model are estimated by the method and no further preprocessing such as filtering is needed in the segmentation process. The segmentation problem consists of estimating the hidden segmentation map, X, from the observed image: $P(X|Y)$, knowing that $P(Y|X)$ is the likelihood of the observed image Y knowing the hidden map X.

$$P(X|Y) = \frac{P(Y|X)P(X)}{P(Y)} \qquad (30.3)$$

For the implementation of the fuzzy model, finite number of fuzzy levels and two hard classes are considered. This model allows the uncertainty of the classification and that voxels may contain both classes. The application can be adapted for PET images since they are noisy and have low resolution. This method segments the lesions less than 2 cm more accurately than fuzzy Hidden Markov Chain (FHMC) and it is less dependent on the noise as opposed to thresholding methods. However, in the case of strong heterogeneity, the two-class modeling (background and lesion) is not adequate to differentiate between multiple regions inside the tumor. Therefore, as far as homogeneous spheres or slightly heterogeneous and nonspherical tumors are concerned, FLAB is shown to be robust.

Hatt et al. [24] proposed a method which is an extension of their previous work FLAB. Their new approach gives better results for the delineation of inhomogeneous tumors by allowing up to three classes, as opposed to the FLAB, which considers only a binary segmentation. Clinical tumors may be characterized by heterogeneous uptake, which requires a nonbinary approach to account for different activity concentrations of the

multiple regions inside the tumor. They evaluated the accuracy of their approach on both real and simulated data sets containing inhomogeneous tumors. Based on the Bayesian framework from Equation 30.3, it is assumed that $P(X|Y)$ is the probability of each voxel belonging to class X, knowing the image Y. $P(Y|X)$ is estimated for each class, whereas $P(X)$ is estimated using a sliding cube of $3 \times 3 \times 3$ voxels, hence each voxel classification is influenced by its neighbors. An iterative approach using stochastic expectation maximization (SEM) technique is employed to estimate the mean and the variance of each class and the spatial probability of each voxel. This method performs well for heterogeneous lesions with good performance. In adaptive thresholding technique [7], 70% threshold is acquired for the initial estimation of the tumor-to-background contrast in the case of heterogeneous uptake, which may results in incorrect results by only retaining the high uptake region. For small regions, 70% threshold may lead to overestimation of the volume of the tumor.

Based on unsupervised estimation and noise modeling, some approaches such as the FCM clustering method [25] and the FHMC [26] attempt to find large groupings within the intensity distributions obtained from the PET image.

Hatt et al. [26] proposed an FHMC algorithm for lesion delineation in PET and compared its performance with thresholding methodologies currently used in clinical practice.

The HMC model is an unsupervised Bayesian-based methodology. X and Y are defined to be two random variables that represent the hidden map and the observed image, respectively. Based on the Bayesian formula (Equation 30.3), $P(Y|X)$ is the likelihood of the image Y, X is the ground truth map, and $P(X)$ is the prior knowledge concerning X. X is defined to be a Markov chain as follows:

$$P(x_t|x_1, \dots, x_{t-1}) = P(x_t|x_{t-1}) \text{ for } 1 < t \ll T \qquad (30.4)$$

Let T be a finite set corresponding to the voxels of an image. According to this definition, the probability of the next state depends only on the current state and not on the sequence of the events that preceded it. The distribution of X is then defined by the distribution of the x_1, which is called the initial distribution for each class c ($P(x_1 = c)$), and the transition matrix $P(x_{t+1} = d|x_t = c)$. In FHMC, they present a fuzzy model within the described Bayesian framework to allow the coexistence of voxels belonging to one of the two hard classes and voxels belonging to a fuzzy level. This adds the uncertainty regarding the hidden map (X) as opposed to classical HMC, which only models the uncertainty of the observed image data (Y). To apply this method to image segmentation, an a priori model of the initial and transition probabilities as well as the noise model of each class of the observed that can fit a Gaussian distribution are assumed. In order to achieve the estimation of the parameters of the models, they use the stochastic iterative procedure called SEM. They compared their algorithm with thresholding using 42% of the maximum uptake value in the lesion and reported that FHMC gave superior results for lesions < 28 mm, considering the S/B ratio of 4:1. Furthermore, FHCM was shown to be more robust than T42 (42% of the maximum uptake), where it is shown to be greatly influenced by the level of noise in the images.

The segmentation results of these fuzzy-based methods show better tumor delineation with respect to the thresholding-based methods. However, they usually require an estimation of the initial class and they consider only the PET modality in their implementations and anatomical information of CT is not considered.

There are other techniques proposed for automatic lesion detection in PET data sets such as edge detection and watershed [27]. These methodologies require some necessary preprocessing steps. For example, a filtering pass is required in the case of the watershed algorithm to smooth the image, and in a postprocessing step resulting regions from the over-segmentation are needed to get fused.

Numerous studies have presented more complex segmentation methodologies [23,28–35]. Tylski et al. [31] performed a phantom study to evaluate the morphological watershed algorithm for image segmentation. The segmentation is a 3D interactive marker-controlled algorithm that involves the user to place markers in the object to be segmented and in the background. Original watershed algorithm simulates flooding coming from the markers on the gradient image. Thus, the image is partitioned into two regions of the object and the background. The contour detected using this algorithm, does not fit with the contour of the object in the PET, which is due to the PVE. They modified the watershed method, in the way that they determine the contour to be the median contour between the contour detected by watershed on the image gradient and the contour detected on the positive part of the image Laplacian.

They compared their method with the results obtained from a segmentation using maximum intensity thresholding. They adapted the threshold to find out the known volumes of the tumors. For both homogeneous spheres and heterogeneous cylinders in their phantoms, they showed that they got results as good as adaptive volume thresholding with a p value greater than 0.5.

Montgomery et al. [33] proposed a statistical spatial segmentation approach from PET data. Their method has the following three steps:

1. A thresholding process to eliminate the artifacts within the background
2. k-Mean clustering algorithm in an EM-based model is performed as the initial segmentation to compute the optimal marginal segmentation
3. Using a multiscale Markov random field (MRF) model, the marginal segmentation achieved in the previous steps refined to segment the data based on the spatial information

They compared their method with the standard k-means and the spatial domain MRF model and reported that their methodology reduces the relative error in the actual tumor volume to less than 8% for small lesions (7 mm radii) and less than 3.5% for larger lesions (9 mm radii).

Demirkaya [28] proposed an algorithm to segment lesions in whole body images based on the MRF model. Their proposed segmentation method is performed in two steps. First, an initial map is obtained manually and then using maximum a posteriori estimation, the maximum likelihood, they solved for the Bayesian model defined. This method is evaluated on phantom and whole body images, and reported that, based on their preliminary results, their method can successfully segment lesions.

Li et al. [34] is an adaptive region growing method that extracts the tumor boundaries using deformable models in PET. Avazpour et al. [36] is also a region growing approach that is employed on co-registered PET/CT for exclusion of collapsed lung. [37] and Woods et al. incorporated textural and structural features in their proposed segmentation method. To summarize, the approaches presented for the segmentation of lung nodules from PET images, Table 30.1 briefly describes for each study the number of the patients enrolled in the study and the type of the nodule delineation approach with respect to the methodology, the approach dimension, and the approach automation level.

30.2.1 PET/CT Fusion

The use of PET for nodule segmentation has improved the accuracy of outlining the tumor contour in lung. However, there are some drawbacks to using PET alone. As PET acquisition takes several minutes, it is influenced by the patient's breathing and motion. These respiratory movements and cardiac actions result in the target motion that creates significant image blur

TABLE 30.1

Summary of Lung Nodule Segmentation Approaches from PET Images

Study	Patients	Delineation Approach	Dim	AL
Mah et al. [12]	30	Thresholding	3D	A
White et al. [30]	26	Thresholding	2D	A
Erdi et al. [7]	11	Thresholding	NA	A
Nestle et al. [9]	34	Visual	NA	NA
Deniaud-Alexandre et al. [14]	101	Visual	NA	NA
Ashamalla et al. [7]	19	Thresholding	3D	A
Hatt et al. [23]	NA	Fuzzy classification	NA	A
Hatt et al. [24]	38	Fuzzy classification	NA	A
Hatt et al. [26]	NA	Fuzzy hidden Markov chain	2D	A
Avazpour et al. [36]	11	Region growing	2D	A
Kiffer et al. [40]	15	Co-registration	2D	A
Munley et al. [41]	35	Manual registration	NA	NA
van Der Wel et al. [42]	21	Visual	NA	NA

For each study, the table summarizes the number of the patients enrolled in the study and the type of the nodule delineation approach with respect to the methodology, the approach dimension, and the automation level.

Note that Dim denotes the approach dimension (2D, 3D, or 4D) and AL denotes automation level (A: automatic, UI: user interactive, or NA: nonapplicable).

that affects the accuracy of GTV estimation. On the other hand, using CT only implies a large uncertainty in the result of target volume delineation, especially in NSCLC [38,39]. There are reported cases, in which the GTV delineated based on CT, including abnormalities that appear totally devoid of FDG activity and can safely be removed from the GTV. Thus, the combination of PET and CT information has been studied in order to improve the target volume definition especially in NSCL and cases with atelectasis. In this regard, the recent studies have shown that the integration of PET information in the treatment planning has significantly reduced the interobserver contouring variability [38,39].

To combine PET and CT information, a fusion technique should be applied to integrate the PET and CT images. The fusion techniques can be classified into one of the three categories: (1) visual fusion in which both imaging modalities are simply considered side by side, (2) software fusion, and (3) hardware fusion. Using visual vision, Kiffer et al. [40] showed that by using PET information, the outlined volume has changed in

26.7% of the cases. They conclude that the variability on the volume estimation is due to the detection of abnormal mediastinal nodes on PET which cannot be detected on CT. Nestle et al. [9] and Munley et al. [41] used software fusion techniques that reported a significant change in the target volume extraction when compared to CT-defined volume. Nestle et al. [9] has documented that in 6 out of 17 patients with dystelectasis or atelectasis, the size of the delineated target was reduced with a median change of 19.3%. Munley et al. [9] reported an increase in the GTV in 34% of the cases when compared with CT. Erdi et al. [10] performed a study on patients who received CT and PET scanning using the same device. They analyzed the contribution of PET in radiotherapy planning for patients with confirmed lung cancer. GTV, PTV, and normal tissues were initially contoured on the CT and then CT and PET were registered in a treatment planning system. There was an average increase of 19% in the PTV volume in 7 out of 11 patients and an average decrease of 18% in the PTV in the other 4 patients. In their study, they found that for all the patients with dystelectasis and atelectasis, the difference between the PTV outlined from CT and PET were significantly more frequent. For the patients without atelectasis, size and shape of the tumor obtained from PET correlated better with topographic information given by CT scans.

Mah et al. [12] performed a treatment simulation with PET/CT and CT alone and compared the results impact on radiation therapy target volume definition and toxicity profiles. FDG images were obtained with a coincidence gamma camera and fused to the CT images with use of external fiducial markers.

The tumor is delineated in both CT and fused PET/CT by a radiation therapist. Before tumor delination, PET data set was reviewed by a nuclear radiologist. A second physician contoured the GTV and PTV from the CT data sets, without knowing the PET results.

In result, radiation targeting with PET/CT images created alternation in radiation therapy planning in over 50% of the cases by comparing with CT alone. Furthermore, in all the patients with atelectasis, PET helped to distinguish the tumor. Their simulation study is not controlled for interobserver variation, which is a considerable factor for differences in tumor contours.

van Der Wel et al. [42] showed that the GTV decreased significantly when shifting from the CT only to the fused PET/CT in 21 patients, thus allowing dose escalation. Further studies on the rate of recurrence when PET is used showed that only 1 out of 44 patients developed the tumor recurrence [43]. Steenbakkers et al. [38] and Fox et al. [39] used software fusion methods and analyzed the observer variation in two phases, one with CT only and the other with fused PET/CT. The two

TABLE 30.2

Assessing Effect of PET/CT on GTV

Study	Patients	PET/CT Fusion Method	GTV Increase	GTV Decrease
Mah et al. [12]	30	Software	22%	NA
Brady et al. [30]	26	Software	46%	12%
Erdi et al. [7]	11	Software	64%	36%
Nestle et al. [9]	34	Visual side-by-side	9%	26%
Deniaud-Alexandre et al. [14]	101	Software	26%	23%
Ashamalla et al. [17]	19	Hardware	26%	26%
Avazpour et al. [36]	11	Software	NA	NA
Kiffer et al. [40]	15	Graphical co-registration	27%	NA
Munley et al. [41]	35	Visual	34%	NA
van Der Wel et al. [42]	21	Visual	14%	52%

For each study, the number of patients, the PET/CT fusion method, and the increase and decrease in the GTV as a percentage of the total number of the study cases is reported.

studies addressed the issue of interobserver variation reduction using matched PET and CT and concluded that the PET/CT software fusion is superior to visual fusion. Table 30.2 summarizes the published studies on the effect of PET on GTV as a complementary to CT. For each study, the number of patients, the PET/CT fusion method, and the increase and decrease in the GTV as a percentage of the total number of the study cases are reported. These studies reported that the PET/CT fusion has improved the GTV estimation and thus is preferable for the treatment optimization in NSCLC. However, some well-known technical issues such as the resolution of PET, the exact tumor edge definition, and the misregistration between PET and CT images need further investigations.

30.3 PET/CT Nodule Diagnosis

Since the incorporation of PET information into CT has shown a significant improvement in outlining the lung nodule contours and estimating the volume of interest, higher diagnostic accuracy using noninvasive imaging modalities is achieved.

CT provides anatomic information and can suggest the likelihood of malignancy of a solitary pulmonary

TABLE 30.3

Evaluation of Nodule Malignancy in PET

Study	Cases	A/PPV	Sensitivity	Specificity
Lowe et al. [46]	89	A = 91%	92%	90%
Gupta et al. [45]	61	PPV = 92%	93%	88%
Lee et al. [49]	71	PPV = 86%	95%	82%
Dewan et al. [44]	30	PPV = 90%	95%	80%
Herder et al. [50]	36	PPV = 72%	93%	77%
Halley et al. [51]	28	NA	94%	89%

A: accuracy, PPV: positive productive value.

nodule (SPN). SPNs are single, spherical, well-circumscribed, radiographic opacity that measures ≤3 cm in diameter.

In PET images, the malignant cells have unregulated metabolism that results in having higher FDG uptake that permits malignancy to be detected. Reported studies [44–51] used this characteristic to detect malignant SPNs in PET. Provided a visually validated diagnostics of the SPNs in PET images, these studies reported an SPN diagnostic accuracy with a sensitivity of 88%–96% and a specificity of 70%–90% for malignant cells. It is clear that PET is highly sensitive and less specific compared with CT (see Table 30.3 for more details). Furthermore, PET has shown to have a higher rate of detection of mediastinal lymph-node and extra-thoracic metastases [52–54].

Using PET alone without incorporation of CT in the diagnosis of lung cancer has some limitations. PET has limited spatial resolution that leads to providing imprecise information on the exact location of focal abnormalities [55]. In general, it has been considered to give less-accurate diagnostic results for tumors smaller than 10 mm [56]. Furthermore, FDG is not a cancer-specific agent, and lesions with low 18F-FDG uptake value may be diagnosed as benign resulting in false negative error results [46,57,58]. False negative results are mainly reported in patients with bronchioloalveolar carcinomas and carcinoids that are due to small size or well-differentiated malignancies. Lesions less than 0.5 cm in diameter may be falsely negative because of poor resolution of the PET images and PVEs. That being said, false positive results are more likely to happen. Using PET alone for malignancy detection can result in a high false positive error rate in patients with active tuberculosis, histoplasmosis, granulomus, chronic inflammation, sarcoidosis, Aspergillus infection and rheumatoid nodules [59,60].

Annema et al. [57] reported the false positive findings of PET to be up to 39%, despite the high negative predictive value of PET, suggesting that the PET positive mediastinal lymph nodes were further biopsied in order to confirm or rule out metastasis.

Recently, PET/CT fusion has been widely considered in lung cancer applications such as the tumor staging and pulmonary nodules diagnostics in lung, which remains a difficult task for radiologists. PET/CT combines the advantage of both morphological and functional imaging and it was shown to be more accurate for T-staging and N-staging of lung cancer than CT or PET alone.

To investigate the integration of PET and CT information on the accuracy of the malignancy detection, Nie et al. [61] developed an artificial neural networks (ANNs) based on CT alone, PET alone, and both CT and PET for distinguishing benign and malignant pulmonary nodules. Their results show that the accuracy of PET/CT (Az = 0.95) is higher than the CT (Az = 0.83) and PET (Az = 0.91).

Kim et al. [62] studied the diagnosis accuracy of side-by-side PET/CT compared with PET and CT alone. CT and PET images were interpreted separately. If the classification results of the PET and CT were concordant, then the fused PET/CT classification result would be the same. In the case of discordant, based on score of malignancy in PET and CT, they followed predefining rules based on the score of the malignancy in both CT and PET to classify the image. According to their results, PET/CT maintained the sensitivity of CT and the specificity of PET, resulting in significant improvement in the accuracy.

Nakamoto et al. [63] compared the diagnosis accuracy of CT, side-by-side PET/CT, and software-fused PET/CT. They documented that the software fusion of PET/CT resulted in the highest accuracy on patients with lung cancer. Tozaki et al. [64] proposed a computer-aided diagnosis of cancer method using whole body FDG-PET images. In their method, first they divide the PET images into some regions based on the intensity levels, and Gaussian curvature and mean curvature of the images are calculated. Next, the positive of Gaussian curvature and the negative of the mean curvature regions are extracted as the candidate regions for cancer. Finally, using defined diagnosis criteria such as the intensity, size, and the intensity difference between the interesting peak surface region and its circumference organ, and the existence position, candidates are evaluated to check for the cancer. As the result, they have shown the comparison between their method and a doctor's diagnosis on two cases. They have reported that their result is as good as the doctor's.

Keidar et al. [65] compared the diagnosis performance of PET/CT and PET alone. Using PET alone resulted in a higher false positive error rate. A higher specificity was achieved using PET/CT, suggesting that the anatomical information on CT is an independent crucial variable in determining malignancy. Yi et al. [58] investigated the sensitivity, specificity, and accuracy for predicting malignant nodules on helical dynamic CT and PET/CT. They documented that all malignant nodules were interpreted correctly using dynamic helical CT or PET/CT. Lardinois et al. [55] investigated tumor staging in 50 patients with proven or suspected NSCLC using PET/CT versus PET or CT alone. Their results showed that the PET/CT fusion is a trustworthy means of nodule diagnosis that has significantly improved the accuracy of the tumor staging.

In a study on 276 patients with newly diagnosed lung lesions by Pauls et al. [66], the performance of each modality of integrated PET/CT, CT, and PET for differentiating malignancy of the lung lesions is presented. It is reported that PET/CT was given more accurate result than CT but the same as PET. Incorporating PET led to an increase in the specificity and is therefore recommended to accurately specify the newly diagnosed lung lesions.

Table 30.4 summarizes PET/CT results. The experiments involved in these studies have shown that using PET/CT achieved a higher diagnostic power than CT or PET alone, suggesting that the PET/CT fusion may present an advance in lung cancer applications.

Another useful technique for lung nodule diagnosis in PET is dual time-point PET imaging. Especially for patients whose nodules have shown an SUV of around 2 to 2.5 g/ml. In this technique, FDG uptake is measured at two different intervals, for example at 1 hour and again at 2 hours after the injection. If the nodule is malignant, the FDG uptake tends to increase in the time between the two measurements, whereas in the case of benign nodules, the FDG uptake tends to remain the same or decreases [67].

TABLE 30.4

Evaluation of Nodule Malignancy in Fused PET/CT

Study	Cases	A/PPV	Sensitivity	Specificity
Nie et al. [61]	92	A = 95%	NA	NA
Nakamoto et al.	53	A = 87%	94%	75%
Keidar et al.	42	PPV = 89%	96%	82%
Kim et al. [62]	42	A = 93%	97%	85%
Lardinois et al. [55]	40	A = 88%	NA	NA
Pauls et al. [66]	276	A = 94% (assuming equal lesions are benign)	96%	87%
Yi et al. [58]	119	A = 93%	96%	88%

References

1. Siegel, R., E. Ward, O. Brawley, A. Jemal. "Cancer statistics, 2011." *CA Cancer J Clin* 61, no. 4 (2011): 212–36.
2. Van de Steene, J., N. Linthout, J. de Mey, V. Vinh-Hung, C. Claassens, M. Noppen, A. Bel, G. Storme. "Definition of gross tumor volume in lung cancer: inter-observer variability." *Radiother Oncol* 62, no. 1 (2002): 37–49.
3. Greco, C., K. Rosenzweig, G. L. Cascini, O. Tamburrini. "Current status of PET/CT for tumour volume definition in radiotherapy treatment planning for non-small cell lung cancer (NSCLC)." *Lung Cancer* 57, no. 2 (2007): 125–34.
4. Leong, T., C. Everitt, K. Yuen, S. Condron, A. Hui, S. Y. Ngan, A. Pitman et al. "A prospective study to evaluate the impact of FDG-PET on CT-based radiotherapy treatment planning for oesophageal cancer." *Radiother Oncol* 78, no. 3 (2006): 254–61.
5. Krak, N. C., R. Boellaard, O. S. Hoekstra, J. W. Twisk, C. J. Hoekstra, A. A. Lammertsma. "Effects of ROI definition and reconstruction method on quantitative outcome and applicability in a response monitoring trial." *Eur J Nucl Med Mol Imaging* 32, no. 3 (2005): 294–301.
6. Kim, C. K., N. C. Gupta, B. Chandramouli, A. Alavi. "Standardized uptake values of FDG: body surface area correction is preferable to body weight correction." *J Nucl Med* 35, no. 1 (1994): 164–7.
7. Erdi, Y. E., O. Mawlawi, S. M. Larson, M. Imbriaco, H. Yeung, R. Finn, J. L. Humm. "Segmentation of lung lesion volume by adaptive positron emission tomography image thresholding." *Cancer* 80 (1997): 2505–9.
8. "Johnstone, P. A., A. C. Paulino. "FDG-PET in radiotherapy treatment planning: pandora's box?" Int J Radiat Oncol Biol Phys 59, no.1 (2004): 4–5."
9. Nestle, U., K. Walter, S. Schmidt, N. Licht, C. Nieder, B. Motaref, D. Hellwig, M et al. "18F-deoxyglucose positron emission tomography (FDG-PET) for the planning of radiotherapy in lung cancer: high impact in patients with atelectasis." *Int J Radiat Oncol Biol Phys* 44, no. 3 (1999): 593–7.
10. "Giraud, P., D. Grahek, F. Montravers, M. F. Carette, E. Deniaud-Alexandre, F. Julia, J. C. Rosenwald et al. "CT and (18)F-deoxyglucose (FDG) image fusion for optimization of conformal radiotherapy of lung cancers." Int J Radiat Oncol Biol Phys 49,no.5 (2001): 1249–57."
11. Erdi, Y. E., K. Rosenzweig, A. K. Erdi, H. A. Macapinlac, Y. C. Hu, L. E. Braban, J. L. Humm et al. "Radiotherapy treatment planning for patients with non-small cell lung cancer using positron emission tomography (PET)." *Radiother Oncol* 62, no. 1 (2002): 51–60.
12. Mah, K., C. B. Caldwell, Y. C. Ung, C. E. Danjoux, J. M. Balogh, S. N. Ganguli, L. E. Ehrlich, R. Tirona. "The impact of (18)FDG-PET on target and critical organs in ct-based treatment planning of patients with poorly defined non-small-cell lung carcinoma: a prospective study." *Int J Radiat Oncol Biol Phys* 52, no. 2 (2002): 339–50.
13. Bradley, J., W. L. Thorstad, S. Mutic, T. R. Miller, F. Dehdashti, BA. Siegel, W. Bosch, R. J. Bertrand. "Impact of FDG-PET on radiation therapy volume delineation in non-small-cell lung cancer." *Int J Radiat Oncol Biol Phys* 59, no. 1 (2004): 78–86.
14. Deniaud-Alexandre, E., E. Touboul, D. Lerouge, D. Grahek, J. N. Foulquier, Y. Petegnief, B. Grs et al. "Impact of computed tomography and 18f-deoxyglucose coincidence detection emission tomography image fusion for optimization of conformal radiotherapy in non-small-cell lung cancer." *Int J Radiat Oncol Biol Phys* 63, no. 5 (2005): 1432–41.
15. Daisne, J. F., M. Sibomana, A. Bol, T. Doumont, M. Lonneux, V. Grgoire. "Tri-dimensional automatic segmentation of PET volumes based on measured source-to-background ratios: influence of reconstruction algorithms." *Radiother Oncol* 69, no. 3 (2003): 247–50.
16. Black, Q. C., I. S. Grills, L. L. Kestin, C. Y. Wong, J. W. Wong, A. A. Martinez, D. Yan. "Defining a radiotherapy target with positron emission tomography." *Int J Radiat Oncol Biol Phys* 60, no. 4 (2004): 1272–82.
17. Ashamalla, H., S. Rafla, K. Parikh, B. Mokhtar, G. Goswami, S. Kambam, H. Abdel-Dayem,. Guirguis, A., P. Ross, A. Evola. "The contribution of integrated PET/CT to the evolving definition of treatment volumes in radiation treatment planning in lung cancer." *Int J Radiat Oncol Biol Phys* 63, no. 4 (2005): 1016–23.
18. "Nestle, U., S. Kremp, A. Schaefer-Schuler, C. Sebastian-Welsch, D. Hellwig, C. Rbe, C. M. Kirsch. "Comparison of different methods for delineation of 18F-FDG PET-positive tissue for target volume definition in radiotherapy of patients with non-small cell lung cancer." *J Nucl Med* 46, no. 6 (2005): 1342–8.
19. Biehl, K. J., F. M. Kong, F. Dehdashti, J. Y. Jin, S. Mutic, I. El Naqa, B. A. Siegel, J. D. Bradley. "18F-FDG PET definition of gross tumor volume for radiotherapy of non-small cell lung cancer: is a single standardized uptake value threshold approach appropriate?" *J Nucl Med* 47, no. 11 (2006): 1808–12.
20. Davis, J. B., B. Reiner, M. Huser, C. Burger, G. Szkely, I. F. Ciernik. "Assessment of 18F PET signals for automatic target volume definition in radiotherapy treatment planning." *Radiother Oncol* 80, no. 1 (2006): 43–50.
21. Caldwell, C. B., K. Mah, M. Skinner, C. E. Danjoux. "Can PET provide the 3D extent of tumor motion for individualized internal target volumes? a phantom study of the limitations of CT and the promise of PET." *Int J Radiat Oncol Biol Phys* 55, no. 5 (2003): 1381–93.
22. "Pham, D. L., C. Xu, J. L. Prince. "Current methods in medical image segmentation." *Annu Rev Biomed Eng* 2, no. 1 (2000). : 315-37"
23. Hatt, M., C. Cheze le Rest, A. Turzo, C. Roux, D. Visvikis. "A fuzzy locally adaptive bayesian segmentation approach for volume determination in PET." *IEEE Trans Med Imaging* 28, no. 6 (2009): 881–93.
24. Hatt, M., C. Cheze le Rest, P. Descourt, A. Dekker, D. De Ruysscher, M. Oellers, P. Lambin, O. Pradier, Visvikis D. "Accurate automatic delineation of heterogeneous functional volumes in positron emission tomography for oncology applications." *Int J Radiat Oncol Biol Phys* 77, no. 1 (2010): 301–8.

25. Bezdek, J. C., L. O. Hall, M. C. Clark, D. B. Goldgof, L. P. Clarke. "Medical image analysis with fuzzy models." *Stat Methods Med Res* 6, no. 3 (1997): 191–214.

26. Hatt, M., F. Lamare, N. Boussion, D. Visvikis. "Fuzzy hidden markov chains segmentation for volume determination and quantitation in PET." *Phys Med Biol* 52, no. 12 (2007): 3467–91.

27. Reutter, B. W., G. J. Klein, R. H. Huesman. "Automated 3D segmentation of respiratory-gated PET transmission images." *IEEE Trans Nucl Sci* 44, no. 6 (1997): 2473–76.

28. Demirkaya, O. "Lesion segmentation in whole-body images of PET." *IEEE Nuclear Sci Symp Conf Record* 4 (2003): 2873–76.

29. "Zhu W., T. Jiang. "Automation segmentation of PET image for brain tumors." IEEE Neurosci Symp Conf Record 4 (2003): 2627–9. "

30. "White, C. J., J. M. Brady. "A semi-automatic approach to the delineation of tumour boundaries from PET data using level sets." June 18–22, Toronto, *Soc Nuclear Med Ann Meeting*, 2005."

31. "Tylski, P., G. Bonniaud, E. Decencire, J. Stawiaski, J. Coulot, D. Lefkopoulos, M. Ricard. "18F-FDG PET images segmentation using morphological watershed: a phantom study." *IEEE Neurosci Symp Conf Record* 4 (2006): 2063–67."

32. Geets, X., J. A. Lee, A. Bol, M. Lonneux, V. Grgoire. "A gradient based method for segmenting FDG-PET images: methodology and validation." *Eur J Nucl Med Mol Imaging* 34, no. 9 (2007): 1427–38.

33. Montgomery, D. W., A. Amira, H. Zaidi. "Fully automated segmentation of oncological PET volumes using a combined multiscale and statistical model." *Med Phys* 34, no. 2 (2007): 722–36.

34. Li, H. W., L. Thorstad, K. J. Biehl, R. Laforest, Y. Su, K. I. Shoghi, E. D. Donnelly, D. A. Low, W. Lu. "A novel PET tumor delineation method based on adaptive region-growing and dual-front active contours." *Med Phys* 35, no. 8 (2008): 3711–21.

35. Yu, H., C. Caldwell, K. Mah, D. Mozeg. "Coregistered FDG PET/CT based textural characterization of head and neck cancer for radiation treatment planning." *IEEE Trans Med Imaging* 28, no. 3 (2009): 374–83.

36. Avazpour, I., R. E. Roslan, B. Bayat, M. I. Saripan, A. J. Nordin, R. S. A. R. Abdullah. "Segmenting CT images of bronchogenic carcinoma with bone metastases using PET intensity markers approach." *Radiat Oncol* 43, no. 3 (2009): 180–6.

37. Mohamed, S. S., A. M. Youssef, E. F. El-Saadany, M. M. A. Salama. "Artificial life feature selection techniques for prostate cancer diagnosis using TRUS images." *Proceedings of 2nd International Conference on Image Analysis and Recognition*, 2005: 903–13.

38. Steenbakkers, R. J., J. C. Duppen, I. Fitton, K. E. Deurloo, L. J. Zijp, E. F. Comans, A. L. Uitterhoeve et al. "Reduction of observer variation using matched CT-PET for lung cancer delineation: a three-dimensional analysis." *Int J Radiat Oncol Biol Phys* 64, no. 2 (2006): 435–48.

39. Fox, J. L., R. Rengan, W. O'Meara, E. Yorke, Y. Erdi, S. Nehmeh, S. A. Leibel, K. E. Rosenzweig. "Does registration of PET and planning CT images decrease interobserver and intraobserver variation in delineating tumor volumes for nonsmall-cell lung cancer?" *Int J Radiat Oncol Biol Phys* 62, no. 1 (2005): 70–5.

40. Kiffer, J. D., S. U. Berlangieri, A. M. Scott, G. Quong, M. Feigen, W. Schumer, C. P. Clarke, S. R. Knight, F. J. Daniel. "The contribution of 18F-fluoro-2-deoxy-glucose positron emission tomographic imaging to radiotherapy planning in lung cancer." *Lung Cancer* 19, no. 3 (1998): 167–77.

41. Munley, M. T., L. B. Marks, C. Scarfone, G. S. Sibley, E. F. Jr. Patz, T. G. Turkington, R. J. Jaszczak, D. R. Gilland, M. S. Anscher, R. E. Coleman. "Multimodality nuclear medicine imaging in three-dimensional radiation treatment planning for lung cancer: challenges and prospect." *Lung Cancer* 23, no. 2 (1999): 105–14.

42. van Der Wel, A., S. Nijsten, M. Hochstenbag, R. Lamers, L. Boersma, R. Wanders, L. Lutgens et al. "Increased therapeutic ratio by 18FDG-PET CT planning in patients with clinical CT stage N2-N3M0 non-small-cell lung cancer: a modeling study." *Int J Radiat Oncol Biol Phys* 61, no. 3 (2005): 649–55.

43. De Ruysscher, D., S. Wanders, E. van Haren, M. Hochstenbag, W. Geeraedts, I. Utama, J. Simons et al. "Selective mediastinal node irradiation based on FDG-PET scan data in patients with non-small-cell lung cancer: a prospective clinical study." *Int J Radiat Oncol Biol Phys* 62, no. 4 (2005): 988–94.

44. Dewan, N. A., N. C. Gupta, L. S. Redepenning, J. J. Phalen, M. P. Frick. "Diagnostic efficacy of PET-FDG imaging in solitary pulmonary nodules. Potential role in evaluation and management." *Chest* 104, no. 4 (1993): 997–1002.

45. Gupta, N. C., Maloof J, Gunel E. "Probability of malignancy in solitary pulmonary nodules using fluorine-18-FDG and PET." *J Nucl Med* 37, no. 6 (1996): 943–8.

46. Lowe, V. J., J. W Fletcher, L. Gobar, M. Lawson, P. Kirchner, P. Valk, J. Karis et al. "Prospective investigation of positron emission tomography in lung nodules." *J Clin Oncol* 16, no. 3 (1998): 1075–84.

47. Erasmus, J. J., H. P. McAdams, J. E. Connolly. "Solitary pulmonary nodules: part II. evaluation of the indeterminate nodule." *Radiographics* 20, no. 1 (2000): 59–66.

48. Goo, J. M., J. G. Im, K. H. Do, J. S. Yeo, J. B. Seo, H. Y. Kim, J. K. Chung. "Pulmonary tuberculoma evaluated by means of FDG PET: findings in 10 cases." *Radiology* 216, no. 1 (2000): 117–21.

49. Lee, J., J. M. Aronchick, A. Alavi. "Accuracy of F-18 fluorodeoxyglucose positron emission tomography for the evaluation of malignancy in patients presenting with new lung abnormalities: a retrospective review." *Chest* 120, no. 6 (2001): 1791–7.

50. Herder, G. J., R. P. Golding, O. S. Hoekstra, E. F. Comans, G. J. Teule, P. E. Postmus, E. F. Smit. "The performance of (18) F-fluorodeoxyglucose positron emission tomography in small solitary pulmonary nodules." *Eur J Nucl Med Mol Imaging* 31, no. 9 (2004): 1231–6.

51. Halley, A., A. Hugentobler, P. Icard, E. Porret, F. Sobrio, J. P. Lerochais. "Efficiency of 18F-FDG and 99mTc-depreotide SPECT in the diagnosis of malignancy of solitary pulmonary nodules." *Eur J Nucl Med Mol Imaging* 32, no. 9 (2005): 1026–32.

52. Steinert, H. C., M. Hauser, F. Allemann, H. Engel, T. Berthold, G. K. von Schulthess, W. Weder. "Non-small cell lung cancer: nodal staging with FDG PET versus CT with correlative lymph node mapping and sampling." *Radiology* 202, no. 2 (1997): 441–6.

53. Weder, W., R. A. Schmid, H. Bruchhaus, S. Hillinger, G. K. von Schulthess, H. C. Steinert. "Detection of extrathoracic metastases by positron emission tomography in lung cancer." *Ann Thorac Surg* 66, no. 3 (1998): 886–92.

54. Dwamena, B. A., S. S. Sonnad, J. O. Angobaldo, R. L. Wahl. "Metastases from non-small cell lung cancer: mediastinal staging in the 1990s—meta-analytic comparison of PET and CT." *Radiology* 213, no. 2 (1999): 530–6.

55. Lardinois, D., W. Weder, T. F. Hany, E. M. Kamel, S. Korom, B. Seifert, G. K. von Schulthess, H. C. Steinert. "Staging of non-small-cell lung cancer with integrated positron-emission tomography and computed tomography." *N Engl J Med* 348, no. 25 (2003): 2500–7.

56. Nomori, H., K. Watanabe, T. Ohtsuka, T. Naruke, K. Suemasu, K. Uno. "Evaluation of F-18 fluorodeoxyglucose (FDG) PET scanning for pulmonary nodules less than 3 cm in diameter, with special reference to the CT images." *Lung Cancer* 45, no. 1 (2004): 19–27.

57. Annema, J. T., O. S. Hoekstra, E. F. Smit, M. Veseli, M. I. Versteegh, K. F. Rabe. "Towards a minimally invasive staging strategy in NSCLC: analysis of PET positive mediastinal lesions by EUS-FNA." *Lung Cancer* 44, no. 1 (2004): 53–60.

58. Yi, C. A., K. S. Lee, B. T. Kim, J. Y. Choi, O. J. Kwon, H. Kim, M. J. Shim, Y. M. Chung. "Tissue characterization of solitary pulmonary nodule: comparative study between helical dynamic CT and integrated PET/CT." *J Nucl Med* 47, no. 3 (2006): 443–50.

59. Fischer, B. M., J. Mortensen. "The future in diagnosis and staging of lung cancer: positron emission tomography." *Respiration* 73 (2006): 267–76.

60. Baxte, C. G., P. Bishop, S. E. Low, K. Baiden-Amissah, D. W. Denning. "Primary aspergillosis: an alternative diagnosis to lung cancer after positive 18F-FDG positron emission tomography." *Thorax* 66, no. 7 (2011): 638–40.

61. Nie, Y., Q. Li, F. Li, Y. Pu, D. Appelbaum, K. Doi. "Integrating PET and CT information to improve diagnostic accuracy for lung nodules: a semiautomatic computer-aided method." *J Nucl Med* 47, no. 7 (2006): 1075–80.

62. Kim, S. K., M. Allen-Auerbach, J. Goldin, B. J. Fueger, M. Dahlbom, M. Brown, J. Czernin, C. Schiepers. "Accuracy of PET/CT in characterization of solitary pulmonary lesions." *J Nucl Med* 48, no. 2 (2007): 214–20.

63. Nakamoto, Y., M. Senda, T. Okada, S. Sakamoto, T. Saga, T. Higashi, K. Togashi. "Software-based fusion of PET and CT images for suspected recurrent lung cancer." *Mol Imaging Biol* 10, no. 3 (2008): 147–53..

64. Tozaki, T., M. Senda, S. Sakamoto, K. Matsumoto. "Computer assisted diagnosis method of whole body cancer using FDG-PET images." *Proc. IEEE Int. Conf. Image Processing (ICIP)* 2 (2003): 1085–8.

65. Keidar, Z., N. Haim, L. Guralnik, M. Wollner, R. Bar-Shalom, A. Ben-Nun, O. Israel. "PET/CT using 18F-FDG in suspected lung cancer recurrence: diagnostic value and impact on patient management." *J Nucl Med* 45, no. 10 (2004): 1640–6.

66. Pauls, S., A. K. Buck, G. Halter, F. M. Mottaghy, R. Muche, C. Bluemel, S. Gerstner et al. "Performance of integrated FDG-PET/CT for differentiating benign and malignant lung lesions—results from a large prospective clinical trial." *Mol Imaging Biol* 10, no. 2 (2008): 121–8.

67. Padma, S., P. S. Sundaram, S. George. "Role of positron emission tomography computed tomography in carcinoma lung evaluation." *J Cancer Res Ther* 7, no. 2 (2011): 128–34.

68. Eakin, R., J. Foster, G. Hanna, A. Hounsell, T. Lynch, J. McAleese, O. McNally, W. Page, D. Stewart, Y. Summers. "The role of PET/CT in radiotherapy planning." *Imaging* 1, no. 6 (2007): 13–15."

Index

Printed and bound by CPI Group (UK) Ltd, Croydon, CR0 4YY

18/10/2024

01776210-0016